Procedural Pediatric Dermatology

ANDREW C. KRAKOWSKI, MD, FAAD

Chair of Dermatology
Program Director of the Residency in Dermatology
St. Luke's University Health Network
Easton, Pennsylvania

Associate Editors:

John C. Browning, MD, MBA, FAAD, FAAP
Craig N. Burkhart, MD, MS, MPH, FAAD, FAAP
Lucía Z. Díaz, MD, FAAD
Amanda A. Gosman, MD, FACS
Kristen M. Kelly, MD, FAAD
H. Peter Lorenz, MD, FACS
Harper N. Price, MD, FAAD, FAAP

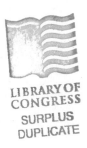
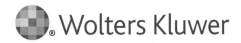
. Wolters Kluwer

Philadelphia · Baltimore · New York · London
Buenos Aires · Hong Kong · Sydney · Tokyo

Acquisitions Editor: Nicole Dernoski
Development Editors: Carole Wonsiewicz and Eric McDermott
Editorial Coordinators: Sean Hanrahan, Annette Ferran, and Kerry McShane
Marketing Manager: Phyllis Hitner
Production Project Manager: Catherine Ott
Design Coordinator: Elaine Kasmer
Manufacturing Coordinator: Beth Welsh
Prepress Vendor: S4Carlisle Publishing Services

9 8 7 6 5 4 3 2 1

Printed in China

Library of Congress Cataloging-in-Publication Data

Names: Krakowski, Andrew C., editor.
Title: Procedural pediatric dermatology / [edited by] Andrew Krakowski ;
    associate editors, John C. Browning, Craig N. Burkhart, Lucia Z. Diaz,
    Amanda A. Gosman, Kristen M. Kelly, H. Peter Lorenz, Harper N. Price.
Description: Philadelphia : Wolters Kluwer Health, [2021] | Includes
    bibliographical references and index.
Identifiers: LCCN 2020016690 | ISBN 9781975112448 (paperback)
Subjects: MESH: Dermatologic Surgical Procedures | Skin Diseases—surgery |
    Child | Infant
Classification: LCC RJ511 | NLM WS 265 | DDC 618.92/5—dc23
LC record available at https://lccn.loc.gov/2020016690

shop.lww.com

Associate Editors

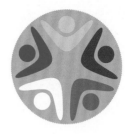

John C. Browning, MD, MBA, FAAD, FAAP
Assistant Professor of Pediatrics and Dermatology
Baylor College of Medicine
University of Texas Health Science Center
Chief of Dermatology, Children's Hospital of San Antonio
Texas Dermatology and Laser Specialists
San Antonio, Texas

Craig N. Burkhart, MD, MS, MPH, FAAD, FAAP
Adjunct Professor of Pediatric Dermatology
University of North Carolina School of Medicine
Chapel Hill, North Carolina
Burkhart Pediatric & Adolescent Dermatology
Cary, North Carolina

Lucía Z. Díaz, MD, FAAD
Chief, Division of Pediatric Dermatology
Assistant Professor of Internal Medicine and Pediatrics
Associate Program Director, Dermatology Residency
    Program
Dell Children's Hospital and Dell Medical School
Austin, Texas

Amanda A. Gosman, MD, FACS
Professor and Chief of Plastic Surgery
Director of Craniofacial and Pediatric Plastic Surgery
University of California, San Diego
Chief of Plastic Surgery
Rady Children's Hospital San Diego
San Diego, California

Kristen M. Kelly, MD, FAAD
Professor of Dermatology and Surgery
Vice Chair of Dermatology
University of California, Irvine
UCI Health Beckman Laser Institute
Irvine, California

H. Peter Lorenz, MD, FACS
Professor of Surgery
Division of Plastic and Reconstructive Surgery
Department of Surgery
Stanford University School of Medicine
Stanford, California
Service Chief, Plastic Surgery,
Director, Craniofacial Surgery Fellowship
Department of Surgery
Lucile Packard Children's Hospital
Palo Alto, California

Harper N. Price, MD, FAAD, FAAP
Clinical Assistant Professor
Department of Child Health
University of Arizona College of Medicine
Assistant Professor of Dermatology
Mayo Clinic College of Medicine and Science
Division Chief, Dermatology
Program Director, Pediatric Dermatology Fellowship
Phoenix Children's Hospital and Phoenix Children's
    Medical Group
Phoenix, Arizona

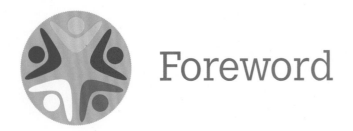

Foreword

Children are not small versions of adults—they have remarkably different physiology, endocrine status, metabolism, peripheral and central nervous system development, skin morphology, response to medications, and response to the surgical and nonsurgical injuries that constitute most therapeutic procedures. Clinical and histopathologic diagnosis is also different between children and adults. It makes no sense to treat children as little adults, and yet there has been a dearth of evidence, or even learned opinion, about how dermatologic procedures should best be performed in children.

Therefore, this is a landmark textbook that starts to fill the void about pediatric dermatology procedures. Moreover, this book illustrates our strong need for new evidence, new strategies, and new technologies in the field. In particular, newborns pose challenges and unique opportunities to achieve best outcomes. An example I see every week is the gratifying response of facial port-wine birthmarks when treated with pulsed dye laser during the first 6 months of life, as discussed herein. After about 1 year of age, however, treatment efficacy decreases. After age 1, children also become much more fearful, general anesthesia is often necessary, and with that comes major expense and the potential risk of blunting cognitive development. Clearly, laser treatment of port-wine birthmarks should be given soon after birth for patients who need it. However, the classic teaching in pediatrics is to avoid all elective procedures until children are at least 3 years old—exactly the opposite of best practice in this setting.

Clinicians have a front-row seat to Mother Nature's human drama. This book sets the stage for those of us who earnestly want to help children with important skin problems. While this is the first book to dive deeply into pediatric skin procedures, I doubt it will be the last. It will probably stimulate much-needed communication and inquiry about how we diagnose and treat neonates, prepubertal children, and teenagers. We can and should do a better job taking care of children. This is a wonderful starting point for that.

This book also exposes how little we really know. In the example above, *why* do neonatal port-wine birthmarks respond so much better than those of older children? Neonatal dermis is thinner and more translucent, which may allow better light penetration; the neonatal neural, immune, and inflammatory systems are naïve and still under development; neonates have fetal hemoglobin, which evolved to mitigate hypoxia in the fetus and might therefore limit hypoxia and rebound angiogenesis after laser treatment—maybe all of these are important factors, maybe none, we just don't know.

The past decade has seen an explosion of so-called biologic drugs, affordable and rapid DNA sequencing, sophisticated imaging devices, and the beginning applications of artificial intelligence. Each of these is changing medical and surgical practices at an exciting, amazing, and sometimes alarming pace. While our capability to prevent, predict, diagnose, and treat disease has blossomed, so has the uncertainty about when to deploy these new things. This is especially true for treatment of children, who are usually not the primary subjects of biomedical innovation. Treating kids poses different ethical challenges, a subject touched on herein. Seventy years ago, Danish politician Karl Steincke quipped, "It is difficult to make predictions, especially about the future." Maybe artificial intelligence will do a better job of that (I doubt it). We are compelled to help children with life-altering skin problems, and equally compelled to be cautious about it. In the midst of rapid-paced change, books like this one are precious. Enjoy!

Prof. R. Rox Anderson, MD
Lancer Endowed Chair in Dermatology
Director, Wellman Center
Massachusetts General Hospital
Harvard Medical School
Boston, Massachusetts

Preface

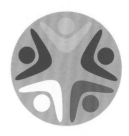

As procedural pediatric dermatologists, we find ourselves at a crossroads. On the one hand, we can choose to remain on a narrow trail, cut by past experiences and anecdotes, where "innovation" is simply rehashing what has been done in the adult world and applying it to children. This is the status quo and the easiest course. Where deference to "the way we've always done it" takes us only so far and, perhaps for some, far enough.

Alternatively, we can choose to blaze a trail of our own. One in which the next generation of experts offers fresh perspectives and collaborations that propel the field of procedural pediatric dermatology forward. One in which technical precision partners with technological innovation to evolve new kid-specific tools essential to completing the delicate tasks at hand. Where scientific method helps light the way to more effective approaches. This path leads to the point where the evolution of a new subspecialty becomes a reality and the standard of procedural care of pediatric patients is raised across the board.

Procedural Pediatric Dermatology represents a great stride toward this ultimate destination. This comprehensive textbook is unusual, if not unique, in its focus on the surgical and procedural approach to managing conditions of the skin, hair, and nails in a pediatric population. Even the textbook itself is physically arranged in an original fashion, with frontloaded, "core" content serving as reference sections designed to teach the basics and expand your comfort zone. The bulk of the book then follows with "A to Z" chapters that detail the procedural approach for over 100 conditions, with lesion-specific technique pitfalls and pearls. Chapter "call-outs" help guide readers to choose their own adventures, and instructional videos help supplement what photographs and manuscript text cannot easily convey.

It is critical to note that contributors to this inaugural edition have been invited from multiple disciplines, across a spectrum of care. From a specialty standpoint, our authors include nurses, pediatric dermatologists, pediatric plastic surgeons, Mohs surgeons, general dermatologists, cosmetic dermatologists, and laser surgeons. From a professional perspective, they include cutting-edge thought leaders, inventors, division directors, department chairs, institutional leaders, esteemed scientific investigators, and Academy and Society presidents—past, present, and future! Many of the authors' names will be immediately recognizable to some, but perhaps as-yet little known to others. That is, to be blunt, the point. Contributors were not chosen based on name recognition alone but, rather, on their ability to perform a procedure expertly and to teach the approach to our readers.

For procedural pediatric dermatologists, the ultimate goal is to be "out of a job" because all pediatric conditions could now be managed medically—without cold steel or light. What a great day that will be! For now, however, the reality is that we must be able to do our best each and every time for each and every pediatric patient because our results may, literally, last a lifetime.

We have much to learn from one another, and only through a multidisciplinary, multimodal approach may optimal treatment regimens be achieved. It is this communal sharing of knowledge and a hope to better serve our patients that inspired this textbook.

Andrew C. Krakowski, MD, FAAD

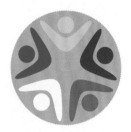

Acknowledgments

Among the most rewarding aspects of this textbook endeavor is the opportunity to collaborate with esteemed and generous colleagues across a spectrum of specialties and expansive geographies.

My associate editors, in particular, have performed a yeoman's effort to deliver the final product you are now holding in your hands. I would like to personally thank—in reverse alphabetical order, for a change!—Harper N. Price, H. Peter Lorenz, Kristen M. Kelly, Amanda A. Gosman, Lucía Z. Díaz, Craig N. Burkhart, and John C. Browning. Each and every one of you stepped up to the plate and knocked my curveballs right out of the park.

My colleagues at St. Luke's University Health Network must also be recognized for providing the opportunity and resources to deliver this tome.

- To Robby Wax, Jeff Jahre, Justin Psaila, Ed Nawrocki, Carol Kuplen, Hal Folander, Jared King, Joel Fagerstrom, and Rick Anderson: Thank you for taking a chance on a new Dermatology program and for living the vision of making Allentown-Bethlehem-Easton a hotspot for medical innovation and superlative clinical care.
- To Steve Senft, Alan Westheim, Laura Huang, Farhaan Hafeez, Carla Errickson, Ryan Johnson, Joseph Zaladonis, and Greg Brady: You are the *original* "St. Luke's Dermatology faculty," and we literally could not have a training program without you. Thank you for making every day fun, exciting, and collaborative, and thank you for striving to be the best.
- To the Derm Dream Team that supports all of our clinical services, including Danielle Margelot, Emily Cordaro, Betzaida Santiago, Ruddy Burgos, Missy Drayton, Cindy Yearwood, Christine Clarke, Allison Sabotta, Karina Rosel, Trevor Roberts, Tiffany Dieter, and Maria Gonzalez: Thank you for caring for our patients like you would for your own family members. Win the skin!

- To our St. Luke's Dermatology Residents: Ultimately, this is all for your benefit. As you take the reins, keep our amazing specialty on an ethical path and remember to make decisions based not on what is easy but, rather, on what you would want for your own loved ones.
- To the Graduate Medical Education crew that supports our burgeoning Residency in Dermatology, including Sandi Yaich, Michael Lilley, and James "Jimmy D" Dalkiewicz: Thank you for righting our ship from year to year and for exceeding all expectations.
- And, last but certainly not the least, thank you to the gentleman-scholar who brought me to St. Luke's and who reaffirms for me every day that there is no place I would rather be. My brother-in-arms. My paisano (or the Polish equivalent). The one and the only Dr. James P. Orlando. JP, you truly embody what it means to be a *connector* and a *facilitator*, and your enthusiasm for education knows no bounds. We are all lucky to have you at the helm.

Many thanks to the entire professional staff at Wolters Kluwer. The publication of this inaugural edition of *Procedural Pediatric Dermatology* was a huge undertaking. Because of the unique format (ie, the number of contributors, chapters, photographs, illustrations, and videos), there was an inordinate amount of planning and tracking that had to be done right from the very beginning. Specifically, I owe a debt of gratitude to the following individuals: Carole Wonsiewicz (who somehow made sense of every "comment" and formatting request), Robin Najar (who never gave up on the project, even when I came close), Sean Hanrahan (who picked up the pieces and made us whole again), Eric McDermott (who handled the multimedia, helped with content review, and helped protect patient privacy), and Nicole Dernoski (who ensured that we get this project over the finish line).

This book is dedicated to the following people who have changed my life for the better.

To my dad, Frank, who as a physician taught me how to treat perfect strangers like family and to be there at someone else's greatest time of need. You were there when I started this project, but you did not get to see the finished product. Your memory lives on within these pages, which hopefully will inspire generations of clinicians to come.

To my mom, Carol, who as a teacher made learning fun and who never wavered in her confidence in me, even when I was unsure of myself. Your light and optimism have touched so many people, and I would not be the person I am without your guidance and love.

To my loving and enduring wife, Carlisle (my "life editor"), and my two greatest accomplishments, Nate and James, around whom my world now revolves. Thanks for allowing me the weekend mornings and late nights needed to complete this book. You will never know just how much you mean to me and how absolutely lost I would be without you. Literally. As you know, I have zero sense of direction.

To all the preemies, infants, toddlers, children, preteens, and adolescents that have given me the privilege of caring for them and that have endured my "practice" of pediatric medicine. You constantly inspire me to do more. I do, honestly, hope to one day be out of a job.

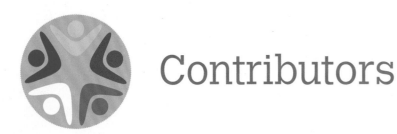

Contributors

Shehla Admani, MD
Assistant Clinical Professor
Stanford University School of Medicine
Palo Alto, California

Maggi Ahmed, MD, MSc
Postdoctoral Clinical Research Fellow
Department of Dermatology
University of Massachusetts Medical School
Worcester, Massachusetts

Murad Alam, MD, MSCI, MBA
Professor
Department of Dermatology
Northwestern University
Vice-Chair, Department of Dermatology
Northwestern Memorial Hospital
Chicago, Illinois

Morgan Albert, BS
College of Osteopathic Medicine
University of New England
Biddeford, Maine

Smita Awasthi, MD
Director of Pediatric Dermatology
Associate Professor
Department of Dermatology and Pediatrics
University of California, Davis
UC Davis Children's Hospital
Sacramento, California

Sarah Azarchi, MD, MSc
Research Assistant
Department of Dermatology
New York University School of Medicine
NYU Langone Medical Center
New York, New York

Folawiyo Babalola, BSA
University of Texas at San Antonio Health Science Center
San Antonio, Texas

Kellie Badger, BS, RN
Clinical Research Nurse Dermatology
Epidermolysis Bullosa Clinic
Phoenix Children's Hospital
Phoenix, Arizona

Emily M. Becker, MD
Clinical Assistant Professor
Department of Dermatology
University of Texas Health Science Center at San Antonio
San Antonio, Texas

Jane Sanders Bellet, MD, FAAD
Professor
Departments of Dermatology and Pediatrics
Duke University School of Medicine
Durham, North Carolina

Latanya T. Benjamin, MD, FAAD, FAAP
Associate Professor, Department of Integrated Medical Science
Co-director, Foundations of Medicine Course
Director, Communication, Compassion and Collaborative Care Thread
Florida Atlantic University
Boca Raton, Florida

Lionel Bercovitch, MD
Professor
Department of Dermatology
Warren Alpert Medical School of Brown University
Director of Pediatric Dermatology
Department of Dermatology
Hasbro Children's Hospital
Providence, Rhode Island

Guilherme Canho Bittner, MD
Mohs Micrographic Fellow
Department of Dermatology
Hospital do Servidor Publico Muncipal
São Paulo, Brazil

Mimi R. Borrelli, MBBS, MSc
Postdoctoral Research Scholar
Department of Surgery
Stanford University
Palo Alto, California

Jeremy A. Brauer, MD
Clinical Associate Professor
Ronald O. Perelman Department of Dermatology
NYU Langone Health
New York, New York

John C. Browning, MD, MBA, FAAD, FAAP
Assistant Professor of Pediatrics and Dermatology
Baylor College of Medicine
University of Texas Health Science Center
Chief of Dermatology, Children's Hospital of San Antonio
Texas Dermatology and Laser Specialists
San Antonio, Texas

Craig N. Burkhart, MD, MS, MPH, FAAD, FAAP
Adjunct Professor of Pediatric Dermatology
University of North Carolina School of Medicine
Chapel Hill, North Carolina
Burkhart Pediatric & Adolescent Dermatology
Cary, North Carolina

Samantha Casselman, RN, DNP
Nurse Practitioner
Department of Dermatology
Phoenix Children's Hospital
Phoenix, Arizona

Giselle Castillo, BS
Department of Dermatology
San Antonio Long School of Medicine
University of Texas Health
San Antonio, Texas

Audrey Chan, MD
Assistant Professor
Dermatology/Pediatric Dermatology
Baylor College of Medicine
Texas Children's Hospital
Houston, Texas

Carol E. Cheng, MD
Assistant Clinical Professor
Division of Dermatology
Department of Medicine
David Geffen School of Medicine
University of California, Los Angeles
Santa Monica, California

Alexander Choi, BS
Department of Medicine
University of Texas Health Science Center at San Antonio
San Antonio, Texas

Kimberly Ann Chun, MD
Department of Dermatology
University of California, San Diego
San Diego, California

Caryn B.C. Cobb, AB
Brown University Warren Alpert Medical School
Providence, Rhode Island

James J. Contestable, MD
Department of Dermatology
Naval Medical Center San Diego
San Diego, California

Colleen H. Cotton, MD
Assistant Professor
Department of Dermatology and Dermatologic Surgery
Department of Pediatrics
Medical University of South Carolina
Charleston, South Carolina

Catherine A. Degesys, MD
Mohs Micrographic Surgeon
MetroDerm, P.C.
Atlanta, Georgia

Lucía Z. Díaz, MD, FAAD
Chief, Division of Pediatric Dermatology
Assistant Professor of Internal Medicine and Pediatrics
Associate Program Director, Dermatology Residency
    Program
Dell Children's Hospital and Dell Medical School
Austin, Texas

Wesley Andrews Duerson, MD
Department of Surgery, Division of Otolaryngology – Head
    and Neck Surgery
Yale School of Medicine
New Haven, Connecticut

Jonathan A. Dyer, MD
Professor
Department of Dermatology
University of Missouri
Interim Chair, Department of Dermatology
University of Missouri Health Care
Columbia, Missouri

Dawn Z. Eichenfield, MD, PhD
Chief Resident
Department of Dermatology
University of California, San Diego
San Diego, California

Lawrence F. Eichenfield, MD
Professor of Dermatology and Pediatrics
Vice Chair, Department of Dermatology
Chief, Pediatric and Adolescent Dermatology
University of California, San Diego
Rady Children's Hospital, San Diego
San Diego, California

Hao Feng, MD, MHS
Assistant Professor
Department of Dermatology
University of Connecticut Health Center
Farmington, Connecticut

Joan Fernandez, BS
Department of Dermatology
Baylor College of Medicine
Houston, Texas

Sheila Fallon Friedlander, MD
Clinical Professor
Department of Dermatology
Rady Children's Hospital San Diego
San Diego, California

Roy G. Geronemus, MD
Director
Laser and Skin Surgery Center of New York
Clinical Professor
Ronald O. Perelman Department of Dermatology
New York University School of Medicine
New York, New York

Dori Goldberg, MD
Assistant Professor, Department of Dermatology
University of Massachusetts Medical School
Mohs Micrographic Surgery Fellowship
Vitiligo Clinic and Research Center
UMass Memorial Medical Center
Worcester, Massachusetts

Madeline L. Gore, BS
Loyola University Chicago Stritch School of Medicine
Maywood, Illinois

Amanda A. Gosman, MD, FACS
Professor and Chief of Plastic Surgery
Director of Craniofacial and Pediatric Plastic Surgery
University of California San Diego
Chief of Plastic Surgery
Rady Children's Hospital San Diego
San Diego, California

Emmy Graber, MD, MBA
President
The Dermatology Institute of Boston
Affiliate Clinical Instructor
Northeastern University
Boston, Massachusetts

Venkata Anisha Guda, BS
Department of Medicine
Long School of Medicine
University of Texas Health, San Antonio
University Hospital
San Antonio, Texas

Deepti Gupta, MD
Assistant Professor
Department of Pediatrics and Division of Dermatology
Seattle Children's Hospital
Seattle, Washington

Allison Han, BA
Research Associate
Department of Pediatric and Adolescent Dermatology
Rady Children's Hospital San Diego
San Diego, California

Nelise Ritter Hans-Bittner, MD
Pediatric Dermatology Fellow
Department of Dermatology
Hospital das Clínicas da Faculdade de Medicina da
    Universidade de São Paulo
São Paulo, Brazil

John E. Harris, MD, PhD
Associate Professor
Department of Dermatology
University of Massachusetts Medical School
Vice-Chair, Department of Dermatology
University of Massachusetts Memorial Healthcare
Worcester, Massachusetts

Asra Hashmi, MD
Assistant Professor
Department of Plastic Surgery
Loma Linda University
Loma Linda, California

Shauna Higgins, MD
Clinical Research Fellow
Department of Dermatology
Nebraska Medicine
Omaha, Nebraska

George Hightower, MD, PhD
Assistant Professor
Department of Dermatology
University of California, San Diego
Rady Children's Hospital
La Jolla, California

Kathryn S. Hinchee-Rodriguez, MD, PhD
Department of Internal Medicine
Baylor College of Medicine
Houston, Texas

Marcia Hogeling, MD
Assistant Professor
Department of Dermatology
David Geffen School of Medicine
University of California, Los Angeles
Los Angeles, California
Director of Pediatric Dermatology
Department of Dermatology
UCLA Medical Center
Santa Monica, California

Kristen P. Hook, MD
Associate Professor
Department of Dermatology and Pediatrics
University of Minnesota
Minneapolis, Minnesota

Sun Hsieh, MD
Assistant Professor
Department of Surgery
University of Minnesota
Pediatric Cleft and Craniofacial Surgeon
Department of Surgery
University of Minnesota Masonic Children's Hospital
Minneapolis, Minnesota

Laura Huang, MD
Academic Staff Dermatologist
Department of Dermatology
St. Luke's University Health Network
Easton, Pennsylvania

Marla N. Jahnke, MD, FAAD
Assistant Professor
Department of Dermatology
Wayne State University School of Medicine
Staff Physician, Department of Dermatology
Henry Ford Health System
Detroit, Michigan

Sara M. James, MD
Department of Dermatology
University of North Carolina at Chapel Hill
Chapel Hill, North Carolina

Puneet Singh Jolly, MD, PhD
Associate Professor
Department of Dermatology
University of North Carolina at Chapel Hill
Chapel Hill, North Carolina

Krystal M. Jones, MD
Instructor
Department of Dermatology
Harvard Medical School
Attending Dermatologist
Dermatology Program, Department of Medicine
Boston Children's Hospital
Boston, Massachusetts

Howard Kashefsky, DPM
UNC Director Podiatry
Department of Vascular Surgery
UNC Hospital, Chapel Hill
Chapel Hill, North Carolina

Nisrine Kawa, MD
Research Fellow
Wellman Center for Photomedicine
Massachusetts General Hospital
Department of Dermatology
Harvard Medical School
Boston, Massachusetts

Kristen M. Kelly, MD, FAAD
Professor of Dermatology and Surgery
Vice Chair of Dermatology
University of California, Irvine
UCI Health Beckman Laser Institute
Irvine, California

Garuna Kositratna, MD
Instructor
Department of Dermatology
Massachusetts General Hospital
Boston, Massachusetts

Andrew C. Krakowski, MD, FAAD
Chair of Dermatology
Program Director of the Residency in Dermatology
St. Luke's University Health Network
Easton, Pennsylvania

Ayan Kusari, MD, MAS
Department of Dermatology
University of California, San Francisco
San Francisco, California

Samuel H. Lance, MD, FACS
Assistant Clinical Professor Plastic Surgery
Department of Plastic and Reconstructive Surgery
University of California, San Diego
Associate Director of Plastic Surgery Residency
Department of Plastic and Reconstructive Surgery
Rady Children's Hospital and UC San Diego Health
San Diego, California

Diana H. Lee, MD, PhD
Assistant Professor
Pediatrics and Dermatology
Albert Einstein College of Medicine
Director of Pediatric Dermatology
Medicine (Dermatology)
Montefiore Medical Center
Bronx, New York

Larissa Marie Lehmer, MD
Department of Dermatology
UCI Health
Irvine, California

Richard L. Lin, MD, PhD
Department of Dermatology
New York University School of Medicine
New York, New York

H. Peter Lorenz, MD, FACS
Professor of Surgery
Division of Plastic and Reconstructive Surgery
Department of Surgery
Stanford University School of Medicine
Stanford, California
Service Chief, Plastic Surgery
Director, Craniofacial Surgery Fellowship
Department of Surgery
Lucile Packard Children's Hospital
Palo Alto, California

Elyse M. Love, MD
Clinical Professor
Department of Dermatology
Mount Sinai
New York, New York

Nicholas Ryan Lowe, MD
Department of Dermatology
Baylor College of Medicine
Houston, Texas

Maria Cecília Rivitti Machado, MD, MA
Department of Dermatology
Universidade de São Paulo
São Paulo, Brazil

Bassel H. Mahmoud, MD, PhD, FAAD
Associate Professor
Department of Dermatology
Director, Teledermatology
Vitiligo Clinic and Research Center
University of Massachusetts Medical School
Worcester, Massachusetts

Jamie R. Manning, MD
Department of Medicine (Dermatology)
Albert Einstein College of Medicine
Montefiore Medical Center
Bronx, New York

Shari Marchbein, MD
Assistant Clinical Professor
Ronald O. Perelman Department of Dermatology
NYU Langone Health
New York, New York

Renata S. Maricevich, MD, FACS, FAAP
Assistant Professor
Department of Surgery
Baylor College of Medicine
Plastic Surgeon
Department of Surgery
Texas Children's Hospital
Houston, Texas

Brent C. Martin, MD
Department of Dermatology
University of California, Irvine
Irvine, California

Catalina Matiz, MD
Pediatric Dermatologist
Department of Dermatology
Southern California Permanente Medical Group
San Diego, California

Julia Roma May, BS
University of Illinois College of Medicine
Chicago, Illinois

Bradley G. Merritt, MD
Associate Professor
Director of Mohs Micrographic Surgery
Department of Dermatology
University of North Carolina at Chapel Hill
Chapel Hill, North Carolina

Denise W. Metry, MD
Associate Professor of Dermatology and Pediatrics
Baylor College of Medicine
Texas Children's Hospital
Houston, Texas

Paul A. Mittermiller, MD
Chief Resident
Division of Plastic and Reconstructive Surgery
Department of Surgery
Stanford University School of Medicine
Palo Alto, California

Deborah Moon, BA
Department of Dermatology
University of California, Los Angeles
David Geffen School of Medicine
Los Angeles, California

Nisma Mujahid, MD, PhD
Department of Dermatology
University of Utah School of Medicine
Salt Lake City, Utah

Girish S. Munavalli, MD, MHS, FACMS
Clinical Assistant Professor
Department of Dermatology
Wake Forest University, School of Medicine
Winston Salem, North Carolina

Sheena Nguyen, DO
Pediatric Dermatology Fellow
Department of Pediatrics and Division of Dermatology
Seattle Children's Hospital
Seattle, Washington

Talia Noorily, BA
Department of Dermatology
Baylor College of Medicine
Houston, Texas

Manisha Notay, MBBS
Department of Dermatology
University of California, Davis
Sacramento, California

Judith O'Haver, PhD, RN
Nurse Practitioner
Department of Dermatology
Phoenix Children's Hospital
Phoenix, Arizona

Zilda Najjar Prado de Oliveira, MD, PhD
Department of Dermatology
Universidade de São Paulo
São Paulo, Brazil

Jennifer Ornelas, MD
Department of Dermatology
University of California, Davis
Sacramento, California

Karina M. Paci, MD
Department of Family Medicine
University of North Carolina School of Medicine
Chapel Hill, North Carolina

Jessica Parappuram, MS
University of Texas at San Antonio
San Antonio, Texas

Kavina Patel, MS
Department of Medicine
University of Texas Health Science Center at San Antonio
San Antonio, Texas

Eileen Peterson, RN
Patient Service Manager
Department of Dermatology
University of North Carolina at Chapel Hill
Chapel Hill, North Carolina

Eugênio Raul de Almeida Pimentel, MD, PhD
Department of Dermatology
Universidade de São Paulo
São Paulo, Brazil

Mark Popenhagen, PsyD
Clinical Director—Inpatient Psychology Services
Director of Mental Health Services
Department of Psychology
Phoenix Children's Hospital
Phoenix, Arizona

Harper N. Price, MD, FAAD, FAAP
Clinical Assistant Professor
Department of Child Health
University of Arizona College of Medicine
Assistant Professor of Dermatology
Mayo Clinic College of Medicine and Science
Division Chief, Dermatology
Program Director, Pediatric Dermatology Fellowship
Phoenix Children's Hospital and Phoenix Children's
    Medical Group
Phoenix, Arizona

Michael C. Raisch, MD
Mohs Micrographic Surgeon and Dermatologist
Private Practice
Boulder, Colorado

Brian Z. Rayala, MD
Associate Professor
Department of Family Medicine
University of North Carolina School of Medicine
Chapel Hill, North Carolina

Christopher Rizk, MD
Dermatologist
Elite Dermatology
Houston, Texas

Danielle H. Rochlin, MD
Department of Surgery
Stanford University School of Medicine
Stanford, California

Ashley M. Rosa, MD
Division of Dermatology
Department of Internal Medicine
Dell Medical School
The University of Texas at Austin
Austin, Texas

Tara L. Rosenberg, MD
Assistant Professor, Department of Otolaryngology
Baylor College of Medicine
Surgical Director, Vascular Anomalies Center
Texas Children's Hospital
Houston, Texas

Mohammed D. Saleem, MD, MPH
Department of Medicine
University of Florida
Gainesville, Florida

Luciana Paula Samorano, MD
Department of Dermatology
Universidade de São Paulo
São Paulo, Brazil

Christopher J. Sayed, MD
Assistant Professor
Department of Dermatology
University of North Carolina School of Medicine
Chapel Hill, North Carolina

Samantha L. Schneider, MD
Department of Dermatology
Henry Ford Health System
Detroit, Michigan

Jennifer J. Schoch, MD
Assistant Professor
Department of Dermatology
University of Florida
Gainesville, Florida

Stephen C. Senft, MD
Academic Staff Dermatologist
Department of Dermatology
St. Luke's University Health Network
Easton, Pennsylvania

Clifford C. Sheckter, MD
Chief Resident
Division of Plastic and Reconstructive Surgery
Department of Surgery
Stanford University School of Medicine
Palo Alto, California

Megan E. Shelton, MD
Department of Internal Medicine, Division of Dermatology
Dell Seton Medical Center
Austin, Texas

Peter R. Shumaker, MD, FAAD, FACMS
Voluntary Associate Clinical Professor
Department of Dermatology
University of California, San Diego
Dermatologic Surgeon
Department of Dermatology/Medicine
VA San Diego Healthcare System
San Diego, California

Gaurav Singh, MD, MPH
Ronald O. Perelman Department of Dermatology
NYU Langone Health
New York, New York

Austin Carter Smith, BS
San Antonio Long School of Medicine
University of Texas Health
San Antonio, Texas

Jessica Sprague, MD
Assistant Clinical Professor
Division of Pediatric and Adolescent Dermatology
Department of Dermatology
University of California, San Diego School of Medicine
Rady Children's Hospital, San Diego
San Diego, California

Alexa Beth Steuer, MD, MPH
Research Fellow
Ronald O. Perelman Department of Dermatology
New York University School of Medicine
New York, New York

Caroline Stovall, MD
Department of Dermatology
University of North Carolina Hospitals
Chapel Hill, North Carolina

Angel J. Su, MD
Baylor College of Medicine
Diagnostic Radiology
University of Texas Health Science Center, Houston
Houston, Texas

Kelly Jo Tackett, MPH
School of Medicine
University of North Carolina at Chapel Hill
Chapel Hill, North Carolina

Jesalyn A. Tate, MD
Department of Dermatology
University of Florida
Gainesville, Florida

Joyce M. C. Teng, MD, PhD
Professor of Dermatology and Pediatrics
Department of Dermatology
Stanford University School of Medicine
Palo Alto, California

Ruth Tevlin, MB, BCh, BAO, MRCS, MD
Plastic Surgery Resident
Stanford University Medical Center
Palo Alto, California

Megha M. Tollefson, MD
Associate Professor
Department of Dermatology and Department of Pediatrics
Mayo Clinic College of Medicine and Science
Consultant (Joint Appointment)
Departments of Dermatology and Pediatric and Adolescent
    Medicine
Mayo Clinic
Rochester, Minnesota

Megan A. Trainor, MD
Division of Dermatology
Department of Internal Medicine
Dell Medical School
The University of Texas at Austin
Austin, Texas

Thanh-Nga T. Tran, MD, PhD
Instructor
Department of Dermatology
Harvard Medical School
Staff
Department of Dermatology
Massachusetts General Hospital
Boston, Massachusetts

Allison Truong, MD, FAAD
Dermatologist
Cedars-Sinai Health System
Los Angeles, California

Nathan S. Uebelhoer, DO
Laser and Cosmetic Surgery Consultant
Compass Dermatopathology
Coronado Dermatology
San Diego, California

Andrea R. Waldman, MD
Department of Medicine (Dermatology)
Albert Einstein College of Medicine
Montefiore Medical Center
Bronx, New York

Catherine Gupta Warner, MD
Department of Dermatology
Atlanta West Dermatology
Austell, Georgia
Pediatric Dermatology Consultant
Department of Pediatric Dermatology
Children's Hospital of Atlanta
Atlanta, Georgia

Ashley Wysong, MD, MS
Chair and Associate Professor
Department of Dermatology
University of Nebraska Medical Center
Medical Director
Department of Dermatology
Nebraska Medicine
Omaha, Nebraska

Kevin Yarbrough, MD
Staff Physician
Department of Dermatology
Kaiser Permanente North West
Clackamas, Oregon

Danielle Yeager, MD
Department of Dermatology
Henry Ford Health System
Detroit, Michigan

Molly J. Youssef, MD
Instructor
Department of Dermatology
Mayo Clinic
Rochester, Minnesota

Christopher B. Zachary, MBBS, FRCP
Chairman, Department of Dermatology
University of California Irvine
Irvine, California

Allison Zarbo, MD
Department of Dermatology
Henry Ford Health System
Detroit, Michigan

Alexandra Zeitany, MD
Department of Dermatology
University of North Carolina at Chapel Hill
Chapel Hill, North Carolina

Contents

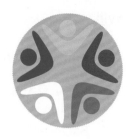

Associate Editors   iii
Foreword   iv
Preface   v
Acknowledgments   vi
Contributors   viii

SECTION I: Preprocedural Approach

1 Quality of Life 2
Kelly Jo Tackett and Craig N. Burkhart

2 Ethical Dilemmas 7
Caryn B.C. Cobb and Lionel Bercovitch

3 Molecular and Cellular Differences Between Children and Adults 11
George Hightower

4 Billing and Coding in Procedural Pediatric Dermatology 14
Murad Alam

5 Surgical Procedure Room Setup 18
Asra Hashmi and Amanda A. Gosman

6 Antiseptics and Aseptic Technique 22
Samantha L. Schneider, Danielle Yeager, and Marla N. Jahnke

7 Surgical Instruments 27
Asra Hashmi and Amanda A. Gosman

8 Sutures 33
Asra Hashmi and Amanda A. Gosman

9 Anatomy and Superficial Landmarks of the Head and Neck 37
Catherine A. Degesys and Craig N. Burkhart

SECTION II: Procedural Approach

10 Hemostasis 47
Jesalyn A. Tate and Jennifer J. Schoch

11 Simple Wound Repair 52
Mimi R. Borrelli, Ruth Tevlin, and H. Peter Lorenz

12 Complex Wound Repair 63
Sun Hsieh and Amanda A. Gosman

13 Special Site Surgery 69
Samuel H. Lance and Amanda A. Gosman

14 Injectables 77
Kavina Patel and John C. Browning

15 Injectable Corticosteroids (Intralesional Kenalog, Intramuscular) 82
Eileen Peterson, Stephen C. Senft, and Craig N. Burkhart

16 Cryosurgery 85
Andrea R. Waldman and Diana H. Lee

17 Electrosurgery/Hyfrecation 88
John C. Browning and Giselle Castillo

18 Laser Surgery 92
Larissa Marie Lehmer and Kristen M. Kelly

19 Laser Treatment of Vascular Lesions 107
Larissa Marie Lehmer and Kristen M. Kelly

20 Phototherapy and Photodynamic Therapy 114
Sara M. James and Craig N. Burkhart

21 Chemical Peels 120
Angel J. Su, Alexander Choi, and John C. Browning

22 Dermabrasion 124
Michael C. Raisch and Bradley G. Merritt

23 Autologous Fat Transfer 127
Amanda A. Gosman, Samuel H. Lance, and Sun Hsieh

SECTION III: Diagnostic-Specific Procedures

MANEUVERS

24 Acquired Keratoderma 132
Jessica Sprague, Catherine Gupta Warner, Kimberly Ann Chun, and Sheila Fallon Friedlander

25 Aquagenic Wrinkling 133
Jessica Sprague, Catherine Gupta Warner, Kimberly Ann Chun, and Sheila Fallon Friedlander

26 Bacterial Culture 135
Jessica Sprague, Catherine Gupta Warner, Kimberly Ann Chun, and Sheila Fallon Friedlander

27 Dermatographism 137
Jessica Sprague, Catherine Gupta Warner, Kimberly Ann Chun, and Sheila Fallon Friedlander

28 Dermoscopy 138
Jessica Sprague, Catherine Gupta Warner, Kimberly Ann Chun, and Sheila Fallon Friedlander

29 Fungal Culture 140
Jessica Sprague, Catherine Gupta Warner, Kimberly Ann Chun, and Sheila Fallon Friedlander

30 Hair Biopsy 142
Jessica Sprague, Catherine Gupta Warner, Kimberly Ann Chun, and Sheila Fallon Friedlander

31 Hair Pull Test 143
Jessica Sprague, Catherine Gupta Warner, Kimberly Ann Chun, and Sheila Fallon Friedlander

32 Nail Matrix Biopsy 144
Jane Sanders Bellet

33 Patch Testing for Allergic Contact Dermatitis 150
Catalina Matiz and Shehla Admani

34 Pinworm Examination 154
Jessica Sprague, Catherine Gupta Warner, Kimberly Ann Chun, and Sheila Fallon Friedlander

35 Polymerase Chain Reaction 155
Jessica Sprague, Catherine Gupta Warner, Kimberly Ann Chun, and Sheila Fallon Friedlander

36 Skin Biopsy Techniques 156
Samantha L. Schneider, Danielle Yeager, and Marla N. Jahnke

37 Viral Culture 161
Jessica Sprague, Catherine Gupta Warner, Kimberly Ann Chun, and Sheila Fallon Friedlander

38 Wood's Lamp Skin Examination 163
Jessica Sprague, Catherine Gupta Warner, Kimberly Ann Chun, and Sheila Fallon Friedlander

MICROSCOPY

39 Demodex Examination 165
Jessica Sprague, Catherine Gupta Warner, Kimberly Ann Chun, and Sheila Fallon Friedlander

40 Hair Microscopy 167
Jessica Sprague, Catherine Gupta Warner, Kimberly Ann Chun, and Sheila Fallon Friedlander

41 Immunofluorescence 169
Jessica Sprague, Catherine Gupta Warner, Kimberly Ann Chun, and Sheila Fallon Friedlander

42 Fungal Examination or Potassium Hydroxide (KOH) Preparation 171
Jessica Sprague, Catherine Gupta Warner, Kimberly Ann Chun, and Sheila Fallon Friedlander

43 Scabies Examination 173
Jessica Sprague, Catherine Gupta Warner, Kimberly Ann Chun, and Sheila Fallon Friedlander

44 Tzank Smear 175
Jessica Sprague, Catherine Gupta Warner, Kimberly Ann Chun, and Sheila Fallon Friedlander

SECTION IV: Lesion-Specific Procedures

45 Abscess 178
Venkata Anisha Guda and John C. Browning

46 Acanthosis Nigricans 181
Giselle Castillo, Andrew C. Krakowski, John C. Browning, and Nathan S. Uebelhoer

47 Accessory Nipple 183
Samuel H. Lance and Amanda A. Gosman

48 Accessory Tragus 186
Samuel H. Lance and Amanda A. Gosman

49 Acne Comedones 188
Emmy Graber and Shari Marchbein

50 Acne Cyst 190
Emmy Graber and Shari Marchbein

51 **Acne Scarring** 191
Gaurav Singh, Elyse M. Love, and
Jeremy A. Brauer

52 **Acrochordons** 196
Megan A. Trainor and Lucía Z. Díaz

53 **Actinic Keratosis** 198
Puneet Singh Jolly

54 **Alopecia Areata** 202
Venkata Anisha Guda, Stephen C. Senft, and
John C. Browning

55 **Angiofibromas** 205
Andrew C. Krakowski, Kristen M. Kelly, Nathan
S. Uebelhoer, and Girish S. Munavalli

56 **Angiokeratoma** 207
Ayan Kusari, Allison Han, and Sheila Fallon
Friedlander

57 **Angioma, Spider** 209
Ayan Kusari, Allison Han, and Sheila Fallon
Friedlander

58 **Aplasia Cutis Congenita** 211
Laura Huang, Angel J. Su, Alexander Choi, and
John C. Browning

59 **Arthropod Bites and Stings** 213
Laura Huang, Angel J. Su, Alexander Choi, and
John C. Browning

60 **Basal Cell Carcinoma** 216
Guilherme Canho Bittner and Nelise Ritter
Hans-Bittner

61 **Basal Cell Nevus Syndrome** 218
Guilherme Canho Bittner and Nelise Ritter
Hans-Bittner

62 **Becker's Nevus** 221
Laura Huang, Angel J. Su, Alexander Choi, and
John C. Browning

63 **Blister** 223
Madeline L. Gore and Kristen P. Hook

64 **Blue Rubber Bleb Syndrome** 226
Shehla Admani and Joyce M. C. Teng

65 **Burns** 229
Deborah Moon, Shauna Higgins, and Ashley
Wysong

66 **Café au Lait Macules** 234
Dawn Z. Eichenfield and Lawrence F. Eichenfield

67 **Calcinosis Cutis** 236
Jonathan A. Dyer

68 **Callus** 238
Brian Z. Rayala and Howard Kashefsky

69 **Chalazion** 239
Austin Carter Smith and John C. Browning

70 **Circumcision Adhesions** 243
Austin Carter Smith and John C. Browning

71 **Condyloma Acuminatum** 246
Kevin Yarbrough

72 **Cutaneous Larva Migrans
(Creeping Eruption)** 249
Caroline Stovall and Craig N. Burkhart

73 **Depigmentation** 251
Nisrine Kawa, Julia Roma May, Morgan Albert,
and Thanh-Nga T. Tran

74 **Dermal Melanocytosis
(Mongolian Spot)** 257
Dawn Z. Eichenfield and Lawrence F. Eichenfield

75 **Dermatofibrosarcoma Protuberans** 259
Guilherme Canho Bittner and Nelise Ritter
Hans-Bittner

76 **Dermoid Cysts** 261
John C. Browning and Folawiyo Babalola

77 **Epidermal Inclusion Cysts
and Pilar Cysts** 264
Austin Carter Smith and John C. Browning

78 **Epidermal Nevi** 267
Allison Zarbo and Marla N. Jahnke

79 **Epidermolysis Bullosa** 271
Madeline L. Gore and Kristen P. Hook

80 **Epstein's Pearl** 275
Emily M. Becker and Jessica Parappuram

81 **Fibroma (Subungal or Periungal)** 276
Mimi R. Borrelli, Ruth Tevlin, and H. Peter Lorenz

82 **Deep Fungal Infection** 278
Talia Noorily, Joan Fernandez, Christopher Rizk,
Renata S. Maricevich, and Audrey Chan

83 **Granuloma Annulare** 281
Jennifer Ornelas and Smita Awasthi

84 **Infantile Hemangioma** 283
Ayan Kusari, Allison Han, and Sheila Fallon
Friedlander

85 **Hematoma** 286
Mimi R. Borrelli, Ruth Tevlin, and H. Peter Lorenz

86 **Hidradenitis Suppurativa
(Acne Inversa)** 289
Christopher J. Sayed and Karina M. Paci

87 **Hyperhidrosis** 292
Jane Sanders Bellet

88 Hyperpigmentation 294
Nicholas Ryan Lowe, Nisma Mujahid, Tara L. Rosenberg, Denise W. Metry, and Audrey Chan

89 Hypertrichosis 298
Deborah Moon, Shauna Higgins, and Ashley Wysong

90 Hypertrophic Scars and Contractures 306
James J. Contestable and Peter R. Shumaker

91 Hypopigmentation 312
Mohammed D. Saleem and Jennifer J. Schoch

92 Onychocryptosis (Ingrown Nail) 313
Jane Sanders Bellet

93 Juvenile Xanthogranuloma 318
Jennifer Ornelas and Smita Awasthi

94 Keratosis Pilaris 320
Manisha Notay, Jennifer Ornelas, and Smita Awasthi

95 Labial Adhesion 323
John C. Browning and Giselle Castillo

96 Laceration Repair 325
Samuel H. Lance and Amanda A. Gosman

97 Lichen Planus 327
Alexandra Zeitany and Craig N. Burkhart

98 Lipoma 330
Mimi R. Borrelli, Ruth Tevlin, and H. Peter Lorenz

99 Lymphatic Malformations 332
Shehla Admani and Joyce M. C. Teng

100 Mastocytoma 334
Allison Truong, Latanya T. Benjamin, Carol E. Cheng, and Marcia Hogeling

101 Median Raphe Cyst 337
Paul A. Mittermiller, Clifford C. Sheckter, and H. Peter Lorenz

102 Melanoma 338
Mimi R. Borrelli, Ruth Tevlin, and H. Peter Lorenz

103 Milium 340
Allison Truong, Latanya T. Benjamin, Carol E. Cheng, and Marcia Hogeling

104 Miliaria 342
Allison Truong, Latanya T. Benjamin, Carol E. Cheng, and Marcia Hogeling

105 Molluscum Contagiosum 344
Allison Truong, Latanya T. Benjamin, Carol E. Cheng, and Marcia Hogeling

106 Mycosis Fungoides 347
Laura Huang and Andrew C. Krakowski

107 Myiasis 351
Jamie R. Manning and Diana H. Lee

108 Neurofibromas 354
Laura Huang

109 Nevi 356
Shauna Higgins, Deborah Moon, and Ashley Wysong

110 Nevus of Ota and Nevus of Ito 362
Dawn Z. Eichenfield and Lawrence F. Eichenfield

111 Nevus Sebaceous 365
Samuel H. Lance and Amanda A. Gosman

112 Nevus Simplex 368
Molly J. Youssef and Megha M. Tollefson

113 Pigmentary Mosaicism 369
Nisrine Kawa, Garuna Kositratna, and Thanh-Nga T. Tran

114 Pilomatricoma (Pilomatrixoma) 374
Ashley M. Rosa and Lucía Z. Díaz

115 Port-Wine Birthmarks 377
Hao Feng and Roy G. Geronemus

116 Psoriasis 379
Kevin Yarbrough and Andrew C. Krakowski

117 Pyogenic Granuloma 383
Molly J. Youssef and Megha M. Tollefson

118 Perianal Pyramidal Protrusions 385
Kathryn S. Hinchee-Rodriguez

119 Rosacea 387
Krystal M. Jones and Lucía Z. Díaz

120 Scabies 389
Craig N. Burkhart

121 Solitary Fibrous Hamartoma of Infancy 392
Paul A. Mittermiller, Danielle H. Rochlin, and H. Peter Lorenz

122 Squamous Cell Carcinoma 393
Guilherme Canho Bittner and Nelise Ritter Hans-Bittner

123 Supernumerary Digits 396
Samuel H. Lance and Amanda A. Gosman

124 Tattoo Removal 398
Richard L. Lin, Alexa Beth Steuer, Wesley Andrews Duerson, Sarah Azarchi, and Jeremy A. Brauer

125 Telangiectasia 400
Brent C. Martin and Christopher B. Zachary

126 Umbilical Granuloma 403
Venkata Anisha Guda and John C. Browning

127 Venous Malformations 405
Shehla Admani and Joyce M. C. Teng

128 Human Papillomavirus Wart (Verruca) 408
Jennifer Ornelas and Smita Awasthi

129 Vitiligo 414

Part I: Overview and Phototherapy and Excimer Laser Procedures 414
Sheena Nguyen, John E. Harris, and Deepti Gupta

Part II: Surgical Transplantation 417
Maggi Ahmed, Dori Goldberg, and Bassel H. Mahmoud

130 Xeroderma Pigmentosum 420
Nelise Ritter Hans-Bittner, Luciana Paula Samorano, Maria Cecília Rivitti Machado, Zilda Najjar Prado de Oliveira, and Eugênio Raul de Almeida Pimentel

SECTION V: Postprocedural Approach

131 Wound Dressings 425
Kellie Badger and Harper N. Price

132 Wound Care and Optimizing Healing 434
Harper N. Price and Kellie Badger

133 Postprocedure Antibiotics 443
George Hightower

134 Pain Management 448
Harper N. Price and Mark Popenhagen

135 Photoprotection 456
Venkata Anisha Guda and John C. Browning

136 Surgical Complications 460
Megan E. Shelton and Lucía Z. Díaz

137 Wet Wrap Therapy 468
Samantha Casselman, Judith O'Haver, and Harper N. Price

138 Bleach Baths 472
Judith O'Haver, Samantha Casselman, and Harper N. Price

139 Patient and Family Resources 475
Colleen H. Cotton

 Appendix Common Dilutions of Triamcinolone Acetonide (Kenalog)

Index 479

To view the Appendix please access the eBook bundled with this text. Instructions are located on the inside front cover.

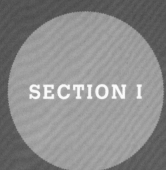

SECTION I

Preprocedural Approach

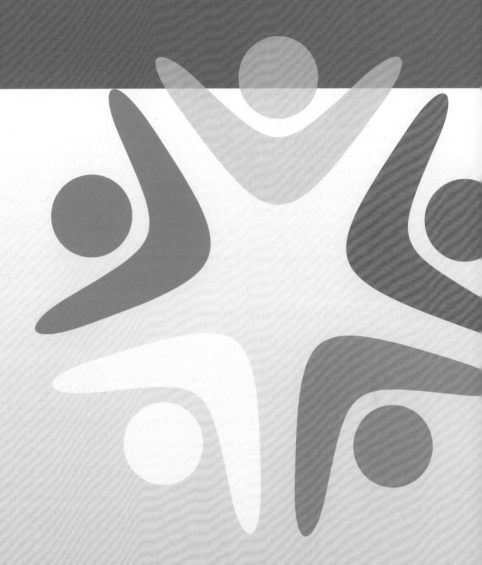

1 Quality of life

2 Ethical Dilemmas

3 Molecular and Cellular Differences Between Children and Adults

4 Billing and Coding in Procedural Pediatric Dermatology

5 Surgical Procedure Room Setup

6 Antiseptics and Aseptic Technique

7 Surgical Instruments

8 Sutures

9 Anatomy and Superficial Landmarks of the Head and Neck

CHAPTER 1

Quality of Life

Kelly Jo Tackett and Craig N. Burkhart

Quality of life (QoL) encompasses numerous components of general well-being, including physical, functional, emotional, social, and family well-being.[1] The inclusion of multiple aspects of well-being in the definition of *health* is a growing movement that coincides with new medical and public health advances that seek to not only delay mortality but also improve quality of lives among patients. The World Health Organization (WHO) embraces this concept by considering mortality and QoL together and by defining health as "a state of complete physical, mental and social well-being and not merely the absence of disease or infirmity."[2] Traditionally, the United States has defined health from the narrower *deficit perspective*, relying solely on measures of morbidity or mortality; however, the focus on QoL continues to gain momentum. As an example, even the Centers for Disease Control and Prevention (CDC) now regularly measures QoL through the National Health and Nutrition Examination Survey (NHANES)[3] and Behavioral Risk Factor Surveillance System[4] (see Table 1.1).

The concept of QoL is particularly emphasized in dermatology as most dermatologic conditions do not shorten life expectancy. Accordingly, clinical trials and health policy evaluations within dermatology often quantify the burden of most disease through QoL measurements.[6] Another important measure related to QoL that is used in some dermatology studies is called QALYs (quality-adjusted life years). A QALY is a measure that combines QoL and length of life into one number and may be seen in adult dermatology trials that assess cost-effectiveness or in some clinical trials.[7] However, one must interpret studies using QALYs in pediatric populations with extreme caution as there is extensive variation in the methods used to calculate QALYs between studies in pediatrics.[8] It is also important to remember that QoL is a subjective measure and can be influenced by many contextual factors including severity of disease, gender, age, culture, ethnicity, social class, personality type, level of anxiety, and education.[9-11] Therefore, numerical QoL measures in dermatology may be most useful as a tool to identify changes after interventions and should be complemented with an understanding of the qualitative patient experience.

This chapter will review several features of QoL that may be useful to clinicians, educators, and researchers in pediatric dermatology. Where possible, we will discuss QoL as it relates to skin conditions that are treated with procedures and QoL issues related to the procedures themselves. To balance the quantitative measures, a qualitative description of the patient experience will precede the quantitative QoL discussion.

TABLE 1.1 : Quality of Life Definitions/ Assessments

- **World Health Organization (WHO) definition of health:** "a state of complete physical, mental and social well-being and not merely the absence of disease or infirmity"
- **WHO definition of quality of life:** "the individuals' perception of their position in life, in the context of the cultural and value system in which they live and in relation to their goals, expectations, standards and concerns"
- **Pediatric-specific definition of quality of life:** "a measure of how a child views his/her life in relationship to how they could reasonably expect or desire it to be"[5]
- **Health-related quality of life:** "an individual's or group's perceived physical and mental health over time"
- **Quality-adjusted life years (QALYs):** a measure that combines length of life and quality of life into a single number
- **Disability-adjusted life years (DALYs):** a measure representing the total number of years lost to illness, disability, and premature death within a given population
- **Cost-effectiveness analysis:** a technique in which the costs of an intervention are compared with a predefined health outcome.
- **Cost-utility analysis:** a type of cost-effectiveness analysis utilizing QALYs as an outcome measure

Sources: World Health Organization. WHOQOL Measuring Quality of Life from Division of Mental Health and Prevention of Substance Abuse. Geneva, Switzerland; 1997; Centers for Disease Control and Prevention. Measuring Healthy Days: Population Assessment of Health-Related Quality of life. Atlanta, Georgia: Centers for Disease Control and Prevention; 2000; Griebsch I, Coast J, Brown J. Quality-adjusted life-years lack quality in pediatric care: a critical review of published cost-utility studies in child health. *Pediatrics*. 2005;115(5):e600–e614; World Health Organization. Metrics: Disability-Adjusted Life Year (DALY). http://www.who.int/healthinfo/global_burden_disease/metrics_daly/en/. Accessed May 14, 2018.

QUALITATIVE EXPERIENCE: WHAT CHILDREN, ADOLESCENTS, AND FAMILIES SAY

Very few qualitative studies have been performed on the parent, child, and adolescent experience of skin disease. The majority of current qualitative studies for childhood skin disease only represent a small number of conditions, including atopic dermatitis, psoriasis, and epidermolysis bullosa.[12] To gain context behind the numbers and statistics of these studies, it is important to understand the effects skin disease has on children, adolescents, and their families in their own words. The following is an overview of the dermatologic patient experience from available qualitative publications.

Children and Adolescent Perspective

In a recent review of qualitative data, three themes emerge from the child and adolescent's perspective related to skin disease: (1) wanting to be normal versus needing to be different, (2) the importance of others' understanding, and (3) powerlessness.[12]

Young people felt a *sense of being different* from others because of their skin condition.[12] Sometimes the children and adolescents developed this awareness of difference based solely on the comments of others. The skin condition resulted in feelings of isolation for some children and a sense that teasing and other negative interactions would be reduced or prevented if the condition was not visible. In addition to feeling different, some children sensed a *need to approach their environment differently* because of their skin condition. For example, some children had physical limitations because of their skin disease, impeding their ability to participate in activities with other children. Some adolescents avoided activities, such as engaging in intimate behaviors, because of embarrassment about their appearance.

In children without visible skin conditions, children reported that others did not appreciate the impact that skin disease had on their lives. They felt a *need to educate others* because of a lack of sympathy or correct misunderstandings such as others' beliefs that the skin condition might be contagious. Misunderstandings also occurred with medical professionals who underestimated the impact of the skin condition on the child's life or did not offer sufficient support.

Lastly, some children and adolescents felt a sense of *powerlessness* as a result of having a skin condition. Discrimination and name-calling are often experienced by children with visible skin conditions. Strangers were also more likely than friends and family to ask children and adolescents openly about their skin condition. Parents spent large amounts of time "policing" how children took care of their skin condition, and many children with skin conditions were viewed as having "special needs" at school. Being separated and labeled this way led to reduced self-esteem and high levels of distress for some children, which contributed to a sense of powerlessness and vulnerability.

Parental Perspective

Parents' QoL may also be significantly impacted by their children's skin conditions. In the same review of qualitative research, three themes emerged for the parental perspective: (1) skin conditions interfere with having a "normal" family life, (2) feeling the stresses that their child feels, and (3) feeling an impact on the parent-child relationship.[12]

Many parents noted that skin conditions can *affect many areas of life.* Often, treatments were noted to be time consuming, which took time away from spending with spouses or other family members. This caused some parents to choose jobs that allowed more flexibility. In some families, the parents felt a sense of isolation and depressed mood because of the impact of the skin condition. In more extreme cases, relationships were severed because of the child's skin condition.

Parents often felt many of the *psychological effects* of the skin condition experienced by the child. Parents felt psychological strain when strangers made comments about their child's skin condition or when the child underwent painful treatments for it. Parents also worried about their child's skin condition getting worse in the future, appearance-related teasing, and their child's ability to make friends.

The *parent-child relationship* may be affected in multiple ways. Some skin conditions required parents to apply treatments that the child dislikes or are painful, leading to a sense of needing coercion or having to restrain the child to apply the treatment. Based on unhelpful comments from medical professionals and relatives, some parents felt blamed for either causing their child's skin condition or not being able to prevent the skin condition or behavioral problems resulting from the skin condition.[12] Parents often felt like they had gained a level of expertise related to their child's skin condition, occasionally leading to an added burden that they felt unable to leave their child with other adults who could not provide adequate care.

Burden of the Treatment Versus Burden of the Condition

Pediatric dermatologic procedures may be used to improve both physical function and improve psychological well-being. Procedural interventions are often assumed to improve the psychological well-being of children with visible skin diseases by increasing their self-esteem, reducing stigmatization, and reducing marginalization within the community.[13] However, empirical evidence challenges this assumption even when patients and families are extremely pleased with the outcome immediately following surgery.[13] This is discussed in the following paragraphs, where research reveals that there is actually a mixture of positive and negative QoL outcomes that may occur at the same time in children who undergo procedural interventions for craniofacial differences.

The positive outcomes reported by patients following reconstructive surgery for craniofacial differences include an improved self-esteem and reduced stigmatization.[13] In patients with craniofacial differences, the primary goal for treatment was to improve QoL by looking more "normal," which they expected to reduce stigmatization, questioning, staring, and teasing. Several patients noted an improvement in self-esteem after surgery.[13]

The negative outcomes reported by patients who had reconstructive surgery for craniofacial differences include: (1) addiction to attaining the "perfect surgical face", (2) missing school for treatments, (3) adjusting to an evolving appearance, (4) wondering when the treatments will end, and (5) experiencing stigma related to undergoing surgery.[13] Many patients were affected by the number of surgeries required during their youth, which sometimes led to being held back grades. Additionally, the multiple facial transformations added to teenage stress and social withdrawal. The period immediately following surgery was often the most difficult time as patients perceived increased social stigmatization in which they had to explain their absences from school and changing appearance. The parent-child relationship was also sometimes affected by the surgical process. Although some patients did not mind their parents' desire for them to have surgery, some resented their parents' suggestion that there was something about their appearance that needed to be changed.

QUANTITATIVE EXPERIENCE: NUMERICAL MEASURING OF THE EFFECTS ON CHILDREN, ADOLESCENTS, AND FAMILIES

As the qualitative studies earlier have revealed, QoL may be difficult to measure, as a person's sense of overall well-being includes physical, psychological, emotional, social, and spiritual dimensions. To aid in measurement, QoL has been defined in a variety of more narrow ways to assess functional health, physical disability, clinical symptoms, psychological well-being, and mood.[14] However, the optimal scale of QoL would include evaluation of physical, psychological, emotional, and social domains.[14] There is no perfect QoL instrument, making it imperative to understand the purpose and limitations of the specific QoL instrument chosen to study a given disease. When making comparisons about disease burdens, QoL measurement tools should be evaluated to ensure that the instruments used encompassed the major features of the diseases being studied.

QoL scales can be divided into generic or disease-specific instruments. *Generic scales* are designed to study any health condition and are therefore useful for making comparisons across diverse populations and diseases. Disease-specific scales are designed to assess the effect of a specific health condition on an individual's perceived QoL. This type of scale is useful for evaluating outcomes in clinical trials related to a specific condition; however, they are not as useful in evaluating QoL as a global construct that includes all major aspects of a person's life. Combining the qualitative experience with one of these quantitative scales could provide a more authentic picture of the effect of dermatologic disease on QoL.

Dermatologic diseases are unique as their significant psychosocial influence often results in a higher burden of disease than expected based on clinical manifestations.[15,16] This is reflective of the fact that living with disease is more complex than clinical findings alone. Skin disease tends to have an increased impact on many nonphysical aspects of a person's life (social, psychological, economic, and sense of community). Therefore, we can be more helpful to patients and families by having an understanding of the qualitative experience and ensuring that clinical trial QoL instruments are valid and reliable. Otherwise, investigators may risk recommending an intervention with no significant benefit to the patient and family or, conversely, recommending against an intervention that actually could have benefited the affected population. Several of the properties related to validity and reliability that should be considered before using a QoL instrument in a clinical trial have been reviewed by Frew et al.[17]

QUALITY OF LIFE INSTRUMENTS IN CLINICAL DERMATOLOGY

Although QoL instruments are designed for use in clinical trials and health policy, they can potentially be used in clinical practice.[6,18] In the right setting, a QoL instrument may improve patient-physician communication, allowing physicians to pick up on other diagnoses (depression) or problems (increasing pain or itch).[19] Use of QoL instruments in oncology resulted in an increased discussion of chronic symptoms, awareness of the impact of disease on patients, and an improvement in patients' well-being.[20] However, a systematic review on the use of patient-reported outcome (PRO) assessments in clinical practice, including QoL instruments, highlighted many challenges to their implementation. The authors noted that PRO assessments can be time consuming; both patients and physicians perceived PRO instruments as burdensome; additional resources are needed to interpret PRO scores in a meaningful way; and the implications for treatment were difficult to determine.[19] To ensure a positive experience for patients and providers, dermatologists should be thoughtful about their patient population and purpose before integrating a QoL instrument in their practice.

Purpose of Quality of Life Instruments

Van Cranenburgh et al.[18] have provided a detailed overview of potential applications of QoL instruments in a clinical dermatology practice. Potential reasons to include a QoL instrument include:

- *Increasing patient self-awareness and empowerment* as patients may gain more insight into the impact of skin disease on components of their overall well-being.

- *Improving patient-centered care* as the dermatologist may better understand the impact of skin disease and/or its treatment on the patient.
- *Helping to guide the optimal choice of treatment* as dermatologists can help adjust the intensity of treatment based on the impact on patients' QoL. Additionally, dermatologists may be able to better recognize when supplemental care (such as psychiatry or social work) may be beneficial.
- Monitor treatment over time.
- Improve treatment outcomes.

Target Population

It is important to remember that QoL instruments may not apply to (or be able to be applied to) every patient. QoL instruments are most suited for patients with chronic disease; thus, the results from a QoL instrument will have limited relevance for patients who only require a single consultation or short-term treatment. Additionally, QoL instruments should not be used with patients who find them unnecessary, intrusive, or inappropriate.[18] Many dermatologists already inquire about patient well-being, which prompts some patients to discuss the impact of their skin disease on mood, work, school, and family life without the need for quantitative assessment.[18] Thus, a QoL instrument may often be most useful when a clinician needs to collect data in a more quantitative and systematic way.

TREATMENT TO IMPROVE QUALITY OF LIFE

Interventions to improve QoL depend on the condition being treated. In many cases, treatment of the cutaneous disease is the only requirement to improve QoL. Many self-limited conditions fit into this category such as molluscum contagiosum, warts, pyogenic granulomas, or ingrown nails. Other diseases that are chronic with additional systemic symptoms or diseases that may not have good treatment options for cure have increased need for QoL measures, such as genodermatoses, giant congenital melanocytic nevi, or large vascular malformations. For these diseases, QoL would be best approached by addressing psychosocial factors alongside medical treatment.

A strong patient-physician relationship is the foundation for addressing psychosocial issues. It is important to remember that parents tend to be natural advocates for their children's medical care and symptom relief who may not be receptive to additional counseling on stress and psychosocial support.[21] Without a strong relationship between parents and providers, any mention of psychological, social, or psychiatric interventions may be met with indifference, disdain, or hostility.[21] Nevertheless, dermatology visits should include some level of screening for emotional state and functional status. If the dermatologist detects a decrease in function during the course of treatment (school, socialization, extracurricular activities, isolation), a referral to a psychiatrist, mental health worker, or social worker may be helpful. Additionally, detection and treatment of comorbid mood disorders, anxiety disorders, or attention-deficit/hyperactivity disorder may improve outcomes and compliance.

The close tie between self-esteem and body image in adolescents and children makes it imperative to maintain a positive and hopeful attitude throughout treatment.[21] Reasonable hope (but not false hope) should also be presented to children and families with difficult-to-treat diseases. The emotional toll of body image

TABLE 1.2 ⋮ Quality of Life Resources for Children with Skin Conditions

- *Positive Exposure* (www.positiveexposure.org): uses visual arts to present the humanity and dignity of individuals living with genetic, physical, behavioral, and intellectual differences
- *Changing Faces* (www.changingfaces.org.uk): advocacy and support group for individuals with facial differences
- *Surgically Shaping Children: Technology, Ethics, and the Pursuit of Normality, edited by Erik Parens* Johns Hopkins University Press. (https://jhupbooks.press.jhu.edu/content/surgically-shaping-children)
- *Basal Cell Carcinoma Nevus Syndrome:* Basal Cell Carcinoma Nevus Syndrome/Gorlin Syndrome Life Support Network (www.bccns.org)
- *Ichthyosis:* Foundation for Ichthyosis and Related Skin Types (FIRST) (www.firstskinfoundation.org)
- *Alopecia Areata:* National Alopecia Areata Foundation (NAAF) (www.naaf.org)
- *Melanocytic Nevi:* Nevus Outreach, Inc. (www.nevus.org)
- *Psoriasis:*

  National Psoriasis Foundation (www.psoriasis.org)
  The Psoriasis Association (www.psoriasis-association.org)
  Psoriasis Help Organization (www.psoriasis-help.org.uk)
  Psoriasis and Psoriatic Arthritis Alliance (www.papaa.org)
  Sparklestone Foundation (sparklestone.org/skinfire.org)

- *Vascular Anomalies:*

  The Sturge-Weber Foundation (www.sturge-weber.org)
  Vascular Birthmark Foundation (www.birthmark.org)
  National Organization of Vascular Anomalies (www.novanews.org)

- *Vitiligo:*

  Vitiligo Support International (VSI) (www.vitiligosupport.org)
  Vitiligo Info (www.vitiligoinfo.org)
  Vitiligo Society (www.vitiligosociety.org.uk)

- *Xeroderma Pigmentosa:* Xeroderma Pigmentosum Family Support Group (www.xpfamilysupport.org)

---

issues, particularly during adolescence, can be lessened by physicians who provide hope for improvement.[21] As bullying is often directed at body variations, dermatologists should inquire about and protect children by informing parents and school officials (such as guidance counselors or school nurses) as appropriate. Finally, a social worker or patient support/advocacy group may be able to help children and families find social supports in children's communities to help them reach their full potential.

Table 1.2 includes a list of several resources useful for children with skin conditions. Surgically Shaping Children by Erik Parens[22] is a volume of in-depth essays useful for providers and families who want to further explore ethical and social issues related to the burden of having a condition versus the burden of treatment. The other resources are websites linked to condition-specific support groups, advocacy, and education.

RESOURCES FOR QUALITY OF LIFE INSTRUMENTS

An excellent review on the use of QoL instruments in pediatric dermatology can be found in a paper by Brown et al.[23] (Table 1.3). As reviewed by Brown et al., many dermatology QoL instruments can be accessed through Cardiff University (https://www.cardiff.ac.uk/medicine/resources/quality-of-life-questionnaires), the Patient-Reported Outcome and Quality of Life Instruments Database (https://eprovide.mapi-trust.org), and TNO Innovation for Life (https://www.tno.nl/en/focus-areas/healthy-living/roadmaps/youth/questionnaires-to-measure-health-related-quality-of-life/).

TABLE 1.3 ⋮ Quality of Life Instruments

INDICATION	INSTRUMENTS
Pediatric skin disease	CDLQI: Children's Dermatology Life Quality Index DLQI: Dermatology Life Quality Index HRQoL: Health-related Quality of Life MHI: Mental Health Inventory NHP: Nottingham Health Profile Skindex-29 Skindex-Teen SF-36 TNO-AZL Quality of Life Questionnaire
Acne vulgaris	CADI: Cardiff Acne Disability Index ADI: Acne Disability Index Acne QoL Index
Atopic dermatitis	CADIS: Child Atopic Dermatitis Impact Scale QoLPCAD: Quality of Life in Primary Caregivers with Atopic Dermatitis PIQoL: Parent's Index Atopic Dermatitis Quality of Life DFI: Dermatitis Family Impact Questionnaire
Psoriasis	PLSI: Psoriasis Stress Life Inventory
Vitiligo	Skin Discoloration Impact Questionnaire

Source: Reprinted from Brown MM, Chamlin SL, Smidt AC. Quality of life in pediatric dermatology. *Dermatol Clin.* 2013;31(2):211-221. Copyright © 2013 Elsevier. With permission.

REFERENCES

1. Schipper H, Clinch J, Olweny C. Quality of life studies: definitions and conceptual issues. In: *Spilker B, ed. Quality of Life and Pharmacoeconomics in Clinical Trials.* 2nd ed. Philadelphia, PA: Lippincott-Raven; 1996:11–23.
2. World Health Organization. Constitution of the World Health Organization. http://apps.who.int/gb/bd/PDF/bd47/EN/constitution-en.pdf. Accessed May 14, 2018.
3. Centers for Disease Control and Prevention. National Health and Nutrition Examination Survey. https://www.cdc.gov/nchs/nhanes/index.htm. Accessed May 14, 2018.
4. Centers for Disease Control and Prevention. Behavioral Risk Factor Surveillance System. https://www.cdc.gov/brfss/index.html. Accessed May 14, 2018.
5. Collier J, MacKinlay D, Phillips D. Norm values for the generic children's quality of life measure (GCQ). *Qual Life Res.* 2000;9:617–623.
6. Chen SC. Health-related quality of life in dermatology: introduction and overview. *Dermatol Clin.* 2012;30:205–208.
7. Centers for Disease Control and Prevention. *Measuring Healthy Days: Population Assessment of Health-Related Quality of Life.* Atlanta, Georgia: Centers for Disease Control and Prevention; 2000.
8. Griebsch I, Coast J, Brown J. Quality-adjusted life-years lack quality in pediatric care: a critical review of published cost-utility studies in child health. *Pediatrics.* 2005;115(5):e600–e6014.
9. Eiser C, Morse R. A review of measures of quality of life for children with chronic illness. *Arch Dis Child.* 2001;84:205–211.
10. Annett RD, Bender BG, Lapidus J, et al. Predicting children's quality of life in an asthma clinical trial: what do children's reports tell us? *J Pediatr.* 2001;139:854–861.
11. Sawyer MG, Spurrier N, Kennedy D, Martin J. The relationship between the quality of life of children with asthma and family functioning. *J Asthma.* 2001;38:279–284.
12. Ablett K, Thompson AR. Parental, child, and adolescent experience of chronic skin conditions: a meta-ethnography and review of the qualitative literature. *Body Image.* 2016;19:175–185.
13. Bemmels H, Biesecker B, Schmidt JL, Krokosky A, Guidotti R, Sutton EJ. Psychological and social factors in undergoing reconstructive surgery among individuals with craniofacial conditions: an exploratory study. *Cleft Palate Craniofac J.* 2013;50(2):158–167.
14. Anderson KL, Burckhardt CS. Conceptualization and measurement of quality of life as an outcome variable for health care intervention and research. *J Adv Nurs.* 1999;29:298–306.
15. Cohen JS, Biesecker BB. Quality of life in rare genetic conditions: a systematic review of the literature. *Am J Med Genet Part A.* 2010;152A:1136–1156.
16. Both H, Assink-Bot ML, Busschbach J, Nijsten T. Critical review of genetic and dermatology-specific health related quality of life instruments. *J Invest Dermatol.* 2007;127:2726–2739.
17. Frew JW, Davidson M, Murrell DF. Disease-specific health related quality of life patient reported outcome measures in Genodermatoses: a systematic review and critical evaluation. *Orphanet J Rare Dis.* 2017;12:189.
18. van Cranenburgh OD, Prinsen CAC, Sprangers MA, Spuls PI, de Korte J. Health-related quality-of-life assessment in dermatologic practice: relevance and application. *Dermatol Clin.* 2012;30:323–332.
19. Valderas JM, Kotzeva A, Espallargues M, et al. The impact of measuring patient-reported outcomes in clinical practice: a systematic review of the literature. *Qual Life Res.* 2008;17:179–193
20. Velikova G, Booth L, Smith AB, et al. Measuring quality of life in routine oncology practice improves communication and patient well-being: a randomized controlled trial. *J Clin Oncol.* 2004;22:714–724.
21. Perry M, Streusand WC. The role of psychiatry and psychology collaboration in pediatric dermatology. *Dermatol Clin.* 2013;31:347–355.
22. Parens E., ed. *Surgically shaping children: technology, ethics, and the pursuit of normality. Baltimore,* MA: Johns Hopkins University Press; 2005. https://jhupbooks.press.jhu.edu/content/surgically-shaping-children.
23. Brown MM, Chamlin SL, Smidt AC. Quality of life in pediatric dermatology. *Dermatol Clin.* 2013;31:211–221.

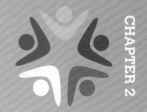

CHAPTER 2

Ethical Dilemmas

Caryn B.C. Cobb and Lionel Bercovitch

INTRODUCTION

Procedures in pediatric dermatology differ from those performed on adults in that they involve a third party, the parent or legal guardian, in the decision process. Although the ethical principles of beneficence, nonmaleficence, autonomy, and justice that govern care rendered to minors are essentially the same as those for adults, the inclusion of a third person (parent or guardian) in the decision-making dynamic introduces new tensions and complexity. The role of the third party can be influenced by the age and maturity of the minor, the nature of the procedure and gravity of the condition being treated, the laws of the jurisdiction in which care is being rendered, and cultural factors.

The requirement of a surrogate decision-maker in procedural pediatric dermatology can lead to ethical conflicts and dilemmas if the interests of the child, parents or guardian, and dermatologist do not align. Although the Best Interests Standard (as defined by Kopelman[1]) is considered a reasonable benchmark for guiding decision-makers in choosing the option(s) that are best for the child, what is considered "best" may be affected by religious, cultural, and social factors; the needs of the family; the maturity of the patient; and sometimes by conflicts of interest, poor relationship with the health care provider, bias, or misinformation.[1] Physicians and caregivers have legal, moral, and ethical responsibilities to the minor patient that may be subject to different perspectives. The dermatologist should be prepared with knowledge of relevant local laws and a moral/ethical framework to handle conflicts when they occur.

Legal Definitions

The concept of a minor is based in common law. A *minor* is an individual under 18 years of age, unless legally designated otherwise (eg, mature or emancipated minor). By legal definition, minors are a *vulnerable population* and are not considered autonomous for purposes of medical decision-making. Because minors do not possess the legal right to make medical decisions and may also not have the requisite decision-making capacity, the American Academy of Pediatrics Committee on Bioethics developed the concepts of *informed permission* and *assent of the patient*.[2]

In *informed permission*, the parent or surrogate makes medical decisions for the minor patient utilizing a framework identical to informed consent.[2] It is assumed that the parent is using his/her best judgment and is acting *in the best interests of the patient*, even though the decision may conflict with the child's wishes. However, several factors can influence this process, including previous medical knowledge and/or experience (eg, input from the Internet, well-meaning relatives and friends), emotional distress, the seriousness of the condition being treated, religion and faith, how the information is presented by the clinician, and the quality of the provider-surrogate-patient relationship.

Assent is the process of obtaining the minor's agreement to undergo the recommended intervention, even though the child may lack both legal authority and the decision-making capacity and maturity to provide standard informed consent.[2] It is routinely obtained as a formal written document in pediatric clinical research, whereas the process in procedural dermatology tends to be informal. Nevertheless, it makes children feel part of the process and that they have some control over what is done to their bodies. Respect for the child's right to assent or dissent to the extent maturity permits is essential to the development of the child's trust in the clinician. The process of assent should be delivered at a pace and level that are developmentally appropriate. This includes assessing the patient's understanding of the intervention and any factors that may unduly influence the patient's assent, such as fear and anxiety, anticipation of reward or punishment, and deferring to the parent's wishes.[2] Indeed, decisions by minor patients are often not truly voluntary, and it is often the parent/surrogate and health care provider who make the decision for the minor. Surrogates are expected to *maximize benefits and minimize risks or harms to the patient, taking the best interests of the minor child and the family into consideration.* Regardless, providers must identify a harm threshold above which parental wishes will not be tolerated. Furthermore, if the child is put at risk of harm or neglect by a parental decision, the state may exert its interest in protecting the child and challenge parental authority.

Adolescent patients constitute a special class. Developmentally, they are at the intersection of childhood and adulthood. They do not consider themselves to be children, and parents do not consider them to be adults. Although often able to make informed and fairly sophisticated decisions, they often lack impulse control and the ability to factor risks into their decisions. Many states have *mature minor* statutes that allow the courts to permit adolescents who possess the maturity to comprehend proposed interventions, as well as their risks, benefits, and alternatives, to make health care decisions independently, without the agreement of their parents or guardians.[2,3] *Emancipated minors* are defined in most states as those who are married, parents themselves, living independently and financially independent of their parents, in the military, or incarcerated as adults.[4] Emancipated minor statutes grant them, unrelated to decision-making capacity, the ability to make independent health care decisions, in contrast to mature minors.

The triangular doctor-patient-parent relationship works well when the adult parties can agree regarding what is in the best interests of the child, or the pediatric dermatologist respects the right of parents and older children to make decisions for themselves (and "agree to disagree" with the decision). However, at times disagreements may be so deep that it is necessary to terminate the provider-parent-patient relationship or, in certain extreme cases, to notify state child protective services and advocate for the child's best interests against the choices or preferences of the parents.

CASE SCENARIOS

The following are a variety of potential scenarios illustrating ethical conflicts that can arise involving procedures in pediatric dermatology practice:

Uncooperative Child (Child's Best Interest Conflicts with Child's Dissent)

Situations arise in which a child refuses to allow an essential minor procedure, such as removal of a bleeding pyogenic granuloma (see Chapter 117. Pyogenic Granuloma) or a diagnostic skin biopsy (see Chapter 36. Skin Biopsy Techniques). Although the parent recognizes the clinical utility of the tests and gives informed permission, the child is not providing assent or cooperating. The child lacks the capacity or legal authority to consent to or refuse the procedure. In situations such as these, the health care provider needs to evaluate the harm/benefit ratio to weigh the child's dissent. In the two scenarios above, the benefits clearly outweigh the brief and minimal physical discomfort as well as the brief psychological trauma of physical restraint. Restraint, "supportive holding," distraction strategies, or attempts to mitigate discomfort, for example, the use of topical lidocaine-prilocaine cream, may be needed. The opposite would be the case if the situation involved cryotherapy of harmless molluscum contagiosum lesions or warts from an otherwise asymptomatic child who will not assent to or cooperate with the procedure. In this situation, the benefits do not justify the emotional and physical trauma being inflicted on the child.

In contrast, the situation is somewhat more complex when it involves an adolescent, particularly one approaching majority. The patient in that situation has the capacity to dissent and is likely too old and/or too big to restrain. Although benefits may clearly outweigh potential harms, autonomy comes into play. Strategies to mitigate pain and anxiety, such as the use of topical anesthetic cream or mild sedation or anxiolytic medication, may help, but ultimately the patient's dissent will have to be respected.

Authoritarian Parental Decision Conflicts With a Minor Patient's Dissent

Consider the situation where a 7-year-old child is brought to the pediatric dermatologist with multiple periungual and digital warts. The parent is upset about their appearance and potential contagion to siblings and demands treatment. After explaining the treatment options (including no treatment or topical keratolytics, which the parents have already tried half-heartedly), the parent feels that the child "can handle it" and she will hold the child for cryotherapy. The mother asks if the child wants the warts gone and she nervously nods "yes." However, after the first application of liquid nitrogen, it becomes apparent that the child cannot tolerate the pain and neither wants the procedure nor will allow it to proceed without forceful restraint. Her mother insists on proceeding further.

In this scenario, the child is incapable of fully comprehending the consequences of the procedure (pain, blistering, need for multiple treatments), and assent is not truly informed. It is doubtful that a child this young is mature enough to provide informed assent for this procedure, and, in any event, assent here is tainted by parental coercion or the child's fear of the consequences of not going along with her mother's wishes. Although parents usually have the best interests of the child in mind, the child may be at risk of unintentional psychological and physical harm resulting from the parent's insistence on the procedure.

The pediatric dermatologist will have to weigh the wishes and interests of both parties and reach a decision that respects both the integrity and limited autonomy of the child and the authority and wishes of the parent or legal guardian. In a situation such as this, where the condition being treated poses no significant threat to either the health or well-being of the child, great weight must be given to the child's dissent.

Situations such as this may also arise when the patient is an adolescent. In such situations, the challenge is to engage both the parent and the patient in shared decision-making that respects the parent's moral and legal authority to make medical decisions that are in the best interest of the child while respecting the adolescent child's right to have his or her wishes taken into consideration. Adolescents seek more independence in all aspects of their lives as they mature, including medical decisions, and they should take a greater role in medical decision-making whenever possible. It is the position of the American Academy of Pediatrics that each patient's assent should be assessed based on the level of maturity as well as the understanding of risks, benefits, and alternatives.[2]

Parent Who Demands Unnecessary Medical Treatment Against the Dermatologist's Best Judgment and Best Interests of the Child

A 10-year-old girl presents with an acquired nevus of the shoulder that has recently become slightly elevated. It is a 5-mm dome-shaped uniformly pigmented papule with a globular pigment network, consistent with a benign-appearing dermal nevus. Her father is reassured, but insists on having the mole removed because his brother was recently diagnosed with melanoma. The patient becomes tearful and agitated at the mention of surgery, stating the mole does not bother her.

In this case, the risks of surgical excision (pain, infection, scar) outweigh the risks of monitoring what is clearly a benign-appearing nevus, for which there is no medical indication for removal. The primary legal, ethical, and moral obligation of the physician and the moral and legal obligation of the parent or guardian is the best interest of the child. Ultimately, the parent has the legal authority to give or withhold permission for the procedure, even if the child does not assent. Regardless, the dermatologist is under no obligation to perform a procedure that she feels is either medically unnecessary or not in the child's best interests. In such situations, the dermatologist should explore in depth what underlies the parent's motivation in demanding (or refusing) a procedure. Sometimes, parental anxiety may arise from misinformation gathered online or from a well-meaning friend, and sometimes it arises from an adverse experience of a friend or relative. In such situations, a reasoned explanation may allay the parent's fears. Should the parent and physician not be able to reach either a compromise or mutual understanding of what is in the child's best interest, a second opinion can be recommended.

Adolescent Demands Unreasonable Surgery That Conflicts With the Dermatologist's Medical Judgment

A 15-year-old presents with his parent. He is upset about several dark brown nevi on his face, none of which appears atypical clinically or is symptomatic. He wants them all removed because he hates them. The dermatologist explains to his parent that there will be multiple facial scars, some of which, especially on the chin, nose, and near the lip, could be more conspicuous than the nevi he wants removed. In addition, his parents' health insurance will likely not cover the procedure because of its cosmetic indication. Nevertheless, he is emphatic. He says, "I want them off. I don't care about scars!" The parent is conflicted. Clearly, their son is unhappy about the moles, but exercising poor judgment in regard to the final outcome and potential scarring.

Situations such as this are not unusual in treating adolescents. There is likely a biologic basis for risk-taking and impulsive behavior in teenagers. The centers for impulse control rest in the ventrolateral prefrontal cortex, and myelination of the fibers connecting it with the subcortical ventral striatum that are involved in responses to emotional cues and reward occurs long after maturation of the subcortical reward centers. Adolescent behavior, particularly risk-taking behaviors, is often affected by the tension in the neural circuitry between centers involved in reward processing and control processing.[5]

The dermatologist must also assess whether the patient has the maturity to factor risks and consequences in conjunction with assessing the medical soundness and reason of the adolescent's request. The parent must also walk the fine line and find a balance between giving the teenager some autonomy in making the decision and exercising parental moral authority. In this situation, the adolescent appears to lack the ability to factor the risks into his decision-making. The dermatologist is not obligated to suspend good professional judgment, nor is the parent expected to forego authoritative (as opposed to authoritarian) parenting. Sometimes the dermatologist can offer a compromise which can defuse such a "standoff," in this case removing just one lesion to evaluate the results/potential scarring, but such compromise solutions require a well-thought-out approach and assurance that all parties understand the end result.

Parent Refuses Dermatologist's Recommended Treatment/Medical Judgment, Which Also Conflicts With Minor Patient's Best Interests or Wishes

Consider a similar case in which the patient is a 14-year-old girl with a conspicuous facial pigmented birthmark, likely a segmental café au lait macule (see Chapter 66. Café au Lait Macules). She has been the object of teasing and bullying at school and desperately wants laser treatment that has been recommended because it is causing her to be socially isolated and withdrawn. Her parents refuse. In this case, the parents are reluctant to allow the treatment because of their own fears and concerns about the procedure. They also fail to grasp the extent of impact the lesion is having on her emotional state and school performance. In this case, the child's autonomy (to the extent that it is recognized) and the physician's clinical judgment do not align with the parents' decision-making. Clearly, the parents have their own agenda, which may be based on irrational fear, anxiety, or skepticism about the procedure or may be a manifestation of an authoritarian parenting style, or a combination of these. In a situation such as this, especially where there is a reasonable expectation of efficacy and a low risk of adverse outcome, the physician should advocate for the patient, consistent with her best interests. Parents usually make judgments that reflect the best interests of their child, but in this scenario something is clearly wrong here. The dermatologist should initiate a dispassionate, unbiased discussion of benefits and risks of the treatment, the impact of the birthmark's stigma on the child's psyche, and the consequences of nontreatment at this crucial time in her life. In the end, the parents have both

the legal and moral authority to make these medical decisions for their children, and absent a *practical* legal remedy, the only option for the physician is to suggest a second opinion and to keep the door open for follow-up evaluation and discussion. When the patient reaches *the age of maturity*, she will be able to make her own decision.

Parents Request a Particular Treatment for Punitive Reasons (Tattoo Removal)

Chheda et al.[6] describe a (presumably) hypothetical situation in which a parent brings an unwilling teenager to the dermatologist to have a tattoo excised to attempt to teach him a lesson by employing the most invasive way of removing it. The likelier scenario is when a teenager acquires a tattoo without parental permission and then parents come to the dermatologist for laser removal. The dermatologist needs to determine whether the patient's apparent willingness to have it removed is real or coerced. This may require interviewing the patient away from the parents and conducting a detailed assent procedure. If the patient dissents and the parent remains insistent, then an ethical dilemma exists. This patient is old enough to be permitted some degree of autonomy in making decisions about health care and too old to restrain or coerce. Forcing a nonemergent medically unnecessary procedure on an unwilling minor can have adverse psychological consequences for the patient and is an unpleasant experience for the entire health care team. The physician is ethically obligated to act in the best interests of the minor and, in this case, to advocate for the patient. Ideally, a discussion should occur involving all parties to outline the treatment options, alternatives, risks, benefits, costs, and possible outcomes and to arrive at a common decision that respects the adolescent's autonomy and integrity, if possible. Physicians and medical procedures should never be instruments of parental punishment. Performing a medically unnecessary procedure forcibly on an unwilling minor because of parental coercion is morally indefensible.

Divorced Parents Disagree on Treatment for Their Child

When the parents are divorced, the therapeutic triangle becomes a quadrilateral. Consider a case in which a 13-year-old girl is brought by her mother for consultation regarding removal of a congenital nevus of the face. The lesion has been the focus of teasing and bullying and is beginning to cause the patient to develop school phobia. Her parents have joint legal and physical custody, and although her mother gives informed permission for the lesion to be removed, her father refuses consent for vague reasons relating to whether the patient is "just going through a phase." The dermatologist needs to know who has the right to give or withhold permission in this case and the custody arrangements spelled out in the divorce decree. *Legal custody* refers to the right to make decisions regarding education, religious upbringing, and health care, among other issues. On the other hand, *physical custody* refers to what portion of the time the child lives with each parent. It is possible to have joint legal custody, even if one parent has primary physical custody. The divorce decree may spell out which parent can break the tie in the event they cannot agree on, for example, a health care decision such as this. If one parent is clearly not acting in the best interests of the child, a family court judge can intervene and change the custody arrangement in the divorce decree, even terminating one parent's legal custody rights, an expensive and time-consuming process. In a clinical scenario such as the above, the physician can, and should, work to get the parents to agree on what is in the child's best interests and move forward accordingly. Primary care physicians often have a copy of the divorce decree in the medical record, and specialists such as dermatologists should also make themselves aware of formal custody arrangements before proceeding with procedures.

Adolescent Request for Cosmetic Procedures Such as Neurotoxins and Fillers

There is a robust body of published work in the plastic surgery literature on cosmetic procedures such as otoplasty, rhinoplasty, augmentation mammoplasty, and labiaplasty in children and adolescents. However, little has been published about less invasive cosmetic procedures in teenagers that are more likely to be encountered in dermatologic practice, such as injection of botulinum toxin or use of fillers for cosmetic rather than medical or reconstructive indications. An article in the *New York Times* in 2010[7] highlighted the increasing use of botulinum toxin for "perceived imperfections from a too-gummy smile to a too-square jaw." The same article cited the widespread erroneous perception among teenagers in the United Kingdom undergoing "Teen Toxing" that botulinum toxin prevents wrinkles and natural aging. A variety of reasons may underlie a teen's request for such procedures, such as teasing or bullying from peers or adults, difficulty in socializing or establishing friendships, peer influence, the desire to please a boyfriend or to conform to an idealized image of beauty gleaned from mass media[8] or social media, poor self-esteem and body dissatisfaction, the "selfie complex,"[9] or body dysmorphic disorder.

The dermatologist is confronted with the ethical conflict of allowing the adolescent some increased autonomy and decision-making versus acting in the patient's best interest (beneficence) and avoiding harm (nonmaleficence). The dermatologist needs to adopt an objective rather than a visceral approach to evaluating the patient's request and perform an objective evaluation that includes the following questions:

- How mature is the patient and how well-thought-out is the request?
- What is the reason for the request?
- Is the procedure being requested to please someone else or to conform to an unattainable ideal?
- Is the defect the patient wishes corrected conspicuous to most observers?
- Is parental consent truly informed?
- Are expectations realistic?
- Is the procedure reversible?
- Is the patient's self-confidence or self-esteem being negatively affected to the point it is interfering with normal social functioning or impacting quality of life?
- Is the defect causing the child to be teased or bullied?

There are rare instances in which botulinum toxin or injectable filler may be indicated and generally deemed acceptable for the cosmetic correction of minor defects in adolescents (as opposed to disease-related defects such as facial hemiatrophy secondary to morphea for which there is little to no ethical or medical controversy). In general, treatments with these injectable substances carry risks that teenagers and their parents may fail to consider in their decision-making. In contrast, laser hair removal for synophrys and hirsutism in children and adolescents seems to be widely accepted without ethical concerns.

Although there is general agreement that most filler and neurotoxin injection procedures are inappropriate in children and adolescents, each patient deserves an objective evaluation and individual consideration. If the dermatologist's screening of the patient raises suspicion of depression, suicidal ideation, or body dysmorphic disorder, beneficence dictates arranging timely mental health intervention (a thorough discussion of this topic is beyond the scope of this chapter). It should also be noted that body image often improves as adolescents mature into young adulthood, and defects regarded by patients as catastrophic during their teenage years may become acceptable a few years later.[10] Furthermore, normalizing the defect for the patient may actually (although not always) be reassuring and alleviate the demand for treatment.

REFERENCES

1. Kopelman LM. The best interests standard for incompetent or incapacitated patients of all ages. *J Law Med Ethics.* 2007;3:187–196.
2. Katz AL, Webb SA, Committee on Bioethics. Informed consent in decision-making in pediatric practice. *Pediatrics.* 2016;138:e20161485.
3. Coleman DL, Rosoff PM. The legal authority of mature minors to consent to general medical treatment. *Pediatrics.* 2013;131:786–793.
4. Michon K. Emancipation of minors: the ins and outs of minor emancipation—what it means and how it can be obtained. https://www.nolo.com/legal-encyclopedia/emancipation-of-minors-32237.html. Accessed November 17, 2018.
5. Casey B, Caudle K. The teenage brain: self control. *Curr Dir Psychol Sci.* 2013;1;22:82–87.
6. Chheda K, Yates B, Makkar H, Grant-Kels JM. The tattoo removal ethical conundrum: should a physician be part of a minor patient's punishment? *J Am Acad Dermatol.* 2017;77:385–387.
7. Saint Louis C. This teenage girl uses Botox. No, she's not alone. *New York Times*, August 11, 2010. https://www.nytimes.com/2010/08/12/fashion/12SKIN.html?_r=1&ref=catherine_saint_louis Accessed November 18, 2018.
8. Wiseman CV, Sunday SR, Becker AE. Impact of the media on adolescent body image. *Child Adolesc Psychiatr Clin N Am.* 2005;14:453–471.
9. Berros P, Armstrong BK, Foti P, Mancini R. Cosmetic adolescent filler: an innovative treatment of the "selfie" complex. *Ophthal Plast Reconstr Surg.* 2018;34:366–368.
10. Holsen I, Carlson Jones D, Skogbrott Birkeland M. Body image satisfaction among Norwegian adolescents and young adults: a longitudinal study of the influence of interpersonal relationships and BMI. *Body Image.* 2012;9:201–208.

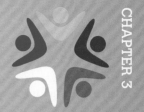

CHAPTER 3

Molecular and Cellular Differences Between Children and Adults

George Hightower

Studying embryonic and fetal development has provided important insights into how the skin maintains itself against a harsh outer environment. When the skin is damaged, whether in utero or ex utero, wound repair entails a complex immunologic and physiologic response.

DEVELOPMENT AND AGING

Starting at 3 weeks of gestation, a single layer of flattened epithelial cells covers the human embryo. At 4 weeks, two distinct layers of cells can be visualized. The outer layer is a permeable barrier: the periderm. The inner portion, the basal germinative layer, is the primordial epidermis and overlays an undifferentiated collection of mesenchymal cells that will give rise to the dermis. Keratinization of the epidermis begins at about 9 weeks of gestation and is synchronized with the shedding of the periderm. This also corresponds with the formation of the vernix caseosa, a coating made of sloughed-off cells, sebum, and lipids that is unique to fetal life—present at birth but soon shed. By 14 weeks of gestation, the epidermis resembles infant skin, and expression patterns of basement membrane proteins, blood

vessels, and certain keratin proteins (K10, K14, K16) appear similar to those in adult skin.[1] At around 33 weeks of gestation, the skin is functionally mature and covered completely by a protective layer of keratin. Following delivery, keratinocytes, the most abundant cells in the epidermis, continue to mature, and a notably thin epidermis steadily increases in thickness until about 2 years of age (Figure 3.1).

The dermis at 6 weeks of gestation is clearly distinguishable from the epidermis and subcutaneous tissue. This "living scaffolding" is made up of an array of cells in a gel-like matrix. To date, most of the observed differences between fetal and adult skin at the molecular level involve the dermal extracellular matrix (ECM).[1] The major components of the ECM are synthesized by fibroblasts and include collagen, elastin, and glycosaminoglycans (GAGs). During fetal growth, fibroblast production of collagen outstrips its destruction, resulting in a progressive thickening of the dermis. Most of this collagen production is centered on collagen type I, the principal component of the ECM.[2] Collagen type I is predominant throughout the fetal period and postnatal life; however, fetal skin has relatively

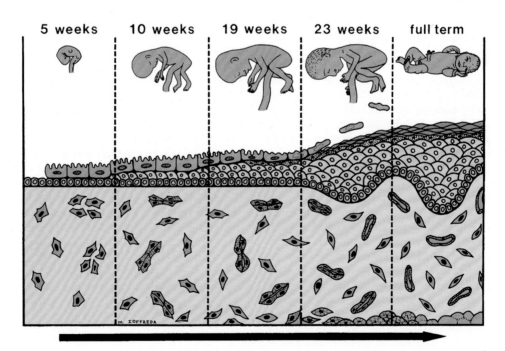

FIGURE 3.1. Schematic overview of embryonic development of the human skin. Reprinted from Elder DE. *Lever's Histopathology of the Skin.* 11th ed. Philadelphia, PA: Wolters Kluwer Health/Lippincott Williams & Wilkins; 2014. Figure 3.1. Courtesy of Dr. Michael Ioffreda.

higher levels of collagen types III and V. The presence of type I collagen not only is thought to provide strength and rigidity but also promotes scarring. Fetal dermis is also defined by the absence of elastin (up to week 22 gestation), which accounts for the resiliency and elasticity of adult skin as well as 2% to 4% of its dry weight.

Mirroring the epidermis, the dermis is functionally mature at birth but development is not complete. There is a steady increase in the thickness of the dermis, and skin appendages such as sweat glands, hair follicles, sebaceous glands, and nails continue to undergo dramatic changes throughout the first year to 2 years of life. Again in puberty, there are important development changes that take place, including a steady increase in the thickness of the dermis and epidermis. Eventually, with aging, thinning and atrophy of the skin are observed, characterized on the molecular level by collagen fragmentation and the buildup of abnormal elastin.[3] Both intrinsic forces and extrinsic factors such as UV radiation feed into a destructive loop that accelerates fibrocyte-mediated degradation of collagen and elastin by matrix metalloproteinases (MMPs), which reduce fibroblast binding and trigger further breakdown of the ECM.[4]

WOUND HEALING

In humans, scarring is part of the normal wound healing process starting around 24 weeks of gestation. Prior to 24 weeks, the fetal dermis when wounded regenerates normal dermal structures (ie, hair follicles) and a collagen matrix identical to nonwounded fetal skin.[1] In children and adults, injury to the skin triggers a structured process of wound repair that is clearly fundamentally different from that in fetal skin; however, there are relatively few human studies that have examined differences in healing by age from infancy through adulthood. Postnatal wound repair is often divided into three overlapping phases: inflammation, proliferation, and ECM remodeling.[5] In the inflammatory phase, following hemostasis, leukocyte recruitment to the wound is essential. First neutrophils and then monocytes are recruited to phagocytose foreign materials, bacteria, and damaged tissue. The recruitment time for peak function for neutrophils and macrophages appears to decrease with age, which may at least in part explain why children heal faster than adults.[6,7] Neutrophils eventually undergo apoptosis and when engulfed by macrophages signal the end of the inflammatory response. By contrast, in scarless fetal wound healing, there are relatively few neutrophils and the inflammatory response appears muted. This apparent paradoxical role of neutrophils highlights the complexity of the human immune response. In the proliferative phase of wound healing, keratinocytes migrate from the wound edge. For injury involving the dermis, regardless of age, "scar" not "regeneration" is the rule.[8] Fibroblasts and endothelial cells are the principal cellular components of granulation tissue. In the proliferative phase of wound healing, the greater number of and activity of fibroblasts observed in pediatric patients are seen as a positive factor influencing wound healing.[9] One of the trade-offs appears to be the potential formation of keloids, which are unlikely before the age of 5 years but occur with notable frequency in the first and second decades of life but rarely in the elderly.[10] Signaling mediated by transforming growth factor-β1 (TGF-β1) appears central to this process through its role in regulating collagen formation and fibroblast apoptosis and differentiation.[11] In fetal wounds, collagen type III appears to predominate in contrast to type I collagen in children and adults. Collagen type III may be optimal for cellular migration,

whereas collagen type I provides strength and rigidity but limits the regenerative capacity of the skin. An overabundance of dermal collagen is seen in both hypertrophic scar (primarily type III) and keloids (mix of types I and III).[12]

BIRTHMARKS

Regardless of perceived deformation or the potential to cause psychosocial distress, nonclinicians often see lesions limited to the skin as amenable to surgical intervention.

We now know that many common birthmarks (eg, congenital melanocytic nevi, epidermal nevi, nevus sebaceous, port-wine birthmarks, and congenital dermal melanocytosis) are the result of post-zygotic activating mutations. Although, clinically, these lesions may appear essentially static, they are maintained by a dynamic interplay of molecular signaling. Recent clinical use of targeted therapeutics provides proof of concept that certain lesions that result from mutations in the RAS pathway such as giant congenital melanocytic nevus might one day be amenable to novel nonsurgical interventions.[13] Currently, standard of care relies on excision, with considerations given to the size, location, and age of the patient. Because of concern for potential malignancy and the importance of continued monitoring (especially lesions >20 cm), laser treatment is generally avoided.[14] Epidermal nevi also result from mutations in the RAS pathway but are benign and can be observed, shaved flat, excised, or treated with laser ablation, each treatment with various risks of recurrence and scarring.[15] Historically, nevus sebaceous, which also result from mutations in the RAS pathway, historically, were excised owing to concern for future malignancy.[16] Although the true incidence of basal cell carcinoma arising within nevus sebaceous is debatable, it is certainly lower than initially reported, and for small lesions strong consideration should be given to clinical observation. By contrast, q-switched laser is the treatment of choice for dermal melanocytosis of the eye (aka nevus of Ota) and upper back (nevus of Ito); these pigmented lesions result from mutations encoded by GNAQ/GNA11 and have a low risk of associated melanoma.[17] Unlike congenital dermal melanocytosis involving the lower back and buttocks, nevi of Ota and Ito tend not to fade on their own.

CONCLUSION

The ability of some gestational human fetal wounds to heal through regeneration rather than scarring reminds us of the limitations of our current tools and what might be possible in the future. Our willingness and ability to physically manipulate the skin with the aid of new treatment modalities such as lasers will likely continue to outpace our understanding of how these interventions truly impact the skin at the molecular and cellular level. Our growing understanding of the biology of pediatric skin offers the ability to improve the tools we currently employ and to develop new approaches that will ultimately allow us to offer better clinical outcomes for our patients.

REFERENCES

1. Coolen NA, Schouten KCWM, Middelkoop E, Ulrich MMW. Comparison between human fetal and adult skin. *Arch Dermatol Res.* 2009;302:47–55.
2. King A, Balaji S, Keswani SG. Biology and function of fetal and pediatric skin. *Facial Plast Surg Clin North Am.* 2013;21:1–6.
3. Cole MA, Quan T, Voorhees JJ, Fisher GJ. Extracellular matrix regulation of fibroblast function: redefining our perspective on skin aging. *J Cell Commun Signal.* 2018;12:35–43.

4. Hornebeck W. Down-regulation of tissue inhibitor of matrix metalloprotease-1 (TIMP-1) in aged human skin contributes to matrix degradation and impaired cell growth and survival. *Pathol Biol.* 2003;51:569–573.

5. Velnar T, Bailey T, Smrkolj V. The wound healing process: an overview of the cellular and molecular mechanisms. *J Int Med Res.* 2009;37:1528–1542.

6. Pajulo OT, Pulkki KJ, Alanen MS, et al. Duration of surgery and patient age affect wound healing in children. *Wound Repair Regen.* 2000;8:174–178.

7. Viljanto J, Raekallio J. Wound healing in children as assessed by the CELLSTIC method. *J Pediatr Surg.* 1976;11:43–49.

8. Krakowski AC, Totri CR, Donelan MB, Shumaker PR. Scar management in the pediatric and adolescent populations. *Pediatrics.* 2016;137.

9. Fisher GJ, Shao Y, He T, et al. Reduction of fibroblast size/mechanical force down-regulates TGF-β type II receptor: implications for human skin aging. *Aging Cell.* 2015;15:67–76.

10. Lane JE. Relationship between age of ear piercing and keloid formation. *Pediatrics.* 2005;115:1312–1314.

11. Ashcroft GS, Horan MA, Herrick SE, Tarnuzzer RW, Schultz GS, Ferguson MW. Age-related differences in the temporal and spatial regulation of matrix metalloproteinases (MMPs) in normal skin and acute cutaneous wounds of healthy humans. *Cell Tissue Res.* 1997;290:581–591.

12. Lichtman MK, Otero-Vinas M, Falanga V. Transforming growth factor beta (TGF-β) isoforms in wound healing and fibrosis. *Wound Repair Regen.* 2016;24:215–222.

13. Kinsler VA, O'Hare P, Jacques T, Hargrave D, Slater O. MEK inhibition appears to improve symptom control in primary NRAS-driven CNS melanoma in children. *Br J Cancer.* 2017;116:990–993.

14. Kinsler VA, O'Hare P, Bulstrode N, et al. Melanoma in congenital melanocytic naevi. *Br J Dermatol.* 2017;176:1131–1143.

15. Hafner C, van Oers JMM, Vogt T, et al. Mosaicism of activating FGFR3 mutations in human skin causes epidermal nevi. *J Clin Invest.* 2006;116:2201–2207.

16. Moody MN, Landau JM, Goldberg LH. Nevus sebaceous revisited. *Pediatr Dermatol.* 2012;29:15–23.

17. Van Raamsdonk CD, Griewank KG, Crosby MB, et al. Mutations in GNA11 in uveal melanoma. *N Engl J Med.* 2010;363:2191–2199.

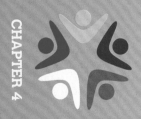

Billing and Coding in Procedural Pediatric Dermatology

Murad Alam[*†]

INTRODUCTION

To be able to perform pediatric dermatology procedures you wish to code for, you will need specialized equipment. When starting out, you may need to buy several types of equipment, including surgical instruments, lasers and energy devices, and office furniture and supplies. When purchasing surgical instruments, you may be guided by one of at least three schools of thought. One says you should buy the least expensive instruments that meet your needs to keep costs down. Another says you should go for the middle priced, which may be the best value. The last suggests you should splurge for the best that you can afford. If you are skilled at bargaining and getting deals and are constantly motivated to minimize your expenses, then the first route may be preferable. If you like as little hassle as possible and want instruments that last forever and are repaired and sharpened for free by the manufacturer, then the final approach may be for you.

As for buying lasers and energy devices, less is usually more when you are starting out. It is unlikely you would need more than a vascular laser, a pigment laser, and possibly a nonablative or ablative resurfacing device. Sometimes these can be found on the same platform—meaning one big box with several arms or handpieces. This can be more cost-effective than buying three entirely separate devices and also helps you save on service contracts. On the contrary, when your single platform goes down, you are temporarily without any devices at all.

Once you have acquired the hardware you need, as well as any necessary training, you will also need to learn how to correctly code the work you perform. The remainder of this chapter is intended to help you with coding and to minimize your coding errors.

CURRENT PROCEDURAL TERMINOLOGY CODE PROCESS

Current Procedural Terminology (CPT) codes are updated annually and are five-digit designators that describe medical procedures performed in the United States.[1-3] Code descriptors explain the procedure, and so-called code vignettes characterize how it is typically performed. CPT codes, and the definitions for each, are created, updated, and altered three times a year at face-to-face meetings of the CPT Panel, which is managed by the American Medical Association and includes members of medical specialty societies and payer groups. The CPT Panel is the voting body that decides to approve or decline so-called code change proposals (CCPs). At each CPT Panel meeting, there are present representatives of major medical professional societies called CPT Advisors who can offer testimony on behalf of particular CCPs and answer Panel questions about clinical practice relevant to their specialties before the Panel votes. CCPs can be submitted by any interested group, including members of industry or the general public. Most successful CCPs (ie, those that are approved by Panel vote) are supported and edited by the CPT Advisors of the relevant specialty societies.

CPT codes for medical procedures performed by physicians are typically Category I or Category III codes. Category I codes represent routine, noninvestigational procedures. Once approved, Category I codes are sent to the Relative Value Scale Update Committee (RUC), which determines how much physician work effort and practice expense are required for completion of the procedure in question. Thereafter, the Centers for Medicare and Medicaid Services (CMS) usually accepts RUC recommendations and uses these to assign a dollar value to the code. The constituents of code value include physician work effort (ie, the sum of preservice, intraservice, and postservice time, adjusted by the intensity of the effort), practice expense (ie, the cost of disposable supplies, nonphysician staff time, a small fraction of the cost of durable equipment required, and other space and utilities costs), malpractice expense (ie, a minute amount that reflects the malpractice risk per procedure), and any additional adjustments that CMS may deem appropriate. The final code values are published by CMS each year in the Physician Fee Schedule. Private insurers usually use CMS designated relative values, which they can adjust as they deem appropriate. For instance, a third-party insurer may price most procedures at 80% or 120% of Medicare.

Category III codes are new procedure codes that denote experimental procedures or procedures that have not yet been widely adopted. These codes are not valued by RUC or priced by CMS. Instead, they are "carrier priced," meaning individual insurers can choose to cover them, and if they do, they can select a payment amount. Often, procedures associated with Category III codes are redesignated with Category I codes after several years. As code utilization increases and procedures become routine, a CCP may be submitted to the CPT Panel requesting an upgrade to Category I status. Even though Category III codes may not be paid, it is important for practitioners to submit them for consideration so that CMS can track utilization. Increased code use is often a major factor favoring eventual Category I status.

CORRECT CODING AND GETTING PAID

The rule of thumb in selecting CPT codes is that if the right code does not exist, the physician provider should select the code that is the best fit. If no code is a reasonably good fit, then a code ending in -99 that designates an unspecified or miscellaneous service should be submitted, along with detailed documentation regarding the procedure and its medical necessity.

Denials may necessitate the need for an appeal. The treating physician will determine when reasonable efforts to pursue a claim are exhausted and the likelihood of receiving payment is slim. If a practice performs a high volume of scar revisions that result in claims submitted to a particular insurer, for example,

---

*The opinions in this chapter are mine alone and were not vetted or approved by ASDS or AMA-CPT Panel.
†Latanya T. Benjamin provided additional editorial review of this chapter.

it may be fruitful for the treating physician to reach out to the local medical director for that insurer to communicate the importance of his or her specialized practice. Each state also has two dermatology carrier advisory committee (DermCAC) members—practicing dermatologists who volunteer their time to meet with insurer groups several times a year. The Derm-CAC representatives can communicate concerns about reimbursement of particular procedures (eg, scar treatment), discuss problems with the appeals process, and advocate for payment.

Prior authorizations and appeals may reduce the likelihood of denials, but may also consume copious staff time and not be cost-effective. It may be preferable in certain instances to forego precertification, submit well-documented claims with the best-fit diagnosis and procedure codes, and hope for the best. Practice patterns and insurer reimbursement practices vary regionally, so it behooves the physician to do "as is usual and customary" in his or her area.

EVALUATION/MANAGEMENT CODING ISSUES
Coding Evaluation/Management and Procedures When There Is One Diagnosis

Based on current coding guidelines, the fact that someone is a new patient is *not* sufficient to code an Evaluation/Management (E/M) code in combination with a procedure that they received at the same visit. Conversely, it is possible to code an E/M with the same diagnosis as a procedure, but the bar for doing so is very high. Many E/M services perceived by dermatologists as distinct from any procedure are in fact already included in most procedures, so billing separately for these is not appropriate.

If you are seeing a child with warts for the first time, and the child has some other notable or symptomatic lesion or condition, you may wish to also code for these. Otherwise, if you only specify the diagnosis "wart," it is better to not use an E/M concurrently. One exception would be when you spent excessive amounts of time with the patient and family unrelated to the treatment of the wart. In that case, you could code an E/M for time alone, with documentation like: "… in addition to the pre-service, intraservice, and postservice procedure time required for wart identification and destruction, an additional period of more than 30 minutes was spent with the patient and his parents, with most of this on counseling and discussion pertaining to…."

"New" Visits to the Same Practice

In general, when patients are seen repeatedly in the same dermatology practice, they are classified as established patients. One exception is when they are seen by a different specialist or, in the case of a dermatology-only practice, by a different subspecialist. In this case, they would be a new patient again. For instance, if a patient were seen by a general dermatologist and then referred to a board-certified pediatric dermatologist in the same practice, their first visit to the pediatric dermatologist would be as a "new" patient. Keep in mind that this holds for established, recognized specialties and subspecialties and not necessarily self-designated ones, like "specialist in atopic dermatitis."

PROCEDURAL CODING ISSUES
Biopsy Versus Removal or Excision

Biopsies are samples of larger lesions. If your intent is to diagnose an inflammatory or neoplastic lesion and sample a portion of that lesion by any shave, punch, or incision, then it is a biopsy even if the entire lesion is inadvertently removed. If, on the contrary, your intent is to take out all of a particular lesion, or all of the symptomatic part of that lesion, then it is a removal even if the histologic margins, if assessed, are not clear. This removal would be a shave removal if it were partial thickness through the dermis, and it would be an excision if it were through the entire dermis to the subcutaneous fat or other underlying tissue. Notably, the type of instrument used is not relevant, as a scalpel, a flat blade, or a punch device could theoretically be used to achieve any of these outcomes.

Skin Biopsy Coding

The general skin biopsy codes that have been in effect since January 2019 replace the prior skin biopsy codes. Now there are three codes, one for tangential (eg, shave, scoop, saucerization, curettage, etc.) biopsies, one for punch biopsies, and one for incisional biopsies (Table 4.1). Incisional biopsies as well as punch biopsies are all the way through the dermis to the fat or underlying tissue (although they may or may not include fat in the specimen). Incisional biopsies are part of a larger lesion, and hence distinguished from excisions, which remove the entire lesion and should be coded using existing excision codes. Importantly, although there is an "add-on" code for each of the new biopsy codes for coding additional similar biopsies, only *one* "primary" biopsy code can be used per patient per day. For instance, if you do three tangential biopsies and two punch biopsies during a single patient encounter, you would code for the primary punch biopsy code, then one punch biopsy add-on, and three tangential biopsy add-ons. The hierarchy for biopsy coding is such that you would code a primary incision biopsy code if any such biopsies were performed; if not, then you would code a punch biopsy primary code if any punch biopsies were performed; if not, then you would code a tangential biopsy primary code. All other biopsies performed at the same visit would be coded as add-ons of the appropriate type.

Site-Specific Biopsy Coding

A number of "site-specific" CPT codes exist when certain anatomic areas are biopsied, regardless of the technique that is utilized. These codes take into account the additional complexity of biopsy at these anatomic locations and include the following special sites: biopsy of the external ear (CPT 69100); biopsy of the eyelid margin (CPT 67810); biopsy of the vermilion and mucosal lip (CPT 40490); biopsy of the penis (CPT 54100); biopsy of the vaginal mucosa (CPT 57100); biopsy of the vulva or perineum (CPT 56605, 56606); and biopsy of the nail unit (CPT 11755). A nail clipping sent for analysis is not considered a biopsy; instead, it is considered part of the E/M.

Importantly, if you sample several areas within the same lesion, these are counted collectively as one biopsy for coding purposes. If, on the contrary, you sample one area per lesion, even if the lesions are qualitatively similar as long as you view them as distinct from each other, then each of these samples is a different biopsy. The biopsying physician has to determine and document whether the biopsies were of adjacent discrete lesions or if multiple samples were obtained of the same lesion.

Intermediate Versus Complex Repairs

The two types of bilayered linear repairs are "intermediate" and "complex" repairs. Removal of Burow's triangles (ie, "dog ears") does *not* by itself make a repair complex. In dermatologic closures, complex repairs require not only deep sutures but also extensive undermining. Historically, the extent of undermining

TABLE 4.1 : **Skin Biopsy Coding**

CODING HIERARCHY	GENERAL BIOPSY TYPE	INTENT OF PROCEDURE	NOTES	PRIMARY CPT CODE[a]	ADD-ON CPT CODE
1	Incisional biopsy	Obtain a full-thickness tissue sample of a skin lesion for the purpose of diagnostic pathologic examination. This type of biopsy may sample subcutaneous fat, such as when performed for the evaluation of panniculitis.	Requires the use of a sharp blade (but not a punch tool) to remove a full-thickness sample of tissue via a vertical incision or wedge, penetrating the dermis into the subcutaneous layer. Although closure is usually required for incisional biopsies, simple closure may not be separately reported.	11106	11107
2	Punch biopsy	Obtain a cylindrical tissue sample of a cutaneous lesion for the purpose of diagnostic pathologic examination.	Requires a punch tool to remove a full-thickness cylindrical sample of skin. Simple closure of the defect, including manipulation of the biopsy defect to improve wound approximation, is included in the service and may not be separately reported.	11104	11105
3	Tangential biopsy	Remove a sample of epidermal tissue with or without portions of underlying dermis for the purpose of diagnostic pathologic examination.	Performed with a sharp blade, such as a flexible biopsy blade, obliquely oriented scalpel, or a curette, to remove a sample of epidermal tissue with or without portions of underlying dermis. Includes scoop, shave, saucerization, and curette biopsy techniques. Results in a superficial sample and does not involve the full thickness of the dermis, such that portions of the lesion could remain in the deeper layers of the dermis. Consequently, this is not considered an "excision."	11102	11103

[a]Only one primary code can be billed per patient per day.
CPT, Current Procedural Terminology.

has not been well-defined; however, starting January 2020, this will be clarified as a "distance greater than or equal to the maximum width of the defect, measured perpendicular to the closure line along at least one entire edge of the defect." So, at least one side of the defect must be undermined, and undermining must be at least as much as the maximum width of the defect. If undermining is performed but it is less than this amount, then the repair is an intermediate repair.

An important requirement when extensive undermining is performed is whether this is medically appropriate and necessary for the closure. The surgeon needs to make a determination that undermining is needed.

Coding Procedures at Different Anatomic Site or by Different Techniques

For some procedures, like excisions and removals, site-specific codes are available. So, a shave removal on the face and one on the leg would be billed with different codes, and not a primary code with an add-on. In many other cases, site-specific codes are not available. For example, if tangential biopsies were performed on the back, leg, and chin, respectively, these would

be billed with the primary code for tangential biopsy plus two times the add-on code because none of these sites is associated with a site-specific biopsy code. In general, if a more specific code exists, then that code should be used.

Excision of Soft Tissue Tumors

Most skin excisions that include subcutaneous tissue are coded using the standard excision codes. However, lesions that are confined to the subcutis and do not communicate with or originate in the overlying skin can be appropriately coded using soft tissue tumor excision codes. Lipomas are one of the very few dermatologic diagnoses that qualify. The soft tissue excision codes are site-specific and are in different parts of the CPT manual. For each anatomic site, there are codes for removal of subcutaneous tumors and subfascial tumors, respectively, and these should be used as appropriate for the relevant type of lipoma. Additionally, once the subcutaneous or subfascial location is specified, there are codes for smaller tumors (eg, less than 2, 3, or 5 cm in diameter, depending on the anatomic site) and larger tumors. Most lipomas removed in dermatology will be subcutaneous and small.

Cysts of all types, including epidermoid and pilar cysts, are excluded from the soft tissue tumor excision code set. This is because they protrude into the dermis or above and are not exclusively located in the subcutis, regardless of how large or complex they may be.

Multimodal Procedural Treatment of Warts and Molluscum

Many destruction codes do not specify method, so the total number of lesions is counted and billed collectively—without consideration for the type of specific destruction technique. In uncommon cases, there may be exceptions and you may be able to bill for more than one treatment method, particularly when diagnostically similar lesions at different anatomic sites are treated with different methods. For instance, if treating a wart on the face with cryotherapy while also injecting another on the finger with Candida antigen, it may be possible to bill for benign destruction as well as for injection. It would be necessary to clearly document which warts were frozen and which were injected, and that these were different lesions receiving different treatments. If such documentation is not possible or such distinctions cannot be made, it may be preferable to bill just the destruction code.

Treatment of Atrophic Scars, Hypertrophic Scars, and Keloids

When they are symptomatic, the intralesional injection of keloids and hypertrophic scars is often covered. For such injections, CPT coding includes a J-code for the material injected (eg, triamcinolone acetonide—per 10 mg) as well as the number of lesions, which may be "up to and including 7" (CPT 11900) or "more than 7" (CPT 11901).

In less common instances, a symptomatic scar may need to be surgically excised, and appropriate excision, shave removal, and reconstruction (eg, simple repair, intermediate repair, complex repair, or adjacent tissue transfer) codes may be used. Although codes do exist for chemical peels and dermabrasion, these are rarely paid when submitted for scar treatment. There are now Category III codes for fractional ablative laser treatment of burn and traumatic scars to improve function, but these may not be paid for by Medicare and other providers.

Laser Treatment of Vascular Proliferative Lesions

A vascular proliferative lesion is typically a port-wine birthmark or hemangioma. The general rule is that this is a congenital vascular anomaly. Other vascular proliferative lesions, such as evolving telangiectasia in a patient with scleroderma, or bleeding telangiectasia in a patient with Osler-Weber-Rendu syndrome, are not specifically included but do appear to meet the definition. Telangiectasia, spider angiomas, and diffuse centrofacial redness associated with rosacea, photodamage, or cystic acne are certainly *not* appropriate to code as vascular proliferative lesions. Treatment of the red or thickened component of hypertrophic scars and keloids is also not covered as neither hypertrophic scars nor keloids would meet criteria for vascular proliferative lesions. If many serial treatments are required to address a port-wine birthmark or hemangioma, each of these should be billed separately, in accordance with the area treated at that visit. Some payers may be more inclined to pay for a series of visits if they first receive a doctor letter and photographs documenting the problem, outlining a treatment plan, and estimating the number of treatments that may be required.

When treating vascular proliferative lesions with laser, the cumulative treated area determines coding. If there are multiple discrete lesions treated at one visit, then adding up the total area of the individual lesions leads to the correct area for coding. Areas should be added up even if they are on different anatomic sites, such as the face, neck, and torso. Needless to say, only the area that is actually treated with laser and the treated parts of a vascular proliferative lesion should be included in the surface area computation. Many sessions, weeks or months apart, may be required for laser treatment of hemangiomas and port-wine stains. For each of these, coding starts anew (ie, the original area should not simply be carried through from previous documentation), and the combined area treated is added up and coded.

Use of "17999" Code

The United States Department of Justice has successfully prosecuted several dermatologists for fraud for using destruction codes for intense pulsed light treatment of actinic keratoses in the context of photodamage, redness, and poikiloderma. This suggests that the dermatologists should be very careful when coding for laser and light procedures. If in doubt, consider using a 17999 code and filing paperwork with the payer to explain what was done and why it was necessary. This may be the best route when treating a medical condition or genetic condition with laser. For instance, there is no specific code for laser hair removal that appears to be medically necessary or needed to correct a genetic condition, as in the case of a pilonidal cyst or Cornelia de Lange syndrome.

REFERENCES

1. *Current Procedural Terminology: Professional Edition*. Chicago, IL: American Medical Association; 2019.
2. Zalla JA. CPT coding and reimbursement issues in dermatology. *Semin Cutan Med Surg.* 2005;24(3):117–123.
3. Alam M. Integrating scar management into clinical practice. In: Krakowski AC, Shumaker PR, eds. *The Scar Book*. Philadelphia, PA: Wolters Kluwer; 2017:349–356.

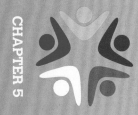

CHAPTER 5

Surgical Procedure Room Setup

Asra Hashmi and Amanda A. Gosman

The main objectives behind all steps undertaken prior to a surgical procedure are to set the stage for a safe and efficient execution of the surgical procedure as well as to minimize the risk of postoperative adverse events (including surgical site infection [SSI]). Surgical setups vary with the type of operation being performed. Following are the steps for operating room setup for a minor procedure.

BEFORE SURGERY

It is estimated that nearly 50% of SSIs are preventable, which is significant considering the medical and financial implications.[1] A targeted systematic review of literature was conducted from 1998 through 2014 to provide guidelines for reducing SSIs. Based on recommendations provided by this review, patients should shower or bathe (full body) with soap (antimicrobial or nonantimicrobial) or an antiseptic agent at least the night before surgery.[1]

MAINTAINING NORMOTHERMIA

Hypothermia is known to contribute to SSI through several mechanisms including peripheral vasoconstriction, impaired neutrophil and macrophage function, and delayed wound healing.[2-4] It is particularly important to maintain normothermia for preemies, neonates, infants, and underweight pediatric patients. Blanket warming devices (Figure 5.1) and body

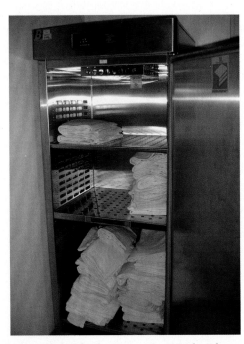

FIGURE 5.1. Blanket/fluid warmer. Reprinted with permission from Britt LD, Peitzman AB, Barie PS, et al. *Acute Care Surgery*. Philadelphia, PA: Wolters Kluwer Health/Lippincott Williams & Wilkins; 2012. Figure 53-2A.

warming systems are used for this purpose. Once the patient is appropriately positioned, minimizing exposure of the body ensures maintenance of normothermia.

PERIOPERATIVE ANTIBIOTICS

Factors that should be considered in the risk-benefit equation for administration of prophylactic perioperative antibiotics include potential for and significance of surgical infection; cost, adverse effects, and ease of administration of antimicrobial agents; development of resistant microorganisms and of superinfection; and improper reliance on antimicrobial agents with resulting disregard for aseptic technique.[5] Most antibiotics should be given within 60 minutes of a surgical incision. For clean and clean-contaminated procedures, additional prophylactic antimicrobial agent doses are not necessary following closure of the surgical incision, even in the presence of a drain.[1]

HAIR REMOVAL

Hair removal may be required to facilitate adequate exposure to the site, preoperative skin marking, suturing, and application of dressing. If necessary, hair removal should be done using surgical clippers, immediately before surgery. Shaving should be avoided, because of the likelihood of causing cuts, nicks, and abrasions. A Cochrane review, published in 2009, found no statistically significant effect of hair removal on SSI rates; however, use of razors resulted in higher SSIs compared to clipping of hair.[6]

PATIENT POSITIONING

Patients should be positioned with all pressure points appropriately padded; this includes anticipating "hot spots" caused by prolonged pressure from supportive equipment such as surgical tables and endotracheal tubes (Figure 5.2). For head and neck surgeries, shoulder roll is often used to lift the shoulders and slightly extend the neck. This allows better exposure of the entire face, especially the lower half of the face. Shoulder roll may also be made out of a rolled-up blanket or saline-filled bag covered with operating room towels. If the patient is placed in lateral decubitus position, an axillary roll should be placed under the thorax, caudal to the axilla, to support the patient's chest and minimize the risk of compression of the dependent brachial plexus. In prone position, the pressure points to be padded include toes, patella, genitalia (especially in males), breast in females, and cheek and ear if head is turned to the side. Patient position should promote the ability to position surgical equipment (eg, laser) for ease of use by the surgical team. Lastly, it is also important to optimize the setup to allow for best ergonomics for the operating surgeon.

SURGICAL LIGHTING

Good quality lighting is essential for every operating room. Light-emitting diode (LED) surgical lights are preferred because they provide appropriate illumination, natural color, and

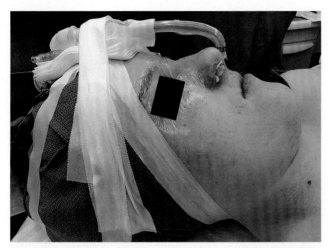

FIGURE 5.2. Example of well-secured and correctly padded nasal endotracheal tube useful for invasive procedures in and around the mouth. A surgical towel is wrapped as a head drape and secured with silk tape to the head as shown. The tube is then resecured to the head drape with gauze padding making sure the endotracheal tube is not applying pressure to the nasal ala. Reprinted with permission from Chung KC, Disa JJ, Gosain A, et al., eds. *Operative Techniques in Plastic Surgery*. Philadelphia, PA: Wolters Kluwer; 2020. Part 2, Figure 37.1B.

minimal shadow. For smaller procedures, regular examination lights or even floor lamps could be utilized for illumination.

SURGICAL CHECKLIST

For surgical success, it is imperative to maintain excellent communication among all personnel involved in surgery. Surgical checklists are implemented to reinforce accepted safety practices and foster better communication and teamwork between clinical disciplines. The checklist divides the operation into three phases. The first phase is before the induction of anesthesia or the "sign-in" phase. During this phase, safety of the procedure is established. The identity of the patient is confirmed, consent is obtained, and surgical site is marked. Additionally, during this phase, anesthetic risks are identified by the anesthesia team including known allergies, difficult airway/aspiration, and anticipated blood loss. The second phase of the checklist is the "time-out," which is performed in the operating room, prior to skin incision. During this phase, a momentary pause is taken by the team to confirm patient's identity, site, and procedure. Furthermore, anticipated critical events, patient-specific concerns, sterility, adequate equipment, and antibiotic prophylaxis are also confirmed during this phase. The last phase is the "sign-out" phase, which is completed before removing the patient from the operating room. During this phase, instrument count and specimen labeling are performed and confirmed. Additionally, the surgeon, anesthesia professionals, and operating room nurse review the key concerns for recovery and management of the patient.[7]

SKIN PREPARATION

Because the source of pathogens for most SSIs is the endogenous flora of the patient's skin, mucous membranes, or hollow viscera, optimization of preoperative skin antisepsis is important to decrease the risk of postoperative infections.[1] The two most common antiseptic agents currently in use are povidone-iodine and chlorhexidine-alcohol. According to a recent large prospective randomized controlled study, for clean-contaminated cases, preoperative cleansing of the patient's skin with chlorhexidine-alcohol is superior to cleansing with povidone-iodine for preventing SSIs.[8] Another meta-analysis performed around the same time also confirmed the efficacy of chlorhexidine over iodine for prevention of SSI.[9] The 2017 Centers for Disease Control and Prevention (CDC) guidelines for the prevention of SSIs also recommended skin preparation using an alcohol-based agent unless contraindicated. Skin preparation should be done widely, in concentric circles moving toward the periphery.[1] (See Chapter 6. Antiseptics and Aseptic Technique, for further information.)

DRAPING

Following prepping, surgical site can then be squared off using surgical towels. For surgeries performed on the head and neck area, a head drape can be used by wrapping sterile towels around the head and clamping the ends of the towel to each other using towel clamps or surgical tape (Figure 5.2). This ensures that hair is kept out of the surgical field. Several commercially available site-specific surgical drapes are available to facilitate the draping process.

SURGICAL INSTRUMENTS REQUIRED FOR MINOR PROCEDURES

Organizing surgical instruments correctly and in the order of use during the procedure facilitates efficient execution of a surgical procedure. See the following list and position of surgical instruments typically required for the performance of a minor procedure (eg, excision of nevus on the face).

SURGEON'S MENTAL PREPARATION

Whether the procedure is minor or major, it is important to sequentially think through the steps of the operation to anticipate potential complications and to minimize operative time. This practice also allows the surgeon to make sure that all adequate instruments are available before starting the surgical procedure. For more complex procedures, it is also important to have an alternative plan of action, in the event that the surgeon encounters unexpected findings during the surgery.

 Clinical Pearls for Surgical Success

- Get to the procedure room early.
- Make sure the room and equipment are set up the same way for each procedure.
- Be aware of your stance.
- Know all equipment better than anyone.
- Know the location of all supplies.
- Optimize your team.
- Consider mental imagery exercises.
- Observe other high-performing surgeons.

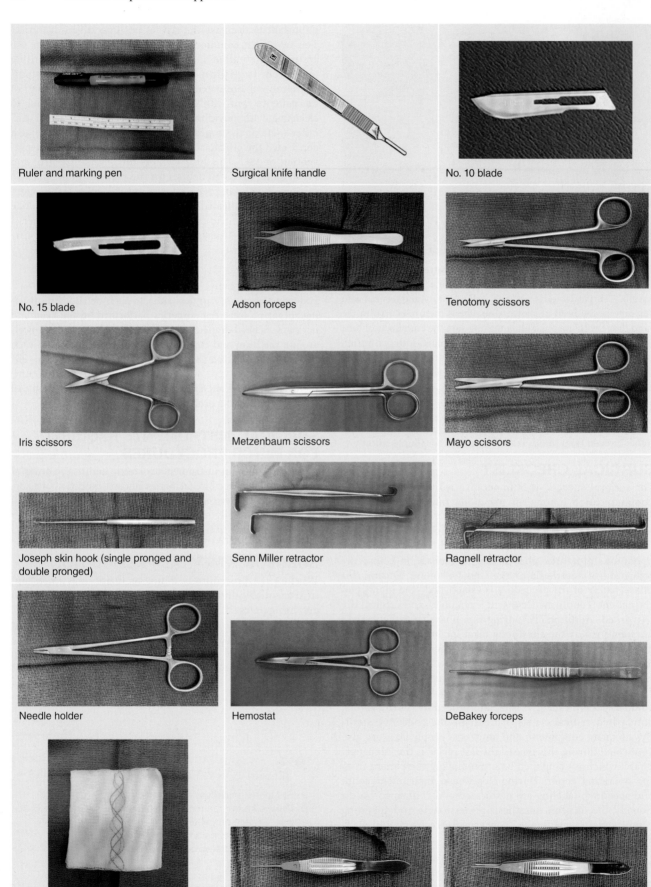

Ruler and marking pen

Surgical knife handle

No. 10 blade

No. 15 blade

Adson forceps

Tenotomy scissors

Iris scissors

Metzenbaum scissors

Mayo scissors

Joseph skin hook (single pronged and double pronged)

Senn Miller retractor

Ragnell retractor

Needle holder

Hemostat

DeBakey forceps

Raytech sponges

0.3 mm forceps

0.5 mm forceps

REFERENCES

1. Berrios-Torres A, Umscheid CA, Bratzler DW, et al. Centers for Disease Control and Prevention guideline for the prevention of surgical site infection, 2017. *JAMA Surg.* 2017;152(8):784–791. doi:10.1001/jamasurg.2017.0904.
2. Smith CE. Prevention and treatment of hypothermia in trauma patients. *Trauma Care.* 2004;14(2):68–79.
3. Tsuei BJ, Kearney PA. Hypothermia in the trauma patient. *Injury.* 2004;35(1):7–15.
4. Feinstein L, Miskiewicz M. Perioperative hypothermia: review for the anesthesia provider. *Internet J Anesthesiol.* 2010;27(2).
5. DiPiro JT, Record KE, Schanzenbach KS, et al. Antimicrobial prophylaxis in surgery: part 1. *Am J Health Syst Pharm.* 1981;38(3):320–334.
6. Tanner J, Norrie P, Melen K. Preoperative hair removal to reduce surgical site infection. *Cochrane Database Syst Rev.* 2011:CD004122.
7. World Alliance for Patient Safety. *Implementation Manual Surgical Safety Checklist.* 1st ed. WHO/IER/PSP/2008.05. Geneva, Switzerland: WHO Press. http://www.who.int/patientsafety/safesurgery/tools_resources/SSSL_Manual_finalJun08.pdf.
8. Lee I, Agarwal RK, Lee BY, et al. Systematic review and cost analysis comparing use of chlorhexidine with use of iodine for preoperative skin antisepsis to prevent surgical site infection. *Infect Control Hosp Epidemiol.* 2010;31(12):1219–1229. doi:10.1086/657134.
9. Darouiche RO, Wall MJ, Itani KMF, et al. Chlorhexidine–alcohol versus povidone–iodine for surgical-site antisepsis. *N Engl J Med.* 2010;362:18–26.

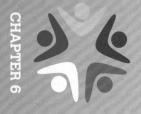

CHAPTER 6

Antiseptics and Aseptic Technique

Samantha L. Schneider, Danielle Yeager, and Marla N. Jahnke

OVERVIEW

Aseptic technique is important in preventing surgical site infections. This technique involves preoperative preparation and maintenance of a semi-sterile environment throughout cutaneous surgical procedures. Specific details related to infection prevention and infection risk in the pediatric population are noted where applicable, but the majority of research available is from adults and inferred for the pediatric population. Children, nonetheless, have fewer comorbidities compared with those of adults, which may contribute to lower rates of infection. Conversely, they also tend to be more active postoperatively, and wound care recommendations should be highlighted for patients and families to minimize postoperative infections. Regardless, aseptic technique applies at any age in the primary prevention of cutaneous wound infections.

Procedures are broadly categorized as clean, clean-contaminated, contaminated, and dirty and/or infected (Table 6.1). Most dermatologic procedures are either clean or clean-contaminated.

- *Clean procedures* are performed under sterile technique in noninflamed tissues.
- *Clean-contaminated procedures* have small breaks in aseptic technique or enter into the gastrointestinal, respiratory, or genitourinary tracts.
- *Contaminated wounds* are those where major breaks in aseptic technique have occurred or there is inflammation but no frank purulence.
- *Dirty wounds* contain frank purulent fluid or include perforation of a viscus or fecal contamination.

GUIDELINES TO PREVENT AND CONTROL INFECTION

The Centers for Disease Control and Prevention (CDC) has published guidelines to prevent and control infection.[1] They include recommendations on the following: hand hygiene, environmental infection control, disinfection and sterilization, and

isolation precautions. We will discuss hand hygiene, environmental infection control, and disinfection and sterilization as these all relate to dermatologic surgery. We have not addressed isolation precautions as this is not frequently employed in dermatologic surgery; the vast majority of dermatologic surgery for all ages occurs in a clean ambulatory setting, where contact precautions generally do not apply.[1]

Hand Hygiene

One of the most important ways that dermatologists maintain aseptic technique is through hand hygiene. Preoperatively, surgical personnel should keep their fingernails short and clean and wash their hands thoroughly with soap and water or alcohol-based sanitizers before the procedure. Alcohol-based sanitizers are commonly accepted as appropriate and effective methods of hand hygiene (Figure 6.1). Alcohol functions as an antiseptic by denaturing the organisms' cell membranes. Soap and water is the classic choice for hand hygiene. Soap functions as a detergent that removes dirt and other skin contaminants and, as such, should be utilized in place of alcohol-based sanitizers for visibly soiled hands. When cleansing their hands, providers should make sure to cover all surfaces of their hands and fingers. With alcohol-based sanitizers, these surfaces should be covered until the hands are dry. If using soap and water, a minimum of 15 seconds is recommended. Some providers may choose to use surgical scrub or chlorhexidine (Figure 6.2); however, there is no difference in the risk of postoperative infections with these techniques, and these may contribute to irritant and allergic contact dermatitis more so than soap- or alcohol-based cleansers.

Environmental Infection Control

The surgical environment is an additional important consideration to limit potential contamination (see Chapter 5. Surgical Procedure Room Setup). The environment consists of the medical personnel, the procedural room, and patient characteristics. The ambulatory setting, where the majority of skin

TABLE 6.1 : Surgical Wound Classification

CLASSIFICATION	CHARACTERISTICS	EXAMPLE
Clean	Immaculate sterile technique Noninflamed site	Melanoma re-excision under sterile technique
Clean-contaminated	Small breaks in sterile technique Involvement of oral mucosa, axillae, gastrointestinal or genital tract but without gross contamination[a]	Biopsy of higher risk areas such as oral mucosa, axillae, or groin
Contaminated	Major breaks in sterile technique Gross spillage from gastrointestinal tract Acute, nonpurulent inflammation is encountered	Animal bite Incision and drainage
Dirty	Involves existing clinical infection or perforated viscus	Bowel resection due to perforation

[a]See discussion. May be appropriate for all or most dermatologic surgeries.

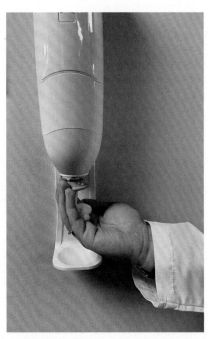

FIGURE 6.1. Alcohol-based cleansers are a widely accepted hand-washing technique. One must be sure to rub all surfaces of the hands for optimal distribution.

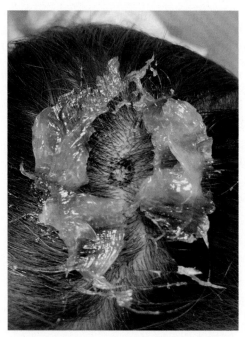

FIGURE 6.3. Petrolatum can be used to help secure hair away from the surgical site in lieu of or lessen the need for excessively cutting or trimming the hair.

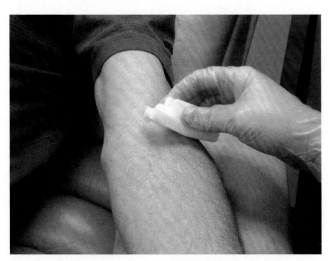

FIGURE 6.2. Example of chlorhexidine being used to clean the surgical field prior to the procedure. Reprinted with permission from *Lippincott's Visual Encyclopedia of Clinical Skills*. Philadelphia, PA: Wolters Kluwer Health/Lippincott Williams & Wilkins; 2009.

surgery occurs, provides an environment with a generally low risk of infection.[2]

Medical personnel should wear appropriate surgical attire to prevent contamination of the surgical environment. In clean-contaminated procedures, this may include wearing surgical gloves and face masks. Sterile gloves are often used during excisions and nail procedures, although there is increasing evidence that nonsterile gloves may be equally appropriate. At this point in time, the studies are inconclusive—some argue that the use of sterile gloves is more important for patient perception and, in the case of pediatric dermatology, parent perception than actual risk

prevention and that this practice contributes to increased costs with minimal benefit.[3,4] Although no studies specifically evaluate wound infections in pediatric skin surgery, wound infections in dermatologic surgery are extremely rare, with multiple studies citing the risk to be under 2.5%, regardless of whether sterile or nonsterile gloves are used.[5-8] In general, surgical gowns are not necessary, but may be worn to provide additional barrier protection for the surgeon from fluid and microbial transmission.

For patients, street clothes do not need to be removed as they do not affect infection rates; a gown, however, may be preferred to allow adequate exposure of the procedural site. When performing procedures involving hair-bearing areas, multiple techniques may be utilized to prepare the field. Hair should not be shaved prior to procedures as this actually increases the infection rate when performed immediately prior.[2] The patient's hair should be secured away from the sterile field, when able, with hair ties or headbands. If hair needs to be removed from the surgical field, trimming with a clipper is preferred.[9] Additionally, clinicians could consider the use of petrolatum as a means of securing hair away from the surgical field (Figure 6.3).

Advanced preparation of the surgical environment and the patients themselves improves the patient's and the physician's experience, aids in safety, and controls as many aspects of the environment as possible. In pediatric procedures, the patient may be somewhat unpredictable and setup is especially important to help maintain aseptic technique. Additionally, when preparing the procedural room between patients, special attention should be taken to ensure that rooms are promptly cleaned and that soiled items are discarded appropriately.

Disinfection and Sterilization

The final key step in aseptic technique for the dermatologic surgeon involves disinfection and sterilization. In addition to ensuring safe and clean personnel and surroundings, patients should be disinfected via the surgical prep. Prepping the surgical site decreases skin debris and dirt as well as transient microorganisms. The most commonly used antiseptics include chlorhexidine gluconate (hibiclens), povidone iodine, and alcohol-based products. There are special considerations for each

of these, which are detailed further in Table 6.2. Chlorhexidine is likely the most widely used surgical preparation on the skin for larger procedures because of its broad-spectrum antiseptic activity, rapid onset, long-lasting antimicrobial effect, and low cost. Chlorhexidine, however, must be used with caution as it

TABLE 6.2 ⋮ Antiseptics

ANTIMICROBIAL AGENT	MECHANISM OF ACTION	ONSET	RESIDUAL ACTIVITY	ADVANTAGES	DISADVANTAGES
Alcohol (isopropyl and ethanol)	Denatures cell membrane	Immediate *(fastest)*	None	Very broad spectrum (gram +/−, mycobacteria, most viruses)	Inactive against spores and nonenveloped viruses Best for short procedures only Not effective for soiled hands *Flammable*! Caution with lasers/electrosurgery
Chlorhexidine (2%-4%)	Disrupts cell membranes	Rapid	Longest acting, >6 h	Broad spectrum (gram +/−, viruses, fungi, mycobacteria) *Not* inactivated by body fluids	Inactive against spores *Avoid* around ears/eyes (ototoxicity, keratitis, and conjunctivitis) Risk of absorption in premature infants Risk of immediate and delayed hypersensitivity reaction
Chloroxylenol (parachlorometaxylenol)	Inactivates enzymes and affects cell wall	Slow	Good	Fairly broad spectrum (gram positive greater than gram negative, viruses, mycobacteria)	Not as broad spectrum, fast acting, or long lasting as chlorhexidine Decreased efficacy with body fluids Ineffective against pseudomonas (unless combined with EDTA)
Hexachlorophene	Inactivates enzymes	Slow	Modest	Effective against staph	Ineffective against gram negative, fungi, mycobacteria Neurotoxicity and teratogenic; do not use in infants *Not used*
Iodine and iodophors (betadine)	Oxidation leads to disruption of protein synthesis and cell membrane	Rapid	Minimal	Very broad spectrum (gram +/−, mycobacteria, fungi, viruses, *bacterial spores*)	Skin irritation, contact allergy, discoloration Inactivated by body fluids Must wait for it to dry to be effective Risk of absorption in premature infants
Quaternary ammonium compounds (benzalkonium)	Punctures cytoplasmic membranes	Slow	Good	Gram positive and lipophilic viruses	Ineffective against gram negative, mycobacteria, fungi Inactivated by body fluids and cotton gauze
Triclosan	Affects cytoplasmic membrane and interrupts synthesis of proteins	Rapid	Good	Gram positive, mycobacteria, candida Not inactivated by body fluids	Ineffective against gram negative and filamentous fungi Skin irritation, contact allergy

Abbreviation: EDTA, ethylenediaminetetraacetic acid.

may cause keratitis when used periocularly and ototoxicity when used around the ear. Additionally, there is concern about the allergenicity of chlorhexidine as both immediate and delayed type hypersensitivity have been reported, likely because of increasing exposure.[10,11] In 2017, the Food and Drug Administration (FDA) issued a warning regarding the use of chlorhexidine and advised that physicians ask patients, prior to its use, if they have a history of reactions.[12] If a history of reactions is known, an alternative should be sought as described in Table 6.2.

There are several other noteworthy considerations when choosing among the most common other surgical preps (Figure 6.4A-D). Iodine's mechanism of action involves oxidation, and it must be completely dry to become fully effective; consequently, it may become inactivated by bodily fluids. Additionally, iodine is a relatively common cause of contact dermatitis, making it a less-than-ideal option. If using an alcohol-based cleanser, it is important to remember that alcohol is flammable and should not be used in close proximity to electrocautery. Additionally, alcohol-based preps are effective only while still wet and are thus reserved for short procedures.

It is also critical that surgical instruments are appropriately cleansed. Surgical equipment should be sterilized, and personnel should be trained on proper sterilization techniques. The most commonly used sterilization technique in office-based settings is the steam autoclave. Autoclaving is a sterilization technique that uses a combination of high pressure (2 atm) and high temperature (121°C) to kill any organisms present. The steam autoclave technique is inexpensive and does not require toxic chemicals for implementation. The main drawback in utilizing a steam autoclave for sterilization is the eventual dulling

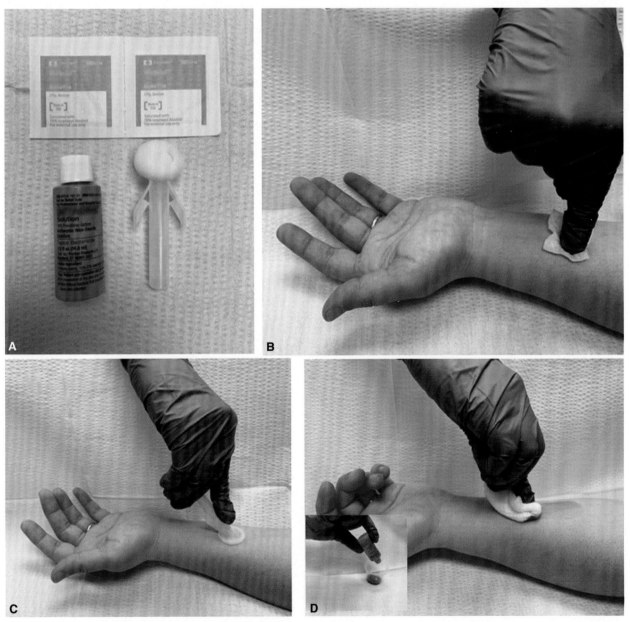

FIGURE 6.4. There are multiple options for skin disinfection (A), including alcohol swabs (B), chlorhexidine (C), and povidone iodine (D). Povidone iodine is available as premoistened swabs and in a bottle to be applied on gauze (inset to D).

of the surgical instruments after repetitive use because of the moist nature of the heat-inducing corrosion. Other less commonly used sterilization techniques include heated chemical vapor, dry heat, gas sterilization, and chemical immersion. After sterilization, instruments should be handled in a manner to maintain sterility. When not in use, instruments on the surgical tray should be covered with a sterile drape. Trays should be kept orderly to allow for easy identification during procedures and for optimal safety.

Surgical site infection is defined by the CDC as any surgical wound that produces pus within 30 days of the procedure. Fortunately, these events are uncommon in dermatologic surgery.[13] As such, both clean and clean-contaminated procedures do not typically require antibiotic prophylaxis. Although the diagnosis of a surgical site infection does not require positive cultures,[14] it is helpful to obtain wound cultures from any wounds suspected to be infected to aid in diagnosis and to guide antibiotic treatment (see Chapter 133. Postprocedure Antibiotics). Prevention of infection is key, and a well-prepared surgical environment is critical in aseptic technique.

REFERENCES

1. Centers for Disease Control and Prevention. Infection control: basic infection prevention and control. 2015. https://www.cdc.gov/infectioncontrol/guidelines/index.html. Accessed March 22, 2019.
2. Elliott TG, Thom GA, Litterick KA. Office based dermatological surgery and Mohs surgery: a prospective audit of surgical procedures and complications in a procedural dermatology practice. *Australas J Dermatol.* 2012;53(4): 264–271.
3. Futoryan T, Grande D. Postoperative wound infection rates in dermatologic surgery. *Dermatol Surg.* 1995;21:509–514.
4. Rhinehart BM, Murphy ME, Farley MF, Albertini JG. Sterile versus nonsterile gloves during Mohs micrographic surgery: infection rate is not affected. *Dermatol Surg.* 2006;32: 170–176.
5. Rogers HD, Desciak EB, Marcus RP, Wang S, MacKay-Wiggan J, Eliezri YD. Prospective study of wound infections in Mohs micrographic surgery using clean surgical technique in the absence of prophylactic antibiotics. *J Am Acad Dermatol.* 2010;63: 842–851.
6. Xia Y, Cho S, Greenway H, Zelac D, Kelley B. Infection rates of wound repairs during Mohs micrographic surgery using sterile versus nonsterile gloves: a prospective randomized pilot study. *Dermatol Surg.* 2011;37:651–656.
7. Perelman V, Francis G, Rutledge T, Foote J, Martino F, Dranitsaris G. Sterile versus nonsterile gloves for repair of uncomplicated lacerations in the emergency department: a randomized controlled trial. *Ann Emerg Med.* 2004;43:362–370.
8. Rogues AM, Lasheras A, Amici JM, Guillot P, et al. Infection control practices and infectious complications in dermatological surgery. *J Hosp Infect.* 2007;65:258–263.
9. Tanner J, Norrie P, Melen K. Preoperative hair removal to reduce surgical site infection. *Cochrane Database Syst Rev.* 2011;(11):CD004122.
10. Aalto-Korte K, Mäkinen-Kiliunen S. Symptoms of immediate chlorhexidine hypersensitivity in patients with a positive prick test. *Contact Dermatitis.* 2006;55:173–177.
11. Okano M, Nomura M, Hata S, et al. Anaphylactic symptoms due to chlorhexidine gluconate. *Arch Dermatol.* 1989;125:50–52.
12. Food and Drug Administration. FDA drug safety communication: FDA warns about rare but serious allergic reactions with the skin antiseptic chlorhexidine gluconate. 2017. https://www.fda.gov/drugs/drugsafety/ucm530975.htm. Accessed March 22, 2019.
13. Berríos-Torres SI, Umscheid CA, Bratzler DW, et al. Centers for Disease Control and Prevention guideline for the prevention of surgical site infection, 2017. *JAMA Surg.* 2017;152(8):784–791.
14. Polk HC, Simpson CJ, Simmons BP, Alexander JW. Guidelines for prevention of surgical wound infection. *Arch Surg.* 1983;118(10):1213–1217.

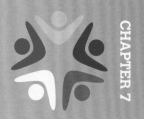

CHAPTER 7

Surgical Instruments

Asra Hashmi and Amanda A. Gosman

INTRODUCTION

This chapter presents photos and uses for commonly used surgical instruments. Instruments are described in the order typically used in the operating room during a simple procedure. Surgical instruments can be broadly classified into six groups based on function. See Table 7.1 for categories and examples of each.

SCALPELS

The surgical scalpel consists of two parts: a blade and a handle. The scalpel handle is held with the index finger guiding the blade, with the handle held between the thumb and the middle finger in the palm of the hand. A variety of blades are available, each with its unique use in the operating room (Figure 7.1). The most commonly used blades and their uses are as follows:

TABLE 7.1 Categories of Surgical Instruments

TYPES OF SURGICAL INSTRUMENTS	EXAMPLES
Cutting and Dissecting	Scalpel, Metzenbaum scissors, Iris scissors, saw
Grasping	Adson forceps, Adson Brown forceps, 0.5 forceps
Retracting	Skin hook, Senn-Miller retractor, Ragnell retractor, Army-Navy retractor
Clamping	Hemostat, Kocher clamp, Mosquito clamp
Suturing	Sutures, needle holders, surgical staplers
Supplementary Instruments	Electrocautery probes and forceps, suction tips, skin adhesives, tapes (see Chapter 17. Electrosurgery/Hyfrecation for further details)

No. 10 Blade: This blade has a curved cutting inferior edge and unsharpened back edge. It is commonly used for making long incisions.

No. 11 Blade: This blade has a sharp triangulated pointed blade with a blunt superior edge and a sharp, straight inferior edge. It is commonly used for incision and drainage of fluid-filled wounds.

No. 12 Blade: This blade has a pointed crescent-shaped blade with a blunt superior edge and a sharp inferior edge. It is used for cutting into deep, difficult-to-access anatomic locations (eg, deep inside the mouth or palate).

No. 15 Blade: This blade is similar to the No. 10 blade but is smaller in size. It is used for making precise smaller incisions (eg, incision for cyst excision on the face).

No. 20 Blade: This blade is similar to the No. 10 blade but is wider and shorter in comparison. It is commonly used in orthopedic surgery.

Beaver Blades: These are smaller blades, designed for enhanced control in more precise incisions (eg, lip, eyelid, nose).

FORCEPS

Adson Forceps (Figure 7.2): These are the most commonly used forceps for tissue handling and suturing and are available with toothed or plain tips. Plain tip Adson forceps are usually used to dissect out delicate tissue such as nerves and vessels. Toothed forceps are used for gripping fine but tougher tissue such as skin, tendon, fascia, and subcutaneous fat.

Adson Brown Forceps (Figure 7.3): This version of the conventional Adson forceps includes broad serrated tips, used to prevent slipping while gripping.

0.3 and 0.5 Forceps (Figure 7.4A and B): These small toothed forceps (with 0.3 mm or 0.5 mm tips) are ideal for handling delicate tissue in the face area (eg, eyelid, nose, lips). Bishop forceps have similar surgical indications but the handle part bears three holes to facilitate grasping.

Debakey Forceps (Figure 7.5): This set of forceps includes long, narrow, blunt tips for atraumatic tissue handling.

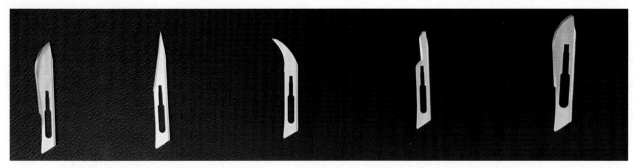

FIGURE 7.1. Commonly used scalpel blades: (left to right) No. 10 blade, 11 blade, 12 blade, 15 blade, and 20 blade.

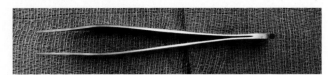

FIGURE 7.2. Adson forceps.

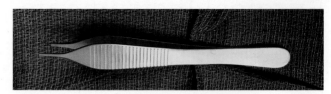

FIGURE 7.3. Adson brown forceps.

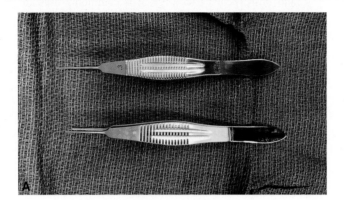

FIGURE 7.4. A and B, 0.3 (top) and 0.5 (bottom) forceps. Copyright © B. Braun Melsungen AG.

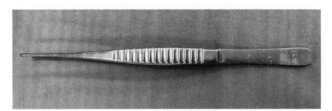

FIGURE 7.5. Debakey forceps.

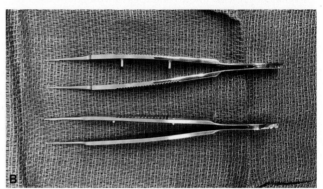

FIGURE 7.6. Electrocautery probe instrument.

ELECTROCAUTERY INSTRUMENTS AND SUPPLIES

Electrocautery applies high-frequency alternating current by a unipolar or bipolar method. The difference between these two methods is that with monopolar electrosurgery, the current passes from the probe electrode (Figure 7.6) to the tissue and through the patient to a return pad to complete the electric current circuit. Bipolar electrocautery passes the current between two tips of a forceps-like tool (Figure 7.7), thus minimizing lateral thermal damage and preventing any disturbance of other electrical body rhythms (such as the heart).[2]

With these devices, electric current is passed through a resistant metal wire electrode, generating heat and achieving hemostasis.[1] A grounding pad is placed on the body before the surgery to protect the person from the harmful

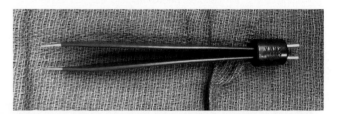

FIGURE 7.7. Electrocautery bipolar forceps.

effects of the electricity. It can be a continuous waveform (yellow button) that cuts tissue or intermittent waveform (blue button) to coagulate tissue. See Chapter 17. Electrosurgery/Hyfrecation.

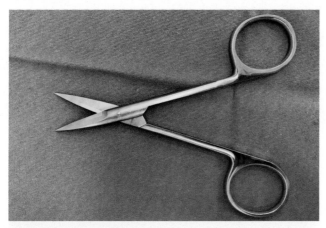

FIGURE 7.8. Iris scissors.

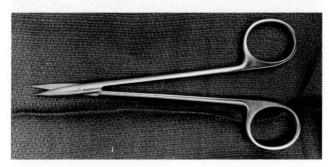

FIGURE 7.9. Tenotomy scissors.

SCISSORS

Iris Scissors: These sharp cutting scissors are available with either curved or straight blades and in various lengths. Straight Iris scissors can often be used as an alternative to knife because of their sharp blades, and curved scissors are useful for dog-ear excisions. Because of the precision required in skin excisions, it is important to prevent blunting of the sharp blades; thus, the surgeon should avoid cutting sutures with Iris scissors (Figure 7.8).

Tenotomy Scissors: These dissecting scissors have blunt tips (in comparison with Iris scissors) and are available in various lengths (Figure 7.9).

Mayo Scissors: These heavy scissors are used to cut suture and dissect dense fibrous tissue, with blades available as either straight or curved (Figure 7.10).

Metzenbaum Scissors: These tissue cutting scissors are available with either curved or straight blades. These scissors are usually used for dissecting through tissue planes (Figure 7.11).

HOOKS

Joseph Skin Hook: This tool is used for retraction of superficial skin edges; it is available as either double pronged or

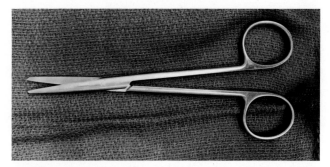

FIGURE 7.10. Mayo scissors.

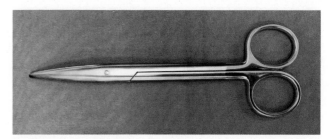

FIGURE 7.11. Metzenbaum scissors.

single pronged and in various lengths. Single-pronged hooks are useful for retraction in small spaces, for example, retraction at the apex of an incision (Figure 7.12). Double-pronged hooks are useful for retraction of skin edges so that the surgeon has an adequate exposure to the next (deeper) layer to be dissected.

Senn-Miller Retractor: This double-ended retractor is used for retraction of superficial tissue deeper than skin, for example, subcutaneous fat and fascia. One side has a three-pronged (sharp or blunt) retractor, used for retraction of tougher tissue, for example, fascia, and the other side has an L-shaped blunt blade facing the opposite direction, typically useful for retraction of softer tissue, for example, subcutaneous fat (Figure 7.13).

Ragnell Retractor: This is another superficial retractor that utilizes double-ended L-shaped blades for retraction of tissue deeper than skin, for example, subcutaneous fat and superficial fascia (Figure 7.14). This retractor has the same indications as the L-shaped blunt side of the Senn-Miller retractor.

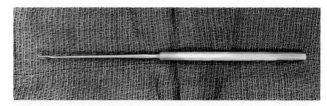

FIGURE 7.12. Joseph skin hook. Copyright © B. Braun Melsungen AG.

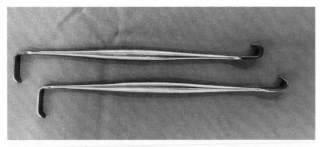

FIGURE 7.13. Senn-Miller retractor.

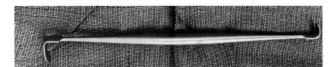

FIGURE 7.14. Ragnell retractor.

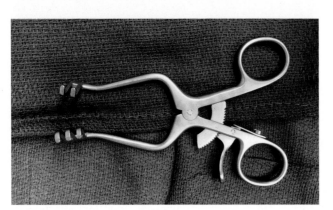

FIGURE 7.15. Weitlaner retractor.

Weitlaner Retractor: This self-retaining retractor is used to hold tissue edges open (Figure 7.15).

Army-Navy Retractor: These retractors are used for wounds of moderate depth (Figure 7.16).

Richardson Retractor: This tool is available in various sizes. The blade of this retractor is wider compared with that of the

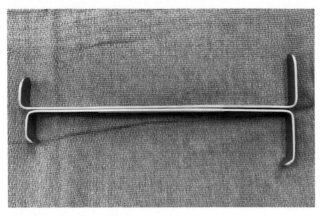

FIGURE 7.16. Army-Navy retractor.

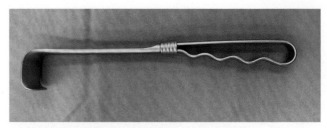

FIGURE 7.17. Richardson retractor.

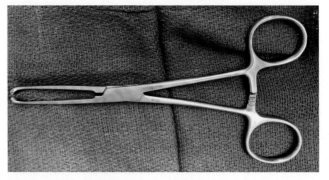

FIGURE 7.18. Allis clamp.

Army-Navy retractor and longer compared with that of the Senn-Miller retractor, so this instrument is usually used for retraction in deep wounds (Figure 7.17).

CLAMPS

Allis Clamp: This instrument has interlocking teeth at the tip and is used for retracting and holding tissue, such as grasping a lipoma during its excision (Figure 7.18).

    Tonsil Clamp: This instrument has long shanks and is used, for example, for dissecting in deeper wounds or passing drains (Figure 7.19).

    Kelley Clamp: This tool is used for grasping and clamping blood vessels before tying them (Figure 7.20).

    Kocher Clamp: This tool is used to grasp tough tissue like fascia. Kocher has serrated teeth at its tip, which makes it useful for grasping fascia (Figure 7.21).

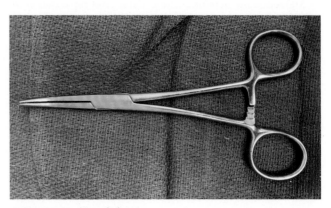

FIGURE 7.19. Tonsil clamp.

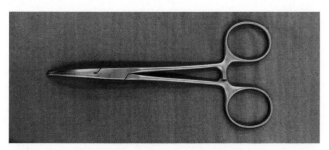

FIGURE 7.20. Kelley clamp.

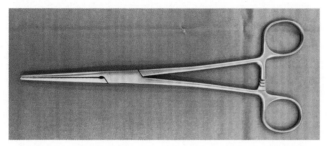

FIGURE 7.21. Kocher clamp. Copyright © B. Braun Melsungen AG.

OTHER MISCELLANEOUS SURGICAL INSTRUMENTS

Needle Holders: These tools are also called needle drivers. Each needle driver has three parts: the jaws, a joint, and clamps. A variety of needle drivers are available, with differences in size and design. Smaller, lighter, and finer drivers are typically used for skin closures, to allow more precision (Figure 7.22).

Periosteal Elevator: This instrument is available in a wide range of shapes and sizes. It is used to lift the periosteum off the bone. This instrument is commonly used in pediatric dermoid excision (Figure 7.23).

Mosquito Clamp: This tool is available as either straight or curved and is used for clamping, holding, dissecting, and ligating vessels in more delicate tissue (Figure 7.24).

Frazier Suction Tip: This suction tip is designed for aspirating fluid from confined spaces. Suction can be controlled with a small hole on the handle (Figure 7.25).

Yankauer Suction Tip: This suction tip utilizes a rounded tip to avoid aspirating tissue and is available in metal or disposable plastic (Figure 7.26).

Rongeur: This tool is used for chipping and cutting bone (Figure 7.27).

Curette: This tool is used for scrapping or debriding tissue and is available as curved or straight, in a wide range of sizes (Figure 7.28).

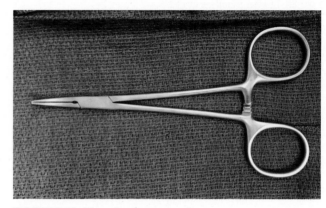

FIGURE 7.24. Mosquito clamp.

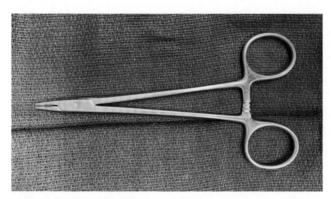

FIGURE 7.22. Needle holder.

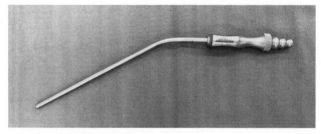

FIGURE 7.25. Frazier suction tip.

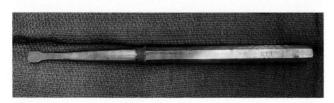

FIGURE 7.23. Periosteal elevator.

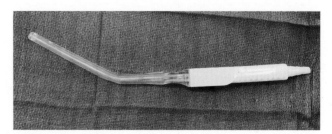

FIGURE 7.26. Yankauer suction tip.

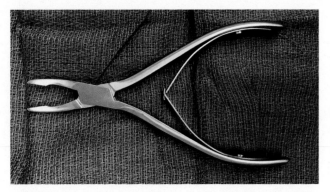

FIGURE 7.27. Rongeur. Courtesy of Integra LifeSciences Corporation.

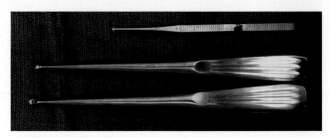

FIGURE 7.28. Curettes.

REFERENCES

1. Pollock SV. Electrosurgery. In: Bolognia JL, Jorizzo JL, Rapini RP, eds. *Dermatology*. 2nd ed. Mosby Elsevier; 2008:chap 140.
2. Sabiston D. *Sabiston Textbook of Surgery*. 19th ed. Philadelphia, PA: Elsevier Saunders; 2012:235.

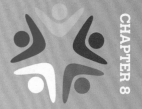

CHAPTER 8

Sutures

Asra Hashmi and Amanda A. Gosman

It is vital to understand the characteristics of suture materials so that the physician is able to select the most appropriate suture for the tissue under consideration and place sutures in a manner consistent with the principles that promote optimum wound healing and scar mitigation. A variety of suture materials, each with unique characteristics, are available, as described in this chapter.[1,2]

SUTURE CHARACTERISTICS

Absorbable Versus Nonabsorbable Sutures

The suture may be classified as absorbable or nonabsorbable depending on the degradation potential. The absorbable type can be further classified into natural absorbable and synthetic absorbable. The degradation process for the two mentioned absorbable suture types is different. The natural absorbable sutures are dissolved via enzymatic degradation and the synthetic ones are absorbed primarily via hydrolyzation. The enzymatic degradation process of the natural sutures produces a relatively higher inflammatory response, in comparison to hydrolyzation of the synthetic sutures.

There is no significant difference in the incidence of wound infection and rates of wound dehiscence between absorbable and nonabsorbable sutures.[3] One advantage of absorbable sutures is that they do not need to be removed and, thus, avoid the need for a return visit and the associated discomfort of suture removal. For this reason, they are often used in children.

Nonabsorbable sutures are, as the name suggests, made from nonbiodegradable materials. Nonabsorbable sutures either require removal in a subsequent procedure or, if left in place, will eventually induce a cell-mediated response and become walled off or encapsulated by the body as the wound heals. For external skin closure, they are typically utilized to minimize inflammation with healing, such as in patients at risk for keloid or hypertrophic scar formation or for cosmetically sensitive areas such as the face. When used for external closure, they should be ideally removed within 5 to 7 days to avoid permanent marks from epithelialization of the suture track.

Nonabsorbable sutures are classified into three types by the United States Pharmacopeia (USP)[1]:

- **Class I:** Silk or synthetic monofilament, where the coating, if any, does not affect the thickness of the suture; example: braided silk, nylon, polypropylene
- **Class II:** Cotton or linen fibers or coated (natural or synthetic) fibers, where the coating, if present, affects the thickness significantly but not the strength of the suture; example: virgin silk sutures
- **Class III:** Monofilament or multifilament metal wires; example: steel suture

Size of Suture

The USP rating system is typically used to refer to the size of the suture. The size of the suture is given either a number (eg, #1 PDS™ [Ethicon US, LLC]) or a number of zeros (eg, 3-0 Monocryl™ [Ethicon US, LLC] or 000 Monocryl suture), based

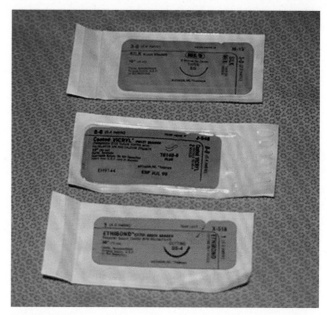

FIGURE 8.1. Several examples of various suture materials supplied in transparent packages, with the size and type clearly labeled on the outside of the packet. The inside of the packet is sterile. Reprinted with permission from Kronenberger J, Ledbetter J. *Lippincott Williams & Wilkins' Comprehensive Medical Assisting.* 5th ed. Philadelphia, PA: Wolters Kluwer; 2016. Figure 22.9.

on breaking strength and suture diameter. A guiding principle is to use the smallest diameter suture that will adequately hold the tissue in the desired place, thus minimizing tissue trauma and foreign body exposure. Figure 8.1 shows sutures of various sizes.

Monofilament Versus Multifilament/Barbed or Unbarbed

Sutures can be classified on the basis of number of strands as monofilament or multifilament. Monofilament sutures pass through the tissue with minimal resistance; however, if any part of the suture is crushed, then it makes the suture more prone to breakage. On the contrary, multifilament sutures (twisted or braided) are generally stronger, but they may have a risk of harboring bacteria within their strands and are associated with a higher risk of infection.

Sutures may also be barbed or unbarbed. The benefits of one-way barbs in the suture include more security, knotless closures, and, hence, faster deployment.[4]

Suture Memory

Memory refers to the tendency of the suture to return to a given shape set by the material's extrusion process or the suture's packaging configuration (ie, the suture's tendency to resist lying flat). The more memory a suture has, the higher the number of throws in a surgical knot that are required to ensure a secure knot. Monofilament sutures generally have more memory compared to polyfilament sutures. So, more knots are generally required in a Monocryl suture compared to a Vicryl™ (Ethicon US, LLC) suture, or a monofilament nylon compared to a polyfilament nylon suture.

Composition and Tensile Strength

Sutures may be prepared from mammalian collagen or synthetic tissue. The following are the commonly used suture types with a description of their composition.[1]

- **Gut sutures:** These sutures are made of purified ribbons of collagen from sheep intestinal submucosa or beef intestinal serosal layer, and hence the named "gut" suture. Mainly, three different types of gut sutures are available: plain gut, fast absorbing gut, and chromic gut sutures. Plain gut sutures typically maintain their tensile strength for 7 to 10 days and are best used where maintenance of excessive strength by the suture material is not necessary. The fast absorbing gut suture is, simply, a plain gut suture that is heat treated to accelerate absorption. The fast gut absorbing suture maintains its tensile strength for only 5 to 7 days and is best used for approximation of the epidermis in cosmetically sensitive areas. The chromic gut suture is named so because it is treated with chromium salt to resist enzymatic absorption by the body. This chromicization process also results in a change of the suture color to tan brown. The chromic gut suture maintains its tensile strength for 10 to 14 days.

- **Glycolide/lactide copolymer (Vicryl):** This is an absorbable synthetic suture made of a copolymer of glycolide and lactide. It typically comes braided; however, a monofilament variety is also available (mainly for ophthalmologic use). In addition to glycolide and lactide, the coating with calcium stearate contributes to the nonflaking lubricant property. This coating of calcium stearate is also postulated to contribute to the suture's nonantigenic property. This suture maintains strong tensile strength for at least 2 to 3 weeks. By 5 weeks postimplantation, the original tensile strength is completely lost, and it is completely absorbed by hydrolysis in approximately 2 months. This property makes Vicryl an ideal suture for approximation of superficial fascia. Coated Vicryl Rapide™ (Ethicon US, LLC) suture is a low-molecular-weight suture that is only available undyed. Vicryl Rapide maintains the benefits of the Vicryl suture but, in addition, gets absorbed more rapidly. It is advised for use only in areas where 7 to 10 days of wound support is required (eg, lip mucosa). Vicryl can also be treated with an antibacterial agent such as Triclosan to provide antimicrobial properties.

  Vicryl (Ethicon US, LLC)

- **Poliglecaprone 25 (Monocryl):** This is another synthetic absorbable monofilament suture composed of copolymer of glycolide and ε-caprolactone. This suture has low reactivity with a half-life of 7 to 14 days, making it an ideal suture for skin closures (eg, deep dermal closure and subcuticular closure techniques). Monocryl completely loses its original tensile strength by 3 weeks postimplantation. It has more memory when compared to Vicryl; however, because of the monofilament configuration, it is less traumatic and easier to pass through tissue.

  Monocryl™ (Ethicon US, LLC)

- **Polydioxanone (PDS II):** This is a nonreactive, slowly absorbing, monofilament suture composed of polyester, p-dioxanone. This suture maintains 70% of its tensile strength at 2 weeks and 50% at 4 weeks and takes about 6 months to dissolve completely. This suture is ideal for approximation of the fascia because of its slow absorption property. Although less commonly used, smaller PDS II sutures (5-0 PDS, etc.) may also be considered for use in superficial tissue approximation, especially in pediatric patients who may be less likely to adhere to postoperative instructions. This suture can hence be used for deep dermal skin closure in the pediatric population.

  Polydioxanone (PDS II®, Ethicon US, LLC 2019)

- **Silk:** Silk suture is one of the oldest surgical sutures available to humans, and it is still used extensively in operating rooms. It is a naturally occurring, nonabsorbable suture, and its filament can be twisted or braided. It is usually dyed black for ease of visibility. This suture is ideal for ligation of blood vessels and it can also be utilized for approximation of tendon or fascial edges. In vivo studies have shown that silk loses its tensile strength 1 year postimplantation.

- **Nylon (Ethilon, Nurolon, Surgilon):** This is a synthetic, nonabsorbable suture, available as monofilament or multifilament. Its inert property makes it an ideal suture for skin closure in cosmetically sensitive areas such as the face, but the suture should be removed in 5 to 7 days to minimize the risk of track marks. Its noninflammatory nature also makes it an ideal suture for closure in areas prone to keloid and hypertrophic scar formation. It can also be used as a retention suture, in areas prone to wound dehiscence and breakdown. The nylon suture loses its tensile strength at the rate of approximately 10% to 20% per year. (Ethilon is a monofilament and Nurolon and Surgilon are multifilament braided nylon sutures.)

  Ethilon® (Ethicon US, LLC 2019), Nurolon® (Ethicon US, LLC) and Surgilon® (Covidien/Medtronic, 2020)

- **Polypropylene (Prolene or Surgipro):** This is a synthetic, monofilament, nonabsorbable suture composed of crystalline stereoisomer of polypropylene. This is a nonreactive suture and is used for a variety of surgical indications. Polypropylene sutures are nonadherent, so they are ideal as "pull out" sutures after subcuticular skin closures in cosmetically sensitive areas. They are also used for vascular anastomosis, fascial closures, tendon and paratendon approximation, and various other surgical indications.

  Prolene™ (Ethicon US, LLC) or Surgipro™ (US Surgical Corporation)

- **Polyester (Mersilene, Ethibond):** Polyester sutures are another group of synthetic, nonabsorbable, braided sutures that maintain their tensile strength indefinitely. Mersilene is uncoated, so it has a higher friction coefficient when passed through tissues. On the other hand, Ethibond is coated with polybutilate, which acts as a suture lubricant, making passage through tissues nontraumatic and ideal for fascial closures as well as for tendon repairs.

  Mersilene® (Ethicon US, LLC) and Ethibond® (Ethicon US, LLC)

- **Steel:** This is a nonabsorbable suture, available as monofilament or multifilament, free wire, or with a swaged needle (a prepackaged eyeless needle with attached suture, used when steel wire is utilized as a suture, eg, suturing cartilage in ear reconstruction, etc.). In addition to the typical uses of steel wire, for example, fixation to bone and bony approximation (eg, sternal closures), it can also be used for keeping a construct stable and intact (eg, ear reconstruction).

CHOOSING THE RIGHT SUTURE AND NEEDLE

Choice of Suture Strength

The basic concept of suture selection in terms of the strength of the suture is to select a suture that will hold the tissue together until it heals with enough strength to endure stress. The strength requirement of a tissue depends on the site and several patient factors. After a procedure, skin strength can be expected to regain 5% of its original strength within a week, nearly 50% within 4 weeks, and 80% within 6 weeks of skin closure. Even after collagen maturation is complete (6 months to 1 year postoperatively), wound tissue will only regain approximately 80% of its original strength.[2,5]

Choice of Suture Needle

A perfect surgical needle is able to penetrate the tissue without much resistance, passes through the tissue atraumatically, and is strong enough to maintain shape with repeated passes, yet flexible enough to bend before breaking. There are three parts to a needle: (1) point, (2) body, and (3) eye. Specific dimensions of the needle are described later.[1,2] The following are the codes and their explanation for some commonly used needle types:

CT (circle taper)
SH (small half circle)
FS (for skin)
FSL (for skin large)
RB (renal bypass)
P (plastic)
PS (plastic surgery)
PC (precision cosmetic)
KS (Keith straight)

Clinical Pearls

For most of our pediatric skin closures, we use 4-0 or 5-0 Monocryl on a P3 needle, especially for closure of small incisions for cosmetically sensitive areas such as the face. Larger needles (3-0 Monocryl on a PS2 needle) may be used for closure of longer incisions in less cosmetically sensitive areas such as the back.

Needle Dimensions (Figure 8.2)

Needle length: Distance between eye and the point of the needle

Needle diameter: Thickness of the needle

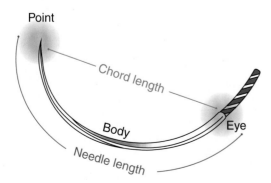

FIGURE 8.2. Needle dimensions.

Needle chord length: Minimum straight line distance between the point and eye of the needle

Needle curvature: Straight needles can be used without instruments, and suturing by hand can be performed when the tissue is easily accessible. There is, however, an increased risk of accidental needle stick injury. Curved needles require the use of a needle holder and forceps and help mitigate this risk. The most common needle curvature used for superficial suturing is 3/8th of a circle. Other curvatures available are 1/4th, ½, and 5/8th of a circle, used for various surgical indications.

Needle Point

Cutting Needles

Cutting needles have at least two opposing sharp edges to make it easy to penetrate through tough tissue, such as the dermis. Two main types of cutting needles are conventional cutting needles and reverse cutting needles (Figure 8.3). The conventional cutting needle has a third sharp edge on the inside of the curvature, where the reverse cutting needle has a third sharp cutting edge on the outside (or convex part) of the curvature of the needle. Conventional cutting needles have a higher risk of cutting through the tissue because of their sharp edge on the convex surface; these needles are typically used for suturing through tough tissue such as the sternum. When using cutting needles (especially conventional cutting needles), it is important to pronate the wrist to follow the curve of the needle because it is driven through the tissue to avoid inadvertently cutting through the tissue. Reverse cutting needles have less risks of cutting through the tissue and are usually used for skin closures as well as for ophthalmic and aesthetic surgery.

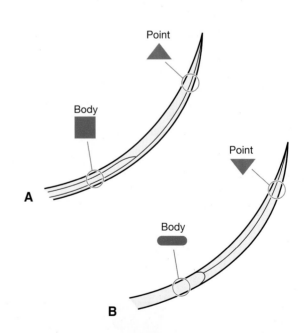

FIGURE 8.3. Triangle shows cross section of needle point. A, Conventional cutting with third cutting edge on the inside of the needle curvature. B, Reverse cutting needle with third cutting edge on the outer curvature of the needle, used for difficult-to-penetrate tissue, such as skin.

Tapered Needle

Tapered or "round-bodied" needles are used for suturing tissues that are easy to penetrate, such as subcutaneous fat, and to avoid cutting more than is necessary. The sharp point of this needle penetrates tissue easily, causing less trauma to structures such as tendons, blood vessels, and the deeper and softer subcutaneous tissue; the rest of the needle spreads the tissue as the needle is driven through it. A tapercut needle is also available for use; this needle has a reverse cutting point with a body that has a tapered configuration. A tapercut needle is ideal for suturing dense connective tissue (eg, fascia, periosteum).

OTHER CLOSURE MATERIALS
Surgical Staples

Surgical staples are sometimes used for temporary skin closure, allowing for alignment of unequal skin edges in the operating room. In this case, the staples are later replaced with sutures. Staples do not crush the skin edges during their approximation, and they are least ischemic to the tissue compared to regular sutures. Hence, they are ideal for scalp closures because of their low risk of causing alopecia, especially if the patient is old enough to be able to cooperate with later removal of staples in 7 to 10 days (see Figure 11.10). Other advantages include the nonreactive nature of the staples and their simple and fast deployment. Staples are not very precise and are inelastic, so they are contraindicated in cosmetically sensitive areas.

Cyanoacrylate Glue

Skin glues can be used for sealing a wound if and when skin edges are well aligned. Some studies also suggest a decrease in postoperative infections with their use.[6,7] They can also be used in simple linear lacerations that are only through the epidermis. In this case, the edges can be gently pushed toward each other and cyanoacrylate glue applied. It is generally best to avoid using petrolatum-based products such as Vaseline™ (Conopco, Inc., US) ointment with cyanoacrylate glue because they can degrade the adhesive properties of the glue (a characteristic that makes them useful for removing or reversing cyanoacrylate glue when necessary).

Cyanoacrylate Glue With Mesh

These closure systems provide a polyester mesh with a cyanoacrylate glue combination (DERMABOND Prineo™ Skin Closure System [Ethicon US, LLC])[8,9] (Figure 8.4). The main advantage of this closure system is that it reduces operating

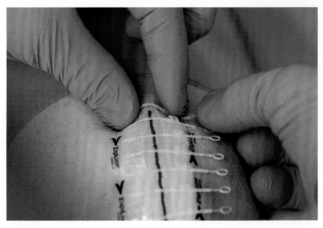

FIGURE 8.5. Closure with Zipline. Reprinted with permission from Stryker.

time (and, in turn, cost) by replacing the subcuticular sutures with this mesh and glue closure system. We typically utilize this device for larger wound closure, where deeper sutures have already been placed and the wound is felt to still have some tension such as in breast wounds or in large abdominal wound closures.

Noninvasive Skin Closure Devices

A variety of noninvasive surgical closure devices are also available,[10,11] with the goal of replacing intracutaneous skin closures. In comparison to intracutaneous skin closures, these devices reduce closure time, are available at lower cost, and offer similar occurrences of postoperative complications. The Zipline device (Figure 8.5) is contraindicated for infected wounds, wounds with high tension, or in areas where adhesion cannot be obtained.

REFERENCES

1. Ethicon. *Wound Closure Manual.* Somerville, NJ: Ethicon; 2005.
2. Law HZ, Mosser SW. Sutures and needles. In: Janis JE, ed. *Essentials of Plastic Surgery.* 2nd ed. New York, NY: Thieme; 2014.
3. Xu B, Wang L, Chen C, Yilmaz TU, Zheng W, He B. Absorbable versus nonabsorbable sutures for skin closure: a meta-analysis of randomized controlled trials. *Ann Plast Surg.* 2016;76:598–606.
4. Rosen A, Hartman T. Repair of the midline fascial defect in abdominoplasty with long-acting barbed and smooth absorbable sutures. *Aesthet Surg J.* 2011;31:668–673.
5. Levenson SM, Geever EF, Crowley LV, et al. The healing of rat skin wounds. *Ann Surg.* 1965;161:293–308.
6. Chambers A, Scarci M. Is skin closure with cyanoacrylate glue effective for the prevention of sternal wound infections? *Interact Cardiovasc Thorac Surg.* 2010;10:793–796.
7. Eymann R, Kiefer M. Glue instead of stitches: a minor change of the operative technique with a serious impact on the shunt infection rate. *Acta Neurochir Suppl.* 2010;106:87–89.
8. Lee JC, Ishtihar S, Means JJ, Wu J, Rohde CH. In search of an ideal closure method: a randomized, controlled trial of octyl-2-cyanoacrylate and adhesive mesh versus subcuticular suture in reduction mammoplasty. *Plast Reconstr Surg.* 2018;142(4):850–856. doi:10.1097/PRS.0000000000004726.
9. Prineo. 2017. DERMABOND® PRINEO® Skin Closure System. www.ethicon.com/na/products/wound-closure/skin-adhesives/dermabond-prineo-skin-closure-system.
10. Zip Surgical. Zipline Medical, Inc. https://www.ziplinemedical.com/zip/. Accessed May 21, 2019.
11. Chen D, Song J, Zhao Y, et al. Systematic review and meta-analysis of surgical zipper technique versus intracutaneous sutures for the closing of surgical incision. *PLoS One.* 2016;11(9):e0162471.

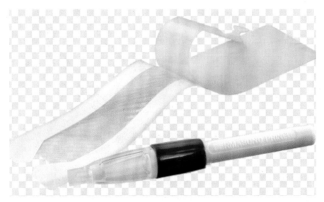

FIGURE 8.4. Prineo skin closure system.

Anatomy and Superficial Landmarks of the Head and Neck

Catherine A. Degesys and Craig N. Burkhart

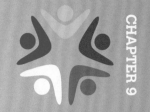

CHAPTER 9

INTRODUCTION

Understanding superficial anatomy is critical to the success of the dermatologic surgeon. When performing closures, one must consider local vasculature, motor and sensory nerves, undermining planes, lines of tension, and cosmetic subunits. Although anatomic landmarks for adults and children are similar, there are age-specific considerations that must be observed by any surgeon to avoid complications.

TOPOGRAPHY OF THE HEAD AND NECK

The bony landmarks of the head can help identify crucial underlying structures when preparing for a surgery of the face. The supraorbital ridges are part of the frontal bone and transmit the supraorbital neurovascular bundle through the supraorbital foramen, which is located 2.5 cm lateral to the midline of the nasal root (Figure 9.1). A vertical line from the supraorbital foramen through the pupils bilaterally will also intersect the infraorbital

foramen 1 cm below the infraorbital rim. The infraorbital foramen transmits the infraorbital neurovascular bundle. The mental foramen falls within the same vertical line on the mandible and transmits the mental neuromuscular bundle.

The zygomatic arch is the most prominent aspect of the cheek and defines the superior aspect of the parotid gland. The anterior aspect of the parotid gland is located on the posterior half of the masseter muscle, which can be palpated by clenching the jaw. The posterior border of the parotid gland is defined by a vertical line from the tragus to the mandible. The facial nerve, superficial temporal artery, and superficial temporal vein course through the glandular tissue before their exit to supply the face. The path of the facial nerve branches is described at length later. The superficial temporal artery and vein exit the superior aspect of the parotid in the preauricular region. The parotid duct (Stensen's duct) drains parotid secretions, and damage to this structure during a surgical procedure can result in a chronic draining sinus that requires surgical repair. The path of Stensen's duct can be visualized by drawing a horizontal line from the tragus to the midpoint of a vertical line connecting the alar rim to the lateral oral commissure. The duct is located in the middle third of this line. It lies superficial to the masseter after its exit from the parotid and makes a sharp turn to enter the buccal mucosa at the second molar after it passes the anterior border of masseter.

The superficial anatomy of the ear is depicted in Figure 9.2. The auricle comprises the underlying cartilage with a minimal amount of subcutaneous tissue, perichondrium, and skin. The only part of the ear without the cartilaginous base is the lobule. The helix and the antihelix form the two major longitudinal components of the ear. The superior and inferior crura of

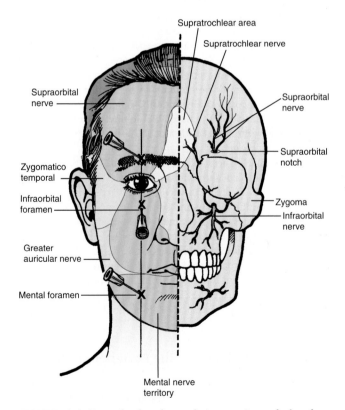

FIGURE 9.1. Bony landmarks and innervation of the face. Supraorbital nerve, infraorbital nerve, and mental nerve. Reprinted with permission from Neal JM, Tran DQ, Salinas F. *A Practical Approach to Regional Anesthesiology and Acute Pain Medicine.* 5th ed. Philadelphia, PA: Wolters Kluwer; 2017. Figure 13.9.

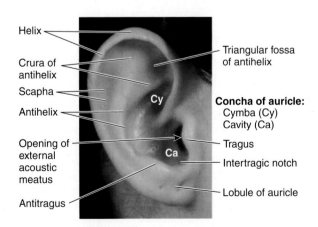

FIGURE 9.2. External anatomy of the ear. Reprinted with permission from Moore KL, Dalley AF, Agur AMR. *Clinically Oriented Anatomy.* 7th ed. Philadelphia, PA: Wolters Kluwer Health/Lippincott Williams & Wilkins; 2014:967. Figure 7.110.

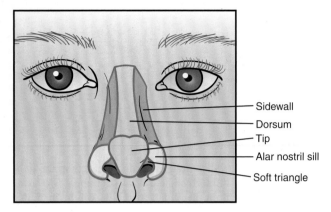

FIGURE 9.3. Nasal aesthetic subunits.

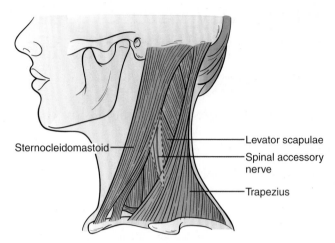

FIGURE 9.4. Sensory nerves of the cervical plexus and the spinal accessory nerve. Triangular *danger zone* of spinal accessory nerve.

the antihelix delineate the triangular fossa. The tragus is the cartilaginous notch located anterior to the external ear canal. Notably, an accessory tragus may appear in the preauricular cheek, but it is recommended that they be removed via elliptical excision, as shave excision may result in exposed, inadequately removed cartilage at risk for chondrodermatitis.[1]

The nose comprises the following subunits: the nasal dorsum, lateral sidewalls, nasal tip, nasal ala, and columella (Figure 9.3). The alar crease serves as the boundary separating the nasal ala from the nasal sidewall. The soft triangles are present bilaterally anterior to the nares and abut the nasal tip. These triangles are a "weak spot" because of the absence of fibrous tissue, and their proximity to adjacent structures may result in deformity of the ala, columella, or tip of the nose if not reconstructed properly. The internal nasal valve of the nose is the triangular area representing the point of greatest resistance in the upper airway. Its borders are defined by the septum medially, the upper lateral cartilage superiorly and laterally, and the inferior turbinate inferiorly.[2] If this area is weakened, the valve can collapse during inhalation, resulting in nasal obstruction.[3]

Similar to the face, understanding the superficial anatomy of the neck allows the surgeon to identify underlying critical structures and "danger zones" to avoid, if possible. The sternocleidomastoid muscle originates from the sternum and clavicle and inserts into the mastoid process and occipital ridge. This muscle divides the neck into its anterior and posterior triangles. The external jugular vein traverses the belly of the sternocleidomastoid muscle. Erb's point is the area posterior to the sternocleidomastoid, around which the cervical plexus and cranial nerve (CN) XI emerge. In order to locate Erb's point, the surgeon should imagine a line extending from the mastoid process to the angle of the jaw. Erb's point is located 6 cm below the midpoint of this line at the posterior aspect of the sternocleidomastoid muscle.[4]

There is inconsistency in the literature when referring to the exit of the spinal accessory nerve. Although many texts suggest that the spinal accessory nerve (CN XI) emerges from the same site as the cervical plexus, others suggest it actually emerges about 2 cm superior to this point.[5,6] One author has suggested recognizing a triangular danger zone for the site of possible damage to the spinal accessory nerve. This zone is created by the following vertices: a point located one-third of the way down the sternocleidomastoid, the midpoint of the sternocleidomastoid, and the point located on the anterior surface of the trapezius muscle two-thirds down its length (Figure 9.4).[7] This is considered a surgical

"danger zone," as damage to the spinal accessory nerve can result in a winged scapula, inability to raise the ipsilateral shoulder, and weakness in turning the head to the contralateral direction against resistance. Table 9.1 summarizes the motor and sensory components of the posterior triangle of the neck.

COSMETIC SUBUNITS AND FREE MARGINS

The boundaries of the cutaneous cosmetic subunits of the face include the nasolabial (melolabial) folds, nasofacial sulcus, mentolabial crease, philtrum, eyebrows, and superior and inferior vermillion borders (Figure 9.5A and B). These separate the face into regions that are similar to each other in contour, skin color and texture, actinic damage, sebaceous content, and hair density. As such, closing surgical defects within the boundaries or utilizing skin from the same or adjacent cosmetic subunits will result in a cosmetically superior outcome. For example, closing a defect within the nasolabial fold will often "hide" the surgical scar without disruption of the aesthetic appearance of the adjacent subunits.

Free margins are areas of the head and neck that are discontiguous with adjacent skin and include the eyelids, helices, lips, and nostrils. As the tension vectors affect free margins differently from continuous skin and soft tissue, special care must be taken in these areas to prevent inadvertent asymmetries. For example, a downward directed tension vector on the inferior eyelid margin can result in ectropion and its associated complications. Similarly, an upward directed tension vector on the nostril will result in a permanent flared appearance. Disruption of the free margin may result from the closure itself or subsequent wound contracture. Therefore, tension vectors should be designed in

TABLE 9.1 ⋮ Contents of the Posterior Triangle of the Neck

Sensory nerves	Transverse cervical (C2-C3) Supraclavicular (C3-C4) Lesser occipital (C2) Greater auricular (C2-C3)
Motor nerves	Spinal accessory nerve

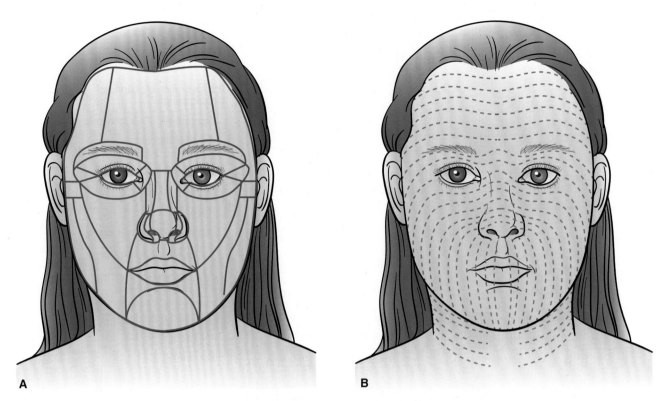

FIGURE 9.5. A, Facial aesthetic subunits. Incisions are designed at the borders of facial aesthetic subunits whenever possible in order to camouflage scarring. B, Relaxed skin tension lines (RSTLs) of the face. Incisions are designed parallel to RSTLs whenever possible.

parallel with free margins and, in most cases, second intention healing around the free margins should be avoided.

SUPERFICIAL MUSCULOAPONEUROTIC SYSTEM

The superficial musculoaponeurotic system (SMAS) is the anatomic feature responsible for orchestrating movement of the facial muscles in concert. It is also responsible for containment of infection and prevention of spread to the deeper structures of the face. It comprises muscle and a thin layer of fascia. The SMAS of the cheek lies superior to deep muscles of mastication and is continuous with the orbicularis oculi muscle. It also has bony attachments in this region.[8] The SMAS is discontiguous on the upper from lower face, due to differential embryogenesis of these muscle groups. The sensory nerves and axial arteries lie within or above the SMAS, whereas the motor nerves lie beneath the SMAS. Understanding these relationships allows the surgeon to utilize a relatively bloodless dissection plane in the sub-SMAS region. This is very helpful in the scalp, where blunt dissection within the scalp SMAS separates the galea aponeurotica from the periosteum. However, dissection beneath the cheek SMAS puts local motor nerves at risk and should only be performed directly above the parotid gland, where the facial nerve is embedded within the parotid parenchyma and is, thus, better protected from transection.

MUSCLES OF FACIAL EXPRESSION

The muscles of the face are paramount in daily functioning (Figure 9.6). They are responsible for mouth and eye function and nonverbal communication via facial expression. They insert directly into the skin and are innervated by the facial nerve, which courses deep to the SMAS prior to innervation of the

muscle at its deep aspect. The muscles are grouped by anatomic region. Table 9.2 includes a comprehensive list of the branches of the facial nerve and the muscles they innervate.

Forehead and Scalp

The muscles of the forehead and scalp include the frontalis, procerus, corrugator supercilii, superior fibers of the orbicularis oculi, occipitalis, and temporoparietalis (auricular) muscles. The frontalis muscle of the forehead is connected to the occipitalis muscle of the scalp by the galea aponeurotica. This whole complex is referred to as the occipitofrontalis muscle or the epicranius, and it allows the skin to slide over the scalp when the muscles contract (Figure 9.6). The occipitalis muscle is innervated by the posterior auricular branch of the facial nerve, but it is not under voluntary control. The frontalis allows for raising the eyebrows and opening the eyelids and is innervated by the temporal branch of the facial nerve. Contraction of this muscle is responsible for horizontal wrinkling of the forehead. The auricular muscles (anterior, posterior, superior) arise from the superficial temporalis SMAS and the lateral galea and are responsible for movement of the ears. The superior and anterior auricular muscles are innervated by the temporal branch of the facial nerve, and the posterior auricular muscle is innervated by the posterior auricular branch. The corrugators and procerus are brow depressors. The corrugators are innervated by the temporal branch of the facial nerve, whereas both the zygomatic and temporal branches have been reported to innervate the procerus.

Eye

The eye region comprises the following muscles: orbicularis oculi, procerus (discussed earlier), and corrugator supercilii (discussed earlier) (Figure 9.6). The orbicularis oculi muscle is situated circumferentially around the orbit and does

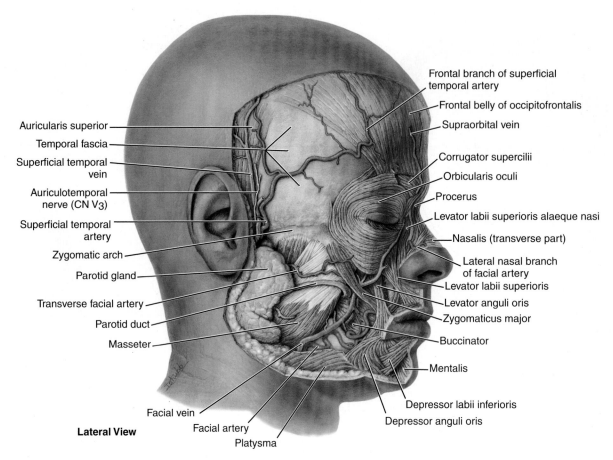

Auricularis superior

Temporal fascia

Superficial temporal vein

Auriculotemporal nerve (CN V₃)

Superficial temporal artery

Zygomatic arch

Parotid gland

Transverse facial artery

Parotid duct

Masseter

Facial vein

Facial artery

Platysma

Lateral View

Frontal branch of superficial temporal artery

Frontal belly of occipitofrontalis

Supraorbital vein

Corrugator supercilii

Orbicularis oculi

Procerus

Levator labii superioris alaeque nasi

Nasalis (transverse part)

Lateral nasal branch of facial artery

Levator labii superioris

Levator anguli oris

Zygomaticus major

Buccinator

Mentalis

Depressor labii inferioris

Depressor anguli oris

FIGURE 9.6. Muscles of facial expression and vasculature of the face. Reprinted with permission from Agur AMR, Dalley AF. *Grant's Atlas of Anatomy*. 15th ed. Philadelphia, PA: Wolters Kluwer; 2020. Figure 7-12A.

TABLE 9.2 : Branches of the Facial Nerve and the Muscle Innervation

Temporal	Frontalis, corrugator supercilii, procerus, orbicularis oculi (upper portion), anterior and superior auricular
Posterior auricular	Occipitalis, posterior auricular
Zygomatic	Orbicularis oculi (inferior portion), nasalis, procerus, levator anguli oris, levator labii superioris alaeque nasi, levator labii superioris, zygomaticus major and zygomaticus minor, buccinator
Buccal	Buccinator, depressor septi nasi, nasalis, zygomaticus major and minor, levator labii superioris, orbicularis oris, levator anguli oris, risorius, depressor anguli oris
Marginal mandibular	Orbicularis oris, depressor anguli oris, depressor labii inferioris, mentalis, risorius, platysma
Cervical	Platysma

From Vidimos A, Ammirati C, Poblete-Lopez C. *Dermatologic Surgery*. Edinburgh, Scotland: Elsevier; 2009:1–39; Robinson JK, Sengelmann RD, Hanke CW, Siegel DM. *Surgery of the Skin: Procedural Dermatology*. St Louis, MO: Mosby; 2005; Robinson J, Arndt K, LeBoit P, Wintroub B. *Atlas of Cutaneous Surgery*. Philadelphia, PA: W. B. Saunders; 1995.

interdigitate with the forehead muscles. It inserts into the medial and lateral canthal tendons and is divided into three main parts: the palpebral, lacrimal, and orbital sections.[9] The upper portion of the orbicularis oculi is innervated by the temporal branch and the lower portion by the zygomatic branch of the facial nerve.

Mouth and Chin

The underlying musculature of the mouth includes the orbicularis oris, zygomaticus major and minor, levator anguli oris, depressor anguli oris, levator labii superioris, levator labii superioris alaeque nasi, depressor labii inferioris, risorius, mentalis, and buccinator (Figure 9.6). The orbicularis oris muscle is circumferentially situated around the mouth orifice and is innervated by the buccal and marginal mandibular branches of the facial nerve. The buccinator contracts with the orbicularis oris muscle to draw the lips together and assist with whistling. The lip elevators are the levator labii superioris alaeque nasi, levator labii superioris, zygomaticus major, zygomaticus minor, levator anguli oris, and risorius. They assist with smiling. The lip depressors are the depressor anguli oris, depressor labii inferioris, and the mentalis muscles. The innervation of these muscles is listed in Table 9.2. Note that several muscles have more than one reported innervation, and therefore, each muscle may be listed under more than one branch of the facial nerve. A comprehensive list is included in Table 9.2 for reference.

VASCULATURE

The external carotid artery supplies much of the central face via the facial artery (Figure 9.7). It can be palpated anterior to the masseter muscle as it crosses the mandible. The facial artery gives rise to the superior and inferior labial arteries, above and below the lips. After giving off the superior labial artery, the facial artery becomes the angular artery. The angular artery anastomoses with a branch of the ophthalmic artery (off the internal carotid artery) called the dorsal nasal artery. It is at this point that the internal carotid and external carotid arteries interface each other. The ophthalmic artery also gives rise to the supratrochlear and supraorbital arteries that supply the central forehead and anterior scalp. The supratrochlear artery exits medial to the supraorbital artery and is isolated in paramedian forehead flaps for nasal defect repairs. Because there are also anastomoses between the facial artery and internal maxillary and superficial temporal (transverse facial) arteries, there remains enough redundancy for perfusion even if its branches are transected during surgery.

The terminal branch of the external carotid artery is the superficial temporal artery, which supplies the lateral face, scalp, and forehead. It gives off the transverse facial artery, which courses medially across the face, beneath the zygomatic arch. The superficial temporal artery then ascends over the zygomatic arch superficial to the auriculotemporal nerve. It lies above the SMAS of the temple and lateral forehead. Perfusion of the posterior scalp is provided by the occipital artery, which is also a branch of the external carotid artery.

Most of the facial veins run parallel in conjunction with their associated arteries (Figure 9.8). Of particular importance, the ophthalmic vein and the pterygoid plexus may communicate with the cavernous sinus of the brain. Therefore, translocation of infection may occur from the skin to the brain, with potentially severe consequences.

SENSORY AND MOTOR INNERVATION OF THE HEAD AND NECK
Motor Innervation

Motor innervation to the muscles of facial expression is provided by the facial nerve (CN VII) (Figure 9.9). It exits the skull at the stylomastoid foramen, where it gives rise to the posterior auricular branch, providing innervation to the occipitalis and posterior auricular muscles. In children, special care must be taken in this region because the mastoid process is not fully developed until age 5. Until that time, the main facial nerve trunk is in the superficial subcutaneous plane and is extremely vulnerable to superficial procedures (Figure 9.10). After this initial bifurcation point, the nerve enters the parotid gland, where it separates into the temporofacial branch and cervicofacial branch. After this point, the five main branches of the facial nerve arise: the temporal, zygomatic, buccal, marginal mandibular, and cervical. These nerves run deep to the SMAS and penetrate the muscle from their ventral surfaces.

The temporal branch of the facial nerve innervates the frontalis, upper orbicularis oculi, corrugator supercilii muscles, procerus, and anterior and superior auricular muscles (Figure 9.9). It usually has four rami and is most vulnerable as it crosses over the mid-zygomatic arch, where it is protected by just the skin, subcutaneous fat, and the SMAS. The temporal branch runs between the deep temporalis fascia and the superficial temporal fascia (the SMAS) until it penetrates the deep aspect of its target muscles. It is deep to the temporal artery and vein. One way to delineate the course of this nerve is by drawing a line connecting the earlobe to the lateral tip of the eyebrow and another line from the earlobe to the lateral tip of the highest forehead crease. The frontalis muscle is often singularly innervated by the temporal branch; therefore, injury to the nerve can have significant cosmetic and functional ramifications, resulting in the inability to raise the eyebrow on the ipsilateral side. Fortunately, there is

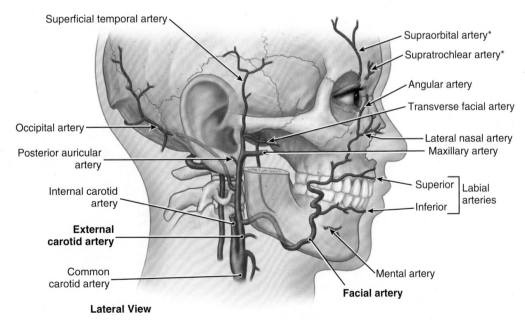

Lateral View

FIGURE 9.7. Arteries of the head and neck. Reprinted with permission from Agur AMR, Dalley AF. *Grant's Atlas of Anatomy.* 15th ed. Philadelphia, PA: Wolters Kluwer; 2020. Figure 7-18B.
*These arteries arise from the ophthalmic artery (instead of the facial artery).

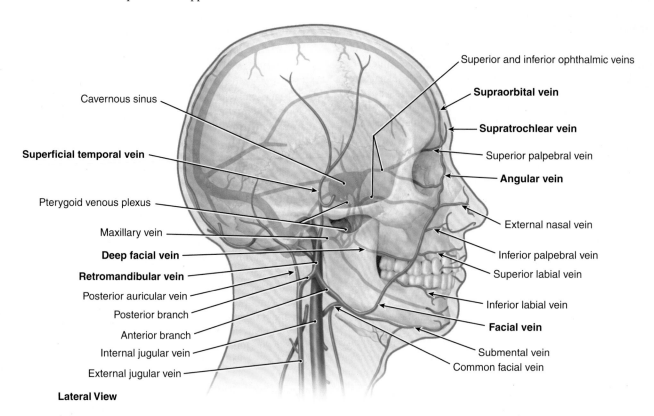

Lateral View

FIGURE 9.8. Veins of the head and neck. Reprinted with permission from Agur AMR, Dalley AF. *Grant's Atlas of Anatomy*. 15th ed. Philadelphia, PA: Wolters Kluwer; 2020. Figure 7-19.

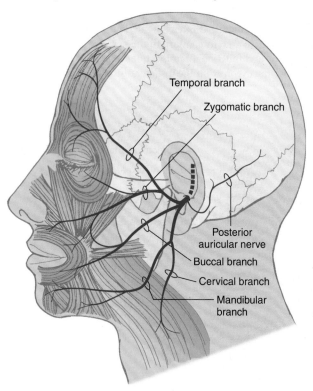

FIGURE 9.9. The facial nerve (cranial nerve VII). The facial nerve gives off the posterior auricular nerve and then its terminal portion divides into several branches: temporal, zygomatic, buccal, mandibular, and cervical. Reprinted with permission from Oatis CA. *Kinesiology: The Mechanics and Pathomechanics of Human Movement*. Philadelphia, PA: Lippincott Williams & Wilkins; 2004. Figure 20.1.

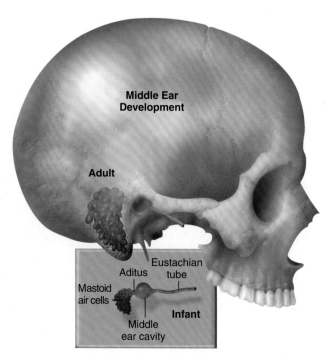

FIGURE 9.10. Middle ear development in adult versus infant. Reprinted with permission from ACC Chart: Middle Ear Conditions.

cross-innervation to the orbicularis oculi (see Table 9.2), and therefore, dysfunction can be minimal in the setting of nerve compromise due to surgery.

The zygomatic branch of the facial nerve innervates the lower orbicularis oculi, procerus, levator labii superioris alaeque nasi, levator labii superioris, levator anguli oris, zygomaticus major, zygomaticus minor, buccinator, and nasalis muscles. It overlies the parotid duct (Stensen's duct), but after its exit from the parotid, it courses horizontally and upward. The buccal branch innervates the buccinator, depressor septi nasi, nasalis, zygomaticus major and minor, levator labii superioris, orbicularis oris, levator anguli oris, risorius, and depressor anguli oris. There are many anastomoses between the buccal and zygomatic branches, making injury to these nerves less problematic and unpredictable than injury to the marginal mandibular or temporal branches. Buccinator dysfunction can result in accumulation of food, and perioral muscle dysfunction may result in difficulty with lip pucker or smile formation. A helpful rule of thumb is that some regeneration and recapitulation of function can be expected if a nerve is injured medial to a vertical line drawn downward from the lateral canthus, due to the extensive cross-innervation of the buccal and zygomatic branches in this region.

The marginal mandibular nerve innervates the orbicularis oris, mentalis, depressor anguli oris, depressor labii inferioris, risorius, and platysma. It generally courses along the inferior border of the mandible; however, in some cases, the marginal mandibular nerve has been observed up to 4 cm inferior to the mandible.[10-12] The marginal mandibular nerve is prone to injury as it crosses the angle of the mandible and ascends upward anterior to the masseter muscle. It lies superficial to the facial vein and artery, which can easily be palpated as a landmark for its location. Damage to the marginal mandibular nerve results in a crooked smile, due to the inability to pull down the ipsilateral lower lip.[13]

Once the facial nerve exits the parotid parenchyma, it is prone to injury during cutaneous surgery. The boundaries of the facial nerve "danger zone" are as follows:

- A horizontal line drawn 1 cm superior to the zygoma, extending to Whitnall's tubercle (in line with the lateral-most aspect of the eyebrow)
- A vertical line from Whitnall's tubercle to the inferior aspect of the mandible
- A curved line 2 cm below the mandible to the angle of the mandible

Additionally, as discussed previously, in children under the age of 5, care should be taken when dissecting posterior to the ear, as the mastoid process is not fully formed and injury to the body of the facial nerve can occur in the superficial subcutaneous fat. The "danger zones," motor nerve, and outcome of injury are reviewed in Table 9.3.

Sensory Innervation

The trigeminal nerve (CN V) provides sensory innervation to the face and is divided into three branches: V1 or ophthalmic, V2 or maxillary, and V3 or mandibular. It courses superficially between the SMAS and subcutaneous fat and is therefore subject to injury during dermatologic surgery. Knowledge of its locations may be helpful in providing regional anesthesia to the face and avoiding injury when possible. The major exit points lie in the midpupillary line bilaterally, from the supraorbital foramen to the mental foramen. It is helpful to have the patient look directly upward, which can lock the eyes centrally when determining these landmarks.[3] The trigeminal nerve also supplies motor innervation to the muscles of mastication.

The ophthalmic branch of the trigeminal nerve (V1) gives rise to the nasociliary, frontal, and lacrimal nerves within the orbit. The nasociliary branch bifurcates into the infratrochlear nerve and the anterior ethmoidal nerve. These nerves innervate the root of the nose and medial canthus, and the nasal dorsum, tip, and columella, respectively. The frontal branch of the ophthalmic nerve gives rise to the supratrochlear and supraorbital nerves. The supratrochlear nerve innervates the medial upper eyelid, medial forehead, and frontal scalp, whereas the supraorbital nerve innervates the forehead, scalp, and upper eyelid. Therefore, a nerve block of the frontal nerve would effectively anesthetize the forehead. Finally, the lacrimal nerve innervates the lateral eyelid.

The maxillary branch of the trigeminal nerve (V2) gives rise to the infraorbital, zygomaticofacial, and zygomaticotemporal

TABLE 9.3 : Outcomes of Nerve Damage in Danger Zones

	TEMPORAL BRANCH OF FACIAL NERVE	MARGINAL MANDIBULAR BRANCH OF FACIAL NERVE	SPINAL ACCESSORY NERVE	FACIAL NERVE TRUNK IN CHILDREN
Danger zone	As it crosses the zygomatic arch within a triangle formed by a line from the earlobe to the lateral eyebrow and from the earlobe to the superior-most forehead crease	Just beneath the superficial musculoaponeurotic system as it crosses the angle of the jaw anterior to the facial artery and vein	Around Erb's point: 6 cm inferior to the midpoint of a line connecting the mastoid process to the angle of the jaw, at the intersection of the posterior SCM *or* ending from the middle one-third to one-half of the SCM and the point located on the anterior surface of the trapezius two-thirds down its length	Exit point from the stylomastoid foramen. (protected by the mastoid process in adults)
Outcome of transection	Inability to raise the forehead on ipsilateral side	Crooked smile/inability to depress ipsilateral lip	Winged scapula—inability to raise ipsilateral arm and weakness in turning head against resistance to contralateral side	Hemifacial paralysis

SCM, sternocleidomastoid muscle.

branches. As discussed previously, the infraorbital nerve exits in the midpupillary line 1 cm below the infraorbital rim. This nerve then supplies the medial cheek, upper lip, nasal sidewall and ala, and the lower eyelid. The zygomaticofacial nerve innervates the malar cheek and the zygomaticotemporal nerve provides innervation to the temple and supratemporal scalp.

The mandibular branch of the trigeminal nerve (V3) gives rise to the auriculotemporal, buccal, inferior alveolar, and lingual nerves. It also carries motor nerves to the muscles of mastication. The auriculotemporal nerve is deep to the superficial temporal artery and ascends from the superior aspect of the parotid gland upward to supply the external anterior ear and auditory canal, temple, temporoparietal scalp, temporomandibular joint, and tympanic membrane. The buccal nerve supplies the cheek, buccal mucosa, and gingiva. The inferior alveolar nerve courses through the mandibular canal, supplying sensation to the lower teeth and ultimately terminates in the mental nerve, which innervates the chin and lower lip. The major branches of the trigeminal nerve and their cutaneous sensory nerves are outlined in Table 9.4.

The cervical plexus comprises the ventral rami of C1-C4. Various anastomoses create the sensory nerves emerging from Erb's point in the posterior triangle of the neck. The greater auricular nerve is formed from anastomosing branches of C2 and C3, the lesser occipital nerve from C2, the transverse cervical nerves from C2 and C3, and the supraclavicular nerve from branches of C3 and C4. The greater auricular nerve (C2, C3) provides sensation to the lateral neck, angle of the jaw, and parts of the ear and postauricular skin. The lesser occipital nerve (C2) innervates the neck, postauricular scalp, and superior portion of the ear. The ear has diverse sensory inputs including the greater and lesser occipital, glossopharyngeal, vagus, facial, and auriculotemporal (CN V3) nerves. The transverse cervical nerve (C2, C3) supplies the anterior neck. The supraclavicular nerve (C3, C4) supplies the lower neck, clavicle, and shoulder. The contents of the posterior triangle of the neck are reviewed in Table 9.1.

LYMPHATIC DRAINAGE

The lymphatic drainage of the head and neck can be variable between patients, but in general the lymphatic vessels run in parallel with the head and neck veins. The major lymph node basins of the face are the parotid, submandibular, and submental regions. The forehead, lateral eyelid, and anterior ear drain into the parotid lymph nodes. The lateral cheek drains into the parotid nodes and the medial cheek drains into the submandibular nodes. The submandibular nodes also collect

lymphatic drainage from the medial canthus and nose. The chin and perioral region drains into the submental basin. The scalp and posterior ears drain into the posterior auricular and occipital lymph nodes.

PERTINENT ANATOMY OUTSIDE OF THE HEAD AND NECK AREA
Gluteal Region

The gluteal region is bordered by the posterior iliac crest superiorly and the inferior border of the gluteus maximus inferiorly. The muscles of this region include the gluteus muscles (maximus, medius, and minimus) and the deeper group of muscles (piriformis, gemellus superior, obturator internus, gemellus inferior, and quadratus femoris). The sensory innervation of the skin is superior cluneal (L1-L3), medial cluneal (S1-S3), and inferior cluneal nerves. The motor innervation is supplied by branches of the sacral plexus. The sciatic nerve is the largest nerve in the body and typically emerges inferior to the piriformis muscle.

The arterial supply is provided by branches of the internal iliac artery. The superficial gluteal artery divides into the superficial and deep branches, which supply the gluteus maximus and gluteus medius and minimus, respectively. The inferior gluteal artery supplies the gluteus maximus, obturator internus, quadratus femoris, and the posterior thigh muscles.[14]

Nipples

The areola is the pigmented area surrounding the nipple. The epidermis of the nipple is 0.5 to 2.0 cm. There is little to no subcutaneous tissue between the skin and glandular tissue beneath the nipple.[15] The vascular supply to the nipple is provided by the internal thoracic and lateral thoracic arteries.[16] About 85% of the time, the second intercostal perforator (off the internal thoracic artery) supplies the nipple complex; ligation of this can result in nipple necrosis.[17] Accessory nipples may occur anywhere along the milk lines (Figure 9.11).

Umbilicus

The umbilicus is a remnant of the fetal umbilical cord. Just below the center of the umbilicus is a fascial layer. Deep to this lies the preperitoneal fatty tissue. In fact, a probe placed deep in the center of the umbilicus can pass freely into the abdominal cavity. This is often utilized in minimally invasive surgery as a portal entry point.[18] Certainly, dissection and undermining should be performed carefully in this area, given the direct entry point to the abdominal cavity.

Median Raphe

The perineal raphe is the dividing line that extends from the anus onto the scrotum and continues to the ventral surface of the penis. It is usually darker than its surrounding skin.[19] The raphe is the presumed effect of the midline fusion of ectoderm along the labioscrotal folds to form the scrotum and the urethral folds that enclose the urethra.[20] The penile blood supply is provided by the internal pudendal artery, which branches into the dorsal artery of the penis, the deep arteries of the penis, and the artery of the bulb of the penis. The innervation of the penis is provided by the pudendal nerve. The layers of the penis are as follows: skin, dartos fascia, Buck's fascia, tunica albuginea, and the corpora cavernosa and spongiosum (the masses of erectile tissue). The skin of the shaft of the penis drains into the superficial inguinal nodes.[21]

TABLE 9.4 : **Major Branches of the Trigeminal Nerve and Main Cutaneous Sensory Branches**

Ophthalmic (V1)	Nasociliary Frontal lacrimal
Maxillary (V2)	Infraorbital Zygomaticofacial Zygomaticotemporal
Mandibular (V3)	Auriculotemporal Buccal Inferior Alveolar

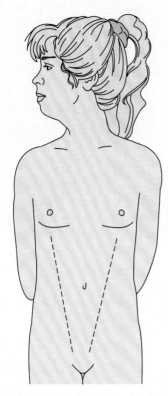

FIGURE 9.11. Accessory nipples may occur anywhere along the milk lines. Reprinted with permission from Silbert-Flagg J, Pillitteri A. *Maternal & Child Health Nursing: Care of the Childbearing & Childrearing Family.* 8th ed. Philadelphia, PA: Wolters Kluwer; 2017. Figure 47.2.

REFERENCES

1. Mehmi M, Balasubramaniam P, Bhat J. Accessory tragus—beware of the preauricular "skin tag". *J Am Acad Dermatol.* 2007;56(2):AB54.
2. Weaver E. Nasal valve stabilization. *Oper Tech Otolaryngol Head Neck Surg.* 2012;23(1):67–71.
3. Chow S, Bennett R. Superficial head and neck anatomy for dermatologic surgery: critical concepts. *Dermatol Surg.* 2015;41(10S):S169–S177.
4. King IJ, Motta G. Iatrogenic spinal accessory nerve palsy. *Ann R Coll Surg Engl.* 1983;65:35–37.
5. Eisele DW, Smith RV. *Complications in Head and Neck Surgery.* 2nd ed. Philadelphia, PA: Mosby; 2009:447–448.
6. Nason RW, Abdulrauf BM, Stranc MF. The anatomy of the accessory nerve and cervical lymph node biopsy. *Am J Surg.* 2000;180:241–243.
7. Breisch EA, Greenway HT. *Cutaneous Surgical Anatomy of the Head and Neck.* London, England: Livingstone Churchill; 1992:106–108.
8. Gosain AK, Yousif NJ, Madiedo G, Larson DL, Matloub HS, Sanger JR. Surgical anatomy of the SMAS: a reinvestigation. *Plast Reconstr Surg.* 1993;92:1254–1265.
9. Thomaidis VK. Forehead. In: Thomaidis VK, ed. *Cutaneous Flaps in Head and Neck Reconstruction.* Heidelberg, Germany: Springer; 2014:77–137.
10. Singh Batra A, Mahajan A, Gupta K. Marginal mandibular branch of the facial nerve: an anatomical study. *Indian J Plast Surg.* 2010;43(1):60–64.
11. Baker DC, Conley J. Avoiding facial nerve injuries in rhytidectomy. Anatomic variations and pitfalls. *Plast Reconstr Surg.* 1979;64:781–795.
12. Nelson DW, Gingrass RP. Anatomy of the mandibular branches of the facial nerve. *Plast Reconstr Surg.* 1979;64:479–482.
13. Thorne C, Chung K, Gurtner G, et al. *Grabb and Smith's Plastic Surgery.* Boston, MA: Little, Brown, and Company; 1991.
14. Moses K, Banks J, Nava P, Peterson D. Gluteal region and posterior thigh. In: Moses K, Banks J, Nava P, Peterson D, eds. *Atlas of Clinical Gross Anatomy.* Philadelphia, PA: Saunders; 2013:526–539.
15. Stone K, Wheeler A. A review of the anatomy, physiology, and benign pathology of the nipple. *Ann Surg Oncol.* 2015;22(10):3236–3240.
16. Skandalakis J. Breast. In: Skandalakis J, ed. *Skandalakis' Surgical Anatomy: The Embryologic and Anatomic Basis of Modern Surgery.* Athens, Greece: PMP; 2004:106–107.
17. Palmer JH, Taylor GI. The vascular territories of the anterior chest wall. *Br J Plast Surg.* 1986;39:287–299.
18. Asakuma M, Komeda K, Yamamoto M, et al. A concealed "Natural Orifice": umbilicus anatomy for minimally invasive surgery. *Surg Innov.* 2019;26:46–49.
19. Wooldridge WE. Congenital anomalies of the median raphe. *Arch Dermatol.* 1955;71:713–716.
20. Thomson J, Itskovitz-Eldor J, Shapiro S, et al. Embryonic stem cell lines derived from human blastocysts. *Science.* 1998;282:1145–1147.
21. Humphrey PA. Male urethra and external genitalia anatomy. In: Brandes S, Morey A, eds. *Advanced Male Urethral and Genital Reconstructive Surgery. Current Clinical Urology.* New York, NY: Humana Press; 2014.

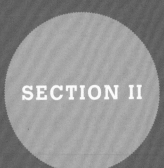

SECTION II

Procedural Approach

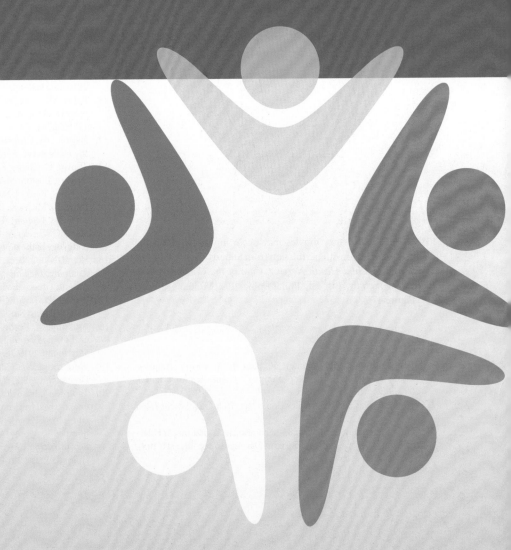

10 Hemostasis

11 Simple Wound Repair

12 Complex Wound Repair

13 Special Site Surgery

14 Injectables

15 Injectable Corticosteroids (Intralesional Kenalog, Intramuscular)

16 Cryosurgery

17 Electrosurgery/Hyfrecation

18 Laser Surgery

19 Laser Treatment of Vascular Lesions

20 Phototherapy and Photodynamic Therapy

21 Chemical Peels

22 Dermabrasion

23 Autologous Fat Transfer

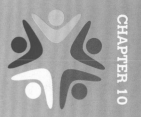
Hemostasis

Jesalyn A. Tate and Jennifer J. Schoch

INTRODUCTION

Hemostasis involves a complex cascade of events, including vasoconstriction, platelet aggregation, platelet plug formation, and fibrin deposition. Achieving adequate hemostasis is a critical component in optimizing patient outcomes in dermatologic surgery. It is a delicate system, and any error can disturb the process. Inadequate hemostasis can lead to prolonged operative time, increased patient anxiety, as well as increased risk of infection, wound dehiscence, and necrosis. Complications of hemostasis may still occur in a small number of patients, despite low risk for bleeding and impeccable surgical technique. This chapter prepares the proceduralist to anticipate issues surrounding hemostasis and to prevent small issues from becoming major problems.

HEMOSTASIS TECHNIQUES

General Principles

A thorough preoperative evaluation with a detailed history and physical examination should be performed to help identify patients at high risk for bleeding complications (Table 10.1). When bleeding occurs, it should be controlled in a systematic manner, starting with the largest vessels and working in a superior to inferior manner to maximize visibility. Hemostasis should be precise and not excessive, because large amounts of charred tissue can increase risks of poor wound healing and infection. The majority of bleeding problems occur in the first 6 hours after surgery; thus, schedule high-risk patients early in the day to allow adequate postoperative monitoring.

Compression is a simple and effective way to achieve hemostasis. Firm pressure applied proximal to a bleeding source allows visibility to identify and ligate the responsible vessel. Circumferential pressure applied around a surgical site (ie, manual pressure or a chalazion clamp; see Figure 10.1 A and B) can temporarily compress vessels and allow a clean and visible surgical field. In a similar manner, a tourniquet fashioned from a rubber glove or Penrose drain (Figure 10.2) can provide hemostasis when performing procedures on the digits or nails. It is critical to remove the tourniquet immediately postoperatively to prevent necrosis.

Decreasing the temperature of the wound bed can also aid in hemostasis through vasoconstriction. Care should be taken to limit time and level of cooling, because significant tissue damage can occur.

Topical Hemostatic Agents

There are a wide variety of topical hemostatic agents available (Table 10.2). For optimal bleeding control, these products are best used in conjunction with other methods of hemostasis such as electrosurgery and suturing. They can be generally grouped into five categories: mechanical agents, caustic agents, physical agents, physiologic agents, and hemostatic dressings.

The mechanical hemostatic agents include bone wax, ostene, and acrylates. Bone wax is applied to bony surfaces for a tamponade effect. It is composed of beeswax and isopropyl palmitate, which can generate a granulomatous foreign body reaction, hinder tissue growth, and serve as a nidus for infection. Ostene is a newer product that is similar to bone wax with a much lower side effect profile. Acrylates are effective physical blockades and are typically used for closure of small wounds under minimal tension.

The most common topical caustic hemostatics are 20% to 70% aluminum chloride, 20% ferric sulfate (Monsel's solution), and 10% to 50% silver nitrate. All of these agents are inexpensive and work well for small, oozing wounds. They are most effective when applied to a dry field.

Physical agents help promote hemostasis by providing a meshwork for platelet adhesion and clot formation. They include gelatins, oxidized cellulose, microfibrillar collagen, microporous polysaccharide spheres (MPHs), and hydrophilic polymers. Gelatins are derived from porcine or bovine animal products and rapidly swell to twice their original volume. Oxidized cellulose has the added benefit of antibacterial properties. Microfibrillar collagen is derived from bovine corium and works especially well for treatment of large or irregular areas. Hydrophilic polymers are not biologically derived and are therefore inexpensive and well tolerated. MPHs are made from potato starch and work by enhancing activity of the natural coagulation cascade. All of the physical agents have the potential disadvantage of causing a granulomatous foreign body reaction.

Physiologic agents are divided into pharmacologic and biologic physical agents. Pharmacologic agents include epinephrine, hydrogen peroxide, and tranexamic acid. Epinephrine is often added to anesthetics to decrease the amount of anesthesia required, prolong duration of anesthesia, and vasoconstrict the wound bed. It is most commonly added in concentrations of 1:100 000 or 1:200 000 and typically takes 15 minutes to achieve maximum vasoconstriction. In the past, there had been significant debate regarding the use of epinephrine in digital blocks, because of concern for vasoconstriction leading to digital necrosis. Most studies have shown that this risk is more likely because of the volume of anesthetic injected, rather than the use of epinephrine. Hydrogen peroxide has minimal hemostatic properties but also can impede wound healing, making it a less attractive choice. Tranexamic acid can be applied topically as an antifibrinolytic agent to help control bleeding.

The biologic physical agents comprise thrombin, hemostatic matrix, fibrin sealants, and platelet gels. Topical thrombin (bovine or human derived) functions the same way as the in vivo coagulation cascade, converting fibrinogen to fibrin. Hemostatic matrix contains thrombin and gelatin, which give this product the added benefit of tamponade for arterial bleeding. Fibrin sealant is a two-part product made of thrombin and fibrinogen. The ingredients are in separate vials and mixed immediately before application. Platelet gels contain bovine collagen and

TABLE 10.1 ⋮ Medications and Substances That Increase Bleeding Risk

GENERIC NAME	COMMON BRAND NAME(S)
Alcohol	
Apixaban	Eliquis
Aspirin	Ascriptin, Aspergum, Aspirtab, Easprin, Ecotrin, Ecpirin, Empirin, Entercote, Genacote, Halfprin, Ninoprin, Norwich AspirinSS
Dabigatran	Pradaxa
Dalteparin	Fragmin
Danaparoid	Orgaran
Diclofenac	Dyloject, Voltaren, Xenaflamm, Zipsor, Zorvolex
Diflunisal	Dolobid
Dipyridamole	Persantine
Echinacea	
Enoxaparin	Lovenox
Fenoprofen	Nalfon
Fish oil	
Flurbiprofen	Ansaid
Garlic	
Ginkgo	
Ginseng	
Heparin	Heparin Sodium
Ibuprofen	Advil, Brufen, Medipren, Motrin, Nurofen
Indomethacin	Indocin
Kava	
Ketoprofen	Orudis
Meclofenamate	Meclomen
Nabumetone	Relafen
Naproxen	Aleve, Anaprox, Naprelan, Naprosyn, Midol, Motrin
Omega-3	
Oxaprozin	Daypro
Pentoxifylline	Trental
Phenylbutazone	Butazolidin
Piroxicam	Feldene
Promethazine	Phenergan, Phenadoz, Promethegan
Propoxyphene	Darvon, Darvon Compound (propoxyphene, ASA, caffeine)
Rivaroxaban	Xarelto

Sodium bicarbonate	Alka-Seltzer
St. John's wort	
Sulindac	Clinoril
Tinzaparin	Innohep
Trilisa	Deertongue
Warfarin	Coumadin
Valerian	
Vitamin E	

COMMON OVER-THE-COUNTER MEDICATIONS CONTAINING ASPIRIN

NAME	INGREDIENTS
Anacin	Aspirin, caffeine
APC	Aspirin, phenacetin, caffeine
Ascriptin	Aspirin, antacid
BC powder	Aspirin, caffeine
Bufferin	Aspirin, antacid
Congesprin	Aspirin, phenylephrine hydrochloride
Cope	Aspirin, caffeine
Excedrin	Aspirin, acetaminophen, caffeine
Fiorinal	Aspirin, butalbital, caffeine
Goody's headache powder	Aspirin, paracetamol, caffeine
Norgesic	Aspirin, caffeine, orphenadrine citrate
Percodan	Aspirin, oxycodone
Robaxisal	Aspirin, methocarbamol
Trigesic	Aspirin, acetaminophen, caffeine
Vanquish	Aspirin, acetaminophen, caffeine

COMMON OVER-THE-COUNTER MEDICATIONS THAT MAY INCREASE BLOOD PRESSURE

NAME	INGREDIENTS
Dristan	Acetaminophen, chlorpheniramine maleate, phenylephrine hydrochloride
Emprazil	Acetaminophen, caffeine, pseudoephedrine hydrochloride, triprolidine hydrochloride
Ephedra	Pseudoephedrine, ephedrine
4-Way Cold Tabs	Phenylephrine
Sine Off	Acetaminophen, phenylephrine
Sine Aid	Acetaminophen, pseudoephedrine

Data Courtesy of Girish S. Munavalli, MD, MHS, Charlotte, North Carolina.

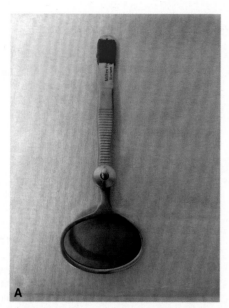

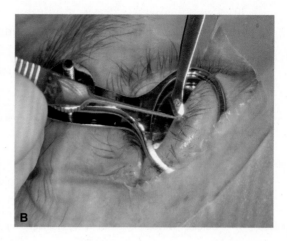

FIGURE 10.1. A, Chalazion clamp. Reprinted with permission from Crowson AN, Magro CM. *Biopsy Interpretation of the Skin*. 2nd ed. Philadelphia, PA: Wolters Kluwer; 2019. Figure 1.6. B, The Chalazion clamp is used for hemostasis during a shave biopsy from the eyelid margin. The proceduralist gently loosens the chalazion clamp. If bleeding is brisk, the ring may be slightly retightened to slow the bleeding so that accurate and specific cautery may be performed. Reprinted with permission from Shields JA, Shields CL. *Eyelid, Conjunctival, and Orbital Tumors: An Atlas and Textbook*. 3rd ed. Philadelphia, PA: Wolters Kluwer; 2016. Figure 15.6.

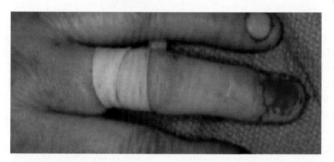

FIGURE 10.2. Use of Penrose drain tourniquet at the base of the digit. Reprinted with permission from Wiesel SW, ed. *Operative Techniques in Orthopaedic Surgery*. Vol 3. 2nd ed. Philadelphia, PA: Wolters Kluwer; 2016. Figure 100.5.

thrombin. The patient's plasma is centrifuged to collect fibrinogen and platelets, which are then combined with the bovine collagen and thrombin, and delivered via a dual chamber syringe delivery system.

Hemostatic dressings provide an additional measure to help control bleeding. These dressings include alginate, chitin/chitosan, mineral zeolite, and dry fibrin. Alginate is inexpensive and also serves as barrier protection for the wound (Figures 10.3 and 10.4). Mineral zeolite (QuikClot) is an inexpensive kaolin-impregnated gauze that activates factor XII in the intrinsic clotting cascade. It may be used for hemostasis briefly, but should not be left in place for more than 24 hours. Chitin and chitosan dressings are derived from crustacean exoskeletons and possess both hemostatic and antimicrobial properties.

TABLE 10.2 ⋮ Overview of Hemostatic Agents

NAME	TRADE NAMES	INDICATIONS	ADVANTAGES	DISADVANTAGES
CAUSTIC AGENTS				
Aluminum chloride (20%-70%)	Drysol, Xerac AC, Certain Dri	Small superficial wounds, healing by secondary intention	Affordable; less risk of dyspigmentation	Tissue irritation; flammable (caution with electrodesiccation)
Ferric sulfate (20%)	Monsel's solution	Small wounds	Affordable; bacteriotoxic; safe for use before electrodesiccation	Dyspigmentation; inflammation; dermal fibrosis
Silver nitrate (10%-50%)		Small wounds, healing by secondary intention	Affordable; bacteriostatic properties	Stinging sensation; rare tattoo; argyria with large application
MECHANICAL AGENTS				
Bone wax	Horsley's bone wax	Limited use in dermatology procedures	Inexpensive; tamponade effect	Granulomatous foreign body reaction; impaired tissue growth; infection

(continued)

TABLE 10.2 ⋮ Overview of Hemostatic Agents (*continued*)

NAME	TRADE NAMES	INDICATIONS	ADVANTAGES	DISADVANTAGES
Ostene		Limited use in dermatology procedures	Does not impair tissue growth or promote infection	Limited utility for skin procedures
Acrylates	DERMABOND, Band-Aid liquid bandage, Tissue-Glue	Small wounds with minimal tension	Mechanical barrier; antimicrobial	Expensive
PHYSICAL AGENTS				
Gelatins	Gelfoam, Gelfilm, Spongostan, Surgifoam	Small-vessel bleeding or oozing	Absorb several times their weight; nonantigenic; absorbable	Tissue damage due to swelling, granulomatous foreign body reactions; infection
Oxidized cellulose	Surgicel, Oxycel	Small-vessel bleeding or oozing	Absorbs several times its weight; antibacterial; absorbable	Granulomatous foreign body reactions; rebleeding common after removal
Microfibrillar collagen	Avitene, Instat, Helistat, Helitene, Collastat, Collatene	Ideal for large surface areas; oozing; effective in patients on aspirin and heparin	Low risk of rebleeding with removal; minimal swelling; more effective than gelatin or cellulose	May bind to neural structures; remove before closure; rare allergic and granulomatous foreign body reactions; less effective in thrombocytopenic patients
Microporous polysaccharide spheres (MPH)	Arista AH, PerClot, Vitasure	Oozing	Plant-based; absorbable	Remove before closure
Hydrophilic polymers	WoundSeal, Pro QR powder	Oozing wounds; can be used during Mohs stages	Inexpensive; over the counter; painless	Remove before closure; rare granulomatous foreign body reactions
PHYSIOLOGIC AGENTS				
Epinephrine (1:1000-1 000 000)	Adrenaline	Added to anesthetic; use for surgeries with anticipated increased bleeding	Prolongs duration of anesthesia	Rare systemic reactions (including arrhythmias); rebound hyperemia
Hydrogen peroxide (3%)		Mild hemostasis for small, superficial wounds	Inexpensive; mildly antimicrobial	Inhibits wound healing
Tranexamic acid		Debrided wounds and grafts		
Thrombin	Thrombostat, Thombin-JMI, Evithrom, Rh Thrombin	Multiple dermatologic procedures including flaps and grafts	Nonreactive; can use in patients on antiplatelet or anticoagulant medications	Expensive; risk of disseminated intravascular clotting if entry into large caliber vessels
Hemostatic matrix	Floseal, Surgiflo	Oozing wounds, arterial bleeding	Effective in patients with platelet dysfunction; added tamponade effect from gelatin	Expensive; must be removed from wound before closure
Fibrin sealants	Tisseel, Evicel, Crosseal	Oozing wounds, skin grafting	Nonreactive; fast acting; effective in heparinized patients	Expensive; alcohol, iodine, and heavy metal ions can denature product, so must clean wound bed before use; difficult application
Platelet gels	Vitagel	Multiple surgical procedures, including laser resurfacing	Platelets improve clot strength; facilitate tissue regeneration	Expensive; centrifugation required
HEMOSTATIC DRESSINGS				
Alginate		Mild low-pressure bleeding; oozing	Inexpensive, wound protective	Not effective for high-pressure bleeding
Chitin/chitosan	Celox, ChitoFlex, HemCon	Emergency field use; minor wounds	Antimicrobial	Expensive; do not use in patients with shellfish allergies
Mineral zeolite	Quickclot/Quikclot	Emergency field use; high- and low-pressure bleeding	Inexpensive	Granulomatous foreign body reactions; remove after hemostasis achieved
Fibrin	Dry Fibrin Sealant Dressings	Large surface abrasions	Can be left in wound; does not require mixing	Expensive; brittle, requires strong packaging

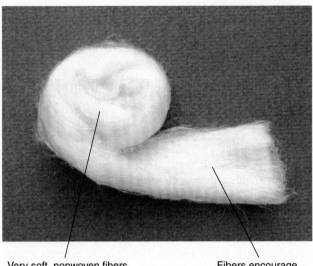

Very soft, nonwoven fibers turn into a biodegradable gel as they absorb exudate.

Fibers encourage hemostasis in minimally bleeding wounds.

FIGURE 10.3. Alginate dressing in rope form. Reprinted with permission from Slachta PA. *Wound Care Made Incredibly Visual.* 3rd ed. Philadelphia, PA: Wolters Kluwer; 2018.

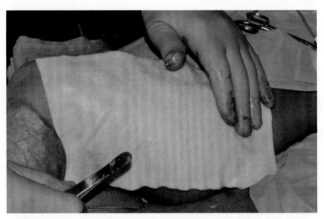

FIGURE 10.4. Applying Kaltostat alginate dressing to a large wound in an operating room setting. Reprinted with permission from Chung KC, Gosain AK. *Operative Techniques in Pediatric Plastic and Reconstructive Surgery.* Philadelphia, PA: Wolters Kluwer; 2020.

Electrosurgery

Electrosurgery is a simple and effective surgical technique for hemostasis in dermatology (see Chapter 17. Electrosurgery/ Hyfrecation for more information).

Suture Techniques

Suture ligation can be particularly useful to control larger bleeding vessels. In general, vessels greater than 2 mm in diameter should be ligated to avoid post-op bleeding complications. An attempt to identify the vessel should be made via compression proximal to the bleeding vessel to temporarily halt bleeding, and further undermining as needed. If this fails, blind ligation can be attempted using a figure-of-eight or purse-string stitch (Figure 10.5). For particularly bloody scalp excisions, an "ex-suture" can be used. In this technique, a running locked

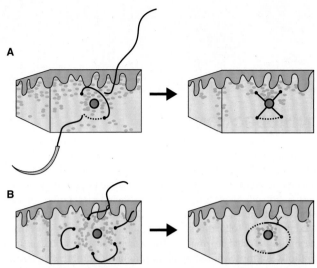

FIGURE 10.5. Control of a bleeding vessel in deep tissue. A, The figure-of-eight stitch. B, The purse-string stitch. Note that these stitches are not tied tightly for the sake of clarity here. In reality, these stitches must be tied tightly to seal the bleeding vessel. Reprinted with permission from Shah K, Egan D, Quaas J. *Essential Emergency Trauma.* Philadelphia, PA: Wolters Kluwer Health/ Lippincott Williams & Wilkins; 2012. Figure 72-2.

suture is placed behind the ellipse as it is being removed. This helps secure hemostasis as the excision is being performed.

Another useful stitch for nonspecific oozing at the wound edge is the standard or fully buried horizontal mattress suture. When excising vascular lesions, hemorrhage is inevitable and sometimes profuse. A simple purse-string suture or a double imbricating suture, consisting of two modified vertical purse-string sutures, can be placed peripheral to the wound to aid in hemostasis. By pulling on the suture ends, vessels are tamponaded as the central area is constricted. This technique is best performed with 3-0 Prolene™ (Ethicon US, LLC) and a PS2 needle.

SUMMARY

Optimal patient outcomes require carefully planned pre-, intra-, and postoperative care. Adequate hemostasis is crucial in avoiding hematoma formation, wound dehiscence, and other surgical complications. Prompt recognition of postoperative complications and appropriate care are essential in reducing patient morbidity.

SUGGESTED READINGS

Achneck HE, Sileshi B, Jamiolkowski RM, Albala DM, Shapiro ML, Lawson JH. A comprehensive review of topical hemostatic agents: efficacy and recommendations for use. *Ann Surg.* 2010;251(2):217–228.

Alam M, Goldberg LH. Utility of fully buried horizontal mattress sutures. *J Am Acad Dermatol.* 2004;50(1):73–76.

Gale AJ. Current understanding of hemostasis. *Toxicol Pathol.* 2011;39(1):273–280.

Glick JB, Kaur RR, Siegel D. Achieving hemostasis in dermatology—part II: topical hemostatic agents. *Indian Dermatol Online J.* 2013;4(3):172–176.

Howe N, Cherpelis B. Obtaining rapid and effective hemostasis: part I. Update and review of topical hemostatic agents. *J Am Acad Dermatol.* 2013;69(5):659.e1–659.e17.

Palm MD, Altman JS. Topical hemostatic agents: a review. *Dermatol Surg.* 2008;34(4):431–445.

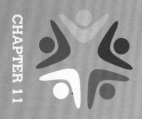

CHAPTER 11

Simple Wound Repair

Mimi R. Borrelli, Ruth Tevlin, and H. Peter Lorenz

INTRODUCTION

A wound is a loss in the integrity of the skin and may arise, most pertinently to this textbook, as an incision—a precise disruption of the tissue by the knife of the surgeon. Unfortunately, skin and soft-tissue wounds are also common pediatric presentations to the emergency department (ED) and include lacerations, abrasions, contusions, and hematomas. Lacerations are wounds created in the skin following blunt or penetrating trauma—they may be simple, beveled, tearing, and burst or stellate types. Stellate lacerations are those caused by blunt trauma or compressive forces and often involve extensive damage around the wound edges, with abrasion of the surrounding skin. (See Chapter 96. Laceration Repair.)

Most wounds heal well naturally because of an innate ability of the body to repair itself; however, certain principles of wound management, including cleansing, repair methods that effectively reapproximate tissue, and excellent post-wound care that minimizes complications, may help optimize cosmetic outcomes. This chapter describes the principles of treating skin and soft-tissue wounds with a specific focus on iatrogenic incisions and traumatic lacerations.

PATIENT EVALUATION

ABC Assessment

Lacerations may present in the context of life-threatening injuries, and patient care starts with an ABC assessment including any necessary treatment following the principles of basic life support (BLS), advanced cardiac life support (ACLS), and advanced trauma life support (ATLS):

- **A**—Check for a patent **airway**.
- **B**—Check for effective spontaneous **breathing** or mechanical ventilation.
- **C**—Check for adequate **circulation**.

Tachycardia and hypotension can suggest significant blood loss. Many children can be tachycardic because of fear and anxiety. Patients must next be assessed for associated injuries and lacerations.

Bleeding from minor incisions and lacerations usually stops spontaneously in patients with normal temperature, adequate platelet count, and normal coagulation parameters. If necessary, bleeding from iatrogenic incisions and lacerations can often be controlled by applying direct digital pressure; electrocautery is also useful in appropriate situations (such as the operating room or procedure room setting). See Chapter 17. Electrosurgery/Hyfrecation.

In life-threatening situations, a tourniquet may be temporarily applied while expediting operative or angiographic intervention. Bleeding from the neck and head as a result of trauma requires immediate and prompt expert attention involving trauma and ENT surgeons, and care should be taken to avoid airway obstruction. Major vascular injuries require consultation with the vascular team. Patients with significant trauma should be transferred to a pediatric trauma center if stable for transport.

Patient History

In cases other than iatrogenic incisions, a thorough history from the child and parents or caregivers is required to understand the specific mechanism of injury, which often will raise concern regarding additional injuries. Different mechanisms and laceration types require different treatment; stellate lacerations, for example, are much more susceptible to infection than are simple lacerations, and higher impact wounds are more likely to be associated with damage to surrounding structures including bones, nerves, and tendons. Details of the patient's tetanus vaccination status, allergies, and past history including that of any conditions that may impair healing (eg, diabetes, immunodeficiency, steroid use, obesity) should be obtained. Nonaccidental injury should remain in the differential, especially when the reported mechanism is inconsistent with the injury. Contamination history is important to help guide debridement and antibiotic use.

Wound Evaluation

Any resultant wound—iatrogenic, traumatic, or otherwise—should be inspected for size, shape, and depth. In the physical assessment of a hemodynamically stable patient, the wound itself should be examined last because it can be distressing to the patient. Exploration of wounds is best performed when patients have been adequately anesthetized to avoid discomfort, especially because exposure of bones, nerves, muscles, or tendons may need to be assessed. Complex wounds are best evaluated in the operating room under appropriate lighting, with the possibility of hemostasis and surgical assistance if necessary. Procedural sedation with ketamine in the ED is typically administered by specifically trained emergency physicians. Anxiolytic medication and procedural sedation can be beneficial. Photographic records of injuries can be helpful for surgical planning, teaching purposes, medical documentation, and may be necessary for medicolegal situations.

PATIENT PREPARATION
Antimicrobial Treatment

Proper debridement and adequate irrigation are the mainstay of wound treatment, and antimicrobial control is an important addition. Wounds contaminated with greater than 10^5 organisms per gram of tissue will, ultimately, undergo dehiscence 70% to 100% of the time. Wounds contaminated with β-hemolytic streptococci fail to heal at even smaller bacterial loads. The Immunization Practices Advisory Committee of the Centers for Disease Control and Prevention (CDC, https://www.cdc.gov/vaccines/vpd/dtap-tdap-td/hcp/recommendations.html) provide guidance for tetanus prophylaxis (Tables 11.1 to 11.3).[1] Clean lacerations are often sufficiently treated with antibiotics covering the common gram-positive skin flora, such as *Staphylococcus aureus*. Dirty lacerations also require gram-negative coverage. Lacerations with high bacterial loads or those involving a contaminating mechanism may

TABLE 11.1 ⋮ CDC Tetanus Wound Management

	CLEAN, MINOR WOUNDS		ALL OTHER WOUNDS[a]	
Vaccination history	Tdap or Td[b]	TIG	Tdap or Td[b]	TIG
Unknown or fewer than 3 doses	Yes	No	Yes	Yes
Three or more doses	No[c]	No	No[d]	No

[a]Such as, but not limited to, wounds contaminated with dirt, feces, soil, and saliva; puncture wounds; avulsions; and wounds resulting from missiles, crushing, burns, and frostbite.
[b]Tdap is preferred to Td for adults who have never received Tdap. Single-antigen tetanus toxoid (TT) is no longer available in the United States.
[c]Yes, if more than 10 years since the last tetanus toxoid–containing vaccine dose.
[d]Yes, if more than 5 years since the last tetanus toxoid–containing vaccine dose.
From Hamborsky J, Kroger A, Wolfe C; National Center for Immunization and Respiratory Diseases (U.S.). *Epidemiology and Prevention of Vaccine-Preventable Diseases.* 13th ed. Atlanta, GA: Centers for Disease Control and Prevention; 2015. https://www.cdc.gov/vaccines/pubs/pinkbook/tetanus.html.

require open wound care and delayed closure. Most of the time with appropriate irrigation and debridement, we try to close simple wounds initially. In the setting of delayed presentation, especially in the setting of animal bites, wounds may be left open depending on their location.

Anesthesia

Minimizing pain and discomfort is essential when caring for children. Lacerations can be particularly tender, and the management of iatrogenic incisions or traumatic wounds can be anxiety inducing and upsetting to young patients. Small children may require sedation or general anesthesia (GA) to reduce movement, pain, and distress associated with the procedure and to enable thorough debridement and precise placement of sutures. There is no hard and fast rule regarding the choice of sedation or GA, and considerations are given to injury, patient cooperativity, and parent preference. Generally, for young children, GA is chosen for elective incisions and sedation for the emergency setting. Anxiolytics, including oral or nasal midazolam, or inhaled nitric oxide, can help calm anxiety.[2,3] Proximity to family members and distraction can also help alleviate patient anxiety.[4]

Local anesthesia or regional blocks can be used to prep iatrogenic incisions or to treat simple, uncomplicated lacerations. Local anesthesia is injected into the surrounding tissue through a small-bore needle (25-gauge or smaller). Digital blocks can be used for planned incisions or lacerations of the

TABLE 11.2 ⋮ DTaP, DT, Td, and Tdap

TYPE	DIPHTHERIA	TETANUS
DTaP, DT	6.7-25 Lf units	5-10 Lf units
Td, Tdap (adults)	2-2.5 Lf units	2-5 Lf units

DTaP and pediatric DT used through age 6 years. Adult Td for persons 7 years and older. Tdap for persons 10 years and older (Boostrix) or 10 through 64 years (Adacel).

TABLE 11.3 ⋮ Tetanus Toxoid

- Formalin-inactivated tetanus toxin
- Schedule
  - Three or 4 doses plus booster
  - Booster every 10 y
- Efficacy
  - Approximately 100%
- Duration
  - Approximately 10 y
- Should be administered with diphtheria toxoid as DTaP, DT, Td, or Tdap

From Hamborsky J, Kroger A, Wolfe C; National Center for Immunization and Respiratory Diseases (U.S.). *Epidemiology and Prevention of Vaccine-Preventable Diseases.* 13th ed. Atlanta, GA: Centers for Disease Control and Prevention; 2015. https://www.cdc.gov/vaccines/pubs/pinkbook/tetanus.html

fingers and involve injection of anesthetic into the adjacent web spaces (Figures 11.1A-D and 11.2). The most common local anesthetic agent used is 1% lidocaine with or without epinephrine. The maximum lidocaine dose depends on body weight in kilograms and concomitant use of epinephrine—where the vasoconstrictive effects of epinephrine keep the lidocaine locally and thereby allow delivery of more lidocaine. *Clark's rule* and the *Rule of 25* are weight-based methods for calculating the maximum recommended dose (MRD) of local anesthetic in the pediatric population.[5] *Clark's rule* states that the dose of local anesthetic should be reduced by the ratio of the child's weight to an adult weight of 150 lb. For example, a child weighing 100 lb is two-thirds the weight of an adult and, thus, the child's MRD for local anesthetic will be two-thirds the established MRD for the 150-lb adult. The *Rule of 25* states that one cartridge of any formulation marketed in the United States can be used for every 25 lb of weight, up to six cartridges maximum per patient for patients more than or equal to 150 lb. Epinephrine (1:100 000) can help control blood loss through its vasoconstrictive effects. A recent review reports that digital blocks can be safely used in healthy patients without risk of poor peripheral circulation.[6] Infiltration with anesthetic itself, however, can be painful and distressing to any child regardless of age.

Topical anesthetics are an attractive anesthetic option in the pediatric population because they are not painful to administer. However, they have less analgesic efficiency compared to conventional lidocaine infiltration for suture repairs.[7] Examples include LMX.4™ (Ferndale Laboratories), EMLA™ (AB Astra Pharmaceuticals, L.P.) cream (eutectic mixture of local anesthetics; 2.5% lidocaine, 2.5% prilocaine) and LET gel (lidocaine [4%], epinephrine [1:2000], and tetracaine [1%]). These topical agents are most effective when applied under occlusive dressings for at least 30 to 60 minutes before a debridement procedure.[8,9] EMLA, however, has been associated with side effects, which may limit its use. Although side effects are mostly mild, transient, and limited to the skin, occasionally life-threatening complications occur. The main concern is systemic absorption of lidocaine and prilocaine, which can cause central nervous system toxicity and methemoglobinemia in overdose.[10-13] Systemic absorption depends on the duration and surface area of application, and great caution should thus be taken when applying these agents to the mucosa and areas where the

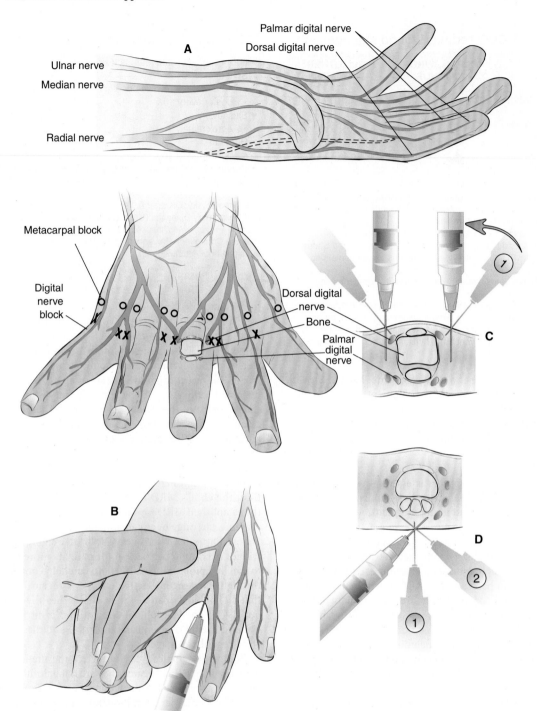

FIGURE 11.1. Dorsal technique for palmar and dorsal digital nerve block. A, Nerve distribution in hand. B, Traditional digital nerve block. C, Dorsal three-sided ring block. D, Volar three-sided ring block. Reprinted with permission from Lewis L, Stephan M. Local and regional anesthesia. In: Henretig FM, King C, eds. *Textbook of Pediatric Emergency Procedures.* Baltimore, MD: Williams & Wilkins; 1997:481. Figure 52-1.

cutaneous barrier is compromised—absorption is faster and toxic plasma concentrations can be reached in these situations. EMLA is contraindicated in patients reporting a prior history of sensitivity to amide-type local anesthetics. To date, there are no reports of toxic complications from the use of LET; however, the mixture of lidocaine and tetracaine theoretically increases the risk of systemic effects.

WOUND PREPARATION

Debridement

All wounds should be judiciously cleaned and debrided of all necrotic or foreign materials from and around the wound. Debridement can involve the removal of large amounts of tissue, and immediate debridement prevents foreign particles

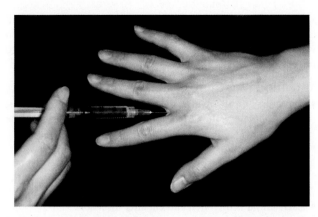

FIGURE 11.2. Traditional digital nerve block. Reprinted with permission from Thorne CH, Bartlett SP, Beasley RW, et al. *Grabb and Smith's Plastic Surgery.* 6th ed. Philadelphia, PA: Wolters Kluwer Health/Lippincott Williams & Wilkins; 2007. Figure 77.4.

becoming fixed in the dermis, reduces the risk of infection from foreign bodies, and can optimize healing of the remaining healthy tissue. Debridement can be conservative at the bedside, or extensive and aggressive in the operating theatre under anesthesia, where wounds can be thoroughly scrubbed with sterile gauze or a moistened scrub brush and sterile saline/mild soap. Ether, acetone, or xylol may be used in small quantities to remove oily substances. Hair-bearing regions may be clipped to facilitate proper cleaning and closure. (See Chapter 5. Surgical Procedure Room Setup.)

Irrigation

Irrigation helps cleanse the wound from contamination by foreign bodies or particulate matter that cannot be removed by debridement and allows for a more thorough inspection of the extent of injury. High irrigation pressures (> 8 psi) can successfully clean wounds of small particulates, soil, and bacteria, and thus decrease infection rates.[14] These pressures can be achieved using a 35-mL syringe with a 19-gauge needle filled with sterile saline at the bedside.[14] An 18-gauge needle, however, may be more universally available and can achieve similar pressures.[15] Irrigation can drive particulates or bacteria deeper into wounds[16] and pressures more than 15 psi may cause damage to wounds, thus impairing healing.[17] Irrigation with antibiotics in cases at risk for contamination can minimize the risk of infection.

Wound Trimming

Once devitalized tissue and debris have been fully removed and the wound has been thoroughly irrigated, the wound edges can be trimmed sharply with care to remove any ragged edges. Sharp edge debridement helps achieve optimal skin closure. Wounds should be trimmed perpendicular to the skin, except in hair-bearing regions where the edges may be beveled in the direction of the hair follicles.

PRIMARY WOUND CLOSURE

The aim of wound closure is to approximate the wound edges to allow for natural healing to occur. Inadequate closure of wounds leaves the injured site at risk for infection and excessive scar formation, with consequent adverse cosmetic outcomes.[18] Primary wound closure is used in the context of iatrogenic incisions and simple lacerations. The wound edges can then be approximated

and closed with sutures using a variety of methods, such as sutures, tissue adhesives, staples, adhesive strips, and hair apposition. (See Chapter 7. Surgical Instruments.) Complicated lesions involving damage to deeper structures may be temporarily closed pending definitive treatment or may be dressed. Complex tissue rearrangement should be avoided in the acute setting. To reduce wound dehiscence, infection, and skin necrosis, the wound should be closed under minimal tension. (See Chapter 8. Sutures.)

Layered Repair

Reapproximation of skin and any of the deeper structures must proceed from deep to superficial to eliminate dead space and reduce tension across the wound margins. Bones should be stabilized first, followed by revascularization, nerve, and tendon repair, before the subcutaneous and cutaneous layers of the skin are addressed. Sutures in the fascial sheets and aligning the deep dermis can help decrease tension across the skin edges.

Suturing Techniques

Suturing is the most commonly used method for wound closure. The aim of suturing iatrogenic incisions and traumatic lacerations is to achieve approximation, alignment, and eversion of the skin edges. Good technique can eliminate dead space, minimize tension, and prevent wound separation.

- The choice of specific sutures depends on the goals of placement (tension, cosmetic considerations, whether closure is in layers, etc.), recipient anatomic location, clinician experience, time to perform the procedure, and patient comfort. (See Chapter 8. Sutures for further details.) Generally, the thinnest, smallest suture possible is best to minimize foreign-body reactions, trauma to the skin, and "track marks," which can leave scars. On the face and nailbeds, thinner sutures, such as 6-0 and 7-0, are used. On the hands, 4-0 and 5-0 are appropriate, whereas on the limbs, scalp, and torso, suture sizes from 5-0 up to 3-0 may be necessary, depending on the thickness of the patient's skin.

- Absorbable sutures (eg, Plain-Gut and Vicryl™ [Ethicon US, LLC]) undergo degradation naturally and do not need to be removed; they save time, reduce patient anxiety and discomfort, and therefore are often used in children. Nonabsorbable sutures (eg, silk, nylon) do not degrade and have high and continued tensile strength. They are unlikely to break and elicit only a minimal inflammatory response; however, they do need to be removed. Time before removal largely depends on anatomic location; generally, sutures on the face are removed after 4 to 5 days, sutures on the arms are removed after 5 to 10 days, and sutures on the lower limbs, torso, or over a joint are removed after 7 to 14 days. There is no difference in long-term cosmetic results between absorbable and nonabsorbable sutures.[19]

- Sutures should be handled carefully; the suture needle should only be grasped with the needle holder two-thirds of the way from the sharp end. The needle should penetrate the epidermis at a perpendicular angle and be passed through the skin along the curvature of the needle. Smooth, fluid pronation of the wrist should be used to drive the needle. As the suture exits, it should be grasped by the forceps to avoid damaging the needle tip. Fine-toothed forceps can be used to grasp and lightly evert the skin to assist visualization and ensure appropriate angle of penetration. The distance from the wound edge should be half the radius of the needle—this will mean the needle naturally exits the contralateral wound edge at equidistance when the curvature of the needle is followed. Sutures should approximate the wound edges appropriately while avoiding strangulation of tissue, which increases the risk of scarring. Strangulation can be avoided by ensuring precise wound approximation and by reducing wound tension. Wrinkling of tissue suggests that a suture is too tight and should be removed and reapplied.

- *Knots* should be used to secure placed sutures; the number of knots depends on the suture material; monofilament nylon, for example, can untie relatively easily. A safe rule is to perform a surgical knot on the first tie, followed by two single knots.
- *Common errors* in suturing techniques include the use of too little or too much tension; too little tension places wounds at risk for infection and is associated with poor cosmetic outcomes, whereas excessive tension puts the wound at risk for skin necrosis.
- *Failure to appropriately evert the skin* can impact healing. This most commonly happens with simple interrupted sutures. The best cosmetic outcomes are achieved with slight wound-edge eversion because scars retract with time.

A number of different suturing techniques can be used for simple repairs.

Simple Interrupted Sutures

Simple interrupted sutures are single loops of suture in series that provide very robust wound closure (Figure 11.3). Each loop takes equal bites wide and deep in the dermis to avoid mismatched heights and overlapping edges after suturing. Large bites can reduce wound tension, and small bites can precisely align wound edges. If there is preexisting asymmetry, this can be corrected using differently sized needle bites on either side.

Although interrupted sutures take time to place and remove, they provide secure closure that remains closed even if one suture breaks. In addition, specific sutures can be removed and/or adjusted to achieve improved esthetic outcomes without opening the entire length of the wound. Interrupted sutures

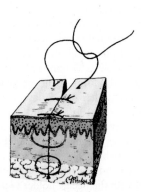

FIGURE 11.3. Simple interrupted sutures. A commonly used suturing technique. The individual stiches are not connected. This can be time consuming to place; however, individual sutures can be easily adjusted and they maintain strength and tissue position if one portion fails. Knots should be tied to one side of the wound to decrease the risk of infection. Reprinted with permission from Rayan GM, Akelman E. *The Hand: Anatomy, Examination, and Diagnosis.* Philadelphia, PA: Wolters Kluwer Health/Lippincott Williams & Wilkins; 2011. Figure 16.2.

achieve mild to moderate tension and fine-tune the wound closure where tension has been shifted. They can be used when wounds are infected because microorganisms are less likely to travel along the series of interrupted sutures.

Technique for Simple Interrupted Sutures

- Typically, sutures are placed 4 to 5 mm from the wound edges; small-diameter sutures (eg, 6-0) may be placed closer to the wound edge.
- Interrupted sutures are placed by entering the epidermis perpendicular to the wound edge, traversing the epidermis and dermis, and exiting perpendicular to the epidermis on the contralateral wound edge.
- Each strand is then tied and cut after insertion.
- Knots should be tied to one side of the wound edge to reduce the risk of infection. Surgical knots, which achieve maximum suture security, can be used to tie the first throw. The stitches should be wider at the base (intradermal) than at the surface to promote eversion of the wound edges.
- The individual sutures in the series should be evenly spaced and positioned close enough to ensure complete closure; typically, intersuture spacing is about 5 mm.
- Simple interrupted sutures are best applied on a reverse cutting needle using silk, because it has excellent knot tying and handling characteristics (Figure 11.4A-D).

Simple Continuous or Running Sutures

A simple running (continuous) suture involves a single suture taking a series of equal bites along the length of the wound (Figure 11.5). Running sutures are associated with less scarring than are interrupted sutures, they help evenly distribute tension across the wound, and they can be placed with ease and speed. Therefore, running sutures are usually used for closures longer than 3 cm or wounds in cosmetically sensitive areas. Owing to the ability of simple running sutures to distribute the tension evenly across a wound, they are also used in areas expected to expand because of edema. A disadvantage of running simple sutures, however, is that the integrity of the whole repair is disrupted if the suture is removed or breaks, which risks wound dehiscence. (See Chapter 136. Surgical Complications.) It is therefore often advised to apply Steri-Strips across the open area and/or to reinforce open areas of the wound with interrupted sutures, especially if the wound is in an area that is not cosmetically sensitive. Interrupted suturing is still a preferred technique for meticulous repair of wounds under moderate tension.

Simple Continuous or Running Suture Technique

- To start, a simple interrupted suture is placed at one end of a wound and only the tail end of the suture is cut—this is the "anchor stitch."
- The long uncut suture thread is then continued as simple uninterrupted sutures placed down the wound length, passing from the epidermis to dermis. This first throw enters the epidermis 4 mm from the initial suture and approximately 2 to 4 mm from the wound edge; in general, smaller diameter sutures (eg, 6-0) may be placed 2 to 3 mm from the wound edge, whereas 4-0 sutures may be placed 4 to 6 mm from the wound edge.
- Similar to simple interrupted sutures, the best cosmetic outcomes are achieved when individual sutures are equal in the separating distance and bite depth to ensure that there are no

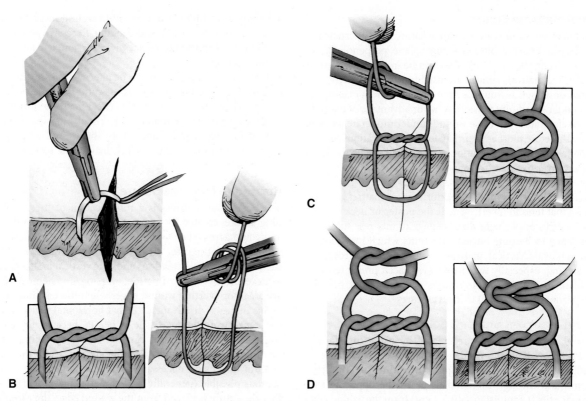

FIGURE 11.4. Placement of a "loop knot" in conjunction with simple sutures of the skin using an eversion technique. A, The needle enters the skin at a right angle in a way that allows somewhat less skin and more subcutaneous tissue to be caught in the passage of the needle. The needle should incorporate the same amount of skin and subcutaneous tissue on each side. The ideal suture material for placing a "loop knot" is 4-0 nylon. One can also use 5-0 nylon. B, The first knot should be a surgeon's knot drawn down gently to barely coapt the skin edges. C, The second tie should be placed to produce a square knot but should be drawn to produce an approximate 2- to 3-mm loop. D, The third tie should be placed to produce a square knot. This third tie can be secured tightly against the second tie, preserving the loop and allowing for some spontaneous loosening of the surgeon's knot as later edema develops. Reprinted with permission from Bachur RG, Shaw KN. *Fleisher & Ludwig's Textbook of Pediatric Emergency Medicine.* 7th ed. Philadelphia, PA: Wolters Kluwer; 2015. Figure 118-5A-D.

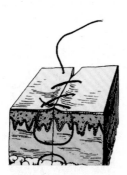

FIGURE 11.5. Continuous or running sutures. An uninterrupted series of simple sutures, with advancing on the underside. One knot is tied at the beginning and at the end. Tension can be easily distributed along the length of the suture if evenly placed in succession. Running sutures are useful to close long wounds that are under minimal tension because of the strategic placement of deeper sutures; however, they cannot be easily adjusted and may compromise blood supply. Reprinted with permission from Rayan GM, Akelman E. *The Hand: Anatomy, Examination, and Diagnosis.* Philadelphia, PA: Wolters Kluwer Health/Lippincott Williams & Wilkins; 2011. Figure 16.2.

overlapping edges after suturing and that tension is equally distributed along the suture line.

- To avoid strangulation, and thus infection scarring or necrosis, *it is essential to ensure that suture tension is not excessive.* One variation of the simple running suture is to "lock" the sutures by passing the needle through the loop of the previous suture as it exits the epidermis. Locking sutures are good for applying continued tension on a wound, but this technique can make it more difficult to distribute tension evenly, which can increase the risk of tissue strangulation.
- A single knot in the suture thread as it exits the skin at the wound edge is sufficient to terminate the running suture.
- Knots should be tied securely enough to ensure the tissue is adequately approximated while avoiding blanching of the skin. If the wound is on a flat immobile area and under minimal tension, the simple running suture can be left unlocked.
- Prolene™ (Ethicon US, LLC) is an ideal suture to use for this stitch because it has low coefficient of friction through skin tissue, and its elasticity and stretch allow for wound edema without risking tissue necrosis or strangulation.
- Sutures should be removed after 5 to 7 days to avoid suture marks remaining in the skin.

Vertical Mattress Suture

Vertical mattress sutures are a series of sutures that alternate between deep and narrow bites in a single plane, perpendicular to the wound edge (Figure 11.6). They can be interrupted or running. Vertical mattress sutures are used to achieve effective approximation as well as wound-edge eversion without placing the wound under significant tension. A major advantage of mattress sutures is their ability to close wounds under moderate tension. They are therefore most appropriate for deep lacerations following punch biopsy or a traumatic laceration and can be used as a secondary layer to assist in wound-edge eversion following the placement of deep dermal sutures.[20,21]

Anatomic locations most suited for vertical mattress sutures are those that tend to invert, such as the posterior neck or concave skin surfaces. A major disadvantage of mattress sutures is the tendency to become buried with time, which may require careful removal. Vertical mattress sutures can also result in crosshatching, especially when they are placed under tension. Monofilament nonabsorbable sutures generally work best for both horizontal and vertical mattress sutures.

Vertical Mattress Suture Technique

- Vertical mattress sutures are created by using the "far-far, near-near" system; the needle is inserted 0.5 to 1 cm perpendicular to the wound margin, down to the depth of the wound, and through the deep tissue to the opposing side where it exits at equidistance (0.5-1 cm) from the wound edge ("far-far").
- The needle is then reversed in the needle holder and reinserted half the distance to the wound edge (1-2 mm) on the side the needle just exited; it is passed superficially (~1 mm depth in the upper dermis) to the opposite wound margin ("near-near"), where it exits at half the distance to the wound edge from where the first deep stich entered.
- The two stiches can then be tied on the side of the wound. The width of the stitch should be increased relative to the tension on the wound; that is, the higher the tension, the wider the stitch.

- Improper techniques may result in wound inversion, uneven distribution of tension, and scarring. Excessive pull on the suture thread can result in excessive eversion, tension, scarring, and necrosis.
- Vertical mattress sutures can be alternated with simple interrupted sutures, and if so, mattress sutures should be removed first. Alternatively, a series of vertical mattress sutures can be placed in series; when this is performed, bites should be equal in depth and equidistance from the wound edge to avoid shelfing of wound edges, which may create scars and an uneven skin surface.

Horizontal Mattress Suture

The horizontal mattress is a modification of the simple running suture, created by forming a box with two parallel loops along and across the wound (Figure 11.7). Horizontal mattress sutures are optimal for areas of skin under increased tension, such as over joints or tendons and, like vertical mattress sutures, achieve effective approximation, eversion, and hemostasis. They are ideal for everting wound edges when there is little subcutaneous tissue. A disadvantage is that horizontal mattress sutures can cause wound-edge tissue ischemia, because the suture is constrictive in design; this can be avoided by taking generous bites, using bolsters when securing sutures, using the minimal amount of tension necessary, and by removing the sutures as soon as possible (generally 5-7 days after placement). The further the suture is placed from the wound edge, the easier it is to remove the suture.

Technique for Horizontal Mattress Sutures

- The skin is penetrated 5 to 10 mm from the wound edge on one side of the wound.
- The needle is passed either dermally or subcutaneously to the opposite wound edge and exits through the epidermis at equidistance (ie, 5-10 mm from the edge).
- The needle then reenters the skin several millimeters laterally on the same side and at the same distance from the wound edge and is passed again dermally or subcutaneously toward the opposite side to exit at equidistance.

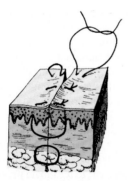

FIGURE 11.6. Vertical mattress sutures. These sutures consist of a suture loop that passes through both sides of the cut edge of the epithelial surface before the knot is tied, using a "far-far, near-near" technique. These sutures can help evert wound edges because they result in good closure strength and can distribute wound tension. They risk the formation of scars and necrosis of the skin on the edge of the wound. Reprinted with permission from Rayan GM, Akelman E. *The Hand: Anatomy, Examination, and Diagnosis.* Philadelphia, PA: Wolters Kluwer Health/Lippincott Williams & Wilkins; 2011. Figure 16.2.

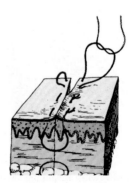

FIGURE 11.7. Horizontal mattress sutures. These are one of the strongest types of suture. They are similar to simple interrupted but with additional parallel bites taken in reverse. They are indicated when there is large distance between wound edges because they can evert wound edges under tension and result in good hemostasis without promoting prominent scars. Reprinted with permission from Rayan GM, Akelman E. *The Hand: Anatomy, Examination, and Diagnosis.* Philadelphia, PA: Wolters Kluwer Health/Lippincott Williams & Wilkins; 2011. Figure 16.2.

Running Subcuticular

The running subcuticular is a single suture taking horizontal bites of the dermal space of either wound edge, along the length of the wound and parallel to the epithelial surface (Figure 11.8). The running subcuticular suture is one of the most critical suturing techniques used in the pediatric population; excellent cosmetic outcomes absent of visible sutures can be achieved when performed correctly. Accurate suture placement, however, is challenging and time consuming. The lacerations most suited for subcuticular sutures are straight, clean, and noncontaminated wounds, with sharp nondevitalized wound edges that have been excised or trimmed such that the wound edges are fresh and straight (eg, a surgical incision). These sutures are therefore rarely used in the emergency setting. Running subcuticular sutures are most easily placed using handheld straight needles; curved sutures are also used but take more time to place.

Body positioning is important in maintaining a good suturing technique, and adjusting the needle loading angle from the traditional 90° to 135° can help execute this technique more effectively and efficiently.

Use of *absorbable sutures* (eg, Monocryl™ [Ethicon US, LLC]) avoids the need for removal and further reduces the possibility of "hatch marks"; however, slow-absorbing sutures may become visible or exposed with epidermal atrophy and increase the risk of a foreign-body reaction or infection. Use of undyed suture material can help improve cosmesis. Prolene (nonabsorbable monofilament) sutures are recommended. *Nonabsorbable sutures* can be removed by pulling on the free suture at one edge of the wound, and, therefore, keeping the length to a maximum can avoid suture snapping. Silk, however, is a braided natural suture and may break, be retained inside, and increase the risk of infection.

Technique for Running Subcuticular Sutures

- Body positioning is important in maintaining a good suturing technique, and adjusting the needle loading angle from the traditional 90° to 135° can help execute this technique more effectively and efficiently.

- To start, the needle is first inserted directly through the epidermis 2 to 5 mm from the apex from one corner of the wound and passed through to the dermis medial to the apex on the interior of the wound on one side.

- A bite is taken through the dermis of the opposite wound edge, and this process is repeated until the length of the wound is closed.

- Cosmetic outcomes are improved and overlapping edges are avoided if the needle trajectory is kept parallel to the incision line at a uniform depth, with spacing between bites. Although spacing between bites is dependent on needle size, a sufficient number should be taken to ensure skin closure and avoid crimping.

- The ends can be buried or free-form ones. Buried sutures avoid the need for removal but increase the chance of infections, and because the ends are not tracked, the epidermis may not be held under stress. This is especially the case with absorbable monofilament sutures. It is advised to use free-form ends and remove sutures roughly 7 days after placement using free-form sutures that can be removed from one end.

- Suture tails can be tacked using adhesive strips, tissue glue, or surgical tape, and this can help minimize skin irritation of sutures. Alternatively, a subcuticular suture can be secured using buried dermal knots at either end, or suture ends can be tied to each other as a bow over the wound if there is sufficient laxity; this approach can, however, risk torque-induced damage or damage from inadvertent pulling.

- Running subcuticular sutures can close the skin alone or may be further reinforced with interrupted sutures.

- *Nonabsorbable sutures* can be removed by pulling on the free suture at one edge of the wound while keeping maximum length to avoid suture snapping.

Steri-Strips

Steri-Strips are adhesive BAND-AID™ (Johnson & Johnson, US) that function to approximate the wound edges by holding the uppermost layers of the skin in place and thereby allow natural healing (Figure 11.9). Steri-Strips are now widely used in the place of sutures for shallow lacerations, because they can be placed by many health care personnel in many settings, including in the ED and in the clinic. Advantages include the minimal time for placement, local anesthetic, and, thus, the cost needed for placement of Steri-Strips, and the fact that patients do not need to return for removal makes them a convenient option. Furthermore, use of Steri-Strips requires minimal training and are thought to have similar cosmetic results, minimal histotoxicity, bacteriostatic properties, and good tensile strength compared to sutures.[22] Steri-Strips are also able to evenly distribute tension over wounds, do not leave suture marks, involve little

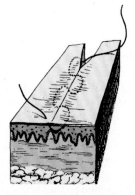

FIGURE 11.8. Running subcuticular suture. A difficult suturing technique with optimal cosmetic results because the suture leaves no entrance or exit marks. All sutures are placed at the same level. Absorbable sutures can be used. This suture is indicated in approximated wounds under minimal tension, with dead space eliminated. Reprinted with permission from Rayan GM, Akelman E. *The Hand: Anatomy, Examination, and Diagnosis.* Philadelphia, PA: Wolters Kluwer Health/Lippincott Williams & Wilkins; 2011. Figure 16.2.

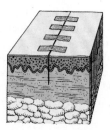

FIGURE 11.9. Adhesive skin tape. Reprinted with permission from Rayan GM, Akelman E. *The Hand: Anatomy, Examination, and Diagnosis.* Philadelphia, PA: Wolters Kluwer Health/Lippincott Williams & Wilkins; 2011. Figure 16.2.

reactions, and can protect against wound infection. They are less appropriate for wounds that are under significant tension or for wounds that are irregular, curved, moist, hairy, and have tissue laxity. They are unable to approximate deeper layers and can be peeled off by children—in which case, they may need to be protected with additional overlying bandages. The ideal lacerations for Steri-Strips are straight wounds under minimal tension. For deeper lacerations, Steri-Strips can be used in conjunction with deep dermal sutures. Steri-Strips can also be used to maintain approximation of wound edges if sutures have been removed prematurely.

Steri-Strip Application Technique

- Wounds are first prepared as described earlier (see Wound Preparation) and hair is removed.
- Steri-Strips are cut to the desired size; most closures can be achieved using ¼- × 3-in strips. Strips should be handled with gloved hands.
- After the skin has dried, the strips can be applied. Forceps can be used to peel the strips off the card. Half of the tape can be placed up until the wound edge, perpendicular in direction, and secured firmly with gentle pressure.
- The opposite wound edge is then opposed and held in position, whereas the remaining half of the tape is continued over this edge.
- The number of strips used should be sufficient to oppose, without totally covering, the length of the wound.
- Steri-Strips can be left in place because they are covered with adhesive bandages to prevent peeling or removal.
- Removal is after 2 weeks or longer by gentle pressure, unless the wound has separated prematurely, or the strips have become moist and soft.

Staples

Staples are the method of choice for pediatric scalp lacerations and can also be used for surgical or traumatic wounds. Staples are safe, inexpensive, and efficient. They can be inserted four times faster than sutures, and they can reduce wound-closure time and length of procedure.[23,24] Infection, patient acceptance, postoperative pain, and cosmetic outcomes do not significantly differ between staples and standard suturing techniques.[23,25] Staples are ideal for lacerations in the scalp because they are thought to cause less hair follicle injury than do sutures.[23] However, staples do not provide extensive hemostasis, and where bleeding is extensive, should be used in conjunction with deep dermal sutures. In addition, staples must be removed, which can be difficult in the uncooperative child. The wounds suitable for staples are straight with relatively sharp edges (Figure 11.10).

Staple Technique

- After wound debridement, the wound edges should be held everted, ideally by another individual. ***Failure to evert the edges is a common error.***
- The stapler should be positioned so that staple points are evenly positioned on either side of the wound edge. The staple machine should be gently placed on the skin to avoid too deep a placement, which can put the wound under pressure and risk ischemia.

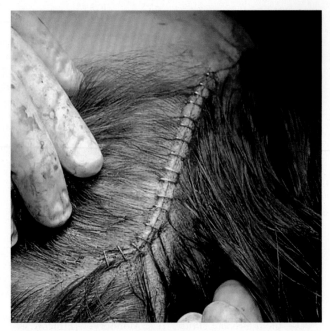

FIGURE 11.10. Staples are used in the scalp. Note the even spacing of the staples and the excellent eversion. Reprinted with permission from Chung KC, Thorne CH, Sinno S. *Operative Techniques in Facial Aesthetic Surgery.* Philadelphia, PA: Wolters Kluwer; 2020. Figure 25.6D.

- Squeezing of the staple trigger automatically advances the staple into the wound. Enough staples should be placed to ensure wound closure and eversion along the length of the wound.
- A dressing and antibiotic ointment can be placed over the laceration, which may be removed after 24 to 48 hours.
- Staples must be removed using a special device that bends the horizontal portion of the staple that traverses the laceration. Cosmetic outcomes and pain can result if staples are left in place for too long. The time to removal depends on the anatomic location.

Tissue Adhesives

Tissue adhesives are compounds or "glue" made from cyanoacrylates (eg, butylcyanoacrylates). Two products have been approved for clinical use in the United States; *N-2*-octylcyanoacrylate (DERMBOND™ Topical Skin Adhesive [Ethicon US, LLC] and *N*-buty-2-cyanoacrylate (INDERMIL® flexifuze™ Topical Tissue Adhesive [Vygon {UK} Ltd]). These products are often applied as liquid monomers that quickly polymerize over an approximated wound to keep approximated wound edges together as they dry. Tissue adhesives are quick to apply, involve minimal discomfort, and do not require any follow-up.[26,27] They can be used in conjunction with, but not in the place of, deep dermal sutures. No dressing is required unless for children who may pick at the glue. Most glues exposed on the surface of wounds naturally come off after 5 to 10 days, and internal glue biodegrades. Tissue adhesives result in no significant differences in short- and long-term cosmetic outcomes compared to standard wound closure,[28] but they give high patient satisfaction and comfort,[29] and are more cost effective.[30] Tissue adhesives are not appropriate for use over mobile areas. The number needed to harm (NNH) is 40—meaning in 40 wounds treated, 1 will dehisce using these products.[31] In addition, tissue adhesives are not recommended for use on animal bite repairs, stellate wounds, infected wounds, mucosal surfaces, or areas of high moisture or dense hair, such as the eyebrow and scalp.[28]

Applying Tissue Adhesive Procedure

- Glue must only be applied to wounds in which adequate hemostasis has been achieved.
- Glue should not typically be applied to hair-bearing surfaces such as the scalp or eyebrow because of the difficulty in removing it.
- To place tissue glue, wound edges are approximated using forceps, hands, or surgical tape and the adhesive is expelled through the applicator at the tip of the container directly onto the wound.
- Glue should be liberally placed along the length of the wound in an adequate amount to approximate 1 to 2 mm in thickness, extending 5 to 10 mm on both sides of the wound edge—the purple color of the glue assists in ensuring adequate coverage.
- Wound edges should be held approximated for at least 1 minute to allow for the glue to dry.
- Wounds can then be covered with a nonadhesive bandage.
- **Do not** apply occlusive dressings, ointments, or surgical tape to wounds closed with glue.
- During the first 4 days following closure, the tensile strength of wounds closed with adhesives is less than that of wounds closed with sutures, but after 1 week the tensile strengths are equivalent.

FOLLOW-UP AFTER SIMPLE WOUND REPAIR

Simple repairs can be covered with a nonadherent dressing, except for facial lacerations, to prevent wound desiccation and wound closure. Dressings should be changed daily. Wound care instructions should be provided and should direct the patient or caregiver to keep the wound dry for 24 to 36 hours; thereafter, the wound area should be gently washed with mild soap and water, while avoiding extensive submersion. Patients should be advised to avoid sunlight for 6 to 12 months to avoid hyperpigmentation, and they should be warned of the potential for infection, scarring, deep structure injury, or wound dehiscence—the complications of iatrogenic incision and laceration repair. Massage can help with the appearance of the scar. The ideal timing for formal scar revision is unknown and should be decided on a case-by-case basis. (See Chapter 90. Hypertrophic Scars and Contractures.)

REFERENCES

1. Kimberlin DW, Brady MT, Jackson MA, Long SS. *Red Book: 2015 Report of the Committee on Infectious Diseases.* Elk Grove Village, IL: American Academy of Pediatrics; 2015.
2. Connors K, Terndrup TE. Nasal versus oral midazolam for sedation of anxious children undergoing laceration repair. *Ann Emerg Med.* 1994;24:1074–1079.
3. Luhmann JD, Kennedy RM, Porter FL, Miller JP, Jaffe DM. A randomized clinical trial of continuous-flow nitrous oxide and midazolam for sedation of young children during laceration repair. *Ann Emerg Med.* 2001;37:20–27.
4. Taddio A, McMurtry CM. Psychological interventions for needle-related procedural pain and distress in children and adolescents. *Paediatr Child Health.* 2015;20:195.
5. Moore PA, Hersh EV. Local anesthetics: pharmacology and toxicity. *Dent Clin.* 2010;54:587–599.
6. Ilicki J. Safety of epinephrine in digital nerve blocks: a literature review. *J Emerg Med.* 2015;49:799–809.
7. Eidelman A, Weiss JM, Baldwin CL, Enu IK, McNicol ED, Carr DB. Topical anaesthetics for repair of dermal laceration. *Cochrane Database Syst Rev.* 2011;(6):CD005364. doi: 10.1002/14651858. CD005364.pub2.
8. Schilling CG, Bank DE, Borchert BA, Klatzko MD, Uden DL. Tetracaine, epinephrine (adrenalin), and cocaine (TAC) versus lidocaine, epinephrine, and tetracaine (LET) for anesthesia of lacerations in children. *Ann Emerg Med.* 1995;25:203–208.
9. Ernst AA, Marvez E, Nick TG, Chin E, Wood E, Gonzaba WT. Lidocaine adrenaline tetracaine gel versus tetracaine adrenaline cocaine gel for topical anesthesia in linear scalp and facial lacerations in children aged 5 to 17 years. *Pediatrics.* 1995;95: 255–258.
10. Rincon E, Baker RL, Iglesias AJ, Duarte AM. CNS toxicity after topical application of Emla cream on a toddler with molluscum contagiosum. *Pediatr Emerg Care.* 2000;16:252–254.
11. Parker JF, Vats A, Bauer G. EMLA toxicity after application for allergy skin testing. *Pediatrics.* 2004;113:410–411.
12. Touma S, Jackson JB. Lidocaine and prilocaine toxicity in a patient receiving treatment for mollusca contagiosa. *J Am Acad Dermatol.* 2001;44:399–400.
13. Yamamoto T, Sawada Y, Minatohara K. Methemoglobinemia and CNS toxicity after topical application of EMLA to a 4-year-old girl with molluscum contagiosum. *Pediatr Dermatol.* 2006;23:592–593.
14. Stevenson TR, Thacker JG, Rodeheaver GT, Bacchetta C, Edgerton MT, Edlich RF. Cleansing the traumatic wound by high pressure syringe irrigation. *JACEP.* 1976;5:17–21.
15. Gall TT, Monnet E. Evaluation of fluid pressures of common wound-flushing techniques. *Am J Vet Res.* 2010;71:1384–1386.
16. Fry DE. Pressure irrigation of surgical incisions and traumatic wounds. *Surg Infect (Larchmt).* 2017;18:424–430.
17. Wheeler C, Rodeheaver G, Thacker J, Edgerton M, Edilich R. Side-effects of high pressure irrigation. *Surg Gynecol Obstet.* 1976;143:775–778.
18. Hollander JE, Singer AJ. Laceration management. *Ann Emerg Med.* 1999;34:356–367.
19. Parell GJ, Becker GD. Comparison of absorbable with nonabsorbable sutures in closure of facial skin wounds. *Arch Facial Plast Surg.* 2003;5:488–490.
20. Moy R, Lee A, Zalka A. Commonly used suturing techniques in skin surgery. *Am Fam Phys.* 1991;44:1625–1634.
21. Zuber TJ. The mattress sutures: vertical, horizontal, and corner stitch. *Am Fam Phys.* 2002;66:2231–2236.
22. Bruns TB, Robinson BS, Smith RJ, et al. A new tissue adhesive for laceration repair in children. *J Pediatr.* 1998;132:1067–1070.
23. Kanegaye JT, Vance CW, Chan L, Schonfeld N. Comparison of skin stapling devices and standard sutures for pediatric scalp lacerations: a randomized study of cost and time benefits. *J Pediatr.* 1997;130:808–813.
24. Mattioli G, Castagnetti M, Repetto P, Leggio S, Jasonni V. Complications of mechanical suturing in pediatric patients. *J Pediatr Surg.* 2003;38:1051–1054.

25. Khan AN, Dayan PS, Miller S, Rosen M, Rubin DH. Cosmetic outcome of scalp wound closure with staples in the pediatric emergency department: a prospective, randomized trial. *Pediatr Emerg Care.* 2002;18:171–173.

26. Applebaum JS, Zalut T, Applebaum D. The use of tissue adhesion for traumatic laceration repair in the emergency department. *Ann Emerg Med.* 1993;22:1190–1192.

27. Quinn J, Drzewiecki A, Li MM, et al. A randomized, controlled trial comparing a tissue adhesive with suturing in the repair of pediatric facial lacerations. *Ann Emerg Med.* 1993;22:1130–1135.

28. Beam JW. Tissue adhesives for simple traumatic lacerations. *J Athl Train.* 2008;43:222–224.

29. Osmond MH, Quinn JV, Sutcliffe T, Jarmuske M, Klassen TP. A randomized, clinical trial comparing butylcyanoacrylate with octylcyanoacrylate in the management of selected pediatric facial lacerations. *Acad Emerg Med.* 1999;6:171–177.

30. Osmond MH, Klassen TP, Quinn JV. Economic comparison of a tissue adhesive and suturing in the repair of pediatric facial lacerations. *J Pediatr.* 1995;126:892–895.

31. Farion K, Osmond MH, Hartling L, et al. Tissue adhesives for traumatic lacerations in children and adults. *Cochrane Database Syst Rev.* 2002;(3):CD003326.

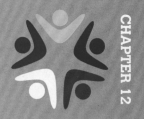
Complex Wound Repair

Sun Hsieh and Amanda A. Gosman

INTRODUCTION

The goal of any primary wound repair is reapproximation of the underlying soft tissue and overlying skin in a tension-free manner. When this can be accomplished in a relatively direct manner with straight line approximation of the defect and minimal manipulation of the surrounding tissue, it is considered a simple wound repair. However, the practitioner can often be faced with a wound in which a direct, straight line repair would be ill-advised owing to the suboptimal long-term aesthetic sequelae of such a repair, distortion of adjacent anatomic structures, or the dimensions and biomechanics of the wound that would preclude apposition of the wound margins in a tension-free setting.

Each wound presents a unique reconstructive challenge, with variability in the healing capacity and medical comorbidities of the patient, physical dimensions of the defect, anatomic location of the wound with respect to vital structures and aesthetic landmarks, and technical expertise of the practitioner. A set of core principles allows for a rational approach to each situation, which may be balanced with heuristic solutions that are gleaned from experience.

The vast majority of wounds benefit from a layered closure, placing greater stress on the dermal closure and minimizing epidermal tension. Optimal dermal approximation minimizes scarring, whereas a single-layer closure may produce a wide scar with higher risk of dehiscence. Wound eversion also minimizes scar width.

Wound closure can be stratified from less complex to more complex methods. Simple wounds such as lacerations without tissue loss may be repaired with primary closure, whereas smaller defects may be repaired via complex closures with wide undermining or elliptical closures. The local tissue flaps described in this chapter represent an increased level of complexity and are often sufficient for moderate defects. However, should these local flaps prove insufficient in providing an aesthetically acceptable closure, alternative adjacent tissue transfer flaps may be employed. Larger wounds may require further escalation up the reconstructive ladder, utilizing skin grafts, regional flaps, axial pattern flaps, and free tissue transfer.

The successful practitioner is able to objectively assess not only the wound at hand but also their own technical limitations and the limitations of a chosen technique.

This chapter describes the multiple factors that must be considered prior to the definitive closure of more complex wounds, the variety of surgical repairs that may be utilized, and the postoperative management. Each of these components must be optimized in order to achieve a successful outcome, resulting in an inconspicuous scar and minimal distortion of the surrounding tissue.

GENERAL CONSIDERATIONS

The appropriate treatment of a surgical defect begins with a comprehensive assessment of the wound and the patient. Optimization of the patient's surgical risk and wound healing ability should be considered prior to any future elective procedures and to whatever extent is possible in an acute setting. Ideal wound healing relies on robust tissue perfusion such that the wound margin may receive adequate oxygenation and the appropriate growth factors to promote each phase of healing. A variety of factors may impair vascular supply to a wound, including active tobacco smoking status, vascular disease, and other medical comorbidities. Tobacco smoking remains one of the most common and controllable risk factors. Nicotine has been associated with a concentration-dependent upregulation of the norepinephrine vasoconstriction pathway. This not only impairs the tissue perfusion at the wound but also limits the vasorelaxation induced by substances such as nitroglycerin. Patients should be counseled on smoking cessation and avoidance of secondhand smoke for at least 6 weeks prior to any surgical intervention. Beyond suboptimal healing, smoking may also increase the risk for developing a postsurgical wound infection.

Patients with significant medical comorbidities such as diabetes mellitus and peripheral vascular disease may also experience decreased tissue perfusion and increased wound healing complications. Medical optimization may be pursued prior to surgical intervention, should time allow. Other factors that may contribute to impaired wound healing include active infections, steroid medications, renal disease, and immunodeficiencies. An in-depth discussion concerning the mechanisms of wound healing and the measures that may be taken to minimize wound healing complications is beyond the scope of this chapter, though the reader is encourage to become familiar with these topics.

Equipment Needed

- Marking pen
- Measuring ruler
- 10-mL syringe
- 25-gauge injection needle
- 18-gauge drawing needle
- Local anesthesia: lidocaine with epinephrine or bupivacaine with epinephrine
- #15 blade or #10 blade scalpel
- Double-hook skin retractors of varying widths
- Electrocautery
- Tenotomy or facelift scissors
- Dermal sutures: 3-0, 4-0, 5-0 Vicryl™ (Ethicon US, LLC) and 3-0, 4-0, 5-0 Monocryl™ (Ethicon US, LLC)
- Epidermal sutures: 5-0, 6-0 fast-dissolving gut, 4-0, 5-0, 6-0 nylon, 5-0, 6-0 Prolene™ (Ethicon US, LLC)
- Needle driver
- Adson forceps, Bishop forceps, or 0.5 mm forceps
- Suture scissors
- ½ or ¼ in Steri-Strips

GENERAL SURGICAL TECHNIQUE

The most crucial component of any complex closure is the surgical marking. Initial assessment of a wound includes the lengths of its dominant axes and its depth. Consideration should

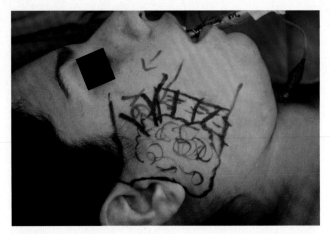

FIGURE 12.1. Operative markings on a patient in the case of a well-planned preauricular incision with a possible submandibular extension; the dashed lines represent the region of the planned skin flap elevation. Reprinted with permission from Chung KC, Gosain AK. *Operative Techniques in Pediatric Plastic and Reconstructive Surgery*. Philadelphia, PA: Wolters Kluwer; 2020. Figure 49.1.

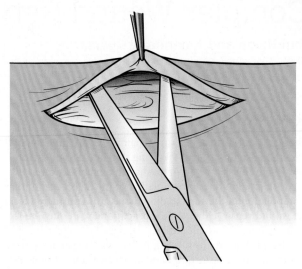

FIGURE 12.2. Blunt tenotomy dissection to circumferentially elevate and undermine the skin flaps about the wound to minimize tension on closure.

then be given to neighboring defining structures. A successful closure approximates the wound edges with minimal tension, avoids distortion of adjacent anatomy, and minimizes scarring. The majority of deliberation then should be directed toward the design and marking of the optimal closure pattern, whether it be by wide undermining, elliptical closures, or local tissue flaps (Figure 12.1). There exists no perfect solution for each case; therefore, what is deemed "best" is dependent on the practitioner's personal experience, aesthetic judgment, and technical limitations.

WIDE UNDERMINING

At times, adjacent soft-tissue attachments may preclude adequate advancement of opposing edges in a tension-free manner. Although it may be technically possible to primarily close the defect without further manipulation, excess tension on the final incision predisposes to wide scarring that the patient may find aesthetically unacceptable. Additionally, the amount of force the sutures exert on the tissue may be sufficient to cause ischemia at the wound edge, which increases the risk of wound dehiscence and infection. One method of relieving such tension is through wide undermining of the adjacent tissue.

After infiltration of local anesthetic with epinephrine, a double-hook retractor is placed on one skin edge, and a vertical retraction force is applied orthogonal to the plane of the underlying wound bed. A tenotomy or facelift scissor is used to sharply dissect the skin flap in the superficial subcutaneous plane (Figure 12.2).

Sharp dissection is preferable because it is less traumatic than blunt dissection. However, blunt dissection by spreading vertically in the superficial subcutaneous plane, deep to the subdermal plexus, can also be effective for mobilizing the skin, especially in areas where there are critical nerves and vessels in the subcutaneous plane. The direction of the tenotomy scissor tips should be parallel to the handle of the double-hook retractor.

The tissue separation may be achieved with both sharp dissection and blunt spreading. Septated attachments between the dermis and the underlying fat may be sharply incised with

scissors or electrocautery. This is completed in a circumferential manner until the entire wound perimeter can be elevated off its underlying subcutaneous base, as shown in Figure 12.2.

Each wound edge may be pulled toward the opposite side with opposing double-hook traction or Adson forceps. If the edges are opposable with minimal tension, then wound closure may proceed; however, if a significant amount of tension remains, then further undermining in the direction orthogonal to the line of closure at the points of maximal tension should be performed.

In addition to relieving tissue stress on closure, wide undermining also serves to minimize bunching of the tissue at the wound margin. Colloquially referred to as "dog-ears," this puckering of the tissue occurs when the preclosure arc length of the wound edge grossly exceeds the straight line length of the eventual closure. Given that soft tissue has a finite distensibility, wide undermining serves to distribute the length discrepancy across a larger area, which may make it less conspicuous.

One must remain cognizant of adjacent anatomic structures and landmarks. Excessive undermining may obliterate anatomic contours, and approximation of wound edges in such a setting may also distort adjacent anatomy. Inability to repair a wound by direct approximation of the edges with wide circumferential undermining may indicate that a local flap should be pursued.

LAYERED CLOSURE

A multilayered closure is often beneficial not only to relieve tension on the epidermal closure but also to optimize scarring. At least two layers should be addressed separately. A series of interrupted buried dermal sutures serves best to align the dermis and evert the wound edge. A second layer of epidermal sutures further aligns the epidermis. In a two-layered closure, the dermis should assume the burden of any residual wound tension. A single-layered closure increases the risk of wound dehiscence should sutures be removed in less than 1 week on the face or 2 weeks on the body as generally recommended. Sutures that remain longer than the recommended duration to compensate for this may, in turn, increase the risk of "train-tracking" or scarring and epithelialization of the suture path through the tissue. Appropriate placement of buried dermal stitches requires meticulous technique. In basic terms, buried sutures have their knots placed beneath the suture loop, minimizing risk of postoperative extrusion, presuming that the suture is placed at an appropriate depth with sufficient intervening soft tissue between the suture and the external environment. For a buried suture, the sequence of needle passes into the tissue is *deep-superficial-superficial-deep*. On the initial side of the wound, the needle enters in a deeper plane and exits in a more superficial dermal layer. The needle then passes onto the opposing wound edge where it enters superficially at exactly the same dermal depth and then exits deeper in the tissue at the same level as the initial entrance point on the original wound edge (Figure 12.3).

There are two divergent schools of thought regarding orientation of the needle path within the tissue. Some advocate for a purely orthogonal passage of the needle with respect to the external plane of the wound, such that, when cinched, the suture loop possesses a perfectly vertical orientation with respect to the skin. This minimizes collateral distortion by avoiding inadvertent capture of adjacent tissue, which, when performed asymmetrically, may produce an uneven wound edge with suboptimal aesthetics.

In contrast, some advocate for an oblique orientation of the needle path such that a single suture loop may function as both a semi-vertical and semi-horizontal mattress stitch. When performed precisely and in a symmetric manner, this may allow for a more efficient coaptation of the wound edge. Once the suture is secured, the loop would lie at a 45-degree orientation to the skin surface, as opposed to a vertical orientation. One key to minimizing adjacent tissue distortion is making symmetric needle passes through the opposing wound edges such that one side of the horizontal mattress is not over-recruiting tissue versus the other.

Eversion of the wound edge on final closure optimizes eventual scarring by maximizing interdermal contact that accelerates

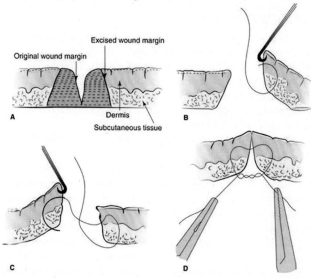

FIGURE 12.3. Diagram of buried dermal suture placement. A, Excisional debridement of chronic wound edges to expose fresh margins which may heal optimally. B, Passage of the suture through the first wound edge, entering deep and exiting superficially. C, Passage of the suture through the second wound edge, entering superficially and exiting deep. Note how the depth of each suture passage mirrors the opposing edge, which optimizes epidermal alignment. D, The final knot is placed deep to the suture loop, minimizing risk of extrusion. Reprinted with permission from Levine MD. *The Washington Manual of Emergency Medicine*. Philadelphia, PA: Wolters Kluwer; 2018. Figure 132-1A-D.

wound healing. A secondary benefit of edge eversion is the tissue redundancy it provides, which minimizes widening of the scar once the wound inevitably flattens with time. With buried dermal sutures, eversion may be maximized by placing the most superficial point of the suture loop lateral to the wound edge; therefore, each of the two superficial needle passes into the wound edge should ultimately be slightly deeper than this lateral, most superficial point. When the suture is tightened, this configuration forces all tissue superficial to the superficial part of the loop to be pushed upward, leading to eversion and tissue redundancy.

ELLIPTICAL CLOSURE

When faced with a circular wound, the geometry of the wound edge does not permit direct straight line closure without the formation of dog-ears. The severity of the dog-ear is proportional to the length discrepancy between the intended line of closure and the original wound arc length. A decision must be made between maintaining the native wound closure length with subsequent dog-earing versus lengthening the scar in order to minimize tissue bunching. The latter choice may result in greater aesthetic outcome, presuming strategic orientation of the closure along Langer's line or relaxed skin tension lines.

Circular-type wounds may then be converted into elliptical "football"-shaped wounds. Converging lines tangent to the wound edge may be drawn at either end to create a wound with a length-to-width ratio of at least 3:1. The angle of the converging tangents should also be less than 45 degrees to minimize the risk of dog-ear formation. This is demonstrated in Figure 12.4A and B. One may choose to begin approximation of the wound starting centrally and excise the dog-ears in a tailor-tacking manner or pre-excise the dog-ears and reapproximate the wound in a standard manner. Figure 12.5 demonstrates one technique of dog-ear excision in which the tissue redundancy is tented and excised. This may be performed with scalpel or scissor excision.

LOCAL TISSUE FLAP

A flap is a piece of tissue with its own blood supply. Local manipulation and detachment of a flap from its neighboring tissue relies on a sufficient, preserved blood supply in order to heal; otherwise, tissue deoxygenation and the lack of growth factors will lead to inevitable necrosis. Historically, local tissue flaps have been categorized based on their method of movement. Advancement, rotation, transposition, and island flaps have been well described in the literature. Although a detailed discussion of each is beyond the scope of this chapter, two pertinent examples are described in the subsequent sections.

RHOMBOID FLAP

When the wound dimension and location preclude apposition of the opposing edges in a direction orthogonal to the major axis, local transposition flaps may be used to reorient the direction of the scar. This not only preserves orientation of nearby structures but also may modify the scar such that future contracture deformities are minimized.

Design of a rhomboid flap begins with outlining of the wound margin. A tangential rhomboid is designed to closely circumscribe the wound. Geometrically, a rhomboid is defined as a quadrilateral of four equal lengths. Equi-length limbs outwardly extending from each vertex are drawn, bisecting each external vertex angle. Equi-length extensions at each of these limbs may be drawn, forming a 60-degree angle in either direction. Eight

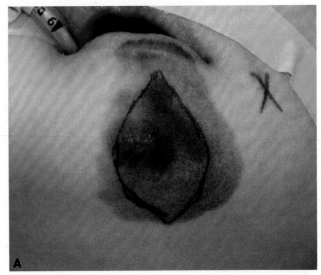

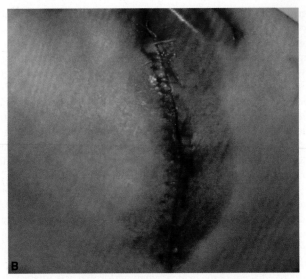

FIGURE 12.4. A, Design of an elliptical partial excision of a sublabial congenital nevus. The acuity of each vertex of the ellipse is designed to minimize bunching at each end. B, Final closure of elliptical excision with minimal tissue bunching. A separate buried dermal layer of sutures was placed prior to the simple running epidermal stitch.

flaps may potentially be drawn from this method. At this point, careful consideration should be given to which rhomboid flap to use. This decision may hinge on the anticipated distortion of nearby tissue with each respective flap in addition to the degree of tissue redundancy in the direction of the flap, the latter minimizing final wound tension. A diagrammatic illustration of the multiple variants of the rhomboid flap is shown in Figure 12.6.

Once the flap design is confirmed, local anesthesia is infiltrated in the form of either lidocaine or bupivacaine with epinephrine. Several minutes may elapse to allow vasoconstriction. The wound edge is freshened with a #15 blade scalpel. The flap marking is then incised with a #15 blade scalpel full thickness through the dermis until the superficial subcutaneous plane

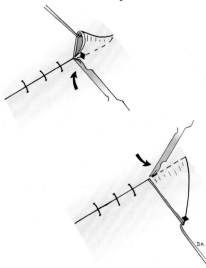

FIGURE 12.5. One technique of dog-ear excision. Note that there exist several methods of minimizing dog-ear deformity (arrows indicates the placement of the scalpel blade and the direction of the incision). Reprinted with permission from Hall JC, Hall BJ. *Sauer's Manual of Skin Diseases.* 11th ed. Philadelphia, PA: Wolters Kluwer; 2017. Figure 6-9.

is visible. The flap is then elevated with gentle double-hook traction. Elevation may be performed with tenotomy scissors, scalpel blade, or electrocautery. Periodically, the flap may be transposed onto the original wound to check for closure tension. Once the appropriate tension is achieved, flap elevation is completed. Wound closure then commences with a series of buried dermal sutures followed by simple interrupted epithelial sutures. Suture choice may be deferred to the practitioner.

BILOBED FLAP

At times, a single transposition flap may produce an untoward outcome, resulting in pincushioning of the rotation point and adjacent tissue distortion. This effect may be obviated by diffusing the burden of the rotation about two transposition flaps. Bilobed flaps are often used for nasal tip defects less than 1.5 cm in diameter; however, their utility may be generalized toward a broad range of soft-tissue defects (Figure 12.7).

The flap design first begins with identification of the soft-tissue defect. The nearby tissue is examined for areas of laxity and redundancy. This orients the source of the intended flap tissue. A pivot point, or center of rotation, is determined, which centralizes the arc of rotation. Typical rotation angles from the distal-most flap to the wound are approximately 100 to 115 degrees.

The first flap is designed immediately adjacent to the defect. The distance between the pivot point and the center of the wound defines the radius of curvature (R). The distance between the pivot point and the distal-most edge of the wound defines the flap height (H). An elliptical primary donor flap is designed with distal tip-to-pivot point distance equal to H, width equal to two-thirds of the wound width (W), and tangent point to the original wound at the radius of curvature.

A secondary donor triangular flap is designed with long axis approximately 45 to 60 degrees rotated from the primary elliptical flap. The base of this triangular flap rests at the radius of curvature, the width of the flap measures one-half the width of the primary elliptical flap, and the height of the flap is approximately 125% to 133% of H. Care must be taken to maintain a

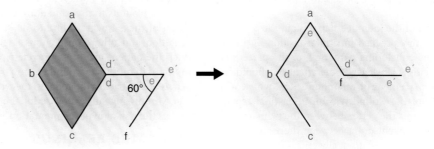

A. Limberg flap

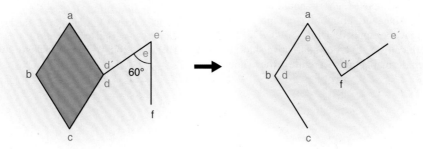

B. Modifications by Dufourmentel

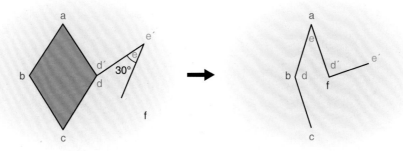

C. Webster 30° modification

FIGURE 12.6. Diagram of multiple variants of the rhomboid flap. Each remains an adjacent tissue transposition flap with variability in the angle of the back-cut. A, Limberg flap. B, Modifications by Dufourmentel. C, Webster 30-degree modification.

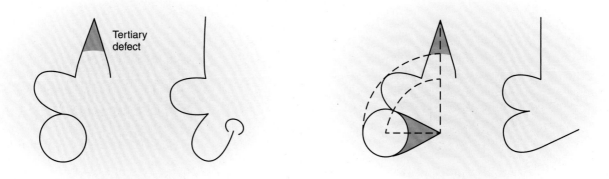

A   B

FIGURE 12.7. Diagram of a bilobed flap design. Note the change in the center of curvature between A and B versions and how the latter minimizes pin cushioning of the tissue at the rotation point. A, Bilobed flap: traditional design. B, Modifications described by Zitelli.

wide enough base at the pivot point to allow tissue perfusion and venous drainage.

Upon confirmation of the intended flap design, the remainder of the procedure may proceed in similar fashion as previously described in the concluding paragraph of the preceding "Rhomboid Flap" section. However, some attention should be devoted towards the placement of the initial stitch, which will assume the majority of the wound tension upon final repair. The first key stitch secures the vertex between the primary and secondary flaps to the tangent point between the wound edge and primary flap. As the flaps are inset, any excess tissue may be trimmed with tenotomy scissors.

POSTOPERATIVE CONSIDERATIONS

Once wound closure has completed, effort should be directed toward minimizing scarring and promoting optimal wound healing. Steri-Strips may be applied. DERMABOND™ Topical Skin Adhesive (Ethicon US, LLC) or alternative skin glue may also be used. If epidermal sutures were used, they should be removed within 1 week for facial wounds and 2 weeks for nonfacial wounds to prevent suture tract marks and epithelialization of these tracts. Failure to do so may lead to hyperpigmentation and other conspicuous stigmata of the procedure, which the patient may not appreciate. Other methods may be employed to minimize wound tension during the healing phase, such as Steri-Strips orthogonal to the wound axis to offload tension. Minimizing sun exposure for the first postoperative year reduces the risk of hyperpigmentation.

SUGGESTED READINGS

Hallock GG, Morris SF. Skin grafts and local flaps. *Plast Reconstr Surg.* 2011;127(1):5e–22e.

Maciel-Miranda A, Morris SF, Hallock GG. Local flaps, including pedicled perforator flaps: anatomy, technique, and applications. *Plast Reconstr Surg.* 2013;131(6):896e–911e.

Taylor IG, Corlett RJ, Ashton MW. The blood supply of the skin and skin flaps. In: *Grabb and Smith's Plastic Surgery.* 7th ed. Baltimore, MA: Lippincott, Williams & Wilkins; 2013:29–42.

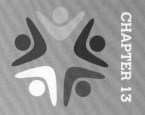
Special Site Surgery

Samuel H. Lance and Amanda A. Gosman

INTRODUCTION

This chapter reviews specialized surgical sites in the pediatric patient, including the scalp, face and head, ear, hand and upper extremity and nail bed, external genitalia, perianal region, and foot. These anatomic locations require specific consideration during preoperative planning and operative execution. High-quality surgical care requires a focused assessment of anatomic location and tissue characteristics prior to intervention. These specialized surgical sites also require consideration of longitudinal pediatric growth and, at times, creativity in preserving the surgical sites postoperatively. A clear understanding of anatomic differences for each location is paramount to achieving surgical success. Also provided are surgical tenets to consider prior to intervention and brief surgical pearls for perioperative and postoperative management.

Careful approach to these sites and appropriate patient education can minimize postoperative morbidity and maximize aesthetic and functional outcomes.

SPECIAL CONSIDERATIONS IN PEDIATRICS

Pediatric Anatomic Growth

Unlike the adult population, the pediatric population presents the unique dynamic of future growth potential; consequently, the pediatric surgeon must consider that the following surgical sites also possess unique functional and anatomic growth potential. The pediatric provider is well served to enhance his or her knowledge of pediatric growth patterns and timing to final adult growth. Elective interventions can often be delayed until adequate growth is achieved, thus lessening growth disturbance with intervention. If urgent or semi-urgent intervention is indicated, measures should be taken to preserve supporting structures and growth centers while minimizing local tissue injury, thereby reducing distortion due to cicatricial formation. Failure to recognize restrictions or alterations in growth potential for these specialized surgical sites can lead to significant future morbidity and anatomic distortion following surgical intervention.

Patient Maturity

Assessment of a pediatric patient's maturity will help guide the surgeon to the most successful outcome. Patient maturity can influence patient involvement with decision-making, anesthetic choices, surgical management, and postoperative care. The mature patient can and should be included during the decision to proceed with surgical intervention (see Chapter 2. Ethical Dilemmas). Active participation of the mature patient will improve overall patient satisfaction and compliance with perioperative care. When addressing surgical care of the immature patient, the surgeon should consider the future repercussions of surgical outcomes once the patient will have reached maturity. The perspective of future repercussions should be conveyed to the parent or guardian and decisions made jointly between parent and provider, bearing the patient's best interest in mind.

From the perspective of surgical planning, maturity of the patient will primarily dictate the appropriate setting in which to perform an intervention. Interventions performed entirely under local anesthesia require sufficient patient maturity, allowing the patient to tolerate the discomfort of local anesthetic infiltration. Even with adequate local anesthesia, patient anxiety and emotional discomfort can negatively impact patient compliance during a surgical intervention. Poor patient cooperation during a procedure can significantly increase the risk of iatrogenic injury to both patient and operator. Further risk of inadequate execution because of patient movement or anxiety during the procedure may lead to poor patient outcomes and suboptimal results. Thus, general anesthesia or sedation should be considered for patients with less than full maturity and for procedures in critical anatomic locations, such as the face or periorbital areas.

Patient maturity can also impact intraoperative and postoperative planning when considering protection of the surgical site and maintenance of surgical site dressing integrity. The pediatric provider should select surgical approaches and postoperative dressings tailored to the needs of each patient. Ease of surgical site care and patient comfort should be balanced with the need to maintain surgical site integrity, often with more aggressive approaches than utilized in the adult population.

Aesthetic Considerations and Scarring

Many of the specialized surgical sites addressed herein are considered unique, given their aesthetic priority. The approaches used for surgical interventions at these sites should reflect an understanding of future scarring and the potential distortion of aesthetic subunits (see Chapter 9. Anatomy and Superficial Landmarks of the Head and Neck).

Surgical scars should be designed to optimize concealment, not only in a child's clothing but also in future adult clothing. Furthermore, scars should be designed to ultimately be incorporated into relaxed skin tension lines or animation folds[1] (see Figure 9.5). Although animation folds are not readily apparent in pediatric patients, assessment and marking of tissue folds during animation or activity will help identify animation folds within the skin, anticipating more discernible development of these skin folds with time.

Anatomic distortions or visible scarring can negatively impact social interactions and social development of a pediatric patient.[2] Thus, every effort should be made to maximize aesthetic outcomes whenever possible. The surgeon should consider his or her limitations and refer to specialists as appropriate to maximize patient aesthetic outcomes when addressing these special sites.

Functional Considerations

Finally, when addressing special surgical sites, it is important to maintain functionality for both social interactions and with dynamic activity. Maintenance of function in the growing child or adolescent should be considered with any intervention in a special surgical site because limitations in function can hinder social progress, delay motor skills, or result in the habitual development of poor motor compensations. Special attention to function is critical when addressing interventions near or directly overlying a joint in the hands, feet, or extremities; near the face; or surrounding the sexual organs. The dynamics of each location should be considered during patient counseling, operative planning, closure choice, and postoperative management. Aggressive physical or occupational therapy should be considered early in the postoperative period to ensure preservation of function whenever possible.

SURGICAL INTERVENTIONS OF THE SCALP

Age and Growth Considerations of the Scalp

Most surgical interventions of the scalp can be safely performed at any age, because growth of the scalp is unlikely to be impaired by minor surgical intervention. More significant surgical interventions resulting in increased tension of closure or pressure to the underlying cranium should be delayed until closure of the fontanelles. Fontanelle closure usually occurs by 18 months of age with some variability between patients.[3] Plagiocephaly due to external pressure results in the distortion of the underlying, mobile cranial bones in the early months of life. Fontanelle closure allows for stability of the cranial bones and can avoid iatrogenic cranial plagiocephaly.

The scalp, while forgiving from a surgical healing perspective, is intrinsically difficult to maintain surgical dressings following operative intervention in the pediatric population. It is paramount to apply surgical dressings, which will be difficult for a child to remove while at the same time preventing airway restrictions and allowing mobility of the mandible. Such dressings can be fashioned from surgical netting or light gauze and can incorporate a chin strap to prevent removal. Care must also be taken to consider postoperative swelling when applying circumferential head dressings. Sufficient padding should be used under any circumferential dressing and care taken to ensure minimal compression during application. Circumferential dressings should only use light materials without elastics or rigidity.

Patient maturity and cooperation should be considered when selecting the method of anesthesia for procedures of the scalp. Routine scalp interventions can safely be performed under local anesthesia in the mature patient.[4] The surgeon should, however, consider the use of a general anesthetic when addressing large posterior scalp lesions as patients often become uncomfortable during prolonged periods in the prone position.

Aesthetic Considerations of the Scalp

Scarring is relatively well tolerated within the hair-bearing areas of the scalp because scars are typically hidden by the overlying hair. Although scalp hair can disguise scars, scar alopecia is an inevitable consequence of surgical interventions to the scalp. When discussing potential scarring within the scalp, the surgeon must inform parents and patients of scar alopecia as this should be considered a permanent result of interventions to the hair-bearing skin. Despite the best efforts of follicular hair grafting into sites of scar alopecia, scar alopecia should be recognized as a permanent and potentially disfiguring result of scarring within the scalp. The surgeon should also consider and discuss the visibility of scalp scars in the male patient because future male pattern baldness may increase the prominence of such scars during adulthood. Unlike most sites of skin closure, a dog-ear is well tolerated in the scalp and will usually resolve with time. The authors recommend that lesion excision in this area be localized to just the margin around the lesion, without excising the dog-ear, to minimize the length of the scar and the resultant scar alopecia.

Functional Considerations of the Scalp

The functionality of the scalp is primarily social because of its large hair-bearing surface. Sensory changes can present some patient discomfort but rarely result in significant functional deficits. Nevertheless, exposed areas of alopecia in large portions of the scalp can present a higher risk of sun exposure. Postoperative sun protection should be addressed with the patient and family in advance of and following surgery.

Surgical Considerations of the Scalp

Total anesthesia of the scalp can be obtained with directed injection into the supratrochlear and supraorbital nerves anteriorly, the auriculotemporal and lesser occipital nerves laterally, and the greater occipital nerves posteriorly.[4] Few indications, though, require total scalp anesthesia. Local anesthesia via field infiltration alone is often sufficient for minor interventions. Local infiltration using epinephrine-containing solutions has the additional benefit of improving local vasoconstriction and further decreasing blood loss during intervention.

The scalp maintains a robust blood supply emanating from 10 primary named vascular bundles, including the paired occipital, posterior auricular, superficial temporal, supraorbital, and supratrochlear vessels.[5] This highly collateralized blood supply allows for rapid healing and infection resistance in the scalp but can lead to frustrating bleeding during surgical intervention. Uncontrolled blood loss during scalp intervention can be significant and lead to continued postoperative blood loss if not appropriately addressed. Liberal use of local anesthetic containing epinephrine should be considered for both intraoperative pain control and minimization of blood loss. Maximum vasoconstriction will vary with differing concentrations of epinephrine used in local anesthetic solutions and site of injection.[6] However, a recommended duration of 15 to 30 minutes should be allowed for maximization of in situ vasoconstriction from epinephrine-containing solutions, thus minimizing blood loss.

Single-layer closures can be performed within the scalp. However, single-layered closures are considered inferior to a multilayer closure where a multilayered closure is possible. The multilayered closure should begin with the galea, also known as the aponeurosis of the frontalis muscle. This layer should be closed using absorbable suture (see Chapter 8. Sutures). Appropriate closure of this layer serves to minimize tension on the overlying skin closure, further improving scar outcomes. Care should be taken to avoid excessive tension when closing the hair-bearing cutaneous layer because such tension can produce ischemia of the hair follicles, leading to further alopecia. Staples can provide a safe and reliable closure to the superficial layers of the scalp. When used in a multilayered closure, staples can be removed at 1 to 2 weeks following surgery, further improving scar appearance.

SURGICAL PROCEDURES OF THE FACE AND NECK

Age and Growth Considerations

Cranial and upper facial growth reaches approximately 85% of final adult growth by 6 to 10 years of age.[7] However, maxillary and mandibular growth continues throughout puberty until approximately age 15 to 16 years in females and 17 to 19 years in males.[8] Although skin excisions are unlikely to influence the underlying skeletal growth, one must consider changes in scar location as the child ages. As mentioned previously, attempts should be made to locate facial scars within relaxed skin tension lines and in future animation folds surrounding the eyelids, perioral, and forehead regions.

Aesthetic Considerations of the Face and Neck

The face is by far the most important structure when addressing the aesthetics of social interaction. When the surgeon encounters patients or families who appear fixated on achieving unrealistic aesthetic outcomes, it is prudent for the surgeon to consider his or her expertise and provide referral to a second opinion as a means of improving patient education in regard to reasonable aesthetic outcomes.[9] The aesthetic subunits of the face provide the surgeon with a useful pattern of facial subdivision and can help direct operative approaches and reconstructive planning (see Figure 9.5A. Facial aesthetic subunits).[10] Care should be taken to avoid distorting or defacing adjacent subunits of the face during intervention.

Functional Considerations of the Face and Neck

Even small scars in the face can distort surrounding structures or present as animation deformities when tethered to the underlying mimetic muscles. Scar atrophy or hypertrophy can further restrict symmetric facial movement and lead to unsightly appearing scars. Scar evolution and potential functional distortions should be addressed with the patient and family prior to facial interventions. No guarantee of final aesthetic outcome should be given prior to intervention as it is impossible to fully predict the natural course of scar healing for each patient. Postoperative care should incorporate scar massage and scar reduction strategies to improve mobility and minimize adhesions of the cutaneous layers with subcutaneous layers (see Chapter 90. Hypertrophic Scars and Contractures).

Surgical Considerations of the Face and Neck

The subcutaneous fatty layers of the face are considerably thinner in pediatric patients when compared to adults. This is most notable within the periorbital, nasal, and temple regions. Beneath the thin layer of subcutaneous fat lay branches of the facial nerve. Understanding the anatomic locations of these superficial branches is critical to avoiding potentially devastating complications during excisions of the facial skin. Within the preauricular tissues, the facial nerve root proceeds in a superficial plane without an intraparotid course in the pediatric patient.[11] This anatomic difference should be thoroughly considered before intervention in the preauricular tissues because damage to the facial nerve root can be a devastating complication (see Figure 9.9). Local anesthesia will inevitably result in temporary loss of nerve function, further masking identification of the nerve branches even in the setting of nerve monitoring. Given the delicate nature of facial interventions in proximity to these vital structures, one should strongly consider a general anesthetic for interventions in these anatomic locations to maximize surgical control and minimize the risk of unwanted intraoperative movement.

EAR

Age and Growth Considerations of the Ear

Growth patterns of the adolescent ear are important when addressing surgical interventions prior to completion of pubertal growth. The adolescent ear reaches approximately 80% of its final growth by age 3 to 4 years.[12] Interventions prior to this age should consider the possibility of growth disturbance when influencing the underlying cartilage structure of the external ear. Although adolescent ear cartilage continues to grow following surgical transection, one must bear in mind the restrictive effects of scar formation to the developing ear. Of note, prior to 2 months of age, circulating maternal estrogens allow for increased playability and molding capability of the neonatal ear.[13] Thus, care should be taken to avoid elective ear interventions prior to 2 months of age and preferably after 4 years of age to minimize potential growth disturbance.

Age and patient cooperation also play a critical part in postoperative recovery. Subcutaneous hematoma formation can result in the development of destructive scaring to the ear identified as the cauliflower-ear deformity with lasting consequences.[14] It is paramount to apply sufficient compression preventing postoperative subcutaneous hematoma formation while minimizing the risk of pressure necrosis. Such a dressing is likely to require a circumferential band securing it around the head. Placement of a secure head wrap following surgery is highly recommended for the immature patient who is unable to cooperate with appropriate postoperative one care. The mature patient may be managed with a removable or replaceable head dressing as indicated.

Aesthetic Considerations of the Ear

The external ear is a critical element of the facial aesthetics (Figure 13.1). It is a three-dimensional structure visible from multiple angles at conversation distance. On frontal view, the extra ear and tragal structures are comparatively evaluated from one side to the other. Ear protrusion and position are readily visible to the patient with differences easily noted by both

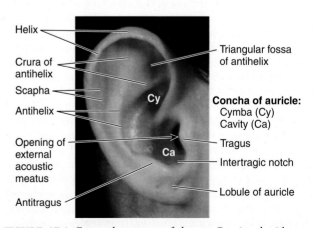

Helix

Crura of antihelix

Scapha

Antihelix

Opening of external acoustic meatus

Antitragus

Triangular fossa of antihelix

Concha of auricle:
Cymba (Cy)
Cavity (Ca)

Tragus

Intertragic notch

Lobule of auricle

Cy

Ca

FIGURE 13.1. External anatomy of the ear. Reprinted with permission from Moore KL, Dalley AF, Agur AMR. *Clinically Oriented Anatomy.* 7th ed. Philadelphia, PA: Wolters Kluwer Health/Lippincott Williams & Wilkins; 2014:967. Figure 7.110.

patient and observer. On the lateral view, the normal anatomic structure, size, and formation of the ear are evaluated. Although less comparison is noted from the lateral view, the subtleties of the underlying cartilaginous framework and thin overlying skin provide a unique geography to the normal ear. This intricate combination of thin skin and underlying cartilage is critical to maintaining normal anatomic configuration and aesthetic appearance of the external ear.[15] Deformities of the external ear have further been shown to significantly impact adolescent psychosocial development.[16] Surgical interventions to the ear should seek to preserve the normal anatomic structure and minimize scarring to both the underlying cartilage framework and overlying skin, thus minimizing distortion of the aesthetic structure.

Functional Considerations of the Ear

The external ear also provides significant functional structure to the face. Changes to the anatomic configuration of the external ear can influence hearing acuity and localization of sound.[12] The normal external ear also provides the structural support for hearing aids and eyeglasses. Changes to the structure of the ear can make use of these devices more difficult. Furthermore, abnormal anatomic structure of the external ear can interfere with the use of protective head equipment, such as helmets.

Surgical Considerations of the Ear

The consistent anatomy of innervation to the external ear makes this structure a prime candidate for regional anesthetic blocks.[4] Sensory innervation to the ear is provided by three major branches, including the auriculotemporal nerve anteriorly, the great auricular nerve from the inferior aspect, and the lesser occipital nerve entering in the posterior aspect of the ear. Regional anesthesia can be achieved using a circumferential ring block focused on directed infiltration at the entry site of the three nerves noted earlier. It is encouraged to use local anesthetic containing epinephrine because this improves surgical visibility and increases the duration of local anesthesia. Anecdotally, the use of epinephrine in the ear has been met with concern. In response to these concerns, several studies have evaluated the safety and efficacy of local anesthetics containing epinephrine without evidence of adverse outcomes.[17]

The blood supply to the external ear also demonstrates important anatomic configurations. The majority of vascularity to the external ear is provided through perforating branches from the posterior auricular artery posteriorly and the superficial temporal artery anteriorly. The rich vascular network of the external ear ensures a strong viability of local flaps for reconstruction of ear defects. With this prominent vascularity, however, comes the risk of postoperative bleeding. Procedures of the ear that require elevation of the skin from the underlying cartilage of the ear increase the risk of bleeding below the skin of the external ear, resulting in hematoma formation. Delayed diagnosis of subcutaneous hematoma can lead to increased fibrosis of the overlying skin, resulting in the formation of the classic cauliflower-ear deformity.[14] Prevention of subcutaneous hematoma formation is improved with either transcartilaginous bolster techniques or adequate overlying compression dressings.

It is the author's recommendation to utilize carefully created, padded dressings designed to conform to the contours of the ear, further preserving the architecture of the cartilage and skin. Additionally, the underlying cartilage structure is not vascularized, but relies on the robust vascular structure of the overlying skin. Minimal vascularity to the cartilage places it at increased risk of infection postoperatively. Should cartilage be exposed, appropriate antibiotics for cartilage penetration are recommended. Additional topical treatments with Sulfamylon can improve infection management in the event of cartilage exposure.

HAND, UPPER EXTREMITY, AND NAIL BED

Age and Growth Considerations of the Hand and Upper Extremity

Growth of the hand in the pediatric patient becomes of critical importance when addressing functionality after surgery. Anatomic studies of pediatric hand growth have demonstrated a linear increase in hand growth from age 2 years until approximately 12 years of age with an expected growth spurt at puberty. Although moderate increases in hand size continue until approximately 17 years old, greater than 80% of final hand length is achieved by 12 years of age.[18] Understanding this dynamic increase in hand size during adolescence, the surgeon should expect significant scarring of the hand to result in restrictions of the natural hand growth. Restricted growth can lead to long-term functional deficits requiring scar revision to maximize future function.

During early childhood development, functional impacts from hand surgery may result in extremity neglect and delays in development of motor skills.[19] Appropriate care following surgery to the hand entails aggressive physical therapy and desensitization protocols to return the hand to appropriate function and maintain full range of motion. Despite these efforts, pediatric patients can demonstrate late restrictions during the pubertal growth phase requiring late revisions to maintain complete range motion.

Aesthetic Considerations of the Hand and Upper Extremity

The hand remains a vital part of daily activities and is often used for both function and communication. Studies outlining the importance of hand appearance as it relates to patient satisfaction and surgical outcomes indicate the importance of aesthetics when addressing surgical procedures of the hand.[20] This element of social satisfaction and hand aesthetics is even more significant in the pediatric population. Hand deformities or congenital differences have clearly been shown to result in increased emotional stress for patients.[19]

Every effort should be made to preserve the aesthetic units of the hand during surgical intervention. This includes reconstructing cutaneous defects with tissue similar in appearance and texture of the native hand tissue. Optimizing postoperative scar care with the use of laser therapies and other scar reduction strategies will further improve the outcome following intervention.

Functional Considerations of the Hand

The hand serves a key role as a functional component of the body. The highly specialized tasks performed by the hand require the maintenance of full mobility within the joints of the hands and upper extremity. Functional considerations should govern the approach and preoperative discussions when contemplating surgery to the hand. The following basic principles of operative hand interventions should be maintained whenever possible:

- Dissection should be limited to avoid damage to critical structures.
- Every effort should be made to avoid incisions crossing perpendicular to joints.
- Postoperative splinting or casting should be utilized when possible to maximize surgical site protection and allow recovery in a position of function.

Surgical Considerations of the Hand

Preoperative consideration of scar placement should include an assessment of the surrounding joints. Whenever possible, scars should be placed away from joints or oriented in such a way to avoid crossing the joint in a perpendicular pattern (Figure 13.2). Orienting scars in this manner will minimize the potential for future scar contractures (see Chapter 90. Hypertrophic Scars and Contractures). The digital neurovascular bundle is very superficial under the palmar skin on the radial and ulnar border of the digit. Excisions in this area should be performed under loupe magnification for adequate visualization of these critical structures. A thorough understanding of the underlying anatomy is essential when preforming excisions on volar aspects of the hand, given the proximity to this critical anatomy. Assistance of a surgical hand specialist is strongly recommended when addressing lesions of the volar aspects of the hand and fingers.

Anesthesia of the hand can be adequately achieved with either local infiltration or directed nerve blocks.[21] Although nerve blocks are effective in achieving regional pain control, a thorough understanding and familiarity of the surrounding

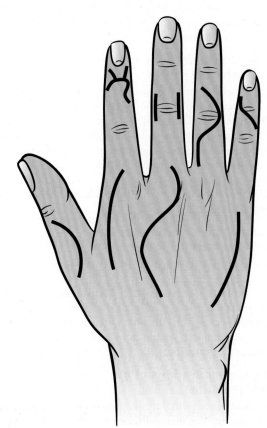

FIGURE 13.2. Dorsal hand incisions avoiding perpendicular incisions crossing the joint creases.

wrist and hand anatomy should be achieved before attempting (see Figure 11.1A. Nerve distribution in hand). There remains historical account of ischemic complications involving the infiltration of local anesthetic containing epinephrine solution into the hand. Since the advent of premixed local anesthetic containing verifiable amounts of epinephrine, local anesthetics containing epinephrine have become widely used within the hand with few reports of complications.[22] The use of epinephrine-containing anesthetics has become routine in hand surgery and is recommended when performing excisions without the assistance of a tourniquet because the vasoconstrictive effects will improve surgical visibility.

Postoperative care of the hand surgical site should take into consideration the patient's age. In younger patients who are unable to participate in appropriate surgical site care, the surgeon should consider applying protective splinting or casting to protect the surgical site. In young patients, the cast or splint should include the elbow and encompass the entire hand or surgical area. Including the elbow will prevent slipping of the cast during recovery. Splinting or casting should be applied over a nonadherent antimicrobial dressing at the site of intervention.

Nail Bed

As a specialized subunit of the hand, specific attention should be directed to reconstruction of the nail during surgical intervention. The fingernail remains a subtle but significant functional and aesthetic feature of the hand (see also Chapter 32. Nail Matrix Biopsy). Although its presence can be taken for granted, the absence of the nail is readily noted. Even with complete length of the digit, a finger with a shortened, malformed or absent nail appears distinctly different from the surrounding digits. This absence is even more significant when cosmetic color is added to the fingernails. These subtle differences can become a source of distraction or social stress as the hands remain a common tool in communication and social interaction for many cultures, including the Western culture. Thus, every attempt should be made to preserve the form of the nail when possible.

A fingernail also provides important functional attributes to the hand. It serves to defend the tips of the fingers against the common injuries and abrasions found in daily activities.[23] It also provides a firm surface dorsal to the sensory pads of the fingertip. This dorsal buttress allows for accurate pressure distinction and fine point discrimination within the fingertip. The absence of the fingernail can result in decreased tactile dexterity making even simple tasks, such as closing a button, difficult.[23]

To perform an accurate operative examination of the nail, the surgeon should possess an understanding of the intimate relationship between the nail and the underlying distal phalanx (Figure 13.3). Nail bed injuries, most notably in children, should raise concern for potential injury to the underlying distal phalanx. X-rays are warranted in the traumatic setting for any nail bed injury prior to repair, as this may diagnose a distal phalanx fracture to be addressed.

The most important anatomy of the nail bed consists of the nail plate, eponychium, and nail matrix. The nail matrix, also identified as the nail bed, is further subdivided into the proximal germinal matrix and distal sterile matrix. The proximal germinal matrix represents the primary growth center of the nail plate. The distal sterile matrix serves primarily as an adherent surface for the overlying nail plate.[24]

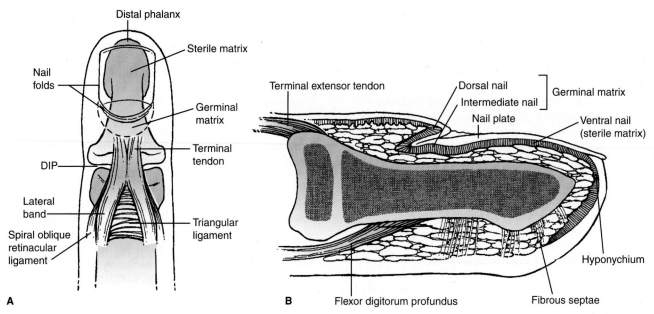

FIGURE 13.3. Anatomy of the distal phalanx and nail bed. A, The skin, nail, and extensor apparatus share a close relationship with the bone of the distal phalanx. B, A lateral view of the nail demonstrating the tendon insertions and the anatomy of the specialized nail tissues. Reprinted with permission from Flynn JM, Skaggs DL, Waters PM. *Rockwood and Wilkins' Fractures in Children.* 8th ed. Philadelphia, PA: Wolters Kluwer; 2014. Figure 10.6.

When addressing surgical intervention at the nail, three critical principles arise:

1. It is imperative to ensure preservation, replacement, or repair of the general matrix following surgical intervention. Inadequate repair or significant deficiencies of the germinal matrix will inevitably result in abnormal nail growth.

2. Removal of the overlying nail plate should be performed with the utmost care preserving the underline nail matrix. Furthermore, careful removal of the nail plate allows for its replacement at the end of the procedure, protecting the nail matrix and preserving the eponychial fold.[25]

3. Protection of the eponychial fold and prevention of scarring to the underlying sterile matrix are crucial to the preservation of normal nail growth. If the native nail plate cannot be salvaged, alloplastic material, such as foil or thin plastic sheeting, should be utilized and sutured in place to preserve the fold until new nail growth displaces the old nail plate or alloplast.

SURGICAL PROCEDURES IN THE EXTERNAL GENITALIA
Age and Growth Considerations of the External Genitalia

When considering the growth phases of the external genitalia, it is critical to evaluate the level of pubertal development in the adolescent patient. The rapid growth of the external genitalia during pubertal development can be restricted by surgical scars and result in poor long-term aesthetic and functional outcomes after reconstruction. Pubertal development can begin as early as 8 years old in females and 10 years old in males. This rapid growth phase continues through adolescence with completion of puberty generally by age 16 years in females and age 18 years in males with some variability.[26] Tanner first described the

clinical stages of pubertal growth in 1962.[27,28] These stages utilize external sexual characteristics of genital or breast development to determine maturation and can provide insight toward the level of pubertal development in the adolescent. Significant growth should be anticipated in any child prior to completion of tanner stage 5 development.

Aesthetic Considerations of the External Genitalia

The aesthetics of the genital region are not routinely addressed in the adolescent population. However, scarring can significantly influence genital aesthetics at sexual maturity and can become a source of serious and often irreversible morbidity. Penial and vaginal or labial tissue maintains little structural support and is especially sensitive to distortion with scarring. Given these risks, it is highly recommended to seek the services of specialized urologic and gynecologic colleagues when excising lesions of the genitals.

Functional Considerations of the External Genitalia

The vagina and penis serve critical urinary and sexual function. Maintenance of this function depends on the preservation of an intricate network of innervation and vascular supply. Furthermore, the specialized tissue of the genitalia allows for expansion and pliability necessary for function. Surgical specialists familiar with the anatomy can serve as a valuable resource to maximize postoperative function.

Surgical Considerations of the External Genitalia

Reconstruction of the genital region presents several challenges following excision. Vascularized tissue transfer in the form of local or free tissue flaps is often required to achieve maximal function. Every effort should be made to preserve sensory innervation and autonomic innervation to the region. Reconstructive options preserving these critical elements of form and function should be considered and addressed with parents and patients in the preoperative setting. Surgical complications of infection and wound dehiscence present an additional challenge to the genital region and should be considered during operative planning and reconstruction. Consultation with specialized reconstructive surgeons can provide valuable support in operative planning and reconstruction.

SURGICAL PROCEDURES IN THE PERIANAL REGION

Age and Growth Considerations of the Perianal Region

Continence or rather the maintenance of continence remains one of the most important age-related aspects of operative intervention in the perianal region. Planned surgical intervention in the perianal region should take into consideration a patient's ability to cooperate with postoperative wound care management to avoid increased risks of infection at surgical site. The surgeon should also consider delaying elective surgical intervention in the incontinent patient when possible. If the procedure is deemed necessary in the incontinent patient, care should be taken to ensure appropriate postoperative dressings and wound care to mitigate the risk of contamination to the surgical site. Careful parental education regarding meticulous surgical site care is necessary to obtain optimal outcomes following surgical intervention to the perianal region.

Aesthetic Considerations of the Perianal Region

Little attention is given to the aesthetics of the perianal region as may be expected. However, the landmarks of the gluteal region and upper thigh region deserve to be addressed as aesthetic components of the perianal region.[29] The gluteal cleft extends from the lower lumbar spine to the anal verge and represents an important aesthetic landmark of the perianal region. Care should be taken to avoid distortion or obliteration of this landmark during surgical intervention. In the event of surgical intervention within the gluteal clefs, care should be taken to reconstruct the normal depth and position of the cleft during the procedure. The second landmark of the perianal region is the gluteal thigh crease outlining the inferior portion of the gluteal region and the superior portion of the posterior thigh. Distortion of this crucial landmark results in poor delineation of the lower gluteal region and a flattened appearance to the lower buttock. This aesthetic landmark is created by dense fibrous connections between the muscle and overlying skin. When possible, disruption of these fibrous connections should be avoided. In the event that destruction of this landmark is necessary, scars should be oriented such that they will lay within the crease, further delineating this anatomic structure and minimizing distortion.

Functional Considerations of the Perianal Region

Perhaps, the most critical functional consideration of the perianal region is the anal sphincter. The anal sphincter is comprised of circumferential muscular bands surrounding the anal verge just beneath the subcutaneous tissue. These muscles receive innervation posteriorly from the pudendal branch of S4 and anteriorly from the inferior hemorrhoidal nerve.[30] It serves a critical function of maintaining continence both voluntary and involuntary. Inadvertent damage to the muscle or innervation

of the anal sphincter can result in the devastating consequence of postoperative incontinence. Thus, the presence of the anal sphincter should be noted during any intervention near the anal verge. It is the author's recommendation to involve a general surgical specialist when considering intervention at or near the anal verge to mitigate potential complications from disruption of the anal sphincter.

Surgical Considerations of the Perianal Region

The perianal region is supplied by a robust vascular network. This enhanced blood supply provides the region with excellent healing capacity and increased resistance to infection. However, this blood supply can also lead to frustrating bleeding and poor visualization during surgical intervention. The use of local anesthetic containing epinephrine is highly recommended to induce vasoconstriction and minimize bleeding during intervention. It is further recommended to maintain electrocautery on hand during any perianal intervention to assist with achieving hemostasis.

Surgical site dressings should be designed to provide protection from fecal or urinary contamination in the incontinent patient. Following closure of surgical incisions, surgical skin glue can provide a temporary watertight closure to the incision. Closure utilizing absorbable suture beneath the skin glue allows for ease of postoperative care as the incision heals. If surgical glue cannot be utilized, one should consider occlusive dressings to provide water-resistant coverage to the incision when possible. If neither of the abovementioned approaches is feasible, perianal wounds can be left without any surgical dressing, presuming meticulous incision care can be performed. Parents should be instructed regarding routine cleaning following fecal or urinary contamination, as this is paramount in preventing infection. The use of Epson salt soaks or sitz baths are also a useful adjunct for wound care if needed in the perianal region.

SURGICAL PROCEDURES OF THE FOOT

Age and Growth Considerations

The adolescent foot length has been shown to grow sequentially with the body until approximately 11 years of age.[31] At this point, a peak in growth is demonstrated, with the end of the accelerated growth phase at approximately age 14 years in female patients and age 16 years in male patients. This accelerated, adolescent growth phase of the foot is important to consider when planning interventions because distortions from scarring can lead to growth disturbance and functional impairment. Plantar scarring of the dense, glabrous skin can lead to development of a flexed foot or toe and limited ability to extend the foot during normal gait. Dorsal scarring can lead to hyperextension of the toes or hammer toe deformities, creating difficulty with footwear and ambulation. These scar deformities can worsen as the foot rapidly increases in length during rapid growth and may require future revisions.

Elective intervention in the foot should take into consideration the difficulties in offloading pressure from the foot following intervention in the immature patient. Elective total contact casting following surgery to the foot can provide excellent protection and mobility restriction for young patients. Mature patients can be managed with surgical dressings and weight-bearing restrictions to allow for optimized healing.

Aesthetic Considerations

Although the aesthetics of the foot are considered less important than those of the hand, maintenance of certain anatomic landmarks remains important to address. The most significant of these landmarks is the first web space. Maintenance of the first web space allows for the use of many specialized footwear and preserves the normal anatomic separation between the great toe and second toe. Should surgical intervention involve the web space, reconstruction with local flaps or skin grafts can preserve the depth of the web space and prevent aesthetic distortion.

Functional Considerations of the Foot

As with the hand, the foot maintains a critical functional role during early childhood development.[32] Distortions of the functional anatomy of the foot can result in an early neglect or, more frequently, development of compensatory gait changes. Prevention of such compensations or delays relies on precise reconstruction of the functional anatomy of the foot and early aggressive physical therapy to maintain mobility.

The specialized glabrous skin of the plantar surface is unique to the body and difficult to replace. The skin provides the ambulatory surface of the foot along with specialized pressure receptors and underlying fibrous attachments to the intrinsic muscles of the foot.[33] Few local tissue options are available for reconstruction of the plantar surface. Small excisions demonstrate excellent healing with minimal postoperative morbidity. In the setting of large excisions, it is the author's recommendation to seek specialized reconstructive care, including distant soft-tissue reconstruction with pedicled or free tissue transfer.

Surgical Considerations of the Foot

Infiltration of local anesthetic can provide excellent regional anesthesia for minor surgical intervention in the foot. Given the multiple dermatomes and deep sensory innervation to the foot, complete nerve block with local anesthetic can be difficult. General anesthesia provides an attractive alternative when considering more significant interventions in the foot.

Postoperative wound care in the foot should focus on management of postoperative edema and maintenance of pressure offloading. Postoperative edema is best managed by persistent foot elevation during recovery. Prolonged periods of dependency to the foot can result in increased edema and stress to surgical incisions. Pressure to the foot in the postoperative setting can decrease perfusion and increase strain to the surgical site. The use of postoperative casting and weight-bearing restrictions is effective management strategies to limit pressure in the postoperative setting.

REFERENCES

1. Baker R, Urso-Baiarda F, Linge C, Grobbelaar A. Cutaneous scarring: a clinical review. *Dermatol Res Pract.* 2009;2009:625376.
2. Kinahan KE, Sharp LK, Seidel K, et al. Scarring, disfigurement, and quality of life in long-term survivors of childhood cancer: a report from the Childhood Cancer Survivor study. *J Clin Oncol.* 2012;30(20):2466–2474.
3. Pindrik J, Ye X, Ji BG, Pendleton C, Ahn ES. Anterior fontanelle closure and size in full-term children based on head computed tomography. *Clin Pediatr (Phila).* 2014;53(12):1149–1157.
4. Davies T, Karanovic S, Shergill B. Essential regional nerve blocks for the dermatologist: part 1. *Clin Exp Dermatol.* 2014;39(7):777–784.
5. Tolhurst DE, Carstens MH, Greco RJ, Hurwitz DJ. The surgical anatomy of the scalp. *Plast Reconstr Surg.* 1991;87(4):603–612; discussion 613–604.
6. Na YC, Park R, Jeong HS, Park JH. Epinephrine vasoconstriction effect time in the scalp differs according to injection site and concentration. *Dermatol Surg.* 2016;42(9):1054–1060.
7. Sgouros S, Goldin JH, Hockley AD, Wake MJ, Natarajan K. Intracranial volume change in childhood. *J Neurosurg.* 1999;91(4):610–616.
8. Mellion ZJ, Behrents RG, Johnston LE, Jr. The pattern of facial skeletal growth and its relationship to various common indexes of maturation. *Am J Orthod Dentofacial Orthop.* 2013;143(6):845–854.
9. Di Blasio A, Mandelli G, Generali I, Gandolfini M. Facial aesthetics and childhood. *Eur J Paediatr Dent.* 2009;10(3):131–134.
10. Choi JH, Kim YJ, Kim H, Nam SH, Choi YW. Distribution of basal cell carcinoma and squamous cell carcinoma by facial esthetic unit. *Arch Plast Surg.* 2013;40(4):387–391.
11. Farrior JB, Santini H. Facial nerve identification in children. *Otolaryngol Head Neck Surg.* 1985;93(2):173–176.
12. Beahm EK, Walton RL. Auricular reconstruction for microtia: part I. Anatomy, embryology, and clinical evaluation. *Plast Reconstr Surg.* 2002;109(7):2473–2482; quiz following 2482.
13. Doft MA, Goodkind AB, Diamond S, DiPace JI, Kacker A, LaBruna AN. The newborn butterfly project: a shortened treatment protocol for ear molding. *Plast Reconstr Surg.* 2015;135(3):577e–583e.
14. Greywoode JD, Pribitkin EA, Krein H. Management of auricular hematoma and the cauliflower ear. *Facial Plast Surg.* 2010;26(6):451–455.
15. Walton RL, Beahm EK. Auricular reconstruction for microtia: part II. Surgical techniques. *Plast Reconstr Surg.* 2002;110(1):234–249; quiz 250–231, 387.
16. Songu M, Kutlu A. Long-term psychosocial impact of otoplasty performed on children with prominent ears. *J Laryngol Otol.* 2014;128(9):768–771.
17. Hafner HM, Rocken M, Breuninger H. Epinephrine-supplemented local anesthetics for ear and nose surgery: clinical use without complications in more than 10,000 surgical procedures. *J Dtsch Dermatol Ges.* 2005;3(3):195–199.
18. Amirsheybani HR, Crecelius GM, Timothy NH, Pfeiffer M, Saggers GC, Manders EK. The natural history of the growth of the hand: I. Hand area as a percentage of body surface area. *Plast Reconstr Surg.* 2001;107(3):726–733.
19. Franzblau LE, Chung KC, Carlozzi N, Chin AY, Nellans KW, Waljee JF. Coping with congenital hand differences. *Plast Reconstr Surg.* 2015;135(4):1067–1075.
20. Johnson SP, Sebastin SJ, Rehim SA, Chung KC. The Importance of hand appearance as a patient-reported outcome in hand surgery. *Plast Reconstr Surg Glob Open.* 2015;3(11):e552.
21. Davies T, Karanovic S, Shergill B. Essential regional nerve blocks for the dermatologist: part 2. *Clin Exp Dermatol.* 2014;39(8):861–867.
22. Mann T, Hammert WC. Epinephrine and hand surgery. *J Hand Surg Am.* 2012;37(6):1254–1256; quiz 1257.
23. Tos P, Titolo P, Chirila NL, Catalano F, Artiaco S. Surgical treatment of acute fingernail injuries. *J Orthop Traumatol.* 2012;13(2):57–62.
24. de Berker D. Nail anatomy. *Clin Dermatol.* 2013;31(5):509–515.
25. Haneke E. Nail surgery. *J Cutan Aesthet Surg.* 2011;4(3):163–164.
26. Lee PA. Normal ages of pubertal events among American males and females. *J Adolesc Health Care.* 1980;1(1):26–29.
27. Marshall WA, Tanner JM. Variations in the pattern of pubertal changes in boys. *Arch Dis Child.* 1970;45(239):13–23.
28. Marshall WA, Tanner JM. Variations in pattern of pubertal changes in girls. *Arch Dis Child.* 1969;44(235):291–303.
29. Centeno RF, Sood A, Young VL. Clinical Anatomy in aesthetic gluteal contouring. *Clin Plast Surg.* 2018;45(2):145–157.
30. Ayoub SF. Anatomy of the external anal sphincter in man. *Acta Anat (Basel).* 1979;105(1):25–36.
31. Liu KM, Shinoda K, Akiyoshi T, Watanabe H. Longitudinal analysis of adolescent growth of foot length and stature of children living in Ogi area of Japan: a 12 years data. *Z Morphol Anthropol.* 1998;82(1):87–101.
32. Price C, McClymont J, Hashmi F, Morrison SC, Nester C. Development of the infant foot as a load bearing structure: study protocol for a longitudinal evaluation (the Small Steps study). *J Foot Ankle Res.* 2018;11:33.
33. Kennedy PM, Inglis JT. Distribution and behaviour of glabrous cutaneous receptors in the human foot sole. *J Physiol.* 2002;538 (Pt 3):995–1002.

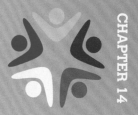
Injectables

Kavina Patel and John C. Browning

INTRODUCTION

From treating acute infections to chronic skin pathologies and for cosmetic purposes, the use of injectables in pediatric dermatology is common. Intralesional and intramuscular (IM) injections of corticosteroids, neuromodulators, fillers, interferons, antibiotics, and other therapies are frequently performed in the pediatric setting. Dermatologists must familiarize themselves with these applications so they can incorporate these techniques into their routine practice and improve patient care.

CORTICOSTEROIDS

Triamcinolone acetonide injectable suspension (Kenalog) is a glucocorticoid corticosteroid with anti-inflammatory properties that may be administered IM and intralesionally. It is used for a wide variety of conditions, including eczema, dermatitis, rashes, and psoriasis to decrease swelling, erythema, and pruritus. Intralesional corticosteroids reduce inflammation, stimulate collagen breakdown, decrease collagen production, and inhibit fibroblast proliferation and vascular endothelial growth factor. (see Chapter 15. Injectable Corticosteroids [Intralesional Kenalog, Intramuscular])

The number of treatments and dosage used depends on the specific underlying pathology of the condition (eg, scar type and thickness), location of the lesion, and concern for site-specific complications. Compared to topical steroids, intralesional corticosteroids are more effective in alleviating conditions deep-seated in the dermis, and the intralesional route of administration has more localized effects than the oral route of administration. Possible adverse events include pain, atrophy of the skin producing depressions, and hypopigmentation. Intralesional corticosteroids should not be injected in an area of active skin infection or in individuals with triamcinolone hypersensitivity. Usage is somewhat limited in clinical practice because of anxiety and pain in pediatric populations. Smaller gauge needles, distraction methods, and use of topical anesthetic creams, such as lidocaine, can be used to diminish discomfort and ease patient stress.[1]

Injection of corticosteroids into the deep dermis and upper subcutis is administered in alopecia areata, an autoimmune condition resulting in hair loss (see Chapter 54. Alopecia Areata). This condition is not unusual in the pediatric population as 11% to 20% of the cases have an age of onset younger than 16 years.[2] Injections are given intralesionally to avoid systemic spread while still maintaining adequate dosing in the affected tissue. For the scalp, typically, Kenalog 10 mg/mL injections are used, with 0.05 to 0.1 mL per injection site, spaced approximately 1 cm apart; maximum volume per session would typically be 2 to 3 mL. For other areas, such as the eyebrows, the Kenalog would typically be diluted to 2.5 to 5 mg/mL.[3]

Hypertrophic scars are optimally treated with intralesional Kenalog 10 to 40 mg/mL 1 month postoperatively because tissues will have advanced to a fibrofatty stage by that time (see Chapter 90. Hypertrophic Scars and Contractures). One conservative approach utilizes *low-dose* Kenalog (0.1 mL at 5-10 mg/mL), which is injected into the scar at the bulkiest region into the level of the dermis or subcutaneous fat. This is repeated approximately every 4 weeks until the scar levels off. For thicker scars,

higher concentrations of Kenalog (ie, 40 mg/mL) may be necessary. Overuse of corticosteroid injections can cause significant atrophy, so side effects (eg, telangiectasia, atrophy, hypopigmentation, local hypertrichosis) should be discussed, and the injections must be used with caution and careful follow-up (Figures 14.1 and 14.2).[4]

Keloids are a skin condition found subsequent to trauma in which the skin grows outside the outline of the original wound. Most keloids appear in individuals between the ages of 10 and 30 years.[5] For keloids, intralesional corticosteroid treatment has a 50% to 100% response rate and a 9% to 55% recurrence rate based on one review.[6] For thick keloid scars, 40 mg/mL should be injected into the mid-dermis every 4 to 6 weeks until the scar flattens (Figure 14.3).[7]

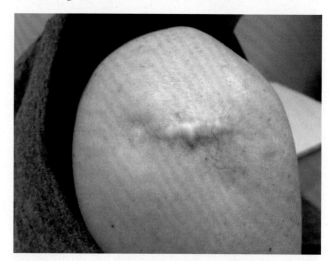

FIGURE 14.1. Hypertrophic scar with surrounding atrophy secondary to corticosteroid causing adverse changes to adjacent normal skin. Reprinted with permission from Krakowski AC, Shumaker PR. *The Scar Book.* Philadelphia, PA: Wolters Kluwer; 2017. Figure 5.4C.

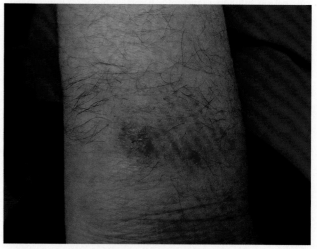

FIGURE 14.2. Telangiectasias and local hypertrichosis at site of corticosteroid injection. Image provided by Stedman's.

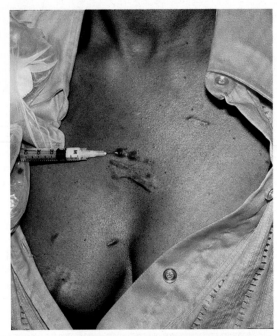

FIGURE 14.3. Intralesional injection of Kenalog 40mg/ml into thick hypertrophic scar. Reprinted with permission from Goodheart H, Gonzalez M. *Goodheart's Photoguide to Common Pediatric and Adult Skin Disorders.* 4th ed. Philadelphia, PA: Wolters Kluwer; 2016. Figure 30.54.

Intralesional corticosteroid injections can also be utilized to treat the onset of acne-induced cysts and nodules (see Chapter 50. Acne Cyst). This therapeutic agent is utilized on an *as-needed* basis and is not meant for preventive or maintenance treatment. It is an option for helping to quickly reduce swelling, erythema, and the appearance of the papule. Kenalog is injected into the papule using a small needle, and within 2 to 4 days, the inflammation and erythema subside. This treatment does not prevent the formation of new papules.[8]

Vitiligo, which is depigmentation of the skin because of loss of melanocytes, usually unveils in childhood, with the average age of onset between 4 and 5 years (see Chapter 129. Vitiligo). In all, 33.33% to 50% of the cases actualize by the age of 20 years, with 25% of the cases manifesting before the age of 8.[9] Vitiligo is usually treated with narrowband ultraviolet B (UVB) phototherapy, topical calcineurin inhibitors, and topical corticosteroids. Unfortunately, these therapies are slow and impotent. Intralesional corticosteroid use as a treatment for vitiligo has been reported with 80% to 90% repigmentation after a 4- to 7-month treatment duration.[10]

Systemic corticosteroids are not recommended as treatment for atopic dermatitis owing to the high risk of adverse events, and topical corticosteroids are more commonly used.[11]

NEUROMODULATORS

Neuromodulators such as BOTOX® (©2020 Allergan, Irvine, CA) and Dysport® (Galderma Laboratories ©2020 US) have been used for many years for cosmetic indications; however, they are not Food and Drug Administration (FDA) approved for cosmetic indications in children. Clinicians have recently begun to explore novel indications for the botulinum neuromodulators. Studies have shown that botulinum can alleviate facial erythema from rosacea, specifically the erythematotelangiectatic rosacea subtype. Acetylcholine is associated with vascular dilation. Thus, hindering acetylcholine discharge with

botulinum can prevent facial erythema in rosacea. Botulinum has also been shown to treat chronic migraine headaches because of the effects the neuromodulator has on neurotransmitter releases other than acetylcholine. Other extracutaneous therapeutic indications of botulinum include depression, pain, obesity, and infectious diseases.[12,13]

Botulinum has also been shown to improve the quality of life in children with hyperhidrosis, a disorder of excess sweating (see Chapter 87. Hyperhidrosis). Although many studies have demonstrated the use of botulinum toxin type A, BOTOX, for adult hyperhidrosis, few studies have been done in children. One study conducted on a 13-year-old girl with palmar hyperhidrosis received 2 U BOTOX injections at 15-mm intervals with 50 injections total per palm. This led to an 80% reduction in sweat production and a significant improvement in the patient's quality of life. A 14-year-old with hyperhidrosis received 150 U of Dysport in each axilla, and significant reduction in sweating was noticed in 3 months. The disadvantage of this therapeutic method is pain at the time of injection, which might require regional anesthesia. Other adverse events include muscle weakness, dry skin, and small hematomas.[13]

FILLERS

In children with atrophic disorders such as lipoatrophy and morphea, poly-L-lactic acid and dermal fillers can be used therapeutically. Morphea has a bimodal age distribution, with adults and children affected equally (Figure 14.4).[14] Additionally, soft-tissue augmentation fillers have been frequently used off-label in the treatment of atrophic scars, including acne scars. For acne, fillers are therapeutically utilized in two ways. First, fillers such as hyaluronic acid (HA) or collagen can be injected beneath each scar for rapid improvement. The filler can be administered employing a cross-hatching or lattice technique and is ideally used for broad, rolling scars that are extendable and soft. It is advised not to inject too much filler, because it is better to inject less and perform additional treatment sessions. Second, volumizing fillers such as poly-L-lactic acid or calcium hydroxylapatite can be injected in areas where a scar is apparent owing to volume loss (ie, atrophic scarring). This is commonly used in deep tissue atrophy of the midface and in human immunodeficiency virus (HIV) lipoatrophy. The filler is injected diffusely into the deep tissue atrophy, causing it to distend.[15]

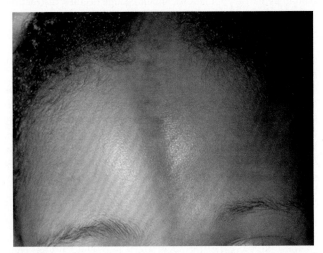

FIGURE 14.4. Linear morphea (en coup de sabre). Reprinted with permission from Burkhart CN, Morrell D, Goldsmith L, et al. *VisualDx: Essential Pediatric Dermatology.* Philadelphia, PA: Wolters Kluwer Health/Lippincott Williams & Wilkins; 2010. Figure 4.99.

WARTS

A wart is a benign skin manifestation caused by a localized infection of human papillomavirus (HPV). Warts come in many different types, such as verruca vulgaris (common wart), plantar warts, flat warts, and filiform warts. They can appear on many different sites of the body and can cause social concerns in many individuals. They are contagious and can be spread from skin to skin contact. Children aged 12 to 16 years have the highest incidence of nongenital warts. Genital warts can be transmitted in children through a variety of methods, such as sexual contact and perinatal transmission.[16,17]

Although the use of injectables may not be first line in the treatment of warts, injectables are particularly useful for treatment-resistant lesions. One of the most common injectable treatment is intralesional *Candida* antigen immunotherapy. One study of treatment with *Candida* antigen demonstrated that in children, there was a 47% efficacy rate following an average of 3.78 treatments in the population of individuals who failed to respond to liquid nitrogen and one other form of therapy. It is recommended that *Candida* antigen should be intralesionally injected as first-line therapy in children with large or numerous warts and as second-line therapy in recurrent warts resistant to other treatment options. Side effects include a delayed-type hypersensitivity reaction with itching at injection site, erythema, and edema in some individuals.

Bleomycin, an antibiotic originating from *Streptomyces verticillus*, is also a common injectable therapy of choice along with *Candida* antigen immunotherapy. The mechanism of action is inhibition of DNA and protein synthesis, triggering apoptosis in squamous cell and reticuloendothelial tissue. It is diluted to 1 mg/mL with normal saline of 1% lidocaine, and 0.1 to 2 mL is injected per session, causing the wart to form a black thrombotic eschar. Injections are given every 3 to 4 weeks until the lesion subsides.[10] Bleomycin has a 92% efficacy; however, side effects include discomfort from injection, flagellate erythema, alopecia, and inflammation.[18]

Intralesional injection of the measles, mumps, and rubella (MMR) vaccine has also been proven effective in resolving resistant warts, with a therapeutic response of around 80%. It has been suggested that the nonspecific inflammatory response to the MMR antigens is the mechanism of action of the immunotherapy.[19]

Interferon α-2b, a less common modality, kills the virus and stimulates the immune system, can be injected to treat genital warts. In one study, 43.8% of patients had their warts subside after treatment with interferon α-2b, whereas 25% of patients had greater than 50% reduction in visibility.[20]

Preventive measures include the HPV vaccination, a safe and effective measure for sexually transmitted warts. The HPV vaccine is a recombinant vaccine with the major viral capsid L1 protein assembled on the exterior of organisms such as a yeast cell, creating a noninfectious HPV-like particle that is immunogenic. The standard HPV vaccine is protective against HPV 6, HPV 11, HPV 16, and HPV 18 and is administered in the midst of preteen years.[21]

PSORIASIS

Psoriasis is a common dermatologic condition and autoimmune disease characterized by erythematous, pruritic, and scaly patches of skin because of overgrowth of skin cells. Onset may occur during childhood for approximately one-third of the psoriasis population and may impair an individual's quality of life.[22]

Initially, therapy starts off with topicals and phototherapy, and persistent psoriasis can be further treated with both biologic drugs and nonbiologic systemic drugs. None of the nonbiologic systemic drugs, such as methotrexate and cyclosporine, are FDA approved for psoriasis in children. Biologic drugs are targeted to control inflammation and can be used clinically in psoriasis patients.

Etanercept, given twice a week by subcutaneous injection of 0.4 mg/kg, is a soluble tumor necrosis factor (TNF) receptor fusion protein that reversibly affixes to TNF and antagonizes its effects. Patients with chronic plaque psoriasis that is resistant to nonbiologic therapy are recommended to undergo treatment with Etanercept.

Adalimumab is a monoclonal antibody against TNFα, administered at 0.8 mg/kg with a maximum dose of 40 mg during weeks 0 and 1 and then once every 2 weeks. It is commonly used for chronic plaque psoriasis that is unyielding to topical treatments and phototherapy in children aged 4 years or older.

Ustekinumab is a monoclonal antibody that appends to the p40 protein subunit on interleukin-12 (IL-12) and IL-23 inflammatory cytokines. There are only a limited number of studies done on pediatric application; however, it has been shown that 78.4% of patients receiving a half dose (0.375 mg/kg) and 80.6% of patients receiving a standard dose (0.750 mg/kg) achieved Psoriasis Area and Severity Index (PASI) 75. Normally, doses are administered at weeks 0 and 4 and then every 12 weeks.

Infliximab is a monoclonal antibody that acts by targeting TNFα, administered at 3 to 5 mg/kg via infusion at weeks 0, 2, and 6 and then every 8 weeks after that. Limited number of studies have been conducted on the pediatric population; however, it has proven to be effective in children with resistant pustular erythrodermic psoriasis.

Side effects of injectable biologics include infections, anaphylaxis, and injection site reaction. Blood count and liver enzymes should be monitored carefully, and a purified protein derivative (PPD) test should be performed annually.[23]

ANTIBIOTICS

For scarlet fever and other manifestations of streptococcal infections, 600,000 units of benzathine penicillin G IM can be given.[24] For newborns with congenital syphilis, crystalline penicillin G 50,000 units/kg is the drug of choice and administered intravenously every 12 hours for the first week of life. This is altered to every 8 hours after the first week, and given for 10 to 14 days. Injection of procaine penicillin 50,000 units/kg/day is another treatment option, which is done for 10 to 14 days. For 10 to 14 days as well, aqueous penicillin G IM can be injected at 50,000 units/kg every 6 hours to treat congenital syphilis.[25]

INTERFERON-γ THERAPY AND 5-FLUOROURACIL THERAPY

Interferon-γ therapy, although not a top-line therapy, has been shown to play a role in the treatment of atopic dermatitis, a chronic inflammatory skin disease with immune system dysfunction. Atopic dermatitis can begin as early as the first year of life and emerges as scaly and pruritic patches and plaques that are generally found on the cheeks, scalp, and forehead. The pathophysiology of this condition is still unknown. However, it has been found to be correlated with hypereosinophilia, high immunoglobulin E (IgE), and IL-4 levels, but low cellular

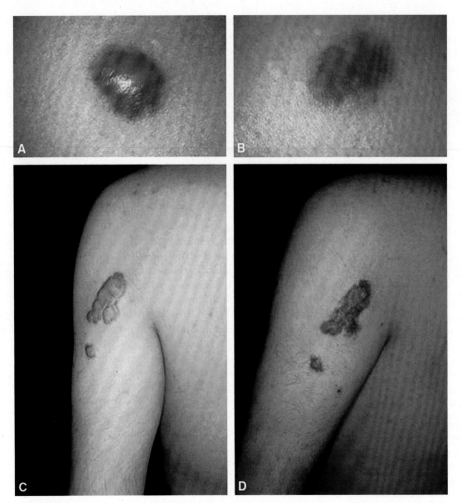

FIGURE 14.5. Use of 5-Fluorouracil to treat keloids. A, C: Keloids were refractory to triamcinolone acetonide and cryotherapy. B, D: After four 5-Fluorouracil intralesional injections at 4-week intervals. Reprinted with permission from Krakowski AC, Shumaker PR. *The Scar Book*. Philadelphia, PA: Wolters Kluwer; 2017. Figure 5.4C.

immunity and interferon-γ levels. Treatment of atopic dermatitis with interferon-γ has been shown to abate white blood cell and eosinophil count, eventuating in improved clinical outcomes. Clinically, patients presented with diminished erythema, pruritus, and dryness subsequent to treatment with interferon-γ. However, the mechanism of these clinical changes with this therapeutic option still remains unknown.[26]

A pyrimidine analog, intralesional 5-Fluorouracil (5-FU), impedes collagen synthesis as it has antimetabolite action by stimulating fibroblast apoptosis without necrosis. It is potent against hypertrophic scars and keloids by decreasing erythema, induration, pruritus, and dimensions of the lesion. It is used *off-label* to treat hypertrophic scars and keloids, and its use in the pediatric population has not been studied (Figure 14.5). Side effects include pain and hyperpigmentation, and it is contraindicated in pregnant women as it is a Pregnancy Category D with potential to cause damage to the fetus.[27]

REFERENCES

1. Krakowski AC, Totri CR, Donelan MB, Shumaker PR. Scar management in the pediatric and adolescent populations. *Pediatrics.* 2016;137(2):e20142065.
2. Schachner L, Hansen R. *Pediatric Dermatology.* Vol 1. 4th ed. London, England: Mosby; 2011.
3. Wang E, Lee JS, Tang M. Current treatment strategies in pediatric alopecia areata. *Indian J Dermatol.* 2012;57(6):459–465.
4. Robinson JK. *Surgery of the Skin, Procedural Dermatology.* Edinburgh, Scotland: Mosby; 2010.
5. Krakowski AC, Totri CR, Donelan MB, Shumaker PR. Scar management in the pediatric and adolescent populations. *Pediatrics.* 2016;137(2):e20142065.
6. Trisliana perdanasari A, Lazzeri D, Su W, et al. Recent developments in the use of intralesional injections keloid treatment. *Arch Plast Surg.* 2014;41(6):620–629.
7. Robles DT, Berg D. Abnormal wound healing: keloids. *Clin Dermatol.* 2007;25(1):26–32.
8. Levine RM, Rasmussen JE. Intralesional corticosteroids in the treatment of nodulocystic acne. *Arch Dermatol.* 1983;119(6):480–481.
9. Kanwar AJ, Kumaran MS. Childhood vitiligo: treatment paradigms. *Indian J Dermatol.* 2012;57(6):466–474.
10. Wang E, Koo J, Levy E. Intralesional corticosteroid injections for vitiligo: a new therapeutic option. *J Am Acad Dermatol.* 2014; 71(2):391–393.
11. Walling HW, Swick BL. Update on the management of chronic eczema: new approaches and emerging treatment options. *Clin Cosmet Investig Dermatol.* 2010;3:99–117.
12. Jagdeo J, Carruthers A, Smith KC. New frontiers and clinical applications for botulinum neuromodulators. *Dermatol Surg.* 2015;41(suppl 1):S17–S18.
13. Gelbard CM, Epstein H, Hebert A. Primary pediatric hyperhidrosis: a review of current treatment options. *Pediatr Dermatol.* 2008;25(6):591–598.
14. Careta MF, Romiti R. Localized scleroderma: clinical spectrum and therapeutic update. *An Bras Dermatol.* 2015;90(1):62–73.

15. Fife D, Zachary C. Combining techniques for treating acne scars. Cosmetic Surgery. https://link.springer.com/content/pdf/10.1007/s13671-012-0011-0.pdf. Published April 8, 2012. Accessed April 10, 2018.

16. Lipke MM. An armamentarium of wart treatments. *Clin Med Res.* 2006;4(4):273–293.

17. Jayasinghe Y, Garland SM. Genital warts in children: what do they mean? *Arch Dis Child.* 2006;91(8):696–700.

18. Shelley WB, Shelley ED. Intralesional bleomycin sulfate therapy for warts. A novel bifurcated needle puncture technique. *Arch Dermatol.* 1991;127(2):234–236.

19. Zamanian A, Mobasher P, Jazi GA. Efficacy of intralesional injection of mumps-measles-rubella vaccine in patients with wart. *Adv Biomed Res.* 2014;3:107.

20. Welander CE, Homesley HD, Smiles KA, Peets EA. Intralesional interferon alfa-2b for the treatment of genital warts. *Am J Obstet Gynecol.* 1990;162(2):348–354.

21. Lipke MM. An armamentarium of wart treatments. *Clin Med Res.* 2006;4(4):273–293.

22. Paller AS, Siegfried EC, Langley RG, et al. Etanercept treatment for children and adolescents with plaque psoriasis. *N Engl J Med.* 2008;358(3):241–251.

23. Napolitano M, Megna M, Balato A, et al. Systemic treatment of pediatric psoriasis: a review. *Dermatol Ther (Heidelb).* 2016;6(2):125–142.

24. Breese BB, Disney FA, Talpey WB. Penicillin in streptococcal infections total dose and frequency of administration. *Am J Dis Child.* 1965;110(2):125–130.

25. Walker GJA, Walker D, Molano Franco D. Antibiotics for congenital syphilis (Protocol). *Cochrane Db Syst Rev.* 2016(2).

26. Chang TT, Stevens SR. Atopic dermatitis: the role of recombinant interferon-gamma therapy. *Am J Clin Dermatol.* 2002;3(3):175–183.

27. Krakowski AC, Totri CR, Donelan MB, Shumaker PR. Scar management in the pediatric and adolescent populations. *Pediatrics.* 2016;137(2):e20142065.

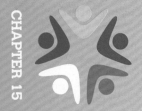

CHAPTER 15

Injectable Corticosteroids (Intralesional Kenalog, Intramuscular)

Eileen Peterson, Stephen C. Senft, and Craig N. Burkhart

INTRODUCTION

Corticosteroids can be injected directly into lesions, intradermally, or intramuscularly (IM) to treat a variety of conditions. Injections often provide quick results for inflammatory conditions and can be useful when strong topical steroids have failed to produce a sufficient response.

Intralesional injections can be used for keloids, hypertrophic scars, infantile hemangiomas, large acne nodules, or inflamed cysts.

Intradermal injections can be used for alopecia areata, discoid lupus erythematosus, hypertrophic lichen planus, lichen simplex chronicus, necrobiosis lipoidica, or other localized inflammatory conditions.

IM injections can be used when a systemic effect is desired, such as when treating widespread allergic contact dermatitis (poison ivy) or diffuse inflammatory skin diseases.

INTRALESIONAL INJECTIONS

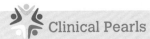 **Clinical Pearls**

- **Guidelines:** No specific treatment guidelines are known to exist for intralesional steroids, and experts vary on injection concentrations, volumes injected, and techniques.
- **Age-Specific Considerations:** Ideally, patients should be old enough to ask for treatment for themselves. Infants and young children are at increased risk for systemic side effects from intralesional injections, and one should ensure that the total dose of steroid is below 2 mg/kg.
- **Anatomic-Specific Considerations:** Inject *away from* anatomic sites, such as the eye. Thin skin areas, such as the face and central chest, typically require less concentrated corticosteroid solutions than other locations.
- **Technique Tips:** Injection pressure is decreased using 1-mL syringes, rather than 3- or 5-mL syringes, which can make injections less painful. Soften keloids by spraying with liquid nitrogen for 5 to 20 seconds before injecting.
- **Skin of Color Considerations:** Darkly pigmented skin is at increased risk for dyspigmentation, especially at higher steroid concentrations or when steroid is injected in the upper dermis.

Contraindications/Cautions/Risks

Cautions

- Side effects are increased when injecting (1) higher concentrations of corticosteroids, (2) at increased volumes and (3) outside the deep dermis (ie, subcutaneously or in the superficial dermis).

Risks

- ○ *Local:* atrophy, dyspigmentation, sterile abscess formation (rarely)
- ○ *Systemic:* menstrual irregularities, adrenal suppression, and reduced blood sugar control (with frequent high cumulative doses of corticosteroids)

Equipment Needed

- Syringe (1 mL, ideally)
- Large-bore needle (19, 21, or 22 gauge) to draw up and dilute the corticosteroid
- Small-bore needle (30, 27, or 25 gauge) to inject the corticosteroid
- Nonsterile gloves
- Alcohol swabs
- 2 × 2 gauze
- Protective eyewear
- BAND-AIDs™ (Johnson & Johnson, US)

Preprocedural Approach

- It is helpful to inquire how the child reacts to vaccinations at the pediatrician's office. The benefits and risks of corticosteroid injections should be strongly considered prior to restraining a child who has prior adverse reaction to injections.
- Gently shake the corticosteroid bottle to resuspend the steroid particles and clean the diaphragm with alcohol before drawing up the corticosteroid with a large-bore needle.
- Dilute the corticosteroid to the desired concentration (Table 15.1) using sterile saline or 0.5% or 1% lidocaine without epinephrine.
- Do not dilute with bupivacaine or other long-acting anesthetics as they will precipitate the corticosteroid.
- Replace the large-bore needle with a small-bore needle. A 30-gauge needle is typically used. However, when injecting into particularly tough tissue (ie, keloids) or using highly concentrated corticosteroid (triamcinolone acetonide 40 mg/mL), a larger needle (27 or 25 gauge) may be helpful.
- Immediately before injecting, gently shake or roll the syringe to ensure that the corticosteroid is evenly suspended for even delivery into the tissue.

Procedural Approach

- Obtain informed consent from the parent/guardian and, when possible, assent from the minor.
- Appropriate protective eyewear should be worn to protect the provider's eyes from potential back-splashing during the injection.
- Prepare the skin by wiping with alcohol.
- Insert the needle at a 45° to 90° angle into the lesion aiming for the mid-dermis; you can decrease the angle (typically, not <15°) for more superficial lesions.
- Inject until the skin is noted to rise slightly and blanch.
- Inject directly into keloids, hypertrophic scars, and inflamed cysts.
- After injecting, apply gauze and light pressure over the site to stop any bleeding. Apply a BAND-AID if the injection site continues to bleed.

TABLE 15.1 ⋮ Concentrations for Intralesional Injections

LESION	TRIAMCINOLONE CONCENTRATION (mg/mL)
Inflamed acne nodule or cyst (face)	1-3
Inflamed cysts (body)	2-5
Psoriasis	2.5-5
Lichen simplex chronicus	5
Prurigo nodularis	5-10
Hypertrophic lichen planus	5-10
Hypertrophic scars	10-20; sometimes up to 40
Keloids	10-40
Aphthous ulcers and oral lichen planus	2-5
Necrobiosis lipoidica	2-10
Alopecia areata	2-5; sometimes up to 10 on the scalp
Chronic cutaneous lupus erythematosus	5-10

Postprocedural Approach

- The site may have a burning sensation for 3 to 5 minutes after the injection.
- Inflammatory lesions typically start to improve within days of the injection. Keloids, hypertrophic scars, and alopecia areata typically respond within a month of each injection.
- Follow-up injection appointments are typically scheduled monthly until the lesion resolves or injections appear to have provided their full benefit.

INTRAMUSCULAR INJECTION

Equipment Needed

- Alcohol wipe
- 2 × 2 gauze
- 1- to 3-mL syringe
- 22- to 25-gauge needle
- BAND-AIDs

Preprocedural Approach

Based on medication, choose the appropriate site. Steroid injections are typically given in the anterolateral thigh (ie, vastus lateralis) or, for older children, the buttocks (ie, dorsogluteal and ventrogluteal). The upper arm (ie, deltoid) may also be used if other sites are not good options (Figure 15.1).

- **Anterolateral thigh injection**—This is an ideal site for injection because it is easily accessible, contains a large muscle mass, and has no major blood vessels or nerves in the target area. It is the most common site of IM injection for children younger than 3 years.
  - Locate the correct thigh IM injection site by forming an imaginary box on the upper leg by the following steps: Locate the groin and measure one hand's width below the groin, and this becomes the upper border of the box. The lower border of the box is one hand's width above the top of the knee. The center of the top of the leg becomes the left border, and the center of the outside of the leg becomes the right border of the box.
  - The IM injection (up to 2 mL of fluid) is given in the middle of this imaginary box.
- **Ventrogluteal injection**—Typically, this technique should *not be used in children younger than 2 years*.
  - Find the trochanter at the superior portion of the proximal leg. Next, find the anterior iliac crest. Place the palm of your hand over the trochanter. Point your index finger toward the anterior iliac crest. Spread your middle finger toward the back, making a "V." The thumb should be pointed toward the anterior leg.
  - IM injection is given between the knuckles of your first and second fingers. Up to about 3 mL of fluid may be given at this site.
- **Deltoid injection**—Locate the correct upper arm IM injection site by forming an imaginary box on the upper arm. Locate the acromion process at the top of the arm; the top border of the box is two finger widths down from the acromion process. The bottom border of the box is an imaginary line running from the crease in the armpit from front to back. To make the two side borders, divide the arm into three equal sections from front to back. The injection site is in the center of the middle third, approximately 3 to 5cm inferior to the acromion process. CAUTION: This is a small injection site, and only 1 mL or less of fluid should be injected at this site.
- **Dorsogluteal injection**—Typically, this technique should not be used in children younger than 2 years because of the risk of damage to the sciatic nerve and gluteal artery. Start by finding the trochanter at the superior portion of the proximal leg. Next, find the posterior iliac crest. Now, draw an imaginary line between the two bones and locate the center of the imaginary line; the target for IM injection is a point 1-in superior to this center point. Up to about 3 mL of fluid may be given at this site.

Procedural Approach

- Check for air by drawing back on the plunger to expose an air space, push plunger slowly until one drop of medication is expelled from the needle tip.
- Wipe site with alcohol swab and allow to dry.
- Spread skin at the site.
- Approach at a 90° angle (or at a 45° angle to the tabletop for the anterolateral thigh technique).
- Inject needle fully into the site. Draw back with the plunger.
  - If blood is noted, then you have likely struck a blood vessel; withdraw without injecting medication. Discard entire syringe and medication. You must redraw using new needle, syringe, and medication.
  - If no blood is noted, then inject slowly to avoid pain. Withdraw quickly and hold pressure to site with 2 × 2 gauze for 1 minute.
- Apply BAND-AID to site.

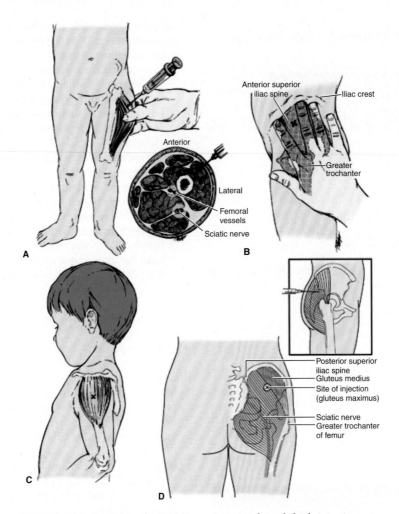

FIGURE 15.1. Intramuscular injections. A, Anterolateral thigh injections are made in the midthigh. The needle should be directed inferiorly and at a 45° angle to the tabletop, which avoids injury to the femoral vessels and sciatic nerve (highlighted areas). B, Site for ventrogluteal injections. C, Site for deltoid injections. D, Site for dorsogluteal injections. Reprinted with permission from McMillan JA, Feigin RD, DeAngelis C, et al. *Oski's Pediatrics: Principles & Practice.* 4th ed. Philadelphia, PA: Lippincott Williams & Wilkins; 2006.

SUGGESTED READINGS

Mathes BM, Alguire PC. Intralesional Injection. *UpToDate.* 2018. https://www.uptodate.com/contents/intralesional-corticosteroid-injection.

Richards RN. Update on intralesional steroid: focus on dermatoses. *J Cutan Med Surg.* 2010;14:19.

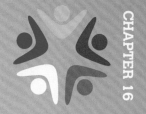

CHAPTER 16

Cryosurgery

Andrea R. Waldman and Diana H. Lee

INTRODUCTION

Cryosurgery represents a highly effective, minimally invasive surgical modality that utilizes the application of a cryogen to induce extremely low temperatures and destroy abnormal tissue. It is most commonly employed for wart destruction, but can be selectively applied to other benign cutaneous lesions, such as molluscum contagiosum, pyogenic granulomas, acne cysts, and acrochordons, as well as malignant lesions such as basal cell carcinoma and squamous cell carcinoma.

Surgical diathermy involves heat transfer from hot matter to cold matter. The larger the temperature differential between the tissue and the cryogen, the faster the heat transfer occurs, enabling the destruction of the target lesion. The most commonly utilized cryogen, liquid nitrogen, which boils at $-196°C$, induces sufficient heat transfer to destroy both benign and malignant cells.

The destructive effects of cryosurgery may be attributed to both direct and indirect tissue injury. Repetitive cycles of fast freezing followed by slow thawing increase the destructive potential of cryosurgery. During the initial freezing period, direct tissue necrosis occurs through extracellular and then intracellular ice crystal formation, ultimately inducing edema and cell lysis. In addition, secondary damage of the vascular endothelium provokes tissue ischemia during the subsequent thawing period. Apoptosis and immunologic destruction also occur in the hours after thawing, creating further tissue injury.

CONTRAINDICATIONS

Cryosurgery is often painful or frightening, and some children, especially those younger than 8 years of age, may not be able to tolerate the procedure. Relative to the spray gun, the use of a cotton-tipped applicator may decrease patient fear or anxiety. Although the child can be restrained to complete the procedure, this is often unfavorable and may be emotionally traumatizing. Thus, it is important to consider alternative treatment modalities in these children.

Contraindications to cryosurgery include undiagnosed lesions, patients with poor circulation, previous sensitivity or adverse reaction to cryosurgery, cold intolerance and other cold-triggered ailments, such as cold urticarial, cryoglobulinemia, or Raynaud's phenomenon. Parents and patients should be informed of the relative risks of cryotherapy compared to other less invasive therapies available. Longer healing times (up to 2 weeks) are involved as second intention healing is required. Scarring and skin retraction represent infrequent complications with deep freezing procedures, especially at free margins. Thus, cryotherapy is not recommended for concave areas (ie, malar surface, corners of the eyes, nasolabial folds). When hair-bearing areas are treated with cryosurgery, alopecia is a potential consequence. Deep freezing of the lateral digits may induce digital nerve damage, because cutaneous nerves are very superficial in these regions. Care must also be taken when performing cryosurgery to treat periungal warts; damage to the nail matrix represents a rare complication. Furthermore, hypo- or hyperpigmentation, especially in individuals with darker skin types, may occur after the therapy.

PREPROCEDURAL CONSIDERATIONS

Before performing cryosurgery, it is important to solidify a cutaneous diagnosis of the targeted lesion. This may be determined via dermoscopy, clinical examination or histopathologic evaluation. Once clinical diagnosis is confirmed and the patient is screened for contraindications to therapy, counseled on the risk–benefit ratio of treatment, and informed consent is obtained, the appropriate cryosurgery technique is then selected.

SPECIFIC TECHNIQUES

Cryosurgery in pediatrics can be categorized into the following techniques:

- Open (spray) technique: This is the most commonly utilized cryosurgery modality. The spray instrument consists of a metal vessel directly attached to a spray tip through which the cryogen in released. This method is suitable for treating a wide variety of cutaneous lesions.
- Frozen forceps technique: This method is ideal for filiform or pedunculated lesions protruding from the skin surface. Utilizing this technique, the lesion is grasped with a prefrozen forceps and held in place for 10 to 20 seconds. The surrounding healthy tissue is spared as the freezing tool is advanced only to the skin surface. This minimized scarring and postinflammatory pigmentary alteration (hypo- or hyperpigmentation).
- Dipstick technique: A cotton-tipped applicator is soaked with cryogen and subsequently placed directly on the cutaneous lesional surface. This modality is often better tolerated by frightened or younger children.
- Intralesional technique: A needle probe attached to the cryogen source is passed through the lesion. This allows freezing to occur from the center of the lesion, sparing epidermal destruction. This technique was originally developed for the treatment of keloid scars.

Equipment Needed

- Liquid nitrogen
- Spray gun, tweezers, cryoneedle probe, or cotton-tipped applicator
- Curette or 15-blade scalpel (optional)
- BAND-AIDs™ (Johnson & Johnson, US) (optional)
- Narrow apertures or disposable plastic ear speculum (optional)
- Protective eyewear
- Gloves

PROCEDURAL APPROACH

Preparation of equipment and medical environment:

- Self-preparation: Apply protective eyewear and gloves.
- Transfer liquid nitrogen or other cryogen of choice into utilized cryosurgery device (for spray method, the cryospray vessel; for cotton-tipped applicator or tweezer methods, a nonpermeable container).

Application of cryogen—the open (spray) technique:
- Wash hands thoroughly and put on medical gloves.
- Select a spray tip of the appropriate size. This is tailored to the individual lesion. Larger spray tips deliver more cryogen and create a temperature differential more rapidly than smaller spray tips. Smaller spray tips allow for more precise targeting and slower freezing of cutaneous lesions. A disposable ear speculum may be utilized to focus the targeted lesion and further increase precision of cryosurgery.
- Prepare the lesion using a 15-blade scalpel or curette to remove excess keratin (optional).
- Apply cryogen with the spray vessel until a white halo appears around the lesion. This timing varies from 5 to 20 seconds.
- Subsequently allow the lesion to thaw for 30 to 45 seconds.
- For thicker lesions, repeat the two previous steps (freeze/thaw) for a second time to allow for two freeze–thaw cycles.

Application of cryogen—frozen forceps technique:
- Wash hands thoroughly and put on medical gloves.
- Place forceps into the nonpermeable cryogen container filled with cryogen for 3 to 5 seconds.
- Grip lesion firmly with forceps and lower to cutaneous surface surrounding lesion. Hold in place for 5 to 20 seconds until a white halo is achieved.
- Allow lesion to thaw for 30 to 45 seconds.
- For thicker lesions, repeat previous two steps to allow for two freeze–thaw cycles.

Application of cryogen—the dipstick (cotton-tipped applicator) technique
- Wash hands thoroughly and put on medical gloves.
- Dip cotton-tipped applicator into the nonpermeable container filled with cryogen and thoroughly saturate.
- Directly place the cotton-tipped applicator on the cutaneous surface of the target lesion and hold in place until a white halo is achieved (5-20 seconds).
- Allow the lesion to thaw for 30 to 45 seconds.
- For thicker lesions, repeat the previous two steps for two freeze–thaw cycles. Cotton-tipped applicators should not be dipped into the cryogen container a second time. New cotton-tipped applicators should be used for subsequent freeze–thaw cycles.

Application of cryogen—intralesional technique:
- Wash hands thoroughly and put on medical gloves.
- Locally anesthetize lesion.
- Attach needle probe to liquid nitrogen source (cryogun).
- Insert cryotherapy needle probe into the center of the cutaneous lesion by gradual twisting motion until penetration through the opposite end of the lesion is achieved.
- Allow cryogen to pass through the needle probe until the lesion is sufficiently frozen.
- Allow the lesion to thaw for approximately 60 seconds.

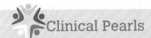

Clinical Pearls

Cryosurgery is a highly efficacious treatment modality for warts and other cutaneous lesions. The cure rate with repeated sessions over several months is documented between 20% and 50% in the literature. A safe, relatively simple, and versatile therapeutic intervention, cryosurgery can be performed on a wide variety of patients with a broad range of cutaneous conditions. The evidence from available randomized control trials, however, is both limited and contradictory.
- The goal of cryotherapy is to produce blister formation after 1 to 2 days above the dermal–epidermal junction, avoiding deep ulceration, scarring, or necrosis of surrounding tissue.
- Liquid nitrogen is applied to the lesion with a spray gun, cotton-tipped applicator, or tweezer until there is a white ring around the lesion.
    - This correlates with a sustained freezing time of approximately 10 to 20 seconds, followed by a thaw time of 30 to 45 seconds.
- Of note, the use of small diameter apertures, including otoscope caps, leads to less peripheral tissue destruction when using the spray technique.
- Treatment may be more efficacious when lesions are prepped with gentle removal of excess keratin with a curette or 15-blade scalpel. More than one treatment is generally required to induce clearance of lesions, with therapy often repeated at 3- to 4-week intervals.

POSTPROCEDURAL APPROACH

Following the procedure, it is essential to inform the patient that the treated area will heal by secondary intention and may blister within a few to 48 hours. Subsequently the blister is replaced by hemorrhagic crusting (a scab) within 48 to 72 hours of blister formation. Bleeding and swelling may occur, and should subside within a few days. Healing time varies according to depth of freezing and anatomic location from 2 weeks to 1 month (distal extremities). Large bullae and/or ulceration rarely develop with deep freezing procedures, and healing times may be increased in such scenarios. A BAND-AID and topical emollient (ie, Vaseline™ [Conopco, Inc., US]) may be placed to enhance healing. Eschars rarely develop in the setting of deep freezing, as a result of cryonecrosis. Debridement facilitates healing of eschars and is often appropriate. Hypopigmentation, hyperpigmention, or scarring may result following site healing. If the patient notices signs of cutaneous infection, such as increased redness or edema of the surrounding skin or discharge of purulent material, they should be notified to contact the provider immediately or report to the emergency department.

TABLE 16.1 ⁞ Benign Pediatric Dermatologic Conditions Responsive to Cryotherapy

Acne cysts—one 5-10 s FTC
Acrochordons—one 5 s FTC with 2-mm margin
Angiofibroma—one 15-20 s FTC
Angiokeratomas—one 10 s FTC with 1-mm margin
Dermatofibromas—one to two 20-60 s FTC with 2- to 3-mm margin
Epidermal nevus—one 5 s FTC with 1-mm margin
Granuloma annulare—one 5-10 FTC
Keloid scars—one 15-30 s FTC with 1-mm margin
Lymphangioma—one 15 s FTC with 1- to 2-mm margin
Milia—one 5-10 s FTC
Molluscum contagiosum—one 5 s FTC
Pearly penile papules—two 15-20 s FTC
Porokeratosis (Mibelli)—one 15 s FTC with 1-mm margin
Prurigo nodularis—one 10 s FTC
Pyogenic granuloma—one 15 s FTC with <1-mm margin
Sarcoidosis—one 10 s FTC
Trichoepithelioma—one 10-15 s FTC
Verruca vulgaris—one to two 10-60 s FTC with 2- to 3-mm margin
Xanthoma—one 10 s FTC

FTC, freeze–thaw cycle.

LESIONS FOR WHICH WE UTILIZE CRYOSURGERY

Cryosurgery is utilized frequently in the management of many benign and malignant pediatric skin conditions. Tables 16.1 and 16.2 outline benign and malignant dermatologic conditions responsive to cryosurgical management.

Cryotherapy is also frequently implemented as an anesthetic modality before other cutaneous surgical procedures. In

TABLE 16.2 ⁞ Malignant Pediatric Dermatologic Conditions Responsive to Cryosurgery

Basal cell carcinoma (superficial)—Two 30 s FTC with 5-mm margin
Squamous cell carcinoma (superficial, well defined)—Two 30 s FTC with 5-mm margin
Melanoma (palliation)—Two 30 s FTC with 5-mm margin

FTC, freeze–thaw cycle.

addition to liquid nitrogen, ethyl chloride is another cryogen widely utilized as an anesthetic agent. Cryogens applied to the cutaneous surface for 3 to 5 seconds before needle insertion or surgical incision may lessen cutaneous discomfort and patient distress.

SUGGESTED READINGS

Dawber R. Cryosurgery: unapproved uses, dosages, or indications. *Clin Dermatol.* 2002;20(5):563–570.
Dvir E, Hirshowitz B. The use of cryosurgery in treating the fibrous papules of tuberous sclerosis. *Ann Plast Surg.* 1980;4(2):158–160.
Goel R, Anderson, K, Slaton, J, et al. Adjuvant approaches to enhance cryosurgery. *J Biomech Eng.* 2009;131:074003.
Guidelines of care for cryosurgery. American Academy of Dermatology Committee on Guidelines of Care. *J Am Acad Dermatol.* 1994;31(4):648–653.
Van Leeuwen MC, Bulstra AE, Ket JC, Ritt MJ, van Leeuwen PA, Niessen FB. Intralesional cryotherapy for the treatment of keloid scars: evaluating effectiveness. *Plast Reconstr Surg Glob Open.* 2015;3(6):e437.
Zimmerman EE, Crawford, P. Cutaneous cryosurgery. *Am Fam Physician.* 2012;86(12):1118–1124.
Zouboulis CC, Blume U, Büttner P, Orfanos CE. Outcomes of cryosurgery in keloids and hypertrophic scars. A prospective consecutive trial of case series. *Arch Dermatol.* 1993;129(9):1146–1151.

CHAPTER 17

Electrosurgery/Hyfrecation

John C. Browning and Giselle Castillo

INTRODUCTION

Electrosurgery uses a multifunction electrosurgical generator with a handpiece and electrode tip to produce high-frequency waves to heat and cut tissue. It is an integral method used in skin surgery. Electrosurgery has a multitude of uses in treating benign and malignant skin growths and provides for the removal of benign and malignant lesions, helps control bleeding, and is useful in cutting and excising tissue.

The general uses of electrosurgery include the following: (1) to excise tissue, (2) to control bleeding, (3) destruction of tissue, and (4) vaporization of tissue fragments. Electrosurgery has many advantages. In addition to being a rapid technique, electrosurgery employs devices that are relatively simple to use and easily mastered with practice. Equipment is compact and affordable for basic devices and can be used to treat a wide variety of skin lesions. Bleeding can be controlled while cutting or destroying tissue, and a sterile field is usually unnecessary when equipment is used only for tissue destruction.

A multifunction electrosurgical generator with a handpiece and electrode tip is used to generate and deliver high-frequency waves with great precision. Varying the wave frequency and the amount of heat produced and the placement of the electrode tip on the tissue helps achieve the desired effect. For example, the amount of heat necessary for tissue destruction is different from the amount of energy/heat needed to cut tissue.

Tissue responds to the amount of heat and the placement of the electrode tip. Adjusting the distance of the electrode tip from the tissue also helps target the depth where heat is delivered. For example, touching the skin with an active electrode tip delivers heat to a different depth than if the electrode tip is inserted into the skin. The following are the four types of electrosurgical techniques:

1. *Fulguration* is conducted by holding the electrode away from the skin and results in the destruction of tissue by heating and charring (Figure 17.1). Fulguration can be used to treat lesions such as skin tags or basal cell carcinoma.
2. *Electrodesiccation* occurs when an active electrode touches the skin and delivers direct energy to the tissue causing the cells to dry out (Figure 17.2). Electrodesiccation is useful in treating lesions such as telangiectasias.

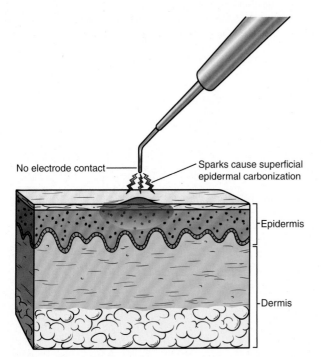

No electrode contact — Sparks cause superficial epidermal carbonization

Epidermis

Dermis

FIGURE 17.1. In fulguration, the electrode is held away from the skin to produce sparking to the skin surface. This produces a high intensity but more shallow tissue destruction that may reach the upper dermis.

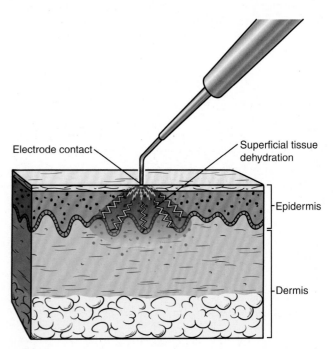

Electrode contact — Superficial tissue dehydration

Epidermis

Dermis

FIGURE 17.2. In electrodesiccation, the active electrode touches or is inserted into the skin and produces destruction deeper into the dermis.

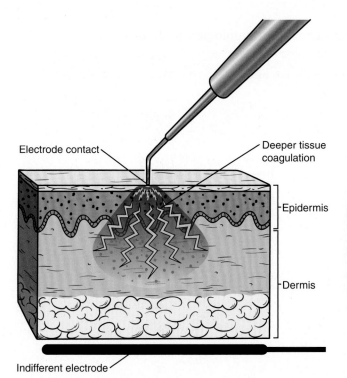

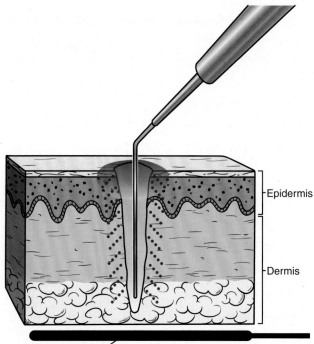

FIGURE 17.3. Electrocoagulation is used to stop bleeding in both superficial and deep surgery.

FIGURE 17.4. In electrosection, a different waveform is used allowing scalpel-like dissection by vaporizing the cellular fluid and causing cellular explosions.

3. *Electrocoagulation* is used to stop bleeding and is often involved in deep and superficial surgery (Figure 17.3).
4. *Electrosection* uses a different waveform that allows for scalpel-like dissection or cutting by vaporizing the cellular fluid and causing cellular explosions (Figure 17.4).

ELECTROSURGICAL DEVICES

Always refer to the manufacturer operator's manual to optimize safety and efficacy when performing electrosurgical procedures as there are differences in the brands of electrosurgical generators on the market. Several electrosurgery devices exist, the most common being the Hyfrecator® 2000 (Conmed, US).

The term "hyfrecator" is often used generically to describe similar devices. These devices are equipped with low and high settings, which allow the user to control the amount of heat delivered to the tissue. The general rule in electrosurgery is to use the lowest amount of heat needed to achieve the desired effect. The current from the electrode can be applied in either a unipolar or bipolar fashion. Most electrosurgical units are unipolar, but bipolar units may be ideal when controlling bleeding because forceps can grasp the site. Electrosurgery procedures can be performed with or without local anesthesia, often without the need of an assistant, and are associated with less bleeding. The site is usually allowed to heal by secondary intention which often occurs after 2 to 3 weeks. Electrosurgery, in combination with curettage, is the recommended procedure for removing most of the skin lesions listed below.

Before beginning electrosurgery, when first turning on the device power, *it is important to check the proper settings for specific use.* Table 17.1 lists the appropriate power settings and type of electrode for common skin lesions. The values listed are starting points and the clinician must find the best setting for each individual patient.

ELECTROSURGERY FOR SPECIFIC LESIONS

Benign Lesions

- **Acrochordon (Skin Tag):** Large skin tags are best shaved off with a scalpel. Small- to medium-sized lesions can be destroyed by electrodesiccation or fulguration. Removal of the remaining char can be accomplished with a gauze pad or curette.
- **Actinic Keratoses:** These precancerous lesions should be removed as soon as they are identified. Most respond well to light electrofulguration. The curette should be sharp and complete electrodesiccation should occur after thorough curettage.
- **Adenoma Sebaceum:** These facial angiofibromas should be treated on a low-power setting. Desiccation should be used for each papule.

TABLE 17.1 ⋮ Suggested Power Settings for Treating Various Dermatologic Conditions.

LESIONS	POWER SETTING (Watts on Low Unless Otherwise Indicated)	TYPE OF ELECTRODE
Benign		
Angiomas (cherry)	2-2.5	Sharp or dull
Angiomas (spider)	2-2.5	Sharp or needle
Condyloma acuminate	12-18	Dull
Dermatosis papulosa nigra	2-2.5	Dull or sharp
Pyogenic granulomas	16-20 (or switch to high)	Dull
Seborrheic keratosis	10-14	Dull
Skin tags (acrochordons)	2-2.5	Sharp
Syringomas	2-2.5	Sharp
Telangiectasias	2-2.5	Sharp or needle
Verrucae vulgaris	12-18	Dull
Verrucae plana	12-18	Sharp or dull
Malignant		
Basal cell carcinoma	16-20	Dull
Squamous cell carcinoma	16-20	Dull

- **Angiokeratoma:** Most can be left alone, but if bleeding is of concern, removal may be achieved with superficial desiccation.
- **Angiomas (Cherry):** Removal by electrosurgery has shown to be an effective treatment option. If the lesion is greater than 4 mm, anesthesia should be considered. Light, superficial desiccation is usually sufficient. The remaining char can be wiped away with a gauze pad or curette.
- **Angiomas (Cavernous):** A similar technique to that used for cherry angiomas may be applied, although multiple needle insertions may be necessary.
- **Angiomas, Spider:** Consider the use of topical anesthetic or no anesthetic at all when treating these lesions. Injecting lidocaine may conceal the lesion because of vasoconstriction. Electrodesiccation at the center, at the central feeding vessel, provides adequate removal.
- **Condyloma Acuminatum (Venereal Wart):** A local anesthetic should first be used. Condylomata respond well to electrofulguration.
- **Fibroma:** Performing light electrodesiccation or fulguration destroys small fibromas.
- **Keratoacanthoma:** A deep shave or "scoop" biopsy should confirm diagnosis before electrosurgery. Electrofulguration destroys the residual tumor and should be aimed at the base of the lesion.
- **Lymphangioma:** Electrodesiccation or fulguration may help treat these tumors.
- **Molluscum Contagiosum:** Most lesions respond well to electrodesiccation.

- **Pyogenic Granuloma:** Treatment with electrofulguration produces adequate results but may require thorough curettage.
- **Seborrheic Keratoses:** These skin tumors associated with old age can be treated with electrosurgery. Fulguration should be performed initially. This allows the charred remains to be wiped away with a gauze pad or curette. Multiple small seborrheic keratoses of the face in young African Americans (dermatosis papulosa nigra) may also be treated with electrosurgery. These lesions may be treated without anesthesia using a low-powered setting.
- **Sebaceous Papules:** These papules are commonly seen in older, oily-skinned patients and may be removed by electrofulguration.
- **Syringomas:** One or two lesions should be tested before beginning electrosurgery. Light fulguration followed by gentle curettage often provides adequate results.
- **Telangiectasias:** Gentle electrodesiccation can treat facial telangiectasias. It is important to note that a low-power setting is usually sufficient. Electrosurgery of these lesions have several advantages over laser treatment that include cost and outcomes. Telangiectasias that occur on the legs, however, must be treated with caution because they are more likely to reoccur.
- **Common Warts (Verrucae Vulgaris):** Most warts encountered in clinic will respond well to electrofulguration with careful curettage of the base. Anesthesia should always be used. If any of the wart remains after curettage, additional electrosurgery should be performed. It is important to note

that deep tissue destruction should be avoided because of painful scarring.

- **Filiform Warts:** Electrodestruction of the pedicle has highly favorable outcomes along with aesthetically pleasing results.
- **Flat Warts (Verrucae Plana):** These warts respond well to light electrofulguration.

Malignant Lesions

A biopsy should be taken first if there is a suspicion of a malignant lesion.

- **Basal Cell Carcinoma:** It is important to obtain a shave biopsy before electrosurgery. Curettage is first performed, followed by fulguration. Removal of debris with additional curettage is often indicated. Curettage and fulguration are typically repeated once or twice.
- **Squamous Cell Carcinoma in Situ (Bowen Disease):** These lesions respond to the same techniques for basal cell carcinomas. Anesthesia should extend 1 to 2 cm beyond the visible lesions because these lesions may extend further laterally than they appear.

- **Squamous Cell Carcinoma:** The same techniques as used for basal cell carcinoma and squamous cell carcinoma in situ (Bowen disease) can be applied. Only lesions that arise in sun-damaged areas should be treated. Lesions in non-sun-exposed skin and in mucous membranes are more aggressive biologically, and for these lesions other removal techniques should be discussed and explored between the clinician and the patient before proceeding.

SUGGESTED READINGS

ConMed. *Hyfrecator 2000 Electrosurgical Unit Operator's Manual.* New York, NY: Utica; 2013.

Ghodsi SZ, Raziei M, Taheri A, Karami M, Mansoori P, Farnaghi F. Comparison of cryotherapy and curettage for the treatment of pyogenic granuloma: a randomized trial. *Br J Dermatol.* 2006;154:671–675.

Soon SL, Washington CV. Curettage and electrodesiccation. In: Robinson JK, Hanke CW, Sengelmann RD, Siegel DM, eds. *Surgery of the Skin.* 2nd ed. New York, NY: Elsevier; 2010.

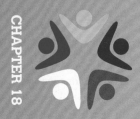

CHAPTER 18

Laser Surgery

Larissa Marie Lehmer and Kristen M. Kelly

INTRODUCTION

Lasers are widely utilized for the treatment of many diagnoses in the pediatric population. When used correctly, lasers can often provide significant benefit with minimal morbidity and should be in the armamentarium of all pediatric surgeons.

"Laser" is an acronym: light amplification by the stimulated emission of radiation (LASER). Laser devices used in the treatment of cutaneous disorders operate on the principle of the wave–particle duality of light conceptualized by physicists Max Planck and Albert Einstein in the first half of the 20th century. Light is a form of energy that comprises photon particles grouped into discrete packets or quanta. The amount of energy carried by each photon is inversely proportional to its wavelength. Therefore, with regard to the optical spectrum of electromagnetic radiation, ultraviolet (100-400 nm) is more energetic than visible (400-750 nm) is more energetic than infrared (750-1000 nm) light. Sunlight defines "broad spectrum" as it emits photons across all wavelengths. Laser devices produce light of a specific wavelength by using electrical energy in the form of an oscillating current to excite the molecules of selected solids (crystals), liquids (dyes), or gasses (argon and carbon dioxide [CO_2]) to generate light of specific wavelengths. Because the electrical current passing through the solid, liquid, or gas media synchronizes the excited molecules, the light discharged is coherent; that is, the photons are aligned in both space and time and collimated (precisely parallel), which allows a laser beam to travel great distances without attenuation.

The very first practical laser was developed by Maiman in 1960 and used a ruby as its medium to generate 694 nm light.[1] The first paper on the clinical applications of lasers in dermatology was published by Goldman in 1963.[2] Until Anderson and Parrish's description of the principle of selective photothermolysis in 1983, the use of lasers in dermatology was confined to conditions that benefitted from nonspecific tissue destruction. The understanding of selective photothermolysis spurred exponential growth in the development of devices that can be tuned to deliver energy precisely to different targets within the tissue based on their characteristic color (ie, chromophore), size, and depth although avoiding or minimizing damage to other nearby structures.

SELECTIVE PHOTOTHERMOLYSIS

Selective photothermolysis allows microscopic laser surgery of histologic targets based on the selection of the following three parameters: (1) a wavelength that provides an absorption coefficient sufficiently distinct from the surrounding tissue, (2) a pulse duration lesser than or equal to the thermal relaxation time of the target structure, and (3) an energy level sufficient to damage the target although limited to prevent nonspecific injury. We discuss the selection of each of these parameters.

Knowledge of the main chromophore(s) present in the targeted condition and target depth within the tissue guides the laser surgeon's selection of the appropriate laser wavelength. Wavelength selection is primarily based on absorption of the energy by three main chromophores: hemoglobin, melanin, and water, present in the skin and its structures. Absorption spectra for the important cutaneous chromophores are summarized in Figure 18.1, whereas the depth of penetration by laser type is depicted in Figure 18.2. Foreign bodies such as tattoo particles or a traumatic tattoo such as asphalt implanted during an injury can also be targeted. Whether the target is tattoo ink, melanin in melanocytes or hair follicles, or hemoglobin in microvessels dictates which wavelength will be best absorbed by the target and thus should be selected. When wavelengths of visible light are used, selection should be complementary to the color of the target chromophore; that is, green light with a wavelength of 532 nm is emitted by the frequency-doubled Q-switched neodymium–yttrium aluminum garnet (Nd:YAG) and can be used for the removal of red tattoo ink, whereas the Q-switched ruby laser discharges red light with a 694 nm wavelength and can be used to break down green pigment (see Chapter 124. Tattoo Removal). To ensure preferential absorption, avoidance of incidental absorption by competing nearby chromophores must be taken into consideration when selecting the laser wavelength. For example, light intended to treat dermal blood vessels must first pass through the epidermis and avoid being absorbed by melanin or being scattered by collagen before reaching its target.

Light energy contacting the skin can either be reflected off of it (scattered) or be transmitted through and absorbed by its tissue target in the form of heat. The higher the energy of the photon or the shorter the wavelength, the more it is scattered when it strikes the tissue and the less deep into the tissue the light will penetrate. For this reason, shorter wavelengths can be used for superficial tissue targeting, whereas longer wavelengths should be used to target deeper structures. For example, Q-switched 532 nm lasers may be used to target epidermal melanin in lentigines, whereas Q-switched 1064 nm devices would be better suited for targeting dermal melanin in nevus of Ota (for further details, see Chapter 110. Nevus of Ota and Nevus of Ito).

The pulse duration (in seconds or portions of seconds) is the time over which laser energy is delivered to the tissue and is set based on the square of the target's diameter in millimeters. In this way, an adequate amount of energy is delivered to effectively heat and destroy the target, which preferentially absorbs the photons emitted, although avoiding excessive collateral heating of nearby structures. Thermal relaxation time (TRT) of a cutaneous structure describes the rate at which the photons are converted to heat and subsequently cool. For example, when considering the wide range of TRTs encompassed by blood vessels, it takes 0.04 seconds for a 0.2 mm telangiectasia to cool whereas it takes only 1 ms (0.001 second) for a 0.03 mm venule in a child's port wine birthmark (PWB) to cool (for further details, see Chapter 115. Port-Wine Birthmarks). By comparison, the target of pigmented lesions is 0.5 μm melanosomes, which carry a 250 nanosecond (ns), that is, 0.000000250 seconds, TRT.[3] This illustrates why the nanosecond Q-switched 755 nm alexandrite laser is effective in addressing pigmented lesions that comprise individual melanocyte cells whereas millisecond pulsed dye lasers (PDLs) are used to address vascular lesions.

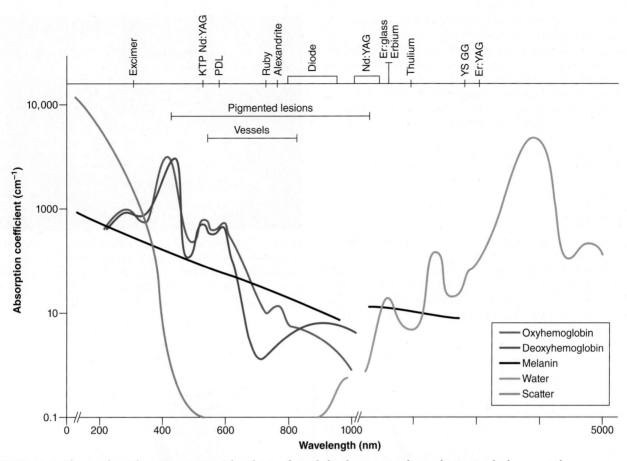

FIGURE 18.1. Chromophore absorption curves. A key driving factor behind appropriate laser selection is whether or not the energy transmitted by the laser will be absorbed by the target chromophore. For pigmented lesions, the chromophore is melanin although hemoglobin residing in varying diameters of vessels is the target pigment in vascular lesions and water is the chromophore target for addressing dermal issues such as scarring. It is important to know the absorption coefficient of the intended target and select a wavelength that will preferentially be absorbed by the target as compared to other chromophores in the surrounding skin.

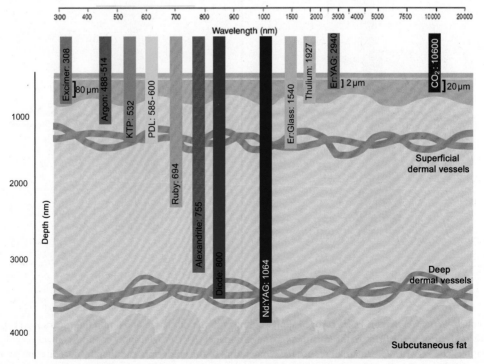

FIGURE 18.2. Relative depth of wavelength penetration. Laser type is arranged in order of wavelength from left (shortest wavelength) to right (longest wavelength). After 1064 nm, depth of penetration is limited by bulk tissue heating through the high absorption of water at longer wavelengths. CO_2, carbon dioxide; Er, erbium; KTP, potassium titanyl phosphate; Nd:YAG, neodymium–yttrium aluminum garnet; PDL, pulsed dye laser.

Finally, an appreciation for laser dosimetry is required for the safe and effective application of light-based technologies. Fluence or energy delivered per unit area in J/cm^2 is the primary component of laser dosing and must take into account the characteristics of the target and the surrounding tissue. For example, increased baseline pigmentation in darker skin types (ie, increased melanin chromophore) may confer an increased risk of skin injury at fluences tolerated in lighter skin types. A laser's power is defined by the amount of energy delivered per second (J/s). If the dose of light energy delivered to the tissue is too low, then no improvement will occur; if the dose is too high, skin injury ranging from dyspigmentation to scarring results (see Figure 18.3).

COOLING

Epidermal cooling, which was introduced in the 1990s, is employed in treatments where the epidermis must be protected from nonselective thermal damage as the laser light passes through on the way to targeted tissues in the dermis (Figure 18.4),[4] for example, millisecond laser light in the visible spectrum traveling through the epidermis to target hemoglobin

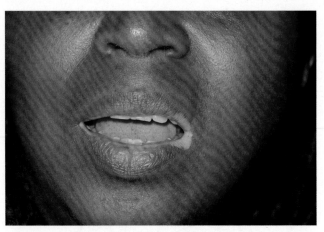

FIGURE 18.3. Illustration of post-inflammatory hypopigmentation, which is an undesired complication that can arise from inappropriate settings in laser hair removal. Reprinted with permission from Hall JC, Hall BJ. *Sauer's Manual of Skin Diseases.* 11th ed. Philadelphia, PA: Wolters Kluwer; 2017. Figure 38.22.

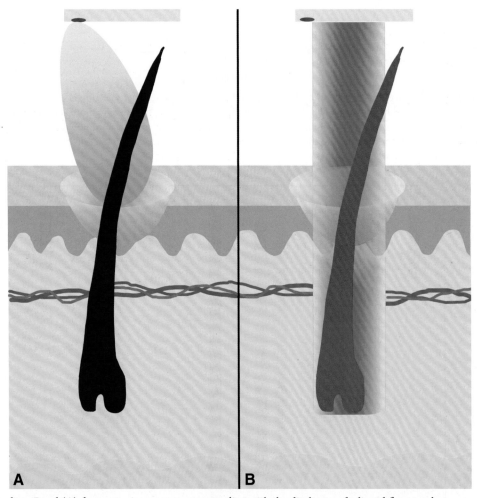

FIGURE 18.4. Cooling. Panel (A) demonstrates cryogen spray cooling with the discharge of a liquid fluorocarbon cryogen spray from the laser device milliseconds prior to the firing of the laser demonstrated in panel (B). Cryogen spray cooling, contact cooling through a cooled handpiece, and parallel cooling with forced air all reduce the temperature of the epidermis and thereby decrease unwanted impact of laser energy passing through the epidermis on the way to deeper targets such as blood vessels and hair follicles.

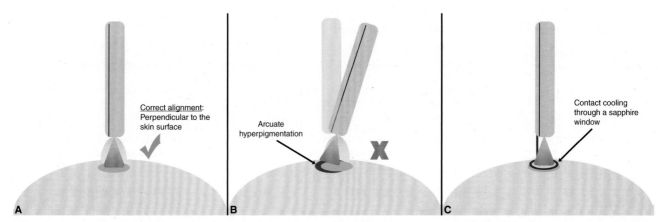

FIGURE 18.5. Laser technique, positioning. Panel (A) demonstrates the appropriate positioning of the laser handpiece perpendicular to the tangent of the curved surface of the skin. B, When using a laser with cryogen spray cooling, failure to continually maintain the handpiece perpendicular to the contour of the skin risks mismatch of the cryogen and laser. Incomplete overlap of the cooling and laser pulses produces characteristic arcuate epidermal burn marks. C, When using contact cooling, it is important to keep desired contact with the cooling handpiece, or cooling effect may be lost resulting in epidermal injury.

in blood vessels or melanin in hair follicles. Epidermal cooling allows the use of higher energies, decreases treatment pain,[5] and allows the treatment of all skin types.[6] Before epidermal cooling was implemented, darker skin type patients with more epidermal melanin were not good candidates for many laser treatments as blistering with subsequent scarring and discoloration would frequently result.

All cooling methods use a cooling agent to extract heat at the skin surface. Cooling is accomplished in one of three ways: cryogen spray cooling, contact cooling, and forced cold air.

Cryogen spray cooling utilizes millisecond spurts of tetra-fluoroethane. This rapidly decreases the epidermal temperature with minimal change to dermal structures. Cryogen spray cooling parameters are described as the millisecond for which the spurt will be delivered/milliseconds of delay between the cryogen spurt and the laser irradiation (eg, 30/30 would be a 30 ms spurt of cryogen with a 30 ms delay between the end of the cryogen spurt and the beginning of the laser irradiation). Companies often provide recommended cryogen settings for different devices and different indications. Longer cryogen spurts are used when the target is deeper. Some examples of setting to demonstrate this point are when treating verrucae, no cooling or 20/10 ms may be used; when treating vascular lesions near the top of the dermis, 30/30 might be used; and when doing laser hair removal, 50/30 might be used. When using devices with cryogen spray cooling, it is important to keep the handpiece perpendicular so that the laser light irradiation area and cryogen spray area remain aligned. If the handpiece is angled, then you can get arcuate scabbing, which may result in arcuate hyper or hypopigmentation from areas of laser irradiation where there is no cooling (Figure 18.5).[7]

Contact cooling utilizes plates made of a variety of materials including sapphire that are kept cold by circulating chilled liquids or cryogen sprayed onto the plate.[8] When using contact cooling, it is important to keep contact with the skin so that cooling occurs. It should also be kept in mind that holding the cooling in place for prolonged periods of time could decrease the temperature of the targeted tissue, which may compromise results. However, in some cases, this is done intentionally to protect the superficial dermis and promote tissue effects in deeper tissues.

Cold air cooling utilizes forced cold air released from a nozzle and is somewhat similar to a hair dryer which emits cold air

(although the nozzle is smaller). This is generally well tolerated[9] although efficiency of cooling may be less. Some patients also may not like the sensation of cold air by an orifice such as the nose, so this should be kept in mind during utilization.

LASER TYPES

We will now review commonly utilized types of lasers used in pediatrics and their indications (Table 18.1).

Millisecond Lasers

Pulsed Dye Laser

This laser will be discussed first because PDL treatment of vascular lesions was the first highly successful application of selective photothermolysis. Although the first PDL emitted yellow light at 577 nm, modern PDL devices emit yellow light with wavelengths from 585 to 600 nm, which generally allows for a 1.2 mm maximum depth of penetration; 595 nm is the wavelength most commonly utilized. Many consider PDL the "go-to" device for treating red-colored lesions, particularly vascular ones such as PWB, facial telangiectasias, superficial infantile hemangiomas (IH) (when laser treatment is performed), and telangiectases. PDL can also be employed to treat erythematous scars, verrucae, inflammatory linear verrucous epidermal nevus (ILVEN),[10] and psoriasis.

The tissue response noted with PDL varies based on pulse duration. Short pulses in the range of 0.45 to 3 ms cause intravascular coagulation/vessel rupture visually evidenced by purpura (see Figure 18.6A). Although the appearance of purpura indicates successful destruction of the vascular target, it can be cosmetically unacceptable to some patients, such as those seeking removal of a facial angioma or telangiectases. Longer 6 to 40 ms pulse durations can be used to achieve vascular removal for these indications without purpura; however, in some cases, multiple treatments may be required.

PDL is a common treatment choice for a variety of pediatric clinical diagnoses including PWB, IH, and spider angiomas.

PWB is a capillary malformation (CM) that affects 0.3% to 0.5% of the population, is present at birth, does not regress, and may become hypertrophic over time with vascular blebs.[11] These are also called "port wine stains," but this term may carry

TABLE 18.1 : Lasers Used in Pediatric Dermatology

LASER	WAVELENGTH (nm)	TARGET	INDICATION	MODE/PULSE DURATION	EXPECTED ENDPOINT
Excimer	308	Nonspecific	UVB phototherapy: atopic dermatitis, psoriasis, vitiligo	ns	Often no immediate tissue change
Pulsed dye laser (PDL)	577-600	Hemoglobin	Port wine birthmark, telangiectasia, warts, red scars	ms	Purpura (short pulsed); vessel disappearance, coagulum in vessel
KTP long-pulsed	532	Hemoglobin	Telangiectasia	ms	Vessel disappearance or coagulum in vessel
KTP QS		Melanin	Ephelides, cafe au lait macules	ns, ps	Immediate whitening
Alexandrite long-pulsed	755	Hemoglobin (weak)	Hypertrophic port wine birthmark, hair removal	ms	Purpura after 5 min or more (port wine birthmark settings); erythema and sometimes mild perifollicular edema at 5 min (hair removal)
Alexandrite QS		Melanin	Nevus of Ota, cafe au lait macules	ns, ps	Immediate whitening
Ruby long-pulsed	694	Melanin	Nevi, hair removal	ms	Erythema and sometimes mild perifollicular edema at 5 min (hair removal)
Ruby QS		Melanin	Dermal pigment; nevus of Ota	ns	Immediate whitening
Diode	800	Melanin DeoxyHb	Hair removal, venous lakes, telangiectasia	ms	Erythema and sometimes mild perifollicular edema at 5 min (hair removal)
Nd:YAG long-pulsed	1064	Melanin	Hair removal in dark skin	ms	Erythema and sometimes mild perifollicular edema at 5 min (hair removal)
Nd:YAG QS		Melanin	Dermal pigment; nevus of Ota	ns, ps	Immediate whitening
Erbium: Glass	1540	Water	Non-ablative dermal remodeling: acne scars, fractional resurfacing	Pulsed: ms	Erythema
Er:YAG	2940	Water	Ablation of epidermal lesions, skin resurfacing, scar revision, acne scars	Pulsed: ms	Pinpoint columns of destruction (fractional); chamois color (full field)
CO_2	10 600	Water	Ablation of lesions, skin resurfacing, scar revision, acne scars	Continuous wave, scanned, or pulsed μs–ms	

Abbreviations: Er, erbium; KTP, potassium titanyl phosphate; ms, millisecond; Nd, neodymium; ns, nanosecond; PDL, pulsed dye laser; ps, picosecond; QS, quality control switched; YAG, yttrium aluminum garnet.

a negative connotation and the use of PWB is preferred by many patients.[12] Development of this type of birthmark is because of a somatic activating mutation in the GNAQ gene (c.548G → A, p.R183Q), which results in the dysregulation of angiogenic signaling during development.[13] The most common location for a PWB is the face; however, they may present on any body location. Laser treatment of PWB is recommended to prevent future disfigurement, associated psychosocial comorbidity, and the development of nodules that may bleed within the malformation.[14] However, before proceeding with treatment, screening for associated syndromes and comorbidities should be performed. Some associated syndromes include Sturge–Weber syndrome (SWS), which necessitates comanagement with ophthalmology for glaucoma surveillance as well as neurology for associated seizures and developmental delay; Klippel–Trenaunay syndrome with associated limb hypertrophy and venous/lymphatic malformations; and capillary malformation/arteriovenous malformation syndrome. Vascular lasers that target hemoglobin, which strongly absorbs light in the 400 to 600 nm wavelength range, such as the PDL are employed in the

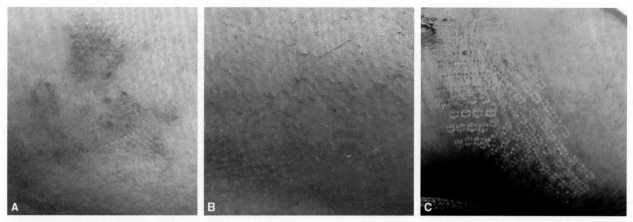

FIGURE 18.6. Examples of laser clinical endpoints. A, Endpoint for pulsed dye laser treatment of PWB is purpura as demonstrated here. *Skin whitening* should be avoided as this is indicative of epidermal damage. B, Laser hair removal clinical endpoints are erythema and, at times, perifollicular edema, that is, accentuation of the hair follicle. More extensive edema or blistering is not a desired endpoint and indicates settings need to be adjusted. C, Ablative fractional resurfacing for scar treatment with Er:YAG demonstrating pinpoint bleeding and pixilated ablation.

treatment of PWB at 4- to 6-week intervals with the expectation of 10 or more total treatments. To ensure vessel targeting and to avoid damage to the surrounding structures, pulse durations should be in the range of the estimated thermal relaxation time for vessels in CMs: 0.45 to 10 ms.

PDL can be used to treat PWB safely in all skin types, although settings may need to be adjusted in darker skin types. Shi et al demonstrated in an 848-patient study that with the implementation of cryogen spray cooling the 595 nm PDL can be safely used in Fitzpatrick skin types III to IV (7 mm spot, 1.5-10 ms, pulse duration, energy 8-12 J/cm^2 with 30/20 ms cryogen spray cooling) with 70% of patients exhibiting at least a 25% improvement after an average of six treatments, with a higher rate of clearance for lesions <20 cm^2.[15] PDL has also been successfully applied in Indian skin of Fitzpatrick types IV to V (spot size of 7-10 mm and settings depending on treatment situation as follows: 0.45 ms at 6.5-8 J/cm^2, 1.5 ms at 8-12 J/cm^2, 3 ms at 8-12 J/cm^2, and 10 ms at 10-15 J/cm^2, cryogen spray cooling 30/10 ms) with 20% of patients experiencing >80% improvement.[16] Of note, this study also commented on the faster rate of clearance with younger age and better overall results when patients underwent nine or more treatments.

IH may affect up to 5% to 10% of children under the age of 1 and constitute the most common tumors of infancy. Most lesions spontaneously regress over years, however, 20% require medical and/or surgical intervention because of complications including obstruction of the eyes, nose, mouth, or auditory canal; painful ulceration; bleeding; or disfiguring scars.[17] Oral and topical β-blockers are the standard of care treatment for IH, but there is evidence that lasers may continue to play a role in the treatment of IH.[18,19]

Spider angiomas are seen in 15% of healthy preschool-aged children on the face, ears, forearms, and hands and usually respond well to treatment with PDL after one to two sessions. A range of settings can be used but one study utilized (585 nm, 5 mm spot, 4.5 ms, 5-7 J/cm^2, with cryogen spray cooling 30/30 ms).[20-22]

Long-Pulsed Frequency-doubled Nd:YAG Laser

The potassium titanyl phosphate (KTP) or frequency-doubled Nd:YAG laser emits a wavelength of 532 nm, which most closely

resembles that of the first hemoglobin absorption peak at 542 nm. It is a solid-state laser where an Nd:YAG crystal is used to first generate a beam of 1064 nm that is then passed through a KTP crystal and results in a beam of photons with half their original wavelength (532 nm), a doubling of the frequency. Longer pulse durations (1.5 – 60 ms) can be employed to treat superficial vascular targets.

The long-pulsed 532 nm KTP laser can be used in Fitzpatrick I to IV skin types for superficial vascular lesions including spider angiomas, telangiectasias, and facial erythema with one large 647-patient review (variable spot size, 12 ms pulse duration, 11 J/cm^2) documenting aggregate rates of 26% "clearance" and 68% "marked improvement" after an average 2.82 treatments (2.3 SD)[23] (for further details, see Chapter 57. Angioma, Spider). The rate of side effects was 5.8% for the KTP study and consisted of swelling, scabbing, and blistering, all of which resolved spontaneously; one patient had one small area of atrophic scarring after seven treatments for a large spider angioma.

The long-pulsed 532 nm KTP laser has also been used successfully for treatment of PWB (see Chapter 115. Port-Wine Birthmarks). In a 44-patient study using the long-pulsed 532 nm laser, all patients achieved a minimum of 25% improvement with the majority (77.3%) experiencing >50% improvement after an average of seven treatments (5-10 mm spot, 5-9 ms pulse duration, 8-11.5 J/cm^2 with contact cooling).[24]

Long-Pulsed Alexandrite Laser

The alexandrite laser emits a 755 nm wavelength. When utilized with pulse durations from 3 to 100 ms, it can be used to treat thicker vascular lesions or vascular lesions with deeper components including venous lakes and hypertrophic PWB. Although it has less affinity for hemoglobin than lasers with wavelengths between 532 and 595 nm, the 755 nm wavelength is still twice as well absorbed by hemoglobin as is the 1064 nm laser and can penetrate 2 to 3 mm into the cutaneous tissue.[25] One study used spot sizes of 8 to 12 mm with 3 ms pulse duration and 35 to 100 J/cm^2 fluences (with majority treated at 60-85 J/cm^2) and cryogen spray of 40 to 60 ms spurt duration and 40 ms delay (40-60/40).[26] Note that the authors may have used longer cryogen spurt durations (compared to settings used for treatment of thinner vascular lesions) to cool the surface of the lesion and to have heat extend deeper into the dermis.

Long-pulsed alexandrite lasers can also be used for laser hair removal, for example, when treating the hair component of Becker's nevi (see Chapter 62. Becker's Nevus).[27] It is important to note that hair removal on these lesions must be performed carefully as the background pigmentation of these lesions makes hair removal more difficult (higher incidence of blistering that could result in scarring or further discoloration).

Long-Pulsed Diode Laser

The long-pulsed diode laser emits 800 to 810 nm, 940 nm, or 980 nm near-infrared energy, where there is less melanin absorption compared to that of the 755 nm alexandrite laser. Less melanin absorption reduces the risk of posttreatment hyperpigmentation in darker skin types. As with the alexandrite laser, the longer wavelength enables deeper tissue penetrance, which also makes this wavelength an option for thicker vascular lesions. Of note, the 980 nm diode laser confers even less absorption by melanin than the alexandrite laser, but there is a trade-off when utilizing diode lasers to treat vascular lesions given the lower absorption by hemoglobin.[25]

Long-pulsed diode lasers have even been successfully deployed percutaneously in conjunction with foam sclerotherapy to address large, symptomatic venous malformations.[28,29] The 980 nm long-pulsed diode laser has been used endovascularly under ultrasound guidance for treating vascular anomalies of the head and neck including high-flow arteriovenous malformations and low-flow venous lesions.[30] Of note, the endovascular approach may require the use of general anesthesia in the pediatric population.

The long-pulsed diode can also be employed for laser hair removal in the treatment of Becker's nevus, as patients often find the hypertrichosis to be more troubling than the underlying hyperpigmentation of these lesions. A Swiss-Israeli study used two sets of settings—(1) 808 nm diode laser (10-12 mm spot, 6 ms pulse duration, 24 J/cm² with contact and level 5/high-flow air cooling); (2) 810 nm diode laser (10-12 mm spot, 20 ms pulse duration, 10 J/cm² with contact and level 5/high-flow air cooling)—to remove hair in Becker's nevi on the shoulder. The treatment interval was every 2 months for eight total treatments and efficacy was assessed at 6- and 12-month follow-up intervals from the final treatment.[31] On a scale of 0 (representing no hair clearance) and 5 (representing complete clearance), subjects' self and independent physician (parentheses) assessment scores were congruent and high with an average of 3.6(3.9) and 3.4(3.5) at 6 and 12 months, respectively.[32]

Long-Pulsed Nd:YAG Laser

The long-pulsed 1064 nm Nd:YAG laser has been utilized for both treatment of vascular lesions and laser hair removal. In the treatment of vascular lesions, the 1064 nm wavelength penetrates relatively deep, with the potential to reach the subcutaneous fat layer, so it can be used to treat deeper vascular lesions and spider veins up to 3 mm in size. Additionally, there is less melanin absorption at 1064 nm than in other lasers previously discussed. However, the 1064 nm wavelength is less specific for hemoglobin compared to the aforementioned PDL, KTP, or even diode. Furthermore, high fluences are required to mitigate the poor coefficient of absorption by hemoglobin in order to produce transmural heating of blood vessels. The higher fluences required at the 1064 nm wavelength increase the potential for

volumetric heating and collateral damage. For these reasons, the window of safety for long-pulsed 1064 nm laser treatment of vascular lesions is very narrow. Furthermore, the endpoint is more difficult to discern and takes several minutes to assess. Graying of the tissue indicates injury that may result in discoloration and scarring. This device can be considered for treatment of blebs on PWB and venous lakes, but in the authors' opinion, there are other options such as the alexandrite laser that should be, first, considered for hypertrophic PWB or other thicker vascular lesions. Those utilizing this laser for vascular lesions should have a good amount of experience with treatment of vascular lesions and these devices to reduce the risk of scarring. Cooling is critical for epidermal protection and pain control.

Long-pulsed Nd:YAG lasers can also be used for laser hair removal and are the preferred choice in patients with darker skin types because of the decreased melanin absorption at 1064 nm wavelength. Rao and Sankar studied 150 individuals with Fitzpatrick IV to VI skin types treated with the long-pulsed Nd:YAG (10-14 mm spot, 30 ms pulse duration, an average of 26.8 J/cm², with air-flow cooling) and demonstrated a mean 54.3% hair reduction after an average 8.9 treatments (range 4-22). They further reported 86% experiencing no complications and only transient, mostly hyperpigmentation, complications experienced by the remainder.[33] Patient satisfaction at follow-up (range 6 months to 5 years) was reported as good or satisfactory in 78.7%.

Long-pulsed Nd:YAG has been used to treat IH with a deep component.[34] However, in the authors' opinion, there is a considerable risk of scarring associated with this approach. IH with a deep component, in our opinion, are best treated with propranolol unless there is a contraindication for a certain patient.

Quality-Switched Lasers

Small targets, that is, pigment granules in melanosomes (approximately 500 μm) or tattoo particles, can be targeted with powerful, nanosecond pulses generated by quality-switched (QS) lasers. QS lasers rely on the principles of variable attenuation and optical resonance to generate very short pulses with high peak intensities. The type of laser used is determined by the color (chromophore) and depth of the lesion being treated. The compact, short pulse of light energy delivered by the laser exerts photothermal, photochemical, and photoacoustic effects on the melanosome causing it to fragment into progressively smaller particles with each subsequent treatment.[35] The photoacoustic effect is the mechanism predominantly responsible for this phenomenon and is described as the rapid thermal expansion of the target chromophore as a result of light energy absorption that results in particle destruction and the production of acoustic waves that disperse into the surrounding tissue.[36] Fragmented pigment particles left behind by the laser are then phagocytosed by macrophages recruited to the site by stimulation of tissue remodeling or passively drain away via cutaneous lymphatic channels.

Quality-Switched 532 nm KTP (Frequency-Doubled Nd:YAG)

The light emitted by the Q-switched 532 nm frequency-doubled Nd:YAG reaches to the level of the papillary dermis. Therefore, it can effectively treat superficial pigmented lesions confined to the epidermis such as ephelides and lentigines in most skin types. Café-au-Lait macules (CALMs) can also be addressed with the QS-KTP. One study utilized 532 nm, 2.0 mm spot, 10 ns pulse duration, 2 to 5 J/cm².[37] Of note, a review by Geronemus et al revealed that CALMs with jagged, "coast of Maine" borders responded better to laser treatment than smooth-bordered "coast of California" lesions (QS-Nd:YAG, picosecond alexandrite, QS-ruby, or QS-alexandrite) (Figure 18.7).[38] Also see Chapter 66. Café au Lait Macules.

Quality-Switched 694 nm Ruby and Quality-Switched 755 nm Alexandrite Lasers

Ruby and alexandrite lasers penetrate to the mid and deep dermis, respectively, making them good modalities for the treatment of nevus of Ota or Ito and other pigmented lesions situated in the mid to deep dermis. As the 694 nm wavelength is most optimally absorbed by melanin, it is advantageous to use this laser when treating pigmented lesion in lighter skin types; however, there is a greater risk of epidermal hypopigmentation with this wavelength compared to longer wavelengths and this needs to be considered especially when treating darker-skinned individuals.

Nevus of Ota is a benign dermal melanocytic nevus that typically presents as unilateral blue-gray macules to patches on the face in the distribution of the second branch of the trigeminal nerve. Starting in 1992,[39] the QS-ruby 694 nm laser has been used to treat nevus of Ota, with one study evaluating 114 patients attaining lesion clearance after four to five treatments (694.3 nm wavelength, 4 mm spot, 30 ns pulse duration, 6 J/cm^2)[40] and with yet another large 150-patient study noting favorable outcomes achieved in all patients treated by 1 year with only eight patients' reports of transient post-inflammatory hyperpigmentation that resolved after 2 months (wavelength 694.3 nm, 6.5 mm spot, 28 ns pulse duration, 4-10 J/cm^2 fluence).[41] Ueda et al observed that darker, blue-green lesions took longer to respond to treatment than brown-colored ones.[41] Importantly, Kono et al found that not only was earlier treatment, that is, in childhood, associated with faster lesion clearance, that is, fewer treatment sessions required (3.5 vs. 5.9), it was also associated with fewer side effects (694 nm wavelength, 4 mm spot, 30 ns pulse duration, 5-7 J/cm^2 fluence at 3-4 month intervals).[42] The QS-alexandrite 755 nm has also been proven effective in treating nevus of Ota and in at least one study (utilizing 2-4 mm

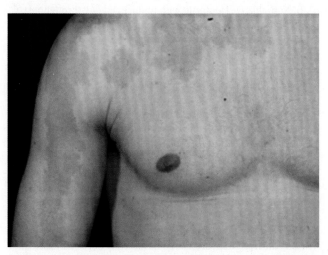

FIGURE 18.7. This young man has a large segmental café au lait with rugged borders reminiscent of the coast of Maine. Reprinted with permission from Weinstein SL, Flynn JM. *Lovell and Winter's Pediatric Orthopaedics*. 7th ed. Philadelphia, PA: Wolters Kluwer Health/Lippincott Williams & Wilkins; 2014. Figure 4.59.

spot, 100 ns pulse duration, 4.2-18 J/cm^2) was shown to be the superior wavelength in addressing lesions in patients with skin phototype IV.[43] Like with the QS-ruby, the most common side effects are transient hyperpigmentation.[44] Some patients who plateau with treatment of nanosecond lasers end up responding to picosecond lasers including the alexandrite laser (one study utilizing 755 nm alexandrite laser, 3-3.5 mm spot, 750 ps pulse duration, 2.08-2.83 J/cm^2, with one to three treatments 8 weeks apart).[45] For further details, see Chapter 110. Nevus of Ota and Nevus of Ito.

The appearance of acquired junctional melanocytic nevi can be improved with either Q-switched or picosecond lasers without scarring; however, treatment response is best with small, flat lesions. Recurrence is not uncommon, which can be frustrating to patients and their treating physicians. In addition, laser treatment of nevi does not allow tissue evaluation and so should be approached with caution. Lasers should not be used to treat any nevi with an atypical appearance or any concern for malignancy. The authors do not treat melanocytic nevi with laser for this reason. See Chapter 109. Nevi.

Quality-Switched 1064 nm Nd:YAG

The QS 1064 nm wavelength can reach to the deeper dermis. This wavelength can again be used to treat nevus of Ota[46] or Ito as well as other pigment targets in the deeper dermis.[47] Liu et al reported on 224 Chinese patients with a nevus of Ota: 99% demonstrated a >75% treatment response in an average of 3.7 sessions with the QS-Nd:YAG. Only eight patients (3.57%) who had achieved complete clearance experienced a recurrence with follow-up range from 2 to 10 years. See Chapter 110. Nevus of Ota and Nevus of Ito. The QS-Nd:YAG is also a good choice for targeting pigment in traumatic tattoos where the pigment may be located more deeply.[48]

ABLATIVE AND NON-ABLATIVE LASER TREATMENTS

Lasers that ablate or vaporize tissue use wavelengths in the infrared portion of electromagnetic energy to target the absorption spectrum of water which accounts for 80% of the skin by weight.

Laser ablation is employed when the desire is to remove either microscopic or macroscopic amounts of tissue "en masse" to normalize the texture of the skin. Ablation is accomplished through the rapid heating of tissue through the targeting of water such that it vaporizes. This requires approximately 2500 J/cm^3 of energy, or roughly 600 times the amount of energy required to raise 1 cm^3 of water by 1°C (4.2 J). Non-ablative lasers transfer energy sufficient to melt or coagulate tissue (Figure 18.8). Whether the target tissue is injured or destroyed, the body is activated to repair and rebuild the area and fill in the damaged areas with new, healthy tissue.

Ablative Lasers

Fully ablative 10 600 nm carbon dioxide (CO_2) and 2940 nm erbium–yttrium argon garnet (Er:YAG) laser treatments have been the gold standard in the arena of skin resurfacing to normalize skin texture as in the case of acne scarring and photorejuvenation in older patients. With fully ablative treatments, recovery time is longer than for fractionated technologies and the risk of adverse effects is higher; however, enhanced results are achieved in one or two treatments.[49] Fully ablative lasers are also very useful when complete removal or debulking of a

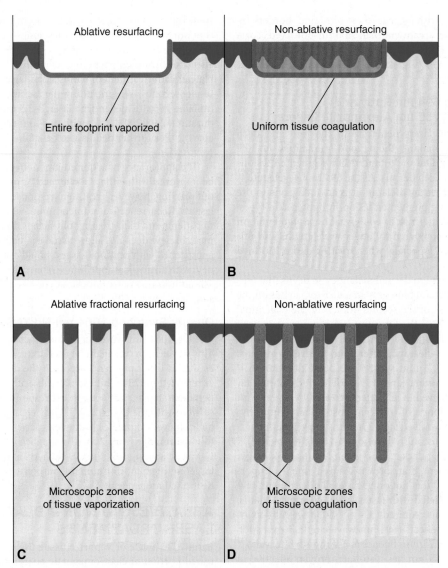

FIGURE 18.8. Ablation is accomplished through rapid heating of tissue by targeting water such that it vaporizes requiring 2500 J/cm^3 of energy, or roughly 600 times the amount of energy required to raise 1 cm^3 of water by 1°C (4.2 J). Non-ablative lasers transfer energy sufficient to melt or coagulate tissue. A, Fully ablative (full footprint vaporized). B, Non-ablative (footprint with uniform energy throughout). C, Fractional-ablative (zones of vaporization). D, Fractional non-ablative (zones of coagulation).

tumor is desired as in lymphangiomas,[50] syringomas,[51] angiofibromas,[52] and xanthomas.[53]

Although tissue is being destroyed, setting parameters to target the level and extent of ablation is necessary to confine tissue effects to the desired region. This is best achieved by reducing the amount of time over which the pulse of energy is delivered. It is safer to deliver high-power, high-energy, short (less than a few milliseconds) erbium and CO$_2$ laser pulses than it is to turn down the power of a device and cause bulk heating, resulting in unwanted injury to the surrounding tissue. Many ablative lasers marketed for dermatologic use have engineered controls to safeguard against errors of dosimetry. However, like all laser procedures, it is important to know the device you are using and monitor for appropriate tissue response.

CO$_2$ lasers remove tissue at a depth of 20 to 120 μm per pass, depending on the fluence and spot size selected, and provide tissue coagulation extending out to the surrounding tissue, which aids in autohemostasis.[54] Collagen remodeling is induced in the treated area.[55] The residual coagulated or charred tissue left by

the first pass of the CO$_2$ laser is removed prior to subsequent passes of the laser; otherwise the desiccated tissue becomes a heat sink leading to less vaporization and increased potential for thermal injury. The clinical endpoint for the CO$_2$ laser depends on the depth of the lesion treated. A chamois color indicates the level of the papillary dermis has been reached, and a "water-logged cotton thread" appearance denotes exposure of the reticular dermis.

The Er:YAG laser is able to vaporize tissue more efficiently, that is, with a narrower zone of coagulation, because the energy it emits at 2940 nm is 15 times better absorbed by water than the 10 600 nm wavelength of the CO$_2$ laser. Although, on the contrary, this feature provides for more rapid tissue clearance without the need to peel charred tissue away between passes and the ability to penetrate deeply into tissue, there is less collagen contraction and hemostasis, which results in increased intraoperative bleeding. Some devices have incorporated "coagulation settings," which involve increasing the pulse duration to induce greater tissue contraction and provide more hemostasis.[56]

Surgeons using ablative lasers should have a good understanding of tissue interactions and desired clinical endpoints in order to use these devices safely without causing scarring.

Fractionated Lasers

Compared with traditional ablative laser devices in which the footprint or spot size defines the smallest possible treatment zone, fractionation takes the laser footprint and divides it into a microscopic checkerboard of alternating treatment and nontreatment zones that extend in columns through the epidermis and dermis down to a calibrated depth. Because there are columns of normal, untreated skin nearby from which tissue healing and remodeling can be instantly activated, the skin surface is able to heal more rapidly post-procedurally and side effects are less common.

Non-ablative Fractional Lasers

Although the first non-ablative fractional laser (NAFL) was the 1550 nm erbium-fiber device (Fraxel ReStore; Valeant Pharmaceuticals), there are many devices available now with wavelengths from 1410 to 1927 nm.[57] The aim of non-ablative fractional photothermolysis is to induce microscopic zones of collagen denaturation or necrosis. Because the "melting" of tissue is a less aggressive form of injury than vaporization, non-ablative lasers have an advantage over ablative forms in faster recovery time; however, tissue remodeling is more subtle. As the skin heals, the microscopic zones of coagulation or necrosis are extruded.[54,58] The more gradual treatment response is mitigated by increasing the number of total sessions. The original U.S. Food and Drug Administration (FDA) clearance for NAFL technology was in the treatment of pigmented lesions, melasma, acne scars, surgical scars, periorbital rhytids, and skin resurfacing.[59] See Chapter 51. Acne Scarring.

NAFL is applied successfully in the treatment of acne[60] and burn scars.[61] A small prospective study using the 1550 nm non-ablative Fraxel ReStore (40-70 mJ/pulse, density of 6%-13% corresponding to 17%-33% tissue coverage) in patients who had suffered deep second- or third-degree burns demonstrated overall improvement in atrophic, hypertrophic, and contracture scars after five treatments in 90% of patients at 6 months posttreatment.[62] Facial acne scarring can have a deep psychosocial impact on an individual, not only in adolescence but into their adult professional lives. NAFR has a relatively favorable safety profile and demonstrated a mean 50% to 75% improvement in a study of 500 patients with mild-to-moderate acne scars after three treatments spaced 4 weeks apart (20-100 mJ/pulse, 100-400 microscopic treatment zone [MTZ] per cm² per pass with total treatment densities of 200-1200 MTZ/cm² depending on treatment location with 33%-66% reduction around the nose and eyelids).[63,64] Notably, this study by Weiss included individuals with skin type up to Fitzpatrick V with no observed post-inflammatory hyperpigmentation (PIH). Subsequently, Mahmoud et al found that even at energies as low as 10 mJ, PIH can occur and it is always advisable to thoroughly assess a patient's recent sun exposure, use caution when selecting treatment settings, and provide thorough counseling on post-procedural sun protection.[65] Larger atrophic scars have been treated successfully with NAFL in combination with autologous fat transfer.

NAFR has also been used in conjunction with the long-pulsed alexandrite in the treatment of recalcitrant hypertrophic PWB to improve preexisting hypertrophic scarring in one of the 20 cases addressed by Izikson et al.[66] As resistant PWB may have

scarring from previous treatments, it can be helpful to treat this complication in addition to addressing the primary lesion.

In general, with pre-application of a topical anesthetic and/or intraoperative forced cool air, NAFL treatments are better tolerated by patients than ablative devices. Expected transient side effects include erythema and edema up to 48 hours posttreatment with fine desquamation occurring days later.[59]

Ablative Fractional Lasers

As with other ablative lasers, the result of ablative fractionated lasers is to vaporize the tissue, but the initial effect is limited to microscopic treatment zones (MTZs). Depending on the system, fractionated CO_2 lasers produce MTZs that are 110 to 150 μm—or more wide and can be tuned to penetrate 50 μm to several millimeters deep. The expected endpoint is pinpoint bleeding in a pixilated pattern (see Figure 18.6C).

Even when fractionated, tissue ablation is quite painful. Therefore, it is advisable to employ some method of anesthesia (see Anesthesia Considerations section). Of note, postoperative pain scores for patients who received treatment under general anesthesia were compared with and without intraoperative opioid administration and no statistical difference was found.[67] When appropriate education and patient selection is used, many older patients are able to tolerate the treatment of hypertrophic scarring with ablative fractional lasers with only local anesthesia.[68] However, when treating younger children or extensive areas, general anesthesia may be beneficial.

In the pediatric population, ablative fractional resurfacing is used in the treatment of hypertrophic scarring, typically sustained in a burn or other traumatic injury, and acne scarring (see Chapter 90. Hypertrophic Scars and Contractures).[69] Particularly exciting are the immediate improvements in postoperative range of motion gained with the use of ablative fractional laser in scars complicated by joint contraction or movement restriction. Short-term gains in function are attributed to the photomechanical fenestration of stiff scar tissue, whereas the long-term effects are attributed to the normalization of dysfunctional scar tissue via gradual dermal remodeling.[70]

Fractionated ablative Er:YAG lasers are also being utilized in early scar treatment (<2 months after primary repair) of facial lacerations to improve aesthetic outcomes (one study utilizing LOTUSII, Laseroptek, Sungnam, Korea, 7 mm spot, 0.35 ms pulse duration, 1.28 J/cm² total fluence with two passes at 400 mJ in short pulse, 0.35 ms, mode and one pass of 800 mJ in long pulse, 1 ms, mode).[71]

Although mild-to-moderate atrophic acne scars respond well to non-ablative fractional laser, patients with moderate-to-severe acne scarring have a higher likelihood of achieving >50% improvement in scar depth and appearance when treated with the ablative fractional CO_2,[72] erbium-yttrium scandium gallium garnet (Er:YSGG), or Er:YAG laser.[73] Of note, You et al found that three consecutive AFL treatments (Fraxel SR 1500; Reliant Technologies, 50 mJ/30 W/150 MTZ/cm²) were as effective as a single fully ablative resurfacing treatment (Coherent Ultrapulse CO_2 laser [Coherent Inc., US]; 10-60 W at 300-500 mJ followed by 250 mJ second pass. Contour Er:YAG; Sciton, in dual mode at 100-200 μm depth with 25-50 μm coagulation) with less downtime and fewer complications.[49] On average, reepithelialization occurs after 4 to 7 days of treatment with fractional ablative lasers (although this does depend on the depth and density of ablation) and there is a lower risk of scarring or infection compared to fully ablative procedures. Transient erythema and PIH are, however, relatively common.[74] Hedelund et al performed a randomized single-blind (assessor) control trial of fractional CO_2 (scanner, single pass with spot diameter 0.5 mm, pulse duration 4 ms, laser power 12-14 W, microbeam energy of 48-56 mJ/pulse, 100 MTZ/cm^2 density of 13%) in patients with atrophic acne scarring that demonstrated significant improvements in the scar texture and atrophy at all assessment time points (1, 3, and 6 months).[75] A 60-patient study on the treatment of acne scarring using fractionated CO_2 laser (Qray-FRX; Dosis, Korea, at 15-25 J/cm^2, density of 100-150 MTZ/cm^2, to a depth of 1.0-1.2 mm) with three to four sessions 6 weeks apart and a 6-month follow-up interval demonstrated that 26 patients had a >50% improvement in scarring with 73% overall patient satisfaction rate.[76] A small study used biopsies at the time of treatment and at follow-up in eight patients who underwent two full-face fractionated Er:YSGG 2790 nm treatments (Cutera; Brisbane, CA, with 6 mm spot, 400 μs pulse duration, 1.5-3.5 J/cm^2, and 20% overlap) 1 month apart and assessed the depth of thermal energy to be 80 μm below the stratum corneum.[77] Another study using fractionated Er:YAG focused on the benefits of this laser technique in addressing acne scarring in Fitzpatrick skin types III to V and demonstrated less transient PIH than fractional CO_2 in this patient population with comparable clinical outcomes (MCL30 Dermablate; Asclepion Laser Technologies, Germany, 9 mm spot with 169 microbeams, delivering 1.5 J per site for a total of 108 J/cm^2).[78,79] Another approach to the improvement of acne scarring is to use superficial full-field Er:YAG to improve skin texture followed by fraction Er:YAG to induce collagen remodeling (zoom mode 2940 nm, 5 mm spot, 1-1.5 J/cm^2, one to three passes on individual atrophic scars; fractional short pulse—350 μs, 8 mm spot, 0.8-1.5 mJ/cm^2, one to two passes on treatment area; fractional long pulse—8 mm spot, 1 ms, 81 MTZs, 0.7-1 J/cm^2, with one pass on treatment area).[73]

Syringomas are benign adnexal neoplasms of eccrine or apocrine origin with a predilection for the periorbital skin[80] with 90% developing in pediatric patients (70% in adolescence, 20% in childhood).[81] Although benign, their abnormal appearance can be a cause of significant psychosocial distress both to patients and parents.[82,83] When there are only a few isolated lesions, surgical or electrosurgical modalities can work well, but these approaches prove impractical if lesions are agminated or disseminated.[84] Of 35 patients who underwent two treatments 1 month apart with fractionated CO_2 laser, three experienced near total clearance (>75%) whereas nearly half of those treated (15) demonstrated >50% improvement. However, 14% of those treated showed a minimal response rate (<25% improvement). This was attributed to the presence of overall larger and flatter syringoma size, that is, less normal tissue to trigger remodeling response.[85] Goldman and Wollina had no recurrence at 12-month follow-up of multiple periocular syringomas treated thrice with two passes of fractionated ablative CO_2 laser at 4-week intervals (600 μm spacing, 800 μs dwell, time, two stack pulses). However, they had notably spot-treated the larger lesions with full-field ablative CO_2 prior to using the fractionated scanner on the entire area.[86]

Fractionated ablative lasers are also used as one part of a multipronged, single-session approach to significantly improve the number, color, and texture of angiofibromas of tuberous sclerosis (see Chapter 55. Angiofibromas). In a series of three cases, in one treatment session under general anesthesia, Weiss

and Geronemus first applied electrosurgery (on low setting) to 100 to 200 of the most elevated lesions, then covered the area with one pass of nonoverlapping 595 nm PDL (10 mm spot, 0.45 ms, 7 J/cm^2, 30 ms duration of cryogen spray cooling), and ended with fractionated ablative CO_2 laser for final resurfacing (15 mm spot, 20-40 mJ/pulse, 40% coverage).[87] Postoperative effects included pinpoint bleeding and oozing for 2 to 3 days, focal crusting at electrosurgical sites for 5 to 7 days, and transient erythema lasting several weeks. Importantly, improvement in lesion number, texture, and color was sustained up to 10-month follow-up. Yet a fourth case has been published employing a combination of electrosurgery, 595 nm PDL, fractional ablative CO_2 laser, and topical 0.2% rapamycin (also called sirolimus) ointment for extensive facial angiofibromas with substantial improvement in number, size, texture, and color of extensive facial angiofibromas.[18] Addition of topical rapamycin once patients are healed can help maintain results.

LASER SAFETY
Eye Safety

Protecting the eyes is important for the laser operator, patient, and anyone else who may be in the room either observing or assisting. It is a sobering realization that it only takes 1% of a reflected beam to cause significant eye injury. A visual inspection that all persons in the room are wearing suitable eye protection should occur prior to removing the laser handpiece from the device. The highest risk of eye injury is from near-infrared (IR) Q-switched (high-energy) lasers; however, each laser type described in this chapter has the potential to cause varying degrees of ocular damage.[88]

Potential Eye Injuries by Laser Type

Wavelengths from 400 to 780 nm that encompass the KTP-Nd:YAG, PDL, and alexandrite devices may cause photochemical damage to the retina resulting in a retinal burn. The diode lasers and Nd:YAG fall in the near-IR range of 780 to 1400 nm and can cause cataracts and retinal burns. The Er:YAG with its high affinity for water may cause an aqueous flare by coagulating proteins in the aqueous humor, a cataract, or corneal burn whereas the CO_2 laser can cause a corneal burn.

Eye Protection for Laser Operator and Observers

After determining the appropriate laser wavelength for the clinical indication treated, laser operators and observers should put on glasses or goggles that correspond to the treatment wavelength and have an optical density (OD) of at least 5. OD is inversely proportional to the logarithm of transmittance or $OD = \log/(1/T)$. Thus, $OD = 5$ implies a transmittance of 10^{-5}; the higher the OD, the lower the transmittance.

Patient Preparation and Protection

If working off the face, the patient could use the same type of protective glasses as the laser operator. However, in young children, these may not fit adequately or the child may try to remove them during the procedure and so often, goggles are not appropriate for young children. If working on the face or for young children where goggles may not fit or it cannot be assured that the patient will keep the goggles on, laser safe adhesive eye pads can be used. These can be gently held in place with gauze eye pads if the patient may attempt to remove them. Importantly, appropriately sized corneal shields must be employed when working around the eyelids.[89] Anesthetic eyedrops are placed immediately before insertion under the eyelid when the patient is awake. Lubricant eye gel can also be applied in the shield to ease application and minimize the risk of a corneal abrasion. There is a low risk of a corneal abrasion with insertion of the eye shield, but there is a greater risk of more serious eye injury if shields are not used when skin within the bony orbit is treated.

MONITORING TISSUE RESPONSE AND CLINICAL ENDPOINTS

Once the proper device, spot size, energy, and pulse duration have been selected based on the characteristics of the pathologic lesion and patient skin type, the fine-tuning of laser treatment occurs intraoperatively dependent on information gained from monitoring the tissue response. When the hemoglobin of vascular lesions is successfully targeted by the PDL, KTP, or long-pulse alexandrite lasers, purpura, durable vessel darkening, and/or vessel disappearance are visible (Figure 18.6A). Gray coloration is a sign of epidermal damage and should be avoided. Blistering or a positive Nikolski sign is a later sign indicative of injury that also should be avoided. The clinical endpoints of melanin-targeting by long-pulsed ruby, long-pulsed alexandrite, diode, or long-pulsed Nd:YAG when used for laser hair removal are erythema and perifollicular edema (Figure 18.6B). It can take 5 minutes or more for this response to be visible. Q-switched lasers used to address melanin and dermal pigmentation cause immediate tissue whitening and provide the additional auditory feedback of a crisp snap or crack as the laser hits its target. An undesired complication is post-inflammatory hyperpigmentation or hypopigmentation (Figure 18.3), which occur fairly commonly in darker-skinned patients. Non-ablative dermal remodeling accomplished by the mid-IR 1320 nm Nd:Yag, 1450 nm diode, 1540 nm Er:glass, and 1927 thulium:YAG is nonselective in nature, that is, targets water, and conveys erythema, edema, and occasionally pinpoint bleeding as its clinical endpoints. Lastly, fully ablative lasers provide signs of diffuse obliteration to a specified depth: CO_2 laser produces a chamois color with bleeding and Er:YAG laser without coagulation eventuates in edema, erythema, and pinpoint bleeding. Fractionated ablative devices yield pinpoint bleeding in a specified pattern depending on the device and settings used (Figure 18.6C).

RISK OF INFECTION AND PROPHYLAXIS

Any treatment that temporarily impairs the barrier function of the skin carries with it the risk of infection. Viral, bacterial, and fungal infections have all been documented following laser procedures. The highest incident infection is that of herpes simplex virus (HSV) with perioral procedures.[90] Although infectious complications are most frequent with ablative resurfacing, overall prevalence is low (5% of procedures), and although even less frequent, HSV infection may also occur with non-ablative treatments (0.6%), QS-lasers, or any other dermatologic treatments that induce breaks or trauma to the skin.[91,92]

Herpes labialis is predominantly caused by HSV-1 with 40% of the population demonstrating seropositivity by age 15.[93] HSV-1 infection is lifelong as it lies dormant in the trigeminal nerve ganglion with 15% to 40% of individuals experiencing recurrences provoked by, but not limited to, emotional stress, physical fatigue, upper respiratory infections, UV-light exposure, local trauma, menses, and immunosuppression.[94] Therefore, it is no surprise that perioral laser resurfacing, with

its intentionally induced cutaneous injury to promote tissue remodeling, has been associated with HSV-1 reactivation. Recurrent HSV-1 may involve the entire treatment area in an eczema herpeticum-like presentation with or without complication by bacterial impetiginization, which may ultimately result in scarring.[95] Because recurrence can be suppressed by antiviral prophylaxis, it is important to ask the patient about prior HSV-1 history prior to treatment of the perioral area. However, as HSV-1 infection is not always symptomatic, it is recommended that all patients undergoing ablative resurfacing procedures on the face and any procedure in the perioral area be considered for prophylaxis, unless there is a contraindication.

HSV prophylactic regimens include the following:
- Valacyclovir 500 mg twice daily for 14 days starting 1 day prior to laser treatment.[96] This approach was also demonstrated to be 100% effective if shortened to 10 days (this study by Beeson and Rachel found that 70% of patients with a negative clinical history had positive serologies).[97]
- Famiciclovir 250 mg (no history of HSV-1) or 500 mg (positive history HSV-1) twice daily for 10 days beginning 24 hours prior to the procedure[98]

ANESTHESIA CONSIDERATIONS

A variety of anesthetic techniques ranging from invasive to noninvasive exist to mitigate the pain and discomfort that can be associated with laser treatment of cutaneous lesions. The "most appropriate" approach is guided by both lesion and patient characteristics, namely the extent of the lesion and patient age, that is, level of comprehension, and patient temperament and/or preference. Noninvasive pain control is appropriate in cooperative patients with localized lesions. Options include pre-treatment with topical medicaments like amide anesthetics such as lidocaine and prilocaine and nonsteroidal anti-inflammatories such as diclofenac and piroxicam.[99] Of note, nonsteroidal anti-inflammatory agents should be avoided during the treatment of vascular lesions as the desired vascular clots may be affected. Skin cooling is another noninvasive way to both reduce pain and protect the epidermis.[5] Additionally, pneumatic skin flattening (PSF), which has been incorporated into some laser handpieces, diminishes pain via the activation of pressure receptors in the skin by a vacuum chamber through which the light is delivered.[100]

Large area treatments in young children involving large vascular lesions where many treatments may be required and the use of ablative fractionated lasers on scars[67] are situations where general anesthesia in an operating room environment with the assistance of trained anesthesiologists may be considered.[101] The Food and Drug Administration has issued a warning about potential effects that may be associated with general anesthesia in young children, and studies are ongoing to clarify risks. When general anesthesia is considered, potential risks and benefits should be discussed with patients and parents so they can make an informed decision.

REFERENCES

1. Maiman T. Stimulated optical radiation in ruby. *Nature.* 1960;187:493–494.
2. Goldman L. Pathology of the effect of the laser beam on the skin. *Nature.* 1963;197:912–914.
3. Anderson RR. Lasers in dermatology—a critical update. *J Dermatol.* 2000;27(11):700–705.
4. Zenzie HH, Altshuler GB, Smirnov MZ, Anderson RR. Evaluation of cooling methods for laser dermatology. *Lasers Surg Med.* 2000;26(2):130–144.

5. Chan HHL, Lam L-K, Wong DSY, Wei WI. Role of skin cooling in improving patient tolerability of Q-switched Alexandrite (QS Alex) laser in nevus of Ota treatment. *Lasers Surg Med.* 2003;32(2):148–151.

6. Tunnell JW, Nelson JS, Torres JH, Anvari B. Epidermal protection with cryogen spray cooling during high fluence pulsed dye laser irradiation: an ex vivo study. *Lasers Surg Med.* 2000;27(4):373–383.

7. Lee S, Park S, Kang J, Kim Y, Kim D. Cryogen-induced arcuate shaped hyperpigmentation by dynamic cooling device. *J Eur Acad Dermatol Venereol.* 2008;22:883–884.

8. Das A, Sarda A, De A. Cooling devices in laser therapy. *J Cutan Aesthetic Surg.* 2016;9(4):215.

9. Tierney EP, Hanke CW. The effect of cold-air anesthesia during fractionated carbon-dioxide laser treatment: prospective study and review of the literature. *J Am Acad Dermatol.* 2012;67(3):436–445.

10. Cordisco MR. An update on lasers in children. *Curr Opin Pediatr.* 2009;21(4):499–504.

11. Brightman LA, Geronemus RG, Reddy KK. Laser treatment of port-wine stains. *Clin Cosmet Investig Dermatol.* 2015;8:27–33.

12. Hagen SL, Grey KR, Korta DZ, Kelly KM. Quality of life in adults with facial port-wine stains. *J Am Acad Dermatol.* 2017;76(4):695–702.

13. Laquer VT, Hevezi PA, Albrecht H, Chen TS, Zlotnik A, Kelly KM. Microarray analysis of port wine stains before and after pulsed dye laser treatment. *Lasers Surg Med.* 2013;45(2):67–75.

14. Geronemus RG, Ashinoff R. The medical necessity of evaluation and treatment of port-wine stains. *J Dermatol Surg Oncol.* 1991;17(1):76–79.

15. Liu, Shi W, Wang J, et al. Treatment of port wine stains with pulsed dye laser: a retrospective study of 848 cases in Shandong Province, People's Republic of China. *Drug Des Devel Ther.* 2014;8:2531.

16. Thajudheen CP, Jyothy K, Priyadarshini A. Treatment of port-wine stains with flash lamp pumped pulsed dye laser on Indian skin: a six year study. *J Cutan Aesthetic Surg.* 2014;7(1):32–36.

17. Kwon SH, Choi JW, Byun SY, et al. Effect of early long-pulse pulsed dye laser treatment in infantile hemangiomas. *Dermatol Surg.* 2014;40(4):405–411.

18. Bae-Harboe YSC, Geronemus RG. Targeted topical and combination laser surgery for the treatment of angiofibromas. *Lasers Surg Med.* 2013;45(9):555–557.

19. Rodríguez-Ruiz M, Tellado MG, del Pozo Losada J. Combination of pulsed dye laser and propranolol in the treatment of ulcerated infantile haemangioma [in Spanish]. *An Pediatr Engl Ed.* 2016;84(2):92–96.

20. Craig LM, Alster TS. Vascular skin lesions in children: a review of laser surgical and medical treatments. *Dermatol Surg.* 2013;39(8):1137–1146.

21. Bencini PL, Tourlaki A, De Giorgi V, Galimberti M. Laser use for cutaneous vascular alterations of cosmetic interest: lasers for cutaneous vascular lesions. *Dermatol Ther.* 2012;25(4):340–351.

22. Tan E, Vinciullo C. Pulsed dye laser treatment of spider telangiectasia. *Australas J Dermatol.* 1997;38(1):22–25.

23. Becher GL, Cameron H, Moseley H. Treatment of superficial vascular lesions with the KTP 532-nm laser: experience with 647 patients. *Lasers Med Sci.* 2014;29(1):267–271.

24. Kwiek B, Rożalski M, Kowalewski C, Ambroziak M. Retrospective single center study of the efficacy of large spot 532-nm laser for the treatment of facial capillary malformations in 44 patients with the use of three-dimensional image analysis. *Lasers Surg Med.* 2017;49(8):743–749.

25. Mccoppin HH, Hovenic WW, Wheeland RG. Laser treatment of superficial leg veins: a review. *Dermatol Surg.* 2011;37(6):729–741.

26. Tierney EP, Hanke WC. Alexandrite laser for the treatment of port wine stains refractory to pulsed dye laser. *Dermatol Surg.* 2011;37(9):1268–1278.

27. Choi JE, Kim JW, Seo SH, Son SW, Ahn HH, Kye YC. Treatment of Becker's nevi with a long-pulse alexandrite laser. *Dermatol Surg.* 2009;35:1105–1108.

28. Levy JL, Berwald C. Treatment of vascular abnormalities with a long-pulse diode at 980 nm. *J Cosmet Laser Ther.* 2004;6(4):217–221.

29. Wales L, Nasr H, Bohm N, Howard A, Loftus I, Thompson M. Paediatric venous malformation: treatment with endovenous laser and foam sclerotherapy. *EJVES Extra.* 2007;14(1):6–7.

30. Tzermias C, Eleftheriadi A, Gkiouzepaki I. Management of vascular lesions using advanced laser technology. *J Surg Dermatol.* 2017;2(t1):115–129. http://www.jsurgdermatol.com/index.php/JSD/article/view/109.

31. Royo J, Urdiales F, Moreno J, Al-Zarouni M, Cornejo P, Trelles MA. Six-month follow-up multicenter prospective study of 368 patients, phototypes III to V, on epilation efficacy using an 810-nm diode laser at low fluence. *Lasers Med Sci.* 2011;26(2):247–255.

32. Lapidoth M, Adatto M, Cohen S, Ben-Amitai D, Halachmi S. Hypertrichosis in Becker's nevus: effective low-fluence laser hair removal. *Lasers Med Sci.* 2014;29(1):191–193.

33. Rao K, Sankar TK. Long-pulsed Nd:YAG laser-assisted hair removal in Fitzpatrick skin types IV–VI. *Lasers Med Sci.* 2011;26(5):623–626.

34. Hartmann F, Lockmann A, Grönemeyer L-L, et al. Nd:YAG and pulsed dye laser therapy in infantile haemangiomas: a retrospective analysis of 271 treated haemangiomas in 149 children. *J Eur Acad Dermatol Venereol.* 2017;31(8):1372–1379.

35. Ahn KJ, Kim BJ, Cho SB. Simulation of laser-tattoo pigment interaction in a tissue-mimicking phantom using Q-switched and long-pulsed lasers. *Skin Res Technol.* 2017;23(3):376–383.

36. Kent KM, Graber EM. Laser tattoo removal: a review. *Dermatol Surg.* 2012;38(1):1–13.

37. Kilmer SL. Treatment of epidermal pigmented lesions with the frequency-doubled Q-switched Nd:YAG laser: a controlled, single-impact, dose-response, multicenter trial. *Arch Dermatol.* 1994;130(12):1515.

38. Belkin DA, Neckman JP, Jeon H, Friedman P, Geronemus RG. Response to laser treatment of café au lait macules based on morphologic features. *JAMA Dermatol.* 2017;153(11):1158.

39. Geronemus RG. Q-switched ruby laser therapy of nevus of Ota. *Arch Dermatol.* 1992;128(12):1618–1622.

40. Watanabe S, Takahashi H. Treatment of nevus of ota with the Q-switched ruby laser. *N Engl J Med.* 1994;331(26):1745–1750.

41. Ueda S, Isoda M, Imayama S. Response of naevus of Ota to Q-switched ruby laser treatment according to lesion colour. *Br J Dermatol.* 2000;142(1):77–83.

42. Kono T, Chan HHL, Erçöçen AR, et al. Use of Q-switched ruby laser in the treatment of nevus of Ota in different age groups. *Lasers Surg Med.* 2003;32(5):391–395.

43. Felton SJ, Al-Niaimi F, Ferguson JE, Madan V. Our perspective of the treatment of naevus of Ota with 1,064-, 755- and 532-nm wavelength lasers. *Lasers Med Sci.* 2014;29(5):1745–1749.

44. Shah VV, Bray FN, Aldahan AS, Mlacker S, Nouri K. Lasers and nevus of Ota: a comprehensive review. *Lasers Med Sci.* 2016;31(1):179–185.

45. Chesnut C, Diehl J, Lask G. Treatment of nevus of ota with a picosecond 755-nm alexandrite laser. *Dermatol Surg.* 2015;41(4):508–510.

46. Yan L, Di L, Weihua W, et al. A study on the clinical characteristics of treating nevus of Ota by Q-switched Nd:YAG laser. *Lasers Med Sci.* 2018;33(1):89–93.

47. Liu Y, Zeng W, Li D, Wang W, Liu F. A retrospective analysis of the clinical efficacies and recurrence of Q-switched Nd:YAG laser treatment of nevus of Ota in 224 Chinese patients. *J Cosmet Laser Ther.* 2018;20:410–414.

48. Gorouhi F, Davari P, Kashani MN, Firooz A. Treatment of traumatic tattoo with the Q-switched Nd:YAG laser. *J Cosmet Laser Ther.* 2007;9(4):253–255.

49. You H-J, Kim D-W, Yoon E-S, Park S-H. Comparison of four different lasers for acne scars: resurfacing and fractional lasers. *J Plast Reconstr Aesthet Surg.* 2016;69(4):e87–e95.

50. Ochsendorf FR, Kaufmann R, Runne U. Erbium:YAG laser ablation of acquired vulval lymphangioma. *Br J Dermatol.* 2001;144(2):442–444.

51. Kitano Y. Erbium YAG laser treatment of periorbital syringomas by using the multiple ovoid-shape ablation method. *J Cosmet Laser Ther.* 2016;18(5):280–285.

52. Fioramonti P, De Santo L, Ruggieri M, et al. Co2/Erbium:YAG/Dye laser combination: an effective and successful treatment for angiofibromas in tuberous sclerosis. *Aesthetic Plast Surg.* 2014;38(1):192–198.

53. Balevi A, Ustuner P, Ozdemir M. Erbium:yttrium aluminum garnet laser versus Q-switched neodymium:yttrium aluminum garnet laser for the treatment of xanthelasma palpebrarum. *J Cosmet Laser Ther.* 2017;19(2):100–105.

54. Omi T, Numano K. The role of the CO2 laser and fractional CO2 laser in dermatology. *Laser Ther.* 2014;23(1):49–60.

55. Preissig J, Hamilton K, Markus R. Current laser resurfacing technologies: a review that delves beneath the surface. *Semin Plast Surg.* 2012;26(03):109–116.

56. Alsaad SMS, Ross EV, Smith WJ, DeRienzo DP. Analysis of depth of ablation, thermal damage, wound healing, and wound contraction with erbium YAG laser in a Yorkshire pig model. *J Drugs Dermatol.* 2015;14(11):1245–1252.

57. Kaushik SB, Alexis AF. Nonablative fractional laser resurfacing in skin of color: evidence-based review. *J Clin Aesthetic Dermatol.* 2017;10(6):51–67.

58. Saedi N, Petelin A, Zachary C. Fractionation: a new era in laser resurfacing. *Clin Plast Surg.* 2011;38(3):449–461, vii.

59. Michael H. Gold. Update on fractional laser technology. *J Clin Aesthetic Dermatol.* 2010;3(1):42–50.

60. Perper M, Tsatalis J, Eber AE, Cervantes J, Nouri K. Lasers in the treatment of acne. *G Ital Dermatol Venereol.* 2017;152(4):360–372. http://www.minervamedica.it/index2.php?show=R23Y2017N04A0360.

61. Krakowski AC, Totri CR, Donelan MB, Shumaker PR. Scar management in pediatric and adolescent populations. *Pediatrics.* 2016;137(2):e20142065.

62. Waibel J, Wulkan AJ, Lupo M, Beer K, Anderson RR. Treatment of burn scars with the 1,550 nm nonablative fractional Erbium Laser. *Lasers Surg Med.* 2012;44(6):441–446.

63. Weiss R, Weiss M, Beasley K. Long-term experience with fixed array 1540 fractional erbium laser for acne scars. Abstract presented at American Society for Laser Medicine and Surgery Conference; April 2008; Kissimmee, FL.

64. Chapas AM, Brightman L, Sukal S, et al. Successful treatment of acneiform scarring with CO2 ablative fractional resurfacing. *Lasers Surg Med.* 2008;40(6):381–386.

65. Mahmoud BH, Srivastava D, Janiga JJ, Yang JJ, Lim HW, Ozog DM. Safety and efficacy of erbium-doped yttrium aluminum garnet fractionated laser for treatment of acne scars in type IV to VI skin. *Dermatol Surg.* 2010;36(5):602–609.

66. Izikson L, Nelson JS, Anderson RR. Treatment of hypertrophic and resistant port wine stains with a 755 nm laser: a case series of 20 patients. *Lasers Surg Med.* 2009;41(6):427–432.

67. Wong BM, Keilman J, Zuccaro J, Kelly C, Maynes JT, Fish JS. Anesthetic practices for laser rehabilitation of pediatric hypertrophic burn scars. *J Burn Care Res.* 2017;38(1):e36–e41.

68. Edkins RE, Hultman CS, Collins P, Cairns B, Hanson M, Carman M. Improving comfort and throughput for patients undergoing fractionated laser ablation of symptomatic burn scars. *Ann Plast Surg.* 2015;74(3):293–299.

69. Werschler WP, Herdener RS, Ross VE, Zimmerman E. Treating acne scars: what's new? Consensus from the experts. *J Clin Aesthet Dermatol.* 2015;8(8, suppl):S2–S8.

70. Krakowski AC, Goldenberg A, Eichenfield LF, Murray J-P, Shumaker PR. Ablative fractional laser resurfacing helps treat restrictive pediatric scar contractures. *Pediatrics.* 2014;134(6):e1700–e1705.

71. Kim SG, Kim EY, Kim YJ, Lee SI. The efficacy and safety of ablative fractional resurfacing using a 2,940-Nm Er:YAG laser for traumatic scars in the early posttraumatic period. *Arch Plast Surg.* 2012;39(3):232.

72. Elsaie ML, Ibrahim SM, Saudi W. Ablative fractional 10 600 nm carbon dioxide laser versus non-ablative fractional 1540 nm erbium-glass laser in Egyptian post-acne scar patients. *J Lasers Med Sci.* 2018;9(1):32–35.

73. Firooz A, Rajabi-Estarabadi A, Nassiri-Kashani MH. Treatment of atrophic facial acne scars with fractional Er:YAG laser in skin phototype III–IV: a pilot study. *J Cosmet Laser Ther.* 2016;18(4):204–207.

74. Hession MT, Graber EM. Atrophic acne scarring. *J Clin Aesthetic Dermatol.* 2015;8(1):50–58.

75. Hedelund L, Haak CS, Togsverd-Bo K, Bogh MK, Bjerring P, Haedersdal M. Fractional CO2 laser resurfacing for atrophic acne scars: a randomized controlled trial with blinded response evaluation. *Lasers Surg Med.* 2012;44(6):447–452.

76. Majid I, Imran S. Fractional CO$_2$ laser resurfacing as monotherapy in the treatment of atrophic facial acne scars. *J Cutan Aesthetic Surg.* 2014;7(2):87.

77. Ross EV, Swann M, Soon S, Izadpanah A, Barnette D, Davenport S. Full-face treatments with the 2790-nm erbium:YSGG laser system. *J Drugs Dermatol.* 2009;8(3):248–252.

78. Al-Saedy SJ, Al-Hilo MM, Al-Shami SH. Treatment of acne scars using fractional erbium:YAG laser. *Am J Dermatol Venereol.* 2014;3(2):43–49.

79. Pai S, Prabhu S, Kudur M, et al. Efficacy and safety of erbium-doped yttrium aluminium garnet fractional resurfacing laser for treatment of facial acne scars. *Indian J Dermatol Venereol Leprol.* 2013;79(2):193.

80. Yates B, Que SKT, D'Souza L, Suchecki J, Finch JJ. Laser treatment of periocular skin conditions. *Clin Dermatol.* 2015;33(2):197–206.

81. Williams K, Shinkai K. Evaluation and management of the patient with multiple syringomas: a systematic review of the literature. *J Am Acad Dermatol.* 2016;74(6):1234–1240.e9.

82. Gómez MI, Pérez B, Azaña JM, Núñez M, Ledo A. Eruptive syringoma: treatment with topical tretinoin. *Dermatology.* 1994;189(1):105–106.

83. Sanchez TS, Daudn E, Casas AP, Garca-Dez A. Eruptive pruritic syringomas: treatment with topical atropine. *J Am Acad Dermatol.* 2001;44(1):148–149.

84. Karma P, Benedetto AV. Intralesional electrodesiccation of syringomas. *Dermatol Surg.* 1997;23(10):921–924.

85. Cho SB, Kim HJ, Noh S, Lee SJ, Kim YK, Lee JH. Treatment of syringoma using an ablative 10,600-nm carbon dioxide fractional laser: a prospective analysis of 35 patients: *Dermatol Surg.* 2011;37(4):433–438.

86. Goldman A, Wollina U. Periocular syringomas—successful treatment with fractional CO$_2$ laser. *J Surg Dermatol.* 2017;2(t1):148–151. http://www.jsurgdermatol.com/index.php/JSD/article/view/145.

87. Weiss ET, Geronemus RG. New technique using combined pulsed dye laser and fractional resurfacing for treating facial angiofibromas in tuberous sclerosis. *Lasers Surg Med.* 2010;42(5):357–360.

88. Sliney DH. Laser safety. *Lasers Surg Med.* 1995;16(3):215–225.

89. Russell SW, Dinehart SM, Davis I, Flock ST. Efficacy of corneal eye shields in protecting patients' eyes from laser irradiation. *Dermatol Surg.* 1996;22(7):613–616.

90. Shamsaldeen O, Peterson JD, Goldman MP. The adverse events of deep fractional CO2: a retrospective study of 490 treatments in 374 patients. *Lasers Surg Med.* 2011;43(6):453–456.

91. Lee SM, Kim MS, Kim YJ, et al. Adverse events of non-ablative fractional laser photothermolysis: a retrospective study of 856 treatments in 362 patients. *J Dermatolog Treat.* 2014;25(4):304–307.

92. Mansur AT, Demirci G, Uzunismail MA, Yildiz S. A rare complication of follicular hair unit extraction: Kaposi's varicelliform eruption. *Dermatol Pract Concept.* 2016;6(1):15–17. http://www.derm101.com/dpc/january-2016-volume-6-no.1/a-rare-complication-of-follicular-hair-unit-extraction-kaposi's-varicelliform-eruption/.

93. Smith JS, Robinson NJ. Age-specific prevalence of infection with herpes simplex virus types 2 and 1: a global review. *J Infect Dis.* 2002;186(s1):S3–S28.

94. Rosen T. Recurrent herpes labialis in adults: new tricks for an old dog. *J Drugs Dermatol.* 2017;16(3):S49–S53.

95. Monheit G. Facial resurfacing may trigger the herpes simplex virus. *Cosmet Dermatol.* 1995;8:9–16.

96. Gilbert S, McBurney E. Use of valacyclovir for herpes simplex virus-1 (HSV-1) prophylaxis after facial resurfacing: a randomized clinical trial of dosing regimens. *Dermatol Surg.* 2000;26(1):50–54.

97. Beeson WH, Rachel JD. Valacyclovir prophylaxis for herpes simplex virus infection or infection recurrence following laser skin resurfacing. *Dermatol Surg.* 2002;28(4):331–336.

98. Alster TS, Nanni CA. Famciclovir prophylaxis of herpes simplex virus reactivation after laser skin resurfacing. *Dermatol Surg.* 1999;25(3):242–246.

99. Greveling K, Prens EP, Liu L, van Doorn MBA. Non-invasive anaesthetic methods for dermatological laser procedures: a systematic review. *J Eur Acad Dermatol Venereol.* 2017;31(7):1096–1110.

100. Kautz G, Kautz I, Segal J, Zehren S. Treatment of resistant port wine stains (PWS) with pulsed dye laser and non-contact vacuum: a pilot study. *Lasers Med Sci.* 2010;25(4):525–529.

101. Namba Y, Mae O, Ao M. The treatment of port wine stains with a dye laser: a study of 644 patients. *Scand J Plast Reconstr Surg Hand Surg.* 2001;35(2):197–202.

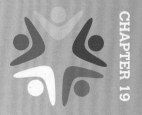

CHAPTER 19

Laser Treatment of Vascular Lesions

Larissa Marie Lehmer and Kristen M. Kelly

INTRODUCTION AND HISTORY

Lasers are commonly utilized for treatment of cutaneous vascular lesions in pediatric patients. Today, laser surgery is the treatment of choice for many vascular lesions, particularly port wine birthmarks (PWBs) and spider angiomas. Other vascular entities found in pediatric patients such as infantile hemangiomas (IHs) and angiofibromas associated with tuberous sclerosis can be treated with medications but may also benefit from laser treatment. Lasers can be used safely in patients of all ages and can provide dramatic benefits.

One of the earliest uses of lasers in dermatology was for the treatment of vascular lesions. Early lasers emitted a continuous wave whereas lasers today can discharge pulses in the millisecond to picosecond range. Ruby and argon lasers, developed in the 1960s, demonstrated improvement in the color of PWB and IH; however, unacceptably high rates of scarring and pigmentary change from collateral nonspecific heating of the skin made these lasers undesirable in clinical practice. The theory of selective photothermolysis (see Chapter 18. Laser Surgery, and Foreword) was proposed in 1983 and marked a major breakthrough for laser development as it provided a foundation of understanding of how to confine thermal injury to the target chromophore.[1]

Selective photothermolysis rests on the following three components: a laser wavelength with preferential absorption of the target chromophore; a pulse duration matched to the target size; and a fluence that destroys the target although minimizing nonspecific thermal injury. For vascular lesions, the classic target chromophore is oxyhemoglobin, which has the greatest absorption peaks at 418, 542, and 577 nm (Figure 19.1). When laser light is absorbed by oxyhemoglobin, it is converted to heat energy that is transferred to the vessel wall causing coagulation and vessel closure or vessel leakage. Depending on the vascular lesion type, other hemoglobin species may also be targeted. For example, wavelengths that target deoxyhemoglobin may be used to treat venous lesions. At 755 nm, the alexandrite laser approximates an absorption peak of deoxyhemoglobin and has been used to address hypertrophic PWB refractory to pulsed dye laser (PDL).[2] Methemoglobin absorption has also been recognized as another potential target chromophore.[3]

In 1986, the PDL became available with an initial wavelength of 577 nm to target the yellow absorption peak of oxyhemoglobin; however, this was only useful for very superficial vessels as the depth of penetration was <1 mm.[4,5] Subsequently, practitioners discovered that selective photothermolysis does not require that the laser wavelength be at the peak absorption of

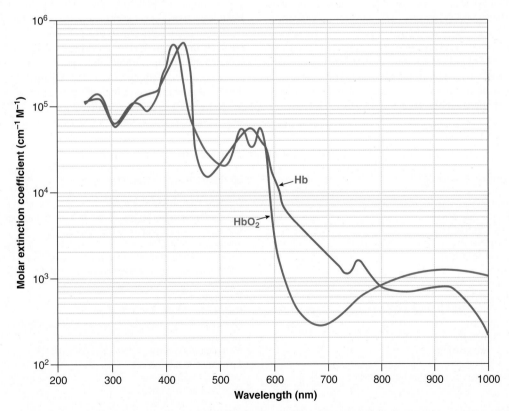

FIGURE 19.1. Hemoglobin absorption spectrum. Peak absorption occurs at 418, 542, and 577 nm. Hb—deoxygenated hemoglobin; HbO$_2$—oxygenated hemoglobin. Reprinted from https://commons.wikimedia.org/wiki/File:Hemoglobin_extinction.png. https://creativecommons.org/licenses/by-sa/3.0/.

107

target chromophore as long as the chromophore preferentially absorbed it over other chromophores in the vicinity. This enabled a shift of PDLs to 585 nm, which increased the depth of penetration to 1.16 mm, and then to 595 nm, which achieved even greater depth of penetration. Longer pulse durations were also incrementally incorporated into PDL devices. Early PDLs had a fixed pulse duration of 0.45 ms, whereas currently available PDLs have pulse durations from 0.45 to 40 ms. A longer pulse duration carries the advantage of treating the target with minimal to no purpura.

The risk of pigmentary side effects and scarring that can accompany laser treatment was significantly reduced with the advent of epidermal cooling in the 1990s. Modern cooling modalities include dynamic spray, contact, and forced cold air. Cooling enables the use of higher fluences, which increases treatment efficacy while simultaneously minimizing patient discomfort.

Given the energy emitted by PDL reaches a depth of only 1 to 2 mm, other lasers have been developed to treat vascular lesions that penetrate deeper. A 50% to 75% increase in depth can be achieved with the use of alexandrite laser at 755 nm or neodymium–yttrium aluminum garnet (Nd:YAG) laser at 1064 nm, respectively. However, to compensate for a lower absolute absorption of hemoglobin at these longer wavelengths, higher fluences are required.

Other vascular lasers and light sources include potassium titanyl phosphate (KTP) (532 nm), other near-infrared long-pulsed lasers such as diode (800-810 nm, 940 nm), and dual wavelength lasers such as PDL combined with Nd:YAG (595 and 1064 nm).

VASCULAR LESIONS

The International Society for the Study of Vascular Anomalies (ISSVA) publishes a widely accepted standard for classification of vascular anomalies that was updated in 2018.[6,7] The two broad categories of vascular lesions include (1) tumors, characterized by a proliferation of blood vessels, and (2) malformations, characterized by vessels with abnormal structure. For example, a hemangioma constitutes a vascular tumor, whereas a PWB is classified as a vascular malformation (Table 19.1).

PORT WINE BIRTHMARKS
Overview

The vast majority of port wine birthmarks (PWBs) are congenital and are present in approximately 0.3% of newborns (see Chapter 115. Port-Wine Birthmarks). PWBs are also called "port wine stains," but the latter term may carry a negative connotation.[8] In rare cases PWB-like lesions can be acquired. Although PWBs may occur anywhere on the body, the head and neck are the most commonly involved locations. Infants go from a relatively oxygen-poor to an oxygen-rich environment, which precipitates a 2- to 3-month hemodynamic transition from an intrauterine hemoglobin concentration of 16 to 18 g/dL to 9 to 9.5 g/dL, that is, physiologic anemia of infancy, which manifests clinically as bright red skin in the first days to weeks of life that gradually fades. In an infant with a PWB, this physiologic fading may be misinterpreted as spontaneous lightening, but spontaneous fading does not occur in PWB.[9]

PWBs are comprised of ectatic capillaries and postcapillary venules in the superficial vascular plexus. Vessels in PWBs vary in size from 7 to 300 μm, with older patients tending to have larger vessels. PWBs grow proportionally with the patient and persist throughout life often increasing in thickness over time. On average, hypertrophy occurs around 37 years with 65% of lesions demonstrating hypertrophy or nodular features by the fifth decade.[10] Associated soft tissue overgrowth may occur and lead to functional impairment if located near the lips, eyelids, or mandibular and maxillary areas (which may lead to tooth and jaw deformation). If present, vascular blebs can bleed easily with minimal trauma. Furthermore, a pruritic eczematous dermatitis may develop within a PWB, that is, the "Meyerson phenomenon," which, although it has been described as a transient finding with PWB laser treatment, also responds to PDL therapy.[11] Notably, the disfigurement of PWB is what prompts many patients to seek treatment.[8]

Various syndromes may present with a PWB. Facial PWBs are seen in Sturge–Weber syndrome (SWS) and may have associated eye and neurologic abnormalities including glaucoma, seizures, and developmental delay. Historically, PWBs in the distribution of the first branch of the trigeminal nerve (V1) were felt to be most highly associated with SWS.[12] More recently, a large review revealed that it is the infants with PWB emanating

---

TABLE 19.1 ⋮ Selected Lesions From ISSVA Classification for Vascular Lesions

BENIGN VASCULAR TUMORS	SIMPLE VASCULAR MALFORMATIONS

• Infantile hemangioma
• Congenital hemangioma (CH)
  • Rapidly involuting (RICH)
  • Non-involuting (NICH)
  • Partially involuting (PICH)
• Tufted angioma
• Spindle-cell hemangioma
• Epithelioid hemangioma
• Pyogenic granuloma (aka lobular capillary hemangioma)
• Hobnail hemangioma
• Microvenular hemangioma
• Anastomosing hemangioma
• Glomeruloid hemangioma
• Intravascular papillary endothelial hyperplasia
	Capillary Malformations (CM)
	• Nevus simplex/salmon patch, "angel kiss," "stork bite"
	• Cutaneous and/or mucosal CM (PWB)
	  • Nonsyndromic CM
	  • CM with CNS and/or ocular anomalies (Sturge–Weber)
	  • CM with bone and/or soft tissue overgrowth
	  • Diffuse CM with overgrowth
	• Reticulate CM
	• CM of CM–arteriovenous malformation
	• Cutis marmorata telangiectatica congenita (CMTC)
	• Telangiectasia
	• Hereditary hemorrhagic telangiectasia (HHT)
	• Lymphatic malformations
	• Venous malformations
	• Blue rubber bleb nevus

Abbreviations: CNS, central nervous system; ISSVA, International Society for the Study of Vascular Anomalies; PWB, port wine birthmark.
Lesions selected from ISSVA classification for vascular anomalies. In: International Society for the Study of Vascular Anomalies; May 2018. http://www.issva.org/UserFiles/file/ISSVA-Classification-2018.pdf.

from skin derived from the embryologic frontonasal placode (forehead and hemifacial phenotypes) that are at the highest risk for underlying SWS.[13] PWBs are the results of somatic mosaicism. Both isolated PWBs and those associated with SWS have been associated with a somatic activating mutation in the gene encoding guanine nucleotide-binding protein G(q) subunit alpha (GNAQ), as detailed in a seminal paper by Shirley et al.[14] Klippel–Trenaunay syndrome (KTS) is yet another condition that involves a PWB on an extremity in association with limb hypertrophy and underlying venous/lymphatic malformations. Rahimi et al reported one case of unilateral KTS in a 2-week-old infant successfully treated with PDL (595 nm, 7 mm spot, fluence 10-11 J/cm^2, 1.5-3 ms pulse duration at 3-week intervals), with improvement of overlying PWB after three treatments, and the infant was found to be stable at 7-year follow-up. Arteriovenous malformations and PWB can co-occur in capillary malformation–arteriovenous malformation syndrome.[15]

Treatment

The aims of PWB treatment are to decrease redness, reduce psychosocial distress, and prevent development of blebs that may bleed or become infected.

As the border of a lesion can become blurred because of treatment-induced erythema, it is helpful to outline the edges of a lesion with yellow highlighter (if using a yellow light laser such as the PDL) prior to the treatment to facilitate consistent visualization of the area of interest.

Laser is the standard of care treatment for PWBs. Overall, PDL is very effective in treating PWBs; however, individual patient response is variable. Although 20% of patients treated experience complete clearance, approximately 80% have a successful decrease in redness or thickness.[16] Three predictors of favorable treatment response include small size (<20 cm^2), location over bony areas, that is, the central forehead, and early treatment. A study of early treatment of PWB in 49 infants who initiated therapy prior to 6 months of age had an average clearance of 88.6% after 1 year.[17] It is felt that early treatment is so effective because skin is thinner in younger patients allowing improved light penetration, younger patients may have less melanin, hemoglobin F is present allowing an additional target, and lesion vessels are not as dramatically dilated. "Redarkening" is a phenomenon occasionally observed when the PWB becomes dark again after initial lightening with laser treatment. However, redarkened areas generally remain improved, that is, lighter than their original untreated color.[18]

The treatment interval for PWB varies but follow up times from 4 to 6 weeks may be considered. It has been proposed that more frequent treatments can provide additional benefit. Multiple treatments are required (10 or more is common), until a plateau is reached or the lesion clears. For the PDL, immediate purpura is the desired clinical endpoint. Evidence that the fluence is too high is a gray color or blister (both of which may not be immediately evident), indicating epidermal injury. Constant careful monitoring for tissue response is essential as tissue response evolves.

✶ Clinical Pearl: Cooling

Ideal pulse duration for PWB treatment is 1 to 10 ms. For a 7 to 10 mm spot size, a pulse duration of 0.45 to 6 ms may be appropriate, with appropriate epidermal cooling, such as cryogen spray cooling of 20 to 30 ms with a 30 ms delay. For treatment in darker skin types, longer pulse durations are more appropriate, but cooling parameters can remain constant.

The targeting of different sizes of vessels can be accomplished via alteration of the pulse duration. In general, the ideal pulse duration for PWB treatment is 1 to 10 ms. For a 7 to 10 mm spot size, a pulse duration of 0.45 to 6 ms may be appropriate, with appropriate epidermal cooling, such as cryogen spray cooling of 20 to 30 ms with a 30 ms delay. When approaching treatment in darker skin types, longer pulse durations are more appropriate. Cooling parameters can remain constant in darker skin types. Initiate treatment at a lower energy with plan to increase as tolerated. Always remember that specific parameters will vary by device, both depending on the manufacturer of each individual device and the different wavelengths that can be used (eg, 532 vs. 595 nm).

Treatment is provided by delivering successive pulses across the lesion with a small amount of overlap (approximately 10%). Depending on the device, the handpiece can be slid across the skin or the handpiece can be stamped across the lesion, with pulses being delivered as the handpiece is moved. Some devices have an option of a hand or foot trigger. Either can be used, depending on what is more comfortable for the operator.

In a prospective study, the 532 nm KTP-Nd:YAG also demonstrated efficacy in lightening PWB (spot 6-10 mm, 3-6 ms pulse duration, fluences 4.8-9 J/cm^2, sapphire tip contact cooling) after a single treatment with histologic evidence of decreased superficial vessels.[19]

Vascular filters can be fitted to intense pulsed light devices and used to treat PWB.[20]

PDL-resistant lesions may be treated with the 755 nm alexandrite laser.[21] The alexandrite laser may be used as a first-line treatment for more hypertrophic or violaceous PWS in adults. The desired endpoint for the alexandrite laser is a transient gray color that transitions to a deeper persistent purpura over several minutes.[22] The operator should avoid overlapping or "stacking" pulses, as this may lead to scarring. The range of appropriate fluences for alexandrite laser is quite broad.[2]

Combined 595 nm and 1064 nm lasers have also been used for PWB.[23] Although the longer wavelengths increase the depth of laser energy penetration, the trade-off is a narrower therapeutic window, that is, a higher risk of scarring. Therefore, these devices should be used for treatment of PWB with caution by experienced laser surgeons.

Nodules or blebs within PWS can be addressed via lasers or excision. With PDL, several pulses, that is, pulse stacking, may be necessary. However, given the penetration depth of PDL is limited, nodules or blebs may be better addressed by the longer wavelengths of the alexandrite or Nd:YAG. There are multiple reports of Nd:YAG, for example, being used with contact cooling with spot sizes ranging from 3, 5, 7, or 10 mm; fluences ranging from 3-300 J/cm^2; and pulse widths ranging from 0.1-300 ms. Ultimately, color (ie, vessel size) and thickness tend to drive lasing parameter selection.[24,25] Alternatively, thick lesions may be ablated with carbon dioxide (CO_2).[26] Again, these longer wavelength devices have a higher risk of resulting in scarring. Blebs can also be treated by excision, especially for larger lesions, or electrocautery. Both of these options often result in some scarring.

Additional gains in treatment efficacy can be achieved with the combination of light-based removal of PWB and posttreatment with antiangiogenic agents such as rapamycin. The synergy is attributed to rapamycin's inhibition of growth-promoting pathways activated by laser-induced vessel damage.[27] Benefit of PDL plus rapamycin has been demonstrated in clinical trials[28-31] but not all patients had augmented response with rapamycin, and future work is likely to identify additional antiangiogenic agents that may be beneficial.[32]

Bruising and swelling are common with laser treatment of PWB and an expected effect.[33] Hyper- or hypopigmentation may occur.[34] Scarring is uncommon with PDL but may occur with any device; however, it is more common when longer wavelengths are used. Treatment in hair-bearing areas may lead to permanent hair loss or decrease, including on the eyelashes, because of the proximity of follicles to the surface.[35] Additionally, the eyebrows and scalp hair of young children, particularly those of darker skin types, are at risk.

SPIDER ANGIOMAS

Spider angiomas (SA) are benign localized lesions with a central feeder vessel, from which multiple small dilated vessels radiate (see Chapter 57. Angioma, Spider). SAs represent the most common type of vascular malformation and are common in healthy individuals. Pulsed dye laser is one of the most common light-based devices used to treat SA, with one large study showing a 89.4% response rate after a single treatment and 91.0% response after two treatments (7 mm spot, 3 ms pulse duration, 40 J/cm^2).[36] The KTP laser is also commonly used for SA. Clark et al treated 102 lesions in 81 patients with a single pulse delivered to the central feeder vessel yielding a 96% response after an average of two treatments (2 mm spot, 10-14 ms pulse duration, 10-12 J/cm^2).[37] Only one patient in the latter study experienced an adverse event of minimal atrophic scarring after seven treatments for a larger-than-average lesion. IPL is a third commonly utilized option (one study utilized 550 nm filter, 25-27 J/cm^2, 5 ms pulse duration in single or double-pulse mode).[38] The footprint for the IPL is often significantly larger than the lesion so areas not requiring treatment can be shielded (ie, covered).

INFANTILE HEMANGIOMAS
Overview

The most common tumor of infancy is the IH, which affects 4% to 10% of all infants (see Chapter 84. Infantile Hemangioma). IHs are proliferations of benign endothelial cells that are three times more common in female than male infants. Prematurity, multiple gestations, advanced maternal age, and family history of hemangiomas are other known risk factors. Histologically, IHs can be distinguished from other vascular tumors and malformations by their expression of GLUT1, a fetal-type endothelial glucose transporter. IHs can be classified as superficial (clinically red), deep (clinically blue or skin-colored), or mixed. IHs characteristically present as whitish, red, or telangiectatic macules that can be present at birth or within the first few weeks of life. Sixty percent of all lesions occur on the head and neck but IHs can occur at any location.[39]

For superficial IHs, the initial proliferative period typically extends for 5 to 8 months whereas deep hemangiomas may progress longer.[40] Involution takes much longer and occurs over a period of years. The formerly cited "rule" was that with each passing year, 10% of hemangiomas regressed, with the majority completing regression by age 10.[41] However, more recent studies suggest that maximal natural diminution is complete at a younger age.[42] Residual fibrofatty tissue, atrophy, or telangiectases may remain after regression and are most common with larger lesions or those with a more angular border (lesions with a sloping border may resolve more completely).

Generally, imaging studies are not required for the diagnosis of IH but there are situations where radiologic investigation may be warranted to assess for possible associated syndromes or visceral involvement.[43] Large segmental facial hemangiomas prompt consideration of PHACES syndrome, which is characterized by posterior fossa malformations, hemangiomas, arterial anomalies, coarctation of the aorta, eye abnormalities, and sternal or supraumbilical raphe. Other concerning findings include a characteristic perineal or lumbar hemangioma that may necessitate radiologic evaluation for related syndromes such as PELVIS (perineal hemangioma, external genital malformations, lipomyelomeningocele, vesicorenal abnormalities, imperforate anus, and skin tags)[44] or LUMBAR (lower body hemangioma, urogenital anomalies or ulceration, myelopathy, bony deformities, anorectal malformations and arterial anomalies, renal anomalies).[45] The presence of multiple skin hemangiomas in multifocal infantile hemangiomatosis (previously referred to under the broad title "diffuse neonatal hemangiomatosis") signifies a potential risk of visceral hemangiomas, with the liver representing the most commonly affected organ followed by the gastrointestinal tract.[46] Workup includes an abdominal ultrasound, complete blood cell count to screen for anemia and thrombocytopenia, stool testing for blood, and imaging of other organs as indicated by IH distribution or specific signs and symptoms.

GLUT1 negative hemangiomas are less common. The two types are known as non-involuting congenital hemangiomas (NICH) and rapidly involuting congenital hemangiomas (RICH).[47] There is now a third category, known as the partially involuting congenital hemangiomas, which begins to regress, but eventually plateaus and persists.[48]

Treatment

Functional impairment and complications of ulceration, infection, and bleeding are all indications for IH treatment. Functional difficulties arise when IHs affect critical anatomical structures and have been known to cause airway compromise, visual obstruction, feeding difficulties, and auditory canal obstruction. Some forms of potential impairment of function by IH including visual obstruction[49] (which can result in permanent visual defects if necessary neural connections are not developed) and airway obstruction[50] are medical emergencies.

Historically, "watchful waiting" (a.k.a. active nonintervention) has been the mainstay of treatment for many IHs that do not impose functional difficulties or complications. However, prevention of long-term scarring and associated psychosocial distress, particularly because the majority of IHs do involve a cosmetically sensitive area, has become a further indication for treatment.[51]

Currently, the main treatment for IH is β-blockers. Propranolol is the first and continues to be the primary β-blocker used with dramatic results.[52] Large studies have demonstrated the benefit of propranolol.[53] A controlled trial of 456 infants between the ages of 35 and 150 days randomized into the treatment: 3 mg/kg propranolol per day (divided into twice-daily dosing) in the 6 month, or placebo, arms demonstrated a 60% versus 4% response, respectively. Hogeling et al placed patients on a regimen of 2 mg/kg/d propranolol divided into three-times-daily dosing for 6 months and noted that patients experienced cessation of IH growth at 4 weeks, reduction in redness at 12 weeks, and reduction in elevation at 24 weeks in the treatment arm.[54] Propranolol is generally well tolerated with risks of bradycardia, hypotension, and hypoglycemia generally easily managed with proper dosing and parent education in otherwise healthy children.[55] Superficial IHs may be addressed topically with timolol.[56]

Laser can play a role in addition to β-blockers in the treatment of IH. Reddy et al demonstrated the benefit of combined propranolol and PDL as superior to monotherapy with either propranolol or PDL as well as superior to sequential treatment with both.[57] The concurrent use of timolol with laser surgery demonstrated an enhanced effect in a randomized, controlled trial, whereby timolol plus PDL was found to be superior to either one as monotherapy for IH.[58] Timolol gel 0.5% or placebo was applied every 12 hours and PDL treatment (585 nm, 5 mm spot, fluence of 9 J/cm^2, pulse duration 0.45 ms with 20% spot overlap) was performed once weekly for 1 month; patients were observed at 6 months after the final treatment with greater improvement in the timolol plus PDL group versus PDL alone (71.79% ± 23.40% and 54.59% ± 25.46%). Ulcerated lesions may respond well to PDL.[59] David et al used a 585 nm PDL to treat 78 infants with ulcerated hemangiomas at 3- to 4-week intervals until cutaneous healing or hemangioma involution occurred for an average of two laser treatment sessions per patient with a 92% response rate measured at 25-month follow-up (5-7 mm spot, 6.6 J/cm^2 fluence, 0.3-0.5 ms pulse duration, Cynosure PhotoGenica V).[59] The authors generally use a 595 nm wavelength, 10 mm spot size, 1.5 ms pulse duration, and 5.0 to 7.0 J/cm^2 with epidermal cooling. Lower energies are preferred when treating ulcerated or proliferating lesions to avoid further injury. Importantly, ulcerated lesions should have supportive local wound care with barrier creams and occlusive dressings to prevent trauma and superinfection. Infection may require topical or oral antibiotics.

The PDL is the most commonly utilized and safest light-based device for the treatment of IH. Superficial IHs respond best to laser treatment because of the laser light's limited depth of penetration. PDL may be implemented to lighten the color of mixed superficial and deep lesions; however, the deeper component will remain unaffected. Propranolol can be used to address the deep component, and as noted earlier, synergistic treatment with propranolol and PDL can be beneficial. Studies suggest early treatment of IH with laser, especially PDL (Kwon et al: 40 infants, PDL 595 nm, 10 mm spot, fluence 7-10 J/cm^2, pulse duration 3-6 ms, dynamic cooling 30/10 ms; Chapas et al: 49 infants, PDL 595 nm, 10 mm spot, 7.75-9.5 J/cm^2 fluence, 1.5 ms pulse duration, dynamic cooling 30/20 ms), may prevent further growth and facilitate a transition to the plateau or involution phase with a favorable side effect profile.[17,60]

Proliferating IHs have been addressed in studies by a broad range of PDL fluences. Given the risk of ulceration with laser treatment of proliferating lesions, it is the opinion of the authors that lower fluences should be used. When treating with PDL, settings to consider include pulse duration 0.45 to 1.5 ms, 10 or 7 mm spot, and appropriate cooling. Multiple treatments are required and should be performed at 2- to 4-week intervals for lesions that are rapidly proliferating versus every 4 to 6 weeks for those that are involuting. As in PWBs, when addressing lesions in darker skin types, lower fluences and longer pulse durations are advised. Specific parameters vary by device. Ulceration, scarring, and hypopigmentation are the main risks of treatment. Rarely, serious bleeding after PDL treatment for IH has occurred, predominantly with older devices without cooling, and in one case with a 595 nm laser with cooling, when higher fluences were used.

Both the 532 nm KTP laser and IPL with vascular filter have also been successfully implemented in the treatment of IHs.[61] The Nd:YAG laser (7 mm spot, 65-120 J/cm^2, 10-30 ms pulse duration) has been used on thick hemangiomas in order to get greater depth of penetration.[62] However, as mentioned in the PWB section, extreme caution is required when using the 1064 nm wavelength as the therapeutic window is incredibly narrow, and significant ulceration and scarring can easily occur. As noted earlier, propranolol is the standard of care for the treatment of IH with a deep component.

Laser surgery can also be performed after IH involution for the treatment of residual telangiectasias or residual fibrofatty tissue. The PDL, long-pulsed 532 nm laser, or IPL can be used to treat telangiectasias, whereas textural changes including fibrofatty residua are best addressed with ablative or non-ablative fractional resurfacing lasers.[63] The fibrofatty residua can be treated with fractional lasers in a manner similar to scarring, with the depth of treatment being based on the depth of lesion. When using ablative fractional lasers (AFLs), the authors have used low density, 5% to 10%, with good results.

ANGIOFIBROMAS

Tuberous sclerosis complex (TSC) is a rare neurocutaneous genetic disorder with a prevalence of 1 in 1600 births (see Chapter 55. Angiofibromas). It is transmitted in an autosomal dominant fashion; however, de novo mutations account for the appearance of two-thirds of all cases. Multiple hamartomas develop in the skin and other organs as a result of uncontrolled cell proliferation caused by mutations in *TSC1* and *TSC2* genes, which regulate mTOR cell signaling.[64] Male individuals with TSC2 mutations tend to have more severe clinical manifestations.[65]

The most common dermatologic manifestation of tuberous sclerosis is angiofibromas, erythematous papules typically located on the central face. It is also one of the earliest signs of the condition as these lesions may appear as early as 2 to 5 years of age. These are highly visible, can enlarge during puberty, can bleed with trauma, and may cause emotional distress.[66]

Several options have been described to treat angiofibromas. PDL may help to treat erythema but this alone is generally not very successful. Papular fibrosis can be targeted with ablative devices, including the AFL. Topical sirolimus, an inhibitor of mTOR, has been reported to improve angiofibromas.[67] A case report by Bae-Harboe and Geronemus used a combination of laser surgery utilizing a 595 nm PDL (10 mm spot, 1.5 ms pulse duration, fluence of 7.5 J/cm^2, and cryogen spray cooling of 30 ms) and an ablative fractional resurfacing laser (15 mm spot size, 70 mJ per pulse, and 40% density). Electrosurgery was also performed on papular lesions with topical 0.2% sirolimus applied twice daily starting post-procedure and continued until follow-up at 3 months. This combination of therapies allowed for a safe and effective way to treat angiofibromas associated with tuberous sclerosis.[68] A series of four cases reported by Park and coworkers underwent topical therapy of 0.1% sirolimus for 2 to 3 months followed by an ablative laser therapy for larger (>4 mm), poorly responsive papules with maintenance three-times-weekly application of sirolimus 0.1% until 3-month post-laser follow-up. This combination regimen enabled successful treatment of larger angiofibromas with added benefit of preventing recurrences after laser treatment.[69]

One case of central facial angiofibromas was successfully addressed by the combination of 595 nm PDL (10 mm spot size, 1.5 ms pulse width, 9 J/cm^2 fluence, cooling parameters not specified) and a macrofractionated 10 600 nm CO$_2$ laser (5 mm spot size, 0.1 second repeat, fluence of 125 mJ/3.5 W, and

5%-6% density). Starting 5 days after laser surgery, topical 0.5% timolol was applied on the right cheek twice daily. At 4-month follow-up, fewer papules and less erythema were found on the timolol-treated area than the control.[70]

REFERENCES

1. Anderson RR, Parrish JA. Selective photothermolysis: precise microsurgery by selective absorption of pulsed radiation. *Science.* 1983;220(4596):524–527.

2. Tierney EP, Hanke WC. Alexandrite laser for the treatment of port wine stains refractory to pulsed dye laser. *Dermatol Surg.* 2011;37(9):1268–1278.

3. Meesters AA, Pitassi LHU, Campos V, Wolkerstorfer A, Dierickx CC. Transcutaneous laser treatment of leg veins. *Lasers Med Sci.* 2014;29(2):481–492.

4. Jasim ZF, Handley JM. Treatment of pulsed dye laser–resistant port wine stain birthmarks. *J Am Acad Dermatol.* 2007;57(4):677–682.

5. Wall TL. Current concepts: laser treatment of adult vascular lesions. *Semin Plast Surg.* 2007;21(3):147–158.

6. Sadick M, Müller-Wille R, Wildgruber M, Wohlgemuth WA. Vascular anomalies (part I): classification and diagnostics of vascular anomalies. *Rofo.* 2018;190:825–835.

7. ISSVA classification for vascular anomalies. In International Society for the Study of Vascular Anomalies; 2018. http://www.issva.org/UserFiles/file/ISSVA-Classification-2018.pdf.

8. Hagen SL, Grey KR, Korta DZ, Kelly KM. Quality of life in adults with facial port-wine stains. *J Am Acad Dermatol.* 2017;76(4):695–702.

9. Cordoro KM, Speetzen LS, Koerper MA, Frieden IJ. Physiologic changes in vascular birthmarks during early infancy: mechanisms and clinical implications. *J Am Acad Dermatol.* 2009;60(4):669–675.

10. Geronemus RG, Ashinoff R. The medical necessity of evaluation and treatment of port-wine stains. *J Dermatol Surg Oncol.* 1991;17(1):76–79.

11. Pavlović MD, Adamič M. Eczema within port wine stain: spontaneous and laser-induced Meyerson phenomenon. *Acta Dermatovenerol Alp Pannonica Adriat.* 2014;23(4):81–83. http://journalhub.io/journals/acta-dermatovenerol-apa/papers/624.

12. Ch'ng S, Tan ST. Facial port-wine stains—clinical stratification and risks of neuro-ocular involvement. *J Plast Reconstr Aesthet Surg.* 2008;61(8):889–893.

13. Zallmann M, Leventer RJ, Mackay MT, Ditchfield M, Bekhor PS, Su JC. Screening for Sturge-Weber syndrome: a state-of-the-art review. *Pediatr Dermatol.* 2018;35(1):30–42.

14. Shirley MD, Tang H, Gallione CJ, et al. Sturge-Weber syndrome and port-wine stains caused by somatic mutation in GNAQ. *N Engl J Med.* 2013;368(21):1971–1979.

15. Eerola I, Boon LM, Mulliken JB, et al. Capillary malformation–arteriovenous malformation, a new clinical and genetic disorder caused by RASA1 mutations. *Am J Hum Genet.* 2003;73(6):1240–1249.

16. Brightman LA, Geronemus RG, Reddy KK. Laser treatment of port-wine stains. *Clin Cosmet Investig Dermatol.* 2015;8:27–33.

17. Chapas AM, Eickhorst K, Geronemus RG. Efficacy of early treatment of facial port wine stains in newborns: a review of 49 cases. *Lasers Surg Med.* 2007;39(7):563–568.

18. Nelson JS, Geronemus RG. Redarkening of port-wine stains 10 years after laser treatment. *N Engl J Med.* 2007;356(26):2745–2746.

19. Reddy KK, Brauer JA, Idriss MH, et al. Treatment of port-wine stains with a short pulse width 532-nm Nd:YAG laser. *J Drugs Dermatol.* 2013;12(1):66–71.

20. Thajudheen CP, Jyothy K, Priyadarshini A. Treatment of port-wine stains with flash lamp pumped pulsed dye laser on Indian skin: a six year study. *J Cutan Aesthetic Surg.* 2014;7(1):32–36.

21. Izikson L, Nelson JS, Anderson RR. Treatment of hypertrophic and resistant port wine stains with a 755 nm laser: a case series of 20 patients. *Lasers Surg Med.* 2009;41(6):427–432.

22. Izikson L, Anderson RR. Treatment endpoints for resistant port wine stains with a 755 nm laser. *J Cosmet Laser Ther.* 2009;11(1):52–55.

23. Alster TS, Tanzi EL. Combined 595-nm and 1,064-nm laser irradiation of recalcitrant and hypertrophic port-wine stains in children and adults. *Dermatol Surg.* 2009;35(6):914–919.

24. Brauer JA, Geronemus RG. Single-treatment resolution of vascular blebs within port wine stains using a novel 1,064-nm neodymium-doped yttrium aluminum garnet laser. *Dermatol Surg.* 2013;39(7):1113–1115.

25. Zhong SX, Liu YY, Yao L, et al. Clinical analysis of port-wine stain in 130 Chinese patients treated by long-pulsed 1064-nm Nd: YAG laser. *J Cosmet Laser Ther.* 2014;16(6):279–283.

26. Tierney EP, Hanke CW. Treatment of nodules associated with port wine stains with CO2 laser: case series and review of the literature. *J Drugs Dermatol.* 2009;8(2):157–161.

27. Gao L, Phan S, Nadora DM, et al. Topical rapamycin systematically suppresses the early stages of pulsed dye laser-induced angiogenesis pathways. *Lasers Surg Med.* 2014;46(9):679–688.

28. Alegre-Sánchez A, Boixeda P. RF-topical rapamycin as an adjuvant to laser treatment in capillary malformations. *Actas Dermosifiliogr.* 2018;109:915–916.

29. Bloom BS, Nelson JS, Geronemus RG. Topical rapamycin combined with pulsed dye laser (PDL) in the treatment of capillary vascular malformations—anatomical differences in response to PDL are relevant to interpretation of study results. *J Am Acad Dermatol.* 2015;73(2):e71.

30. Greveling K, Prens EP, van Doorn MB. Treatment of port wine stains using pulsed dye laser, erbium YAG laser, and topical rapamycin (sirolimus)—a randomized controlled trial. *Lasers Surg Med.* 2017;49(1):104–109.

31. Griffin TD, Foshee JP, Finney R, Saedi N. Port wine stain treated with a combination of pulsed dye laser and topical rapamycin ointment. *Lasers Surg Med.* 2016;48(2):193–196.

32. Lipner SR. Topical adjuncts to pulsed dye laser for treatment of port wine stains: review of the literature. *Dermatol Surg.* 2018;44(6):796–802.

33. Nguyen CM, Yohn JJ, Huff C, Weston WL, Morelli JG. Facial port wine stains in childhood: prediction of the rate of improvement as a function of the age of the patient, size and location of the port wine stain and the number of treatments with the pulsed dye (585 nm) laser. *Br J Dermatol.* 1998;138(5):821–825.

34. Zhu J, Yu W, Wang T, et al. Less is more: similar efficacy in three sessions and seven sessions of pulsed dye laser treatment in infantile port-wine stain patients. *Lasers Med Sci.* 2018;33:1707–1715.

35. Feldstein S, Totri CR, Friedlander SF. Can long-term alopecia occur after appropriate pulsed-dye laser therapy in hair-bearing sites? Pediatric dermatologists weigh in. *Dermatol Surg.* 2015;41(3):348–351.

36. Yang B, Li L, Zhang L, Sun Y, Ma L. Clinical characteristics and treatment options of infantile vascular anomalies. *Medicine (Baltimore).* 2015;94(40):e1717.

37. Clark C, Cameron H, Moseley H, Ferguson J, Ibbotson SH. Treatment of superficial cutaneous vascular lesions: experience with the KTP 532 nm laser. *Lasers Med Sci.* 2004;19(1):1–5.

38. Kumaresan M, Srinivas C. Lasers for vascular lesions: standard guidelines of care. *Indian J Dermatol Venereol Leprol.* 2011; 77(3):349.

39. Munden A, Butschek R, Tom WL, et al. Prospective study of infantile haemangiomas: incidence, clinical characteristics and association with placental anomalies. *Br J Dermatol.* 2014;170(4): 907–913.

40. Craig LM, Alster TS. Vascular skin lesions in children: a review of laser surgical and medical treatments. *Dermatol Surg.* 2013;39(8):1137–1146.

41. Zheng JW, Zhang L, Zhou Q, et al. A practical guide to treatment of infantile hemangiomas of the head and neck. *Int J Clin Exp Med.* 2013;6(10):851–860.

42. Nguyen TA, Krakowski AC, Naheedy JH, Kruk PG, Friedlander SF. Imaging pediatric vascular lesions. *J Clin Aesthetic Dermatol.* 2015;8(12):27–41.

43. Mahady K, Thust S, Berkeley R, et al. Vascular anomalies of the head and neck in children. *Quant Imaging Med Surg.* 2015;5(6):886–897.

44. DeRosa A, Hellstrom WJG, Lang E. Magnetic resonance imaging for the diagnosis and management of perineal hemangiomas in children. *J Urol.* 2008;179(1):324.

45. Yu X, Zhang J, Wu Z, et al. LUMBAR syndrome: a case manifesting as cutaneous infantile hemangiomas of the lower extremity, perineum and gluteal region, and a review of published work. *J Dermatol.* 2017;44(7):808–812.

46. Glick ZR, Frieden IJ, Garzon MC, Mully TW, Drolet BA. Diffuse neonatal hemangiomatosis: an evidence-based review of case reports in the literature. *J Am Acad Dermatol.* 2012;67(5):898–903.

47. Boull C, Maguiness SM. Congenital hemangiomas. *Semin Cutan Med Surg.* 2016;35(3):124–127.

48. Nasseri E, Piram M, McCuaig CC, Kokta V, Dubois J, Powell J. Partially involuting congenital hemangiomas: a report of 8 cases and review of the literature. *J Am Acad Dermatol.* 2014;70(1):75–79.

49. Babiak-Choroszczak L, Giżewska-Kacprzak K, Puchalska-Niedbał L, Walecka A, Gawrych E. Propranolol as an effective treatment for inoperable periocular haemangiomas in children. *Pomeranian J Life Sci.* 2016;62(1):16–20.

50. Haggstrom AN, Skillman S, Garzon MC, et al. Clinical spectrum and risk of PHACE syndrome in cutaneous and airway hemangiomas. *Arch Otolaryngol Head Neck Surg.* 2011;137(7):680–687.

51. Williams EF, Hochman M, Rodgers BJ, Brockbank D, Shannon L, Lam SM. A psychological profile of children with hemangiomas and their families. *Arch Facial Plast Surg.* 2003;5(3):229–234.

52. Bagazgoitia L, Torrelo A, Gutiérrez JCL, et al. Propranolol for infantile hemangiomas. *Pediatr Dermatol.* 2011;28(2):108–114.

53. Léauté-Labrèze C, Hoeger P, Mazereeuw-Hautier J, et al. A randomized, controlled trial of oral propranolol in infantile hemangioma. *N Engl J Med.* 2015;372(8):735–746.

54. Hogeling M, Adams S, Wargon O. A randomized controlled trial of propranolol for infantile hemangiomas. *Pediatrics.* 2011;128(2):e259–e266.

55. Hagen R, Ghareeb E, Jalali O, Zinn Z. Infantile hemangiomas: what have we learned from propranolol? *Curr Opin Pediatr.* 2018;30:499–504.

56. Ng MSY, Tay YK, Ng SSY, Foong AYW, Koh MJA. Comparison of two formulations of topical timolol for the treatment of infantile hemangiomas. *Pediatr Dermatol.* 2017;34(4):492–493.

57. Reddy KK, Blei F, Brauer JA, et al. Retrospective study of the treatment of infantile hemangiomas using a combination of propranolol and pulsed dye laser. *Dermatol Surg.* 2013;39(6):923–933.

58. Asilian A, Mokhtari F, Kamali A, Abtahi-Naeini B, Nilforoushzadeh M, Mostafaie S. Pulsed dye laser and topical timolol gel versus pulse dye laser in treatment of infantile hemangioma: a double-blind randomized controlled trial. *Adv Biomed Res.* 2015;4(1):257.

59. David LR, Malek MM, Argenta LC. Efficacy of pulse dye laser therapy for the treatment of ulcerated haemangiomas: a review of 78 patients. *Br J Plast Surg.* 2003;56(4):317–327.

60. Kwon SH, Choi JW, Byun SY, et al. Effect of early long-pulse pulsed dye laser treatment in infantile hemangiomas. *Dermatol Surg.* 2014;40(4):405–411.

61. Becher GL, Cameron H, Moseley H. Treatment of superficial vascular lesions with the KTP 532-nm laser: experience with 647 patients. *Lasers Med Sci.* 2014;29(1):267–271.

62. Zhong S, Tao Y, Zhou J, Liu Y, Yao L, Li S. Infantile hemangioma: clinical characteristics and efficacy of treatment with the long-pulsed 1,064-nm neodymium-doped yttrium aluminum garnet laser in 794 Chinese patients. *Pediatr Dermatol.* 2015;32(4):495–500.

63. Stier MF, Glick SA, Hirsch RJ. Laser treatment of pediatric vascular lesions: port wine stains and hemangiomas. *J Am Acad Dermatol.* 2008;58(2):261–285.

64. Marchini M, Giglio E. Tuberous sclerosis complex. *N Engl J Med.* 2017;376(20):e42.

65. Shepherd C, Koepp M, Myland M, et al. Understanding the health economic burden of patients with tuberous sclerosis complex (TSC) with epilepsy: a retrospective cohort study in the UK Clinical Practice Research Datalink (CPRD). *BMJ Open.* 2017;7(10):e015236.

66. Cinar SL, Kartal D, Bayram AK, et al. Topical sirolimus for the treatment of angiofibromas in tuberous sclerosis. *Indian J Dermatol Venereol Leprol.* 2017;83(1):27–32.

67. Amin S, Lux A, Khan A, O'Callaghan F. Sirolimus ointment for facial angiofibromas in individuals with tuberous sclerosis complex. *Int Sch Res Notices.* 2017;2017:8404378.

68. Bae-Harboe Y-SC, Geronemus RG. Targeted topical and combination laser surgery for the treatment of angiofibromas: targeted topical and combination laser surgery. *Lasers Surg Med.* 2013;45(9):555–557.

69. Park J, Yun SK, Cho YS, Song KH, Kim HU. Treatment of angiofibromas in tuberous sclerosis complex: the effect of topical rapamycin and concomitant laser therapy. *Dermatol Basel Switz.* 2014;228(1):37–41.

70. Krakowski AC, Nguyen TA. Inhibition of angiofibromas in a tuberous sclerosis patient using topical timolol 0.5% gel. *Pediatrics.* 2015;136(3):e709–e713.

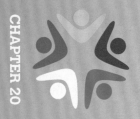

CHAPTER 20

Phototherapy and Photodynamic Therapy

Sara M. James and Craig N. Burkhart

Phototherapy

INTRODUCTION

Phototherapy is a highly effective treatment for a variety of dermatologic conditions including psoriasis, atopic dermatitis, vitiligo, cutaneous T-cell lymphoma (CTCL), localized and systemic sclerosis, and more. Although natural sunlight is beneficial for these diseases, an additional benefit can be reaped from the use of targeted ultraviolet (UV) sources in the office including broadband UVB (290-320 nm), narrowband UVB (nbUVB; 311-313 nm), UVA (320-400 nm), and UVA1 (340-400 nm). The addition of psoralens to UVA (PUVA) for photochemotherapy is particularly useful for the treatment of localized scleroderma, urticaria pigmentosa, and flares of atopic dermatitis.

The mechanism of action of phototherapy is complex, not fully understood, and varies by type of UV therapy in terms of depth of penetration, side effects, and diseases in which they are most effective. In general, UV radiation exerts its effects via absorption by chromophores, for example, nuclear DNA, which leads to the creation of reactive oxidative species and immunologic effects including alteration of cytokines, decrease of Langerhan's cells in the epidermis, and modulation of T-cell activity.

The feasibility of phototherapy is often limited by the patient's ability to come to the office several times per week for treatment sessions. Treatment duration and risk of recurrence vary by disease. Although phototherapy may be covered by insurance, direct out-of-pocket costs can include an individual's copay per each phototherapy session. Indirect costs may include travel expenses related to the appointment and time off from school or work. Adverse effects including pain, burning, and increased risk of carcinogenesis are important considerations for treatment of the pediatric population. In this chapter, we discuss the use of each targeted UV source in the treatment of pediatric patients followed by a discussion of photodynamic therapy (PDT).

Clinical Pearls

- Although phototherapy is a useful treatment modality for many diseases commonly present in infant- and child-aged populations, it is contraindicated in infants and is often reserved for severe or recalcitrant disease in children.
- In general, PUVA is not recommended in children because of pain and the increased risk of carcinogenesis.
- Although there is no standardized age cutoff for phototherapy, the child must be able to sit still unattended in a hot, sometimes fully enclosed environment for 10 minutes or longer.
- Phototherapy can be targeted toward specific sites such as the hands and feet or include the whole body with or without the face.
- Genitals should be shielded because of the increased risk of genital cutaneous malignancy. Goggles should also be worn because of the theoretical risk of cataracts as well as malignancy (eg, ocular melanoma). The risk of cataracts is higher with PUVA because psoralens bind to proteins within the lens.
- Phototherapy can be effective in patients of all skin colors, but extra caution should be taken in patients with lighter skin types or patches of depigmentation because they are more susceptible to adverse effects (eg, burning) when not appropriately dosed. Postinflammatory hyperpigmentation may worsen in patients with darker skin types.

Contraindications/Cautions/Risks

- Relative contraindications include a history of a photosensitizing disorder and use of a photosensitizing drug (see Box 20.1).
  - *Lupus erythematosus and xeroderma pigmentosum (XP) are considered to be absolute contraindications by many practitioners.*
- Current use of immunosuppressive agents, for example, azathioprine or cyclosporine, should also be a strong consideration because of increased risk of carcinogenesis.
- Adverse effects of phototherapy include erythema, xerosis, pruritus, blistering, and reactivation of herpes simplex virus (HSV). The specific adverse effects of each modality are discussed in their corresponding sections.

BOX 20.1. COMMON ORAL PHOTOSENSITIZING MEDICATIONS

- Antihistamines
- Fluoroquinolones
- Nonsteroidal anti-inflammatory drugs (NSAIDs)
- Oral contraceptives
- Phenothiazines
- Sulfonamides
- Sulfonylureas
- Tetracyclines (especially doxycycline)
- Thiazides
- Tricyclic antidepressants

From Comprehensive FDA-approved list of medications that increase sensitivity to light: a 1990 listing. https://www.fda.gov/media/75892/download.

Equipment Needed

- Light source for phototherapy. These can include whole-body panels or hand/foot units. Fluorescent lamps are most commonly used.
- Eye shields and genital shields
- Oral or topical psoralen for PUVA; only 8-methoxypsoralen (8-MOP) is available in the United States.
- Bathtub for bath PUVA
  - The bathtub should be in the office because irradiation must happen immediately owing to the rapid decrease in effectiveness.

ULTRAVIOLET A1 AND ULTRAVIOLET B PHOTOTHERAPY

Broadband UVB therapy (290-320 nm) has historically been used to treat a wide variety of dermatologic diseases, but nbUVB with a targeted wavelength of 311 to 313 nm was designed for optimal clearance of psoriasis. This range was found to be optimal in a study by Parrish and Jaenecke in 1981, which demonstrated that wavelengths longer than 313 nm did not clear psoriatic plaques, whereas wavelengths shorter than 300 nm were erythrogenic and also did not clear plaques. Owing to its longer wavelength, UVA (320-400 nm) penetrates more deeply into the dermis. UVA1 (340-400 nm) is used more often than is broadband UVA because it exerts effects similar to UVB. However, UVA1 therapy is utilized more heavily in Europe, where it is more accessible. Many practitioners feel that nbUVB is the preferred treatment for multiple conditions including psoriasis, vitiligo, and other inflammatory skin diseases.

Preprocedural Approach: Ultraviolet B Therapy

The starting dose can be determined in one of two ways: phototyping or phototesting. Fitzpatrick phototype assigns individuals a number I through VI based on their ability to tan or burn following exposure to UV radiation. Individuals who always burn and do not tan are assigned a I, whereas individuals who never burn are assigned a VI (Table 20.1). Phototesting is not mandatory, but it may be useful as the Fitzpatrick skin type does not always reliably predict response. To perform phototesting, six 1 cm^2 areas of non–sun-exposed skin (eg, lower back, inner forearm) should be exposed to increasing UV doses. For nbUVB, doses of 200, 400, 600, 800, 1000, and 1200 mJ/cm^2 should be used. For broadband UVB, doses of 20, 40, 60, 80, 100, and 120 mJ/cm^2 should be used. Following phototesting, the minimal erythema dose (MED) is determined as the lowest dose to produce minimal uniform erythema 24 hours after exposure. This 24-hour waiting period is recommended because erythema due to UVB typically peaks 24 hours later. A therapeutic dose is considered to be 50% to 70% of the MED. The goal of treatment is to produce minimally perceptible erythema.

TABLE 20.1. : Fitzpatrick Phototype

FITZPATRICK PHOTOTYPE	SKIN TONE AND REACTION TO SUN EXPOSURE	SKIN TONES
I	Light, ivory skin—always burns/peels, never tans	
II	Light, fair complexion—burns quickly, tans rarely	
III	Beige tint to skin—may burn but capable of tanning	
IV	Olive or light brown skin— rarely burns, tans regularly	
V	Dark brown or black skin tone—rarely burns, always tans	
VI	Black/darkest skin tone—never burns, tans quickly/darkly	

Procedural Approach: Ultraviolet B Therapy

Treatments should occur two to five times per week, with subsequent dose increases after each exposure. The dose increase is needed because phototherapy thickens the stratum corneum over time. For UVA1, UVB, as well as PUVA, numerous treatment protocols have been proposed in the literature on the basis of author experience. There are clear guidelines on the AAD website (www.aad.org) for both atopic dermatitis and psoriasis. The manufacturers of the equipment also typically provide dosing guides for the physician, which account for dose increases depending on phototype and contain protocols for resuming treatments after missed sessions. In general, the rate of increase depends on the level of erythema and treatment frequency. For example, for nbUVB treatments three times per week, the dose should be increased by 30% to 40% if there is no erythema. If there is minimal erythema, the dose should be increased by 10% to 20%. However, if there is persistent erythema, the dose should not be increased. If a patient experiences painful erythema, treatments should be held. For broadband UVB, the dose should be increased by 25% for the first 10 treatments and then 10% per treatment. Treatments may be continued until a patient's skin condition is in remission or no further improvement is obtained. The use of maintenance treatments to keep a condition in remission is debatable, but may be most beneficial for diseases such as CTCL.

Pediatric Applications of Ultraviolet B

UVB therapy is used to treat psoriasis, CTCL, atopic dermatitis, and vitiligo. For psoriasis, nbUVB is considered to be more effective than is broadband UVB because of its targeted wavelength. For CTCL, UVB was found to be more effective than was UVA in some studies, and there are no comparison studies between nbUVB and UVB. Phototherapy is felt to be most effective for the patch stage of the disease. For atopic dermatitis, broadband UVB has been used for decades, but UVA in combination with UVB appears to be superior; nbUVB may also be effective. For vitiligo, current studies suggest that nbUVB is as effective as is PUVA with fewer side effects. Intense erythema should be avoided because this may initiate the Koebner effect. More care should be taken with dose increases because of the vulnerability of affected (ie, depigmented) skin. Similar to other treatment protocols, treatment two to three times per week is recommended with a dose increase of 10% to 20% per session.

UVA has been found to be most effective when used in combination with UVB for atopic dermatitis. Other conditions that benefit from UVA1 include urticaria pigmentosa. In addition, UVA1 activates matrix metalloproteinase-3, which leads to collagen breakdown that benefits sclerotic diseases.

Adverse Events of Ultraviolet B

Burns typically appear most evident 12 to 24 hours after UVB treatment, but may present later following UVA1 with peak erythema 72 to 96 hours after exposure. nbUVB is less erythrogenic than is broadband UVB; up to 10× higher doses of nbUVB are required for erythema, edema, and sunburn. When burns occur on limited areas, treatments may be continued with shielding of burned areas (physically or with sunscreen). However, it is important to keep in mind that the dose may need to be lowered when resuming treatments following a burn.

UVB is overall less carcinogenic than is UVA. Patients should not have more than 10 to 15 treatments with UVA per year because it has been shown to cause DNA damage and increase risk of carcinogenesis. For nbUVB, there are several studies that did not find increased carcinogenicity unless more than 300 treatments were performed. nbUVB is newer and long-term effects are less well studied; however, it may be less carcinogenic because fewer treatments are typically required.

PSORALEN ULTRAVIOLET A

PUVA consists of UVA in combination with psoralens, which are naturally occurring furocoumarins found in plants. Psoralens can be administered orally or topically (solutions, creams, baths) (Box 20.2). Available psoralens include 8-MOP, 5-MOP, and 4,5,8-trimethylpsoralen (TMP). Only 8-MOP is available in the United States. Psoralens become activated by wavelengths between 320 and 340 nm.

BOX 20.2. TOPICAL PHOTOTOXIC PLANTS

- Angelica
- Carrot
- Celery
- Cow parsley
- Dill
- Fennel
- Fig
- Gas plant
- Giant hogweed
- Lemon
- Lime
- Meadow grass
- Parsnip
- Stinking mayweed
- Yarrow

Psoralens exert their effects through DNA damage. They react with DNA as follows:

1. Psoralens intercalate into the DNA double strand.
2. Following absorption of the first photon, they form cyclobutane addition products with pyrimidine bases.
3. Following absorption of the second photon, they cross-link the double helix with a bond between pyrimidine bases in each strand.

PUVA results in a decrease in cell division and DNA synthesis, which leads to a reduction in keratinocyte proliferation and also stimulates melanogenesis. Similar to other phototherapy modalities, cytokines are altered, antigen-presenting cells are decreased, and there is a direct phototoxic effect on lymphocytes. The reaction between excited psoralens and oxygen forms reactive oxidative species, which impact other cellular components such as proteins and RNA.

Preprocedural Approach: Psoralen Ultraviolet A

In the United States, we most frequently base the dose of PUVA on phototype, whereas Europeans tend to use the minimal phototoxicity dose (MPD), which is analogous to the MED. Determination of the MPD uses the same process as does MED with ingestion of psoralen followed by increasing doses of UVA. For skin types I and II, 0.5, 1, 2, 3, 4, 5 J/cm² of UVA should be used. For types III and IV and darker, 1, 2, 4, 6, 8, and 10 J/cm² of UVA is recommended. Patches must be read 72 hours after exposure when peak erythema occurs.

Procedural Approach: Psoralen Ultraviolet A

For oral PUVA, 0.6 mg/kg of micronized 8-MOP is given 120 minutes before UVA exposure. Liquid formulations are absorbed faster than are micronized forms and have a more reliable serum level, so the dissolved form is given as 0.4 to 0.6 mg/kg 90 minutes before exposure. The maximum dose of 8-MOP is 70 mg for patients weighing greater than 115 kg. Of note, it has been proposed that body surface area should be used instead (25 mg/m²) because it may provide more reliable serum concentrations. Fatty foods may slow absorption and decrease serum levels. Treatments should occur two to four times per week, but not on consecutive days, and should start at 50% to 70% of the MPD. If dosing by phototype, the starting dose should be 0.5, 1, 1.5, 2, 2.5, and 3 J/cm² for phototypes I to VI, respectively. The rate of UVA dose increase based on phototype is 0.5, 0.5, 1, 1, 1.5, and 1.5 J/cm² for phototypes I to VI, respectively. Of note, oral PUVA should not be used in patients with hepatic or renal disease because it may impair metabolism or excretion of the drug, respectively.

PUVA can also be administered as a bath treatment with the advantage of even distribution of the drug over the entire body. It is highly reproducible and has very low serum levels. A patient should spend 15 to 20 minutes of whole-body immersion in solutions of 1 mg 8-MOP per liter of body temperature bath water. Irradiation must occur immediately because photosensitivity decreases rapidly. Treatments should occur twice weekly for bath PUVA and start at 30% of the MPD. Doses of UVA can be increased by 20% per week.

Topical PUVA formulations such as creams, ointments, and lotions are also available (eg, 1% methoxsalen lotion); however, it can be more difficult to achieve uniform distribution and application is time consuming. Plasma levels are similar to those with oral treatment. Irradiation should be performed 30 minutes after application.

Pediatric Application of Psoralens to Ultraviolet A

Pediatric dermatologists tend to use topical psoralens when performing PUVA. However, PUVA is rarely used because the risks of carcinogenesis and burns usually outweigh the benefit of treatment.

PUVA with 8-MOP is approved by the U.S. Food and Drug Administration (FDA) for the treatment of psoriasis and vitiligo. Topical PUVA with creams, ointments, or lotions may be particularly effective for palmoplantar psoriasis or plaque psoriasis with few, limited areas that are recalcitrant to other treatments. The majority of patients with psoriasis (between 70% and 100%) see significant improvement within 24 treatments, whereas vitiligo typically requires between 150 and 300 treatments. Vitiligo can be treated with topical psoralens for localized disease or systemic psoralens for more diffuse involvement. PUVA can also be used for treatment of lymphoproliferative disorders, such as CTCL, with the same dosimetry as psoriasis treatment. Maintenance treatment has been proposed for these patients. Because CTCL varies by patient, individualized treatment courses are recommended.

Adverse Events of Psoralens to Ultraviolet A

Pruritus following PUVA treatment is common and may be found in up to 10% of patients. Rare effects include polymorphous light-like eruptions, subungual hemorrhages, and onycholysis. Similar to UVA1, burns appear later with peak erythema 72 to 96 hours after exposure. The erythema can persist for up to 1 week and is deeper red or violaceous. When overdosed, PUVA causes a delayed phototoxic response with edema, pruritus, and stinging. PUVA burns may extend deeper in the dermis and may even necessitate burn unit admission when severe.

Oral 8-MOP is often associated with nausea and vomiting, which can be limiting. This side effect is more common with liquid preparations than with micronized forms because of higher serum levels. Taking the medication with food or splitting the dose may improve these symptoms, although food may decrease its effectiveness.

Long-term effects, for example, photoaging and carcinogenesis, should also be considered because PUVA has been shown to cause lentigines, photoaging, and carcinogenesis. The risk of non–melanoma skin cancer (NMSC) and, somewhat debatably, melanoma skin cancer increases in a dose-dependent manner. In particular, the development of cutaneous malignancies of the genitals is significantly increased, which led to the utilization of genital shields during phototherapy. Currently, there is no standard effective genital shield in use. Cataracts are also a consideration because psoralens bind to proteins in the lens when exposed to UVA. This risk may be diminished by the use of UVA-protective glasses during treatment.

Photodynamic Therapy

INTRODUCTION

Photodynamic Therapy (PDT) is FDA approved for the treatment of actinic keratoses and superficial NMSC. PDT may also be used off-label for the treatment of a variety of other conditions including cutaneous infections, acne, psoriasis, photoaging, and vascular lesions.

Similar to PUVA photochemotherapy, PDT consists of a photosensitizing drug in combination with light. The photosensitizing drug can be applied topically, orally, or intravenously (Boxes 20.1 and 20.2). In contrast to PUVA, different chemicals and wavelengths of light (eg, red and blue) are utilized to target alternate chemical pathways. In particular, photosensitizers for PDT are prodrugs of aminolevulinic acid (ALA), specifically 5-aminolevulinic acid (5-ALA) and methyl aminolevulinate (mALA). Only ALA is commercially available in the United States. These prodrugs are converted to protoporphyrin IX (PpIX) within the skin. All of these chemicals are part of the innate heme biosynthesis pathway. With application of an exogenous photosensitizer, regulatory steps are bypassed and there is an accumulation of toxic protoporphyrin by-products. PpIX preferentially accumulates within the sebaceous glands and epidermis.

PDT requires a photochemical reaction with generation of singlet oxygen (Figure 20.1). Light activates the photosensitizer to a higher energy state, and it can then transfer this energy to oxygen molecules, creating singlet oxygen. Singlet oxygen reacts with lipids, nucleic acids, and proteins to create oxidative damage with subsequent cellular damage and apoptosis. Of note, singlet oxygen and other reactive oxidative species can also interact with the photosensitizer, creating the phenomenon of "photobleaching," which helps terminate the reaction loop. The photosensitizer successfully targets the desired tissue because it is more highly absorbed in tissues with higher metabolism, increased vascularity, and lymphatic hyperpermeability. Particular lesions, such as actinic keratoses, NMSC, and psoriasis have increased permeability of ALA-like prodrugs.

Equipment Needed

- Acetone scrub to apply preprocedure
- PDT light source (blue or red light)
- Photosensitizer with applicator (eg, tongue depressor)
- PDT goggles for eye protection
- Fan ± cool mist spray during light application
- Ice packs or cold compresses

ADVERSE EFFECTS OF PHOTODYNAMIC THERAPY

Intraprocedure pain is a strong consideration for pediatric patients. Patients describe the sensation of pain, stabbing, burning, or stinging during the treatment. Decreasing the irradiance can make the pain more tolerable. It may be beneficial to provide preprocedure analgesia or sedation. Combining PDT with other procedures requiring anesthesia can limit the patient's exposure to general anesthesia. Application of ice cubes on or near treatment sites during the treatment is also beneficial.

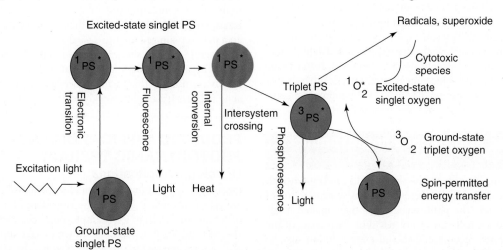

FIGURE 20.1. Graphical illustration of the photophysical and photochemical mechanisms of photodynamic therapy. Reprinted from Castano AP, Demidova TN, Hamblin MR. Mechanisms in photodynamic therapy: part one-photosensitizers, photochemistry and cellular localization. *Photodiagnosis Photodyn Ther.* 2004;1(4):279-293. Copyright © 2005 Elsevier. With permission.

Spraying cold water, using a fan, or interrupting light exposure may prove helpful.

Photosensitization is a common side effect, and it is generally worse with systemic photosensitizers than with locally applied topical photosensitizers. This is characterized by edema, blistering, pain, burning, and stinging. Photosensitizing medications may make patients more sensitive to PDT; these include thiazides, tetracyclines, sulfonamides, methotrexate, fluconazole, griseofulvin, quinolones, chlorpromazine, azathioprine, and many more (see most common in Boxes 20.1-20.4). Sunscreens have little utility because the action spectrum extends beyond those of sunscreens, even physical blockers. Indoor light exposure can take advantage of the process of "photobleaching" to decrease the duration of photosensitivity. Postprocedure inflammation, scarring, and postinflammatory pigment changes may also occur.

BOX 20.3. TOPICAL PHOTOALLERGENIC COMPOUNDS

- Antiseptics (chlorhexidine, hexachlorophene)
- Fragrances (methylcoumarin, musk ambrette)
- Phenothiazines
- Salicylanilides
- Sulfonamides
- Sunscreens (benzophenones, cinnamates, dibenzoyl-methanes, para-aminobenzoic acid, para-aminobenzoic acid esters)

BOX 20.4. TOPICAL PHOTOTOXINS

- Psoralens (methoxypsoralen, trimethylpsoralen)
- Tars (creosote, pitch)
- Dyes (eosin, methylene blue)
- Medications (phenothiazines, sulfonamides)

Preprocedural Approach: Photodynamic Therapy

Preprocedure analgesia should be provided (eg, acetaminophen). Stronger pain medications should be considered for aggressive treatments. If there is a history of HSV infection, it is recommended that the patient begins an oral antiviral either the day before or on the day of treatment for 3 to 5 days.

When selecting the light source, there are a number of sources that can be utilized to achieve the desired effect. Red light (longer wavelength) produces a deeper dermal effect with better tissue penetration compared to blue light (shorter wavelength) with increased porphyrin absorption. Currently, FDA approval encompasses red light with mALA and blue light with ALA.

Procedure Approach: Photodynamic Therapy

On the day of the procedure, the skin should be cleansed with a gentle cleanser followed by acetone to increase penetration of the photosensitizer. The photosensitizer is then applied to affected skin and a small rim of normal skin. Two coats of the photosensitizer are recommended, and extra solution may be used to "spot treat" thicker areas as needed. It is important to get close to the eyes because the orbital skin will not be adequately treated otherwise. However, care should be taken to avoid the eyelids, cornea, and ocular canthi.

The standard incubation time is 1 to 3 hours. During incubation, the patient should be kept away from sunlight and direct or reflected light sources. Avoidance of light is crucial to prevent premature activation of the photosensitizer and phototoxic reactions. The face should be washed again following incubation to decrease the risk of pain and superficial skin burning if excess photosensitizer remains on the skin.

The exposure time can be calculated by dividing the fluence (J/cm^2) by the irradiance (W/cm^2). Dose can be determined by the fluence of light as well as by the amount of photosensitizer. Topical photosensitizers are limited by the maximum amount that can be absorbed transepidermally. Dose can also be affected by the amount of time between application of the photosensitizer and PDT; a longer incubation time leads to higher prodrug concentration.

For treatment of thin actinic keratoses and superficial lesions, the standard fluence of blue light ranges between 10 and 48 J/cm^2. For treatment of acne, thicker actinic keratoses, and deeper lesions, the standard fluence of red light ranges between 34 and 96 J/cm^2. Manufacturers of photosensitizers often recommend lower fluences (15 J/cm^2 for blue light and 34 J/cm^2 for red light), but many experts recommend higher fluences. During treatment, patients may experience minimal erythema and edema, which will respond very rapidly to cold compresses or ice packs.

Postprocedural Approach: Photodynamic Therapy

Following treatment, patients may apply ice packs to any uncomfortable areas to improve pain and swelling. Swelling is most notable around the eyes. Patients may take anti-inflammatories, for example, ibuprofen, if necessary. In general, topical products other than bland emollients are not recommended, but mild topical steroids may be used if needed. Longer downtime is expected with longer incubation periods.

Patients should limit outdoor exposure for the first 48 hours following treatment. They should avoid direct sunlight for 1 week following treatment and wear a sunscreen with SPF 30 or greater. Even reflected light, for example, light coming through a car window, can induce phototoxicity. Scarves and hats may be useful during this period. Patients' skin may feel tight and dry. A nonscented, gentle moisturizer should be applied on the day of treatment and daily throughout the rest of the week. The treated area may remain red for 1 to 2 weeks.

Several treatments may be needed to reach goals of treatment for each patient. For photorejuvenation and associated actinic keratoses, monthly treatments, as needed, are recommended. For acne vulgaris treatments, weekly or biweekly treatments may be used. The treatment plan must be individualized for each patient.

PEDIATRIC APPLICATIONS OF PHOTODYNAMIC THERAPY
Oncologic Applications

Oncologic applications are limited in pediatric patients. There are rare cases when PDT can be considered for the treatment of NMSC in children, for example, basal cell nevoid syndrome (BCNS) and XP. PDT has been shown to have superior cosmetic outcomes compared to surgery or cryotherapy. Red or blue light can be used to treat actinic keratoses, but red light is typically chosen to treat NMSC. For children with XP and BCNS, PDT is typically performed in the operating room (OR) for pain control

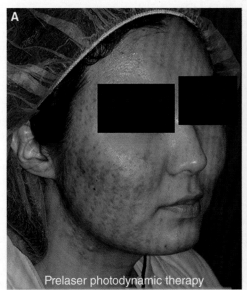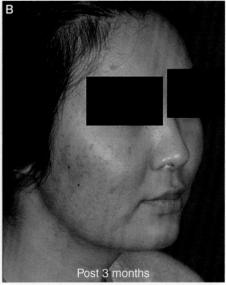

FIGURE 20.2. Combination treatment for acne scar treatment. A 22-year-old skin type IV patient with active acne and numerous erythematous and atrophic acne scars. A, Baseline. B, 3 months' status post combination photodynamic therapy utilizing red and blue light sources, and use of spironolactone and topical benzoyl peroxide. Reprinted from Krakowski AC, Shumaker PR. *The Scar Book*. Philadelphia, PA: Wolters Kluwer; 2017. Figure 17.15. Courtesy of Sabrina Guillen Fabi, MD.

and is combined with other physical and topical therapies (ie, curettage, topical chemotherapy, excisions) to limit anesthesia exposure. When red or blue light is not available, the light in the OR can be used to activate the porphyrins, although it is not as effective or able to be controlled as accurately.

Mycosis fungoides, which is a rare diagnosis in pediatric patients, can also be managed with PDT because ALA has been found to accumulate within activated T cells.

Nononcologic Applications

Because PpIX accumulates within the pilosebaceous unit, acne is another condition in which PDT has utility in treatment (Figure 20.2). However, PDT is not commonly used because of significant downtime and pain associated with each treatment. Of note, exposure to blue light alone without a photosensitizing agent has been shown to improve inflammatory acne. This improvement is due to the fact that *Propionibacterium acnes* produces endogenous porphyrins. Similarly, singlet oxygen's antibacterial effects can help treat cutaneous infections, for example, condyloma, verruca vulgaris, and leishmaniasis.

Psoriasis is another condition that responds to PDT; however, there is a high accumulation of PpIX in treated plaques and

pain is often limiting, particularly for pediatric patients. Pain along with the widespread nature of psoriasis make nbUVB a superior therapy compared to PDT.

SUGGESTED READINGS

Bolognia J, Jorizzo JL, Schaffer JV. *Dermatology*. Philadelphia, PA: Elsevier Saunders; 2012.

Goldsmith LA, Katz SI, Wolff K. *Fitzpatrick's Dermatology in General Medicine*. 8th ed. New York, NY: McGraw-Hill; 2012.

Krutmann J, Honigsmann H, Elmets C, eds. *Dermatological Phototherapy and Photodiagnostic Methods*. 2nd ed. Berlin, Germany: Springer; 2009.

Menter A, Korman NJ, Elmets CA, et al. Guidelines of care for the management of psoriasis and psoriatic arthritis. Section 5: Guidelines of care for the treatment of psoriasis with phototherapy and photochemotherapy. *J Am Acad Dermatol*. 2010;62(1):114–135.

Parrish JA, Jaenicke KE. Action spectrum for phototherapy of psoriasis. *J Invest Dematol*. 1981;76:359–362.

Sidbury R, Davis DM, Cohen DE, et al. Guidelines of care for the management of atopic dermatitis. Section 3: Management and treatment with phototherapy and systemic agents. *J Am Acad Dermatol*. 2014;71(2):327–349.

CHAPTER 21

Chemical Peels

Angel J. Su, Alexander Choi, and John C. Browning

INTRODUCTION

Chemical peels are a widely used noninvasive tool in the enhancement of facial rejuvenation and aesthetics. Chemical peels can treat a wide variety of dermatologic lesions and can be utilized in multiple different ways. They are designed to cause well-controlled damage at a designated depth, promote facial resurfacing of the skin through exfoliative properties, and stimulate the regeneration of the underlying epidermis, providing smoother skin. Common indications for using chemical peels in pediatrics include hyperpigmentation (ie, melasma), acne vulgaris and subsequent scarring, lentigines, photodamage, or dyschromias.

PREPROCEDURE PREPARATION

Patient Assessment

A general treatment sequence begins with assessing the patient's dermatologic condition and expected clinical outcome. Significant criteria for determining the type of peel used include the patient's ethnicity, skin type, depth of lesion, oiliness, and thickness. Asian descent and inflammatory skin conditions are traits that would call for use of a more superficial peel or decreased concentrations of chemicals because of the increased proclivity for dyspigmentation.

Relative contraindications to chemical peel therapy include recent peel therapy in the past week, shaving in the past 24 hours, and open sores/lesions on the area of treatment. For patients with a history of herpes simplex virus, prophylaxis with either acyclovir or valacyclovir is recommended. The antiviral is typically taken starting 1 to 2 days before the chemical peel. The specific dosages range by patient's immune status, age, medication, and physician preference. The antiviral is typically continued up to 1 week following superficial and medium-depth peels, whereas deep peels require 2 weeks. In the past, the use of oral isotretinoin was a contraindication to chemical treatments and required a period of 1 to 2 years after completing therapy to safely receive a peel. Recent updates have cited that chemical peels are safe starting 3 months after completion oral isotretinoin therapy.

Priming

After the patient assessment, the next step is priming. Priming is an important step in preparing the skin for chemically induced damage and has resulted in enhanced peel effects; decreased side effects, particularly postinflammatory hyperpigmentation (PIH); and uniform penetration of the chemical to the cutaneous layers. Priming techniques vary but predominantly involve depigmentation via topical pretreatment therapy such as tretinoin, hydroxychloroquine, or glycolic acid. The priming period can range between 2 weeks and 1 month or more before treatment. This technique is becoming more widely used in chemical peel therapy.

Immediate Patient Preparation and Anesthesia

Immediately before the procedure, prepare the face using facial cleansing agents to rid of debris, oils, and fats to facilitate peel-to-skin contact. Cleansing agents can be alcohol, acetone, a combination of the two, or chlorhexidine gluconate.

Depending on the type of peel, appropriate anesthetic agents can be utilized to lessen the patient's pain and facilitate the procedure. A superficial peel generally does not require an anesthetic agent. Topical anesthetic agents such as a combination of benzocaine, lidocaine, and tetracaine can be used for medium-depth chemical peels. The medium-depth and deep peels are painful and may require oral anesthetic medication such as Demerol or morphine.

The final step in preprocedure preparation is to prepare the desired chemicals at appropriate concentrations for the specific type of peel discussed later.

TYPES OF CHEMICAL PEELS AND CHOOSING THE APPROPRIATE TREATMENT

There are three major types of chemical peels: superficial, medium-depth, and deep peels. Superficial peels affect only the epidermis, whereas medium-depth peels affect the epidermis as well as the papillary dermis. Deep peels are able to penetrate down to the mid-reticular dermis. In addition, each category has a variety of chemicals and concentrations to utilize for the desired effect. The combination of peel type, chemical used, concentration of chemical, and duration of peel-to-skin contact are important measures to ensure optimal results with minimal adverse effects.

The side effect profile of chemical peels is dependent on the depth classification of the chemical peel. Furthermore, the adverse effects can vary depending on the training and expertise of the physician performing the peel. It is important to receive adequate education on peels as well as complete a thorough assessment of the patient's skin type and desired outcome before choosing the proper treatment.

The type of peel to be used depends on the desired clinical outcome. In general, the amount of skin damage increases with the type and concentration of the peel; however, the drawback to "deeper" peels is increased healing time and more possible side effects.

Superficial Chemical Peels

Superficial chemical peels are especially useful for mild skin discoloration and mild acne scarring. For mild scars that do not distort the surface of the skin, acne, photoaging, and mild pigmentation such as melasma, multiple rounds of superficial chemical peels may be considered as first-line treatment. Superficial chemical peels include the α-hydroxy acids (AHA), β-hydroxy acids (BHA), and Jessner's solution. The most common AHA used is glycolic acid and the most common BHA used is salicylic acid (SA). Jessner's solution is a mixture of 14% SA, 14% lactic acid, and 14% resorcinol suspended in ethanol designed to minimize the toxicity of each individual acid while maintaining potency. The treatment process takes a minimum of 6 months and requires multiple rounds of treatment, but the side effects are minimal and recovery is swift.

Glycolic Acid Peel

Glycolic acid peels are associated with minimal pain and side effects. During the procedure, patients feel a slight burning or itching sensation that resolves soon after the procedure is finished. Occasionally, these symptoms may persist, lasting up to 2 to 5 days after the procedure. Treatment to alleviate these symptoms includes application of ice, topical calamine lotion, and emollients. Topical analgesics are typically not used for superficial peels because they increase the absorption of the acid and cause a deeper peel than desired.

Before starting the procedure, the patient's skin is cleansed and defatted with acetone-soaked gauze. The glycolic acid peel of desired strength (usually between 30% and 70%) is applied in a thin layer onto the patient's skin, carefully avoiding the eyes and lips. The peel is applied quickly to the face to avoid uneven exposure. Application of the peel in skin areas with thin stratum corneum such as around the nose and lips is performed last. A neutralizing agent with alkaline properties such as sodium bicarbonate is applied over the acid peel when the patient's skin is noted to be uniformly erythematous. All AHAs need to be neutralized to stop epidermolysis. The endpoint of the glycolic acid peel is around 3 minutes, but this is subject to the discretion of the operator. The entire solution is then rinsed off the face with tap water. A gentle moisturizer, such as a neutral lotion, is applied to the treated area and sunscreen is applied over the moisturizer.

Salicylic Acid Peel

The SA peel is another superficial peel that has minimal associated pain during the procedure. As with the glycolic acid peel, the patient may experience some burning or itching during the peel. The desired area of skin is cleansed and defatted (ie, degreased) with acetone-soaked gauze before application. The SA peel is applied with either gauze or a cotton-tipped applicator. The applicator is dipped into the solution and excess solution is wiped away to avoid dripping the solution on an unwanted area. The solution is evenly spread across the skin, avoiding sensitive areas such as the eyes and lips. Unlike the glycolic acid peel, the SA peel self-neutralizes by precipitating into a frost, indicating the endpoint, which takes around 3 to 5 minutes. Neutralization of the acid is not necessary, but it can be rinsed off of the patient's skin using water. A gentle moisturizer and sunscreen is applied to the patient's face afterwards.

Trichloroacetic Acid Superficial Peel

When utilizing trichloroacetic acid (TCA) peels, the level of penetration is dependent on the concentration of TCA in the chemical peel solution. Concentrations of 10% to 25% TCA are used for superficial peels. Two weeks prior, pretreatment to the area using 0.05% tretinoin cream helps accelerate healing and cell turnover. Preparation of the treated area can be done using degreasers and "depth-enhancing agents" such as alcohol and Jessner's solution, respectively. The TCA is applied in an even manner, with either gauze or a cotton-tipped applicator. The endpoint of the superficial TCA peel is a speckled white frost. TCA does not need to be neutralized because it neutralizes itself by binding with proteins within the skin. After 3 to 5 minutes, the patient may use cool water splashes to rinse the treated area.

Postpeel care begins immediately, with instructions to avoid picking, peeling, or scratching the treated skin. For superficial peels, patients should avoid direct sunlight for at least 1 week.

Sunscreen and hypoallergenic lotions can be applied 4 hours after the procedure for sun protection and moisture control.

Medium-Depth Chemical Peels

Medium-depth chemical peel is used for moderate scarring with slight textural changes in skin such as rolling acne scars, small ice pick scars, and small boxcar scars. In contrast to superficial peels, medium-depth peels can be quite painful for the patient. An oral sedative such as a benzodiazepine with an analgesic may be used to decrease the discomfort. The most common medium-strength peel is the 35% to 50% TCA. The TCA peel is used with or without Jessner's solution. Jessner's solution acts as a primer to the TCA treatment by removing the stratum corneum and allowing the solution to achieve a deeper peel.

Patients undergoing TCA peel treatment are placed on prophylactic oral antibiotics and antivirals 2 days before the procedure and continuing until the fifth day after the procedure. Before the start of the procedure, the patient's skin is cleansed and defatted using acetone-soaked gauze. Jessner's solution can be applied before the TCA peel at this time, if desired. A cotton-tipped applicator is used to dip into the TCA solution and the excess acid is removed by pressing against the side of the container to avoid spilling droplets on the skin. The solution is applied to the skin until the skin achieves a generalized, even white frosting over a layer of erythema. This signifies appropriate penetration of the acid (Figure 21.1). Although the frosting process continues, a cool compress can be applied to the skin to decrease discomfort. The frosting will dissipate without further intervention and does not need to be neutralized. When the frosting is no longer visible, an ointment containing 1% hydrocortisone or a nonmedicated emollient, such as Aquaphor® (Beiersdorf AG, US), can be applied to the skin to keep it moist.

Once reepithelialization has occurred, the patient can resume a normal skin care routine of moisturizing cream or lotion. The patient may experience swelling of the skin and can be prescribed oral prednisone at 40 mg for 2 days and 20 mg for 3 days to decrease edema (Figure 21.2). Patients receiving medium-depth to deep peels should avoid direct sun

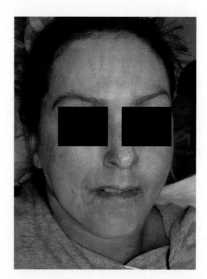

FIGURE 21.1. Patient after two coats of 30% trichloroacetic acid with a dense white frost representing keratocoagulation. Reprinted from Krakowski AC, Shumaker PR. *The Scar Book.* Philadelphia, PA: Wolters Kluwer; 2017. Figure 17.4. Courtesy of Joseph Niamtu, III Cosmetic Facial Surgery Richmond VA.

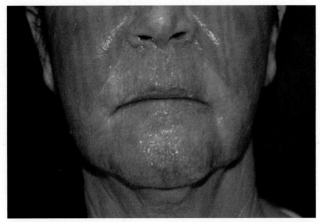

FIGURE 21.2. Erythematous neoepithelialization has replaced the sloughed chemoexfoliated skin in this adult patient who underwent a Hetter (phenol-Croton oil) chemical peel. Reprinted with permission from Johnson J. *Bailey's Head and Neck Surgery.* 5th ed. Philadelphia, PA: Wolters Kluwer Health/Lippincott Williams & Wilkins; 2013. Figure 193.2.

exposure for 3 weeks and continue to limit sun exposure for at least 6 months to lessen the chance of hyperpigmentation and sunburn.

Deep Chemical Peel

For multiple deep scars with abundant textural changes or congenital nevi, a much more potent deep chemical peel is necessary. The most common deep chemical used is the Gordon-Baker phenol peel, which is composed of 88% phenol, 2 mL of distilled water, eight drops of Septisol, and three drops of Croton oil. Septisol and Croton oil are added into the solution to aid in the penetration of the oil into skin.

Anesthesia and Patient Monitoring for Deep Chemical Peels

For phenol peels, the patient is given intravenous (IV) sedation because of the pain and discomfort experienced. In addition to IV sedation, local anesthesia such as lidocaine may also be necessary. *Patients with hepatorenal or cardiac disease require preoperative clearance.* Phenol is metabolized in the liver and excreted through the kidneys and can be toxic in patients with hepatorenal disease, and patients typically require IV hydration before and during the procedure. Phenol has been known to cause arrhythmias and the patient needs continuous cardiac monitoring during the procedure and for 2 hours postoperatively. Intraoperative steroids are typically given to minimize skin edema.

Deep Chemical Peel Procedure Approach

To begin, the patient's face is washed and defatted with acetone-soaked gauze over the desired area. The patient's head is placed at a 35° angle until the end of the procedure to decrease facial swelling and to prevent the acid from dripping down into the neck area. The desired preparation of phenol acid is created and thoroughly mixed. Using a cotton-tipped applicator, the skin is treated in small patches. The application of phenol should change the skin to a frosty white color to indicate proper peeling. Approximately 30 minutes should elapse before moving onto a different patch of skin to prevent phenol accumulation and subsequent toxicity. After the application is complete and the frosting disappears, an occlusive wet dressing can be used to cover the treated areas.

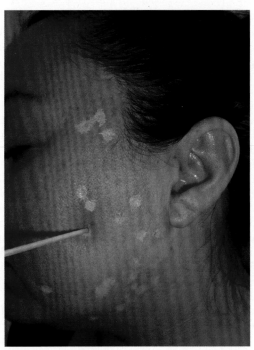

FIGURE 21.3. The CROSS technique or "dot peeling," being applied to acne scars. Reprinted from Krakowski AC, Shumaker PR. *The Scar Book.* Philadelphia, PA: Wolters Kluwer; 2017. Figure 17.6. Courtesy of Joanna G. Bolton, MD.

CROSS Technique or Dot Peeling

The CROSS technique, or "dot peeling," may be applied as a very effective solo or adjunctive treatment for ice pick and small boxcar acne scars, as well as in the treatment of atrophic postvaricella (chickenpox) scarring (Figure 21.3). Up to about 25% improvement in atrophic scars may be noted with one CROSS session, with up to 70% or more after three to six treatments at intervals of 2 to 4 weeks. The major advantage of the CROSS technique is that adjacent normal tissue and adnexal structures are spared, promoting more rapid healing with less complications. The technique entails stretching the skin and using a fine wooden toothpick or needle to apply a high-strength TCA (65%-100%) directly to the bottom of the atrophic scar, which leads to destruction of the epithelial tract. TCA is applied for a few seconds until the scar displays the characteristic white frosting. Neocollagenesis ensues in the subsequent healing phase (2-6 weeks), helping to gradually fill in the depressed scar sites. Transient mild to moderate burning pain is typical with application; however, local anesthesia or sedation is not necessary, making this an effective in-office procedure.

Postprocedural Management of Deep Chemical Peel

After an hour, an emollient is applied to the treated area to keep it moist, and this should be reapplied every 3 to 4 hours. After a week, the ointment can be switched to a less occlusive, gentle cream. Once reepithelialization of the treated area has occurred, the patient can, according to personal preference, start applying lotion to the face instead of cream. Because of the depth of the peel, postprocedural erythema can last several weeks to months and requires careful sun protection and attentive skin care. Patients receiving medium-depth to deep peels should avoid direct sun exposure for 3 weeks and continue to limit sun exposure (ie, practice excellent sun protection and sun avoidance) for at least 6 months to lessen the chance of hyperpigmentation and sunburn.

POSTPROCEDURE CARE

Posttreatment care incorporates standard facial cosmetic care. Moisturizers and sunscreen are imperative to providing proper skin hydration and photoprotection. Specific posttreatment care varies depending on the type of peel, but the following are general patient instructions:

Patient Instructions for Care After Chemical Peels
- Refrain from peeling or picking at the skin because this may cause scarring and infection.
- Avoid direct sun exposure for at least 1 week for superficial peel and for medium-depth and deep peels for 3 weeks and limited sun exposure for 6 months.
- Physical sun blockers such as hats, umbrellas, and clothing and avoidance of direct sun are preferred over chemical sunscreen to help prevent hyperpigmentation.
- Sunscreen of SPF 30 or greater must be used for at least 1 month after the procedure.
- Sweating can cause skin irritation, so avoid any strenuous exercise that causes sweating for several weeks after the procedure.
- Discontinue over-the-counter or prescription moisturizers containing retinoids or AHAs until the skin has completely regenerated.
- Moisturizing the skin is very important. Follow dermatologist's instructions about when and what type of moisturizer/emollient to use.
- For deep peels, further care also includes debridement soaks of a dilute vinegar solution to remove necrotic epidermal tissue and to prevent extensive crusting and application of mupirocin ointment for moisture retention and prevention of bacterial infections.
- Superficial chemical peels can be repeated as often as every 2 weeks, and medium-depth peels can be repeated every several months. Deep peels are generally not repeated but can be repeated after a year has elapsed.

COMPLICATIONS

Possible complications of chemical peels are missed areas, postinflammatory pigmentation as discussed earlier, skin infection, acneiform eruption, keloids, hypertrophic scars, and atrophic scars (Figure 21.4). Postinflammatory pigmentation is mitigated by priming and careful adjustment of the chemical peel concentration.

The anatomic variations and topographic features of the skin of the face create *facial cosmetic units* (see Figure 9.5A). Chemical peels and resurfacing techniques generally respect these zones as demarcation lines, because the edges of the treatment areas can be effectively disguised by the boundary between cosmetic units. Special care should be taken when applied to the eyelid skin, which has an extremely thin epidermis and dermis, and to the skin of the mandibular border and neck, which is both thin and sparsely populated by appendages. Both areas are at greater risk of scarring.

Skin infections usually occur after a deep peel, and infection is treated with the appropriate oral and topical medication.

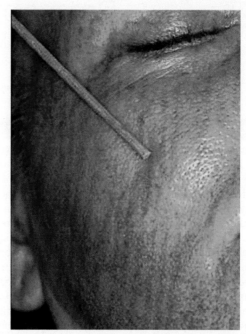

FIGURE 21.4. This demonstrates the clear line of hyperemia that occurs at the periphery of a peeled area. This hyperemic skin has not been peeled. Care must be taken to peel this area so as to not leave a discrete line of unpeeled skin. Reprinted with permission from Johnson J. *Bailey's Head and Neck Surgery*. 5th ed. Philadelphia, PA: Wolters Kluwer Health/Lippincott Williams & Wilkins; 2013. Figure 193.1.

Commonly seen skin infections are caused by gram-positive bacteria (ie, *Staphylococcus* and group A *Streptococcus*), *Pseudomonas*, *Escherichia coli*, herpes, and *Candida*. The signs of skin infection include fever, pain, redness or excessive warmth of the skin, discharge, and skin crusting. Acneiform eruptions often occur immediately after the chemical peel and are best managed with an oral antibiotic as in acne vulgaris. Hypertrophic and keloid scars are treated with either injected or topical corticosteroids.

Most side effects of chemical peels arise as a consequence of poor postprocedural care, so it is important for the patient to thoroughly understand instructions to refrain from picking at flaking skin and hypervigilance about sun protection. Sunscreen can be applied immediately after the procedure if the patient will be exposed to sunlight. For superficial peels, patients should avoid direct sunlight for at least 1 week and for medium-depth to deep peels direct sun exposure avoided for 3 weeks and limited sun exposure for at least 6 months to lessen the chance of hyperpigmentation and sunburn. Other severe possible side effects include renal failure, toxic shock syndrome, and laryngeal edema. Any other issues during recovery should be brought up during follow-up appointments with the physician.

SUGGESTED READINGS

Clark E, Scerri L. Superficial and medium-depth chemical peels. *Clin Dermatol.* 2008;26:209–218.

Landau M. Chemical peels. *Clin Dermatol.* 2008;26:200–208.

Rendon MI, Berson DS, Cohen JL, et al. Evidence and considerations in the application of chemical peels in skin disorders and aesthetic resurfacing. *J Clin Aesthet Dermatol.* 2010;3(7):32–43.

Tung RC, Rubin MG. *Procedures in Cosmetic Dermatology Series: Chemical Peels*. 2nd ed. Philadelphia, PA: Saunders; 2011.

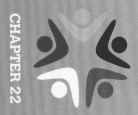

CHAPTER 22

Dermabrasion

Michael C. Raisch and Bradley G. Merritt

Introduction

Manual dermabrasion with sandpaper is an inexpensive, safe, and highly effective technique that is best used to improve contour deformities of the epidermis and/or superficial dermis. Dermabrasion is most often done for improvement of postsurgical and acne scars. It serves to plane irregularly contoured edges, thereby decreasing the contrast of light and shadow they induce. Pilosebaceous units serve as the reservoir for epidermal stem cells, which regenerate the epidermis after dermabrasion. Therefore, thicker, more sebaceous skin, such as that on the nose, responds best to dermabrasion. Prepubescent children have immature sebaceous glands and there is the potential risk of increased scarring. Given the relative inefficiency of this technique and need for patient cooperation, it is likely better utilized in adolescents when performed in the office setting.

Mechanical rotating abraders, such as wire brushes and diamond fraises, allow for deeper penetration and larger treatment areas. However, this technique is highly operator dependent, carries greater risk of scarring and dyspigmentation, poses a patient safety hazard when used around hair and free margins, and can splatter blood droplets risking blood-borne pathogen exposure. Mechanical rotating dermabrasion has largely been replaced by manual dermabrasion and other treatments with more favorable effect and risk profiles.

The advantages of manual dermabrasion are its simplicity, low cost to perform, good efficacy for appropriately selected sites, and predictable side effect and healing profiles. Its disadvantages are its operator dependence, need for local anesthesia, and tendency to be less time efficient to perform than is laser for focal scar revision.

Clinical Pearls

- **Guidelines:** No formal guidelines exist for manual dermabrasion, which is the subject of this chapter. The American Academy of Dermatology published guidelines for mechanical dermabrasion in 1994.
- **Technique Tips:**
    - Best used for small regional scar revisions where scars have shadow-casing edges and irregular contour.
    - Sites with ample pilosebaceous units respond with greater efficacy and less probability of scarring.
    - The objective is to blend the scar with surrounding skin rather than to remove it. A 50% improvement is generally considered a good result. Occasionally, dermabrading an entire cosmetic unit in which the area of concern is located can provide additional concealment.
    - Dermabrasion can be performed in one to three sessions spaced at a minimum of 3-month intervals. Each subsequent session generally has diminished returns relative to the one prior.
    - Dermabrasion can cause acne to flare and acne should be well controlled before dermabrasion.
- **Skin of Color Considerations:**
    - When performed too deeply, dermabrasion can cause hypopigmentation, which will be cosmetically unacceptable in darker skin types and is likely permanent.

- Bony prominences such as the zygoma and jawline provide greater opposing resistance and are more easily abraded deeper than intended, increasing the risks of scarring and hypopigmentation. Skin at the jawline shares characteristics with neck skin, and further caution should be taken when dermabrading this area because of the risk of scarring.
- Postinflammatory hyperpigmentation is more common in darker skin types but is rarely permanent.

Contraindications/Cautions/Risks

Contraindications
- Dermabrasion is contraindicated in patients with active acne, active herpes simplex virus (HSV), and keloidal or hypertrophic scarring.
- Although the package insert for isotretinoin states that dermabrasion should not be done within 6 months of taking isotretinoin, recent consensus statements have affirmed the safety of localized, manual dermabrasion in the setting of isotretinoin use and shortly thereafter. In contrast, mechanical dermabrasion and fully ablative laser procedures remain contraindicated in patients on isotretinoin or with recent use (<6-12 months).

Cautions
- Sites with limited adnexal structures such as the neck, chest, back, areas of hypertrophic scars, radiation fields, scleroderma, morphea, and burn scars should be approached with caution because of the increased risk of complications.
- Patients with vitiligo can develop depigmentation in dermabraded sites.

Risks
- Anticipated risks include bleeding, crusting, edema, mild discomfort, and a period of erythema generally lasting fewer than 6 months.
- Other possible complications include scarring, infection, hypopigmentation, postinflammatory hyperpigmentation, prolonged skin erythema, acne flare, and milia formation.

Equipment Needed
- Lidocaine 0.5% to 1% with epinephrine 1:100 000
- 3-mL syringe capped with either 30- or 33-gauge needle to deliver lidocaine
- 2 × 2 inch gauze
- A 60 to 150 grit silicon carbide sandpaper cut into 3 × 5 cm strips and autoclaved or gas sterilized. This can be obtained from a hardware store. Alternatively, a Bovie ESSP Disposable Electrosurgical Scratch Pad is a presterilized and relatively inexpensive option if in-office sterilization is unavailable.
- 3- or 10- mL syringe on which to roll the sandpaper (optional)

Preprocedural Approach

- A complete history and examination of the affected area should be taken. Attention should be paid to factors that might increase risk of complications such as history of HSV, use of isotretinoin, history of hypertrophic/keloidal scarring, or factors that limit wound healing ability.
- Counseling to provide the patient and family with a reasonable expectation of the effects of dermabrasion. Dermabrasion will lessen a scar's appearance and help blend it with the surrounding skin, but will be unlikely to achieve complete resolution of the scar. In general, a 50% improvement in the area is considered a success.
- Informed consent to include the expected recovery and effects of dermabrasion as well as possible unintended complications.

Procedural Approach

- Dermabrasion is painful and local anesthesia is recommended. For extensive areas or for individuals who cannot tolerate local anesthesia, sedation may be needed. Local anesthesia can be achieved by slowly infiltrating lidocaine into the subcutaneous tissues of the treatment area in a manner that approximates tumescent anesthesia. This technique is less painful and the tumescence provides additional firmness to the treatment area, which assists in dermabrasion.
- If the treatment site includes a depressed scar, such as an atrophic acne scar, it can be helpful to perform subscision at the end of anesthesia delivery. This is done by moving the needle back and forth beneath the scar to create a potential space that is filled with lidocaine and blood, which helps lift the scar base when wound healing occurs.
- Once adequate anesthesia is obtained, manual dermabrasion with sandpaper is undertaken by wrapping sandpaper around either a 3- or 10-mL syringe or the surgeon's gloved finger (Figure 22.1). Care should be taken to avoid ridges in the sandpaper, because these can gouge furrows deeper than intended. Sandpaper grit used ranges from 60 to 150 with rougher grit (ie, the lower the grit rating, the coarser the grit) providing greater removal. A handheld diamond fraise can also be used.

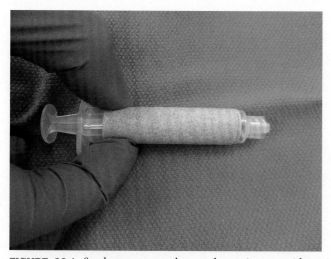

FIGURE 22.1. Sandpaper wrapped around a syringe provides a smooth, firm surface for dermabrasion.

- Short, rapid, back-and-forth strokes are most effective. Particular attention should be paid to applying firm traction–countertraction to the surrounding skin to enable the abrading effect of the sandpaper rather than allowing the skin to oscillate along with the sandpaper.
- Although dermabrasion should be performed to the level needed to correct the contour abnormality, it should never be deeper than the level of adnexal structures, which will provide the source for reepithelialization. Dermabrasion too deep will induce undesirable scarring and dyspigmentation.
- If scarring is deeper than can be addressed with dermabrasion alone, such as with ice pick acne scars, then punch grafting or excision can be done concurrently. A general stopping depth in dermabrasion is when multiple sites of pinpoint bleeding are produced, signifying the papillary dermis is reached.
- Postprocedure bleeding in the absence of a bleeding diathesis can easily be addressed with pressure dressing, topical aluminum chloride, or light electrocautery, if needed.
- Any loose sandpaper grit should be rinsed from the wound with saline to prevent potential granuloma formation. However, this is rarely necessary when sandpaper of sufficient quality is used.

Postprocedural Approach

- Counseling
  - Patients should be counseled that reepithelialization takes about 5 to 10 days. The newly generated skin will be more erythematous than is the surrounding skin and this erythema should fade in 6 to 12 weeks.
  - Makeup can help camouflage erythema and can be applied after reepithelialization is complete.
  - In general, postprocedure pain is minimal and can be best managed with low-dose acetaminophen or ibuprofen.
  - Regular activity can be resumed after 24 hours of relative rest.
  - Patients should also be counseled regarding potential signs of infection such as increased pain and pruritus, although this is rare. Areas not epithelialized in 10 days should be reevaluated for potential complications.
- Wound Care
  - Initial bandage: Petrolatum ointment covered by nonstick gauze and affixed with medical tape. For wounds with difficult hemostasis, a 4 × 4 gauze can be folded over repeatedly, placed over the nonstick gauze, and affixed with medical tape to form a pressure dressing.
  - After 24 hours, the initial bandage is removed and the area can either be cleansed with mild soap and water or a solution of dilute acetic acid; 0.5% acetic acid can be made by adding 1 tablespoon of white vinegar in 1 cup of distilled water. Crusting can be removed by soaking in 0.5% acetic acid solution for 5 to 10 minutes and gently wiping away the crusts. After cleansing, the site is dressed with petrolatum and a nonstick bandage.
  - Moist wound care is continued until no scabs or crusts form and the skin is reepithelialized.
  - Postprocedure erythema and hyperpigmentation are worsened by sun exposure, and use of a moisturizer with at least SPF 30 is recommended.
  - Follow-up should occur in 2 to 3 months to determine whether additional sessions or complementary treatments are needed.

SUGGESTED READINGS

Guidelines of care for dermabrasion. American Academy of Dermatology Committee on Guidelines of Care. *J Am Acad Dermatol.* 1994;31(4):654–657.

Spring LK, Krakowski AC, Alam M, et al. Isotretinoin and timing of procedural interventions: a systematic review with consensus recommendations. *JAMA Dermatol.* 2017;153(8):802–809.

Waldman A, Bolotin D, Arndt KA, et al. ASDS Guidelines Task Force: consensus recommendations regarding the safety of lasers, dermabrasion, chemical peels, energy devices, and skin surgery during and after isotretinoin use. *Dermatol Surg.* 2017;43(10):1249–1262.

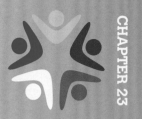
Autologous Fat Transfer

Amanda A. Gosman, Samuel H. Lance, and Sun Hsieh

INTRODUCTION

Initially described over a century ago, autologous fat transfer, colloquially referred to as "fat grafting," remains one of the most versatile techniques for addressing soft-tissue contour deformities, with an ever-expanding list of applications limited only by practitioner creativity. Soft-tissue deficits may arise secondary to a panoply of etiologies, whether it be via congenital malformation, postoncologic extirpation, iatrogenic injury, developmental hypoplasia, or traumatic injury resulting in scarring and fat necrosis. Survival of grafted fat is variably dependent on the recipient bed and practitioner technique. Although autologous fat transfer offers numerous benefits, application of improper technique and inadequate consideration of the relevant anatomy may lead to catastrophic complications and mortality.

We present a safe, methodical approach to autologous fat harvest and transfer. Although the principles of tissue handling remain universal, the structural, anatomic considerations of the donor and recipient sites are very much case dependent and outside the purview of this book. The importance of understanding the surrounding neurovascular and vital structures at each site cannot be understated and merits repeating. Fat transfer is oftentimes an elective procedure that may produce an appreciable outward change for the patient; however, the risk versus benefit ratio may easily skew toward the former if one does not appropriately respect the tissue and the potential morbidity of imprecise technique.

Clinical Pearls

- **Donor sites:** Common donor sites include the abdomen and medial thigh.
- The percentage of fat that survives transfer is oftentimes unpredictable, ranging from less than 50% to 90%. Consequently, multiple transfers may be required to achieve the desired outcome. Patients should be counseled to set appropriate expectations.
- Conversely, compensatory overgrafting is not recommended. Greater than expected survival, also referred to as "take," may require suction-assisted lipectomy or surgical excision to correct.
- Fat should always be transferred in the smallest aliquots achievable in a homogeneous distribution to maximize the surface-area-to-volume ratio of the fat. This optimizes survival of the grafted tissue via nutrient diffusion. Large boluses of fat are predisposed to avascular resorption or conversion to fat cysts.
- **Technique Tips:** Following fat transfer, some gentle massaging of the recipient will facilitate softening of irregular graft contours.

Contraindications/Cautions/Risks

Contraindications

- ○ Active soft-tissue infection at the recipient or donor site would preclude any successful graft survival.
- ○ Unstable recipient wound environment. The site should be in a state of static quiescence for at least 6 months before autologous fat transfer to maximize predictably of the aesthetic outcome.
- ○ Inadequate donor site fat volume
- ○ Inappropriate patient expectations

Cautions

- The maximum dose of tumescent lidocaine is 55 mg/kg. Practitioners should remain cognizant of the amount of tumescent solution—more specifically lidocaine—infiltrated at a time. Peak absorption occurs 8 to 16 hours following initial infiltration. Early symptoms of lidocaine toxicity include circumoral numbness, tongue paresthesia, and dizziness, which may eventually transition to agitation, paranoia, and seizures. Severe cases may result in coma and cardiovascular instability including hypotension, bradycardia, arrhythmia, atrioventricular blockade, ventricular tachycardia, ventricular fibrillation, and, possibly, death.

Risks

- Undercorrection of the contour deformity
- Overcorrection
- Infection
- Patient dissatisfaction with results
- Iatrogenic fat emboli. Intravascular injection
- Blindness when injecting near the nose
- Death

Equipment Needed

- Tumescent cannula (Figure 23.1A)
- Fat harvesting cannula (Figure 23.1A)
- Fat transfer cannula (Figure 23.1B)
- 10-mL (or smaller volume) fat transfer syringe
- 30-mL (or larger volume) tumescent cannula
- Tumescent solution: Mixture of 1 L of lactated Ringer's, 30 to 50 mL of lidocaine, 1 ampule 1:100 000 epinephrine
- Filtration system for washing fat graft before injection: PureGraft™ (SUNEVA® Medical, San Diego, CA) filtration bag or fine mesh gauze secured over basin with rubber bands
- #11 or #15 blade scalpel
- 6-0 Nylon suture
- Needle driver
- Adson forceps
- Curved hemostat or mosquito
- ½ or ¼ in Steri-Strips
- Mastisol
- 2 × 2 gauze
- Tegaderm® (3M, US) dressing

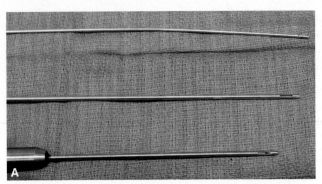

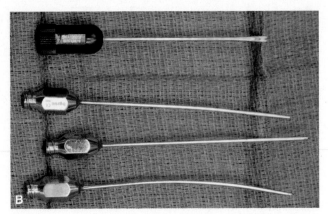

FIGURE 23.1. A, Tumescent cannula (top) and two fat harvesting cannulas (below). B, Fat grafting cannulas; forked cannula (top) which may be used to disrupt scar tissue during or before fat injection.

Preprocedural Approach

- During the preoperative visit, an extensive discussion should be entered into regarding the goals of care for the intended procedure. Deliberate counseling should be completed regarding the possible need to do serial fat transfers to accomplish these goals in a staged manner.
- A thorough history and examination is useful in ensuring that the patient is medically well and stable for this procedure, because autologous fat transfer is frequently done on an elective basis and any operative risk should be minimized.
- To maximize fat graft survival, patients who smoke should complete 6 weeks of smoking cessation before the surgical date.
- The donor should be marked in a standing position for the planned donor site of the fat graft. The areas or prominence should be marked for the margin of the fat harvest area and the most protruding portion (Figure 23.2A).
- The recipient's planned injection should also be marked with the patient awake and upright to identify all of the dynamic and static anatomic landmarks of the site (Figure 23.2B).

Procedural Approach

- Informed consent should be obtained after discussing the risks and benefits of surgery.
- General anesthesia is oftentimes utilized to limit patient motion during fat harvest and transfer.

- Appropriate protective eyewear should be worn if transferring in proximity to the eye or on the face. Corneal shields lubricated with moisturizing ointment such as Lacri-Lube should be used.
- A small stab incision may be made with a #11 or #15 blade scalpel. If using an abdominal donor site, this incision may be hidden within the upper and lower umbilical hoods (Figure 23.3). If using the medial thigh donor site, orient the stab incision along Langer's lines or relaxed skin tension lines to minimize scar prominence.
- Use the tumescent cannula to carefully infiltrate the tumescent solution into the donor site in a subcutaneous plane. This may be done with a 30-mL or larger syringe or with an infusion pump depending on the size of the donor region and the intended volume of tumescence. This should be done in an evenly distributed, fan-shaped manner including all marked areas. Apply even pressure to the syringe plunger throughout each pass. At least 15 minutes should elapse to allow vasoconstriction from the epinephrine to minimize blood loss.
- The fat harvesting cannula may be used to retrieve the donor site fat (Figure 23.3). This may be done with the tulip cannula and syringe system, a Luer-Lok® cannula and syringe system (Becton-Dickinson and Company, Franklin Lakes, NJ), or with a liposuction machine connected to a graft processing receptacle such as the Revolve system. For the syringe-based harvest systems, a "Johnnie Lok" can be used to help maintain the syringe plunger in a position that will generate negative

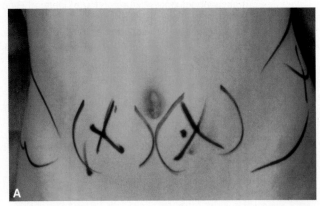

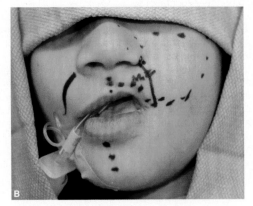

FIGURE 23.2. Preprocedure patient and donor sites marked (A) donor site and (B) recipient site with dotted circumscribed region highlighting the area of relative soft-tissue deficiency.

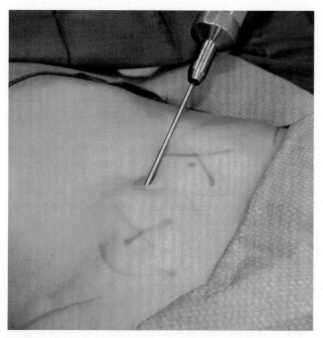

FIGURE 23.3. Fat harvesting from abdominal donor site.

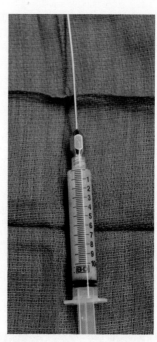

FIGURE 23.4. Processed lipoaspirate transferred into 10-mL fat grafting syringe with a luer-locked fat grafting cannula.

pressure. To start harvesting, the cannula is inserted into the subcutaneous plane that was previously tumesced with the plunger maximally compressed. Retract the plunger such that vacuum pressure may be formed within the syringe. The plunger can then again be held in place with a "Johnnie Lok" to maintain negative pressure. Make even, reciprocating passes with the cannula in a homogeneously distributed, fan-shaped pattern, taking care not to create any contour irregularities or indentations. If the cannula tip portal is accidentally pulled outside the skin, suction may be lost. Simply invert the syringe and recompress the plunger, taking care not to spray the retrieved fat. Reintroduce the cannula into the donor site, retract the plunger, and continue as before.

- Once the fat is harvested, it should be washed with lactated Ringer's to remove excess blood and oil. The fat can be filtered and washed through commercially available systems such as the PureGraft system, which requires that the harvested fat is transferred into a filtration bag, washed with lactated Ringer's, and then withdrawn from the bag to be transferred into injection syringes (Figure 23.4).

- Fat grafts can also be washed with lactated Ringer's using fine mesh gauze over a basin before transfer. Once the fat is washed, it should be transferred into small syringes for transfer into the site.

- The appropriate cannula volume is dependent on the intended transfer site. Cannulas as small as 0.3 to 1 mL may be utilized to precisely monitor the volume of fat transferred.

- Make a stab incision with a #11 or #15 blade scalpel adjacent to, but not within, the recipient site. Multiple incisions may be used to facilitate cross-hatching of the transferred fat. Orient the incision inconspicuously within Langer's lines or relaxed skin tension lines. A curved hemostat or mosquito may be bluntly introduced through this incision to break up connective tissue, facilitating entry of the transfer cannula. Forked cannulas can also be used to help break up scar tissue before or during fat injection.

- Luer lock the fat transfer cannula onto the appropriate fat-loaded syringe (Figure 23.4). Introduce the cannula into the recipient in a subcutaneous or subdermal plane.

- Inject the fat carefully while pulling back the cannula (Figure 23.5). Injecting fat while pushing the cannula in under positive pressure increases the risk of intravascular fat emboli. Multiple passes in separate planes with distribution of tiny amounts of fat along a variety of orientations should be used to maximize take and minimize contour irregularities.

- Once fat transfer has concluded, the donor site and recipient site incisions should be closed with suture of choice (eg., simple interrupted 6-0 nylon suture) (Figure 23.6).

- Dress the incisions with Steri-Strips and Mepilex® (2019 Mölnlycke Health Care AB) dressings.

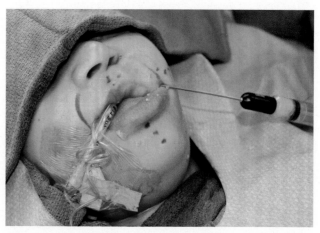

FIGURE 23.5. Fat transfer into preprocedure-marked left cheek region to address soft-tissue deficiency.

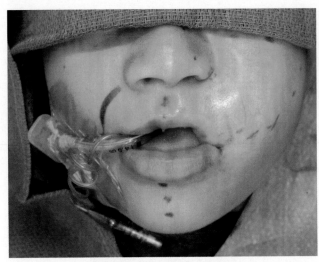

FIGURE 23.6. Immediate posttransfer result with markedly improved fullness to left cheek. There is intentional slight overcorrection in anticipation of partial resorption of grafted fat.

Postprocedural Approach

- The outer dressing may be removed after 48 hours.
- Patients may shower and allow the Steri-Strips to fall off on their own.
- The postoperative appointment should be made 1 week following fat transfer for future removal.

- At this point, patients should be counseled on the expected edema and ecchymosis at both recipient and donor sites.
- Patients should be followed up at least 1 month following fat transfer to evaluate the amount of fat graft survival.
- Patients should be advised not to manipulate the recipient site, because any shear injury or trauma in the acute healing phase may compromise graft take.
- Massaging of the recipient site may occur 2 weeks following fat transfer to smoothen any contour irregularities.
- Postoperative downtime is moderate. Patients should expect to be absent from school or work for 1 week and possibly longer depending on the severity of bruising.
- Serial photography may be used at each office visit to document preoperative, immediate postoperative, and longer postoperative outcomes.
- If further fat transfer is required, wait at least 6 months from most recent transfer to allow appropriate tissue healing and incorporation.

SUGGESTED READINGS

Coleman SR, Katzel EB. Fat grafting for facial filling and regeneration. *Clin Plast Surg.* 2015;42(3):289–300.

Ross RJ, Shayan R, Mutimer KL, Ashton MW. Autologous fat grafting: current state of the art and critical review. *Ann Plast Surg.* 2014;73(3):352–357.

Strong AL, Cederna PS, Rubin JP, Coleman SR, Levi B. The current state of fat grafting: a review of harvesting, processing, and injection techniques. *Plast Reconstr Surg.* 2015;136(4):897–912.

Diagnostic-Specific Procedures

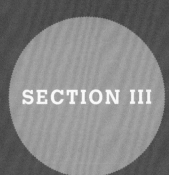

Maneuvers

24 Acquired Keratoderma

25 Aquagenic Wrinkling

26 Bacterial Culture

27 Dermatographism

28 Dermoscopy

29 Fungal Culture

30 Hair Biopsy

31 Hair Pull Test

32 Nail Matrix Biopsy

33 Patch Testing for Allergic Contact Dermatitis

34 Pinworm Examination

35 Polymerase Chain Reaction

36 Skin Biopsy Techniques

37 Viral Culture

38 Wood's Lamp Skin Examination

Microscopy

39 Demodex Examination

40 Hair Microscopy

41 Immunofluorescence

42 Fungal Examination or Potassium Hydroxide (KOH) Preparation

43 Scabies Examination

44 Tzanck Smear

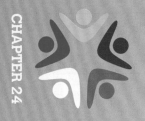

CHAPTER 24

Maneuvers
Acquired Keratoderma

Jessica Sprague, Catherine Gupta Warner, Kimberly Ann Chun, and Sheila Fallon Friedlander

OVERVIEW

Acquired keratoderma (AK) is also referred to as terra firma-forme dermatosis, Duncan's dirty dermatosis, and retention hyperkeratosis. AK is considered to be along a spectrum of hyperkeratotic diseases with dermatosis neglecta at one end and retention hyperkeratosis at the other. AK is characterized by light to dark brown hyperkeratotic plaques with accentuation of the normal skin lines resulting in a speckled, mottled, or reticulated appearance. AK can occur anywhere on the body, and it is most commonly seen around the neck or along the trunk. Although not life-threatening, AK can be cosmetically troublesome to patients who cannot achieve clean-appearing skin. Although AK is often misinterpreted to be secondary to poor hygiene (dermatosis neglecta), these "dirty" plaques are actually resistant to regular washing with soap and water and are easily rubbed off with 70% isopropyl alcohol or an alcohol pad (Figures 24.1 and 24.2).

Differential Diagnosis

Differential diagnosis includes dermatosis neglecta, acanthosis nigricans, tinea versicolor, seborrheic keratoses, and confluent and reticulated papillomatosis. In contrast to AK, dermatosis neglecta is due to inadequate cleaning or scrubbing of the skin with resulting thickened and hyperpigmented plaques. These plaques can be removed with vigorous rubbing and are typically seen in patients with physical disabilities or in those who do not have access to regular bathing. History and clinical course can help differentiate dermatosis neglecta from retention hyperkeratosis over time.

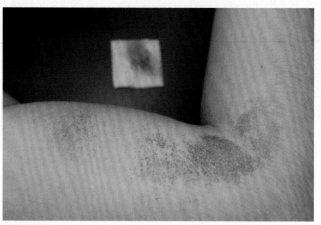

FIGURE 24.2. Brown plaque has been removed and appears on alcohol gauze pad. Photo courtesy of Catherine Gupta Warner, MD.

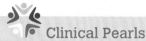 Clinical Pearls

- Removal of the plaques with an alcohol swab is both diagnostic and therapeutic.
- In the case of recurrence, weekly application of isopropyl alcohol to the affected site is generally sufficient treatment.

Contraindications/Cautions

No specific contraindications or cautions.

Equipment Needed

- Alcohol swab or isopropyl 70% alcohol-soaked gauze

Procedural Approach

- Rub an alcohol pad or gauze soaked with isopropyl 70% alcohol over the affected area until the brown pigmentation is removed.

SUGGESTED READING

Weintraub G, Craft N, Goldsmith LA, et al. Terra firma-forme dermatosis. In: Goldsmith LA, ed. *VisualDx*. Rochester, NY: VisualDx; 2018.

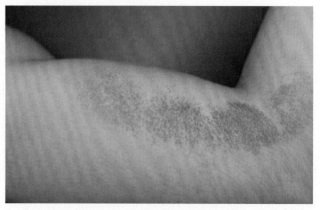

FIGURE 24.1. Light to dark brown hyperkeratotic plaques of acquired keratoderma. Photo courtesy of Catherine Gupta Warner, MD.

Aquagenic Wrinkling

Jessica Sprague, Catherine Gupta Warner, Kimberly Ann Chun,
and Sheila Fallon Friedlander

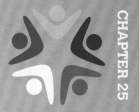

CHAPTER 25

INTRODUCTION

Aquagenic wrinkling or "hand-in-the-bucket" sign is an exaggerated response of normal skin wrinkling that occurs when the hands are soaked in water for prolonged periods of time (Figure 25.1A and B). Aquagenic wrinkling is a rare condition that has been observed in patients with cystic fibrosis or in those who carry the cystic fibrosis mutation. It has also been associated with nephrotic syndrome, marasmus, focal hyperhidrosis, atopic dermatitis, and to the use of COX-2 inhibitors and other medications. It may also be idiopathic. In addition to skin wrinkling, small translucent or white papules that coalesce into plaques occur on the palms after a brief exposure to water. In addition, patients may complain of itching, burning, or a feeling of tightness of their skin. Patients with cystic fibrosis typically experience a quicker onset after exposure to water (~2-3 minutes) versus carriers who may develop the eruption after about 7 minutes following exposure. The soles of the feet are unaffected. Wrinkling usually resolves 10 to 60 minutes after drying of the skin, although the palmar eruption may persist for longer periods of time.

The etiology of aquagenic wrinkling is related to sweating; however, the pathogenesis is not fully known. It is thought to be due to salt imbalance and subsequent increased retention of water within the skin cells resulting in higher transepidermal water loss.

Clinical Pearls

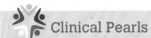

- Some patients have success with nightly application of 20% aluminum chloride.

Contraindications/Cautions/Risks

- No specific contraindications for the procedure

Equipment Needed

- Container large enough to fit one or both hands
- Enough water to fully submerse the palms of the hands

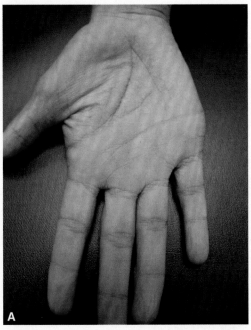
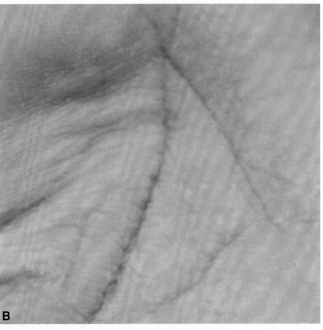

FIGURE 25.1. A, Clinical example of aquagenic wrinkling of hands. B, On close examination, note the white papules that coalesce into confluent plaques. Photos courtesy of Andrew C. Krakowski, MD.

Procedural Approach ▶

- Immerse hand in water for 10 minutes.
- Observe whether clinical signs and symptoms occur, such as confluent white papules and wrinkling with pain, itching, or tight sensation.

SUGGESTED READINGS

Garçon-Michel N, Roguedas-Contios AM, Rault G, et al. Frequency of aquagenic palmoplantar keratoderma in cystic fibrosis: a new sign of cystic fibrosis? *Br J Dermatol*. 2010;163(1):162–166. doi:10.1111/j.1365-2133.2010.09764.x.

Katz KA, Yan AC, Turner ML. Aquagenic wrinkling of the palms in patients with cystic fibrosis homozygous for the ΔF508 CFTR mutation. *Arch Dermatol*. 2005;141(5):621–624. doi:10.1001/archderm.141.5.621.

Park L, Khani C, Tamburro J. Aquagenic wrinkling of the palms and the potential role for genetic testing. *Pediatr Dermatol*. 2012;29(3):237–242. doi:10.1111/j.1525-1470.2011.01609.x.

Weibel L, Spinas R. Images in clinical medicine. Aquagenic wrinkling of palms in cystic fibrosis. *N Engl J Med*. 2012;366(21):e32.

Bacterial Culture

Jessica Sprague, Catherine Gupta Warner, Kimberly Ann Chun, and Sheila Fallon Friedlander

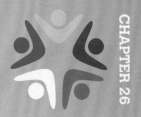

CHAPTER 26

OVERVIEW

Bacterial cultures are used to determine the presence of pathogenic bacteria and antibiotic susceptibility and can serve a variety of purposes in dermatology. They can be used to assess for superinfection in eczema, determine the causative bacteria in impetigo, folliculitis, furuncles, and other crusted or purulent skin lesions and are commonly used to tailor antibiotic regimens in known bacterial infections or superinfections. Antibiotic susceptibility testing is especially important in the age of high bacterial resistance to traditional antibiotics. Bacterial culture is also a useful tool to rule out infection in the case of sterile pustulosis, such as that seen in pustular psoriasis and eosinophilic pustular folliculitis. Wound cultures are of highest yield when they are taken from tissue directly; however, this is often not feasible in the clinic. More commonly, bacteria cultures are obtained via swab, which tends to collect a small fraction of a milliliter of specimen. This greatly reduces the amount of bacteria that can be recovered for culture and can be especially limiting if multiple types of cultures are requested from a single swab (eg, mycobacterial, fungal, anaerobic).

Wound cultures are plated using a "semiquantitative method" in which the cultures are inoculated onto the media with sequential dilution. Results are then reported as 1+, 2+, 3+, etc. depending on which dilution demonstrates bacterial growth. Bacterial cultures generally require between 36 and 48 hours before results are reported. Clinical judgment must be used to determine whether cultured bacteria are truly pathogenic or merely represent colonization.

 Clinical Pearls

- If sampling a skin surface, do not prep skin with disinfectant before obtaining specimen because this can result in a falsely negative culture.
- If sampling an intact lesion such as a pustule, gently swab the surface with disinfectant and allow it to dry before puncturing the lesion to sample its contents.
- Highest yield areas are those with intact pustules or a moist base.
- Cultures should ideally be obtained before initiation of any antimicrobial therapy when the diagnosis is uncertain or when there is concern for potential antibiotic resistance (eg, MRSA).

Contraindications/Cautions/Risks

Contraindications
- No specific contraindications

Cautions
- In infants and young children who are likely to move during the procedure, make sure to secure the body area you are scraping and brace your hand against the patient to avoid potentially cutting the patient with the blade or needle while deroofing intact pustules.

Equipment Needed (Figure 26.1)
- Sterile #15 blade, #11 blade, or 18-gauge needle
- Bacterial culture including associated culture swab
- Sterile gloves
- Alcohol prep, sterile gauze, and plastic adhesive bandage

Procedural Approach

- Always wear gloves to avoid contamination.
- The culture medium should be labeled with the patient's pertinent identifying information before collection.
- When obtaining a specimen from a nonintact pustule, crusted lesion, or otherwise dry skin, wet the swab by inserting it into

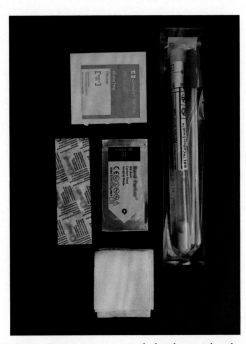

FIGURE 26.1. Equipment tray includes bacterial culture with swab; sterile #15 blade, #11 blade, or 18-gauge needle; alcohol prep; sterile gauze pad; and plastic adhesive bandages. Photo courtesy of Jessica Sprague, MD.

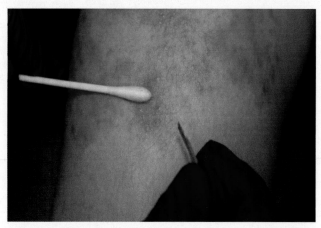

FIGURE 26.2. When obtaining a specimen from an intact pustule, puncture the pustule with a sterile blade or needle and rub the swab on the newly exposed lesion base and collect any purulent discharge on the swab. Photo courtesy of Catherine Gupta Warner, MD.

the culture medium and then rub the moistened swab vigorously over the target area.

- When obtaining a specimen from an intact pustule, puncture the pustule with a sterile blade or needle and rub the newly exposed lesion base with the swab as well as collecting any purulent discharge on the swab (Figure 26.2).
- Place the swab in the culture medium and place the cap on the tube.

SUGGESTED READINGS

Kallstrom G. Are quantitative bacterial wound cultures useful? *J Clin Microbiol.* 2014;52(8):2753–2756.

Lagier JC, Edouard S, Pagnier I, Mediannikov O, Drancourt M, Raoult D. Current and past strategies for bacterial culture in clinical microbiology. *Clin Microbiol Rev.* 2015;28(1):208–236.

Lim JS, Park HS, Cho S, Yoon HS. Antibiotic susceptibility and treatment response in bacterial skin infection. *Ann Dermatol.* 2018;30(2):186–191.

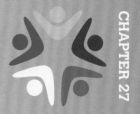

CHAPTER 27

Dermatographism

Jessica Sprague, Catherine Gupta Warner, Kimberly Ann Chun, and Sheila Fallon Friedlander

Introduction

Dermatographism literally means "the ability to write on the skin" and represents an exaggerated response to pressure. It is seen in 3% to 5% of the normal population; however, the prevalence is up to 24% in the pediatric population. Dermatographism is diagnosed by stroking the skin with a blunt object, such as a tongue depressor, causing first a white line and then a red line, which then produces a wheal. Urtication typically peaks within 5 to 10 minutes and resolves within 1 hour. Most dermatographism is asymptomatic, termed "simple dermatographism" and does not require intervention. Symptomatic dermatographism manifests with itching, widespread burning, and a larger area of involvement. First-line treatment is usually antihistamines.

White dermatographism is not a true form of dermatographism but instead represents a blanching response resulting from capillary vasoconstriction after skin stroking. It manifests as a persistent white line without evidence of urtication, which replaces the initial red line produced by skin stroking, generally within 10 seconds. White dermatographism is seen with a particularly high incidence in individuals with atopic dermatitis.

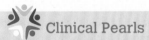

Clinical Pearls

- **Age-Specific Considerations:** When performing on nervous toddlers and young children, tell them you are going to "tickle" the skin, which usually does not sound threatening to the patient. The procedure can also be demonstrated on a parent first to relieve anxiety.

Contraindications/Cautions/Risks

- No specific contraindications

Equipment Needed

- Tongue depressor, cotton-tipped applicator, or ballpoint pen

Procedural Approach

- Determine an uninvolved area of skin on the patient to test. The back usually works well; however, if the back is clinically involved, the forearm can be used as a substitute.
- Use the wooden tip (ie, noncotton side) of the cotton-tipped applicator, the bottom of a ballpoint pen, or the end of a tongue depressor and stroke the patient's skin with light but steady pressure (Figure 27.1).
- Draw several parallel lines, a hash mark, or an "X" to best demonstrate the effect to the patient (Figure 27.2).
- Continue to monitor the patient's skin over the next 5 minutes for the characteristic white line, followed by a red line and then a wheal.

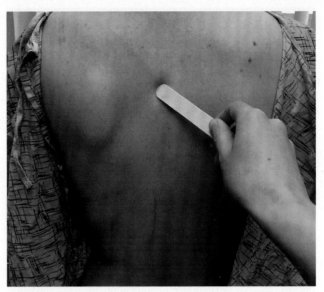

FIGURE 27.1. Use the wooden tip (noncotton side) of the cotton-tipped applicator, the bottom of a ballpoint pen, or the end of a tongue depressor and stroke the patient's skin with light but steady pressure. Photo courtesy of Jessica Sprague, MD.

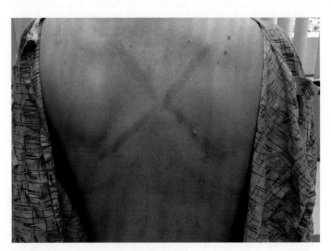

FIGURE 27.2. Draw several parallel lines, a hash mark, or an "X" to best demonstrate the effect to the patient. Photo courtesy of Jessica Sprague, MD.

SUGGESTED READINGS

Paller A, Mancini AJ. (2016). *Hurwitz Clinical Pediatric Dermatology: A Textbook of Skin Disorders of Childhood and Adolescence.* 5th ed. Edinburgh, Scotland: Elsevier.

Taskapan O, Harmanyeri Y. Evaluation of patients with symptomatic dermatographism. *J Eur Acad Dermatol Venereol.* 2006;20(1):58–62.

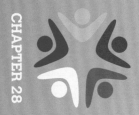

CHAPTER 28

Dermoscopy

Jessica Sprague, Catherine Gupta Warner, Kimberly Ann Chun, and Sheila Fallon Friedlander

Overview

Dermoscopy is the examination of the skin using skin surface microscopy and allows for assessment of the macroscopic and microscopic morphology of skin lesions. Traditionally used to evaluate pigmented lesions, its use has expanded to include a wide array of cutaneous malignancies and inflammatory and infectious skin diseases. Different types of dermoscopy exist. Traditional dermoscopy involves placing a dermatoscope with nonpolarized light directly on the skin with a liquid interface, which allows for better visualization of the superficial layers. Dermoscopy with polarized light does not require contact with the skin and allows for better visualization of the deep epidermal and superficial dermis as well as improved ability to visualize vascular structures.

Dermoscopy is a noninvasive procedure, causing neither physical discomfort nor emotional distress; thus, it is ideally suited to pediatric patients. In pediatric dermatology, dermoscopy is most commonly used to diagnose and monitor melanocytic lesions, particularly identification of Spitz nevi and identification of atypical features of acquired and congenital melanocytic nevi.

Although dermoscopy is an inexpensive and efficient auxiliary tool for clinical diagnosis and monitoring, accuracy is contingent on appropriate training. When used appropriately, it can increase diagnostic accuracy and reduce the number of unnecessary biopsies; however, if used by inexperienced providers, it could lead to inaccurate diagnosis and poor clinical outcome.

Clinical Pearls

- **Age-Specific Considerations:** When using dermoscopy in infants and very young children, make sure to cover/protect the child's eyes while evaluating lesions on the face.
- **Technique Tips:**
  - A dermatoscope can also be used as a pocket flashlight to allow for visualization of the oral cavity or to provide side lighting.
  - If mineral oil is not easily available, an alcohol swab can be used to provide a liquid layer for contact dermoscopy; however, be aware the alcohol will evaporate quickly and may need to be reapplied.

Contraindications/Cautions/Risks

- No specific contraindications

Equipment Needed

- Dermatoscope
  - Pocket dermatoscopes range in price from $300 to over $2000.
  - Popular dermatoscope models include the DermLite DL100, DermLite DL200 Hybrid, DermLite DL4, and the DermLite II Pro HR.
- Alcohol swab
- Mineral oil or other oil for contact dermoscopy

Procedural Approach

- Clean the dermatoscope with an alcohol swab before use in each patient; certain dermatoscope models now support the use of a physical barrier to help prevent cross-contamination between patients.
- When using contact dermoscopy, apply a drop of mineral oil or other oil directly to the skin lesion of interest and then place the dermatoscope directly on the oil, making sure to eliminate all air bubbles and thus enhance visualization (Figure 28.1).
- When using noncontact dermoscopy, hold the dermatoscope approximately 1 cm away from the skin for best visualization (Figure 28.2).

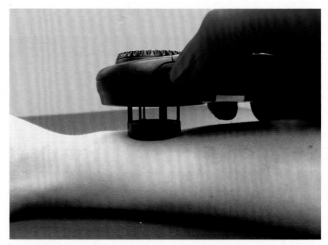

FIGURE 28.1. For contact dermoscopy, a drop of mineral oil or other oil is applied directly to the skin lesion. The dermatoscope is then placed directly on the oil, making sure to eliminate all air bubbles and thus enhancing visualization. Photo courtesy of Jessica Sprague, MD.

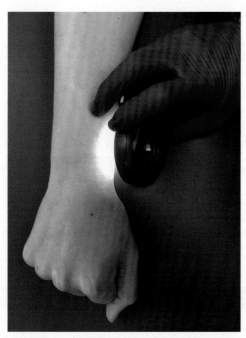

FIGURE 28.2. For noncontact dermoscopy, hold the dermatoscope approximately 1 cm away from the skin for best visualization. Photo courtesy of Jessica Sprague, MD.

LESION-SPECIFIC FINDINGS

Scabies: Dermoscopy has been shown to have equal or greater sensitivity compared to traditional microscopic examination of skin scrapings for identification of scabies infestations. Burrows can be visualized as thin serpiginous tracts of whitish scale with a small, dark-brown, delta-shaped structure at the leading end of the burrow, which represents the body of the female mite.

Verruca: Although most verruca are easily diagnosed clinically on the basis of their verrucous surface characteristics, plantar verruca can be mistaken for a callus or corn. Dermoscopy can be used to distinguish verruca on the basis of the presence of small black dots, representing thrombosed capillary loops, and by interruption of dermatoglyphs (skin lines) in the lesion.

Angiomas: Angiomas can occasionally be mistaken for melanocytic nevi or inflammatory lesions. Dermoscopy can usually help distinguish angiomas on the basis of the presence of red-purple lacunae and lack of pigment.

Melanocytic nevi: Dermoscopy is most frequently employed to classify melanocytic nevi including congenital nevi, acquired nevi, and blue nevi and evaluate for atypical or concerning features. Benign melanocytic nevi typically present with benign dermatoscopic patterns and lack any melanoma-specific structures.

  Dermatoscopic patterns associated with benign melanocytic nevi include the following:
  - Diffuse reticular pigment network: most common pattern seen in acquired nevi
  - Patchy reticular network interspersed with homogenous areas

  - Peripheral reticular network with central hypo- or hyperpigmentation
  - Diffuse globules: most commonly seen in congenital nevi
  - Peripheral reticular pattern with central globules: most commonly seen in congenital nevi
  - Peripheral globules with central reticulate pattern or homogenous area: represents an acquired growing nevus
  - Homogeneous brown pigmentation: seen in congenital nevi
  - Homogeneous tan pigmentation: seen in acquired nevi in fair skin phenotypes
  - Homogeneous blue pigmentation: seen in blue nevi

Spitz nevus: Dermoscopy is particularly useful for identifying Spitz nevi because 50% have a characteristic "starburst pattern" on dermoscopy, with outwardly radiating streaks of pigment around the perimeter of the lesion. Spitz nevi can also display a negative pigment network; globular pattern, consisting of regular or irregular brown dots, globules, or both; or a homogeneous pigment pattern, which exhibits a featureless pink papule with polymorphous vessels. These varying patterns can make Spitz nevi more difficult to identify.

Melanoma: Dermoscopy can be a useful tool to identify lesions concerning for melanoma, although even with dermoscopy it can be difficult to distinguish from Spitz nevi that lack the characteristic "starburst pattern." Identification of any "melanoma-associated features" on dermoscopy should prompt consideration of biopsy. Accurate identification requires significant clinical dermatoscopic training and experience.

  Dermatoscopic patterns associated with melanoma include the following:
  - Atypical pigment network: broad/thickened lines
  - Focal peripheral streaks
  - Negative pigment network
  - Crystalline structures—fine white shiny lines visible with polarized dermoscopy
  - Atypical dots and globules of varying sizes
  - Asymmetric dark diffuse areas of pigmentation
  - Blue-white coloration overlying thicker areas of a lesion
  - White scarlike areas overlying thinner areas of a lesion
  - Atypical vascular structures—dotted, linear, or twisted red vessels of varying sizes
  - Peripheral light brown structure less areas

SUGGESTED READINGS

Benvenuto-Adrade C, Dusza SW, Agero AL, et al. Differences between polarized light dermoscopy and immersion contact dermoscopy for the evaluation of skin lesions. *Arch Dermatol.* 2007;143(3):329–338.

Haliasos EC, Kerner M, Jaimes-Lopez N, et al. Dermoscopy for the pediatric dermatologist. Part I: dermoscopy of pediatric infectious and inflammatory skin lesions and hair disorders. *Pediatric Dermatol.* 2013;30(2):163–171.

Haliasos EC, Kerner M, Jaimes N, et al. Dermoscopy for the pediatric dermatologist. Part II: Dermoscopy of genetic syndromes with cutaneous manifestations and pediatric vascular lesions. *Pediatric Dermatol.* 2013;30(2):172–181.

Haliasos EC, Kerner M, Jaimes N, et al. Dermoscopy for the pediatric dermatologist. Part III: Dermoscopy of melanocytic lesions. *Pediatric Dermatol.* 2013;30(3):281–293.

Marghoob AA, Usatine RP, Jaimes N. Dermoscopy for the family physician. *Am Fam Physician.* 2013;88(7):441–450.

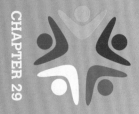

CHAPTER 29

Fungal Culture

Jessica Sprague, Catherine Gupta Warner, Kimberly Ann Chun, and Sheila Fallon Friedlander

Introduction

Samples collected from hair, nails, or skin can establish or confirm a diagnosis of fungal infection. In addition, the results can optimize selection of the most appropriate therapy. Fungal culture is considered the gold standard in the diagnosis of fungal infections because it is the only technique that allows identification of the fungal species. However, fungal culture may take 3 weeks or longer to identify the causative organism. Therefore, alternative evaluations, including periodic acid–Schiff (PAS) stain of infected tissue or polymerase chain reaction (PCR), are alternative options in some institutions.

Clinical Pearls

- Sampling of the nail should be done at least 3 months after withdrawal of oral antifungals. Topical antifungals and over-the-counter antifungal medications should also be discontinued.
- Subungual debris is preferable to distal nail clippings because nail clippings may contain contaminants or bacteria that can outgrow the pathogenic organism on culture medium.
- Multiple noninvasive techniques for sampling hair have been utilized, including using a cotton-tipped applicator, toothbrush, or hairbrush. The hairbrush method is the most accurate noninvasive procedure; however, sterile plastic hairbrushes are not readily available in an office. The cotton swab method is a simple, yet effective and noninvasive method of fungal culture. Wet the cotton swab with the transport medium, then roll over affected area as well as over the other unaffected three quadrants of the scalp surface.
- Friction generated in the hairbrush and toothbrush methods causes the bristles to become negatively charged, attracting hair and scale. Wetting the cotton swab with the collection liquid medium causes the scales and hair to adhere to the swab.

Contraindications/Cautions/Risks

Contraindications
- No specific contraindications

Cautions
- In infants and young children who may move during the procedure, secure the area you are scraping to avoid cutting the patient with any blade while obtaining the sample. Cotton swab sampling may be the safer alternative for young or anxious children.

Equipment Needed
Nail
- Sterile container (such as sterile urine cup)
- Isopropyl alcohol
- Nail clipper

Hair
- Sterile cotton-tipped applicator (often available in swab/transport culturette)/plastic hairbrush/toothbrush
- Sterile container or bag

Skin
- Sterile container (such as sterile urine cup)
- Isopropyl alcohol
- Cotton-tipped applicator, preferably in transport culturette system

Procedural Approach

NAIL
- Thoroughly clean the nail with isopropyl alcohol or soap and water.
- Clip distal nails as close as possible without causing discomfort (Figure 29.1).
- Be sure to include subungual debris with the specimen by gently scraping with a 1-mm curette.
- Place nail clipping and subungual debris in sterile container.

HAIR
- Before culture, a high-yield target area should be identified, such as an area of erythema, scaling, or hair loss (Figure 29.2).

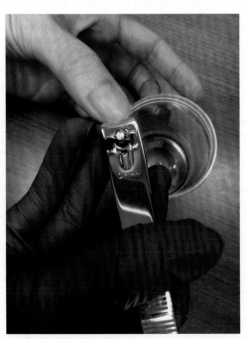

FIGURE 29.1. For nail sampling, clip distal nails as close as possible without causing discomfort. Photo courtesy of Catherine Gupta Warner, MD.

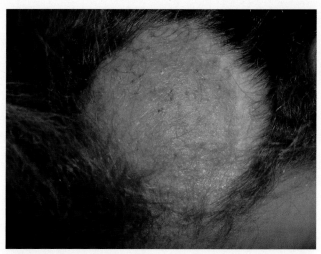

FIGURE 29.2. For hair sampling, identify a high-yield target area such as this area of erythema, scaling, or hair loss as seen in this case of tinea capitis. Photo courtesy of Andrew C. Krakowski, MD.

Cotton-Tipped Applicator Method

- Moisten a sterile cotton-tipped applicator with the transport medium in the bottom of the culturette tube.
- Rub target area vigorously while rotating the surface of the cotton-tipped applicator for 15 seconds (Figure 29.3).
- Repeat sampling of the other three unaffected quadrants of the scalp.
- Place cotton-tipped applicator in a sterile container or bag.

Hairbrush Method

- Rub brush on target area for 15 seconds.
- Place brush in a sterile bag.

Toothbrush Method

- Rub toothbrush on target area for 15 seconds.
- Place brush in a sterile bag.

SKIN

- Gather and ready all equipment before initiating skin scraping in any patient.
- Before scraping, a high-yield target area should be identified, such as a leading scaling border of an annular plaque, or, if present, pustules.
- Wipe the area to be scraped with alcohol to help control the scraping of the scale and minimize loss of the scale.
- Using the belly of a #15 blade, scrape the scale or pustule sideways at an angle to obtain the sample.
- Place scrapings in a sterile container.

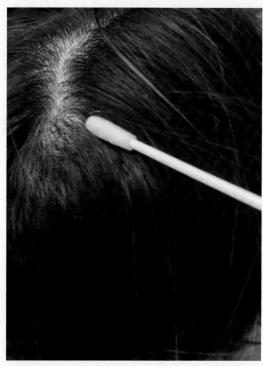

FIGURE 29.3. Rub target area vigorously while rotating the surface of the cotton-tipped applicator for 15 seconds. Photo courtesy of Catherine Gupta Warner, MD.

SUGGESTED READINGS

Akbaba M, Ilkit M, Sutoluk Z, Ates A, Zorba H. Comparison of hairbrush, toothbrush and cotton swab methods for diagnosing asymptomatic dermatophyte scalp carriage. *J Eur Acad Dermatol Venereol.* 2008;22(3):356–362. doi:10.1111/j.1468-3083.2007.02442.x.

Friedlander SF, Pickering B, Cunningham BB, Gibbs NF, Eichenfield LF. Use of the cotton swab method in diagnosing tinea capitis. *Pediatrics.* 1999;104(2, pt 1):276–279.

Ghannoum M, Mukherjee P, Isham N, Markinson B, Rosso JD, Leal L. Examining the importance of laboratory and diagnostic testing when treating and diagnosing onychomycosis. *Int J Dermatol.* 2018;57(2):131–138. doi:10.1111/ijd.13690.

Gupta AK, Mays RR, Versteeg SG, et al. Tinea capitis in children: a systematic review of management. *J Eur Acad Dermatol Venereol.* 2018;32(12):2264–2274. doi:10.1111/jdv.15088.

Hull PR, Gupta AK, Summerbell RC. Onychomycosis: an evaluation of three sampling methods. *J Am Acad Dermatol.* 1998;39(6): 1015–1017.

Jordan CS, Stokes B, Thompson CT. Subungual debris cytopathology increases sensitivity of fungus detection in onychomycosis. *J Am Acad Dermatol.* 2016;75(1):222–224.

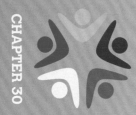

CHAPTER 30

Hair Biopsy

Jessica Sprague, Catherine Gupta Warner, Kimberly Ann Chun, and Sheila Fallon Friedlander

Introduction

Alopecia is a common dermatologic condition that often requires both clinical and pathologic information for diagnosis. Although submitting biopsies to aid in diagnosis can be helpful, a good understanding of the hair biopsy process is required to yield accurate results.

Hair biopsies can be evaluated in two ways—via a horizontal section or a vertical section. Several studies have been performed to address the question of horizontal versus vertical sectioning; however, both techniques have their own advantages and limitations. Most studies conclude that examination of both horizontal and vertical sections maximizes the diagnostic yield compared to either section alone. Histologic sectioning methods such as the Hovert or Tyler techniques exist to obtain both horizontal and vertical sections from one punch biopsy specimen. However, many studies and institutions advocate for two separate biopsies to be performed, one for horizontal sectioning and one for vertical sectioning. This decreases the possibility of sectioning or laboratory error that can lead to tissue loss, increased turnover time, and decreased cost-effectiveness.

In general, vertical sectioning is preferred for diagnosis of nonscarring alopecias, whereas horizontal sectioning is favored for diagnosis of scarring alopecias. The one exception to this is lichen planopilaris, which is a scarring alopecia with a higher diagnostic yield with vertical sections. A Hair Research Society consensus meeting concluded that horizontal sectioning is preferred if a single biopsy is received. In many cases, however, both types of sectioning may be complementary and even synergistically helpful for diagnosis.

Clinical Pearls

- Because significant pathologic overlap exists between various types of alopecia, it is imperative to submit as much clinical information as possible to the pathologist, such as clinical scarring versus nonscarring process, presence of inflammation or pustules, distribution, duration, and pattern.
- For scarring alopecias, biopsies taken from the peripheral edge of the affected area are more likely to be diagnostic.
- For nonscarring alopecias, biopsies taken from an area with a positive hair pull test or active loss are more likely to be diagnostic.
- For evaluation of possible androgenic alopecia or telogen effluvium, two biopsies, one from involved (generally vertex) and one from uninvolved (generally occiput) skin, can be helpful.
- Vertical sectioning is useful for evaluation of alopecia with interface change or lichenoid infiltrates, as well as to assess all levels of the skin and the complete hair profile. The disadvantage of vertical sectioning is the low number of follicles per vertical section, typically 10% of the overall follicles from the sample. This may lead to sampling error or missed pathology.

- Horizontal sectioning allows for evaluation of all follicles, but may prevent full assessment of patterns of inflammation within the sample or changes along the dermal–epidermal junction. Evaluation of the numbers and types of hair can aid in the diagnosis of scarring or androgenic processes.
- In certain scenarios, a specimen may also be sent for direct immunofluorescence (DIF; see Chapter 41. Immunofluorescence). A differential that includes lupus of the scalp would be one example.

Contraindications/Cautions

- No specific contraindications
- Risks are the same for any typical biopsy (ie, risk of bleeding, scar, infection, recurrence, and lack of diagnosis), although the scalp tends to bleed more vigorously than do other areas of the body. Precautions may include having electrocautery available and/or allowing the patient to sit for 10 to 15 minutes after lidocaine with epinephrine has been injected.

Equipment Needed

- All tools needed for a typical 4-mm punch biopsy (see Chapter 36. Skin Biopsy Techniques)
- Detailed pathology requisition form with adequate clinical history and type of sectioning desired depending on number of biopsies performed (one or two)

Procedural Approach

- Because the scalp has a dense vascular plexus and often bleeds more than do other parts of the body, it is recommended that an anesthetic with epinephrine be injected and be allowed to dwell for 5 to 10 minutes before initiation of the biopsy.
- Before biopsy is performed, a decision must be made as to the type of sectioning required. If both horizontal and vertical are desired, a decision must be made as to whether both sectioning will be performed on the same section (ie, a "split" specimen) versus one separate biopsy for each sectioning type (ie, one section for horizontal sectioning and one section for vertical sectioning).
- On the basis of the type of alopecia, chose and mark your biopsy site(s). Perform one or two 4-mm punch biopsies for pathology submission.
- Pathology requisition forms should be filled out with all relevant clinical information and specific sectioning requests.

SUGGESTED READINGS

Elston DM, McCollough ML, Angeloni VL. Vertical and transverse sections of alopecia biopsy specimens: combining the two to maximize diagnostic yield. *J Am Acad Dermatol.* 1995;32:454–457.

Olsen EA, Bergfeld WF, Cotsarelis G, et al. Summary of North American Hair Research Society (NAHRS)-sponsored workshop on cicatricial alopecia, Duke University Medical Center, February 10 and 11, 2001. *J Am Acad Dermatol.* 2003;48:103–110.

Stefanato, CM. Histopathology of alopecia: a clinicopathological approach to diagnosis. *Histopathology.* 2010;56(1): 24–38.

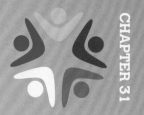

CHAPTER 31

Hair Pull Test

Jessica Sprague, Catherine Gupta Warner, Kimberly Ann Chun, and Sheila Fallon Friedlander

Introduction

Excessive shedding of hair resulting in hair loss can be examined using a hair pull test. When 50 to 60 hairs are grasped and firmly but slowly pulled from the scalp to the distal end, normally zero to two telogen hairs (Figure 31.1) will pull loose from the scalp. Telogen implies hairs in the resting phase of the hair cycle, which are identified under the microscope by a rounded bulb or a club-shaped proximal end. In contrast, anagen hairs, or hairs in the growth phase, have attached root sheaths with a distorted and pigmented bulb. Up to two telogen hairs is considered within normal limits; however, more than two telogen or any anagen hairs is considered abnormal. The hair pull test is ideally used for monitoring acute cases of telogen effluvium or anagen effluvium, loose anagen syndrome, and the active edge of alopecia areata.

 Clinical Pearls

- If the hair pull test is positive in more than one area of the scalp, consider anagen or telogen effluvium, as well as loose anagen syndrome.
- Earlier guidelines recommended having patients avoid washing their hair at least 1 to 5 days before the test. However, a recent study has shown no significant difference in the number of hairs removed regardless of when the hair was last washed or brushed.
- Loose anagen syndrome has anagen hairs that show a ruffled cuticle.

Contraindications/Cautions/Risks

Contraindications
- There are no specific contraindications for the procedure.

Equipment Needed
- Microscope

Hair Pull Test Procedure

- Select 50 to 60 hairs and grasp the bundle close to the patient's scalp using your thumb, index finger, and third finger.
- Firmly pull on the hair, slowly sliding your fingers down the hair shaft. Avoid pulling forcefully or too quickly (Figure 31.1).

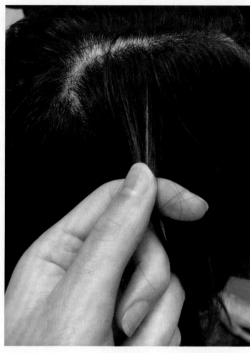

FIGURE 31.1. Firmly pull on the hair, slowly sliding your fingers down the hair shaft. Avoid pulling forcefully or too quickly. Photo courtesy of Catherine Gupta Warner, MD.

- Count the loose hairs. Any broken hairs should be discarded.
- If more than two loose telogen hairs are present, the hair pull test is positive.
- Repeat the steps so that the test is performed at the vertex, bilateral parietal, and occipital scalp.
- Examine loose hairs under the microscope using a clear tape to hold the hairs in place. The presence of two or more telogen hairs or one or more anagen hairs is positive (see Chapter 40. Hair Microscopy).

SUGGESTED READINGS

Gordon KA, Tosti A. Alopecia: evaluation and treatment. *Clin Cosmet Investig Dermatol*. 2011;4:101–106.

Hillmann K, Blume-Peytavi U. Diagnosis of hair disorders. *Semin Cutan Med Surg*. 2009;28:33–38.

McDonald KA, Shelley AJ, Colantonio S, Beecker J. Hair pull test: evidence-based update and revision of guidelines. *J Am Acad Dermatol*. 2017;76(3):472–477.

Towersey L. Hair disorders. *InnovAiT*. 2011;4:63–74.

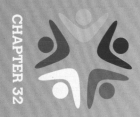

CHAPTER 32

Nail Matrix Biopsy

Jane Sanders Bellet

Introduction

A nail matrix biopsy is undertaken to diagnose conditions arising in the nail matrix. Longitudinal melanonychia is the most common indication. Psoriasis involving the matrix, lichen planus, erythronychia, and onychomatricoma can also be diagnosed with a nail matrix biopsy. A longitudinal pigmented band of the nail plate can arise at any age. In children, this almost always signifies a nevus; however, melanoma is the concern and a biopsy distinguishes between the two. There are two primary methods to obtain a nail matrix specimen: punch biopsy or matrix shave biopsy. Matrix shave can be used in any circumstance; however, the punch technique should only be employed for lesions less than 3 mm wide.

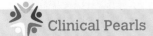

Clinical Pearls

- **Guidelines:** No specific biopsy guidelines exist for melanonychia.
- **Age-Specific Considerations:** Local versus general anesthesia. As a general rule, children younger than age 12 will require general anesthesia and, in certain circumstances, even older adolescents may also require general anesthesia. Some physicians do these procedures on young children with the initial use of topical anesthetic under occlusion for 2 hours.
- **Technique Tips:**
  - To decrease risk of ischemia, use minimal anesthetic volume.
  - Bandage in a "longitudinal" manner to avoid ischemia.
  - Removal of tourniquet should be done only by the operating surgeon to ensure removal.

Contraindications/Cautions/Risks

Cautions
- Nail dystrophy may result from nail matrix biopsy; however, superficial and distal matrix procedures usually heal quite well. In a worst-case scenario, if the matrix is fully ablated, a fully split nail will occur.

Risks
- Pain, dysesthesia, bleeding, ischemia that leads to gangrene and possible amputation, infection, drainage, septic arthritis or osteomyelitis if the joint space is violated, flexor or extensor tendon injury (should not be encountered in usual matrix biopsies), scarring, nail dystrophy.

Equipment Needed
- Local anesthetic (ropivacaine or lidocaine)
- Ethyl chloride spray and/or vibrating massager
- Sterile scrub, such as chlorhexidine (surgical scrub brush is easy to use)
- Tourniquet (T-ring tourniquet or Penrose drain and hemostat)

- Sterile drapes
- Freer nail elevator
- English anvil action nail splitter
- 15 blade scalpel (preferably Teflon coated)
- Forceps (Adson or Castro-Viejo)
- Needle driver
- Suture (5-0 rapidly absorbing suture)
- Hemostat
- Scissors to cut suture (iris, Gradle, etc.)
- Cotton-tipped swabs
- 4 × 4 gauze
- Pathology cassette with nail map, sponges, mesh bag ("tea bag")
- Formalin container
- Gel foam (potentially)
- Electrocautery (usually not needed)
- Hypafix tape (or other strong tape)
- 2 × 2 gauze
- Mastisol (or other adhesive)
- Stockinette (small sizes)
- Splint (potentially)

Preprocedural Approach

- Examination of all 20 nails is critical because this may aid in diagnosis even without a biopsy.
- If the condition affects more than one nail, then a toenail should typically be selected over a fingernail, and a smaller nail (fourth or fifth) should typically be selected over a larger nail (first, second, and third). Such an approach should pose less of a functional problem and should help mitigate issues of cosmesis postoperatively.
- Photographs before the procedure to document the lesion as well as the appearance of the entire nail unit are useful.

Procedural Approach

- Informed consent should be obtained from the parent/guardian before any nail procedure.
- Often, both a digital and wing block are placed, although for most procedures a wing block is sufficient (see Chapter 11. Simple Wound Repair for traditional digital nerve block, dorsal three-sided ring block, and volar three-sided ring block). These blocks are placed using local anesthetic. Some providers prefer plain 1% lidocaine; some prefer 1% lidocaine with epinephrine or ropivacaine 0.2% to 1%. Still others prefer a mixture of short- and long-acting local anesthetics such as 0.5% lidocaine and 0.25% bupivacaine, which provides for further anesthesia after the procedure. The actual volume of local anesthetic injected must be monitored carefully because there is a risk of ischemia due to pressure created by the given volume itself, especially if the anesthetic is inadvertently infiltrated as a total ring block. The smallest volume possible should be used. Most digital and wing blocks are fully functional with 1 mL or less of local anesthetic. If more anesthesia is needed, very careful attention should be paid to the total volume.

- For awake patients, the injections of a digital and wing block are much better tolerated with the use of ethyl chloride spray before each injection, as well as the use of a vibrating massager, which uses the gate theory in reducing pain perception.
- There are multiple techniques for digital blocks. One of the simplest and safest is to use a 30-gauge needle on a 3-mL syringe, with the first injection of the digital block placed in the interdigital web space into the subcutaneous fat in the middle of the proximal phalanx. This then is repeated on the other side of the digit.
- A *wing block* can be placed in addition to a digital block or as a stand-alone block (Figure 32.1). A wing block is placed with the first injection 2 to 3 mm proximal to the lateral proximal nail fold; this is then repeated on the opposite side. Then, a point 1 to 2 mm proximal to the center of the proximal nail fold is infiltrated. Each side of the lateral nail fold more distally is injected and then finally the eponychium in three separate sites. At this point, the functionality of the block should be checked in an awake patient.
- Once the digit is fully anesthetized, the entire hand or foot is cleansed with surgical scrub. A chlorhexidine surgical scrub brush works well.
- The hand or foot is then draped sterilely. In an older child or adolescent, a sterile glove can be pulled over the entire hand; however, this technique does not work well in smaller patients, nor very well for toenails. A fenestrated drape is often useful to isolate the single digit on which the procedure will be done.
- Marking the nail lesion (melanonychia, etc.) with a marking pen on the proximal and distal cutaneous skin is often useful because sometimes no lesion, pigment, or other identifying features can be seen once the overlying nail plate has been removed.
- Nail surgery must be performed in a bloodless field; therefore, a tourniquet is often needed. There are a number of different ways in which to apply a tourniquet. One method: snip the tip of the sterile glove that is already in place on the patient's hand

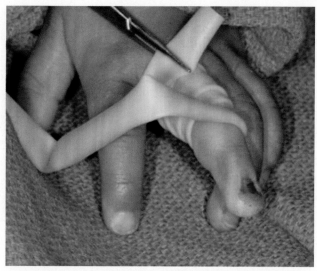

FIGURE 32.2. Tourniquet using a Penrose drain and hemostat.

and roll back the finger of the glove to the base of the digit. The residual material of the glove finger can then be clamped with a hemostat. Alternatively, the flat side of a small Penrose drain can be wrapped from the most distal aspect of the digit to the base of the digit and then clamped using a mosquito or Halsted hemostat (Figure 32.2). The more distal portion is then unwrapped, effectively exsanguinating the digit. Even more effective is the proprietary "T-ring" tourniquet (Figure 32.3) (Precision Medical Devices, LLC, Thousand Oaks, CA), which provides equal pressure circumferentially, as well as a more predictably bloodless field. The biggest risk with tourniquet use is ischemia due to lack of oxygen delivery leading to acidosis. The shortest amount of time a tourniquet is in place, the better. Monitoring the exact amount of time a tourniquet is in place is very important; therefore, an assistant should mark the starting and ending time. In general, 20 minutes should be sufficient for a matrix biopsy and clinically important ischemia is unlikely at times less than this as

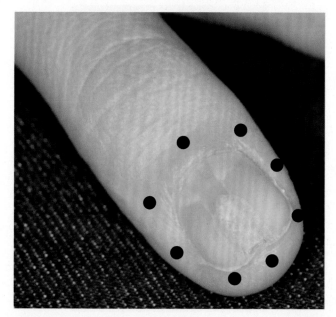

FIGURE 32.1. Wing block. The black circles indicate the injection points for a full wing block. Starting at a proximal lateral corner and then alternating side to side, the anesthetic will diffuse, allowing for less pain with each subsequent injection. The final injection is at the central tip of the digit, just distal to the free edge of the nail plate.

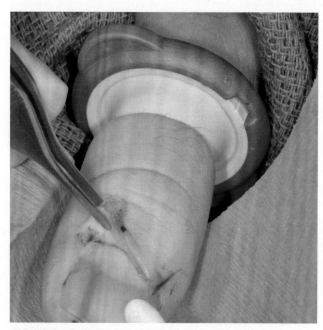

FIGURE 32.3. T-ring tourniquet.

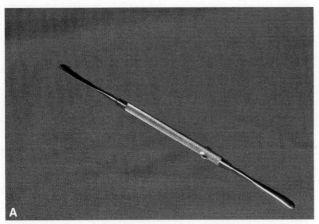

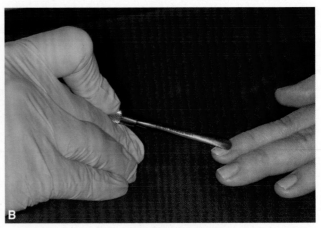

FIGURE 32.4. A, Freer nail elevator. B, A Freer nail elevator is used to separate (elevate) soft tissues from hard surfaces. In this instance, the proximal and lateral nail folds from the nail plate.

long as a small volume of local anesthetic was used. Procedure times longer than 30 minutes often require release of the tourniquet and then reapplication, often at 20 minutes into the procedure.

There are two primary methods to obtain a nail matrix specimen: punch biopsy or matrix shave biopsy.

PUNCH BIOPSY

This can be done with or without nail avulsion. Sometimes it is preferable to submit the nail plate for histopathologic evaluation, in which case a punch biopsy directly through the nail plate to the matrix or bed is performed. Otherwise, to visualize the matrix, bilateral reflecting incisions at the junction of the proximal and lateral nail folds are often required. These incisions run from the lateral proximal nail fold more proximolaterally either straight or on a diagonal. The proximal nail fold is then gently loosened, first, with a Freer nail elevator (Figure 32.4) and then with a 15 blade scalpel or iris scissors; a skin hook can then be used to reflect the proximal nail fold and visualize the matrix. A 3-mm trephine is used for a punch biopsy of the matrix or bed to a superficial depth of less than 1 mm, although often specimens are taken down to bone, because there is no subcutaneous fat in this location (Figure 32.5). Closure of this small defect is usually not required, especially when the site is more distal. If reflecting incisions were placed, then the skin flaps should be returned to anatomic position and each side sutured using either 5-0 polypropylene or 5-0 fast-absorbing 910 polyglactin suture. Absorbable suture is usually preferable because the patient does not need to return for suture removal. A larger trephine size runs the risk of causing permanent dystrophy, especially if taken from the proximal matrix without careful approximation of the edges. If the lesion is larger than 3 mm, the matrix shave technique should be used.

MATRIX SHAVE BIOPSY

For lesions larger than 3 mm, the matrix shave is often a good option, because the nail matrix can be very superficially excised using the nail matrix shave technique as described by Haneke. To visualize the entire matrix without full nail avulsion, partial proximal nail plate avulsion is needed. The proximal nail fold is reflected as described earlier. A Freer nail elevator is used to loosen both the proximal and lateral nail folds (Figure 32.4). An

English anvil-action nail splitter is then placed in the lateral sulcus underneath the nail plate (Figure 32.6). A horizontal cut of the nail plate is then made. This can go across one quadrant, or the entire width of the nail. A hemostat is then attached laterally and then "rolled" over the bed, allowing excellent visualization of the matrix as well as the proximal nail bed (Figure 32.7). If needed for histopathologic evaluation, this piece of plate can be removed completely. The matrix to be sampled is scored in a very shallow manner ($<$1 mm), in a rectangular shape, using a Teflon-coated 15 blade scalpel and then the specimen is cut at the base using the scalpel in a manner parallel to the specimen (Figure 32.7) while gentle pressure is applied with a cotton-tipped applicator. The specimen is then oriented either directly on a nail diagram and/or inked and placed in a pathology cassette so that the orientation is preserved (Figure 32.8).

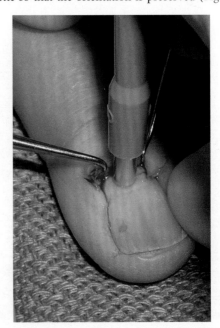

FIGURE 32.5. Punch biopsy of nail matrix. Reprinted from Jellinek N. Nail matrix biopsy of longitudinal melanonychia: diagnostic algorithm including the matrix shave biopsy. *J Am Acad Dermatol.* 2007;56(5):803-810. Copyright © 2007 American Academy of Dermatology, Inc. With permission.

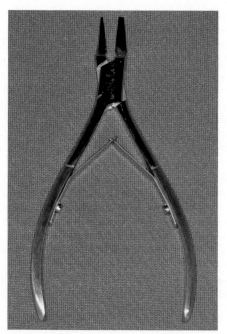

FIGURE 32.6. An English anvil-action nail splitter.

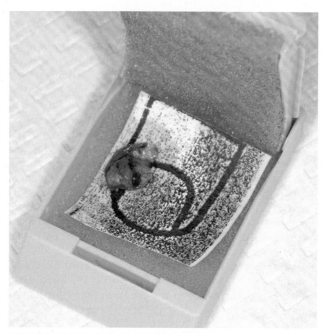

FIGURE 32.8. Pathology cassette with nail map for specimen orientation.

No suture placement of the defect is required. The specimen is so superficial (<1 mm) that there is not usually resultant nail dystrophy, particularly if the location is in the distal matrix. The nail plate should be replaced into anatomic position and sutured with either 5-0 polypropylene or 5-0 fast absorbing 910 polyglactin suture (Figure 32.9), taking care to suture the skin side first and then through the nail plate to avoid the possibility of a foreign body reaction secondary to nail plate being embedded in the skin. Alternatively, Steri-Strips and Mastisol (Ferndale

Laboratories Inc., Ferndale, MI) can be used to secure the plate. The patient/parent should be advised that this nail will eventually be shed. Replacement of the nail into anatomic position allows for greater comfort, protects the underlying tissue, and leads to more rapid healing. The reflecting incisions should be

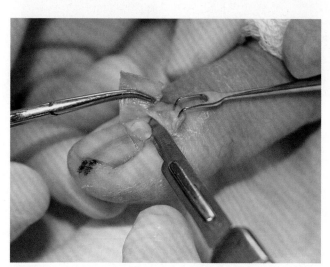

FIGURE 32.7. Nail matrix shave. A hemostat is attached laterally and "rolled" over the bed, providing excellent visualization of the matrix as well as the proximal nail bed. A Teflon-coated no. 15 blade is used to score around the matrix pigment in a very shallow manner (<1 mm) and then cut parallel to the specimen. Reprinted from Jellinek N. Nail matrix biopsy of longitudinal melanonychia: diagnostic algorithm including the matrix shave biopsy. *J Am Acad Dermatol.* 2007;56(5):803-810. Copyright © 2007 American Academy of Dermatology, Inc. With permission.

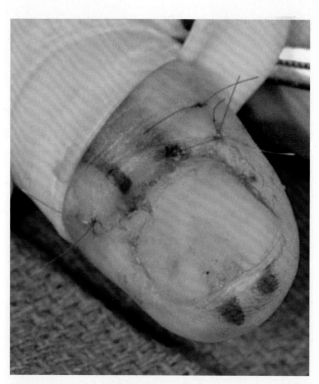

FIGURE 32.9. The nail plate and proximal nail fold are carefully returned to their original anatomic positions and suturing is performed "skin side first" and then through the nail plate to avoid the possibility of a foreign body reaction.

sutured using either 5-0 polypropylene or 5-0 fast absorbing 910 polyglactin suture.

- Once the nail procedure is complete, the tourniquet is released by the surgeon and the time noted for "tourniquet time." Blood flow should be immediate. Depending on the extent of the procedure, and whether or not epinephrine was used, bleeding may be significant or not. Electrocautery is to be avoided if possible, because destruction of the nail matrix can cause nail dystrophy. Even with active bleeding, the digit can usually be bandaged. This is in contrast to cutaneous excisional surgery. If the bleeding seems excessive, pressure can be held for 10 minutes before bandaging and then a piece of Gelfoam (Pharmacia and Upjohn Company, Kalamazoo, MI) can be placed over the site and then bandaging can proceed. Pressure should be held by compressing the distal interphalangeal (DIP) joint laterally on both sides, so that the digital arteries are occluded.

- For procedures of the nail unit, many different bandaging methods exist. One method includes application of a small piece of petrolatum gauze or bismuth tribromophenate-impregnated gauze (Xeroform™ [Covidien/Medtronic]), followed by regular gauze, and then tape. Another technique includes application of plain petrolatum, then a nonstick pad such as Telfa (Covidien LP, Mansfield, MA), then regular gauze, and then tape. Tape application often requires an adhesive such as Mastisol and should only be done in a longitudinal manner to prevent postoperative ischemia of the digit (Figure 32.10A and B). Because the patient is either under general anesthesia or cannot sense how much pressure is being applied because of a block, circumferential bandaging is not advisable. Tubular gauze or stockinette can provide a snug cohesive final layer (Figure 32.10C). The patient is then monitored for approximately 15 to 20 minutes to ensure there is no bleeding through the bandage. Patients given general anesthesia are rechecked in recovery before discharge. If there is excessive bleeding through the bandage at this point, a new bandage should be reapplied. If there is just a small area of bleeding, that part of the bandage can be reinforced with more gauze.

- Finger or toe splints can also be used and in certain situations are more useful a few days after the procedure to help protect the digit from unintended trauma. An orthopedic shoe can be used for toenail procedures.

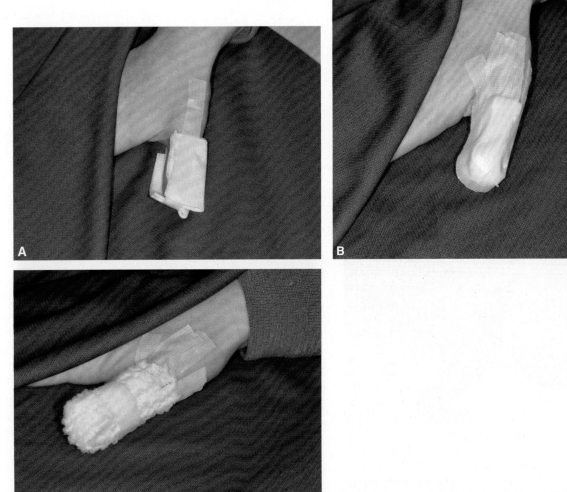

FIGURE 32.10. A, B, Longitudinal bandaging with Mastisol, gauze, and tape. C, Bandage with stockinette. Final appearance.

Postprocedural Approach

- Patients should keep their hand or foot elevated on the way home. For those older adolescents who may be able to drive, it is important that someone else drive them home.
- Sometimes there is already bleeding through the bandage on the day of the procedure, in which case the patient should either reinforce that portion of the bandage if possible or re-apply the entire bandage.
- Postoperative pain management is very important. Nail procedures can be very painful postoperatively as the blocks wear off. Acetaminophen should be given on arrival at home. Ibuprofen alternating with acetaminophen can be used and is often quite effective. Narcotic pain medications such as oxycodone may be required for 1 to 3 days, because there can be significant throbbing for the first 36 hours postoperatively. Alternating these two agents often works well. If pain is not under good control and continues to be significant, the patient should be evaluated to assess for causes of pain, including subungual hematoma. For 1 to 3 weeks postoperatively, there can be dull pain at the surgical site.
- Daily wound care is required, usually starting 48 hours after the nail matrix biopsy. Soaking the bandage off in a bath or bowl of warm water facilitates the process. Epsom salts or regular table salt can be added to the water if desired.
- Bleach or vinegar soaks are not needed. The finger or toe should be gently dried and Vaseline™ (Conopco, Inc., US) applied to the nail unit.
- The entire nail unit should then be rebandaged. At this point, this can be done circumferentially because the patient has full sensation and can sense if the bandage is too tight and potentially causing ischemia. Bandaging daily is done for a number of reasons: to prevent infection; collect drainage; and to provide protection from inadvertent trauma and subsequent pain.
- More padding will be required in the first week because there usually is more drainage; this diminishes with time. Often, bandaging is necessary for 3 to 4 weeks, because of drainage, especially of the great toe.

SUGGESTED READINGS

Collins SC, Cordova K, Jellinek NJ. Alternatives to complete nail plate avulsion. *J Am Acad Dermatol.* 2008;59(4):619–626.

Jellinek J. Nail matrix biopsy of longitudinal melanonychia: diagnostic algorithm including the matrix shave biopsy. *J Am Acad Dermatol.* 2007;56(5):803–810.

Richert B, Theunis A, Norrenberg S, Andre J. Tangential excision of pigmented nail matrix lesions responsible for longitudinal melanonychia: evaluation of the technique on a series of 30 patients. *J Am Acad Dermatol.* 2013;69(1):96–104.

CHAPTER 33

Patch Testing for Allergic Contact Dermatitis

Catalina Matiz and Shehla Admani

INTRODUCTION

Allergic contact dermatitis (ACD) is a type IV T-cell-mediated hypersensitivity reaction that occurs following an initial allergen exposure with subsequent sensitization. ACD occurs mainly from contact exposure through the skin; however, reactions through systemic exposure (eg, oral ingestion, medical devices, and injections) can also be seen.

Patch testing is the gold standard for diagnosing ACD. The goal of this procedure is to reproduce the effects of topical exposure to the suspected allergen by generating a skin reaction with erythema, edema, and, occasionally, vesiculation.

Although patch testing is the gold standard for the diagnosis of ACD, it can be quite cumbersome to perform in children, especially in those younger than 6 years of age. The main areas of concern regarding patch testing in the pediatric population include poor tolerability of the procedure, small back space for placement of patches, length of patch application, risk of sensitization, and worsening of existing dermatitis.

T.R.U.E. TEST® VERSUS COMPREHENSIVE PATCH TESTING

Patch testing can be performed using either commercially available premanufactured Thin-layer Rapid-Use Epicutaneous (T.R.U.E. test® [Allerderm, Phoenix, AZ]) test panels (SmartPractice, Phoenix, AZ) or through comprehensive patch testing (Figure 33.1). There are advantages and limitations to the use of either test.

The T.R.U.E. test, which was recently granted U.S. Food and Drug Administration (FDA) approval to be used in children older than 6 years of age, has the advantage that it is commercially available and is easy to use; however, it has a limited number of allergens (currently 35). Some of the common allergens in children (eg, propylene glycol and cocamidopropyl betaine) are not present in the T.R.U.E. test panels and, as a result, this test can fail to detect up to 40% of the reactions in children, as noted by Jacob et al.[1]

The greatest advantage of comprehensive patch testing is that the allergens included in the testing can be tailored to each child, knowing their individual exposure history and pattern of

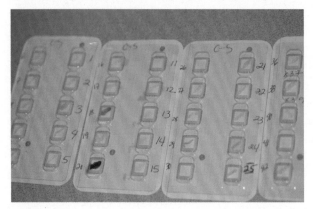

FIGURE 33.1 An example of comprehensive patch testing using panels tailor-made to the child based on individual exposure history and pattern of dermatitis.

dermatitis. This custom approach allows avoidance of allergens that the child has not yet been exposed to, which can decrease the potential risk of sensitization. A recent panel of experts in pediatric patch testing proposed a 38-allergen "baseline" pediatric series; all included allergens are listed in Table 33.1.[2] In addition to commercial allergens, it is also best to test the patients' own products to increase the yield of a positive reaction.

PREPATCH TEST COUNSELING

The success of patch testing in children is dependent on the prepatch test counseling. Parents and children may not have an adequate understanding of the procedure, resulting in anxiety and failure to follow through with the testing process. Risks of the procedure, including the possibility of sensitization, exacerbation of dermatitis, postinflammatory pigmentation, persistent inflammatory reactions, infection, and the possibility of a negative result, need to be fully discussed with the parents as part of the informed consent process. In addition, a detailed explanation of the patch testing procedure is essential in obtaining successful results. For example, systemic immunosuppressants and topical medications such as corticosteroids and calcineurin inhibitors must be discontinued at least 3 days before patch test application because of the risk of false-negative reactions.[3] Also, the patient should not shower nor participate in any intense physical activity while the patches are in place to avoid wetting the patches and altering the chemical concentrations.

Procedural Approach

- The allergen concentration recommended for use in children is the same as that used in adults, with the exception of formaldehyde, nickel, and rubber chemicals, which should be applied in lower concentrations to decrease atypical skin reactions, as suggested by some experts.[4]
- During the application process, it is important to keep the child distracted and comfortable. The use of tablets, smart phones, and other such devices can help distract the child at the time of patch application and removal[5] (Figure 33.2).
- If the patient has areas of dermatitis on the back, the authors recommend that those be marked with a marking pen and avoid application of the allergens on these areas to prevent false-positive reactions (Figure 33.3).
- Patches should be applied to the upper back whenever possible because this body site has been shown to have the least false-negative reactions. Because children have smaller backs than do adults, this can limit the number of chemicals that can be tested, and in certain circumstances, application of additional patches on the arms or legs may also be needed.
- It is advised to mark the location of the patches on the patient's back with a skin marking pen as well as creating a map with the location of the allergens. This is extremely important to prevent confusion in case the patches are inadvertently moved.
- Once the patches are in place, it is also recommended to secure them with an extra layer of hypoallergenic tape, such as Hypafix (Figure 33.4).

TABLE 33.1 ⁝ Proposed Pediatric 38-Allergen "Baseline" Panel

Metals
Nickel sulfate
Cobalt chloride

Antibiotics
Neomycin
Bacitracin

Fragrances
Balsam of Peru
Fragrance mix I
Fragrance mix II
Cinnamic aldehyde

Formaldehyde releasing preservatives
Quaternium 15
DMDM hydantoin
Formaldehyde
Diazolidinyl urea
Imidazolidinyl urea
Bronopol

Other nonformaldehyde preservatives
Methylchloroisothiazolinone/methylisothiazolinone (MCI/MI)
Methylisothiazolinone (MI)
Propylene glycol
Iodopropynyl butylcarbamate
Paraben mix

Surfactants
Amidoamine
Cocamidopropyl betaine
Dimethylaminopropylamine
Decyl glucoside

Corticosteroids
Tixocortol-21-pivalate
Hydrocortisone-17-butyrate budesonide
Clobetasol 17 propionate
Budesonide

Sunscreen
Benzophenone 3

Dyes
Carmine

Emollients
Amerchol L101

Rubber accelerators
Carba mix
Thiuram mix

Adhesive
p-tert-Butylphenol formaldehyde resin

Plant derived "natural" allergens
Compositae mix
Sesquiterpene lactones
Propolis
Tea tree oil
Colophony

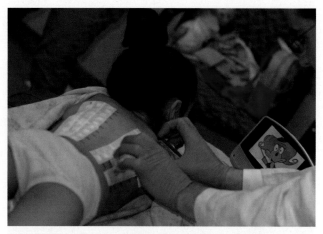

FIGURE 33.2. The use of tablets, smart phones, and other such devices can help distract the child at the time of patch application and removal.

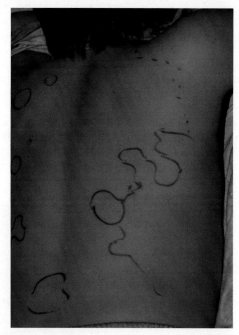

FIGURE 33.3. If the patient has dermatitis on the back, it is recommended to mark the affected areas and to avoid application of the allergens within the affected boundaries in order to prevent false-positive reactions.

PEDIATRIC PATCH TESTING PROTOCOL

- Patches should be left in place for 48 hours, except in very young children in whom it is advisable to remove patches after 24 hours.[6]
- After removal of the patches, the authors advise that the locations of the patches be marked a second time with a yellow fluorescent marker with the help of a Wood's lamp (see Chapter 38. Wood's Lamp Skin Examination) to enable allergen identification on reading day (Figure 33.5).
- Immediately after patch removal, it is best to wait a couple of minutes for any erythematous reactions caused directly by tape removal to fade before performing the first diagnostic interpretation (ie, the "read").

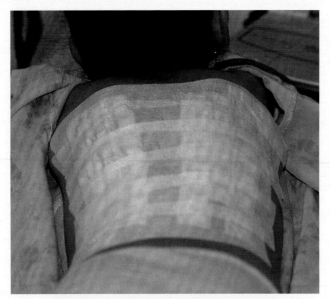

FIGURE 33.4. Also recommend securing patches with an extra layer of hypoallergenic tape, such as Hypafix.

- A second reading is performed after 72 to 96 hours and a third reading at 7 days is strongly advised because late delayed reactions can occur.
- Reactions that are noticed on patch test removal day and persist in a crescendo (ie, worsening) pattern are most likely allergic rather than irritant in nature. Irritant reactions tend to fade subsequent to patch removal.

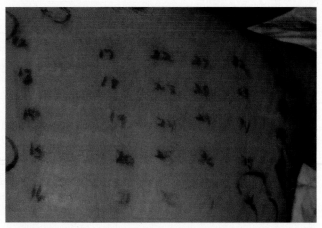

FIGURE 33.5. After removal of patches, mark the patch locations a second time with a yellow fluorescent marker with the help of a Wood's lamp to enable allergen identification on reading day.

GRADING OF PATCH TEST REACTIONS

Patch test reactions are graded as negative (−), doubtful (?), weak positive (+), strong positive (++), extreme positive (+++), and irritant (IR) following the International Contact Dermatitis Group (ICDRG) scoring system (Figure 33.6).

ACD is defined as a positive patch test reaction that is clinically relevant to the patient's exposure history and dermatitis and that can be reproduced after reintroducing the causative allergen. After determining a positive reaction, the patient's products should be reviewed to identify the source of exposure.

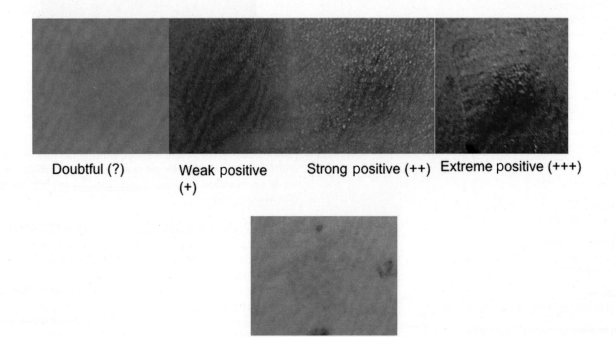

FIGURE 33.6. Patch test reactions are graded as negative (−), doubtful (?), weak positive (+), strong positive (++), extreme positive (+++), and irritant (IR) following the International Contact Dermatitis Group (ICDRG) scoring system.

TABLE 33.2 ⦂ Allergic Contact Dermatitis Resources for Patient/Parents

Chemotechnique	www.chemotechnique.se
T.R.U.E. Test	www.truetest.com
Smart Practice	www.allergeaze.com
American Contact Dermatitis Society (ACDS)	www.contactderm.org
Preventice	www.allergyfreeskin.com
Videos	www.mypatchlink.com
CAMP	www.acdscamp.org

Also, the patient's home environment and hobbies need to be explored because exposure in these settings may occur. Once the source of exposure to the positive allergen has been identified, education on proper avoidance, other possible sources for the allergen(s), as well as cross-reactors should be discussed. Safe alternatives should be reviewed and easy-to-read printed material and online resources should be shared with the patient and parents to achieve compliance (Table 33.2). The authors recommend providing the patient with a copy of the safe allergen alternative product list from the contact allergen management program, better known as CAMP, available at the American Contact Dermatitis Society website (www.contactderm.org).[7]

TREATMENT APPROACH TO POSITIVE TEST REACTIONS

The authors recommend treatment of positive reaction(s) and active dermatitis with topical corticosteroids, and in cases of severe reactions/dermatitis, systemic corticosteroids should be considered at the conclusion of patch testing. Improvement of the dermatitis after avoidance and adequate treatment may take up to 6 to 8 weeks. It is best to see the patient again in clinic 8 to 12 weeks after patch testing to address improvement and compliance. If the patient has not noticed improvement or has worsening of his or her dermatitis, depending on the putative allergen, other sources of exposure such as diet or medications should be investigated. The relevance of dietary allergen exposure has been highlighted in cases of nickel, cobalt, balsam of Peru, and propylene glycol, among others, which can cause systemic contact dermatitis and in which limiting oral intake of the allergen may improve the patient's symptoms.[8]

REFERENCES

1. Jacob SE, Brankov N, Kerr A. Diagnosis and management of allergic contact dermatitis in children: common allergens that can be easily missed. *Curr Opin Pediatr.* 2017;29(4):443–447.
2. Yu J, Atwater AR, Brod B, et al. Pediatric baseline patch test series: initial findings of the pediatric contact dermatitis workgroup. *Dermatitis.* 2018;29:206–212.
3. Green C. The effect of topically applied corticosteroid on irritant and allergic patch test reactions. *Contact Dermatitis.* 1996;35:331–333.
4. Mortz C, Andersen KE. Allergic contact dermatitis in children and adolescents. *Contact Dermatitis.* 1999;41:121–130.
5. Jacob, SE. Avoid the shriek with Shrek: video-distraction assist for pediatric patch testing. *Dermatitis.* 2007;18(3):179–180.
6. Worm M, Aberer W, Agathos M, et al. Patch testing in children—recommendations of the German Contact Dermatitis Research Group (DKG). *J Dtsch Dermatol Ges.* 2007;5(2):107–109.
7. Scheman A, Severson D. American Contact Dermatitis society contact allergy management program: an epidemiologic tool to quantify ingredient usage. *Dermatitis.* 2016;27(1):11–13.
8. Veien NK. Systemic contact dermatitis. *Int J Dermatol.* 2011; 50(12):1445–1456.

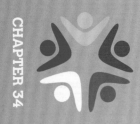

CHAPTER 34

Pinworm Examination

Jessica Sprague, Catherine Gupta Warner, Kimberly Ann Chun, and Sheila Fallon Friedlander

Introduction

Pinworms, also known as *Enterobius vermicularis*, are small nematodes living in the lower gastrointestinal tract of humans. Infestation of pinworms most commonly occurs in young children, affecting those aged 5 to 10 years of age. Most patients are asymptomatic; however, infestation can also cause restlessness or irritability. In addition, *E. vermicularis* can cause pruritus ani (itching around the anus). The itching, caused by an inflammatory reaction in response to the worm and its eggs on the skin, is typically worse at night and may cause difficulty sleeping. The nighttime pruritus is a result of the female adult pinworm leaving the anus at night to lay eggs onto the perianal skin. Occasionally, the adult worms migrate to the vagina, leading to vaginitis. Scratching the skin may lead to superimposed bacterial infections, such as impetigo, and severe infestations may rarely result in abdominal pain, nausea, and vomiting. Pinworms are spread when the eggs are lodged underneath fingernails after scratching the anus. Individuals who unknowingly ingest the eggs then become infested.

Clinical Pearls

- **Technique Tips:** The sticky tape test is best performed at night when the female worms are most active.
- **Treatment includes the following:**
  - Prevention of infection is accomplished by frequent handwashing with soap and water, taking a shower or bath daily, frequently trimming fingernails, washing bedsheets and clothing, and avoidance of scratching.
  - Mild infestations may be self-limiting; however *E. vermicularis* infections are typically treated with 2 doses of albendazole, mebendazole, or pyrantel pamoate, 2 weeks apart. Bedsheets should be washed and bedroom vacuumed after each dose.
  - Because reinfection is common, the whole family can be treated at the same time to prevent spread of infection and recurrence.

Contraindications/Cautions/Risks

- No specific contraindications

Equipment Needed

- Clear adhesive tape
- Glass slide
- Specimen bag
- Microscope

Procedural Approach

- Because the female worms are most active at night, it is recommended to teach parents to perform the tape test at home.
- Using a 2 × 6-cm-sized rectangle of transparent tape, the adhesive side of the clear tape is placed on perianal skin and pulled off.
- Place the adhesive side down on the glass slide and place in specimen bag to be transported.
- The glass slides are examined under the light microscope for the presence of pinworm eggs.

SUGGESTED READINGS

Amiri SAN, Rahimi MT, Mahdavi SA, et al. Prevalence of *Enterobius vermicularis* infection among preschool children, Babol, North of Iran. *J Parasit Dis.* 2016;40(4):1558–1562. doi:10.1007/s12639-015-0727-4.

Cinotti E, Labeille B, Cambazard F, Dupuis F, Rubegni P, Perrot JL. Noninvasive skin imaging for the diagnosis of myiasis. *J Eur Acad Dermatol Venereol.* 2017;31(8):e365–e366.

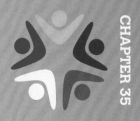

CHAPTER 35

Polymerase Chain Reaction

Jessica Sprague, Catherine Gupta Warner, Kimberly Ann Chun, and Sheila Fallon Friedlander

Introduction

Polymerase chain reaction (PCR) is a molecular biology technique used to amplify a DNA sequence. PCR was developed in 1983 by Kary Mullis, who subsequently won a Nobel Prize in Chemistry in 1993 for this discovery. This technique of DNA amplification has since been applied to numerous fields within modern science. Because significant amounts of a sample of DNA are usually necessary for molecular and genetic analyses, studies of isolated pieces of DNA are almost impossible without PCR. Common applications of PCR include diagnosis of many genetic diseases and the detection of bacterial, viral, and fungal pathogens.

PCR has proved to be a more sensitive and specific method to diagnose many types of infections because only small amounts of DNA are required for testing. Moreover, PCR is often a faster modality than is culture, allowing for earlier diagnosis and treatment of infectious diseases.

 Clinical Pearls

- PCR in dermatology is often performed on skin (herpes simplex virus [HSV], varicella zoster virus [VZV], human papilloma virus [HPV]) or mucosal lesions (upper respiratory pathogens such as cytomegalovirus [CMV], Epstein–Barr virus [EBV], adenovirus, rhinovirus, enterovirus, and parvovirus).
- PCR may also be used as a fast and reliable way to identify *Mycobacterium* species versus the 1 to 2 months it often takes for culture confirmation.
- Other pathogens that may be evaluated by PCR include *Borrelia*, *Leishmania*, *Toxoplasma*, *Treponema*, *Chlamydia*, and *Neisseria*.
- A respiratory viral panel PCR test may be performed to help diagnose many viral-induced rashes in dermatology, including viral exanthem, hand, foot and mouth, herpangina, erythema infectiosum, erythema multiforme, Stevens–Johnson, Giannoti Crosti, as well as others.
- Other newer commercially available panels, such as the Karius test, are able to detect more than 1000 pathogens with one sample.
- The use of alcohol to cleanse the lesion may lead to PCR amplification failure and should be avoided.
- PCR specimens are generally collected using a cotton or Dacron swab with a plastic shaft, which are placed into a tube with a universal or viral transport medium (see Chapter 37. Viral Culture). These mediums contain buffered, isotonic, and balanced salt solution, as well as antibiotics to prevent bacterial contamination.

Contraindications/Cautions

- No specific contraindications
- **Cautions:** In infants and young children who are likely to move during the procedure, make sure to secure the body area from which you are obtaining your sample (either skin or mucosa).

Equipment Needed

- Universal or viral transport medium (used interchangeably)
- Dacron or cotton swab with plastic shaft
- A #15 blade or sterile needle if culture requires unroofing of a vesicle

Procedural Approach

- Acquire the appropriate swab and transport medium bottle needed for testing.
- The tube should be labeled with the patient's pertinent identifying information before collection.
- Choose your desired skin or mucosal (oral, nasal, anal or vaginal/urethral) site.
- Remove the sterile swab from its packaging and rub it along the active lesion.
- If an intact vesicle exists, then use a sterile needle or a #15 blade to unroof the lesion and expose the base. If enough vesicle fluid is available, aspirate the fluid with a fine gauge needle and tuberculin syringe, and place the fluid into cold viral transport medium. Then, use the Dacron or cotton swab with plastic shaft to rub the exposed base vigorously.
- Once the sample has been collected, the swab should be inserted into the transport bottle.
- The swab shaft should then be broken and the cap placed on the tube.
- Collected specimens should be stored immediately in a refrigerator set to 4°C and transported to the laboratory within 24 hours of collection.
- Information that should accompany the sample includes patient name and date of birth, date of collection, specimen source, clinical symptoms or suspected diagnosis, and tests requested by numerical order code and test name.
- During transport, the specimen should be protected from heat with use of a cold or ice pack in a sealed plastic bag.

SUGGESTED READING

Lo AC, Feldman SR. Polymerase chain reaction: basic concepts and clinical applications in dermatology. *J Am Acad Dermatol*. 1994;30(2, pt 1):250–260.

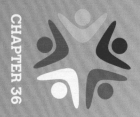

CHAPTER 36

Skin Biopsy Techniques

Samantha L. Schneider, Danielle Yeager, and Marla N. Jahnke

INTRODUCTION

The skin biopsy is an essential part of the diagnosis and management of cutaneous disease. It allows the physician to correlate histologic findings with the physical examination when there is diagnostic uncertainty, and it may provide direct tissue sampling that guides future treatments. Despite the anxiety and discomfort a biopsy may create for pediatric patients, the procedure may be necessary. With the proper preparation of the patient, family, and medical team, nearly all pediatric skin biopsies can be performed in the office utilizing local anesthesia with minimal stress and unwanted sequelae.

BIOPSY SITE AND CHOICE OF BIOPSY TECHNIQUE

The ability to interpret a biopsy depends on the quality of the biopsy sent and the skill of the pathologist interpreting the specimen. Therefore, it is essential that the physician performing the biopsy chooses the site that most accurately reflects the clinical pathology and that this site has not been altered or manipulated by the patient. Furthermore, he or she must perform the appropriate type of biopsy to answer the clinical question at hand. The physician performing the procedure must have an understanding of the differential diagnosis when making these decisions. When a provider does not consider the differential diagnosis before the biopsy, unnecessary additional procedures may follow; for example, a pink papule on the trunk of a child could represent a bite or pyogenic granuloma, but it could also be a Spitz nevus, among other diagnoses. If Spitz nevus is not considered in the differential diagnosis or the provider performing the biopsy does not understand the implications of the potential results, a superficial shave biopsy might be performed, which makes the pathologic interpretation challenging and may lead to significant controversy in management. Pathologists may identify the lesion as having a positive margin requiring a larger, more complicated reexcision, which could have been avoided with conservative excisional biopsy from the outset.

There are multiple biopsying techniques to consider when confronting a lesion in the pediatric patient including curettage, snip excision, saucerization, punch, and incisional or excisional biopsies (see Chapter 4. Billing and Coding in Procedural Pediatric Dermatology).

- *Curettage* can be performed on small, superficial benign lesions involving only the epidermis, such as in verrucae or epidermal nevi (Figure 36.1).
- Alternatively, for pedunculated lesions such as acrochordons or filiform warts, *snip or scissor biopsy* should be considered.
- *Shave or saucerization biopsies* may be performed when lesions involve the epidermis and superficial dermis. Both curettage and shave biopsy can heal by secondary intention with petroleum-based ointment and bandages.
- *Punch biopsies* should be performed when the underlying process is suspected to involve the dermis or subcutaneous fat. This type of biopsy often results in primary closure with simple interrupted sutures, although some providers may prefer

to allow the lesion to heal by secondary intention for small (<2 mm) biopsy sites. Gel foam may be used for hemostasis.
- *Incisional biopsies* allow deeper visualization of the dermis, subcutaneous fat, and, when needed, fascia as well. Indications for incisional biopsies include large tumors and subtle deep disorders of the connective tissue, such as eosinophilic fasciitis.
- Finally, *excisional biopsies* are performed to achieve definitive removal of a lesion and to provide deep visualization down to the level of the subcutaneous fat. An excisional biopsy might be performed when there is suspicion for cutaneous malignancy or for the removal of benign lesions such as epidermoid or pilar cysts. Both incisional and excisional biopsies typically require primary closure, often with deep and superficial layered sutures (Figure 36.2).

In certain situations, multiple biopsies are employed at the same time. A second biopsy, for example, may be performed to send a specimen for direct immunofluorescence (DIF) in addition to standard hematoxylin and eosin (H&E) staining. DIF is helpful in diagnosing blistering disorders in children, such as linear immunoglobulin A (IgA) bullous dermatosis of childhood. In addition, DIF may be performed to aid in the diagnosis of vasculitis, such as Henoch–Schönlein purpura and autoimmune connective tissue diseases such as lupus. When obtaining a specimen for DIF in cases of blistering disorders such as pemphigus foliaceus, the sample should be perilesional. This is in contrast to the specimen obtained for H&E, which is preferred at the edge of a fresh vesicle or bulla. Uniquely,

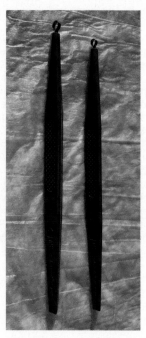

FIGURE 36.1. Instruments for curette biopsy. Photo courtesy of Andrew C. Krakowski, MD.

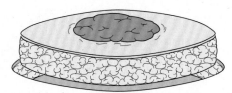

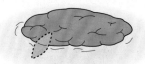

Excisional biopsy   Incisional biopsy

FIGURE 36.2. Excisional biopsy versus incisional biopsy. Excisional biopsy completely excises the lesion with a rim of normal tissue. It extends down to the subcutaneous tissue to be able to measure the depth of the lesion. Incisional biopsy excises a portion of the margin of the lesion with a segment of normal tissue. Reprinted with permission from Jarrell B. *NMS Surgery Casebook*. 2nd ed. Philadelphia, PA: Wolters Kluwer; 2015. Figure 10.1.

when assessing for dermatitis herpetiformis with DIF, the biopsy is performed from nearby normal skin, not necessarily perilesional. In contrast, when evaluating for vasculitis or autoimmune connective tissue disorders, DIF can be sent from biopsies of lesions directly. It is recommended that biopsies for DIF are obtained from more proximal lesions to avoid distracting changes that may occur in sites of high hydrostatic pressure. In addition, in vasculitis, it is important to sample "fresh" lesions that developed, ideally, within the last 24 to 48 hours. All DIF specimens should be placed in Michel's transport medium (or something similar) or sent "stat" to the laboratory on saline-soaked gauze.

PATIENT PREPARATION AND PREPROCEDURE STRATEGIES

Taking the time to properly prepare for a procedure on a child ensures safety and allows for efficiency.

- Before performing any procedure, *it is important to discuss the risks, benefits, technique, and potential complications with parents and patients*, when applicable. An important consideration in the pediatric population is a discussion of visible scarring, prompting an important discussion about realistic expectations. After a thorough discussion, consent should be obtained from the parent or legal guardian of the child. When possible, assent should be obtained from the patient, as well.
- It is the authors' opinion that *preoperative photos should be taken in all cases after obtaining verbal parental consent*. An in-focus "away" photo that provides anatomic location and a well-lit, in-focus "close" photo that provides morphologic detail and regional landmarks are a minimum. These photographs allow for better clinical pathologic correlation and aid in appropriate monitoring at follow-up. They also help ensure optimum patient safety (ie, confirming the correct anatomic site for a procedure) and are helpful if and when a photograph is required for a future publication.
- The *biopsy site should be clearly marked* to ensure sampling of the correct area. Critically, all marking should be completed before delivery of local anesthesia because lesions may become less apparent—even obscured—after infiltration.
- *Strong consideration should be given to patient comfort and positioning*. Although not all physicians prefer parents to remain in the room, it can be helpful for calming the patient. With pediatric patients, it is helpful to position them lying down comfortably with their parents in sight, often at the head of the examination table for comfort and distraction. This technique eases procedural anxiety for the patient and allows parents to assist in keeping the child static during the procedure. Some pediatric dermatologists and surgeons recommend the

use of a papoose board to safely secure children temporarily during the procedure; this, however, is physician and patient dependent. Likewise, patients who are likely to move or become uncooperative can be wrapped with sheets "burrito" style.

- Another consideration involves *where to place the surgical tray*. The surgical tray, with its various sharp-bladed instruments and pointy needles, may itself cause significant anxiety in the pediatric patient. Instruments are best kept under a drape and out of immediate reach of children, and anesthesia is best kept out of the patient's sight until the moment it is ready to be administered (Figure 36.3).
- Once the patient and room are prepared, the *next step is a procedural "time out" to confirm the patient identity and biopsy site*. The surgical team should confirm that everyone and everything is in place before injecting anesthesia to ensure safety and optimize clinical outcomes. Teamwork is critical to this process, and staff should be well trained and well prepared.

ANESTHESIA

Topical anesthetics may be used before the injection of local anesthesia to reduce the discomfort and anxiety of needle penetration in children. To maximize their efficacy, topical anesthetics can be used under occlusion at least 1 hour before the procedure. The most commonly used topical anesthetics are lidocaine and eutectic mixtures of lidocaine and prilocaine. Potential adverse effects of prilocaine to note include methemoglobinemia. Topical anesthetics are considered safe for use when applying to limited body surface areas, but caution should be used if applying large amounts or if treating skin with impaired barrier function. This is especially a concern in neonates and in young children who are at greatest risk for methemoglobinemia. Lidocaine 4% is not U.S. Food and Drug Administration (FDA) approved in children younger than 2 years of age; however, it is commonly used "off label" for this purpose.

Clinical Pearls

- Lidocaine is the most commonly used injectable local anesthetic and can be safely used in children. It is important to keep in mind its onset of action, duration of efficacy, and maximum dosage in pediatric patients to ensure optimal benefit and minimum side effects. Buffering the lidocaine with sodium bicarbonate helps reduce pain associated with infiltration of anesthesia; typically, the ratio that is used for this purpose is 1 mL of 8.4% sodium bicarbonate to 10 mL of 1% lidocaine with epinephrine (1:100 000).

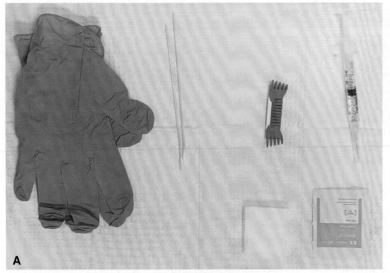
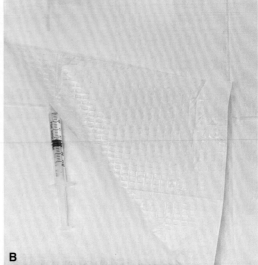

FIGURE 36.3. A, A typical instrument tray used for shave excision or biopsies with all of its sharp instruments can cause tremendous anxiety for patients new to the experience. B, It is recommended to keep the instruments covered and out of reach until the moment they are needed. Photo courtesy of Missy Drayton, DCA.

Other helpful techniques include slowing the rate of infiltration and/or using tactile distraction such as tapping, vibration, or skin cooling with ice or ethyl chloride spray.

For superficial procedures such as curettage and saucerization, care should be taken to ensure superficial infiltration of anesthetic in the dermis noted by the creation of a wheal. Deep subcutaneous infiltration may be needed if a punch biopsy or incisional or excisional biopsy is required. To minimize patient discomfort, deep injections should be performed initially to anesthetize the area with continued injection of the anesthetic as the needle is withdrawn from "deep" to "superficial." Gentle massage may help spread and distribute the anesthetic agent. Stabilization of the patient and distraction are also essential during the injection.

BIOPSY PROCEDURAL TECHNIQUES

The specific procedural technique varies depending on the type of biopsy being performed. Once the patient is positioned and anesthetized, the actual biopsy may be performed. It is critical to keep sharp objects out of sight of the patient as much as possible and to perform the procedure efficiently. For all biopsy procedures, the area should first be cleansed with an antiseptic agent. Then, one of the following biopsy procedures is performed:

- *Curettage:* Use the nondominant hand to stabilize the surrounding tissue and the dominant hand to hold the curette to scrape away the lesion.
- *Snip excision:* Use forceps to handle the specimen and a sharp, curved iris scissor to remove it (Figure 36.4A and B).
- *Shave/saucerization:* Use the nondominant hand to pull the skin taut (for countertraction) and the dominant hand manipulates the blade or scalpel to remove the lesion (Figure 36.5A-C).
- *Punch:* The punch tool rotates between the first and second finger of the dominant hand to remove the skin plug. Angling the tool while pulling it out helps the tissue fall outside of the surrounding skin. Once the skin plug has been freed from the surrounding tissue, gently handle the tissue with forceps,

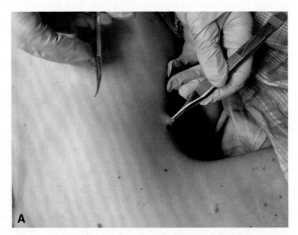
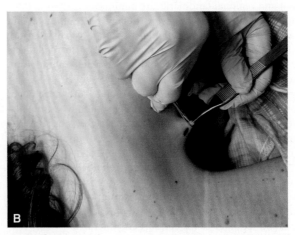

FIGURE 36.4. Snip biopsy technique. A, After cleansing, the skin is anesthetized with 1% lidocaine with 1:100 000 epinephrine and the skin lesion is gently pulled away from the skin surface using forceps. B, The skin lesion is snipped with a pair of Gradle scissors. Reprinted with permission from Crowson AN, Magro CM. *Biopsy Interpretation of the Skin.* 2nd ed. Philadelphia, PA: Wolters Kluwer; 2019. Figure 1-4 B,C.

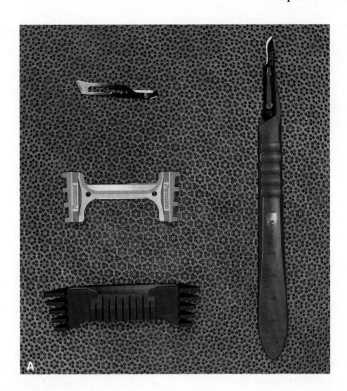

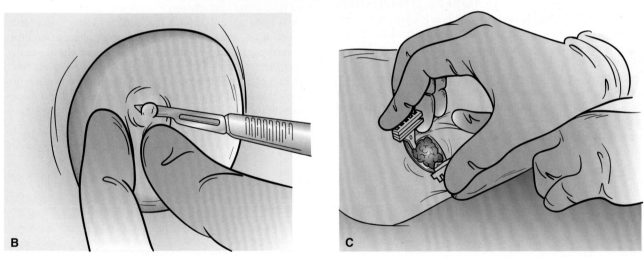

FIGURE 36.5. A, Various instruments, including scalpel blades and flexible blades, are available to aid the clinician in performing a shave biopsy. Photo courtesy of Missy Drayton, DCA. B, Use the nondominant free hand to pull the skin taut (for counter traction) and the dominant hand manipulates the blade/scalpel parallel to the skin surface under the lesion to remove. C, Shave biopsy can also be performed using a flexible blade. Holding the blade tangentially to the skin surface, the blade can remove a sample of the epidermis and dermis. A deeper saucerization requires a sharper angle to the skin, allowing the blade to scoop deep into the dermis.

making sure to avoid crushing the specimen. Iris scissors are then used to free the deep margin (Figure 36.6A and B).

○ PRO TIP: The otherwise round wound that would result from a punch biopsy can be "converted" to something more elliptical in nature by stretching the skin perpendicular to the natural skin tension lines before performing the biopsy. This allows for an oval-shaped defect with minimized redundant skin (Figure 36.6A and B).

○ PRO TIP: If biopsying a pigmented lesion, one can press lightly with the tool before performing the biopsy to score it first to ensure that the entire lesion will reside within the skin plug.

○ PRO TIP: When the biopsy specimen remains tethered at the skin base, the specimen can be stabilized with a needle to allow the specimen to be extruded then snipped at the base with iris scissors.

● *Incisional and excisional:* A scalpel is used to remove a small elliptical wedge of either part of the lesion in question (incisional) or of the entire lesion (excisional). Be sure to hold the scalpel at a 90° angle to the tissue for straight edges that can be cleanly approximated with sutures. Then, either a scalpel or iris scissors can free the deep margin with care taken to ensure an even excision plane.

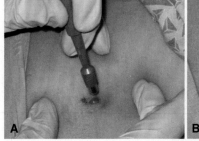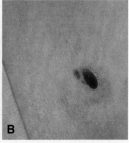

FIGURE 36.6. A, B, Punch biopsy technique for optimal closure. In this clinical scenario, a 6-mm trephine has been selected as the punch biopsy tool. The trephine is held in the dominant hand, as shown, while the middle finger and thumb of the nondominant hand are used to stretch the skin perpendicular to the natural skin tension lines. A circular punch performed with the trephine in this manner results in an oval-shaped (ie, not circular) defect, which will close with minimized redundant/puckered skin ("dog ears"). Reprinted with permission from Schalock PC, Hsu JT, Arndt KA. *Lippincott's Primary Care Dermatology*. Philadelphia, PA: Wolters Kluwer Health/Lippincott Williams & Wilkins; 2010. Figure 3-7.

Labeling and Specimen Storage

After any sample is obtained, it should be placed directly into the properly labeled specimen jar. The jar should be labeled with patient identifiers and the biopsy site. It is helpful to prepare the specimen requisition in a single standardized format. For example, specimen letter (eg, "specimen A"); tissue type (eg, "skin"); specific anatomic site (eg, "hypothenar eminence of left hand"); specific technique utilized to provide the specimen (eg, "shave biopsy"); size and morphologic description of lesion (eg, "3-mm violaceous, blanchable dome-shaped papule with a collarette of scale"); and differential diagnosis (eg, "suspect pyogenic granuloma versus infectious process"). This provides crucial information to the pathologist and helps minimize errors.

Cessation of Bleeding, Wound Closure, and Wound dressing

After securing the specimen, the provider must tend to the surgical site. For curettage, saucerization, and often snip excisions, aluminum chloride or electrocautery is usually sufficient to stop any residual bleeding. Once bleeding has ceased, the lesion should be dressed with petroleum jelly and a bandage. For punch, incisional, and excisional biopsies, the defect should be sutured to allow for faster wound healing and optimal cosmesis. One can consider fast-absorbing or nonabsorbable sutures depending on the location and the age of the child. After suturing is complete, the lesion should be dressed with petroleum jelly and a bandage.

AFTERCARE AND INSTRUCTIONS

After any procedure, parents and the patient should be counseled on appropriate aftercare. Biopsy wounds are often cared for by washing with soap and water once to twice daily starting 24 hours after the procedure, followed by the immediate application of petroleum jelly and any appropriate bandages. With larger procedures requiring sutures, patients should be counseled regarding light activity to avoid possible wound dehiscence. Areas such as the upper back and thighs are highly mobile and thus are at risk of dehiscence and scar spread. Parents and patients should also be counseled against swimming until the wound has fully reepithelialized.

It is imperative to inform the family of when to expect biopsy results. Once the results have returned, correlation of the clinical presentation with the histopathologic results is essential. In pediatric patients, especially, a pathologist's experience may vary in reading pediatric specimens. If the results do not return as expected or if diagnostic uncertainty remains, a direct discussion with the pathologist is often helpful.

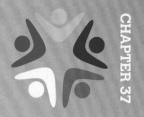

CHAPTER 37

Viral Culture

Jessica Sprague, Catherine Gupta Warner, Kimberly Ann Chun, and Sheila Fallon Friedlander

Introduction

Viral culture has historically been the gold standard for the diagnosis of many viral infections. However, not every virus can effectively be detected via viral culture. Detectable viruses include herpes simplex virus (HSV), varicella zoster virus (VZV), cytomegalovirus (CMV), adenovirus, enterovirus, influenza virus, respiratory syncytial virus (RSV), parainfluenza virus, and rhinovirus. Nondetectable viruses include coxsackie A, hepatitis, arbovirus, parvovirus, human papillomavirus, retroviruses, measles virus, and gastrointestinal viruses (rotavirus, coronavirus, astrovirus, and Norwalk virus). Viral culture of skin lesions is most often performed to evaluate for HSV and VZV.

Viral cultures use a combination of primary cell lines (eg, human fibroblast) and continuous cell lines (eg, human lung carcinoma) to promote replication of a wide variety of clinically relevant viruses. Collected specimens are inoculated onto these culture cell lines and monitored by light microscopy for cytopathic effect, which is the visible cellular change that occurs in response to a viral infection. On the basis of the specimen source, time to cytopathic effect, quality of cytopathic effect, and specific cell lines showing cytopathic effect, a preliminary viral identification can be made. The presence of a specific virus is then confirmed by immunofluorescent staining using virus-specific, fluorescently labeled antibodies (also known as direct fluorescent antibody or DFA test).

With the advent of newer diagnostic techniques such as polymerase chain reaction (PCR; see Chapter 35. Polymerase Chain Reaction), viral culture is often no longer the most sensitive test. For example, HSV is rarely detected via cerebrospinal fluid (CSF) viral culture in HSV encephalitis cases (<5% in adults and <50% in pediatrics); conversely, HSV DNA in CSF is detected by PCR in greater than 98% of cases. PCR also provides results more rapidly than does culture, often within 24 hours. When available, PCR has rapidly become the diagnostic method of choice.

Clinical Pearls

- Specimens should be collected in the acute stage of the illness, ideally within the first few days, and not more than 7 days after symptom onset.
- Dacron or cotton swabs dispensed with the commercially available viral culture mediums should always be used.
- Often a moist sample source, such as the contents of a vesicle or mucosal ulcer, will yield better results than that from a crusted lesion. Once crusting and healing have begun, rates of HSV recovery starts to drop rapidly.
- Ideally, more than one lesion should be sampled.
- Avoid the use of alcohol to cleanse the lesion because this may inactivate the virus.
- Specimens are unstable at room temperature. They are stable for about 72 hours in a refrigerator (4°C). Ideally, specimens should be transported to a laboratory within 24 hours.
- The shelf life of viral transport medium kept at 4°C is 6 months. It can be stored for 1 year at −20°C.

Contraindications/Cautions

Contraindications
- No specific contraindications

Cautions
- In infants and young children who require unroofing of a vesicle, make sure to secure the body area you are sampling and brace your hand against the patient to avoid potentially cutting the patient with the blade.

Equipment Needed
- Viral transport medium including Dacron or cotton swab with plastic shaft (Figure 37.1)
- A #15 blade or sterile needle if vesicle requires unroofing

Procedural Approach

- Acquire the appropriate swab and viral transport medium tube needed for viral culture.
- Label the tube with the patient's pertinent identifying information before collection.
- Remove the sterile swab from its packaging.
- If an intact vesicle exists, then use a sterile needle or a #15 blade to unroof the lesion and expose the base. If enough vesicle fluid is available, aspirate the fluid with a fine gauge needle and tuberculin syringe, and place the fluid into cold viral transport medium. Then, use the Dacron or cotton swab with plastic shaft to rub the exposed base vigorously. If no intact vesicle exists, then rub the target lesion vigorously.

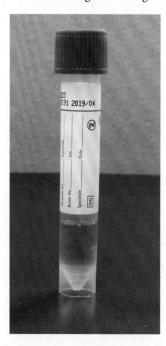

FIGURE 37.1. Viral transport medium.

- Once the sample has been collected, the swab should be inserted into the viral transport tube and the swab shaft broken so the cap can be placed onto the tube.
- Collected specimens should be stored immediately in a refrigerator set to 4°C and transported to the laboratory within 24 hours of collection.
- Patient information that should accompany the viral culture includes patient name and date of birth, date of collection, specimen source, clinical symptoms or suspected diagnosis, and tests requested by numerical order code and test name.
- During transport, the specimen should be protected from heat with use of a cold or ice pack in a sealed plastic bag.

SUGGESTED READINGS

Lakeman FD, Whitley RJ. Diagnosis of herpes simplex encephalitis: application of polymerase chain reaction to cerebrospinal fluid from brain-biopsied patients and correlation with disease. National Institute of Allergy and Infectious Diseases Collaborative Antiviral Study Group. *J Infect Dis.* 1995;171(4):857.

Quest Diagnostics. Herpes simplex/Varicella-zoster virus culture. https://www.questdiagnostics.com/testcenter. Accessed May 3, 2018.

Singh A, Preiksaitis J, Ferenczy A, Romanowski B. The laboratory diagnosis of herpes simplex virus infections. *Can J Infect Dis Med Microbiol.* 2005;16(2):92–98.

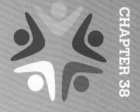

CHAPTER 38

Wood's Lamp Skin Examination

Jessica Sprague, Catherine Gupta Warner, Kimberly Ann Chun, and
Sheila Fallon Friedlander

Introduction

A Wood's lamp emits ultraviolet light at a wavelength of 320 to 400 nm (peak 365 nm), and can be used as a diagnostic test when examining the skin and hair. Wood's light can accentuate pigmentary alterations in the skin as well as certain bacterial and fungal infections. Melanin absorbs light emitted by the Wood's lamp; therefore, when melanocytes (and hence, melanin) are absent, such as observed in the skin depigmentation caused by vitiligo, the skin fluoresces.

Wood's lamp examination is also helpful to identify colorful fluorescence, sometimes indicative of certain fungal and bacterial infections (Figure 38.1A and B). However, a negative finding in Wood's lamp examination with negative fluorescence does not exclude a bacterial or fungal infection. Most tinea capitis in North America is caused by *Trichophyton tonsurans*, which unfortunately does not fluoresce under Wood's light. However, *Microsporum canis* (transmitted by dogs and cats) does fluoresce green or yellow-green.

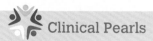 Clinical Pearls

- **Technique Tips**:
  - The examination room should be completely dark, with windows covered by drapes or blinds.

- The Wood's lamp should be allowed to warm up for at least 20 seconds.
  - Avoid washing the area before examining because this may minimize the fluorescence.
- **Fluorescence Results:**
  - *Vitiligo:* Depigmented patches on the skin appear bluish white under Wood's lamp.
  - *Fungal infections:* Fluorescence color may vary, but certain *Microsporum* infections fluoresce bright green or yellow-green (Figure 38.1A and B).
  - *Erythrasma:* Fluoresces red owing to *Corynebacterium minutissimum*
  - *Tinea versicolor:* The pityrosporum causing Tinea versicolor produces yellow–orange fluorescence, likely due to the presence of pteridines.

Contraindications/Cautions/Risks

- No specific contraindications

Equipment Needed

- Wood's lamp

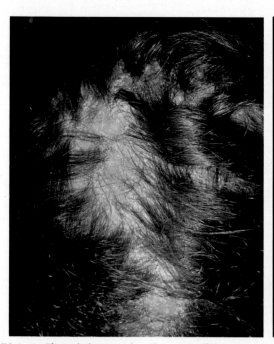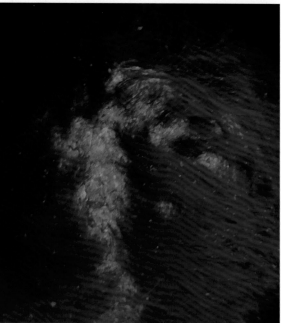

FIGURE 38.1. A, Clinical photograph without Wood's lamp reveals scaly erythematous plaques with various degrees of alopecia throughout the scalp of a young girl. There were several large lymph nodes detected in the posterior neck and occipital scalp areas. B, Same patient's scalp observed under Wood's lamp demonstrating blue–green fluorescence. Fungal culture confirmed the presence of *Microsporum canis*. Photo courtesy of Andrew C. Krakowski, MD.

Procedural Approach

- Darken examination room and allow the Wood's lamp to warm up for at least 20 seconds.
- Hold the light source approximately 4 to 5 in from the area examined.
- Observe whether fluorescence occurs.

SUGGESTED READINGS

Kaliyadan F, Kuruvilla J. Using a hand-held black-light source instead of a Wood's lamp. *J Am Acad Dermatol.* 2015;72(6):e153–e154. doi:10.1016/j.jaad.2015.02.1096.

Klatte JL, van der Beek N, Kemperman PM. 100 years of Wood's lamp revised. *J Eur Acad Dermatol Venereol.* 2015;29(5):842–847. doi:10.1111/jdv.12860.

Pinto M, Hundi GK, Bhat RM, et al. Clinical and epidemiological features of coryneform skin infections at a tertiary hospital. *Indian Dermatol Online J.* 2016;7(3):168–173. doi:10.4103/2229-5178.182351.

Sharma S, Sharma A. Robert Williams Wood: pioneer of invisible light. *Photodermatol Photoimmunol Photomed.* 2016;32(2):60–65. doi:10.1111/phpp.12235.

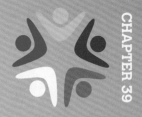
Microscopy
Demodex Examination

Jessica Sprague, Catherine Gupta Warner, Kimberly Ann Chun, and Sheila Fallon Friedlander

Introduction

Demodex spp. mites are considered commensal organisms that occupy the hair follicles in humans; however, they may play a pathogenic role when they are present in an excessive number or when they penetrate into the dermis. Demodex infestation is associated with rosacea, steroid-induced dermatitis, seborrheic dermatitis, and primary irritation dermatitis, and it should be considered in any erythematous facial eruption that is not improving with standard treatment (Figure 39.1). Demodex infestation is seen more frequently in patients older than 30 years of age, although it can occur in any age group and in those with mixed or oily skin as compared to neutral or dry skin. In the pediatric population, Demodex folliculitis is more commonly seen in immunocompromised patients, such as HIV-positive individuals and leukemic patients post chemotherapy. Skin scraping is an inexpensive and efficient method for determining the presence of Demodex mites. Initial treatment of Demodex infestation is usually with a topical antiparasitic agent such as metronidazole or ivermectin cream.

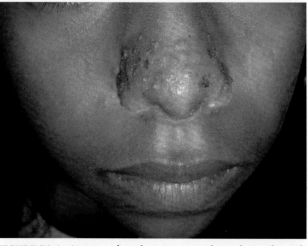

FIGURE 39.1. Agminated erythematous papules and pustules with crusting on the nose of a young female. Photo courtesy of Andrew C. Krakowski, MD.

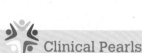 Clinical Pearls

- **Age-Specific Considerations:** If possible, providers should try to avoid obtaining skin scrapings from the face of infants and young children because this may be traumatic, with a relatively higher risk of accidental injury to the child with sudden movement. When scraping the face of infants and young children who are likely to move during the procedure, make sure to secure the body area you are scraping and brace your hand against the patient to avoid potentially cutting the patient with the blade.
- **Technique Tips:**
  - Wet the #15 blade with mineral oil before scraping the skin to increase adherence of material to the blade edge.
  - The skin can be gently squeezed between thumb and forefinger before scraping because this may facilitate detection of *Demodex* spp. mites by extruding them from the hair follicles.
  - Some investigators utilize cyanoacrylate glue application to identify mites.

Contraindications/Cautions/Risks

- No specific contraindications or cautions

Equipment Needed (Figure 39.2)

- A sterile #15 blade
- Mineral oil
- Microscope
- Glass slide
- Slide cover

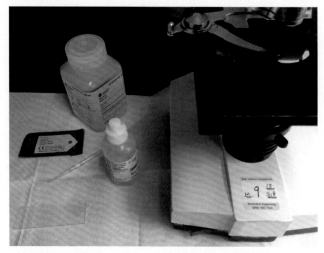

FIGURE 39.2. Equipment required for Demodex specimen include #15 sterile blade, mineral oil, glass slide, slide cover, and microscope. Courtesy of Delasco.

Procedural Approach

- Gather and prepare all equipment before initiating skin scraping in any patient.
- Apply a drop of mineral oil to the slide surface.
- Gently squeeze the skin surrounding a pore because this may increase the yield.
- Wet the #15 blade with mineral oil before scraping the skin to increase adherence of material to the blade edge.
- Use the belly of the #15 blade and gently scrape sideways at an angle to obtain sample.
- Scrape multiple areas to increase yield; all areas can be evaluated on a single slide.

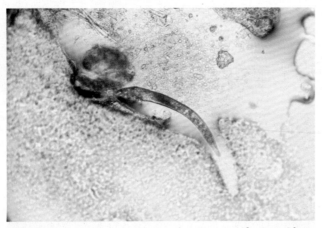

FIGURE 39.3. Demodex mite viewed at 10x magnification. Photo courtesy of Andrew C. Krakowski, MD.

- Smear obtained specimen onto center of slide and place a slide cover over the top; additional liquid medium can be added if necessary.
- View the slide on the microscope; scan the entire slide in a methodical manner under 4× or 10× magnification (Figure 39.3).

SUGGESTED READINGS

Bunyaratavej S, Rujitharanawong C, Kasemsarn P, et al. Skin scraping versus standardized skin surface biopsy to detect Demodex mites in patients with facial erythema of uncertain cause—a comparative study. *Indian J Dermatol Venereol Leprol.* 2016;82(5):519–522.

Zhao YE, Peng Y, Wang XL, et al. Facial dermatosis associated with Demodex: a case-control study. *J Zhejiang Univ Sci B.* 2011;12(12):1008–1015.

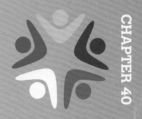

CHAPTER 40

Hair Microscopy

Jessica Sprague, Catherine Gupta Warner, Kimberly Ann Chun, and Sheila Fallon Friedlander

Introduction

Light microscopy of the hair can help in the evaluation of primary hair abnormalities or of secondary hair abnormalities caused by diseases affecting the scalp. Hair abnormalities may also be seen in association with various genodermatoses. An outline of the types of hair defects and associated diseases are noted here.

INFECTIOUS DISEASES OF THE HAIR

Tinea capitis: Dermatophyte infection of the scalp and hair whereby fungal hyphae grow along the stratum corneum and exterior or interior of the hair shaft

Pediculosis capitis: Head louse infection whereby nits (eggs) are attached strongly to the hair shaft and through which louse nymphs emerge

Piedra: Superficial mycosis characterized by black or white nodes along the shaft of the hair. These are difficult to remove in contrast to dandruff or hair casts.

Trichomycosis axillaris: Superficial *Corynebacterium* infection of the axillary or pubic hair characterized by yellow–brown nodules that are adherent to the hair shaft

STRUCTURAL DEFECTS OF THE HAIR

Monilothrix: Autosomal dominant condition of hair keratins resulting in beaded hair

Pili torti: Flattened and irregularly twisted hairs seen in isolation as an autosomal dominant condition as well as in association with other genodermatoses

Pohl-Pinkus constrictions: Similar to Beau's lines of the nails, these areas of decreased shaft diameter result from an acute stressor such as illness or death of a loved one. Generally, there will be one discrete area of decreased diameter that grows out with the hair.

Spun glass hair: Also known as wooly hair, this autosomal dominant disorder leads to hairs growing in all directions because of a triangular cross section and longitudinal grooving.

Trichostasis spinulosa: Hyperkeratosis of the follicular infundibulum leading to retention of vellus hairs with an open comedone-type appearance

Trichorrhexis invaginata: Classically associated with Netherton's syndrome, bamboo hair is due to a defect in keratinization of the hair cortex.

Hair casts: Remnants of the inner root sheath that slide easily along the hair shaft

Bubble hair: Air spaces within the hair caused by thermal damage

TYPES OF FRACTURE OF THE HAIR

Trichoptilosis: Longitudinal splitting of the distal end of the shaft due to trauma; more commonly known as "split ends"

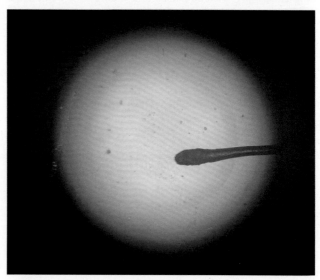

FIGURE 40.1. Telogen effluvium. Increased numbers of hair being shed in the telogen phase that demonstrate white bulbous hair root. Photo courtesy of Catherine Warner, MD.

Trichoclasis: Transverse fracture of the shaft seen in a variety of congenital and acquired fragile hair disorders

Trichoschisis: Clean transverse fracture through the cuticle and cortex

Trichorrhexis nodosa: Response of the hair shaft to injury resulting in a broomstick appearance

DISEASES OF THE HAIR BULB

Telogen effluvium: Increased numbers of hair being shed in the telogen phase that demonstrate white bulbous hair root (Figure 40.1)

Loose anagen syndrome: Rumpled sock appearance of the hair bulb due to anagen hairs that are loosely anchored and easily removed from the scalp

DISEASES LEADING TO BANDING OF THE HAIR

Trichothiodystrophy: Although normal in appearance on light microscopy, this brittle hair with an abnormally low sulfur content demonstrates alternating bright and dark bands with polarized light.

Pili annulati: Light and dark banding of the hair, causing a sandy appearance

Kwashiorkor: Alternating pale and dark bands of the hair known as the flag sign due to periods of poor nutrition

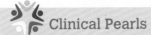

Clinical Pearls

- Clipping of the hair may be performed when hair shaft anomalies are suspected, whereas extracted hairs should be used when evaluation of the hair bulb is required.
- When a fungal infection is suspected, plucked hairs or scrapings should be placed onto a slide followed by the addition of potassium hydroxide (KOH) and a cover slip.
- For tinea capitis, KOH prep will demonstrate fungal spores on the outside of the hair shaft in ectothrix and on the inside of the hair shaft in endothrix. These spores are often in a longitudinal box-car formation.
- Normal hair shafts are cylindrical, with uniform pigmentation.
- The root of a hair in anagen is deeply pigmented, whereas the tip of a hair in telogen is nonpigmented or white.

Contraindications/Cautions

- No specific contraindications

Equipment Needed

- Glass slide
- Cover slip (optional)
- Clear tape (optional)

Procedural Approach

- Obtain the appropriate hair sample via plucking, clipping, or extraction of the hair.
- If forceps is used to pluck the hair, deformity of the hair may be induced at the site of pressure.
- Hairs should be placed onto the slide with or without a cover slip.

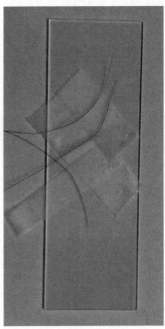

FIGURE 40.2. Placement of clear tape along the edge of the slide can help secure the hairs to the slide. Photo courtesy of Catherine Warner, MD.

- Often the use of clear tape along the edge of the slide can help secure the hairs to the slide (Figure 40.2). Alternatively, slide mounting adhesive can be purchased online.
- Evaluate the shaft of the hair or the hair bulb under the microscope.

SUGGESTED READING

Adya KA, Inamader AC, Palit A, Shivanna R, Deshmukh NS. Light microscopy of the hair: a simple tool to "untangle" hair disorders. *Int J Trichology*. 2011;3(1):46–56.

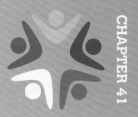

CHAPTER 41

Immunofluorescence

Jessica Sprague, Catherine Gupta Warner, Kimberly Ann Chun, and Sheila Fallon Friedlander

Introduction

Immunofluorescence (IF) is a histologic technique used to detect antigen-bound antibodies in the tissue or in the circulating body fluids. The technique involves linking antibodies to a specific fluorochrome that will "light up" when visualized under an ultraviolet microscope. For all autoimmune bullous diseases, it is best to employ a salt-split skin technique. Salt-split skin is skin tissue that has been incubated with 1 M solution of sodium chloride for 24 hours, which results in an artificial split of the skin at the level of the lamina lucida in the basement membrane and allows for more accurate diagnosis of basement membrane diseases.

Although newer blood antibody testing has become available, IF tests continue to be invaluable in the accurate diagnosis and management of immune-mediated dermatologic conditions. They are used as an adjuvant to clinical and histochemical diagnosis, particularly for vesiculobullous and connective tissue diseases such as bullous pemphigoid, pemphigus vulgaris, dermatitis herpetiformis, porphyria cutanea tarda, and lupus erythematosus. Accurate interpretation of IF results requires both familiarity with testing techniques as well as knowledge of the structure of the basement membrane and expected patterns of IF seen in dermatologic disease.

IF is divided into direct immunofluorescence (DIF) and indirect immunofluorescence (IIF).

DIF is used to identify antibodies bound in vivo to antigens in the skin or along mucosal surfaces. A punch biopsy specimen is required from *perilesional* skin in bullous diseases. Specimens obtained from lesional skin can give falsely negative results because in vivo antigens are consumed by inflammation. DIF specimens should ideally be taken from a new lesion because antibodies in older lesions may undergo degradation. Biopsy specimens must be placed in either Zeus' or Michel's media for examination because formalin exposure renders the specimen unusable. DIF identifies the class of immunoglobulin (IG) as well as the location, distribution, and density of IGs. The pattern of IF is then used in conjunction with the clinicopathologic presentation to make an accurate diagnosis.

Examples of DIF patterns in dermatologic diseases include the following:

- Bullous pemphigoid: Linear deposition of IgG and C3 along the basement membrane (roof of salt-split skin)
- Epidermolysis bullosa acquisita: Linear deposition of IgG and C3 along the basement membrane (floor of salt-split skin)
- Dermatitis herpetiformis: Granular deposition of IgA in the dermal papillae
- Henloch–Schönlein purpura: Deposits of IgA in vessel walls
- Linear IgA bullous dermatosis: Linear deposition of IgA along the basement membrane
- Pemphigus vulgaris: Deposition of IgG throughout the epidermis in an intercellular "chicken wire" pattern
- Porphyria cutanea tarda: Linear IgG, C3, and fibrinogen along the basement membrane and around superficial vessels
- Systemic lupus erythematous: Granular deposition of IgM > IgG and C3 along basement membrane in lesional and nonlesional skin

IIF is used to identify the presence of circulating antibodies to a specific antigen in the patient's serum. Although less commonly used than is DIF, IIF can provide useful adjunctive information in complex cases. In IIF, serial dilutions of the patient's sera are incubated with frozen sections of a suitable substrate to identify both the presence and quantity of a specific antibody. In general, IIF is less sensitive than is DIF and accuracy depends on the substrate used. For example, monkey esophagus is highly sensitive to pemphigus vulgaris antibodies, whereas rat bladder is best used for paraneoplastic pemphigus. The use of multiple substrates can increase diagnostic accuracy. In addition to diagnosis, IIF titers may also correlate with disease severity and thus can be used to both predict disease prognosis and monitor treatment response.

Examples of IIF substrates include the following:

- Pemphigus vulgaris: Monkey esophagus—titers correlate with disease activity.
- Paraneoplastic pemphigus: Rat bladder
- Pemphigus foliaceous: Guinea pig esophagus—titers correlate with disease activity.
- Connective tissue diseases: Hep2 cells

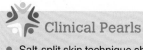

Clinical Pearls

- Salt-split skin technique should be requested for any suspected disease that involves the basement membrane (bullous pemphigoid, epidermolysis bullosa, pemphigus gestationis, etc.).
- If in doubt of best location to biopsy for bullous diseases, then two samples should be sent for DIF evaluation: one from perilesional skin and the second one from normal skin.
- When performing biopsy for DIF and biopsy for conventional histopathologic diagnosis at the same time, obtain the sample for DIF first to avoid contamination of sample with formaldehyde (formalin).

Contraindications/Cautions/Risks

- No specific contraindications

Equipment Needed

- Supplies for punch biopsy—DIF (see Chapter 36. Skin Biopsy Techniques)
- Zeus' or Michel's media—DIF
- Phlebotomy supplies—IIF
- Access to a laboratory with capability of performing IF—specimens can be sent to a specialty laboratory if not available locally; examples include Beutner Laboratories in Buffalo, New York, and Mayo Medical Laboratories in Rochester, Minnesota.

Procedural Approach

DIRECT IMMUNOFLUORESCENCE

- Perform a 3- to 4-mm punch biopsy on normal, lesional, or perilesional skin depending on the suspected disease (see Chapter 36. Skin Biopsy Techniques):
  - Fresh lesional skin (lesion present <48 hours)
    - Leukocytoclastic vasculitis, Henoch–Schönlein purpura
  - Two-thirds normal skin and one-third edge of a lesion
    - Bullous pemphigoid, epidermolysis bullosa acquisita, pemphigus, diseases with non–disease-specific immune deposits, that is, lichenoid, psoriasiform, or allergic eruptions
  - One-third normal skin and two-thirds edge of a lesion
    - Porphyria, pseudoporphyria
  - Normal skin approximately 3 mm away from edge of lesion
    - Dermatitis herpetiformis
  - Exposed normal skin
    - Systemic lupus erythematosus
  - Lesional exposed skin
    - Discoid lupus erythematosus, subacute lupus erythematosus, Sjögren's syndrome, scleroderma
- Place specimen in appropriate media (Zeus' or Michel's media).
  - Biopsies can be placed in physiologic saline if they are shipped on the same day for next-day delivery.
  - Biopsies can be frozen immediately with liquid nitrogen and transported to the laboratory on dry ice via overnight carrier service if the appropriate media are not available.
- Send specimen to a laboratory with the appropriate test request form that identifies the suspected disease, requested test, and request for salt-split skin (if suspected disease involves the basement membrane).

INDIRECT IMMUNOFLUORESCENCE

- Patient's blood is drawn via conventional phlebotomy.
- 5 to 8 mL of whole blood should be collected in a dry tube or a red-top vacutainer or serum separator tube.
- Allow blood to clot, centrifuge blood, and place into tube for laboratory transport.
- Specimen is sent to laboratory with correct test request form that identifies the suspected disease, requested tests, and ideal substrate.

SUGGESTED READINGS

Beutner Labs. Specimen collection. http://www.beutnerlabs.com/request/collection.php. Accessed May 8, 2018.

Mutasim DF, Adams BB. Immunofluorescence in dermatology. *J Am Acad Dermatol.* 2001;45(6):803–822.

Shetty VM, Subramanian K, Rao R. Utility of immunofluorescence in dermatology. *Indian Dermatol Online J.* 2017;8(1):1–8.

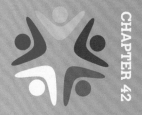

Fungal Examination or Potassium Hydroxide (KOH) Preparation

Jessica Sprague, Catherine Gupta Warner, Kimberly Ann Chun, and Sheila Fallon Friedlander

Introduction

Potassium hydroxide (KOH) preparation is an inexpensive and rapid bedside technique to diagnose fungal infections; results are interpreter dependent and correct interpretation requires training and experience. KOH is used to help dissolve excess skin cells for improved visualization of hyphae or yeast forms.

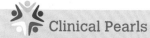

Clinical Pearls

- **Technique Tips:** If no other dissolving agents, such as dimethyl sulfoxide (DMSO), are used along with the KOH, gently heating the slide will help facilitate the dissolution of keratinocytes. However, overheating will cause crystal formation, which may preclude an accurate diagnosis.

Contraindications/Cautions/Risks

- **Contraindications:** There are no specific contraindications for the procedure.
- **Cautions:** In infants and young children who may move during the procedure, secure the area you are scraping, to avoid cutting the patient with the blade while obtaining the sample. Some practitioners will utilize two glass slides and scrape scale from the skin with one, depositing it on the other. Although some feel this is a safer method, others argue it does not provide as high a yield as using a blade.

Equipment Needed

- #15 blade
- KOH (± DMSO)
- Flame source (lighter or match) can be used.
- Microscope
- Slide(s)
- Cover slip

Procedural Approach

- Gather and prepare all equipment before initiating skin scraping in any patient.
- Before scraping, a high-yield target area should be identified, such as a leading scaling border of an annular plaque or pustules, if present.
- Wipe the area to be scraped with alcohol to help control the scraping of the scale and minimize loss of the scale.
- Using the belly of a #15 blade or a glass slide, scrape the scale or pustule sideways at an angle to obtain the sample (Figure 42.1).
- Apply the scale to a focal area of a glass slide.
- Apply one drop of KOH and add cover slip. If KOH contains 40% DMSO, then heating is unnecessary to facilitate dissolution of epithelial cells. If heating, heat gently with the flame of a lighter or match for less than 5 seconds, taking care to avoid

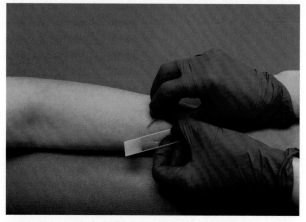

FIGURE 42.1. Using the belly of a #15 blade or a glass slide, scrape the scale or pustule sideways at an angle. Photo courtesy of Jessica Sprague, MD.

boiling the specimen. If a heat source is not available, it is usually sufficient to wait 3 to 5 minutes before examining the slide.

- To improve the contrast of the slide and to better visualize the fungal elements, lower the microscope's condenser until skin cells are seen clearly.
- For thick scale, gently push on the cover slip with the back of a pen in order to help flatten out the obtained specimen.
- Scan through the entire slide looking for skin cells at 4× magnification. Once a collection of scale is seen, increase magnification to 10×, 20×, or 40× to identify hyphae or yeast forms.
- To facilitate identification of hyphae, turn up and down the microscope's focus knob. Hyphae appear as branching or filamentous tubes that appear to change brightness when the focus is changed or may appear with a green tint. In addition, hyphae will cross epithelial cell lines, whereas artifact will not (Figure 42.2).

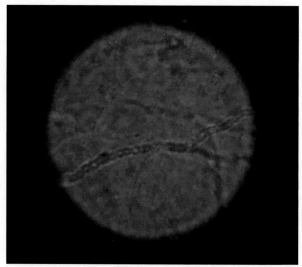

FIGURE 42.2. Branched hyphae visualized at 40x magnification with microscope's condenser lowered. Photo courtesy of Jessica Sprague, MD.

SUGGESTED READINGS

Wanat, KA, Dominguez AR, Carter Z, Legua P, Bustamante B, Micheletti RG. Bedside diagnostics in dermatology. *J Am Acad Dermatol.* 2017;77(2):197–218.

Wilkison BD, Sperling LC, Spillane AP, Meyerle JH. How to teach the potassium hydroxide preparation: a disappearing clinical art form. *Cutis.* 2015;96(2):109–112.

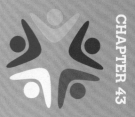

CHAPTER 43

Scabies Examination

Jessica Sprague, Catherine Gupta Warner, Kimberly Ann Chun, and
Sheila Fallon Friedlander

Introduction

Scabies is a common, highly contagious infestation caused by
the parasite *Sarcoptes scabiei var. hominis.* Skin lesions are intensely pruritic, generally presenting as nonspecific papules,
vesicles, and excoriations secondary to an intense inflammatory
response in the skin. Typical areas of involvement include the
wrists, hands, axillae, abdomen, buttocks, inframammary folds,
and genitalia. Although adults do not generally exhibit involvement of the head and neck, infants and young children may
have involvement of these areas. Mites burrowing within the
superficial skin cause specific lesions, aptly coined "burrows."
These burrows represent the highest yield area for obtaining a
scabies mite via scraping. They are commonly seen in the interdigital web spaces and along the wrists.

Scabies should be considered in any patient with widespread
pruritus and skin lesions, particularly those who also have close
contacts with individuals complaining of itch. Diagnosis is usually clinical and is made on the basis of the history, physical examination findings, and positive skin scraping. Dermoscopy can
also be used to identify the presence of mites under a burrow;
if this is present, skin scraping is not required (see Chapter 28.
Dermoscopy). First-line treatment is topical permethrin to be
applied to the patient and all close contacts, with repeat application 1 week later (see Chapter 120. Scabies). Reapplication is
required because the eggs are not destroyed by permethrin and
thus any newly hatched mites must be addressed by a second
treatment course. All bedding, towels, and clothing should be
washed at time of treatment or can be sealed in an airtight bag
for 1 week to prevent reinfection.

Clinical Pearls

- **Age-Specific Considerations:** When evaluating infants,
  consider scraping the caretaker instead of the child because lesions are frequently found on the hands/wrists of
  those in frequent contact with the child.
- **Technique Tips:**
  - Use of mineral oil or sterile saline can facilitate identi-
    fication of the scabies mite because they can be seen
    moving on the slide.
  - Use of potassium hydroxide (KOH) kills the mite and
    lack of movement can make them more difficult to dis-
    cern; however, KOH will help dissolve hemorrhagic
    crust and other debris obscuring scabies mites and
    eggs in scrapings with significant debris.
  - Mites can be identified on the basis of their character-
    istic large (0.25-0.4 mm) oval appearance with a pair
    of legs immediately adjacent to each side of the head
    and posteriorly located long hairs.
  - Eggs can be identified as smooth oval, thick-walled
    structures measuring 0.10 to 0.15 mm in length (4× to
    5× the size of a typical epidermal cell).
  - Scybala (mite fecal matter) can be identified as small
    solid yellow-brown smooth oval structures that are of-
    ten clumped together.
  - Scybala can only be identified when using mineral
    oil because KOH preparations will dissolve the fecal
    matter.
  - Scybala identification is more difficult than is identifi-
    cation of mites or eggs and requires an experienced
    practitioner for diagnosis in the absence of concom-
    itant eggs or mites.

Contraindications/Cautions/Risks

- No specific contraindications
- **Cautions:** In infants and young children who are likely to
  move during the procedure, make sure to secure the body
  area you are scraping and brace your hand against the patient
  to avoid potentially cutting the patient with the blade while
  obtaining the sample.

Equipment Needed (Figure 43.1)

- A #15 surgical blade
- Mineral oil, sterile saline, or KOH 10%
- Microscope
- Glass slide
- Slide cover slip
- Surgical gloves

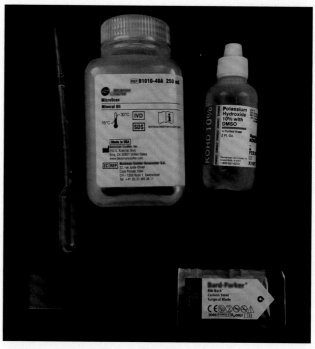

FIGURE 43.1. Equipment required includes #15 surgical blade,
mineral oil, sterile saline, or KOH 10%, microscope, glass slide, and
slide cover slip.

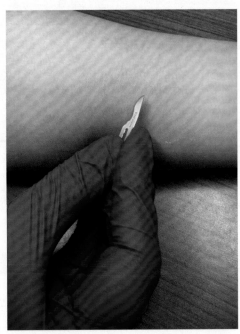

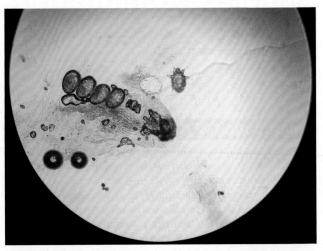

FIGURE 43.3. The "triple crown" of scabies examination: mite + eggs + scybala. Photo courtesy of Andrew C. Krakowski, MD.

FIGURE 43.2. Use the belly of the #15 blade to gently scrape sideways at an angle to obtain sample; some mild bleeding should be anticipated. Photo courtesy of Catherine Gupta Warner, MD.

Procedural Approach

- Gather and prepare all equipment before initiating skin scraping in any patient.
- Always wear gloves to avoid transmission of infestation.
- Apply a drop of mineral oil, sterile saline, or KOH to the slide surface.
- Wet the #15 blade with mineral oil or sterile saline before scraping the skin to increase adherence of material to the blade edge.
- Use the belly of the #15 blade to gently scrape sideways at an angle to obtain some mild bleeding should be anticipated (Figure 43.2).
- Scrape/unroof any vesicles or pustules.

- Scrape multiple areas to increase yield; all areas can be evaluated on a single slide. Highest yield areas include burrows on wrists, ankles, and interdigital web spaces, and intact pustules and vesicles.
- Smear specimen onto center of slide and place a slide cover slip over the top. Additional liquid medium can be added if necessary.
- View the slide on the microscope. Scan the entire slide in methodical manner under 10× to 40× magnification.
- Visualization of mite, egg, or scybala is sufficient for diagnosis (Figure 43.3).

SUGGESTED READINGS

Chouela E, Abeldaño A, Pellerano G, Hernández MI. Diagnosis and treatment of scabies: a practical guide. *Am J Clin Dermatol.* 2002;3(1):9–18.

Golant AK, Levitt JO. Scabies: a review of diagnosis and management based on mite biology. *Pediatr Rev.* 2012;33(1):e1–e12.

Kandi V. Laboratory diagnosis of scabies using a simple saline mount: a clinical microbiologist's report. *Cureus.* 2017;9(3):e1102.

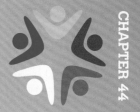

CHAPTER 44

Tzank Smear

Jessica Sprague, Catherine Gupta Warner, Kimberly Ann Chun, and Sheila Fallon Friedlander

Introduction

The Tzanck smear was named after the French doctor Arnault Tzank, who was the first to use the microscopic appearance of cells (cytology) to evaluate skin diseases, starting in the 1940s. Classically, the Tzanck smear is a process by which cells are obtained, fixed to preserve the specimen histologically, and then stained, most commonly with Giemsa (May-Grunwald Giemsa or Wright-Giemsa). Generally, these stains contain a combination of methylene blue, eosin, and/or azure B. Other stains such as methyelene blue alone, toluidine blue, or even hematoxylin eosin may also be used. Fixation occurs either with alcohol (generally methanol) or heat. Often methanol is included in the stains themselves to allow for self-fixing. Since the 1940s, cutaneous cytology has been used in the diagnosis of various vesiculobullous, erosive, tumoral, and granulomatous diseases; however, the Tzanck smear is best known for its use in the diagnosis of herpes simplex virus (HSV) or varicella zoster virus (VZV).

HSV and VZV are common viral infections worldwide. HSV is classically characterized by grouped vesicles on an erythematous base on the orolabial or genital mucosa, often diagnosed by clinical examination without the need for confirmatory testing. In atypical presentations, rapid confirmation allows for earlier treatment and monitoring. Although viral culture or polymerase chain reaction can take days to result, a Tzanck can be performed within 10 to 15 minutes of collecting a sample. See also Chapters 35. Polymerase Chain Reaction and 37. Viral Culture.

Although the classic presentation in neonates is the same as that in adults, lesions may sometimes be more discrete or diffuse, making diagnosis more difficult. This diagnosis carries a high mortality and significant morbidity in neonates, so care should be taken to initiate diagnosis and treatment early to prevent or treat associated central nervous system (CNS) disease.

Clinical Pearls

- The typical features of HSV or VZV on Tzanck smear include multinucleated keratinocytes, acantholytic cells, and nuclear margination. Balloon degeneration is a term used to describe the virally infected cells that appear as if they have been inflated (Figure 44.1).
- Tzanck smear cannot differentiate between HSV types or VZV.
- The stained nuclei may vary in color from reddish blue to purple to pink. The cytoplasm stains bluish.
- Studies have shown Tzanck smears to be about 80% to 90% sensitive and specific for diagnosing viral change, especially when performed on early vesicular lesions; however, results are interpreter dependent.
- Samples taken from an intact blister rather than from a crusted one are more likely to yield virally infected cells.
- Numerous stains are commercially available as kits. Different stains result in variable coloring, but the nuclear features are the same.

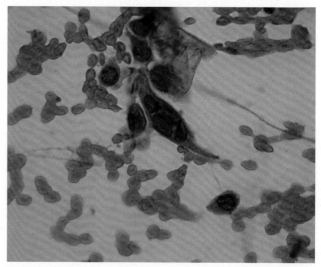

FIGURE 44.1. The typical features of herpes simplex virus (HSV) or varicella zoster virus (VZV) on Tzanck smear include multinucleated keratinocytes, acantholytic cells, and nuclear margination. Balloon degeneration is a term used to describe the virally infected cells that appear as if they have been inflated. Photo courtesy of Catherine Gupta Warner, MD.

Contraindications/Cautions

- No specific contraindications
- **Cautions:** In infants and young children who are likely to move during the procedure, make sure to secure the body area you are scraping and brace your hand against the patient to avoid potentially cutting the patient with the blade while obtaining the sample.

Equipment Needed

- Glass slide
- A #15 surgical blade
- Giemsa stain and methanol or Giemsa solution
- Light microscope

Procedural Approach

- In the case of a vesiculobullous lesion, the lesion should be incised along one side with a blade and folded back (ie, "unroofed") to expose the base of the lesion.
- Using a #15 blade, scrape the floor of the lesion and spread the cellular material as a thin layer onto a clear glass microscope slide.
- After the slide has been prepped, it should be air-dried quickly and then fixed and stained.
- Fixation may be performed before staining or in conjunction with it.
- After staining, the slide is washed with water and allowed to dry before examination under a light microscope.

SUGGESTED READINGS

Cordero AA. The man behind the eponym. Arnault Tzanck, his work and times. *Am J Dermatopathol*. 1985;7:121–123.

Coscia-Porrazzi L, Maiello FM, Ruocco V, Pisani M. Cytodiagnosis of oral pemphigus vulgaris. *Acta Cytol*. 1985;29:746–749.

Durdu M, Baba M, Seçkin D. More experiences with the Tzanck smear test: cytologic findings in cutaneous granulomatous disorders. *J Am Acad Dermatol*. 2009;61:441–450.

SECTION IV

Lesion-Specific Procedures

45 Abscess

46 Acanthosis Nigricans

47 Accessory Nipple

48 Accessory Tragus

49 Acne Comedones

50 Acne Cyst

51 Acne Scarring

52 Acrochordons

53 Actinic Keratosis

54 Alopecia Areata

55 Angiofibromas

56 Angiokeratoma

57 Angioma, Spider

58 Aplasia Cutis Congenita

59 Arthropod Bites and Stings

60 Basal Cell Carcinoma

61 Basal Cell Nevus Syndrome

62 Becker's Nevus

63 Blister

64 Blue Rubber Bleb Syndrome

65 Burns

66 Café au Lait Macules

67 Calcinosis Cutis

68 Callus

69 Chalazion

70 Circumcision Adhesions

71 Condyloma Acuminatum

72 Cutaneous Larva Migrans (Creeping Eruption)

73 Depigmentation

74 Dermal Melanocytosis (Mongolian Spot)

75 Dermatofibrosarcoma Protuberans

76 Dermoid Cysts

77 Epidermal Inclusion Cysts and Pilar Cysts

78 Epidermal Nevi

79 Epidermolysis Bullosa

80 Epstein's Pearl

81 Fibroma (Subungal or Periungal)

82 Deep Fungal Infection

83 Granuloma Annulare

84 Infantile Hemangioma

85 Hematoma

86 Hidradenitis Suppurativa (Acne Inversa)

87 Hyperhidrosis

88 Hyperpigmentation

89 Hypertrichosis

90 Hypertrophic Scars and Contractures

91 Hypopigmentation

92 Onychocryptosis (Ingrown Nail)

93 Juvenile Xanthogranuloma

94 Keratosis Pilaris

95 Labial Adhesion

96 Laceration Repair

97 Lichen Planus

98 Lipoma

99 Lymphatic Malformations

100 Mastocytoma

101 Median Raphe Cyst

102 Melanoma

103 Milium

104 Miliaria

105 Molluscum Contagiosum

106 Mycosis Fungoides

107 Myiasis

108 Neurofibromas

109 Nevi

110 Nevus of Ota and Nevus of Ito

111 Nevus Sebaceous

112 Nevus Simplex

113 Pigmentary Mosaicism

114 Pilomatricoma (Pilomatrixoma)

115 Port-Wine Birthmarks

116 Psoriasis

117 Pyogenic Granuloma

118 Perianal Pyramidal Protrusions

119 Rosacea

120 Scabies

121 Solitary Fibrous Hamartoma of Infancy

122 Squamous Cell Carcinoma

123 Supernumerary Digits

124 Tattoo Removal

125 Telangiectasia

126 Umbilical Granuloma

127 Venous Malformations

128 Human Papillomavirus Wart (Verruca)

129 Vitiligo

130 Xeroderma Pigmentosum

CHAPTER 45

Abscess

Venkata Anisha Guda and John C. Browning

Introduction

An abscess is a localized collection of purulent material. It forms during an infection when the body tries to protect itself by creating a wall. Abscesses can occur anywhere in the body. Often in the skin an abscess may develop within a hair follicle and is called a furuncle. Multiple adjoining furuncles are called a carbuncle. Common types of bacteria within an abscess include *Staphylococcus aureus* and *Streptococcus pyogenes*. People generally carry these bacteria on their skin but do not usually develop an infection unless their immunity is lowered or they come in contact with a more virulent strain. Cutaneous abscesses often occur in the axilla, rectal, and groin areas but can be located anywhere. They are round and firm with pus inside and characterized by overlying erythema, edema, and pain. Occasionally, there may be an opening (punctum) in the center.

SEVERAL TECHNIQUES HAVE BEEN UTILIZED TO MANAGE ABSCESSES:

- Conventional "incision and drainage" (I&D) is the most common and most effective technique for the procedural treatment of an abscess. The simple procedure entails incising an abscess to express (and drain) the pus (Figure 45.1A and B). Empiric antibiotic therapy may be initiated postoperatively when there is concern about a rapidly progressing infection.
- The "loop technique" has been shown to be effective, with outcomes similar to I&D. This technique consists of making a small stab incision on each side of the abscess, followed by wound exploration, irrigation, and drainage. A vessel loop drain is then introduced through one incision and pulled out the other, tied to itself, and left in place until the drainage stops and the loop can be removed.
- Ultrasound-guided needle aspiration, which is less invasive and painful, is a third option; however, this technique may not be as readily available or as reliable as I&D.

Clinical Pearls

- Although abscesses can develop in any individual, they are more common in those who are immunosuppressed or are on steroid therapy, chemotherapy, dialysis, or otherwise at increased risk.
- Cellulitis, lymphangitis, regional lymphadenopathy, fever, and leukocytosis can occur along with an abscess; consider systemic antibiotics and hospitalization in the appropriate setting.
- Patients with persistent lesions or recurrent lesions should be evaluated for possible colonization by organisms such as *S. aureus*.
- A bacterial culture may be helpful for identifying a specific causative organism; do not use sodium bicarbonate in the local anesthetic (if one is used) because it may impede bacterial growth.
- Sufficient local anesthesia allows for better disruption of any loculations.
- The incision should encompass the whole diameter of the abscess cavity so that the cavity can be evacuated easily.
- Postoperative warm water soaks to the abscess site hasten resolution of the inflammatory process and promote healing.

Contraindications/Cautions

- There are few contraindications to the procedure, but physicians should be cognizant of certain situations. These include large or complex abscesses, abscesses in sensitive areas, or in regions with close proximity to blood vessels.

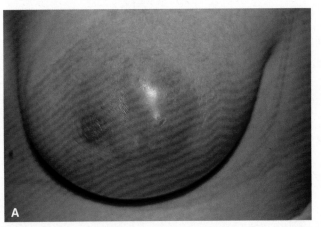
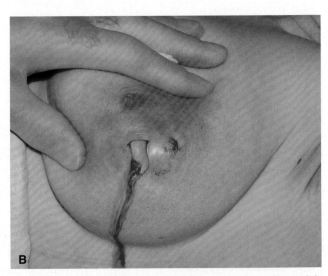

FIGURE 45.1. A, Peripheral abscess: Note the shiny thin skin. This abscess was treated by min-incision and drainage with resolution (B). Reprinted with permission from Harris JR, Lippman ME, Monica M, et al. *Diseases of the Breast*. 5th ed. Philadelphia, PA: Wolters Kluwer Health; 2014. Figure 5-12A & B.

- Abscesses that do not resolve despite repeated drainage should prompt consideration of a foreign body, osteomyelitis, septic arthritis, or an unusual organism.
- Adverse events include infection, bleeding in patients taking blood thinners, and reactions to anesthesia. Recurrent episodes of abscess formation can also occur, although warm compresses can help encourage continued drainage. Sterile tools should be used to prevent contamination.

Equipment Needed

- Clean examination gloves are necessary; in the appropriate setting, sterile gloves, drapes, and surgical gowns may be required.
- Antiseptic cleansing solutions such as chlorhexidine, povidone-iodine, or isopropyl alcohol
- Syringe containing 0.5% or 1% lidocaine with epinephrine (avoid the use of sodium bicarbonate if performing a bacterial culture)
- Disposable 3 or 10 mL syringe (depending on the size of the abscess)
- Sterile saline solution
- ¼- or ½-in iodoform gauze (if desired)
- Disposable 25 gauge needle
- For large abscesses, iodoform or plain sterile gauze packing may be considered.
- 4-in by 4-in gauze pads for dressing
- Nonallergenic adhesive tape for dressing
- Electric razor for shaving if abscess is in a hair-bearing area
- Scalpel with a #11 blade
- Hemostat (curved or straight)
- Plain forceps
- Surgical scissors
- Cotton-tipped sterile applicators
- Culture swabs

Preprocedural Approach

- Before performing incision and drainage, the provider should consider the depth of the abscess and its proximity to a sensitive or vulnerable anatomic location (eg, blood vessels, nerves, etc).
- Pain management must be considered. Local anesthetic may be necessary, and in some cases, a regional block may be helpful. In children, procedural sedation may be necessary in the appropriate setting.
- Perioperative use of antibiotics has the advantage of reducing the surrounding cellulitis, localizing the abscess, and sharply defining the incision site. Antibiotics may also help prevent bacteremia and should be considered on an individual basis.

Procedural Approach

- The abscess area and surrounding skin should be properly prepared before the procedure. The area should be shaved, if necessary, to visualize the wound. The area should be washed and prepared with chlorhexidine, povidone-iodine, or isopropyl alcohol.
- The area should be draped.

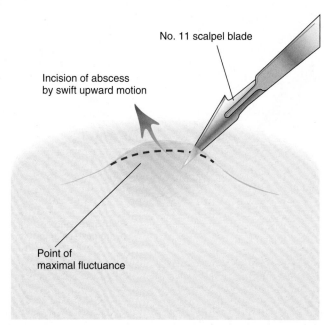

No. 11 scalpel blade

Incision of abscess by swift upward motion

Point of maximal fluctuance

FIGURE 45.2. Linear incision of a cutaneous abscess using a #11 scalpel blade. Reprinted with permission from Young GM. Incision and drainage of a cutaneous abscess. In: Henretig FM, King C, eds. *Textbook of Pediatric Emergency Procedures.* Baltimore, MD: Williams & Wilkins; 1997:1202. Figure 70.3.

- Local anesthetic (0.5% or 1% of lidocaine with epinephrine) should be infiltrated into the incision site over the abscess. The area should be anesthetized well beyond the incisional portion so that better disruption of any loculations may be achieved without pain.
- The incision should be delayed for several minutes after the injection to ensure that there is a complete anesthesia and vasoconstriction.
- Using a #11 blade, incise the abscess deeply from one side of the fluctuant area to the opposite side of the lesion. This is essential to ensure complete evacuation of the purulent drainage (Figure 45.2).
- Express purulent material from the wound.
- Obtain bacterial culture from the drainage.
- Perform an intracavity exploration to disrupt any loculations; blunt spreading with a hemostat clamp is useful for this purpose. For smaller abscesses, a cotton-tipped applicator may be soaked with hydrogen peroxide. The cavity should be explored and any pus, debris, or exudative material should be removed (Figure 45.3).
- After exploration, clean the cavity with four to six hydrogen peroxide-soaked, cotton-tipped applicators. You can also irrigate the cavity with a sterile saline solution.
- Observe the incision for hemostasis. Hemostasis should occur spontaneously; it will be aided by subsequent packing.
- The abscess can be loosely packed with 1/4 or 1/2 in iodoform or plain gauze packing. This helps in keeping the cavity open, permitting adequate drainage (Figure 45.4).
- If necessary, loosely apply a sterile gauze dressing and secure the dressing with nonallergenic adhesive tape.

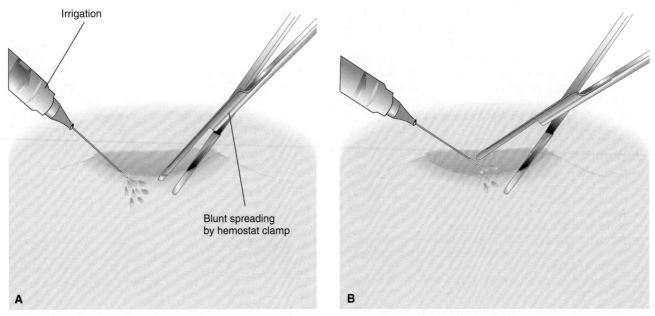

FIGURE 45.3. Removal of loculations and irrigation of an abscess. A, Use of irrigation to help break up adhesions and loculations within an abscess. B, Movement of blunt forceps in an abscess will help open up the abscess to allow drainage. Reprinted with permission from Young GM. Incision and drainage of a cutaneous abscess. In: Henretig FM, King C, eds. *Textbook of Pediatric Emergency Procedures*. Baltimore, MD: Williams & Wilkins; 1997:1203. Figure 70.4.

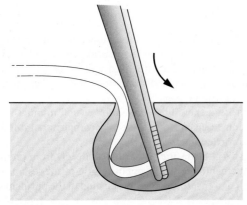

FIGURE 45.4. If the cavity is large enough, pack it with plain or iodoform gauze to promote drainage and prevent premature closure. Reprinted with permission from Zuber TJ, Mayeaux EJ, Jr. *Atlas of Primary Care Procedures*. Philadelphia, PA: Lippincott Williams & Wilkins; 2004. Figure 1.4.

Postprocedural Approach

- Patient education should be provided postoperatively.
- The initial dressing should be left in place until the next day.
- The affected extremity, if applicable, should be elevated to promote drainage and to decrease edema.
- Analgesics are usually not necessary.
- Starting the day after surgery, the patient should remove the external dressing but leave the packing in place (if the abscess was packed). A warm compress should be applied or the site should be soaked with warm water or in a tub bath for 20 to 30 minutes. The site should be submerged during the soak. A sterile dressing should be reapplied after each soak.

- If the packing falls out, it should not be reinserted.
- The physician should reevaluate the patient 36 to 48 hours after the incision and drainage procedure to complete the following steps:
  ○ Remove the external dressing.
  ○ Gently remove the packing from the healing abscess cavity.
  ○ Cleanse the abscess cavity with a cotton-tipped applicator soaked in hydrogen peroxide. Anesthesia is not necessary, but analgesics may be provided to the patient if necessary.
  ○ For larger cavities, repack once or twice per day both to debride and to help prevent abscess recurrence. This typically continues until the cavity has healed to the extent repacking is no longer possible (ie, when the cavity is less than 0.5 cm in diameter).
  ○ Reapply a sterile gauze dressing to the open wound site.
  ○ The patient should continue applying warm compresses or soaking three to four times daily. Warm compresses or soaks should be continued for 5 to 7 days or until the incision has healed. The patient should be reminded to remove the dressing before each warm compress or soaking, to pat the area dry, and to reapply the dressing.
- If the abscess was sufficiently drained, then the abscess cavity will close spontaneously through secondary intention within 5 to 7 days of the procedure. Wound healing by secondary intention depends on the size of the wound. A small puncture wound may heal in 7 days. A wound that requires packing can take 3 weeks or longer to heal completely.

SUGGESTED READINGS

Baiu I, Melendez E. Skin abscess. *JAMA*. 2018;319(13):1405.
Hughey M. *Surgical Methods*. 200th ed. Wilmette, IL: Brookside Associates; 2015.
Thornton J, Hellmich T. Current management of abscesses. *Prim Care Rep*. 2016;22(6):65-75.

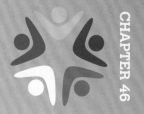
Acanthosis Nigricans

Giselle Castillo, Andrew C. Krakowski, John C. Browning, and Nathan S. Uebelhoer

Introduction

Acanthosis nigricans (AN) is a hyperpigmentation disorder that is characterized by dark, velvety skin, chiefly in body folds such as the neck, axilla, and groin (Figure 46.1). The exact prevalence is unknown; however, the condition appears to affect patients with darker skin more frequently, often presenting before 40 years of age. Multiple "clinical variants" exist and are commonly related to genetics, obesity, endocrine disorders, drug administration, or malignancy; these are summarized in Table 46.1.

In children with an inherited variant, the onset of the skin condition may be as early as infancy or childhood and can intensify in adolescence. A malignant variant rarely presents in childhood and is classified by a rapid onset and progression and extensive lesions. Idiopathic AN is the most common variant found in clinical practice. Although idiopathic, the disorder is commonly found in individuals who are at risk for developing type 2 diabetes. These individuals may present with insulin resistance and obesity. Additional risk factors include race and ethnicity, with an increased prevalence in Hispanic, African-American, and Native American individuals.

Treatment of AN should, primarily, focus on addressing the underlying cause of the condition. For example, if drug-induced AN is suspected, then the culprit medication should, if permissible, be discontinued. The most successful improvement has been noted in individuals who succeed at weight loss. Medications are generally not indicated. However, topical lactates (eg, ammonium lactate 12%), topical vitamin A, topical vitamin D analogs (eg, calcipotriol 0.005% cream), topical keratolytics, and/or topical or systemic retinoids may improve cosmetic appearance and help decrease symptoms such as pruritus.

Because AN is characterized by a thickened stratum corneum, acanthosis, hyperkeratosis, and papillomatosis—with minimal dermal involvement—it would seem that the condition would lend itself to a procedural approach. So far, however, a reliably

TABLE 46.1 : Classification of Acanthosis Nigricans

TYPE	CHARACTERISTICS
Type 1: hereditary benign AN	Inherited as an autosomal dominant disorder Can present at any age: infancy, childhood, or adulthood No associated endocrine disorder
Type 2: benign AN	Also referred to as acral acanthotic anomaly Endocrine disorders associated with insulin resistance: insulin-resistant type 2 diabetes mellitus, Cushing's disease, hypothyroidism
Type 3: pseduo-AN	Associated with obesity Obesity produces insulin resistance. More common in dark-skinned people
Type 4: drug-induced AN	Uncommon but can be the result of nicotinic acid in high-dosage, protease inhibitors, systemic corticosteroids, oral contraceptives, and insulin
Type 5: malignant AN	Rare in pediatric AN Usually adenocarcinoma of gastrointestinal or genitourinary tract

AN, acanthosis nigricans.

effective approach remains elusive. Dermabrasion, chemical peels (eg, trichloroacetic acid), electrodesiccation, curettage, simple excision, and cryotherapy are treatment modalities; however, the side effects of hypopigmentation and local recurrence have limited their uses. Pulsed-dye laser has not demonstrated an acceptable response. This chapter details two approaches: one using the long-pulsed alexandrite laser and another utilizing a combination macro- and microfractionated carbon dioxide laser protocol.

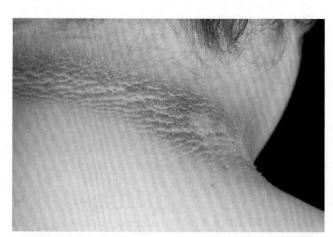

FIGURE 46.1. Acanthosis nigricans on the posterior aspect of the neck. Reprinted with permission from Baranoski S, Ayello EA. *Wound Care Essentials.* 3rd ed. Philadelphia, PA: Wolters Kluwer Health/Lippincott Williams & Wilkins; 2011. C Fig 21.

Clinical Pearls

- **Guidelines:** No known procedural treatment guidelines exist for this condition.
- **Age-Specific Considerations:**
  - A workup for insulin resistance in a child presenting with AN is warranted.
  - Malignancy-associated AN is rare in children but should be considered.
  - Young children (ie, younger than 10 years of age) typically require sedation.
- **Technique Tips:**
  - The plaques of AN are almost always symmetrical and, unlike acquired keratoderma, do not rub off with an alcohol wipe (see Chapter 24. Acquired Keratoderma).
  - Weight loss remains the most important treatment in patients with associated obesity.
- **Skin of Color Considerations:** Hypopigmentation is a likely side effect of most procedural treatments that should be considered in darker skin types.

Contraindications/Cautions/Risks

Contraindications
- Active, local skin infection (especially herpes labialis or impetigo)
- Inability to care for postoperative wounds

Cautions
- Presence of a suntan may increase dyspigmentation.

Risks
- Dyspigmentation (especially hypopigmentation in darker skinned patients), death (from infection or anesthesia), scarring, pain, bleeding, local recurrence of lesions

Equipment Needed
- Topical anesthesia (eg, LMX.4™ [Ferndale Laboratories] or eutectic mixture of local anesthetics [EMLA™ {AB Astra Pharmaceuticals, L.P.}] ± ice)
- Wavelength-specific eye shields
- Long-pulsed alexandrite (755 nm) laser (Approach #1)
- Fractional carbon dioxide laser (Approach #2)
- Smoke evacuator
- Sterile cotton-tipped applicators
- Sterile water
- Petrolatum-based ointment
- Ice

Preprocedural Approach

- Six to 8 weeks before surgery, we ask that patients minimize sun exposure and maximize sun protection so that their skin is as light (ie, untanned) as possible; although this may be somewhat seasonally and geographically dependent, the approach reduces melanin in the skin as a competing chromophore.
- If appropriate, consider having patients utilize hydroquinone 4% for 2 to 6 weeks before treatment to help reduce postinflammatory hyperpigmentation.
- Prophylaxis for herpes simplex is started 1 to 2 days before laser surgery, if indicated.
- Patients should bathe either the evening before or on the morning of their surgery.

Procedural Approach

- Informed consent from the parent/guardian and, when possible, assent from the minor are obtained.
- Anesthesia can vary from case to case and generally consists of either "topical plus local" or general anesthesia. Young children (ie, younger 10 years of age) typically require sedation; owing to controversial literature on risks and long-term sequelae from general anesthesia in pediatric patients, referral to a tertiary care center is recommended.
  - Because these procedures are associated with significant discomfort when performed in outpatient clinics, higher percentages of topical lidocaine, that is, up to 30% compounded ointment or mixture of lidocaine and tetracaine, are often used.
  - When using higher percentages of lidocaine, it is important to be mindful of the body surface area (BSA) being treated and limiting application to less than 1% BSA for less than 30 minutes.
  - Before application of topical lidocaine or injection of local lidocaine, risks of potential systemic absorption should be considered.
  - Maximum allowed local anesthetic dosing should be calculated on the basis of the patient's weight.

- Isopropyl alcohol should be utilized to remove residue chemicals on the skin.
- Appropriate protective eyewear should be worn, and patients should have eye pads (disposable adhesive eye shields offering full eye protection from medical lasers with wavelengths between 190 and 11 000 nm at an optical density >7; OD 7@190-11 000 nm) or correctly fitted metal eye shields in place.

Procedural Approach #1—Long-Pulsed Alexandrite Laser

- Long-pulsed alexandrite (755 nm) is employed to treat the affected areas using either a 10- or 12.5-mm spot size, fluences of 16 to 23 J/cm^2, and 5-ms pulse width, depending on skin type and clinical response. Pulses are single stacked, and overlapping should be avoided.

Postprocedural Approach #1

- Cold compress/ice can be applied as tolerated for the first 24 hours.
- Alternating over-the-counter acetaminophen and ibuprofen is generally sufficient for pain control. However, some patients may also benefit from schedule III narcotic pain medication for breakthrough pain during the first 2 to 3 days.
- Dressing should be applied after the treatment and left in place for the first 24 hours. The treated area can then be cleansed with gentle soap and water daily. If the treated areas are at risk for infection, dilute vinegar or dilute bleach soaks can also be used daily.
- Petrolatum-based ointment is recommended in the immediate postoperative period and also for continued use until the treatment area is fully healed.
- It is important to protect the treatment sites from trauma and friction during the healing process. Protective dressings can be used for 1 to 2 weeks postoperatively. Compression garments can also be helpful to decrease postoperative edema and reduce risks of recurrence with continued use.
- Patients can typically return to school or daily activities within 2 to 3 days.
- Clinic follow-up is recommended 6 to 8 weeks after the treatment to assess response and determine additional management plans. Longer treatment intervals are often preferred for school-aged children to minimize school absences and to reduce the frequency of general anesthesia (if it is being used).
- Serial photography to document treatment response is always helpful.
- Multiple treatment intervals should be anticipated at 4- to 8-week intervals.

Procedural Approach #2—Combination Macro- and Microfractionated Carbon Dioxide Laser

- The affected areas of the skin are treated as a single "sheet," using a macrofractionated 10 600-nm CO_2 laser (Active FX™ [Lumenis, Yokneam, Israel]). A single-pulse, nonoverlapping "stamping" technique is utilized at the following settings (adjusted for skin type and overall thickness of lesions): 100 to 125 mJ/3.5 W/size 3 to 5/density 5 to 6/spot size fixed at 300 μm. These parameters result in nonfractionated, focal full-field ablative resurfacing in the desired areas. We would expect other CO_2 laser devices to achieve similar results if a uniform sheet of nonoverlapping pattern of ablation is created to a depth of approximately 100 μm with minimal collateral thermal damage. As with most CO_2 laser treatments, bleeding is minimal.

- Sterile water is then applied to the treatment area, and sterile cotton-tipped applicators are rubbed vigorously over the surgical field to remove acanthotic skin to the superficial papillary dermis. Scarring is more likely at increasing depths, so a conservative approach is favored.
- After completing the macrofractionated treatment, an ablative microfractionated 10 600-nm carbon dioxide laser (UltraPulse) may be utilized. The entire wound area may be treated with a single-pulse, nonoverlapping stamping technique at a pulse energy of approximately 10 to 20 mJ and treatment density of 10% to 20%.
- Immediately after surgery, a petrolatum-based ointment is liberally applied.
- Ice may be applied to help decrease discomfort and limit edema.

Postprocedural Approach #2

- Generally, swelling and pain should decrease quickly with time.
- Patients should complete any herpes prophylaxis for a total of 7 to 10 days.
- At least three times a day, patients are instructed to gently cleanse the treated areas using a mixture that consists of 1 capful of acetic acid (ie, food-grade white distilled vinegar) combined with 1 L of distilled water. Gauze is soaked in this mixture and, with patients lying supine, left in place on the treated areas for 10 minutes. Then, the gauze is removed, and the area is rinsed gently with fresh water. Petrolatum-based ointment is immediately reapplied and maintained until reepithelialization has occurred—typically 5 to 7 days after laser surgery.
- Patients should be vigilantly monitored for signs and symptoms of infection, with special consideration paid to viral, fungal, and atypical mycobacterial infections, as well as to the more typical bacterial culprits. For example, posttreatment *Candida* or fungal infections tend to evolve as bright red eruptions that may be intensely itchy.
- Postoperative downtime is significant, and patients should expect to be absent from school or work for at least 1 week.
- After a follow-up appointment to directly assess reepithelialization, about 7 to 10 days after laser surgery, topical retinoid may be applied to the treated areas in an effort to mitigate recurrence.
- Patients are encouraged to contact the physician directly for concerns, and we often provide our cell phone numbers for direct contact and reassurance.
- Serial photography (ie, "selfies") are always helpful.

SUGGESTED READINGS

Brickman WJ, Binns HJ, Jovanovic BD, et al. Acanthosis nigricans: a common finding in overweight youth. *Pediatr Dermatol.* 2007;24(6):601–606.

Rosenbach A, Ramin, R. Treatment of acanthosis nigricans of the axillae using a long-pulsed (5-msec) alexandrite laser. *Dermatol Surg.* 2004;30(8):1158–1160.

Sinha S, Schwartz RA. Juvenile acanthosis nigricans. *J Am Acad Dermatol.* 2007;57(3):502–508.

CHAPTER 47

Accessory Nipple

Samuel H. Lance and Amanda A. Gosman

The accessory nipple is a benign condition presenting in both male and female patients. The accessory breast tissue is present from birth; however, it may remain undiagnosed until puberty. With the onset of pubertal hormones, the lesions may increase in size, darken in color, or become symptomatically painful. Because the incidence of breast cancer is one in eight women, surgical excision of ectopic breast tissue is recommended because it is difficult to screen it for cancer risk during adulthood.[1] Accessory breast tissue is associated with the natural milk line. The milk line is an embryologic line of mammary origin extending from the axilla to the groin bilaterally. Accessory nipples or accessory breast tissue may present at any point along the entirety of the milk line[2] (Figure 47.1). Accessory nipples with associated underlying breast tissue may demonstrate the most significant growth, namely, in pubertal female patients. This palpable breast tissue often lies at the base of the breast and may be a source of discomfort when wearing supporting breast garments (Figure 47.2). A male patient with accessory nipples may desire excision to prevent social or psychological stigma associated with overt nipple duplication.

Clinical Pearls

- **Guidelines:** No specific treatment guidelines are known to exist for this condition.
- **Age-Specific Considerations:**
  - Continued growth or recurrence in growth during puberty should be addressed with the prepubertal patient.
  - Patient and parent should be counseled regarding the relative risk of growth during puberty and consider delaying the intervention until breast development is complete. Following breast development, the underlying breast tissue can be better visualized during excision.
- **Technique Tips:**
  - Excision can be achieved with a relatively simple surgical setup. Although smaller lesions may be excised in the office under local anesthesia, larger lesions—most notably those with underlying breast tissue—may best be excised in the operating room setting. The use of general or monitored anesthesia care can be utilized

in the operative setting to decrease patient discomfort and minimize local anesthetic toxicity for larger lesions.
- Although these lesions rarely present the potential for malignant transformation, they are, in fact, breast tissue and should be analyzed pathologically after resection.
- Patients should be informed of the potential for malignant transformation in the future at the same frequency of native breast tissue.
- Patients should be encouraged to proceed with breast cancer screening at the appropriate age depending on their family history.
- Despite excision, microscopic remaining elements of breast tissue may continue to demonstrate growth during the pubertal growth phase or with mammary hypertrophy during pregnancy.

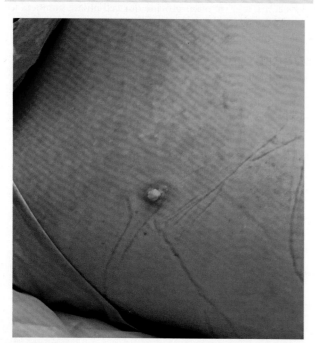

FIGURE 47.1. Accessory nipple on the left medial thigh, along the *milk line*. Photo courtesy of Andrew C. Krakowski, MD.

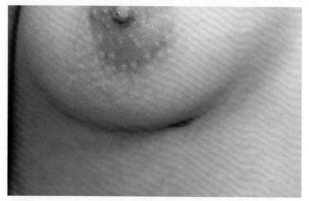

FIGURE 47.2. Accessory nipple inferior to the normal breast.

Contraindications/Cautions/Risks

- History and physical examination concerning for active breast neoplasm remain the only firm contraindication to elective excision. In this setting, patients should be referred to the appropriate oncologic specialist.

- Active anabolic steroid use or endocrine disturbance, most notably in the male population, is considered a relative contraindication and should be addressed in the preoperative setting before excision.

Equipment Needed
- 1% lidocaine with epinephrine 1:100 000
- Scalpel #15
- Electrocautery
- Toothed Adson forceps
- Needle driver
- Suture: 3-0 Monocryl™ (Ethicon US, LLC) suture
- 4-0 Monocryl suture
- 5-0 Prolene™ (Ethicon US, LLC) suture
- ½ in Steri-Strips
- 2 × 2 gauze
- Tegaderm® (3M, US) bandage dressing

Preprocedural Approach

- Scarring associated with excision and the risk of recurrent growth should be addressed with the patient preoperatively.
- Scarring following this procedure should be addressed specifically with the female patient given the nature of the intervention in relation to the form and function of the female breast.
- A discussion is held with the patient and parent regarding the aesthetic and sexual function of the chest wall surrounding the breast. Although excision is unlikely to distort the native breast or interfere with breast growth, scarring in the peribreast area may be of concern to the patient and should be specifically addressed.

Procedural Approach

- To prevent the risk of misidentification of the accessory nipple, the lesion should be marked and confirmed with the patient and family before the procedure.
- The areola or pigmented tissue should be marked with an approximately 1- to 1.5-mm margin.
- The presence of any underlying palpable breast tissue should then be marked to encompass the greatest dimensions of the underlying tissue (Figure 47.3).

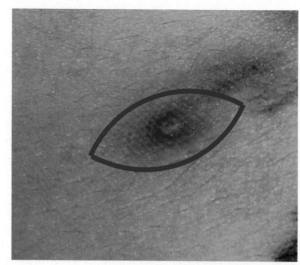

FIGURE 47.3. Preprocedure marked area to be excised.

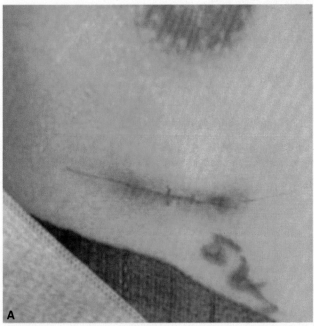
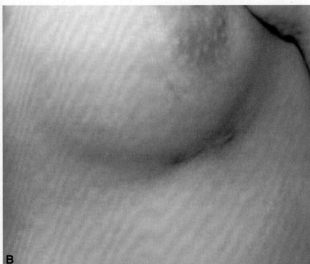

FIGURE 47.4. A, Closure after excision. B, Well-healed surgical scar 6 months after the procedure.

- Following marking, the patient is provided either with appropriate general anesthesia or proceeds directly to infiltration with local anesthetic. Care should be taken to avoid overinfiltration of local anesthetic into the area of palpable breast tissue because this may distort the underlying breast tissue and prevent precise excision.
- Incision should be made through the skin utilizing a #15 scalpel. It is the author's preference to excise only the marked lesion with margins, as noted earlier, and allow for dog-ear excisions during closure. Alternatively, an elliptical excision can be designed encompassing the pigmented area.
- Once the pigmented tissue is incised, tissue scissors or cutting electrocautery may be utilized to dissect the underlying breast tissue free from the surrounding adipose tissue.
- An indistinct plane between these two tissue types is sometimes visible and can be utilized to direct this dissection. Care should be taken to excise only breast tissue because overresection of the subcutaneous fat can result in significant distortion of the soft tissue.
- Following resection, hemostasis can be achieved with electrocautery.
- Closure is then performed in a multilayer manner depending on the depth of resection.
  - With resections extending into the subcutaneous fat, it is recommended that closure of the superficial fascia layer be performed with 3-0 monofilament absorbable suture. This deep closure should relatively approximate the level of the deep dermis.
  - At this point, a deep dermal closure may be performed utilizing either interrupted 3-0 or 4-0 monofilament absorbable suture.
  - During the dermal closure, visible dog-ears at the margins of the incision may be excised utilizing triangular excisions as necessary to allow for a more level closure.

- It is the author's preference to proceed with skin closure utilizing a running subcuticular 5-0 Prolene suture to minimize the superficial reaction from suture absorption at the epidermal level (Figure 47.4A and B). Of note, this nonabsorbable suture should be removed within 5 to 7 days of the procedure. Alternatively, a running 4-0 monofilament absorbable suture may be utilized for the epidermal closure.
- Steri-Strips and a nonpermeable occlusive dressing should be placed following closure.

Procedural Approach

- Activity should be limited to noncontact sports and light activity only for duration of 4 to 6 weeks following intervention.
- In the setting of the female patient, breast-supporting garments with underwire or restrictive elastic overlying the incision should be avoided until approximately 4 weeks following intervention.
- Should nonabsorbable sutures be utilized for skin closure, removal is recommended in 5 to 7 days following intervention to prevent epithelialization along the suture filament.
- Occlusive dressings can be removed 1 week following surgery and the area can be washed gently with soap and water.
- Scar management with silicone gel or sheeting and scar massage is recommended after 2 weeks.

REFERENCES

1. Patel BK, Jafarian N, Abbott AM, Khazai L, Lee MC. Imaging findings and management of primary breast cancer in accessory axillary breast tissue. *Clin Breast Cancer.* 2015;15(4):e223–e229.
2. Patel PP, Ibrahim AM, Zhang J, Nguyen JT, Lin SJ, Lee BT. Accessory breast tissue. *Eplasty.* 2012;12:ic5.

CHAPTER 48

Accessory Tragus

Samuel H. Lance and Amanda A. Gosman

Introduction

Preauricular lesions containing cartilaginous and cutaneous redundancy are often described as an accessory tragus (Figure 48.1A and B). The terminology describing these lesions as an accessory tragus is accurate given the shared first branchial arch origin of these accessory structures and the native tragus.[1] Although these structures may be composed only of excess cutaneous material, there is often underlying cartilage stalk supporting the protrusion of the accessory tragus (Figure 48.2). Surgical treatment will focus on management of both cutaneous and cartilaginous structures to optimize outcomes.

The accessory tragus often presents in isolation. However, development of structures along the first and second branchial arch may demonstrate additional abnormalities that are associated with the accessory tragus. The most commonly associated syndrome with accessory tragus is oculoauriculovertebral syndrome, also known as Goldenhar syndrome. Additional findings associated with the accessory tragus include hemifacial microsomia, microtia, and Treacher Collins syndrome.[1] Complete or partial facial nerve dysfunction may be present with the findings of an accessory tragus or associated syndromes. A complete facial nerve examination is helpful in identifying underlying facial nerve deficits before intervention. Any associated abnormalities found in a patient with accessory tragus should be investigated and an appropriate workup performed before intervention.

Clinical Pearls

- **Guidelines:** No specific treatment guidelines are known to exist for this condition.

- **Age-Specific Considerations:** A key element during excision of an accessory tragus includes an understanding of the proximity of facial nerve branches in the pretragal area of the pediatric patient because this anatomy differs when compared to that of the adult patient. The course of the facial nerve in pediatric patients is considerably more superficial and lies just below the subcutaneous fascial layers of the face compared to the extensive intraparotid course of the nerve in the adult patient.[2] The parotid gland is significantly smaller in children and covers less of the facial nerve branches at the pretragal area compared to that in adults. Most notably, the superior branches of the facial nerve are the most superficial in pediatric patients and demonstrate less parotid coverage compared to lower facial nerve branches.[2] Care should be taken to avoid iatrogenic damage to these branches during dissection of the cartilage structures in the accessory tragus.

- **Technique Tips:** The accessory tragus is rarely composed of skin and subcutaneous fat only. Frequently, an underlying cartilage structure is present and may connect to the cartilage of the auricle. The cartilage stalk must be addressed during excision. Failure to perform adequate excision of the underlying cartilage can result in increased recurrence rates and a continued palpable deformity after excision.

Care should be taken to avoid distortion of the native tragus during closure of the surgical site. Anterior displacement of the native tragus under the tension of a skin closure can result in increased exposure of the external auditory canal. These aesthetic distortions of the native tragus can be difficult to correct and should be avoided at the onset of intervention when possible.

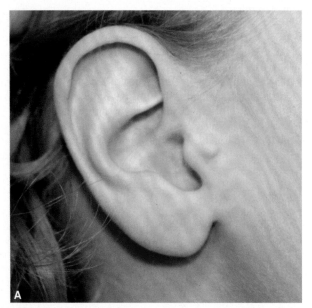
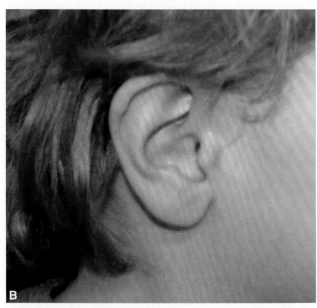

FIGURE 48.1. Excision of accessory tragus with cartilaginous stalk. A, Preprocedure photo. B, Postprocedure photo demonstrating well-healed scar.

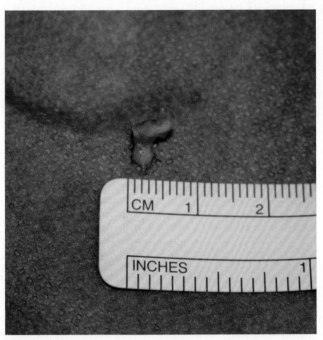

FIGURE 48.2. Excised accessory tragus with cartilaginous stalk.

Preprocedural Approach

- Complete history and physical examination should be performed focusing on signs of preexisting facial nerve dysfunction. Any abnormal findings should be documented and discussed with parents before intervention.

Procedural Approach

- Planned excision of the accessory tragus should be marked as an ellipse at the base of the lesion. Redundancy of the overlying tissue within the base should be preserved and excised as necessary during closure to provide a tension-free closure.
- Following induction with general anesthesia or achieving local anesthesia with infiltration, incision can be made in an elliptical manner at the base of the accessory tragus. Incision is made only through the dermis to allow for preservation and identification of the underlying cartilage.
- Tenotomy scissors are then utilized to dissect bluntly overlying the cartilage while placing gentle traction to the cartilage. The risk of nerve injury is decreased with the use of blunt dissection directly overlying the cartilaginous structure.
- Circumferential dissection of the cartilage should be performed to a level approximately 0.5 to 1 cm below the skin. At this level, the cartilage is then sharply excised under direct visualization (Figure 48.2).
- Hemostasis can be achieved utilizing direct pressure. Bipolar electrocautery should be minimized in the deep tissue to avoid iatrogenic nerve injury.
- The skin can then be closed utilizing interrupted 5-0 Monocryl suture in a deep dermal manner followed by interrupted 6-0 nylon suture to the epidermal layer.

Postprocedural Approach

- The area can be dressed with antibiotic ointment and covered with a light gauze dressing. Dressings can be removed the day following surgery to proceed with incision care.
- Wound care overlying incisions can be performed with light daily washing using soap and water followed by patting the area dry and application of antibiotic ointment.
- Patients should be reevaluated at 1 week post the procedure for assessment of appropriate wound healing.
- Nonabsorbable sutures should be removed at 5 to 7 days following the procedure, thus avoiding epithelialization along the monofilament suture.
- Following suture removal, patients may be transitioned to daily incision care with washing and drying followed by application of nonallergenic, petroleum-based, moisturizing ointments.
- Scar reduction techniques including silicone application, scar massage, and protection with sunscreen are initiated at 2 weeks following intervention.

Contraindications/Cautions/Risks

- As with most elective surgical interventions, active infection remains the most definitive contraindication to excision of the accessory tragus.
- Planned future ear reconstruction of associated microtia is considered a relative contraindication to excision of accessory tragus. The utility of preserving the accessory cartilage and the creation of scars at the site of a future ear reconstruction should be carefully planned by the reconstructive surgeon.
- Unrealistic parental expectations of scarring and surgical outcomes should also be considered relative contraindications for excision.
- Risk of facial nerve injury is considered a rare but significant risk of this procedure. Anatomic differences in the facial nerve of a pediatric patient have been addressed earlier. A thorough anatomic understanding of the pretragal soft-tissue anatomy and careful technique can mitigate this risk and decrease the possibility of iatrogenic injury.

Equipment Needed

- Surgical marking pen
- Local anesthesia 1% lidocaine with epinephrine 1:100 000
- Scalpel #15 blade
- Tenotomy scissors
- Bipolar cautery
- Fine-toothed forceps
- Fine needle driver
- Suture: 5-0 Monocryl™ (Ethicon US, LLC) and 6-0 Nylon

REFERENCES

1. Bahrani B, Khachemoune A. Review of accessory tragus with highlights of its associated syndromes. *Int J Dermatol.* 2014;53(12):1442–1446.
2. Farrior JB, Santini H. Facial nerve identification in children. *Otolaryngol Head Neck Surg.* 1985;93(2):173–176.

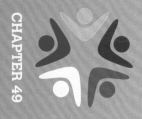

CHAPTER 49

Acne Comedones

Emmy Graber and Shari Marchbein

Introduction

Acne is an exceedingly common condition, especially in adolescence, affecting 85% of teenagers. Significant physical and psychological damage may occur from acne, resulting in skin scarring, low self-esteem, and depression.

Although individual acne comedones tend to be diminutive in terms of their physical size, they can still result in inflammation that leads to scarring, anxiety, and distress. They are also direct targets for picking behaviors, which can lead to infections on the face. Therefore, they may need to be treated. Although topical medications are first-line treatment for acne comedones, other procedurally based treatments may provide more rapid results. Although topical creams may take 6 to 8 weeks for significant improvement, comedone extraction can improve lesions immediately. This treatment option does not prevent the development of future comedonal acne; however, extraction provides fast results that can be desirable for patients not wanting to wait weeks for improvement. When done by an experienced practitioner, comedone extraction is a safe and minimally painful treatment.

Chemical peels (see Chapter 21. Chemical Peels) may also provide some improvement in comedones, but large, multi-centered, double-blinded clinical trials are lacking. There is a plethora of agents utilized for chemical peels, of varying strengths and performed in different ways. Acne consensus work groups recognize that chemical peels "may result in mild improvement in comedonal acne," but given the lack of evidence and absence of standard chemical peel procedural guidelines, they are not addressed here. Similarly, there are some small studies and anecdotal reports of lasers improving acne, although there is more evidence that lasers and light devices improve noncomedonal lesions, such as pink inflammatory papules and pustules. Given the lack of evidence for lasers improving acne comedones and the variability in lasers and treatment protocols, this modality is not addressed here. Cryotherapy is a technique for treating acneiform lesions that was more commonplace years ago; however, given its propensity to leave scarring and dyspigmentation, it is rarely utilized today. Herein, we focus on the technique of manual extraction.

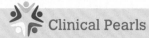

Clinical Pearls

- **Guidelines:** Despite its long-standing clinical use, there is limited evidence published in peer-reviewed medical literature that addresses the efficacy of comedone removal. No specific guidelines are known to exist, although acne consensus groups recognize that it is "helpful in the management of comedones that are resistant to other therapies."
- **Age-Specific Considerations:** Ideally, patients should be old enough to ask for treatment, understand the risks and benefits, and be able to cooperate for the procedure.
- **Technique Tips:** Different comedone extractor tools have been used for removal, with various shaped loop tips that encircle the comedo. Applying excessive pressure with these extractors can result in purpura or prolonged erythema. It is the experience of the authors that extraction is best performed utilizing an 18 G needle to gently nick the comedone, followed by manual pressure on each side of the comedone utilizing two cotton-tipped wooden applicators.
- **Skin of Color Considerations:** Darker skin types may have higher risks of hyperpigmentation after extraction.

Contraindications/Cautions/Risks

Contraindications
- Skin infection on area where treatment is to be performed

Cautions
- Overly forceful extraction may result in purpura, prolonged erythema, or hyperpigmentation.

Risks
- Purpura, prolonged erythema, or hyperpigmentation. Very rarely, infection may result after excessive pressure.

Equipment Needed (Figure 49.1A and B)
- 18 G needle or 11-blade
- Comedone extractor or two cotton-tipped wooden applicators

Preprocedural Approach
- None

Procedural Approach
- Informed consent from the parent/guardian and assent from the minor are obtained. For this minor procedure, consent is usually in the form of verbal consent, although some practitioners may opt for written consent.

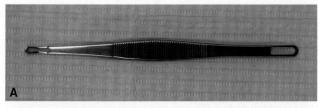

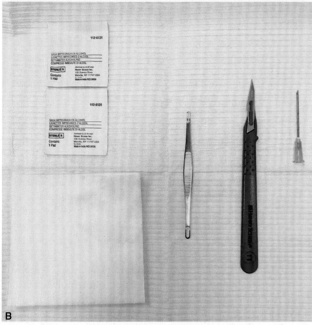

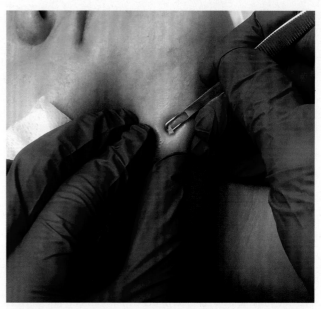

FIGURE 49.2. Holding the comedone extractor comfortably in the hand at the textured midshaft, the correctly sized wire loop is placed over a comedone, encircling it fully. Gentle downward force is, then, applied using slow, even pressure as the tool is gently "dragged" across the skin. Once extraction is complete, the comedone extractor must be cleaned and disinfected.

FIGURE 49.1. A, Comedone extractor. This handy tool is basically a tiny lever with thin wire loops on both ends. It provides the user enhanced mechanical leverage to make comedone extraction easier. B, Setup for comedone extraction, demonstrating an 11-blade or an 18-gauge needle, rubbing alcohol prep pads, and gauze. The 11-blade or 18-gauge needle may be used to nick the surface of the comedo so that extraction is facilitated.

- Clean the area to be treated with an alcohol prep pad swab; extraction should not be attempted in areas of active infection.
- Typically, anesthesia is not utilized given that the pain of the procedure is minimal. However, should the patient be apprehensive about any discomfort, a topical numbing agent can be applied before the procedure. Alternatively, ice or a forced air-cooling device could be utilized to anesthetize the area just before treatment.
- Either one of two approaches may be utilized:
  - Utilizing the mechanical advantage afforded by a comedone extractor (ie, it acts as a lever), place the looped end of the instrument around the comedo and apply pressure perpendicularly to the skin. As the comedo begins to extrude from the skin, the comedone extractor is gently "dragged" (ie, pulled) across the skin firmly and slowly toward the practitioner to further encourage extrusion of the comedo (Figure 49.2).
  - Utilizing either an 18G needle or an 11-blade, nick the surface of the comedo (so that there is minimal or no bleeding). Gentle pressure from opposite sides of the comedo is performed with two cotton-tipped wooden applicators. Alternatively, a comedone extractor may be utilized instead of the two cotton-tipped wooden applicators. However, it is the opinion of the authors that the comedone extractor is a more traumatizing instrument and often leaves residual erythema or purpura.
  - If the practitioner experiences difficulty extruding the lesions, do not continue to apply force on the lesion. Bleeding should be very minimal.

Postprocedural Approach

- Makeup should not be applied to the area immediately after treatment, but no other postoperative instructions are needed.
- Topical products, including retinoids and chemical exfoliants (α- and β-hydroxyl acids), may be continued.

SUGGESTED READINGS

Wise EM, Graber EM. Clinical pearl: comedone extraction for persistent macrocomedones whole on isotretinoin therapy. *J Clin Aesthet Dermatol.* 2011;4(11):20–21.

Zaenglein AL, Pathy AL, Schlosser BJ, et al. Guidelines of care for the management of acne vulgaris. *J Am Acad Dermatol.* 2016;74:945–973.

CHAPTER 50

Acne Cyst

Emmy Graber and Shari Marchbein

Introduction

Acne is an exceedingly common condition, especially in adolescence when it affects 85% of teenagers. Acne cysts, in particular, are often cosmetically distressing to patients, may be painful, and are associated with subsequent scarring that is permanent. Although topical and oral medications are the mainstay of acne management, most of these treatments require weeks to months to adequately reduce inflammation. With a fast onset of action, intralesional corticosteroid injections can provide near-immediate relief from symptoms for acutely inflamed acne cysts. It should be stressed that intralesional corticosteroid injections are not suitable as a long-term acne management, and correct injection technique is not as easy as it may first appear.

Clinical Pearls

- **Guidelines:** No specific consensus guidelines exist for acne cysts in particular, and for use of intralesional corticosteroid treatments, although acne consensus groups recognize that this is a "commonly used technique" that provides "rapid improvement and decreased pain."[1]
- **Age-Specific Considerations:** Ideally, patients should be old enough to ask for treatment, understand the risks and benefits of the procedure and be able to cooperate for an injection.
- **Technique Tips:**
  - Various corticosteroids have been used for intralesional injection, although the most commonly used and published is triamcinolone acetonide.
  - Always inject in a direction "away from" the eye.
- **Skin of Color Considerations:** The technique is best suited for lighter skin types, because there is a risk of hypopigmentation that would be more pronounced in darker skin types, should it occur.

Contraindications/Cautions/Risks

Contraindications
- Allergy to corticosteroids
- Inability to sit still for injection or assent to injection

Cautions
- Smaller lesions have an increased risk of atrophy after injection and hypopigmentation would be more pronounced in darker skin types.
- Always inject in the direction "away from" the eye.

Risks
- Death (infection, anaphylaxis to corticosteroids), systemic absorption of corticosteroids and adrenal suppression, skin atrophy, skin hypopigmentation

Equipment Needed (Figure 50.1)

- Syringe
- 30 G ½-in needle
- 18 G needle
- Triamcinolone acetonide 10 mg/mL injectable suspension
- Normal saline
- Alcohol wipe
- Sterile gauze

Preprocedural Approach

- Draw up the desired concentration of triamcinolone acetonide by diluting it with normal saline (or other suitable diluent) for injection (see Chapter 15. Injectable Corticosteroids [Intralesional Kenalog, Intramuscular] and Appendix. Common Dilutions of Triamcinolone Acetonide [Kenalog]). Most facial cysts will respond to a concentration of 2.5 mg/mL. For example, to obtain 1 mL volume of triamcinolone acetonide (Kenalog) diluted to a concentration of 2.5 mg/mL, one would first draw up 0.75 mL of normal saline (utilizing the 18 G needle) and then draw up 0.25 mL of "stock" triamcinolone acetonide 10 mg/mL (utilizing the same syringe and 18 G needle). The resulting solution should be manually mixed by shaking the syringe, and the 18 G needle should be replaced with a 30 G needle before proceeding with the injection.

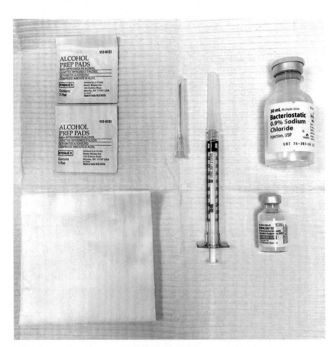

FIGURE 50.1. Acne cyst intralesional corticosteroid set-up.

Procedural Approach

- Informed consent from the parent/guardian and assent from the minor are obtained. For this minor procedure, this is usually in the form of verbal consent, although some practitioners may opt for written consent.
- Typically, anesthesia is not utilized given that the pain of the procedure is minimal. However, should the patient be apprehensive about any discomfort, a topical numbing agent can be applied before the procedure. Alternatively, ice or a forced air-cooling device could be utilized to anesthetize the area just before injection.
- It is recommended that the practitioner wear a mask and protective eyewear during the injection.
- Gently cleanse the area to be treated with ethyl alcohol.
- Next, insert the needle so that the tip is in the middle of the cyst (Figure 50.2). Pressure is applied slowly and steadily to the syringe to inject enough corticosteroid into the cyst until the lesion blanches.
- Upon blanching of the lesion, the needle is withdrawn and firm pressure is applied with a gauze. Pressure is usually adequate to stop minimal bleeding and a small bandage is often not necessary, but it can be placed if needed.
- During injection, the patient will experience a burning sensation. Given that fluid (corticosteroid) is injected into the cyst, the patient may have an increased sense of pressure in the area just after injection, as well.

Postprocedural Approach

- Makeup should not be applied to the area immediately after treatment, but no other postoperative instructions are needed.
- It is expected that the lesion will be significantly smaller and less painful in 12 to 24 hours.
- If local atrophy develops, this may be improved with sterile saline injections into the area.

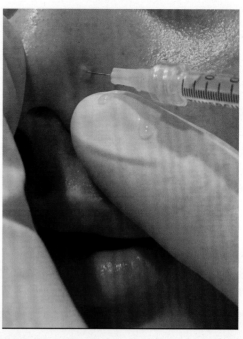

FIGURE 50.2. Intralesional corticosteroid injection of an acne cyst. Note the blanching that occurs as the volume of corticosteroid is delivered correctly into the lesion. Photo courtesy of Nathan S. Uebelhoer, DO.

REFERENCE

1. Zaenglein AL, Pathy AL, Schlosser BJ, et al. Guidelines of care for the management of acne vulgaris. *J Am Acad Dermatol.* 2016;74:945–973.

SUGGESTED READING

Levine RM, Rasmussen JE. Intralesional corticosteroids in the treatment of nodulocystic acne. *Arch Dermatol.* 1983;11(6):480–481.

Acne Scarring

Gaurav Singh, Elyse M. Love, and Jeremy A. Brauer

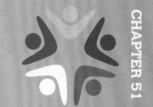

CHAPTER 51

Introduction

Acne vulgaris is a disorder of the pilosebaceous unit that affects 85% of individuals between 12 and 24 years of age, with increasing impact in 7- to 11-year-olds.[1] Increased risk in children can be associated with several conditions including XYY karyotype, polycystic ovarian syndrome, hyperandrogenism, hypercortisolism, and precocious puberty. All ethnicities and both genders are affected; however, Caucasian males are the most prone to developing severe nodulocystic acne, with severe scarring in 30% of all patients with acne, and at least mild scarring is noted in 95%.[1] Scarring can have not only physical but also psychological implications in these patients, especially in the pediatric population.

Fortunately, multiple modalities are available in the treatment of acne scarring depending on individual patient and scar characteristics. These procedures are generally focused on the improvement of texture and appearance, including redness and/or pigmentation. Most acne scars are atrophic, including boxcar, ice pick, and rolling scars (Figure 51.1), whereas 10% to 20% are hypertrophic.[1] Acne scars are often erythematous compared to unaffected skin (Figure 51.2). Lasers and energy devices, chemical peels, needling, injectables including intralesional steroids and fillers, and platelet-rich plasma (PRP) are often employed in the correction of textural concerns (see further details in Chapters 14. Injectables, 15. Injectable Corticosteroids [Intralesional Kenalog, Intramuscular], and 21. Chemical Peels).

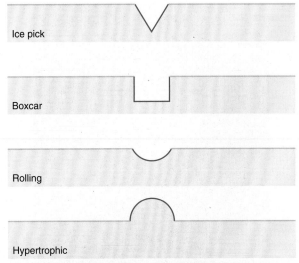

FIGURE 51.1. Morphologic description of scars that typically may result as a consequence of inflammatory acne vulgaris.

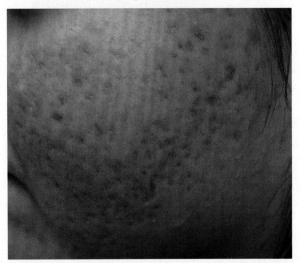

FIGURE 51.2. Adolescent female with scarring that resulted from her severe inflammatory acne; this photograph demonstrates the atrophic nature of her scarring and the erythema specifically associated with the scars (ie, sparing "normal" skin). Photo courtesy of Andrew C. Krakowski, MD.

Clinical Pearls

- **Guidelines**
  - Although formal guidelines do not exist, treatment regimens should be individualized by considering patient characteristics such as skin type, expectations, budget, and tolerance for pain and downtime, and scar characteristics such as changes in texture and pigmentation (Table 51.1).
- **Laser and Energy Devices**
  - Ablative fractional 10 600-nm CO_2, nonablative fractional 1550/1927-, and 755-, and 532/1064-nm picosecond lasers with diffractive lens and holographic beam splitter are recommended for atrophic scars; the 755- and 1064-nm wavelengths in the latter devices are preferred in skin of color.[2] Ablative fractional CO_2 and nonablative fractional 1550-nm lasers are effective for hypertrophic scarring. Scars with erythema or prominent telangiectasias can be treated with 595-nm pulsed-dye laser (PDL) and 532-nm potassium titanyl

phosphate (KTP) lasers. Hyperpigmented scars can be treated with Q-switched nanosecond lasers including 532-, 694-, 755-, and 1064-nm wavelengths; picosecond lasers, including 532-, 755-, and 1064-nm wavelengths; or nonablative fractional 1927-nm lasers. The 1064-nm nanosecond, 755-, and 1064-nm picosecond, and the low-energy, low-density 1927-nm nonablative fractional lasers are safe and effective in skin of color patients. Radiofrequency microneedling is also effective in treating atrophic scars, particularly in skin of color.
- **Chemical Peels**
  - Although the authors do not routinely utilize chemical peels for treatment of acne scarring, there have been successful reports in the literature for use of this modality in the treatment of both texture and pigmentation of acne scarring.
- **Microneedling**
  - This modality, as a standalone or with other therapies, has been demonstrated to be effective for atrophic scarring in all skin types.
- **Injectables**
  - The authors do not routinely use injectables in adolescent patients. However, fillers are effective in improving the appearance of atrophic (particularly rolling and boxcar) scars, often requiring multiple sessions with temporary results unless a permanent filler, such as silicone, is used. Silicone, although not routinely used by the authors, can be injected to improve and eliminate depressed, broad-based acne scars. Although multiple hyaluronic acid fillers can be utilized, to date, only Bellafill® (Suneva Medical Inc., US 2020. Note: Bellafill was previously known as ArteFill) has received U.S. Food and Drug Administration (FDA) approval for the correction of moderate to severe atrophic acne scarring in adults. Intralesional triamcinolone and/or intralesional 5-fluorouracil are used in the treatment of hypertrophic scarring. Platelet-rich plasma (PRP) is effective in treating atrophic scars as standalone therapy or when combined with other modalities such as microneedling, chemical peels, and carbon dioxide or erbium fractional laser.

Contraindications/Cautions/Risks

Contraindications

- Active infection such as herpes or impetigo, excoriated acne lesions, or open wounds
- Patients on isotretinoin should not undergo mechanical dermabrasion or fully ablative laser until 6 to 12 months after therapy is complete. Other procedures do not need to be avoided, contrary to prior dogma.[3]
- It is the belief of the authors that filler injection should not be performed in children, patients with autoimmune disorders, or in patients with known allergy to filler material.
- Dental procedures should not be performed for a minimum of 2 weeks before or after filler injection because of potential increased risk of biofilm formation.

Cautions

- Parental/legal guardian consent is required for the care of minors in these circumstances.
- Patients should be of an appropriate age to express desire for treatment and report symptoms of complications such as fevers and pain.
- Scarring and dyspigmentation are more likely to occur in skin of color and in individuals with suntanned skin undergoing laser treatment.

TABLE 51.1 : Acne Scar Treatment Options, Determined by Scar Morphology and Safety Profile

ACNE SCAR TYPE	LASER AND ENERGY DEVICES	OTHERS
Atrophic	• Ablative fractional 10 600-nm CO_2 • Nonablative fractional 1550/1927 nm • 755- and 532/1064-nm picosecond	• Radiofrequency • Microneedling • Dermal fillers • Platelet-rich plasma
Hypertrophic	• Ablative fractional 10 600-nm CO_2 • Nonablative fractional 1550-nm	
Erythematous	• 595-nm pulsed-dye laser • 532-nm potassium titanyl phosphate	
Hyperpigmented	• 532-, 694-, 755-, or 1064-nm Q-switched nanosecond • 532-, 755-, or 1064-nm picosecond • Nonablative fractional 1927-nm	
Preferred in skin of color patients	• 1064-nm nanosecond • 755- or 1064-nm picosecond • Low-energy-density 1927-nm nonablative fractional	• Radiofrequency • Microneedling

Risks

○ Laser resurfacing: Infection, scarring, koebnerization of certain existing skin conditions, changes in pigmentation (specifically, hyper- or hypopigmentation), contact dermatitis, prolonged erythema
○ Chemical peels: Change in pigmentation, scarring, infection, and, rarely, systemic toxicity
○ Needling (including radiofrequency [RF]): Edema,. infection, milia, change in pigmentation, scarring
○ Injectables: Bruising/swelling, nodules, vascular compromise with skin necrosis, granulomas, and infection

Equipment Needed

● Laser and energy devices
  ○ Wavelength-specific eye shields
  ○ Smoke evacuator for ablative fractional procedures
  ○ Lasers (including but not limited to 532-nm KTP, 595-nm PDL; 755- and 532/1064-nm picosecond lasers with or without diffractive lens array/holographic beam splitter; Q-switched nanosecond 532-, 694-, 755-, and 1064-nm lasers; ablative fractional 10 600-nm and nonablative fractional 1550/1927-nm lasers)
  ○ RF microneedling
● Needling device
● Chemical peels

● Injectables
  ○ Bellafill is the only FDA-approved filler, but a variety of fillers are regularly utilized.
  ○ Reversal agents such as hyaluronidase should be available if hyaluronic acid augmentation is planned.
● Platelet-rich plasma kit

Preprocedural Approach

● Selection of the appropriate patient, treatment modality, and parameters are necessary for successful outcomes. Patients should understand the risks, benefits, alternatives, and expectations, as well as the postoperative course.
● Obtain a comprehensive history (past medical, surgical, and medication/allergy), specifically but not limited to a history of therapeutic radiation exposure or gold therapy, history of abnormal scar formation, medications such as isotretinoin and anticoagulants, as well as prior treatments for the indication.
● Abnormal wound healing and/or therapeutic radiation exposure should raise caution for resurfacing procedures.
● History of gold therapy precludes use of lasers for treatment of pigmented scars.
● Avoid procedures on areas of active infections and open wounds.
● Herpes antiviral prophylaxis should be prescribed for all patients with history of cold sores, as well as those without but are undergoing ablative or nonablative fractional resurfacing, chemical peels, and injectable fillers.
● Topical retinoids should be held 1 week before any procedure.
● Practice of appropriate sun-protective behaviors to minimize tanned skin ahead of laser procedures as well as immediately post the procedure and recovery (see Chapter 135. Photoprotection).
● Dental procedures should be avoided 2 weeks before and after filler injection.

Procedural Approach

A detailed understanding of the procedure is imperative. Incorrect selection of patient candidates, devices, and parameters, as well as poor intraoperative technique increase the chances of common and serious adverse events.

LASER AND ENERGY DEVICES

● Depending on surface area of involvement, focal treatment may be performed on acne scars.
● Everyone in the room, including the patient, operator, assistants, and observers, must wear wavelength-appropriate eye protection for the entirety of the procedure.
● The patient's face should be cleansed of all cosmetics that may interfere with laser absorption.
● Topical anesthesia for a defined period of time will minimize procedure discomfort. Intralesional anesthesia, nerve blocks, opioids, and/or anxiolytics may be preferred for fractional ablative procedures.
● Laser parameters and technique will vary depending on the laser properties and the patient's skin type and scar burden, as outlined here:

Pulsed-Dye Laser

The erythema and vascular component of acne scars can be treated with PDL. An example of this device includes the 595-nm

Vbeam Perfecta™ (Candela Corporation, US). *PDL is not contraindicated in darker skin types, but should be used with extreme caution because of risk of pigmentary alteration and burns.*

- We recommend a 10-mm spot size, fluence of between 6.5 and 7.5 J/cm^2, and pulse duration of 1.5 to 6 ms, depending on patient characteristics. Pulse duration of 1.5 ms will produce moderate purpura as the desired clinical endpoint. Longer pulse duration of 6 ms should be used in patients who desire less downtime, with erythema as the desired endpoint at this pulse duration.
- Pulses should be overlapped by 10% to 20% during treatment, and the device should be held perpendicular to the area treated at all times.
- If ablative laser will be performed on the same day, we advise that PDL be utilized first because ablative devices can alter the vascular target of PDL.
- Treatments can be repeated every 4 to 6 weeks for multiple sessions.

Ablative Fractional CO$_2$ Laser

Fractional lasers, which create pixilated columns of thermal injury that result in collagen production, offer excellent results. The ablative fractional CO$_2$ laser is effective for moderate to severe atrophic scars (Figure 51.3A-C). Side effects can include scarring, dyspigmentation, erythema, and edema. These adverse impacts are minimized by appropriate device parameter and patient skin type selection. Devices that can be used include the UltraPulse™ (Lumenis, Yokneam, Israel).

- Ensure that safe laser practices are followed: All participants should wear masks and a smoke evacuator should be utilized.
- Settings vary depending on patient skin and scar type. Utilize single pulses without overlap in a uniform pattern across the skin to achieve a depth of about 100 μm.
- With a fixed spot size of 120 μm, pulse energies of 20 to 100 mJ/pulse, densities of 100 to 400 MTZ/cm^2 per pass, and total treatment densities of 200 to 1200 MTZ/cm^2 can be used.
- Treatments can be repeated monthly for several months.

CHEMICAL PEELS

- Superficial to medium-depth peels can be applied to the entire face with improvement in overall skin texture, background acne, and treatment of acne scars.
- Treatment protocol will vary depending on chemical peel agent used and the desired depth of penetration.
- Chemical peels typically produce mild discomfort that resolves within minutes of application. For patients with low pain tolerance, topical anesthetic can be applied before the procedure.
- The patient should present with a clean face.

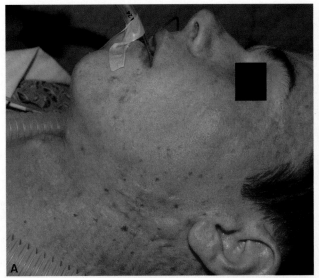
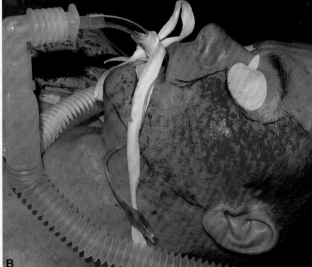
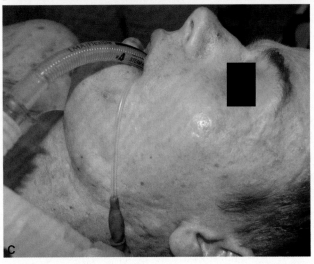

FIGURE 51.3. Adolescent male with a combination of atrophic and hypertrophic scarring as a consequence of severe inflammatory acne. Ablative fractional CO$_2$ laser was utilized to help improve the texture of the cheeks and to help decrease the range-of-motion limitation that the deep scars around the mandible caused. A, Patient required general anesthesia for this procedure. B, Field treatments over entire cosmetic units, showing mild bleeding associated with this device. C, Postprocedure results after three treatments spaced roughly 6 to 8 weeks apart; this patient is prepared for the fourth and final treatment under general anesthesia. Photos courtesy of Andrew C. Krakowski, MD.

- The skin is degreased with acetone to allow even distribution of the peeling solution.
- Concentration and depth of penetration is determined by the applicator used to apply the peeling solution, the saturation of the applicator during application, and the pressure used to apply the peeling solution.
- The need for neutralization will vary by peeling agent.
- Superficial chemical peel agents include glycolic acid, salicylic acid, and 10% to 20% trichloroacetic acid (TCA).
- Medium-depth peels include 40% to 50% TCA.
- Application of Jessner's solution, 70% glycolic acid, or solid CO_2 followed by 35% TCA produces a similar medium-depth effect as does 40% to 50% TCA with decreased risk of dyschromia and scarring. With combination regimens, only one layer of the priming peel agent should be applied.
- For Jessner's solution, a thin layer is applied to the entire face, one cosmetic subunit at a time (see Figure 9.5A). The eyes, nasal mucosa, and lips should be avoided. Level I frosting (mild frosting on a background of erythema) is expected. Neutralization is not needed.
- Application of glycolic acid is similar to that for Jessner's solution but requires neutralization at the presentation of erythema, approximately 3 to 5 minutes after peel application. If frosting occurs earlier, the area should be neutralized immediately.
- TCA is applied in a similar fashion with frosting presenting within 1 minute, depending on the abovementioned technique parameters. Neutralization is not necessary. Medium-depth peeling produces a level II frosting (prominent white frosting on a background of erythema). Level III frosting produces thick white frosting without background erythema and is associated with deeper peels.
- For TCA peels, if only level I or no frosting is present after 4 minutes, the undertreated areas can be focally retreated to obtain the desired treatment effect. Repeat application should not be applied to areas that reached the desired level of frosting, because this increases depth of penetration and risk of complications.
- Cool compresses may be applied to the skin following chemical peels for discomfort relief.
- Deeper ice pick scars may benefit from focal scar treatment with 90% TCA and level III frosting. This technique, termed "CROSS" or "dot peeling" (see Figure 21.3), creates a full-thickness wound that heals over 2 to 3 weeks. It is analogous to ablative full-thickness destruction and should not be applied to the entire face.
  - First, clean the treatment area with a degreasing agent to ensure that the acid penetrates evenly. Dry the area.
  - Then, use a fine wooden toothpick to apply the TCA to the bottom of the scar. A characteristic sheet of white frost should become evident. The peel should be cleaned at this point with either a neutralizing agent or cold water.
  - Patient can expect mild to moderate burning pain, but anesthesia and sedation are not typically required.
  - Neocollagenesis occurs in the ensuing weeks.
  - Postoperatively, sunscreen and moisturizer should be used. Erythema, edema, and scale can be expected and may last days. Scarring or dyspigmentation can occur.
  - Peels can be repeated every 4 to 6 weeks.

MICRONEEDLING

- A lubricant is applied to clean skin. Options include the manufacturer-provided gel, hyaluronic acid, and PRP.

- The needling device is glided over the skin. The specific technique will depend on which needling device is used. Options include manual or powered "pen devices" and more elaborate devices with radiofrequency.
- Depth of penetration is determined by needle length and operator pressure.
- The device produces minimum discomfort. Topical anesthesia is not often needed but may be of benefit for pain control.

INJECTABLES

- The face is cleaned with an antibacterial preparation before filler injection to minimize infection and prevent biofilm formation.
- Technique will be individual; however, a variety of approaches have been used and reported in the literature including threading, fanning, deep bolus, serial punctures, and superficial microdroplet injections.
- Arterial occlusion is a serious adverse reaction that can present with immediate pain and skin blanching. Although occlusion protocols may vary, and this text is not intended to discuss management of complications, the authors suggest the following for hyaluronic acid products: The area should be flooded with the appropriate amount of hyaluronidase; warm compress and/or nitroglycerin paste applied; and massage, oral aspirin, prednisone, and sildenafil administered, if not otherwise contraindicated, to consider hyperbaric oxygen.
- For hypertrophic scarring on the face, intralesional triamcinolone (2.5-5 mg/mL) in combination with 5-fluorouracil (500 mg/10 mL) is often used in conjunction with laser resurfacing

Postprocedural Approach

- Cold compresses, emollients such as petrolatum, and mask and bandage should be applied after the procedure to minimize bruising, swelling, and edema.
- Strict sunscreen use must be encouraged to minimize dyspigmentation and increased risk of photodamage.
- Topical retinoids should be held until inflammation has resolved.
- A short course of topical steroid and/or hydroquinone and nonhydroquinone lightening agents may be a useful adjunct to minimize PIH.
- Patients who received an injectable should be counseled to return immediately if signs of vascular occlusive events such as pain occur. These patients should also avoid dental procedures for at least 2 weeks to minimize the risk of biofilm formation.
- For vascular occlusion, close follow-up with adequate wound care will be necessary over the next weeks.

REFERENCES

1. Bhargava S, Cunha PR, Lee J, Kroumpouzos G. Acne scarring management: systematic review and evaluation of the evidence. *Am J Clin Dermatol.* 2018;19:459–477. doi:10.1007/s40257-018-0358-5.
2. Brauer JA, Kazlouskaya V, Alabdulrazzaq H, et al. Use of a picosecond pulse duration laser with specialized optic for treatment of facial acne scarring. *JAMA Dermatol.* 2015;151:278–284. doi:10.1001/jamadermatol.2014.3045.
3. Spring LK, Krakowski AC, Alam M, et al. Isotretinoin and timing of procedural interventions: a systematic review with consensus recommendations. *JAMA Dermatol.* 2017;153(8):802–809. doi:10.1001/jamadermatol.2017.2077.

CHAPTER 52

Acrochordons

Megan A. Trainor and Lucía Z. Díaz

Introduction

Acrochordons, or skin tags, are common and occur in both the pediatric and adult population. Acrochordons typically present as skin-colored to hyperpigmented, soft, pedunculated papules that are commonly found in areas of friction such as the neck, axilla, and inguinal folds (Figure 52.1). The cause of acrochordons is unknown, but friction is thought to play a role, and some studies have shown increased incidence in patients with obesity and insulin resistance. The majority of acrochordons are asymptomatic; however, they may become painful if irritated or inflamed. The differential diagnosis for acrochordons in children includes basal cell carcinomas such as those seen in nevoid basal cell carcinoma syndrome. Thus, if several acrochordons are present and there is suspicion of basal cell carcinoma, lesions should be removed with the shave or snip technique and the excised tissue should be sent to pathology. We typically discuss the role of pathology with the family and do not routinely send suspected acrochordons for pathology if the clinical diagnosis is not in doubt.

Several methods may be used to remove acrochordons including cryotherapy, electrodesiccation, ligation, shave removal, and snip removal. These treatments have a low rate of recurrence, but the procedures may result in scarring and temporary pain. In addition, it is common for patients to develop new acrochordons in areas of friction.

Herein, we offer step-by-step instructions for the various treatments of acrochordons. It is important to note that acrochordons are benign lesions and removal is not required, but it may be indicated for symptomatic or cosmetically bothersome lesions.

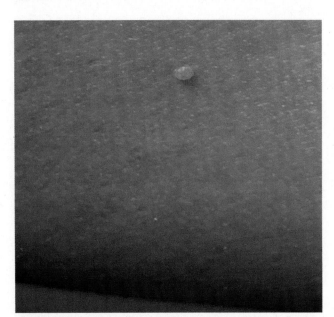

FIGURE 52.1. Acrochordons typically present as flesh-colored to hyperpigmented, soft, pedunculated papules that are commonly found in areas of friction such as the neck, axilla, and inguinal folds.

Clinical Pearls

- **Guidelines:** No specific treatment guidelines are known to exist for this condition.
- **Age-Specific Considerations:** Because acrochordons are benign, lesions should be symptomatic to warrant medical management. A practitioner may consider cosmetic treatment if the patient is old enough to request treatment and has parental consent.
- **Technique Tips:** Smaller acrochordons may be snipped without first injecting lidocaine because the pain associated with injection may be greater than the pain associated with actual removal. Acrochordons may also be sprayed with ethyl chloride immediately before removal to reduce pain associated with the procedure. If you are not planning on sending the specimen for histopathological confirmation, then consider applying aluminum chloride to the lesion *before* a snip removal or shave removal procedure to help reduce bleeding associated with the procedure.

Contraindications/Cautions/Risks

Contraindications
- Active skin infection in the treatment area

Cautions
- Especially large lesions may be referred to surgery; however, most acrochordons seen in children are typically suitable for in-office treatment.
- Cryosurgery and electrodesiccation may not be used if the lesion is being sent to pathology because these processes may affect histopathologic diagnosis.

Risks
- Infection, scarring, pain, and bleeding

Equipment Needed

- Alcohol swab or
- Local anesthetic (reserved for larger lesions): 1% lidocaine or ethyl chloride spray or a eutectic mixture of local anesthetics (EMLA™ [AB Astra Pharmaceuticals, L.P.]) cream
- Cryotherapy
  - Handheld liquid nitrogen canister or
  - Cryospray gun or
  - Liquid nitrogen in foam cup and cotton-tipped applicator or forceps
- Electrodesiccation
  - Hyfrecator 2000™ (Conmed, Utica, NY)
  - Electrode tip
- Ligation
  - Silk suture
- Snip removal
  - Iris scissors
  - Small forceps
- Shave removal
  - Dermablade™ (Accutec Blades Inc., US) or Personna blade or #15 blade

- Aluminum chloride
- Cotton-tipped applicator
- Petrolatum ointment

Preprocedural Approach

- No routine preoperative preparation is required of patients. In cases of larger acrochordons, the practitioner may recommend the patient apply LMX.4™ (Ferndale Laboratories) or EMLA cream to the lesion under occlusion at home an hour before the procedure.
- If you are not planning on sending the specimen for histopathological confirmation, then consider applying aluminum chloride to the lesion *before* a snip removal or shave removal procedure to help reduce bleeding associated with the procedure.

Procedural Approach

- Informed consent from the parent/guardian and, when possible, assent from the minor are obtained.
- Local anesthesia with intralesional lidocaine injected into the base of the lesion or ethyl chloride spray or topical anesthetic cream (LMX.4 or EMLA) may be utilized depending on the size and location of the acrochordon and patient age. We offer intralesional lidocaine for snip removal, shave removal, and electrodesiccation, but do not routinely utilize because the injection may be more painful than the actual procedure.
- Position patient depending on location of the acrochordon.
- Cleanse acrochordon with alcohol swab.

  Several techniques are listed here. We often discuss the treatment options with the patient and family and proceed pending patient preference. We often utilize the snip removal technique in children because it is typically well tolerated, does not often require intralesional lidocaine, and only one treatment session is needed.

- Cryotherapy (three technique variants are offered)
  - Spray the acrochordon with liquid nitrogen, either with a canister holding approximately 1 to 2 cm away from the lesion or with a cryospray gun. Use short, pulsating sprays until lesion has frozen and turns white (typically 5-10 seconds; Figure 52.2). Let thaw completely and then repeat for two additional freeze–thaw cycles.
  - Dip cotton-tipped swab into foam cup filled with liquid nitrogen until cotton tip is frozen and place directly on acrochordon until lesion is frozen and turns white. Let thaw completely and then repeat for two additional freeze–thaw cycles.

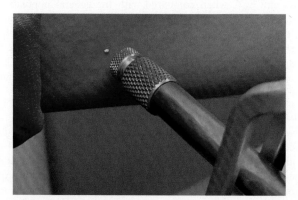

FIGURE 52.2. Liquid nitrogen can be administered by a handheld canister or cryospray gun, using short, pulsating sprays until the lesion is frozen and turns white (typically 5-10 seconds), then allowing to thaw completely, and repeating for two additional freeze–thaw cycles.

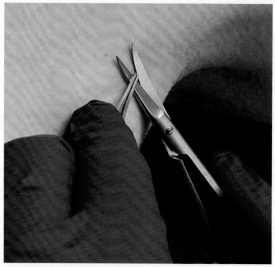

FIGURE 52.3. Snip removal using forceps to hold tip of acrochordon and cutting at the base with iris scissors.

  - Dip small forceps into foam cup filled with liquid nitrogen until tips are frozen and grasp the base of the acrochordon until lesion is frozen and turns white. Let thaw and then repeat for two additional freeze–thaw cycles.
- Electrodesiccation
  - Use electrodesiccation setting on Hyfrecator set to a power setting of 6 to 10. Place electrode in direct contact with the acrochordon for desired destructive effects (typically 2-4 seconds).
- Ligation
  - After cutting needle off suture, use silk surgical suture to tie a knot around the base of the acrochordon. Lesion will necrose after several days and fall off.
- Snip removal
  - Use forceps to hold tip of acrochordon and cut base of acrochordon with iris scissor (Figure 52.3).
  - Apply aluminum chloride to achieve hemostasis if required.
  - Send lesion for pathology pending differential diagnosis.
- Shave removal
  - Use Dermablade or Personna blade or #15 blade to shave acrochordon at the base.
  - Apply aluminum chloride to achieve hemostasis.
  - Apply petroleum ointment to wound and apply adhesive bandage.
  - Send lesion for pathology pending differential diagnosis.

Postprocedural Approach

- Minimal pain is expected after the procedure.
- If the area is dressed with an adhesive dressing, we recommend the patient leave the area dry for 24 hours followed by daily gentle cleaning and daily application of petroleum ointment.
- Counsel patient on signs and symptoms of infection; however, infection is rare post acrochordon removal.
- Larger acrochordons may require more than one treatment with cryotherapy for removal.
- Follow up as needed.

SUGGESTED READINGS

Chiritescu E, Maloney ME. Acrochordons as a presenting sign of nevoid basal cell carcinoma syndrome. *J Am Acad Dermatol.* 2001;44:789–794.

Shaheen MA, Abdel Fattah NA, Sayed YA, Saad AA. Assessment of serum leptin, insulin resistance and metabolic syndrome in patients with skin tags. *J Eur Acad Dermatol Venereol.* 2012;26:1552–1557.

Uzuncakmak TK, Akdeniz N, Karadag AS. Cutaneous manifestations of obesity and the metabolic syndrome. *Clin Dermatol.* 2018;36:81–88.

CHAPTER 53

Actinic Keratosis

Puneet Singh Jolly

Introduction

Actinic keratoses (AKs) are common lesions encountered in most dermatology clinics in the United States as well as in Europe and Australia. These precancerous lesions, which present clinically as scaly erythematous macules, patches, and plaques, are precursors to cutaneous squamous cell carcinomas (SCCs) (Figure 53.1). The etiology includes environmental as well as host factors including fair skin tone, male gender, older age, freckling, and living close to the equator. There is abundant evidence to implicate sun-induced DNA damage, which results in the formation of thymidine dimers. Normally these dimers lead to an arrest in the cell cycle followed by a DNA repair guided by the tumor suppressor p53. Sun-induced DNA damage can also cause mutations in p53 inhibiting normal DNA repair, which leads to the development of AKs and subsequently SCCs. Although there are several clinical scenarios where children are at increased risk of developing SCCs, not all involve the formation of AKs as precursor lesions. For example, sites of radiation, burn scars, or scars from dystrophic epidermolysis bullosa are not preceded by AKs and usually form after decades but can occasionally occur in children.

AKs develop for a variety of reasons including mutagenesis, immunosuppression, chronic inflammation, or oxidative stress. There are some data to suggest that human papillomavirus (HPV) may also play a role. Understanding what is involved in the formation of AKs also provides insight into what circumstances may lead to the development of these lesions in children.

SPECIAL POPULATIONS AND SUN PROTECTION

There are a few special circumstances whereby children develop AKs. It is important for dermatologists to recognize these scenarios in order to intervene using appropriate measures. In

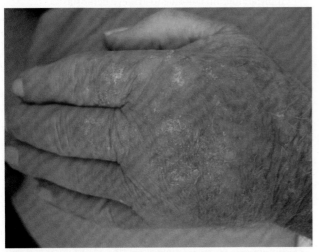

FIGURE 53.1. Clinical presentation of actinic keratoses. Multiple scaly erythematous macules and papules on dorsum of sun-exposed skin on the hand. Image provided by Stedman's Illustrated Guide of Dermatology Eponyms, © Wolters Kluwer.

addition to the treatments reviewed in this chapter, it is imperative that these children practice strict sun-protective measures and are instructed on how to apply sunscreen as well as the importance of sun-protective clothing and wide-brimmed hats and potentially even sun avoidance (see also Chapter 135. Photoprotection). As such, checking vitamin D levels and supplementing appropriately may be necessary. Reducing immunosuppression or avoiding certain immunosuppressive medications that may cause a more significant increase in photocarcinogenesis, such as cyclosporine or azathioprine, should be reviewed with patients and providers. Finally, engaging in frequent skin surveillance examinations ensures the early diagnosis of both precancerous AKs and nonmelanoma skin cancer.

Albinism

One person in 17 000 has some type of albinism. Children with albinism have mutations in genes that are involved in melanin synthesis. Melanin pigment provides a protective barrier for the nuclei of keratinocytes against ultraviolet (UV) radiation. Without this protection, these patients are particularly susceptible to UV radiation. Studies have demonstrated that patients with oculocutaneous albinism show signs of actinic damage even in childhood. A large study in Tanzania examined actinic damage in patients with oculocutaneous albinism.[1] Out of 164 patients examined, all but 4 infants showed signs of actinic damage. Solar elastosis was nearly universal by the age of 10 and actinic cheilitis was seen in greater than 90% of people in the study. Greater than 20% of individuals less than 20 years old had AKs and the majority were on sun-exposed sites such as the face, extremities, and chest. Surprisingly, despite these findings, most people did not practice sun-protective measures, highlighting the need for proper education and prevention.

Xeroderma Pigmentosum

Xeroderma pigmentosum (XP) is a group of rare conditions with the defining feature of hypersensitivity to UV radiation because of a defective DNA repair process (see Chapter 130. Xeroderma Pigmentosum). As a result of this defect, patients with XP have a roughly 1000-fold increase in the incidence of AKs and SCC when compared with the general population. Seven distinct complementation groups exist (A-G) in addition to the XP variant. AKs and SCC typically develop within the first decade of life. Patients must follow strict sun avoidance to reduce their risk of AKs and SCCs (as well as melanoma), but even incidental or indirect sun exposure is enough to precipitate the formation of such lesions.

Immunosuppression

Over the past three to four decades, better immunosuppressive medication combinations have helped to increase survival in both bone marrow and solid organ transplant patients. Most of these medications target T cells in one way or the other. Appropriate T-cell function is necessary for immune surveillance against AKs and skin cancers. A well-known side effect of these medications in adults is a significant increase in the formation of AKs and SCCs. This risk also exists in children and correlates with increasing immunosuppression. Furthermore, certain immunosuppressive medications, such as cyclosporine or azathioprine, confer a greater risk in promoting AKs and skin cancers than tacrolimus or sirolimus. As providers gain familiarity with these medications, we will see greater on- and off-label use. For example, children with severe atopic dermatitis often require steroid-sparing immunomodulators such as cyclosporine or azathioprine to control their disease. As a result, although still rare, development of AKs can occur in patients who are on prolonged immunosuppression.[2]

Medication Use: Voriconazole

Voriconazole is a third-generation triazole family of antifungal medications. This potent drug has activity against a variety of fungal infections including aspergillosis, coccidioidomycosis, and fusarium. It is thought that metabolism by-products of voriconazole may increase photosensitivity and promote formation of aggressive SCCs as well as melanoma. Even a short course of voriconazole can predispose patients to developing skin cancers. There are reports of children who have taken voriconazole for a few months and developed significant actinic skin damage, AKs, and even SCCs.[3] It is also worth noting that alternatives to voriconazole such as posaconazole and itraconazole often have similar antifungal coverage but do not confer the same level of skin cancer risk.

TOPICAL THERAPY

There are several topical agents available to treat AK. The most commonly used are 5-fluorouracil (Efudex), imiquimod (Aldara), as well as ingenol mebutate (Picato) and diclofenac sodium (Solaraze). These are used to treat individual lesions but are more commonly employed as "field treatments" in patients who have larger confluent areas of actinic damage and AK. There are several reports describing the successful clearance of AKs and even skin cancers in children treated using these agents. Care must be taken when using these agents in children because of the potential for developing an exuberant inflammatory reaction (Figure 53.2). Topical 5-fluorouracil is an antimetabolite targeting pyrimidine DNA synthesis. It is approved to treat AKs and superficial basal cell carcinomas (sBCC) that are not amenable to surgery. Off-label use in dermatology includes warts, keloids, and more recently vitiligo (see Chapters 128. Human Papillomavirus Wart [Verruca] and 90. Hypertrophic Scars and Contractures). Imiquimod induces the innate immune response through the activation of toll-like receptor 7 (TLR-7). Cells targeted by imiquimod secrete interferon alpha (IFN-α), tumor necrosis factor (TNF), and interleukin 6 (IL6). It was initially U.S. Food and Drug Administration (FDA) approved to treat genital warts in 1997 but is now also approved to treat AKs and sBCC. Ingenol mebutate (Picato) is approved to treat facial and nonfacial AKs in adults. The mechanism of action includes direct necrosis of the treated tissue as well as neutrophil-mediated antibody-dependent cytotoxicity. There are no known reports of ingenol mebutate used to treat AKs in children, but there are no known restrictions at this time.

CRYOTHERAPY

Destruction of tissue by cryotherapy results from direct effects of freezing tissue as well as vascular stasis. Cryotherapy is used to treat a variety of benign, premalignant, and precancerous lesions in adults and children (see Chapter 16. Cryosurgery). This is by far the most common modality used to treat AK and is quite effective. Cryotherapy is commonly used to treat benign

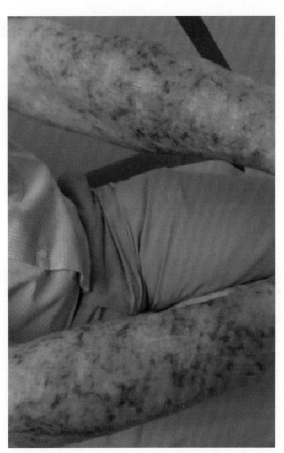

FIGURE 53.2. Inflammatory reaction from topical 5-fluorouracil (5-FU). Erythema, erosions, and crusting after 2 weeks of twice-daily 5-FU cream application. Similar reactions are observed after using imiquimod and ingenol mebutate. Reprinted with permission from Council ML, Sheinbein DM, Cornelius LA. *The Washington Manual of Dermatology Diagnostics.* Philadelphia, PA: Wolters Kluwer; 2016. Figure 15.6.

lesions such as warts and molluscum in children and is very safe and quite well tolerated. For isolated lesions in children who are able to tolerate this modality, it is the treatment of choice.

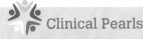

Clinical Pearls

- **Guidelines:** No specific treatment guidelines are known to exist for treating AKs. In general, cryotherapy for AK can be performed using a metal cryosurgery spray device or by applying a cotton swab after it has been submerged in liquid nitrogen (usually by decanting a small amount from a small cryosurgery spray canister into a Styrofoam cup). The target is treated for 5 to 10 seconds with a margin of 1 to 2 mm around the lesion.
- **Age-Specific Considerations:** Younger patients may not tolerate 10-second treatments. Shorter treatment bursts can still be effective.
- **Technique Tips:** In children, use of cotton applicator/cotton swab dipped in liquid nitrogen may be less traumatic and more easily tolerated.
- **Skin of Color Considerations:** The technique is best suited for skin types I and II, as the risk for dyspigmentation increases with darker skin types.

Contraindications/Cautions/Risks

Contraindications

- The procedure should not be performed in a location where circulation is compromised or in a patient previously unable to tolerate the procedure or unwilling to accept risks of the procedure (including hypopigmentation).

Cautions

- Presence of a suntan may increase dyspigmentation.

Risks

- Risks include scarring, pain, blister formation, hemorrhagic crusting, recurrence of lesions, swelling, blister formation, infection, bleeding, hyper- or hypopigmentation.

Equipment Needed

- Topical anesthesia such as LMX.4™ (Ferndale Laboratories)
- Liquid nitrogen
- Cryo container or insulated cup to hold liquid nitrogen
- Cotton-tipped applicators wrapped with gauze

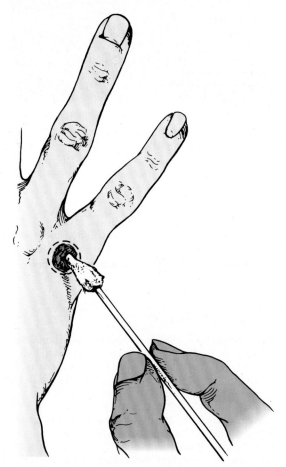

FIGURE 53.3. Cryosurgery. Liquid nitrogen is administered to the tissue in a circular motion around the target extending 2 to 3 mm beyond the edge of the lesion for 10 seconds per lesion. Modified with permission from Arndt KA, Hsu JTS, Alam M, et al. *Manual of Dermatologic Therapeutics.* 8th ed. Philadelphia, PA: Wolters Kluwer Health; 2014. Figure 48.6.

Preprocedural Approach

- We typically do not perform curettage and cryotherapy concomitantly.
- Typically no preprocedure preparation is required.
- Topical anesthesia may be applied.

Procedural Approach

- Target sites are treated with cryotherapy spray using a circular motion with a goal of 10-second frosting, extending about 1 to 2 mm beyond each lesion (Figure 53.3).

Postprocedural Approach

- Generally local swelling and pain should decrease quickly with time.
- Vaseline™ (Conopco, Inc., US) ointment may be applied to the treated area as a skin protectant.
- Pain is typically easily managed with acetaminophen as needed.
- Sun avoidance and sun protection are critical.

PHOTODYNAMIC THERAPY

Photodynamic therapy (PDT) involves using a photosensitizer, light, and oxygen to generate free radicals to induce apoptosis of precancerous or cancerous cells (see Chapter 20. Phototherapy and Photodynamic Therapy). Aminolevulinic acid (ALA; Levulan)-induced PDT is approved to treat facial AKs. Similar to topical agents, PDT is used as "field treatment." It is commonly used as an off-label indication to treat acne in kids.

Clinical Pearls

- **Guidelines:**
  - There are a number of suggested protocols for using PDT for AKs in adults.
  - It is important to note that there are a number of PDT devices, and dosage on one device may not be exactly the same on other devices.
- **Age-Specific Considerations:** There are a few things about PDT that should be considered during use in children.
  - PDT can be uncomfortable. Many patients will describe a burning sensation or heat while under the light source. Topical anesthetics like EMLA™ (AB Astra Pharmaceuticals, L.P.) 30 minutes prior to treatment can be considered but are generally not effective. If small areas are being treated, local injectable anesthetics like 1% lidocaine can be very effective, but this involves an injection that can itself be prohibitive in younger children. Anxiolytics can also be used and be very effective (more effective than topical anesthetics), but some parents are not comfortable using these types of medications.
  - Protective eye goggles are used during the illumination of light. Patients who are claustrophobic typically do not do well during this part of the procedure.
- **Technique Tips:**
  - There are reports of "daylight-activated PDT" being as effective as red or blue light PDT, with the additional benefit of being less painful. There are a few important considerations—there is more variability in ensuring an even, reproducible dose because numerous variables including time of day, season, and cloud cover can

change effective dose. Nonetheless, most protocols recommend broad-spectrum UV sunscreen application followed by ALA or methyl ester cream (MAL) sensitizer. After allowing the sensitizer to sit for 1 to 3 hours (would start with 1 hour in children), patients will sit outside for 30 to 120 minutes (start with 30 minutes).

- In red or blue light PDT, we generally use very light curettage to remove any hyperkeratosis from AKs and then apply the sensitizer.
- For extremities, there are reports of using a space heater to help sensitizer enzymatic conversion into the active intermediate, protoporphyrin 9. We do not use a space heater but will apply sensitizer followed by two Kerlix™ (Covidien/Medtronic, US) bandages and then a coban bandage in an attempt to heat the extremity.
- We also advise against going outside if it is cool because this will inhibit conversion of ALA or MAL to protoporphyrin 9.
- **Skin of Color Considerations:** It may take longer incubation times and dosage in patients with darker complexions as compared with fairer skinned patients. In general, I still start out with the lower dose but increase at greater increments if lower dosage/shorter incubation times are well tolerated.

Contraindications/Cautions/Risks

Contraindications
- An absolute contraindication to PDT is a diagnosis of porphyria.
- I also avoid doing PDT around the time of surgical excision (either immediately before or after) because it can cause significant swelling and could theoretically cause a dehiscence or increase infection risk.

Cautions
- During red or blue light PDT, patients wear protective eye goggles and providers need to wear protective eyeglasses.

Risks
- Common side effects include discomfort during treatment as well as the potential for phototoxic reactions up to 48 hours after treatment.
- Protective eye goggles/glasses are worn in both red and blue light PDT. Because blue light is close to the wavelength of UVA, there is a risk for corneal damage.
- Many patients want to know if PDT increases one's risk for future skin cancers similar to radiation exposure. We know that whereas PDT and external beam radiation therapy (EBRT) work by generating reactive oxygen species (ROS), in PDT, ROS is generated in mitochondria (rather than DNA as in EBRT) and results in apoptosis. This means that PDT is not mutagenic and does not increase skin cancer risk.

Equipment Needed
- Protective eyeshields or goggles
- A sensitizer. The most commonly used sensitizers include 20% ALA solution (Levulan) and 16.8% methyl ALA (Metvixia). Levulan is widely available; Metvixia is no longer commercially available; however, compounded formulations can be utilized. The Levulan solution is packaged as a two-compartment application stick. One end contains the solvent, and the other contains the active ingredient powder (ALA). Each end is cracked and shaken for 3 minutes to facilitate mixing of the two components. One end of the stick has an applicator tip, which can be applied directly to the intended treatment site.
- A light source. There are a number of light sources such as the Blu-U (DUSA), OmniLux (Photomedex), VersaClear (Theralight), Aktilite (Galderma), ClearLight (Lumenis) that can be used in combination with either sensitizer).

Preprocedural Approach
- It may be useful to try a much shorter incubation duration (20-30 minutes) and treatment time (2-3 minutes) in young children who may be anxious. Once the patient, parents, and providers feel comfortable, longer incubation durations and treatment times can be used. An alternative approach could be using daylight PDT (as described earlier).
- Application of the sensitizer is painless. A thin coat of either the ALA solution or the compounded MAL cream is evenly applied to the treatment site. Some providers use vertical strokes followed by horizontal strokes for different facial subunits (ie, forehead, nose, cheeks, chin) for the ALA solution because it is a clear liquid.
- Eye protection in the form of eyeshields or goggles is used during the activation of the sensitizer by the light source.
- Several aspects of the PDT procedure can cause anxiety, which should be mitigated when possible. An anxiolytic like diazepam (Valium) dosed 0.12 to 0.8 mg/kg/d divided over 4 to 6 doses administered 30 to 60 minutes prior to the procedure (1 or 5 mg/mL solution) may be helpful.

Procedural Approach
- After a 1 to 3 hour incubation, the light source is employed.
- In general, using the lowest dose with the shortest incubation time will result in the least discomfort for patients. We use an OmniLux light source, which allows us the flexibility of using either blue or red light (Figure 53.4A-C). Typically, we start off at a dose of 37 J/cm^2 of the red light after a 1 hour incubation with either MAL or ALA sensitizer. If we plan on using blue light, we apply ALA for 1 hour and use a dose of 15 J/cm^2. Both of these doses translate to around 6 minutes of light exposure.

Postprocedural Approach
- We recommend sun avoidance for 48 hours.
- Pain control using acetaminophen or ibuprofen
- Patients follow up in 2 to 6 weeks and depending upon the response (ie, reduction in AKs) and how well the initial treatment was tolerated, we decide whether to repeat at the same dose or incrementally increase the dose (10%-20%).
- We typically plan on a series of three treatments 2 to 6 weeks apart and then may repeat in 6 to 12 months.

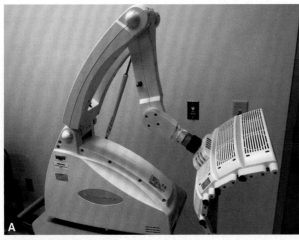
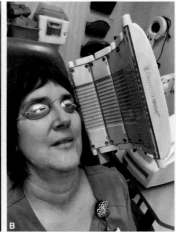
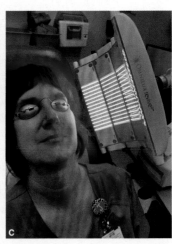

FIGURE 53.4. Photodynamic therapy. A, OmniLux light-emitting diode (LED) light source with both blue and red light capability. B, Light source is positioned about 6 to 8 in away from treatment area and eye protection is used. C, Target area is illuminated using the device for a prescribed period of time and dose.

REFERENCES

1. Lookingbill DP, Lookingbill GL, Leppard B. Actinic damage and skin cancer in albinos in northern Tanzania. Findings in 164 patients enrolled in an outreach skin care program. *J Am Acad Dermatol.* 1995;32:653–658.
2. Balakirski G, Duekers G, Niehues T. A non-healing lesion in a 14 year old boy with primary immunodeficiency: a rare case of actinic keratosis in a child. *J Eur Acad Dermatol Venereol.* 2016;30:1408–1409.
3. Cowen E, Nguyen J, Miller D, et al. Chronic phototoxicity and aggressive squamous cell carcinoma of the skin in children and adults during treatment with voriconazole. *J Am Acad Dermatol.* 2010;62(1):31–37.

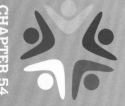

CHAPTER 54

Alopecia Areata

Venkata Anisha Guda, Stephen C. Senft, and John C. Browning

Introduction

Patients with alopecia areata have autoimmune-induced hair loss that occurs in round patches. The hair can fall from the scalp as well as from other areas of the body. The problem often appears with coin-sized, round, smooth, bare patches on the scalp, eyebrows, eyelashes, or beard area (Figure 54.1). A few short hairs are often seen at the edges of the bare spots. These hairs get narrower at the bottom, like an exclamation mark. Over time, some patients lose all of their hair. Alopecia areata can also affect the fingernails and toenails. This is seen as nail pitting or white spots or lines. Alopecia areata can develop at any age but usually occurs during childhood, especially in those individuals with a family history of the disease. Because alopecia areata is an autoimmune disease where the body attacks the hair follicles, people with alopecia areata are at higher risk for developing other autoimmune diseases such as vitiligo (see Chapter 129. Vitiligo) or thyroiditis.

Physicians can diagnose alopecia areata by examining the extent and pattern of hair loss and by analyzing a few hair samples under a microscope. The dermatologist may also perform a scalp biopsy to rule out other conditions that involve hair loss including lichen planopilaris and trichotillomania. Blood tests may be performed if other autoimmune conditions are suspected. These may include tests for C-reactive protein and erythrocyte sedimentation rate (ESR), iron levels, antinuclear antibody (ANA), thyroid hormones, free and total testosterone, and follicle-stimulating and luteinizing hormone. Once the diagnosis is made, there are a variety of therapies that can be used.

Whatever specific treatment option is selected, it is essential to provide emotional support to affected children because the condition can take a toll on their self-esteem. In mild cases, the hair can grow back even without treatment, although it can also fall out again. When the hair loss is widespread, there is a greater chance that the hair will not grow back. For a few people, the condition never returns. For others, the condition recurs. This can be very frustrating for patients. As a result, it is important to discuss the emotional aspects of the disease with the patient and reassure them that this will not impact their overall health. Patients should be encouraged to join a support group, if necessary (see Chapter 139. Patient and Family Resources).

TREATMENT APPROACHES

- There is no cure for alopecia areata, so treatment should focus on management from the perspective of a chronic condition.
- Corticosteroids are considered first-line treatment. They are typically administered either topically or intralesionally

(the focus of this chapter). When successful, they suppress the cutaneous immune system and allow regrowth of hair. Intralesional injections have the advantage of delivering medication directly to the areas affected by hair loss. When successful, patients continue to receive injections every 3 to 6 weeks. In severe cases, oral corticosteroids or other immunosuppressive medications (such as Janus kinase inhibitors) may be considered.

- Minoxidil 5% may help some patients regrow their hair. Both children and adults can use it, but avoid applying it to the face to prevent unwanted hair growth. Minoxidil can be applied twice a day to the scalp and causes new hair growth in about 3 months.
- Anthralin alters the skin's immune function. The patient applies the medicine on the skin and leaves it on for 20 to 60 minutes. After this time, the anthralin is washed off to prevent the skin from being overly irritated, although mild irritation is essential to the treatment process.
- Diphenylcyclopropenone (DPCP) 2% may also be utilized. It is first applied to the arm or leg to sensitize the immune system. A lower concentration (depending on the sensitization reaction) is then applied to the scalp. DPCP causes a low-grade allergic reaction. In severe cases, the patient can have redness, swelling, and itching.
- Studies have shown that corticosteroid injections are the first line of treatment because there is evidence that the therapy stimulated hair growth in 60% to 67% of injection sites. The treatment protocol depends on the age and extent of scalp involvement. For children younger than 10 years, a minoxidil 5% solution or topical corticosteroids or a short-contact anthralin should be used in place of intralesionals because of the likelihood that these children will not tolerate injections. For children older than 10 years who have greater than 50% scalp involvement, topical immunotherapy should be used (ie, DPCP) in

place of intralesional steroids. If the response is poor, then the previously mentioned therapies should be used. For children with less than 50% scalp involvement, intralesional corticosteroids (Kenalog) can be used with topically applied minoxidil 5% solution or topical corticosteroids or a short-contact anthralin.

- Initial research in animals has shown that quercetin, a naturally occurring bioflavonoid found in fruits and vegetables, can protect against alopecia areata and treat existing hair loss. Additional research is needed to demonstrate the efficacy of quercetin in humans. Quercetin can be used as an adjuvant therapy along with the aforementioned treatment ladder.

Clinical Pearls

- Device distractions/techniques are helpful for decreasing anxiety around intralesional injections.
- Use of local anesthetics such as lidocaine before or during infiltration can provide partial relief from pain.
- Dilution of triamcinolone should be done for each patient individually. (See Appendix. Common Dilutions of Triamcinolone Acetonide [Kenalog].)
- When diluting triamcinolone, always draw up the saline first so that you do not contaminate your saline supply with medication (ie, triamcinolone).

Contraindications/Cautions

- Be careful when working with intralesional triamcinolone because it can clog the needle; when this happens, flick the distal end of the syringe to unclog the needle. Do not simply "push harder" on the syringe plunger because this may cause the needle to fly off the syringe under pressure. For the same reason, always try to inject in the direction "away from" the patient's eye when possible.
- Intralesional steroids should not be injected at the site of an active skin infection such as impetigo or herpes simplex.
- Intralesional steroids should not be used if there is a history of hypersensitivity to Kenalog (triamcinolone) or if the area of alopecia is so extensive that injections would be impractical or total dosing would risk adrenal axis suppression.
- Side effects and risks of Kenalog can be separated into "early" and "late" effects. Early effects include pain, bleeding, bruising, infection, contact dermatitis, impaired wound healing, or sterile abscess. Late adverse effects include cutaneous and subcutaneous lipoatrophy, leukoderma or postinflammatory hypopigmentation, telangiectasia, localized hypertrichosis, localized or distant steroid acne, and adrenal axis suppression.

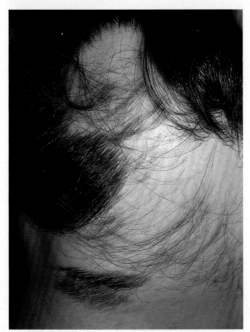

FIGURE 54.1. Alopecia areata. Patchy alopecia characteristic of alopecia areata, ophiasis pattern. Despite the microscopic lymphocytic infiltrate that is sometimes present, the areas lack clinical evidence of inflammation, namely, erythema. Reprinted with permission from Elder DE. *Lever's Histopathology of the Skin.* 10th ed. Philadelphia, PA: Wolters Kluwer Health/Lippincott Williams & Wilkins; 2015. Figure 18-22.

Equipment Needed (Figure 54.2)

- Alcohol wipes
- Injectable steroids (triamcinolone acetonide, 10 and 40 mg/mL)
- 18-Gauge needle ("blunt fill" if available) to draw
- 27-Gauge needle to inject triamcinolone (30-gauge may clog)
- 30-Gauge needle to inject local anesthetic
- Syringes (1 or 3 mL [Luer-Lok® (Becton-Dickinson and Company, Franklin Lakes, NJ) preferable when injections are under pressure])
- Vials of sterile saline for dilution
- Lidocaine 1% or 2% (for anesthetic and/or dilution)
- Distraction devices

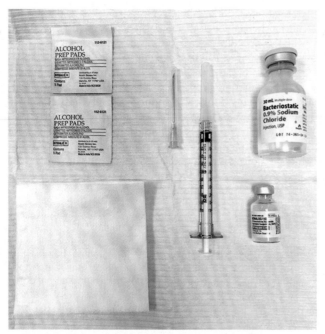

FIGURE 54.2. Intralesional corticosteroid setup for alopecia areata. Photo courtesy of Shari Marchbein, MD.

Preprocedural Approach

- Before the procedure is performed, the physician should ensure that the team is following a "no-touch" technique and that sterile equipment and aqueous solution are being utilized.
- Before the injection, it is important that the patient is positioned correctly and reassured.
- Device distractions and techniques are helpful for decreasing anxiety; allow enough "lead time" so that the patient is fully engaged with the distraction device.
- The main goal is to enter the injection site and provide the steroid agent with limited pain and trauma. Have any local anesthetic ready for use and out of sight of the patient until necessary.
- Proper dilution of triamcinolone is crucial for optimizing outcomes while minimizing side effects. Triamcinolone acetonide suspension is available in 10 and 40 mg/mL concentrations (see Chapter 15. Injectable Corticosteroids [Intralesional Kenalog, Intramuscular]). For alopecia areata, the appropriate strength for triamcinolone is approximately 5 to 10 mg/mL for the scalp and 3 mg/mL for the face. To create a 5-mg/mL concentration, draw 0.5 mL of sterile saline into a 1-mL syringe and add 0.5 mL of 10 mg/mL of triamcinolone. To create a 3-mg/mL concentration, draw 0.7 mL of sterile saline into a 1-mL syringe and add 0.3 mL of 10 mg/mL triamcinolone.
- Triamcinolone is usually diluted with sterile normal saline for injection because the isotonicity and neutral pH of sterile saline makes it preferable. Alternatives to sterile saline include sterile water or lidocaine 1% or 2%.
- Use a blunt fill 18-gauge needle, if one is available, to draw the desired amount of sterile saline into a 1-mL Luer-Lok or tuberculin syringe.
- Next, draw the desired amount of triamcinolone into the same syringe.

- Turn the syringe upside down several times to mix the suspension thoroughly.
- Remove the 18-gauge drawing needle and replace it with a 27-gauge (or 30-gauge) injecting needle.
- Cap the syringes to maintain sterility, and keep the needles and syringes out of sight of the child until necessary.

Procedural Approach

- Position the patient so that he/she is secure.
- Palpate the area and select an injection site.
- Mark the skin with firm pressure using the edge of a nail or a ballpoint pen that has its ink cartridge and point retracted. This will create a temporary "target mark" that lasts for about 5 to 15 minutes.
- Wash your hands.
- Swab the skin with alcohol pads. Do not touch the skin after swabbing.
- If necessary, use a 30-gauge needle to inject local anesthesia to the site. Spraying the site with ethyl chloride can be used as an alternative because its cooling effect can help numb the skin.
- Use a 0.5-in-long 27- or 30-gauge needle to inject the selected site. Ensure that there is no resistance to the injection. The procedure should be halted and the needle repositioned if any resistance is felt. Any pain or paresthesia remote from the injection site should also stop the procedure (Figure 54.3).
- Apply sterile dressing and tell the patient to avoid excess touching of the site where any injections were placed.

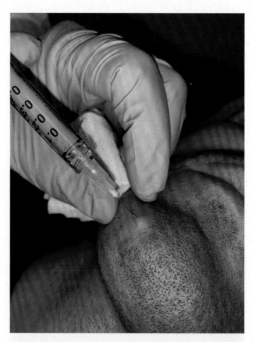

FIGURE 54.3. Intralesional injection of corticosteroid for alopecia areata barbae. Kenalog 2.5 mg/mL is injected using a 1-mL tuberculin syringe with a 30-gauge needle attached by a "Luer-Lok"-style connector. A slight pinch by the clinician at the lateral side of the injection site helps distract the patient and reduce pain. A raised, blanched wheal appears at the site of injection; gentle massage of the area after the injection helps disperse the Kenalog more evenly. Photo courtesy of Andrew C. Krakowski, MD.

Postprocedural Approach

There is generally no specific aftercare protocol other than following up for inspection of the results and analysis of additional forms of treatment. In general, these authors try to follow the "rule of three" for repeat corticosteroid injections: review the patient in 3 to 6 weeks to analyze the efficacy and complications of the injections; repeat injections approximately every 3 to 6 weeks; and do not inject any single lesion more than three times without reconsidering the accuracy of the diagnosis and the progress that has been made up to this point.

SUGGESTED READINGS

Bolduc C. Alopecia areata treatment & management. Medscape. https://emedicine.medscape.com/article/1069931-treatment. Accessed May 8, 2017.

Ho CTK, Lau CS. Intralesional steroid injection: general considerations. *Hong Kong Pract.* 1997;19(8):425–429.

Usatine R, Pfenninger JL, Stulberg DL. *Dermatologic and Cosmetic Procedures in Office Practice.* Philadelphia, PA: Elsevier Saunders; 2012.

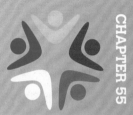

CHAPTER 55

Angiofibromas

Andrew C. Krakowski, Kristen M. Kelly, Nathan S. Uebelhoer, and Girish S. Munavalli

OVERVIEW

Angiofibromas associated with tuberous sclerosis typically arise in childhood and early adulthood (Figure 55.1). Current management strategies include cryotherapy, electrocoagulation, radiofrequency ablation, dermabrasion, lasers such as fully ablative laser skin resurfacing (ALSR), ablative fractional resurfacing (AFR), and pulsed-dye laser (PDL), and topical podophyllotoxin. Although these treatments have proved successful, they can result in scarring, postinflammatory hyperpigmentation, and pain, and the recurrence rate for angiofibromas may be as high as 80%, necessitating serial treatments.

Herein we offer our step-by-step instruction for multimodal treatment of angiofibromas that addresses the unique characteristics of these lesions. Our protocol utilizes PDL and ALSR, gentle vinegar soaks to reduce infection, and postoperative continuous application of topical rapamycin. Our multimodal approach seeks to achieve prolonged clinical improvement while minimizing adverse events. In the authors' experience, long-term (ie, years) lesion remission has been noted. Even with continued use of topical rapamycin, recurrence over time is not uncommon, and repeat treatments may be considered periodically.

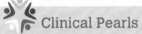

Clinical Pearls

- **Guidelines:** No specific treatment guidelines are known to exist for this condition.
- **Age-Specific Considerations:** Ideally, patients should be old enough to ask for treatment for themselves and be developed enough to assist in detecting and reporting postsurgical complications such as increasing pain, redness, warmth, swelling, and fever/chills.
- **Technique Tips:** At least one author has used a preoperative lead-in with topical timolol to help reduce the "angio" component.
- **Skin of Color Considerations:** The technique is best suited for skin types I and II, because the risk for dyspigmentation increases with darker skin types.

Contraindications

- Active skin infection on face (especially herpes labialis or impetigo)
- Presence of a suntan
- Inability to care for postoperative wounds

Equipment Needed

- Wavelength-specific eye shields
- Pulsed-dye laser
- Smoke evacuator

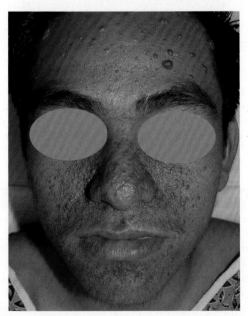

FIGURE 55.1. Preprocedure photograph of angiofibromas associated with tuberous sclerosis. Note the large fibrous lesions on the left forehead.

- CO$_2$ laser
- Sterile cotton-tipped applicators
- Sterile water
- Petrolatum-based ointment
- Ice

Preprocedural Approach

- Six to 8 weeks before surgery, we ask that patients minimize sun exposure and maximize sun protection so that their skin is as light (ie, untanned) as possible; although this may be somewhat seasonally and geographically dependent, the approach reduces melanin in the skin as a competing chromophore.
- Prophylaxis for herpes simplex is started 1 to 2 days before laser surgery.
- Patients should bathe either the evening before or on the morning of their surgery.

Procedural Approach

- Informed consent from the parent/guardian and, when possible, assent from the minor are obtained.
- Typically, general anesthesia is utilized because of pain associated with the procedure.
- Appropriate protective eyewear should be worn, and patients should have eye pads (disposable adhesive eye shields offering full eye protection from medical lasers with wavelengths between 190 and 11 000 nm at an optical density > 7; OD 7@190-11 000 nm) or correctly fitted metal eye shields in place.
- PDL (595-nm Vbeam Perfecta™ [Candela Corporation, US]) is employed to treat the "angio" component of the lesions. PDL is performed before ALSR so that any "wheal and flare" reaction does not alter the vascular target within the lesions. The cheeks, nose, and chin are treated with a 10-mm spot size, fluence of approximately 7 to 9 J/cm^2, and 0.45 to 1.5 ms pulse width, depending on skin type and clinical response. A 10% to 20% overlap of pulses is the goal, and the clinical endpoint is moderate purpura.
- Next, CO$_2$ laser is used and protective goggles must be changed to protect for the 10 600-nm wavelength. A smoke evacuator is necessary to help remove plume smoke, and all present should wear masks. The affected areas of the face are treated as a single "sheet," using a macrofractionated 10 600-nm CO$_2$ laser (Active FX™ [Lumenis, Yokneam, Israel]). A single-pulse, nonoverlapping "stamping" technique is utilized at the following settings (adjusted for skin type and overall thickness of lesions): 100 to 125 mJ/3.5 W/size 3 to 5/density 5 to 6/spot size fixed at 300 µm. These parameters result in nonfractionated, focal full-field ablative resurfacing in the desired areas. We would expect other CO$_2$ laser devices to achieve similar results if a uniform sheet of nonoverlapping pattern of ablation is created to a depth of approximately 100 µm with minimal collateral thermal damage. As with most CO$_2$ laser treatments, bleeding is minimal.
- Sterile water is then applied to the treatment area, and sterile cotton-tipped applicators are rubbed vigorously over the surgical field to remove fibrous lesions to the superficial papillary dermis (Figure 55.2). Scarring is more likely at increasing depths, so a conservative approach is favored (Figure 55.3).
- Immediately after surgery, a petrolatum-based ointment is liberally applied.
- Ice may be applied to help decrease discomfort and limit edema.

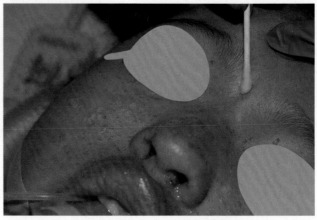

FIGURE 55.2. Intraoperative photo demonstrating use of a sterile cotton-tipped applicator dipped in sterile water to manually debride an angiofibroma after macrofractionated ablation with CO$_2$ laser.

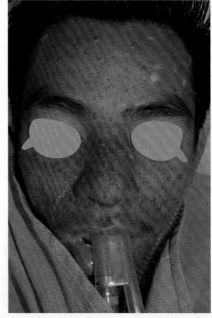

FIGURE 55.3. Intraoperative photo immediately after ablative skin laser resurfacing of cheeks and nose with a macrofractionated CO$_2$ laser. Note that several of the larger fibrous lesions on the patient's left forehead were manually debrided down to the level of the superficial papillary dermis.

Postprocedural Approach

- Generally, swelling and pain should decrease quickly with time.
- Patients should continue herpes prophylaxis for a total of 7 to 10 days.
- At least three times a day, patients are instructed to gently cleanse the treated areas using a mixture that consists of 1 capful of acetic acid (ie, food-grade white distilled vinegar) combined with 1 L of distilled water. Gauze is soaked in this mixture and, with patients lying supine, left in place on the treated areas for 10 minutes. Then, the gauze is removed, and the area is rinsed gently with fresh water. Petrolatum-based

ointment is immediately reapplied and maintained until reepithelization has occurred—typically 5 to 7 days after laser surgery.

- Patients are instructed to sleep with an extra pillow for the first week postoperatively to elevate the head and decrease edema.
- Patients should be vigilantly monitored for signs and symptoms of infection, with special consideration paid to viral, fungal, and atypical mycobacterial infections, as well as the more typical bacterial culprits. For example, posttreatment *Candida* or fungal infections tend to evolve as bright red eruptions that may be intensely itchy.
- Postoperative downtime is significant, and patients should expect to be absent from school or work for at least 1 week.
- After a follow-up appointment to directly assess reepithelialization, about 7 to 10 days after laser surgery, topical rapamycin may be applied to the treated areas. The authors tend to use topical rapamycin 0.1% once daily; however, higher concentrations (up to 1%) and more frequent application (twice daily) have been reported and may be considered depending on availability and the financial situation of individual patients. Less frequent applications do not seem to provide significant results. Typically, if there is scabbing or blistering, then application of topical rapamycin is delayed until resolution. The authors no longer perform any laboratory evaluation as routine monitoring; however, a complete blood count, comprehensive metabolic panel, and urinalysis may be considered. Ointment-based vehicles may be associated with acne, and if this occurs, other vehicles seem to work as effectively. Patients are warned that slow healing may be a risk associated with this medication.

- Patients are encouraged to contact the physician directly with any concerns and may be provided with the physician's cell phone number for direct contact and reassurance.
- Serial photography (ie, "selfies") may be used if the photographs are sent securely.

SUGGESTED READINGS

Bae-Harboe YS, Geronemus RG. Targeted topical and combination laser surgery for the treatment of angiofibromas. *Lasers Surg Med.* 2013;45(9):555–557.

Malissen N, Vergely L, Simon M, Roubertie A, Malinge MC, Bessis D. Long-term treatment of cutaneous manifestations of tuberous sclerosis complex with topical 1% sirolimus cream: a prospective study of 25 patients. *J Am Acad Dermatol.* 2017;77: 464–472.e3.

Webb DW, Clarke A, Fryer A, Osborne JP. The cutaneous features of tuberous sclerosis: a population study. *Br J Dermatol.* 1996;135:1–5.

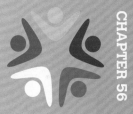

Angiokeratoma

Ayan Kusari, Allison Han, and Sheila Fallon Friedlander

CHAPTER 56

Introduction

Angiokeratomas are a family of vascular lesions associated with capillary dilation in the papillary dermis and, as their name implies, overlying hyperkeratosis. Clinical presentation varies widely. Small solitary angiokeratomas are common in adults (Figure 56.1), as are angiokeratoma of Fordyce (multiple angiokeratomas of the scrotum and vulva) (Figure 56.2). Angiokeratoma circumscriptum, by contrast, typically develops during infancy with a female predilection, and is a much larger lesion with pronounced hyperkeratosis. Angiokeratoma of Mibelli is a rare, familial condition that typically presents in early adolescence with angiokeratomas, acrocyanosis, and, rarely, digital ulceration. In Fabry disease (X-linked α-galactosidase A deficiency), widespread angiokeratomas are commonly seen, particularly in the lower abdomen and groin area; this presentation is known as angiokeratoma corporis diffusum. Removal is usually not necessary, but larger lesions or lesions in high-friction areas (groin, toes, and heel) are more likely to become irritated and/or bleed. Dark, violaceous angiokeratomas can occasionally resemble melanoma, and in this situation, dermoscopy (showing red, black, or blue lacunae) or biopsy may be useful to confirm the diagnosis.

Angiokeratomas do not require treatment unless they are symptomatic or bothersome to the patient. Here, we describe our step-by-step approach to the management of bothersome angiokeratomas that addresses the unique characteristics of these lesions. Our protocol utilizes paring with a 10 or 15 blade, followed by electrocautery and/or pulsed-dye laser (PDL) or ablative laser therapy. Treatment is individualized to the needs of each patient.

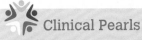

Clinical Pearls

- **Guidelines:** No specific treatment guidelines are known to exist for this condition.
- **Anatomic Considerations:** Multiple small lesions located between the belly and knees raise concern for Fabry disease and should prompt appropriate evaluation.
- **Age-Specific Considerations:** Angiokeratomas are not disabling or life-threatening, and urgent treatment is usually not needed. As such, providers should carefully weigh the need for treatment and strive to avoid unnecessary exposure to general anesthesia. In general, we typically postpone treatment until children are sufficiently mature to tolerate treatment under local anesthesia alone.
- **Technique Tips:** Angiokeratomas vary in size and degree of hyperkeratosis. Lesions with more hyperkeratosis require paring down to the skin surface or CO_2 laser ablation, whereas less hyperkeratotic lesions may not require this measure.
- **Skin of Color Considerations:** Risk for dyspigmentation with laser increases with darker skin types.

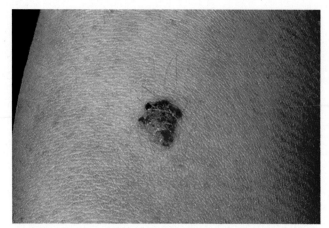

FIGURE 56.1. Solitary angiokeratoma on forearm with characteristic vascular and hyperkeratotic appearance. Reprinted with permission from Requena L, Kutzner H. *Cutaneous Soft Tissue Tumors.* Philadelphia, PA: Lippincott Williams & Wilkins; 2014. Figure 65.1.

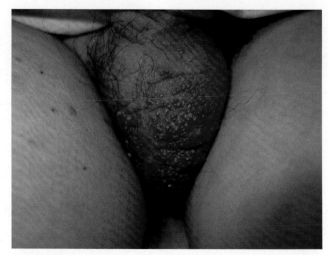

FIGURE 56.2. Angiokeratoma of Fordyce on scrotum. Image provided by Stedman's.

Contraindications/Cautions/Risks

Contraindications
- Active skin infection
- Inability to care for postoperative wounds

Cautions
- Presence of a suntan may increase dyspigmentation with laser therapy. Lesions may not completely resolve, particularly large or hyperkeratotic lesions. Multiple treatments may be required.

Risks
- Scarring, pain, bleeding, recurrence of lesions

Equipment Needed
- Alcohol or iodine prep pads
- A 10 or 15 blade
- Sterile gauze
- Electrocautery
- Wavelength-specific eye shields
- PDL
- Smoke evacuator
- CO₂ laser
- Sterile cotton-tipped applicators
- Sterile water
- Petrolatum-based ointment
- Ice

Preprocedural Approach

- Six to 8 weeks before surgery, we ask that patients minimize sun exposure and maximize sun protection so that their skin is as light (ie, untanned) as possible; although this may be somewhat seasonally and geographically dependent, the approach reduces melanin in the skin as a competing chromophore.
- Patients should bathe either the evening before or the morning of their surgery.

Procedural Approach

- The risks, benefits, and alternatives of treatment are discussed with the patient and family. If all parties are agreeable, informed consent from the parent/guardian and assent from the minor are obtained.
- Local anesthetic, particularly lidocaine cream (LMX.4™ or LMX.5™ [Ferndale Laboratories]; http://www.ferndalepharmagroup.com) is applied to the area to be treated. LMX cream is available over the counter and should be applied to the treatment area 45 minutes to 1 hour before the procedure for maximum effect. A eutectic mixture of lidocaine and prilocaine (Anodyne LPT; Fortus Pharma, LLC, Southaven, MS) also works well and can be obtained via prescription; if this is used, it should also be applied to the treatment site 45 minutes to 1 hour before the procedure.
- The treatment site is sterilized with povidone iodine or chlorhexidine gluconate (Hibiclens; Mölnlycke Health Care, Gothenburg, Sweden; https://hibiclens.com) and marked with a sterile surgical marker.
- If there is a significant hyperkeratotic component to the angiokeratoma, then this component is gently pared down using a 10 blade, within approximately 0.5 mm of or flush with the skin surface. If significant bleeding is noted, then electrocautery (Bovie Aaron 940 [Bovie Medical Corporation, Purchase, NY]; boviemedical.com or Hyfrecator 2000™ [Conmed, Utica, NY]; conmed.com) is used to stanch the flow of blood. If significant paring or cautery is required, intralesional lidocaine would be appropriate.
- Before utilization of laser, appropriate protective eyewear should be worn, and patients should have eye pads (disposable adhesive eye shields offering full eye protection from medical lasers with wavelengths between 190 and 11 000 nm at an optical density >7; OD 7@190-11 000 nm) or correctly fitted metal eye shields in place.
- PDL (595-nm Vbeam Perfecta™ [Candela Corporation, US]; candelamedical.com) is employed to treat the "angio" component of the lesions. A 7- to 10-mm spot size, fluence of approximately 6 to 8 J/cm², and 0.45 to 1.5 ms pulse width are typically used, depending on skin type and clinical response. Cryogen cooling spray should be considered for epidermal cooling when operating the PDL device.

Postprocedural Approach

- Generally, swelling and pain should decrease quickly with time.
- Patients are instructed to leave dressings dry and intact for 48 hours. Patients may remove bandages when bathing. Petrolatum-based ointment is immediately reapplied and maintained for at least 5 to 7 days after treatment.
- Patients should self-monitor for signs and symptoms of infection.
- The authors do not perform any laboratory evaluation as routine monitoring.
- Retreatment may be required.
- Patients are encouraged to contact the physician directly for concerns.
- Serial photography (ie, "selfies") may be used if the photos are sent securely.

SUGGESTED READINGS

Elluru RG. Cutaneous vascular lesions. *Facial Plast Surg Clin North Am.* 2013;21(1):111–126.

Nguyen J, Chapman LW, Korta DZ, Zachary CB. Laser treatment of cutaneous angiokeratomas: a systematic review. *Dermatol Ther.* 2017;30:e12558.

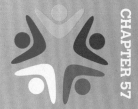

Angioma, Spider

Ayan Kusari, Allison Han, and Sheila Fallon Friedlander

CHAPTER 57

Introduction

Spider telangiectasias (nevi aranei) are small, subtly raised papules with surrounding dilated vessels that may vary in size from 1 mm to 1 cm (Figure 57.1). These lesions are most commonly seen on the face (Figure 57.2), hands, and upper trunk and are sometimes associated with high estrogen states, including pregnancy, oral contraceptive pill (OCP) use, and liver disease.[1] Lesions that arise during pregnancy are more likely to resolve spontaneously, perhaps due to the shorter duration of estrogen exposure. There is no medical indication for treatment of asymptomatic telangiectasias, although medical conditions may underlie their appearance. Some believe they are more likely to occur on sun-exposed areas. Pulsed-dye laser (PDL), intense pulsed-light (IPL), and electrocautery have been shown to effectively treat spider telangiectasias.[2]

Here, we describe our step-by-step approach to the management of spider telangiectasias in pediatric patients that addresses the unique characteristics of these lesions. Our protocol utilizes 595-nm PDL therapy at purpuric fluences and pulse durations.

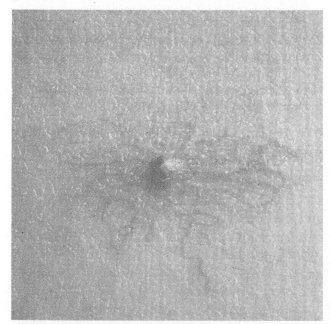

FIGURE 57.1. Spider telangiectasia with characteristic appearance: small central papule with surrounding looped and dilated blood vessels. Reprinted with permission from Smeltzer SC, Bare BG, Hinkle JL, et al. *Brunner & Suddarth's Textbook of Medical-Surgical Nursing.* 11th ed. Philadelphia, PA: Wolters Kluwer Health/Lippincott Williams & Wilkins; 2008. Figure 39.14.

Clinical Pearls

- **Guidelines:** No specific treatment guidelines are known to exist for this condition.
- **Age-Specific Considerations:** Spider telangiectasias that arise during childhood and during pregnancy may resolve spontaneously. If lesions are long standing or bothersome, treatment is reasonable. Clinicians should consider the possibility of underlying disease if many spider telangiectasias are present, particularly if they involve the lips or the tips of the fingers.
- **Technique Tips:** Purpura and bluish coagulum are useful endpoints for treatment of spider telangiectasias.
- **Skin of Color Considerations:** Risk of dyspigmentation with PDL increases with darker skin types. Lower fluences with longer pulse durations and use of epidermal cooling should be used for darker skin types.

Contraindications/Cautions/Risks

Contraindications
- Active skin infection
- Inability to avoid direct sun exposure to the treated site for 10 to 14 days

Cautions
- Presence of sun damage may increase dyspigmentation with laser therapy.

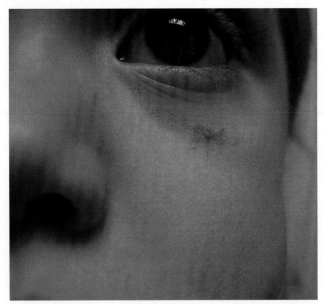

FIGURE 57.2. Spider angioma on cheek of child. Image provided by Stedman's.

Risks

- Scarring, pain, bleeding, recurrence of lesions

Equipment Needed

- Wavelength-specific eye shields
- PDL
- Petrolatum-based ointment
- Ice

Preprocedural Approach

- Six to 8 weeks before surgery, we ask that patients minimize sun exposure and maximize sun protection so that their skin is as light (ie, untanned) as possible; although this may be somewhat seasonally and geographically dependent, the approach reduces melanin in the skin as a competing chromophore.
- Patients should bathe either the evening before or the morning of their surgery.

Procedural Approach

- The risks, benefits, and alternatives of treatment are discussed with the patient and family. If all parties are agreeable, informed consent from the parent/guardian and assent from the minor are obtained.
- Topical anesthetic, particularly lidocaine, cream (LMX.4™ or LMX.5™ [Ferndale Laboratories]) may be applied to the area to be treated. LMX cream is available over the counter and should be applied to the treatment area 45 minutes to 1 hour before the procedure for maximum effect. A eutectic mixture of lidocaine and prilocaine (Anodyne LPT; Fortus Pharma, LLC, Southaven, MS) also works well and can be obtained via prescription; if this is used, it should also be applied to the treatment site 45 minutes to 1 hour before the procedure.
- After this point, appropriate protective eyewear should be worn, and patients should have eye pads (disposable adhesive eye pads offering full eye protection from medical lasers with wavelengths between 190 and 11 000 nm at an optical density >7; OD 7@190-11 000 nm) or correctly fitted metal eye shields in place.
- PDL (595-nm Vbeam Perfecta™ [Candela Corporation, US]) or (585 nm) (Cynergy Laser; CynoSure Corporation, Westford, MA) is employed to treat the "angio" component of the lesions. A 7- to 10-mm spot size fluence of approximately 7 to 12 J/cm^2, and 0.45 to 1.5 ms pulse width are typically used, depending on skin type and clinical response. Depending on the size of the laser utilized, if the spider angioma is less than 5 mm, one can utilize a piece of gauze with an appropriate size hole cut out in the center as a shield to protect surrounding normal skin. The clinical endpoint is moderate purpura, which usually requires double pulsing (Figure 57.3A and B). Cryogen cooling spray should be used for epidermal protection when operating the PDL device. Higher Fitzpatrick skin types are at higher risk for dyspigmentation or blistering. Skin types V and VI may not be optimal candidates.

Postprocedural Approach

- Patients should protect the treated lesions from sun exposure for at least 2 weeks; a small dot bandage will sometimes suffice for this purpose.
- Sun protection is the single most important intervention postoperatively (SPA bandage, hats, sunscreen). See Chapter 135. Photoprotection.

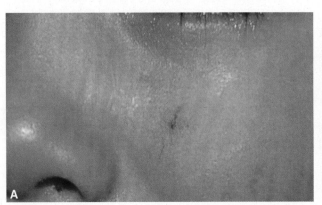
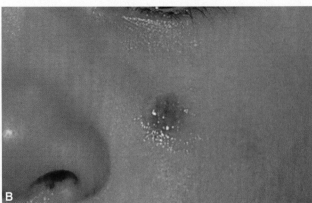

FIGURE 57.3. Single treatment pulsed-dye laser therapy of spider telangiectasia on the left medial cheek in a young child. Before (A) and after with petrolatum ointment applied postoperatively (B) are marked. Photo courtesy of Andrew C. Krakowski, MD.

REFERENCES

1. Luis Requena and Omar P Sangueza. Cutaneous vascular proliferations. Part II. Hyperplasias and benign neoplasms. *Journal of the American Academy of Dermatology*. 1997;37(6): 887–922.
2. Jayne Joo, Daniel Michael, Suzanne Kilmer. Lasers for Treatment of Vascular Lesions. *Lasers in Dermatology and Medicine*. Springer, Cham; 2018:49–61

SUGGESTED READINGS

Habif T, Dinulos J, Chapman MS, Zug K. *Skin Disease E-Book: Diagnosis and Treatment*. Amsterdam, The Netherlands: Elsevier Health Sciences; 2017.

Jeon H, Cohen B. Lack of efficacy of topical timolol for cutaneous telangiectasias in patients with hereditary hemorrhagic telangiectasia: results of a pilot study. *J Am Acad Dermatol*. 2017;76(5):997–999.

Neuhaus, IM, Zane LT, Tope WD. Comparative efficacy of nonpurpuragenic pulsed dye laser and intense pulsed light for erythematotelangiectatic rosacea. *Dermatol Surg*. 2009;35(6):920–928.

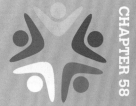

Aplasia Cutis Congenita

CHAPTER 58

Laura Huang, Angel J. Su, Alexander Choi, and John C. Browning

Introduction

Aplasia cutis congenita is a rare congenital absence of normal skin and its associated structures that occurs in 0.5 to 1 in 10 000 births. The etiology of aplasia cutis is multifactorial and occurs in utero. The exact mechanism or cause of the defect is unclear, and no strong genetic or racial correlations have been found. Some cases are associated with intrauterine fetal demise of a twin early in pregnancy (ie, fetus papyraceus) limb abnormalities (ie, Adams–Oliver syndrome), congenital nevi, epidermolysis bullosa, and cleft lip and palate.

Although aplasia cutis lesions may occur anywhere on the body, greater than 85% of patients present with isolated scalp lesions (Figure 58.1). Evaluation for potential surgical intervention is warranted when patients meet certain size and location criteria for aplasia cutis lesions. For example, larger scalp lesions with underlying bone involvement may require immediate intervention because of the possible exposure of brain matter,

hemorrhage and/or thrombosis of the sagittal sinus, and risk of infection. Close collaboration with a skilled radiologist, pediatric plastic surgeon, and neurosurgeon is often necessary in these rare but life-threatening cases.

Clinical Pearls

- **Guidelines:**
    - There is no specific guideline for workup and evaluation of aplasia cutis.
    - No skin biopsy or surgical intervention should be attempted before imaging if the diagnosis and possibility of underlying involvement remain in doubt.
- **Age-Specific Considerations:**
    - Underlying osseous defects may close spontaneously, and allow the clinician—on a patient-by-patient basis—to follow up a child until a few years of age to determine the need for cranioplasty.
- **Technique Tips:**
    - Presence of the "hair collar" sign—distorted hair growth around the lesion—may be a marker for an underlying neural tube defect such as encephalocele, meningocele, and brain tissue outside the skull (Figure 58.2).
    - Small defects that are less than 1 cm on the scalp without potential to cause massive hemorrhage can be treated conservatively in the neonatal setting with ointments such as petrolatum or bacitracin along with an occlusive dressing to aid healing by secondary intention. Simple truncal lesions may be treated with a similar approach.
    - Larger midline defects of the scalp that expose dura, bone, or brain matter require immediate surgical intervention to prevent potentially fatal complications.
    - Large lesions on the body of extremities, more than 3 to 4 cm, will usually require surgical intervention.
    - The decision for emergent versus delayed surgical intervention depends on the potential for associated life-threatening complications; a scalp lesion that communicates from the brain to the skin, for example, is at risk for infection and massive hemorrhage from a cerebral vessel.

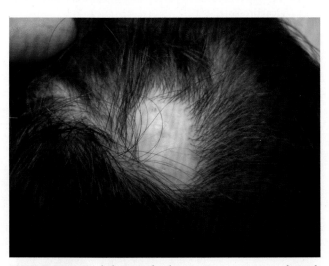

FIGURE 58.1. Healed area of aplasia cutis on vertex scalp with overlying scar.

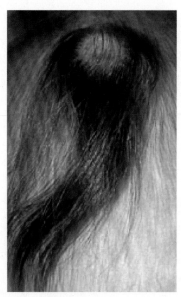

FIGURE 58.2. "Hair collar" sign demonstrating a congenital ring of hair that is denser, darker, and coarser than the normal scalp hair. This lesion requires urgent imaging and, if appropriate, neurosurgical intervention.

Contraindications/Cautions/Risks

Contraindications

- Diagnostic testing and procedural intervention will depend on overall size and severity of the skin defect.

Risks

- Infection, meningitis, sagittal sinus thrombosis, hemorrhage

Equipment Needed

- Varies greatly depending on what imaging is required and what surgical intervention, if any, is chosen

Preprocedural Approach

- Carefully evaluate the affected anatomic site, palpating for any bony defect or pulse or compressible lesion that may reside just inferior to the surface of the skin defect. A thorough physical examination should be performed, looking carefully for any truncal, limb, and oral cavity abnormalities.
- No skin biopsy or surgical intervention should be attempted before imaging if the diagnosis and possibility of underlying involvement remains in doubt.
- To rule out brain-to-skin communication:
  - State the specific anatomic location of the skin defect and the specific rule-out request on the imaging order form so that the radiologist can best decide which protocol will be most useful (Figure 58.3).
  - Ultrasound in the hands of a skilled technician may be used as the initial imaging modality in neonates.
  - If the diagnosis remains in doubt after ultrasound or if the patient is too old for ultrasound to prove effective, then magnetic resonance imaging (MRI) of the brain without and with contrast and magnetic resonance angiogram (MRA) of the head with contrast should be considered.
- To assess for bony involvement, computed tomography (CT) is usually preferred over MRI. Skull radiographs may also be used.

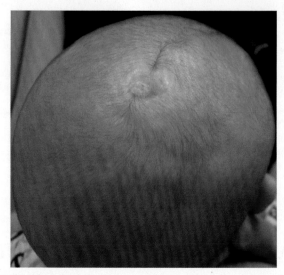

FIGURE 58.3. Healed aplasia cutis in an infant. Imaging with ultrasound or magnetic resonance imaging would be helpful to discern any underlying defect in this midline lesion.

- In cases of suspected fetus papyraceus (Figure 58.4) a placental exam may help to confirm the diagnosis of intrauterine fetal demise of a twin.

Procedural Approach

- Smaller defects (ie, <1 cm) confined to the scalp or trunk may be conservatively managed.
- Larger defects that are only missing skin (ie, no underlying involvement) may utilize a skin flap or skin graft to cover the defect.
  - Generally, patients will require general anesthesia for either procedure.
  - For skin flaps:
    - Either a local flap or regional flap can be used to cover the defect, depending on availability and size.
    - The flap area is marked out before starting the procedure.
    - The flap is incised to create an area large enough to cover the defect with primary closure.
    - The flap is secured in place using stitches, staples, or surgical dressing.

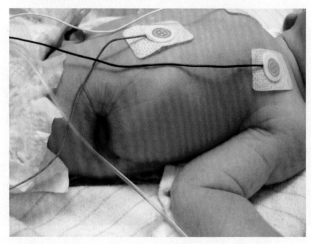

FIGURE 58.4. Large area of aplasia cutis on the trunk of a twin neonate; the other twin did not survive and was born as fetus papyraceus.

- For skin grafts:
  - An acceptable donor site is selected, which is usually the buttocks or the thigh.
  - A dermatome device is used to create an acceptable skin graft from the donor site. For full-thickness grafts, the skin needs to be meshed and then placed over the defect.
  - The defect is closed using sutures, staples, or surgical dressing.

Postprocedural Approach

- Wound care is very important to prevent secondary infection, trauma, and hemorrhage.
- Areas used for skin grafting heal within 10 days without significant scarring. The site of the defect after skin graft placement can recover in as early as a month.
- Consider prophylactic antibiotic therapy in any at-risk patient to reduce chances of contracting serious infections such as meningitis until full closure of the defect has been obtained.

- Following hospital discharge, the infant should be followed up in the outpatient setting at around 1 to 2 months to examine the healing defect. No additional follow-up is necessary if the defect has fully healed and closed without side effects, unless they have an underlying disorder that needs to be addressed.
- Normal pediatric follow-up is recommended for these children unless they have scarring or other remaining concerns:
  - CO_2 laser can help reduce scar tissue.
  - Pulsed-dye laser can help reduce residual erythema.
  - Hair transplant can be utilized when conservative management results in an area of scalp alopecia.

SUGGESTED READINGS

Humphrey SR, Hu X, Adamson K, Jensen JN, Drolet B. A practical approach to the evaluation and treatment of an infant with aplasia cutis congenita. *J Perinatol.* 2008;38:110–117.

Lonie S, Phua Y, Burge J. Technique for management of aplasia cutis congenita of the scalp with a skin allograft. *J Craniofac Surg.* 2016;27:1049–1050.

Silberstein E, Pagkalos VA, Landau D, et al. Aplasia cutis congenita: clinical management and a new classification system. *Plast Reconstr Surg.* 2014;134(5):766–774.

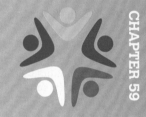

Arthropod Bites and Stings

Laura Huang, Angel J. Su, Alexander Choi, and John C. Browning

CHAPTER 59

Introduction

Arthropods are a phylum of various invertebrates with exoskeletons, encompassing arachnids, insects, centipedes, and millipedes. Arthropod bites are common among all populations and usually create a mild localized reaction on the skin; however, occasionally, they may be associated with more drastic hypersensitivity reactions.

Arthropod venom contains substances such as phospholipase that causes an immunoglobulin (Ig) E–mediated allergic reaction upon exposure. Less than 5% of arthropod bites results in a systemic reaction. One of the more common hypersensitivity reactions is papular urticaria, which is often associated with mosquito, flea, sand fly/midge, or bedbug bites. The presentation of this reaction varies by arthropod but usually involves an erythematous wheal with subsequent firm, brownish-red pruritic papules. Lesions may be distributed in any anatomic distribution depending on exposure at the time; however, some clues are as follows: "above the socks and below the knees" for fleas; any exposed areas of the face, neck, arms and legs for flying insects; and trunk and extremities sparing the underwear area for bedbugs.

The risk of arthropod bites with hypersensitivity reactions increases with warmer weather because outdoor activities, such as hiking, gardening, and camping, increase the chances of arthropod bites. There is no age or gender preference when it comes to these bites. Usually, the diagnosis is clinical and easily suspected by recent exposure history; however, a biopsy may be necessary to convince patients (or, more likely, their families) of the reality of the situation.

For most mild arthropod bites, supportive care is effective. Moderate and severe reactions to bites or stings may necessitate stronger interventions such as topical or oral corticosteroids for reactions such as papular urticaria, epinephrine for several systemic reactions, and possible venom immunotherapy to prevent future attacks.

This chapter focuses on how to properly use epinephrine in the "procedural" setting. Tick and stinger removal are also addressed from a procedural perspective.

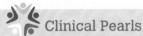

Clinical Pearls

- **Guidelines:** American Academy of Pediatric guidelines on the use of epinephrine in anaphylaxis are reviewed in this chapter.
- **Age-Specific Considerations:** No age-specific considerations; however, epinephrine is weight based (see below).
- **Technique Tips:**
  - If a patient has a systemic reaction, alert emergency services and consider immediate transfer to higher level of care.
  - Immunocompromised patients, from illnesses such as human immunodeficiency virus/acquired immunodeficiency virus (HIV/AIDS) or leukemia, may warrant quick transfer to a higher level of care because the reaction could progress to involve systemic symptoms.
  - Patients with mast cell disorders may have severe reactions. Patients who present with hypotension, shortness of breath, and flushing after an

arthropod bite should be suspected of having possible mastocytosis.
- Any patient with recurrent severe reactions to arthropod bites should be tested for immunologic disease or mastocytosis.
- First-line treatment always centers around prevention of the bite by removing risk factors. Steps to facilitate prevention include limiting outdoor exposure, utilizing correct insect repellent, and minimizing exposed areas for bites to occur.

USE OF EPINEPHRINE

Contraindications/Cautions/Risks

Contraindications
- Per Centers for Disease Control and Prevention (CDC), "there are NO absolute contraindications to epinephrine in the setting of anaphylaxis."

Cautions
- Per CDC, "the most common signs and symptoms are cutaneous (eg, sudden onset of generalized urticaria, angioedema, flushing, pruritus). However, 10% to 20% of patients have no skin findings."
- Per CDC, the danger signs include the following: "Rapid progression of symptoms, evidence of respiratory distress (eg, stridor, wheezing, dyspnea, increased work of breathing, retractions, persistent cough, cyanosis), signs of poor perfusion, abdominal pain, vomiting, dysrhythmia, hypotension, collapse."
- If anaphylaxis is suspected, do not delay the administration of epinephrine. Delays are associated with increased hospitalization and poor outcomes, including death. If the diagnosis of anaphylaxis is not confirmed, it is recommended to err on the side of treating with epinephrine.
- Do not inject this medicine into a vein, into the muscle of the buttocks, or into fingers, toes, hands, or feet.

Risks
- Epinephrine injection can cause anxiety, palpitations, and tremors.

Equipment Needed
- Epinephrine
  - Autoinjector (have at least two at the ready)
    - 15 to 30 kg: EpiPen Jr 0.15 mg (0.15 mg/0.3 mL epinephrine)
    - >30 kg: EpiPen 0.3 mg (0.3 mg/0.3 mL epinephrine)
  - Syringe
    - Dosage: epinephrine 0.01 mg/kg
    - Maximum dosage: 0.3 mg in prepubertal patient
    - Maximum dosage: 0.5 mg in large children (>50 kg) or teenagers

Preprocedural Approach
- Recognize the signs and symptoms of anaphylaxis. It is likely if the patient meets at least one of these three criteria:
  - Acute onset involving skin and/or mucosa with respiratory distress, reduced blood pressure, or symptoms of end-organ dysfunction

  - After exposure to allergen, acute onset of two or more of the following: skin/mucosa involvement, respiratory distress, reduced blood pressure/symptoms of end-organ dysfunction, gastrointestinal symptoms
  - After exposure to allergen, reduced blood pressure
    - Children: low systolic blood pressure or >30% decrease in systolic
    - Teenagers/adults: systolic blood pressure <90 mm Hg or >30% decrease from baseline systolic blood pressure
- Assess patient's airway, breathing, and circulation.
- Alert emergency medical services.
- Calculate appropriate dose.
  - Epinephrine 0.01 mg/kg (0.01 mL/kg of epinephrine 1 mg/mL) to maximum of 0.3 mg in prepubertal patient and up to 0.5 mg in large children (>50 kg) or teenagers
  - OR use epinephrine autoinjector
    - 15 to 30 kg: 0.15 mg dose
    - >30 kg: 0.3 mg dose

Procedural Approach
- Inject intramuscularly in the mid-outer thigh (vastus lateralis muscle). If using autoinjector, follow instructions on injector.
- In an emergency, inject through clothing with avoidance of items in pockets and thick seams.
- If there is no response or the response is inadequate, the injection can be repeated in 5 to 15 minutes (or more frequently).

Postprocedural Approach
- Patient should be transferred to emergency department for further monitoring.
- Patient should be prescribed and advised to carry an epinephrine autoinjector for use in future episodes.
  - Check expiration dates of the medicine and renew as needed.
  - Should be kept between 68°F and 77°F, away from heat, moisture, and direct light. Do not store the medicine in a refrigerator or freezer or in a vehicle's glove box.
- Parents and patients, if possible, should be educated on how to recognize anaphylaxis and how to properly use an autoinjector.
- Consider providing the patient with an autoinjector trainer to practice.
- Triggers should be elucidated and a personalized emergency action plan should be made.

TICK REMOVAL

Ticks are a vector for multiple diseases, so early detection and immediate removal are important for preventing infection. Avoid folklore remedies such as slathering the tick with nail polish or petrolatum or using heat to make the tick voluntarily detach from the skin. The goal is to remove the tick as quickly as possible—not waiting for it to detach.

There are several "tick removal devices" on the market, but a plain set of fine-tipped tweezers works just as well, if not better, and is recommended by the CDC. Manual removal can usually be accomplished as follows:
- Fine-tipped tweezers should be used to grab the tick as close to the patient's skin as possible.

- Then, use gentle steady force pulling upward to extract the tick. Do not twist or jerk the tick because this can cause mouthparts to break off and remain in the skin.
- If any mouthparts remain in the skin, you can try to remove with clean tweezers. If not possible, you can perform a punch biopsy or leave it alone.
- The bite area and the hands of everyone involved should be thoroughly cleansed with rubbing alcohol or soap and water.
- Dispose of the live tick by placing it in alcohol or formalin (useful for future identification if necessary). Do not crush the tick.
- Perform a thorough inspection of the patient, specifically looking for ticks in and around the ears, in and around the hair, in and around the umbilicus, within the axillae, around the waist, in the groin and buttock areas, and within the popliteal fossae.
- Patient should be monitored for systemic symptoms (eg, rash, fever, fatigue, headache, muscle pain, joint swelling and pain, etc) and/or laboratory testing should be considered depending on which geographic region the tick bite occurred.
- If the patient lives in an area where Lyme disease is highly endemic, a single prophylactic dose of doxycycline (200 mg for adults or 4.4 mg/kg for children of any age weighing less than 45 kg) may be used to reduce the risk of acquiring Lyme disease. Consider the benefits of prophylaxis against the risks when all of the following circumstances are met:
  - Doxycycline is not contraindicated.
  - Attached tick can be identified as an adult or nymphal *Ixodes scapularis* tick (Figure 59.1).
  - Estimated time of attachment is ≥36 hours based on the degree of tick engorgement with blood or likely time of exposure to the tick.
  - Prophylaxis can be started within 72 hours of tick removal.
  - Lyme disease is endemic in the county or state where the tick bite occurred. Currently, the CDC reports these following states as "highly endemic": CT, DE, DC, MA, MD, ME, MN, NH, NJ, NY, PA, RI, VA, VT, WI, WV.

STINGER REMOVAL

- Have someone remain with the patient to ensure that he or she does not have an allergic reaction while unsupervised.
- Wash the site gently with soap and water.
- Examine the site with a magnifying glass or dermatoscope to decide whether the stinger is still embedded within the skin.
- If the stinger is embedded within the skin, wipe over the area using clean gauze or gently scrape over the area with the sharp edge of a credit card.
- Never use tweezers or other devices that could squeeze the stinger; doing so could cause more venom to be released into the patient's skin.
- The affected area should again be thoroughly cleansed.
- Apply ice to reduce swelling.

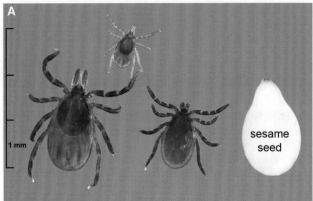

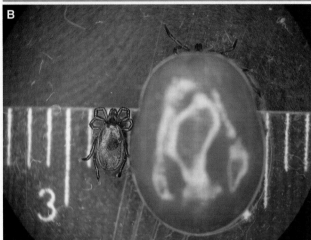

FIGURE 59.1. *Ixodes scapularis*: black-legged deer ticks. *I. scapularis* ticks are the arthropod vectors that transmit the spirochete *Borrelia burgdorferi* to humans, causing Lyme disease. A, From left to right, an unfed *I. scapularis* adult female, nymph, and adult male. The sesame seed demonstrates relative size. B, An unfed *I. scapularis* adult female (left) and a fully engorged *I. scapularis* adult female (right). Reprinted with permission from Engleberg NC, DiRita VJ, Dermody TS. *Schaechter's Mechanisms of Microbial Disease*. 5th ed. Philadelphia, PA: Wolters Kluwer Health/Lippincott Williams & Wilkins; 2012. Figure 25-4.

- Over-the-counter oral antihistamines may help (warn patients that they may cause drowsiness); topical antihistamines are not recommended.

SUGGESTED READINGS
Krakowski AC, Golden DBK. Hymenoptera stings: a practical guide to prevention and management. *Contempor Pediatr*. 2006;8(23):30–37.

Sicherer SH, Simons FER. AAP Section on allergy and immunology. Epinephrine for first-aid management of anaphylaxis. *Pediatrics*. 2017; 139(3):e20164006.

Steen CJ, Carbonaro PA, Schwartz RA. Arthropods in dermatology. *J Am Acad Dermatol*. 2004;50(6):819–842.

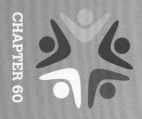

CHAPTER 60

Basal Cell Carcinoma

Guilherme Canho Bittner and Nelise Ritter Hans-Bittner

Introduction

Basal cell carcinoma (BCC) in children is unusual. Cases of BCC in the pediatric population have been reported in association with xeroderma pigmentosum, basal cell nevus syndrome, nevus sebaceous, and after high-dose radiotherapy.[1,2]

Isolated cases of BCC unrelated to one of these causes are seldom reported in pediatric patients. Consequently, clinicians often have a low index of suspicion, leading to delay in diagnosis.[1,2]

Herein we offer our step-by-step instruction for BCC excision in children and tips to make the surgery less traumatic. Our protocol is to perform Mohs micrographic surgery (MMS), but excision with wider margins (5 mm) can be made. We further explain both techniques and how to achieve the best results on both.

 Clinical Pearls

- **Guidelines:** MMS is the treatment of choice for most BCCs, especially on the high-risk area (central face, ears, genitalia, hands, feet, and pretibial).[3]
- **Age-Specific Considerations**: Some patients are mature enough to be aware of the procedure and cooperate with the surgeon. In these patients, the MMS can be done with local anesthesia (Figure 60.1).
- **Technique Tips:** Bupivacaine 0.5% with epinephrine 1:200 000 is a long-lasting anesthestic and well tolerated after lidocaine. It acts as an adjunct in decreasing patients' pain during the procedure.

  Consider sedation with an anesthetist if the child does not understand or is unable to cooperate. The child's response to the biopsy before the surgery is a good indicator. If calm/cooperative during the biopsy, the child will likely be calm during surgery.

- **Skin of Color Considerations:** The technique can be performed in any skin color.

Contraindications/Cautions/Risks

Contraindications
- Active skin infection on surgical site
- Inability to care for postprocedure wounds

Cautions
- History of bleeding and allergic reactions (check family history)

Risks
- Death (infection or anesthesia), scarring, pain, bleeding, recurrence of lesions

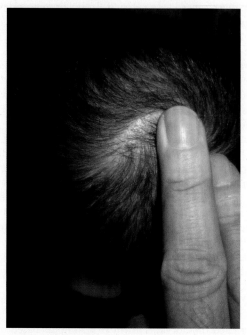

FIGURE 60.1. Basal cell carcinoma of the occipital scalp in a 14-year-old male who had received adjuvant radiation therapy in the area for a brain tumor. The patient was mature enough to perceive that he would not likely tolerate the Mohs procedure ("too long in a chair"), so he opted for a regular excision with margins. Photo courtesy of Andrew C. Krakowski, MD.

Equipment Needed
- Lidocaine
- Saline
- Cleansing antiseptic
- Bupivacaine
- Scalpel
- Scissors
- Clamps
- Hooks
- Hemostatic clamps
- Electrocautery
- Smoke evacuator
- Gauze
- Surgical marker pen
- Tissue stain
- Mohs laboratory (cryostat, hematoxylin and eosin stain)
- Suture of choice
- Petroleum jelly–based ointment
- Micropore Surgical Tape™ (3M™, US)

Preprocedural Approach

- Ask the patient to bring all medications to show the surgeon. Take all regular medicines except those that affect bleeding.
- Clearly instruct patients to avoid supplements (herbs, vitamin E, niacin, fish oil tablets) or nonsteroidal anti-inflammatory medicines (ibuprofen, naproxen, etc) for 1 week before surgery because these substances can cause bleeding.
- Prophylaxis for herpes simplex is not necessary.
- Patients should bathe either the evening before or the morning of surgery.

Procedural Approach

- Informed consent from the parent/guardian and, when possible, assent from the minor are obtained.
- Typically, general anesthesia is utilized because of pain associated with the procedure.
- The surgery site must be cleansed with alcohol 70%.
- The area of the tumor is marked with a permanent pen. The first margin is 1 to 2 mm from the dermoscopy tumor edge.
- Some older patients might be submitted to a local anesthesia with lidocaine 1% with epinephrine 1:100 000.
- To reduce the anesthesia infiltration pain, inject it slowly. Repetitive movements with the fingertip around the needle can help in reducing the pain. Also, good conversation and ambient music always help distract and keep the patient relaxed during the procedure.
- When the patient is anaesthetized, bupivacaine 0.5% with epinephrine 1:200 000 is then infiltrated around the area. Sometimes laboratory work can take several hours depending on the tumor size. It will keep the area numb.
- The surgical field is cleaned again with another antiseptic, either with alcohol 70%, chlorhexidine 2%, or a combination of both as ChloraPrep™ (Becton, Dickinson and Company, US).
- Curettage or a superficial excision of the tumor is now performed.
- A Mohs layer is taken after that, with a second scalpel (preventing tumor contamination), and the tissue is marked with proper tissue stain.
- Good hemostasis is then made with electrocauterization, if necessary.
- A dressing with a small amount of saline and gauze covers the surgical defect until closure or a new Mohs surgery phase.
- The procedure continues for as many phases as needed until all surgical margins are clear.
- After clear margins are obtained, reconstruction is made. Primary closure, when possible, is the best option. Some areas, depending on the tumor size and dimension (oval, circle, or another shape), may require a flap or graft, especially for larger surgical defects.
- Suture the wound always using absorbable deep stitches, such Monocryl™, Vicryl™, or PDS™ (Polydioxanone [PDS II®]) (Ethicon US, LLC).
- External suturing is performed with Prolene™ (Ethicon US, LLC) or Fast-absorbing Surgical Gut Suture (Plain) (Ethicon US, LLC)
- The wound may sometimes be left open to heal by second intention. Head, legs, or small defects in the fingers are the usual areas where this approach could be considered.
- Clean the surgical site with saline and dry well.
- Apply a petroleum-based ointment and dress with gauze and Micropore Surgical Tape.

- In cases where MMS is not an option, a similar approach may be made utilizing excision with wider margins (5 mm) from the tumor edges.
- Conventional surgery can be performed in some cases:
  1. Nonrecurrent BCC in intermediate-risk areas (cheeks, forehead, scalp, and neck) with a healthy, nonimmunocompromised patient and superficial subtype in lesions less than 6 mm[3]
  2. Nonrecurrent BCC in low-risk areas (trunk and extremities, except hands, feet, and pretibial), with a healthy, nonimmunocompromised patient, superficial subtype, or nodular subtype in lesions less than 2 cm[3]
  3. Nonrecurrent BCC in low-risk area (trunk and extremities, except hands, feet, and pretibial), immunocompromised patient, superficial subtype, or nodular subtype in lesions less than 1 cm[3]
- We recommend marking the edge of the specimen with a suture (eg, 12 o'clock "tagged" with one suture and 3 o'clock "tagged" with two sutures) and two cuts at 6 o'clock and 9 o'clock to inform the pathologist of the specimen's orientation.

Postprocedural Approach

- Pain generally increases during the night of the excision. Pain medications such as Tylenol are usually enough to control it. After the second day, pain should decrease; increasing pain may be a sign of infection.
- Swelling and bruising around the surgical site is normal. The bruising will fade in approximately 10 to 14 days. Elevate the area to reduce swelling.
- Keep the bandage in place for 24 to 48 hours. Remove bandaging after this time, clean the wound area daily with saline and gauze, and recover with a BAND-AID™ (Johnson & Johnson, US) or gauze and tape (Micropore Surgical Tape).
- For skin grafts, avoid prolonged exposure to extremely cold temperatures for at least 3 weeks.
- Patients should be vigilantly monitored for signs and symptoms of infection, especially symptoms of worsening pain, fever, or redness.
- Postoperative downtime is significant. Patients should expect to be absent from school or work for 3 days for minor reconstructions and 5 to 7 days for the larger ones.
- When the suture is not absorbable, stitches should be removed after 5 to 7 days.
- At around 1 week after surgery, the area should be cleansed with soapy water using a Q-tip or gauze pad (shower/bathe normally). Dry the wound, apply Vaseline™ (Conopco, Inc., US), Polysporin™ (Johnson & Johnson, US), or bacitracin ointment (do *not* use Neosporin™ [Johnson & Johnson, US]).
- Cover the wound with a nonstick gauze pad and paper tape.
- Repeat wound care once a day for another week.
- Patients are encouraged to contact the physician directly for concerns; we often provide our cell phone numbers for direct contact and reassurance.

REFERENCES

1. Griffin JR, Cohen PR, Tschen JA, et al. Basal cell carcinoma in childhood: case report and literature review. *J Am Acad Dermatol.* 2007;57:S97–S102. doi:10.1016/j.jaad.2006.09.032.
2. LeSueur BW, Silvis NG, Hansen RC. Basal cell carcinoma in children: report of 3 cases. *Arch Dermatol.* 2000;136:370–372. doi:10.1001/archderm.136.3.370.
3. Kauvar AN, Cronin T Jr, Roenigk R, Hruza G, Bennett R. Consensus for nonmelanoma skin cancer treatment: basal cell carcinoma, including a cost analysis of treatment methods. *Dermatol Surg.* 2015;41:550–571. doi:10.1097/DSS.0000000000000296.

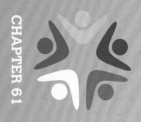
Basal Cell Nevus Syndrome

Guilherme Canho Bittner and Nelise Ritter Hans-Bittner

Introduction

The basal cell nevus syndrome (BCNS) is an uncommon disorder caused by a mutation in the patched, tumor suppressor gene (PTCH). It is mainly characterized by numerous early-onset basal cell carcinomas (BCCs), odontogenic cysts of the jaw, and skeletal abnormalities (Figure 61.1). Owing to the wide clinical spectrum, treatment and management of its modalities are not standardized and should be individualized and monitored by a multidisciplinary team.[1,2]

Herein we offer our step-by-step instruction for BCNS treatment with surgical excisions, tips to make the surgery less traumatic until the postoperative care. Our protocol indicates that Mohs micrographic surgery (MMS) is too high risk, but excision with wider margins (5 mm) can be made. Nonsurgical treatments are also possible; because of the number of lesions some patients have, we will explain photodynamic therapy, cryosurgery, and curettage.

We will further explain all techniques and how to achieve the best results in both.

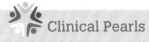

Clinical Pearls

- **Guidelines:** Modalities of treatment are not standardized.
- **Age-Specific Considerations:**
  - Some patients are old enough to be aware of the procedures and cooperate with the surgeon/dermatologist. In these patients, the MMS, photodynamic therapy, and curettage can be done with local anesthesia.
  - Consider sedation with an anesthetist if the child does not understand or collaborate.
  - The biopsy before the surgery is a good indicator. If the patient accepts the biopsy well, he or she will be more likely to tolerate the surgical procedure.
- **Technique Tips:** Bupivacaine 0.5%, in addition to epinephrine 1:200 000, is a long-lasting anesthetic and well tolerated after lidocaine. It acts as an adjunctive and slows the patient's pain during the procedure.
- **Skin of Color Considerations:** Cryotherapy, electrocoagulation, and photodynamic therapy may cause depigmentation.

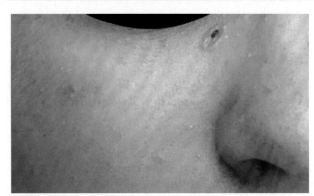

FIGURE 61.1. Adolescent female with basal cell nevus syndrome presented with a basal cell carcinoma (BCC) at the right superior-medial cheek. She was mature enough to understand and assent to the Mohs procedure. Courtesy of Frederico H. Sanchez, MD (Head of the Mohs Micrographic Surgery Center of Rio de Janeiro).

Contraindications/Cautions/Risks

Contraindications
- **Surgery:** active skin infection on surgical site, inability to care for postoperative wounds
- **Cryosurgery:** skin tumor without well-defined borders, lesions on the angle of the mouth, cold contact urticaria
- **Electrocoagulation and curettage:** same as cryotherapy, and periorificial lesions, because of the risk of skin retraction
- **Photodynamic therapy:** nonresponsive tumor, a history of porphyria, systemic lupus erythematosus, photosensitive dermatoses

Cautions
- **Surgery:** history of bleeding and allergic reactions (check family history)
- **Electrocoagulation and curettage:** patients with cardiac devices; avoid alcohol as an antiseptic agent, or allow it to dry completely, because it may ignite
- **Photodynamic therapy:** allergy to the active ingredients in the photosensitizer, which is considerably rare

Risks
- **All procedures:** death (infection or anesthesia), scarring, pain, bleeding, recurrence of lesions

Equipment Needed
Surgery
- Lidocaine 1% with epinephrine 1:100 000
- Saline
- Bupivacaine 0.5% with epinephrine 1:200 000
- Scalpel
- Scissors
- Clamps
- Hooks
- Hemostatic clamps
- Electrocautery
- Smoke evacuator
- Gauze
- Surgical marker pen
- Tissue stain
- Mohs laboratory (cryostat, hematoxylin and eosin stain)
- Suture
- Petrolatum-based ointment
- Micropore Surgical Tape™ (3M™, US)

Cryosurgery
- Lidocaine 1% with epinephrine 1:100 000
- Cryosurgical unit: CRY-AC® (Brymill Cryogenic Systems)
- Liquid nitrogen
- Spray-tip size C

Electrocoagulation and curettage
- Electrosurgical device
- Disposable electrode tips
- Smoke evacuator
- Antiseptic agent (chlorhexidine or povidone-iodine)

- Curette/scoop
- Local anesthetics

Photodynamic therapy
- Lidocaine 1% with epinephrine 1:100 000
- Gauze
- Aluminum foil
- Cling film
- Curette
- 5-Aminolevulinic acid (5-ALA)
- Red light (Aktlight)

Preprocedural Approach

- **Surgery, cryosurgery, electrocoagulation and curettage and photodynamic therapy**
  - Patients must bring all medications to show the doctor, and take all regular medicines except those that affect bleeding.
  - Patients must be advised about avoiding supplements that exacerbate such as herbs (eg, Ginkgo biloba), vitamin E, niacin, fish oil tablets, or nonsteroidal anti-inflammatory medicines (ibuprofen, naproxen, etc) for 1 week before surgery.
  - Prophylaxis for herpes simplex is not necessary.
  - Patients should bathe either the evening before or on the morning of their surgery/procedure.

Procedural Approach

- **Surgery**
  - Informed consent from the parent/guardian and, when possible, assent from the minor are obtained.
  - Typically, general anesthesia is utilized because of pain associated with the procedure.
  - The surgery site must be cleaned with alcohol 70%.
  - The area of the tumor is marked with a permanent pen. The first margin is 1 to 2 mm from the dermoscopy tumor edge.
  - Some older patients might be submitted to local anesthesia. The authors recommend lidocaine 1% with epinephrine 1:100 000.
  - To reduce the anesthesia infiltration pain, apply it slowly. A repetitive tapping movement with the fingertips around the needle can trick the sensitive nervous system and reduce the pain. Also, good conversation and ambient music always help distract the patient and keep him or her relaxed during the procedure.
  - When the patient is anesthetized, bupivacaine 0.5% with epinephrine 1:200 000 is infiltrated around the area. Sometimes, laboratory work can take several hours depending on the tumor size, and this addition will keep the area numb.
  - The surgical site is cleaned again with another antiseptic, either with alcohol 70%, chlorhexidine 2%, or a combination of both such as ChloraPrep™ (Becton, Dickinson and Company, US).
  - Curettage or a superficial excision of the tumor is now performed.
  - A Mohs layer is taken after that, with a second scalpel (preventing tumor contamination) and the tissue is marked with proper tissue stain.
  - Good hemostasis is then made with electrocauterization, using the clamps if necessary.
  - A dressing with a small amount of saline and gauze should be used to cover the surgical defect until the closure or a new Mohs surgery phase.

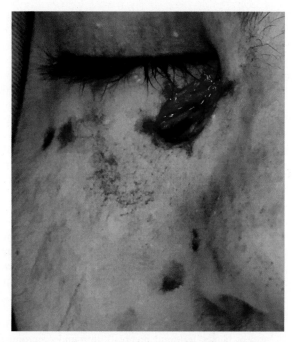

FIGURE 61.2. Intraoperative defect resulting from Mohs surgery. Courtesy of Frederico H. Sanchez, MD (Head of the Mohs Micrographic Surgery Center of Rio de Janeiro).

  - The procedure continues for as many phases as needed until all surgical margins are clear (Figure 61.2).
  - Next, after clear margins, reconstruction is done. In some areas, depending on the tumor size and dimension (oval, circle, or another shape), primary closure when possible is the best option, but flaps or grafts are options for bigger wounds (Figure 61.3).

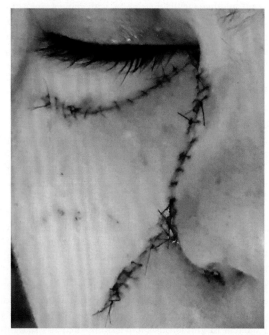

FIGURE 61.3. Rotation flap with periosteal stich on the right lower eyelid was used to repair the defect. Courtesy of Frederico H. Sanchez, MD (Head of the Mohs Micrographic Surgery Center of Rio de Janeiro).

○ Suture the wound always using absorbable inner stiches as Monocryl™, Vicryl™, or PDS™ (Ethicon US, LLC).

○ External suture is performed with Prolene™ (Ethicon US, LLC) or plain gut fast absorbable.

○ The wound sometimes will be left open to heal by second intention. Head, legs, or small defects in the fingers are the usual areas.

○ Clean the surgical site with saline and dry well.

○ After that, a petrolatum-based ointment is applied and a dressing with gauze and Micropore Surgical Tape is then made.

○ Some places where MMS is not an option to treat their patients, a similar approach is made; however, the margins from the tumor edges are wider (5 mm).

○ Conventional surgery can be performed in some cases:

1. Nonrecurrent BCC in an intermediate-risk area (cheeks, forehead, scalp, and neck) with a healthy patient (nonimmunocompromised), superficial subtype with less than 6 mm

2. Nonrecurrent BCC in a low-risk area (trunk and extremities, except hands, feet, and pretibial), with a healthy patient (nonimmunocompromised), superficial subtype, or nodular with less than 2 cm

3. Nonrecurrent BCC in low-risk area (trunk and extremities, except hands, feet, and pretibial), immunocompromised patient, superficial subtype, or nodular with less than 1 cm

○ Personally, I recommend to mark the edge of the specimen with a suture (eg, 12 o'clock one suture and 3 o'clock two sutures) and two small cuts (at 6 o'clock and 9 o'clock) on the specimen when conventional surgery is performed to have an idea where the further approach should be made if a margin is positive to the tumor.

• **Cryosurgery:**

○ Is an option for smaller lesions (1-2 mm)

○ Tumor area is marked with a pen. The margin is 3 to 4 mm from the dermoscopy tumor edge.

○ Surgical site must be cleaned with alcohol 70%.

○ Local anesthesia with lidocaine 1% with epinephrine 1:100 000

○ Open spray technique: spray liquid nitrogen through a cryospray (CRY-AC) directly over the lesion, using spray-tip size C held close to the lesion (approximately 1-cm distance) and perpendicular to the skin surface.

○ First cycle: 90 seconds freezing-time. The white halo of freezing should disappear after 60 to 180 seconds.

○ Repeat this process one more time.

• **Electrocoagulation and curettage:**

○ Smoke evacuator is necessary to help remove plume smoke, and all present should wear masks.

○ The dispersive plate should make good contact with the bare skin of a well-vascularized part of the patients' body.

○ Local anesthetics before the procedure

○ Tumor curettage: use a large curette (4-6 mm) to debulk all friable tissue. Next, use a small curette (2 mm) to scrape across the surface of the treatment site in every direction.

○ Electrosurgical treatment: electrocoagulation current to stop bleeding and potentially remove further tumor

○ Repeat this process for a total of three cycles of curettage and electrosurgery, until all friable tissue has been removed.

• **Photodynamic therapy**

○ Excellent for numerous small lesions, such as 1 to 2 mm

○ Tumor area is marked with a pen.

○ Local anesthesia with lidocaine 1% with epinephrine 1:100 000, because pain is the most common complaint during delivery of treatment.

○ Curettage is performed until the deep dermis. Use a gauze to stop the bleeding before applying 5-ALA.

○ A layer of 5-ALA is placed, with a thickness of 1 mm and 5 to 10 mm around the normal skin.

○ A dressing with cling film covered with aluminum foil is done, to prevent exposition to the light for 3 hours.

○ After 3 hours, the 5-ALA is removed by a gauze with physiologic serum.

○ Lidocaine is then reapplied to prevent pain during the Aktlight application.

○ Red light (Aktlight) is now applied for 7 minutes and 50 seconds.

○ After the Aktlight, a dressing with nonstick gauze and paper tape is made.

○ The procedure needs two sessions. The second is performed after 2 weeks (14 days).

Postprocedural Approach

• **Surgery**

○ Generally, pain should increase during the night of the excision. Pain medications such as Tylenol are usually enough to control it. After the second day, pain should decrease.

○ It is normal to have swelling and bruising around the surgical site. The bruising will fade in approximately 10 to 14 days. Elevate the area to reduce swelling.

○ Leave the bandage in place for 48 hours. Remove after this time, cleaning daily with saline and gauze and closing with a BAND-AID™ (Johnson & Johnson, US) or gauze and tape (Micropore Surgical Tape).

○ For skin grafts, avoid prolonged exposure to extremely cold temperatures for 3 weeks.

○ Patients should be vigilantly monitored for signs and symptoms of infection, especially if there are symptoms of pain, fever, or reddish area.

○ Postoperative downtime is significant, and patients should expect to be absent from school or work for 3 days for minor reconstructions and 5 days to a week for bigger ones.

○ When the suture is not absorbable, the stiches must be removed after 7 days.

○ One week after surgery, the area should be cleaned with soapy water using a Q-tip or gauze pad (shower/bathe normally). Dry the wound, apply Vaseline™ (Conopco, Inc., US), Polysporin™ (Johnson & Johnson, US), or bacitracin ointment (do NOT use Neosporin™ [Johnson & Johnson, US]).

○ Cover the wound with a nonstick gauze pad and paper tape.

○ Repeat wound care once a day for another week.

○ After 1 week, continue to apply ointment until fully healed.

○ Patients are encouraged to contact the physician directly for concerns and are often provided with cell phone numbers for direct contact and reassurance.

• **Cryosurgery and photodynamic therapy**

○ Erythema, local edema, vesicle formation, exudation, and crusting are expected after the procedure, and should disappear within 2 to 4 weeks.

○ The area should be daily cleaned with soapy water using a Q-tip or gauze pad (shower/bathe normally). Dry the wound, apply Vaseline, and cover the wound with a nonstick gauze pad and paper tape.

○ The dressing should be done until the lesion is fully healed.

○ Scar development is expected.

• **Electrocoagulation and curettage**

○ An eschar forms within a few days and separates in about 10 days; deeper wounds should take 2 to 4 weeks to heal (or longer on the lower extremities).

- Generally, pain medications such as acetaminophen are sufficient to prevent discomfort after the procedure.
- The original bandages should be removed within 24 hours.
- The exposed wound area should be cleaned with saline using a gauze pad after showering normally.
- Then, Vaseline or mupirocin ointment with a clean Q-tip should be applied.
- The wound should be covered with a nonstick gauze pad and nonirritating tape.
- The wound care should be repeated once a day until the wound is completely healed.
- The wound should heal faster with a better cosmetic result if kept moist with ointment and covered with a bandage.

- Patients should be vigilantly monitored for signs and symptoms of infection.
- Patients are encouraged to contact the physician directly for concerns.

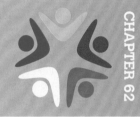

REFERENCES

1. Neves DR, Ramos DG, Magalhães GM, Rodrigues RC, Souza JBA. Photodynamic therapy for treatment of multiple lesions on the scalp in nevoid basal cell carcinoma syndrome: case report [in English, Portuguese]. *An Bras Dermatol.* 2010;85:545–548.
2. Ribeiro PL, Souza Filho JB, Abreu KD, Brezinscki MS, Pignaton CC. Syndrome in question: Gorlin-Goltz syndrome. *An Bras Dermatol.* 2016;91:541–543.

Becker's Nevus

Laura Huang, Angel J. Su, Alexander Choi, and John C. Browning

CHAPTER 62

Introduction

Becker's nevus is a benign skin disorder that appears in the pubertal period as a hyperpigmented, hypertrichotic, or mixed nevus. It has a predilection for males with a prevalence of 0.5% in males and a male-to-female ratio of 5:1. The exact etiology of the condition is unclear; however, the association with males, acne, and appearance during puberty links the condition to an increase in androgen receptors. No clear genetic association has been found for Becker's nevus, so it is considered an acquired nevus especially because the lesions commonly arise after prolonged sun exposure. The lesion usually starts in the upper torso or unilateral upper extremity and gradually spreads, becoming thicker and hairier (Figure 62.1).

As the treatment for Becker's nevus focuses on cosmetics, the best treatment strategy and timing of the intervention depends mostly on patient safety, preference, and convenience. One approach is the Q-switched ruby laser, which utilizes photoacoustic and photothermal effects of high-frequency and high-energy pulses to disrupt melanosomes and established melanin deposits, sparing the overall epidermal structure. Fractional ablative laser resurfacing with either a carbon dioxide or erbium: Yttrium aluminum garnet (Er:YAG) laser is another approach. These devices create thousands of microscopic treatment zones (MTZs) that penetrate into the epidermis and dermis. The penetration results in cutaneous thermal injury but preserves the overall integrity of the epidermis, conferring the benefit of swift healing with complete reepithelialization within 1 week. Multiple sessions are typically required regardless of which laser is utilized.

Laser hair removal is an adjunct treatment for hypertrichotic lesions. The mechanism of action is believed to be related to photothermal, photomechanical, and photochemical injury to the hair follicle. In general, patients with lighter skin types have better response to the 755-nm alexandrite or the 800-nm diode laser and patients with darker skin types have better response to the 1064-nm Nd:YAG.

All laser treatments can cause erythema, pain, hyperpigmentation, or hypopigmentation to the area that is treated. Overall, the use of laser technology in treating Becker's nevus has provided satisfactory results among patients.

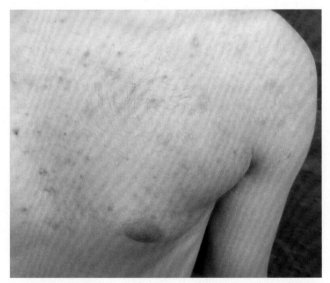

FIGURE 62.1. Becker's nevus on left superior chest of an adolescent male. Note the hypertrichosis located superiorly within the lesion. Photo courtesy of Andrew C. Krakowski, MD.

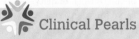

Clinical Pearls

- **Guidelines:** No specific treatment guidelines are known to exist for this condition.
- **Age-Specific Considerations:**
  - The nevus usually first becomes noticeable in the patient's late teens to early adulthood.
  - Because Becker's nevi are benign, the patient should ideally be old enough to decide whether to treat.
- **Skin of Color Considerations:** The technique is best suited for skin types I and II, because the risk for dyspigmentation increases with darker skin types.

Contraindications/Cautions/Risks

Contraindications
- ○ Active skin infection
- ○ Inability to care for postoperative wounds

Cautions
- ○ History of abnormal scarring or keloid formation
- ○ History of herpes simplex

Risks
- Erythema, pain, dyspigmentation, death, scar, recurrence, infection. *Also, patients should be counseled that multiple sessions are usually required to achieve desired result.*

Equipment Needed
- Wavelength-specific eye shields
- Masks
- Smoke evacuator
- Appropriate laser
  - ○ Pigmentation: Q-switched ruby, fractional carbon dioxide or Er:YAG
  - ○ Hypertrichosis: 755-nm alexandrite, 800-nm diode laser, or 1064-nm Nd:YAG
- Topical anesthetic
- Optional cold air cooling system
- Moist gauze
- Sterile water
- Sterile Vaseline™ (Conopco, Inc., US)

Preprocedural Approach

- Avoid sun and maximize sun protection weeks before and after procedure.
- Stop topical retinoids and bleaching creams a few days before treatment.
- For fractional ablative laser resurfacing, antiviral prophylaxis for herpes simplex is typically started 1 to 2 days before laser surgery and continued until reepithelialization.
- Informed consent from the parent/guardian and, when possible, assent from the minor are obtained.
- Apply a topical anesthetic, such as lidocaine, under occlusion for an hour before the procedure to help minimize pain.
- For laser hair removal, the area needs to be shaved prior to treatment.

Procedural Approach

- Appropriate protective eyewear should be worn, and patients should have eye pads (disposable adhesive eye shields offering full eye protection from medical lasers with wavelengths between 190 and 11 000 nm at an optical density >7; OD 7@190-11 000 nm) or correctly fitted metal eye shields in place.
- A cold air cooling system and/or ice applied directly to the treated areas can be utilized intraoperatively to lessen pain.
- Procedural site should be cleaned using alcohol and marked.
- Fractional ablative laser resurfacing: Fluence should be adjusted to target the pigment in the papillary dermis and for pain tolerance. While treatment parameters will vary by device, a "starting point" protocol for the fractionated CO_2 laser (10,600 nm) could be 10-20 mJ; 10-20% density, while the Er:YAG laser (2940 nm) might be single pass; 3 mm spot; 22-28 J/cm^2.
- Q-switched frequency-doubled Nd:YAG (532 nm) and Q-switched ruby (694 nm): These technologies have demonstrated some utility in terms of pigment reduction but recurrence should be expected. An example of treatment parameters for the Q-switched frequency-doubled Nd:YAG (532 nm) is as follows: 3 mm spot size; 8-10 J/cm^2; 3 to 4 treatment sessions.
- Long-pulsed alexandrite (755 nm): Useful for reducing hair density within the lesion. Standard "laser hair removal" protocols apply. For patients with Fitzpatrick skin phototype III to V, one uncontrolled study demonstrated good success using the following parameters: 3 ms; 20 to 25 J/cm^2; spot size 15 to 18 mm.
- Nonablative fractionated erbium-doped fiber laser (1550 nm): Reported to be useful for reduction of hyperpigmentation with one protocol utilizing 8 to 10 passes, 6 to 10 mJ, and 250 to 254 MTZs/cm^2 per pass.

Postprocedural Approach

- Apply a petrolatum-based ointment.
- Edema and pain generally decrease quickly with time. Ice and cold packs can also be applied to reduce both.
- Mild analgesics can be given for pain and oral antihistamines for pruritus.
- For fractional ablative laser resurfacing:
  - ○ Patients should continue herpes prophylaxis for a total of 7 to 10 days, or until reepithelialization.
  - ○ At least two to three times a day, patients are instructed to gently cleanse the treated areas using a mixture that consists of 1 capful of acetic acid (ie, food-grade white distilled vinegar) combined with 1 L of distilled water. Gauze is soaked in this mixture and, with patients lying supine, left in place on the treated areas for 10 minutes. Then, the gauze is removed, and the area is rinsed gently with fresh water. Petrolatum-based ointment is immediately reapplied and maintained until reepithelization has occurred—typically 5 to 7 days after laser surgery.
  - ○ Patients should be vigilantly monitored for signs and symptoms of infection, with special consideration paid to viral, fungal, and atypical mycobacterial infections, as well as the more typical bacterial culprits. For example, posttreatment Candida or fungal infections tend to evolve as bright red eruptions that may be intensely itchy.
  - ○ After the last treatment, patients should have regular follow-up with the first visit at 1 week to assess how the skin is healing. Regular visits at 1, 3, and 6 months, and at 1 year should be scheduled to make sure the lesion has not recurred.
- Patients are encouraged to contact the physician directly for concerns.
- Repeat treatments should be scheduled at least 1 month after treatment to allow sufficient skin healing.
  - ○ Laser hair removal should be spaced at 6- to 10-week intervals.
  - ○ Fractional ablative laser resurfacing generally requires four to five treatments, spaced 4 to 6 weeks apart, to obtain desired results.
- Sunscreen application is imperative for improved wound healing and minimized scar and hyperpigmentation formation.

SUGGESTED READINGS

Momen S, Mallipeddi R, Al-Niaimi F. The use of lasers in Becker's naevus: an evidence-based review. *J Cosmet Laser Ther*. 2016;18(4):188–192.

Patel P, Malik K, Khachemoune A. Sebaceous and Becker's nevus: overview of their presentation, pathogenesis, associations, and treatment. *Am J Clin Dermatol*. 2015;16(3):197–204.

Tanzi EL, Alster TS. Single-pass carbon dioxide versus multiple-pass Er:YAG laser skin resurfacing: a comparison of postoperative wound healing and side-effect rates. *Dermatol Surg* 2003;29(1):80–84.

Blister

Madeline L. Gore and Kristen P. Hook

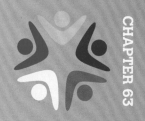

CHAPTER 63

INTRODUCTION

Blistering conditions occur across all ethnicities and sexes. Blisters can form for a variety of reasons, including genetic skin disorders, infection, and trauma or autoimmune etiologies. The distribution, onset, and configuration and depth can all be clues to diagnosis. Traumatic blisters form when layers of the epidermis separate because of friction. The bullae fill with fluid as the upper layer of skin remains intact and may be painful. These types of blisters are often found on the palms, soles, and ankles. In genetic skin disorders, temperature, friction, and moisture may increase the likeliness of blistering. Autoimmune bullous diseases often present with more widespread involvement and/or mucosal involvement and may have pediatric-specific presentations.

Blisters can be filled with clear fluid, blood, or purulent material. When a patient presents with blisters or pustules, it is important to perform specific tests to rule out life-threatening conditions.

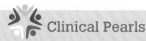

Clinical Pearls

- **Age-Specific Considerations:** Beware of infectious causes of blistering in neonates and infants, especially in the first 6 months of life.
- **Technique Tips:** It is important to first identify potential causes of the infection and rule out life-threatening conditions. Several tests may be performed at the bedside or in-office. For patients with suspected epidermolysis bullosa (EB), biopsy for immunofluorescence mapping (IFM) and electron microscopy (EM) should be done by an experienced clinician. Also, genetic testing is closely approaching as a first-line diagnostic test for EB with lower costs and more rapid turnaround time.
- **Skin of Color Considerations:** Postinflammatory pigment change may be more common in patients with skin of color.
- **Helpful Publications:**
  - Marathe K, Lu J, Morel KD. Bullous diseases: kids are not just little people. *Clin Dermatol.* 2015;33(6): 644–656. doi:10.1016/j.clindermatol.2015.09.007.
  - Hussain S, Venepally M, Treat JR. Vesicles and pustules in the neonate. *Semin Perinatol.* 2013;37(1): 8–15. doi:10.1053/j.semperi.2012.11.005.

Contraindications/Cautions/Risks

Contraindications
- Lancing blisters are indicated for some genetic causes of blistering, mainly epidermolysis bullosa, but may be contraindicated in other causes of blistering.

Cautions
- Carefully monitor local infections to avoid local spread and progression. Several infections in neonates and young infants can be life-threatening and require immediate treatment with antivirals/antibiotics (herpes simplex, neonatal herpes simplex, *Staphylococcus aureus*, and *Streptococcus*). See details in Procedural Approach.

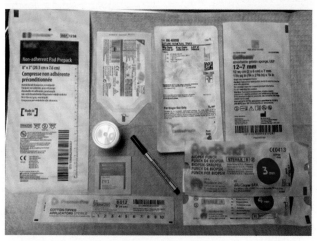

FIGURE 63.1. Sample supply tray for blister care.

- It is imperative to inform the family of signs and symptoms of infection. For localized infections, local antiseptics or bleach and vinegar baths can be helpful. If more severe, parents are instructed to contact a physician immediately.

Risks
- Systemic infection can be life-threatening if not treated.

Equipment Needed (Figure 63.1)
- Culture swabs for bacterial infection
- Viral culture and/or viral polymerase chain reaction (PCR) materials
- KOH (potassium hydroxide) preparation materials
- Alcohol swab or appropriate skin preparation
- Blood test materials
- Biopsy materials
- Lancet or sterile needle
- Sterile gauze
- Bland ointment (Aquaphor® [Beiersdorf AG, US], Vaseline™ [Conopco, Inc., US], etc)

Preprocedural Approach

- For children and neonates presenting with blisters, infection should be immediately ruled out.
  - In a denuded or eroded blister, swab the blister fluid or the base for viral and bacterial culture. If the blister is intact, it can be gently punctured with a lancet to release the fluid to be cultured. See Chapters 26. Bacterial Culture or 37. Viral Culture for more detailed discussion and appropriate techniques for these tests. For candidiasis and other fungal infections, a KOH and fungal culture should be performed (see Chapter 42. Fungal Examination or Potassium Hydroxide [KOH] Preparation).

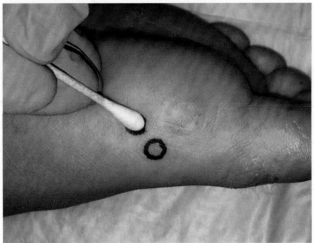

FIGURE 63.2. Use a Q-tip to induce a new blister.

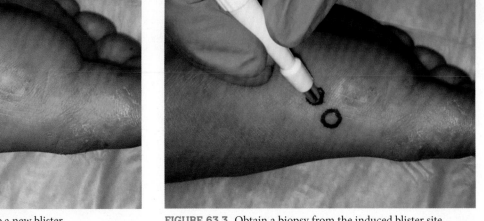

FIGURE 63.3. Obtain a biopsy from the induced blister site.

- Clinical assessment and important questions to ask:
  - Identify whether the blisters are vesicular or pustular in nature.
  - Determine the time of onset and how the blistering has changed over time.
  - Inspect the blister distribution on the skin (linear, groin, generalized, etc).
  - Query the family history, especially that of the mother, for viral infections or skin conditions in past or during pregnancy. Prenatal care should also be reviewed.
  - Identify any associated symptoms the child may be experiencing (fever, lethargy, failure to thrive, etc).
- If EB is suspected, the below steps should be followed if proceeding with skin biopsy for immunofluorescence and EM (see Chapter 79. Epidermolysis Bullosa):
  - Choose an area of the skin that is not blistered, but near affected areas. Palms and soles should be avoided because the skin is too thick for an accurate diagnosis. Also consider wound care postbiopsy and sites more at risk for infection (eg, diaper area).
  - A new blister should be induced before biopsy (Figure 63.2). Twist a cotton swab or the eraser end of a pencil on the skin for about 10 to 20 seconds until the area turns red or an early blister is noted. Stop if the skin tears because this will not be an ideal specimen. A clinical blister may not be recognized, but microscopically it will be present.
  - Wipe area with an alcohol swab and inject with buffered 1% lidocaine with epinephrine until a bleb has formed. Topical anesthetics may also be applied beforehand if preferred (caution should be taken on the basis of age, drug choice, and amount).
  - Perform a 3 or 4 mm punch biopsy at the edge of the blister and place in Michel's solution.
  - Take a 3 or 4 mm punch biopsy from the other edge of the blister and place in 2.5% glutaraldehyde for EM (Figure 63.3).
  - Wound closure: smaller wounds may be left open to heal by secondary intention or Gelfoam placed for hemostasis. For larger wounds, simple interrupted sutures can be placed.
  - Cover wound with bland ointment and nonstick dressing.

Procedural Approach

VIRAL INFECTION

- *Herpes simplex virus (HSV 1, 2)* appears as erythematous, eroding pustules and vesicles typically near mucosal surfaces. Lesions are painful, often grouped, and can be treated with topical or systemic antiviral medications. If viral PCR is available, this is often the most rapid route to diagnosis. A Tzanck smear can also be performed.
- *Neonatal HSV can be life-threatening and must be treated with antivirals immediately if suspected.* The disease includes groups of vesicles on erythematous surfaces that occur in the first month after birth. The patient may also have flu-like symptoms. If viral PCR is available, this is often the most rapid route to diagnosis. A Tzanck smear can also be performed.
- *Varicella zoster virus (VZV)* often presents in infants in the first 5 months of life. The wounds are centered to the trunk and head. They begin as macules, then papules, vesicles, pustules, and then erode and crust. Viral culture for VZV takes 1 to 2 weeks and is not ideal; thus, viral PCR or direct fluorescent antibody (DFA) should be sought. Treatment is with systemic antiviral medications.

BACTERIAL INFECTION

- *Impetigo (bullous or nonbullous) is mainly caused by S. aureus and, in some cases, Streptococcus (often group A beta-hemolytic Streptococcus [GABHS]; group B Streptococcus [GBS] in neonates).* Patients present with red papules/pustules that evolve into vesicles/bullae with rim of erythema: honey-colored crusts are considered pathognomonic for *S. aureus*. Streptococcal impetigo can appear more with hemorrhagic crusts and erosions. Both are best diagnosed by Gram stain and culture and treated on the basis of sensitivities when indicated. Impetigo can be especially dangerous in newborns.
- *Cellulitis* often presents in the setting of malaise, fever, and sometimes lab abnormalities, as warm, red, edematous areas of skin with an infiltrated appearance, and typically occurs on the face or limbs. This is a deeper infection of the skin, often in the subcutaneous tissues, and thus, superficial wound cultures may be negative; blood cultures may be indicated.

- *Staphylococcal scalded skin syndrome (SSSS)* is seen in young children and presents as erythematous and easily desquamated vesicles/bullae in skin folds like the axilla, groin, and neck as well as around the nose, eyes, and mouth. Skin will be painful and appear sunburn-like. Skin cultures should be taken around mucosal areas like the eyes, nose, and mouth or groin. Blood cultures may also be taken.
- *Special note about* Streptococcus *infections causing impetigo, bullous impetigo, or cellulitis in the pediatric population.* Thick pustules and crusts as well as skin pain can be a sign of group A *Streptococcus* (GAS) infections. Patients with GAS are more likely to be hospitalized and have invasive infections with fever. These can be particularly dangerous in young infants and must be treated immediately with systemic antibiotics after skin culture and blood culture (when indicated).

FUNGAL INFECTION

- *Candidal* skin infections can present with pustules and rarely vesicles. A KOH preparation can help with a rapid diagnosis and a fungal culture should be done: There are a wide range of *Candida* infections that may present in infants. However, the most life-threatening form must be ruled out immediately in low birth weight, preterm neonates that present with pustules within the first few days of birth. The benign form usually occurs as pustules in full-term infants on mucosal surfaces (skin folds of the groin) or in folds of the skin.

ACQUIRED AUTOIMMUNE BULLOUS DERMATOSES

- *Bullous pemphigoid (BP)* is rare in children. Pruritic, tense vesicles with overlying plaques tend to appear on the palms, soles, and head of newborns, but will be generalized in children with potential mucosal involvement; there is also a localized form occurring in the vulvar area. Lesional skin biopsy for hematoxylin and eosin (H&E) stain and perilesional biopsy for direct immunofluorescence (DIF) should be performed for immunoglobulin G (IgG) antibodies against BP 180 and BP 230; indirect immunofluorescence for epidermal pemphigoid antibodies will also confirm diagnosis.
- *Pemphigus vulgaris (PV)* patients present with flaccid blisters, erosions, and crusting. The oral mucosa is involved most often, but PV may also involve the genital, ocular, and nasal mucosa. Skin biopsy for DIF and H&E stain should be performed for IgG antibodies against desmoglein 1 and desmoglein 3.
- *Linear immunoglobulin A (IgA) bullous dermatosis* results in blisters distributed in a "string of pearls" or "cluster of jewels" pattern on the abdomen, thighs, and genital area. It is most commonly seen in children 4 to 5 years old and is due to linear IgA along the basement membrane to BP 180, BP 230, linear IgA disease (LAD) 285, or laminin 332. Biopsy of the blister for H&E and DIF is needed to make the diagnosis.

CONGENITAL BULLOUS DERMATOSES

- EB is a complex group of genetic disorders with four main subtypes:
  - *EB simplex (EBS)* is commonly caused by keratin 5 or 14 mutations. Nonscarring blistering occurs in the epidermal layers of the skin and appears as tense bullae, either acral localized or generalized.
  - *Junctional EB (JEB)* is due to laminin 332, collagen 17, and $\alpha_6\beta_4$ mutations, among others. Large and generalized bullae occur in the junction between the epidermis and the dermis. Granulation tissue, nail loss, and hoarse voice may be key findings.
  - *Dystrophic EB* is due to collagen 7 mutation, and blistering occurs between the sublamina densa and basement membrane zone.
    - *Dominant dystrophic EB (DDEB)*: lesions localized to dorsal hands overlying joints, feet, and toes; extensor knees and elbows; or generalized. Common symptoms include scarring, nail deformity or loss, and milia.
    - *Recessive dystrophic EB (RDEB)*: more severe than DDEB and is more often generalized. Complications can include anemia, malnutrition, osteoporosis, esophageal strictures, dental disease, and eventual squamous cell carcinoma development.
  - *Kindler's syndrome (KS)* is caused by $\alpha_6\beta_4$ integrin or plectin mutations. KS presents with generalized blistering among all layers of the skin with photosensitivity. There can be internal involvement that may lead to colitis or anal stenosis.
- *Incontinentia pigmenti (IP)* occurs because of a dominant X-linked mutation in the *NEMO* gene. Patients with IP are most often female or males with mosaic presentation. In neonates, vesicles may be present along the limbs and scalp in a blaschkolinear distribution, followed by verrucous plaques. The verrucous stage may present at birth because of the vesicular phase occurring in the womb. Following this stage, hyperpigmentation develops in the same distribution. Hypopigmented scarring in a streak pattern can begin in adolescence and adulthood as the hyperpigmentation fades. In addition to the skin, hair, teeth, nail, eye, and neurologic abnormalities may also be present and should be monitored. If IP is suspected in a neonate, a skin biopsy can be taken to confirm the diagnosis; white blood cell count may be elevated because of an eosinophilia, leading to initial concern for neonatal infection; the mother should also be examined to look for hypopigmented skin lesions with a Wood's lamp. If IP is suspected, urgent referral for an eye examination should be made.

TRANSIENT BULLOUS DISORDERS IN THE NEWBORN

- *Erythema toxicum neonatorum (ETN)* is common in newborns and presents as small vesicles and pustules overlying pink wheals, often concentrated on the trunk, but can be generalized. ETN usually develops in the first few days of life and will disappear within 1 to 3 days. Examination of the pustules should show a lack of organisms and numerous eosinophils.
- *Neonatal acne (neonatal cephalic pustulosis)* presents as numerous pustules typically on the face of infants and can last for weeks to a few months. Examination of the pustules should show Malazzesia. The condition is benign.
- *Miliaria* presents as pinpoint pustules that develop from blocked sweat ducts, typically in neonates, and will self-resolve. The condition is benign and occurs in warm, moist areas of the skin. Culture and microscopic examination can rule out infectious causes when indicated.

Postprocedural Approach

- Regular follow-up appointments are important to monitor the progress of the disease.
- Patients with acquired and congenital blistering conditions are susceptible to infection. It is imperative to inform the

patient and family of signs of infection. For minor infections, local antiseptics or dilute bleach and vinegar baths can be helpful. If the infection is severe, parents are instructed to contact a physician immediately as systemic treatment may be indicated.

- After diagnosing the patient, educate caretakers and the child about how to care for the blisters and wounds, including infection prevention and wound dressings.
- If the condition is long-lasting, provide the family with information about disease-based support groups.
  - The Dystrophic Epidermolysis Bullosa Research Association of America (debra of America): www.debra.org.
- For psychosocial support for older children and adolescents: Camp Discovery is hosted by the American Academy for Dermatology (https://www.aad.org/public/kids/camp-discovery) every summer in multiple locations for children with various skin conditions. Campers are referred by a

dermatologist and are under the expert care of dermatologists, nurses, and pediatricians while attending camp. This is a great way for children to experience camp adapted to their specific medical needs and allows children to socialize and establish friendships with others who have similar skin conditions.

SUGGESTED READINGS

Dystrophic Epidermolysis Bullosa Research Association of America (debra of America). www.debra.org.

Hussain S, Venepally M, Treat JR. Vesicles and pustules in the neonate. *Semin Perinatol.* 2013;37(1):8–15. doi:10.1053/j.semperi.2012.11.005.

Intong LRA, Murrel DF. How to take skin biopsies for epidermolysis bullosa. *Dermatol Clin.* 2010;28(2):197–200. doi:10.1016/j.det.2009.12.002.

Marathe K, Lu J, Morel KD. Bullous diseases: kids are not just little people. *Clin Dermatol.* 2015;33(6):644–656. doi:10.1016/j.clindermatol.2015.09.007.

Blue Rubber Bleb Syndrome

Shehla Admani and Joyce M. C. Teng

Introduction

Blue rubber bleb nevus syndrome (BRBNS) is a rare disorder characterized by venous malformations (VMs) in the setting of somatic *Tie2* mutations. Malformations of the skin as well as the gastrointestinal (GI) tract can be seen, and, less often, in other organ systems. Morbidity and mortality of BRBNS are mostly attributed by the severity of GI disease. Cutaneous lesions do not need to be treated unless they are symptomatic or in cosmetically sensitive areas (Figures 64.1 and 64.2).

Management options include observation, laser surgery, sclerotherapy, excision, and medical therapy for the malformation

as well as associated complications. For localized small VMs, surgical excision offers a possible definitive treatment option. For complex and extensive VMs, combined medical and surgical interventions may be beneficial. The superficial components of these large VMs can often be treated with laser surgery to improve cosmesis as well as to reduce intermittent bleeding at the affected sites. However, the intradermal and subcutaneous

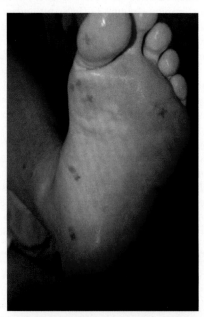

FIGURE 64.2. Blue rubber bleb nevus lesions on an adolescent's foot. The lesions marked with green marker were noted to be painful and interfered with the patient's participation in athletic activities. Photo courtesy of Andrew C. Krakowski, MD.

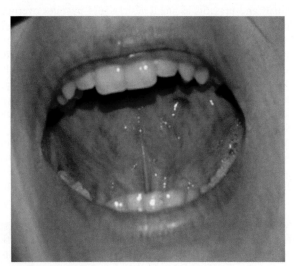

FIGURE 64.1. Sublingual blue rubber bleb nevus lesions. Photo courtesy of Andrew C. Krakowski, MD.

components can often benefit from sclerotherapy by an interventional radiologist. Sclerotherapy can also be performed before surgery to decrease the size of the lesion, surgical complexity, and resultant surgical scar. It can also be performed before or concurrent with laser treatment to optimize the overall outcome. A multidisciplinary approach, therefore, should be employed in the management of complex VMs.

The scope of this chapter is to offer step-by-step instruction for the treatment of VMs in the setting of BRBNS. Our protocol utilizes long-pulsed alexandrite laser (755 nm), often in combination with long-pulsed Nd:YAG laser (1064 nm) depending on the morphology of the vascular malformation. Although pulsed-dye laser (595 nm) can be used as part of a combined treatment regimen to treat VMs in general, it does not tend to be as effective in lesions of BRBNS, and its use is typically reserved for only small lesions (<4-5 mm). We aim to achieve lasting clinical improvement while minimizing adverse events. In the authors' experience, long-term (ie, years) disease remission can be achieved especially when appropriate combination therapies are employed. However, as demonstrated in recent literature, VMs in the setting of BRBNS result from somatic mutations of the *Tie2* gene. Recurrence, therefore, remains a lifelong possibility. Periodic touch-up treatments may be needed, especially in areas where residual lesions remain.

Clinical Pearls

- **Guidelines:** There are no published treatment guidelines for this condition. However, there has been increased evidence about the benefits of using mammalian target of rapamycin (mTOR) inhibitors for disease control.
- **Age-Specific Considerations:** Because these lesions tend to progress over time, early intervention should be considered. However, in cases that require general anesthesia, it is reasonable to postpone elective laser surgery until general anesthesia is considered to be safe. Laser surgery can also be coordinated with other procedures to minimize the overall number of general anesthesia events needed for these treatments.
- **Technique Tips:** Concurrent use of antiangiogenic therapy such as the mTOR inhibitor may reduce disease burden and prevent rebound growth.
- **Skin of Color Considerations:** Laser settings should be adjusted to minimize epidermal pigment damage and strict sun protection is always advised for patients with darker skin.

Contraindications/Cautions/Risks

Contraindications
- Active skin infection
- Inability to care for postoperative wounds (eg, upcoming sporting events, vacations)

Cautions
- Presence of a suntan may increase dyspigmentation after laser surgery.

Risks
- Pain, bleeding, blistering, infection, dyspigmentation, and scarring

Equipment Needed

- Wavelength-specific eye shields (metal eye shields if treating periorbital area)
- Long-pulsed alexandrite laser
- Long-pulsed Nd:YAG laser
- Sterile water
- Gauze (wet and dry)
- Petrolatum-based ointment
- Ice
- Anesthetic, either topical or general anesthesia, followed by injectable local anesthetic (see specific guidelines below)
- Surgical prep (isopropyl alcohol, chlorhexidine, or Betadine followed by sterile water cleansing to remove residue chemicals on the skin)
- Dressing (will vary depending on treatment site)

Preprocedural Approach

- Anesthetic can vary from case to case and generally consists of either topical or general anesthesia followed by injectable local anesthetic. Children younger than 10 years of age typically require sedation. Owing to controversial literature on risks and long-term sequelae from general anesthesia in pediatric patients, referral to a tertiary care center is recommended. Because these procedures are associated with significant discomfort when performed in outpatient clinics, higher percentages of topical lidocaine, that is, up to 30% compounded ointment or mixture of lidocaine and tetracaine, are often used. When using higher percentages of lidocaine, it is important to be mindful of the body surface area being treated and limiting application to less than 1% BSA for less than 30 minutes. Before application of topical lidocaine or injection of local lidocaine, risks of potential systemic absorption should be considered. Maximum allowed local anesthetic dosing should be calculated depending on the patient's weight.
- Sun protection is recommended before the procedure to reduce the risk of epidermal damage and to assure optimal treatment.
- Antiviral prophylaxis should be considered when treating patients with facial VMs and history of herpes labialis.
- Although controlled studies are needed, there is anecdotal experience suggesting the use of antiangiogenic therapy such as mTOR inhibitors can be beneficial before and/or concurrent with laser treatments.

Procedural Approach

- The types of anesthetics used for the laser procedure should be determined depending on age/pain tolerance of the patient, location, and extent of the VM. Although the combined use of topical and local injectable anesthetics may be applicable for adolescents and young adults undergoing these laser procedures, general anesthesia is often needed for young children or those with extensive VMs or VMs involving oral mucosa or genital area. With smaller lesions, it is best to avoid the use of anesthetic with epinephrine because this can cause vasoconstriction, and thereby reduce the efficacy of the treatment. However, in larger lesions, it can be difficult to obtain adequate analgesia to perform the procedure in office without use of epinephrine. Risks and benefits must be weighed and an appropriate regimen should be determined on an individualized basis.

- For oral mucosal lesions, benzocaine 20% spray can be helpful before the injectable anesthetic. When working on focal areas, local infiltration is sufficient; however, when more widespread treatment of multiple lesions is needed, a nerve block (eg, infraorbital nerve block and mental nerve block) is preferred.

- Appropriate protective eyewear should be worn by both care providers and patients during the entire procedure. Disposable adhesive eye shields are easy to use on patients and offer full eye protection from medical lasers with wavelengths between 190 and 11 000 nm at an optical density greater than 7 (OD 7@190-11 000 nm). Correctly fitted metal eye shields should be placed when the periorbital area is being treated. Before the insertion of a metal eye shield, it is important to check its integrity and to make sure there are no obvious scratches on the shield, which can lead to corneal abrasions. For ease of insertion, it is best to lift the upper eyelid and to start by first placing the eye shield inferiorly. After insertion of the shield, it is important to make sure there are no lashes caught under the shield, which may cause injury to the cornea. The placement of metal shields can be challenging for younger children in the outpatient clinic setting.

- To decrease fire risk in the operating room, wet towels should be placed around the treatment area. For short procedures, nasal cannula oxygenation can be a safer alternative. For intraoral procedures, room air ventilation may be used to decrease the percentage of oxygen in the surgical field, and thereby reduce the fire risk. Airway fires are lethal and appropriate precautions should be taken when treating facial/oral lesions.

- A combination of alexandrite (755 nm) and Nd:Yag lasers may be used for treatment of VMs in the setting of BRBNS depending on the epidermal, dermal, and subcutaneous involvement of the malformations. For malformations with obvious epidermal hypertrophic changes, alexandrite and Nd:Yag lasers are usually the better choices. For example, the use of 3-mm spot size, fluence of 44 J/cm^2, and microsecond pulse width of alexandrite laser (Candela, AlexTriVantage) is often effective for VMs with a significant epidermal vascular component and mild hypertrophic changes. It is best to avoid overlap and pulse stacking during initial treatment. Depending on the tissue reaction, a second pass to areas with epidermal hypertrophy is generally well tolerated as long as no blistering is noted during the first pass. The clinical endpoint is dark purpura with minimal whitening. To avoid blistering and excessive epidermal damage, cooling should be used during the entire procedure. Concurrent cooling built into the laser device or a separate cold air cooling unit (Zimmer Medizin Systems, Irvine, CA) can be used. When concurrent cooling is not available, ice should be used with frequent pauses at 10- to 20-second intervals during the procedure.

- For VMs involving subcutaneous tissue, long-pulsed Nd:YAG laser (1064 nm) may be more effective. Spot size and energy (J/cm^2) need to be adjusted depending on patient response as well as on the specific laser model being used. In general, laser setting using a 4- to 6-mm spot size, pulse duration of 20 to 40 μs, and fluence of 35 to 70 mJ/cm^2 may be used. Lower energy settings are recommended for the initial treatment, which can be increased gradually at subsequent treatments. The Nd:YAG laser does not cause significant purpura and the endpoint is often subtle visually with only minimal edema and tissue contraction being seen. Therefore, it is important not to overlap pulses and inform patients of the possibility of significant postoperative edema. For patients with VMs affecting the oral mucosa and lip, it is important to note that the swelling may affect speech as well as the patient's ability to drink from a cup. A short course of systemic steroid may be needed if there is concern for oral edema leading to airway obstruction.

- Of note, if Nd:Yag laser treatment is performed intraoperatively to an open wound bed, much lower fluences should be used.

- Immediately after surgery, a petrolatum-based ointment should be applied liberally.

- Application of intra- and postoperative cooling is very important to help decrease discomfort and minimize edema as well as risk of blistering especially in setting of mucosal treatment.

- Combined sclerotherapy and laser treatment should be used cautiously because excessive tissue destruction can result in localized skin ulceration.

Postprocedural Approach

- Cold compress/ice can be applied as tolerated for the first 24 hours.

- Alternating over-the-counter acetaminophen and ibuprofen is generally sufficient for pain control. However, some patients may also benefit from schedule III narcotic pain medication for breakthrough pain during the first 2 to 3 days.

- Dressing should be applied after the treatment and left in place for the first 24 hours. The treated area can then be cleansed with gentle soap and water daily. If the treated areas are at risk for infection, dilute vinegar or dilute bleach soaks can also be used daily.

- Petrolatum-based ointment is recommended in the immediate postoperative period and also for continued use until the treatment area is fully healed.

- It is important to protect the treatment sites from trauma and friction during the healing process. Protective dressings can be used for 1 to 2 weeks postoperatively. Compression garments can also be helpful to decrease postoperative edema and reduce risks of recurrence with continued use.

- Patients can typically return to school or daily activities within 2 to 3 days.

- Clinic follow-up is recommended 6 to 8 weeks after the treatment to assess response and determine additional management plans. Longer treatment intervals are often preferred for school-age children to minimize school absences and to reduce the frequency of general anesthesia (if it is being used).

- Although additional evidence is needed, early initiation of treatment for extensive VMs may be beneficial because of the lower disease burden overall at younger ages. Once the disease progression is controlled, additional treatments may be offered as in-office procedures later in life.

- Serial photography to document treatment response is always helpful.

SUGGESTED READINGS

Kizilocak H, Dikme G, Celkan T. Sirolimus experience in blue rubber bleb nevus syndrome. *J Pediatr Hematol Oncol*. 2018;40(2):168–169.

Salloum R, Fox CE, Alvarez-Allende CR, et al. Response of blue rubber bleb nevus syndrome to sirolimus treatment. *Pediatr Blood Cancer*. 2016;63(11):1911–1914.

Yuksekkaya H, Ozbek O, Keser M, Toy H. Blue rubber bleb nevus syndrome: successful treatment with sirolimus. *Pediatrics*. 2012;129(4):e1080–e1084.

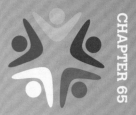

CHAPTER 65

Burns

Deborah Moon, Shauna Higgins, and Ashley Wysong*

Introduction

Burn injuries are a serious cause of morbidity and mortality in children, with at least 440 000 children being medically treated for burn injuries annually.[1] Early evaluation and management is critical for optimal outcomes. First-degree burns, which commonly result from sun exposure in children, involve the epidermis and present as erythematous, warm, and painful lesions expected to heal within 14 days with cleansing and moisturizing. Second-degree burns, which are frequently due to contact with hot liquids in children, involve both the dermis and epidermis and present as erythematous, painful, and blistering or moist skin that may become insensate or pale in deeper burns. Third-degree (full-thickness) burns, often resulting from flame injury, involve the epidermis, dermis, and subcutaneous layer, and may appear dry and leathery with a tan color, and may be insensate centrally but painful peripherally.[1] Fourth-degree burns involve injury to deeper tissues such as muscle, tendons, or bone and can be particularly disfiguring. Prompt referral to a burn center is critical for evaluation and multidisciplinary management.

Appropriate burn wound care, which includes keeping wounds moist, infection prevention, sun avoidance, and timely debridement if needed, plays a critical role in scar management (Table 65.1). First- and second-degree burns

TABLE 65.1 : Burn Wound Care

	PRESENTATION	COMMON CAUSE IN CHILDREN	MANAGEMENT	ANTIBIOTICS	HEALING TIME	REFERRAL AND OTHER SPECIAL CONSIDERATIONS
First degree	Erythematous, warm, painful; no blistering	UV exposure (eg, sunburns)	Cleanse with mild soap and emolliate with ointment; if needed, pain relief with acetaminophen or NSAIDs	No antibiotics needed.	3-6 d	Less commonly, may be admitted for pain relief and hydration.
Second degree (partial thickness)	Erythematous, painful, with intact blisters or moist areas	Scald (spill or splash)	Cleanse with mild soap, lightly debride remnants of already ruptured blisters to prevent infections. Do not rupture thick, intact blisters. Apply topical antibiotics and cover with a nonadherent dressing such as Xeroform™ (Covidien/Medtronic) as well as a bulky gauze dressing to be changed every 12-24 h.	Topical ointment: bacitracin; neomycin often mixed with bacitracin or polymyxin to decrease cutaneous hypersensitivity; silver sulfadiazine; if evidence of infection, start systemic antibiotics.	7-21 d	If burn wound persists >2 wk, consider grafting.
Deep partial thickness	May appear pale or cherry red; may be painful or anesthetic	Scald (spill) Flame Oil Grease	Cleanse, lightly debride, and apply topical antibiotics with dressings as above.	(As above)	>21 d	For deep second-degree burns, refer to burn center for prompt grafting if it covers an extensive area, is located in critical areas (face, hands, and feet), or if burns do not heal within 2 wk.

(continued)

---

*Latanya T. Benjamin provided additional editorial review of this chapter.

TABLE 65.1 ⋮ Burn Wound Care (*continued*)

	PRESENTATION	COMMON CAUSE IN CHILDREN	MANAGEMENT	ANTIBIOTICS	HEALING TIME	REFERRAL AND OTHER SPECIAL CONSIDERATIONS
Third degree (full thickness)	Dry and leathery with a tan color or charred black; may have no sensation centrally but often painful peripherally	Flame injury most common; also scald, steam, oil, grease, chemical, electrical	Cleanse, lightly debride, apply topical antibiotics (cream preferred) with dressings (change every 12-24 h).	Silver sulfadiazine 1% cream most popular for massive burn wounds; also, mafenide acetate 0.5% cream	Rarely to never heals independently; ~3 wk for partial-thickness skin graft, more for full-thickness skin graft.	Prompt referral to a burn center for multidisciplinary evaluation and consideration of grafting. Dressing changes often not well tolerated by children.

d, day; h, hour; NSAIDs, nonsteroidal anti-inflammatory drugs; UV, ultraviolet; wk, week.

often heal without significant scarring; however, scars formed after third-degree burns can be disfiguring and functionally limiting. Treatment of burn scars may include intralesional (IL) corticosteroids for hypertrophy or keloidal scarring (see Chapter 90. Hypertrophic Scars and Contractures), pulsed-dye laser (PDL) for erythema, nonablative fractional laser (NAFL) and ablative fractional laser (AFL) therapy, and surgical excision and revision. For patients with complicated scars, it may be beneficial to employ a multidisciplinary team involving dermatology, plastic surgery, trauma/abuse counseling, wound care, nutrition, behavioral health, physical/occupational therapy, radiology, and social work.

Clinical Pearls

- **Guidelines:** No specific treatment guidelines are known to exist for this condition.
- **Age-Specific Considerations:** Ideally, patients should be old enough to ask for treatment for themselves and be developed enough to assist in detecting and reporting postsurgical complications such as increasing pain, redness, warmth, swelling, and fever/chills.

- **Technique Tips:** At least one author has used a preoperative lead-in with topical timolol to help reduce the "angio" component.
- **Skin of Color Considerations:** The technique is best suited for skin types I and II, because the risk of dyspigmentation increases with darker skin types.

Unlike adults, children may develop scars even from superficial burns and wounds, thus highlighting the importance of preventive measures (eg, appropriate wound care, infection prevention, sun protection).[2] Children who experience painful or pruritic scars may find relief from emollients, silicone gel sheeting, systemic antihistamines, topical corticosteroids, antidepressants, massage, and hydrotherapy (Figure 65.1).[3] When using silicone sheets, counsel parents to wash the covered area twice daily, because several studies in children demonstrated an increased incidence of rash, pruritus, and/or ulceration, which resolved with cessation or when hygienic measures were taken.[4] One study on pediatric burn scars reported safety and efficacy of combination therapy with the 595-nm PDL and the 10 600-nm ablative fractional CO_2 laser.[5] Surgical therapy with adjunctive therapy (eg, silicone gel, corticosteroids) may be considered if

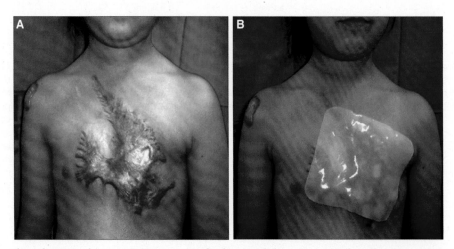

FIGURE 65.1. A, Post-burn hypertrophic scar. B, Treatment with silicone gel sheet. From Goel A, Shrivastava P. Post-burn scars and scar contractures. *Indian J Plast Surg.* 2010;43(suppl):S63-S71. https://creativecommons.org/licenses/by/2.0/.

severe burn scars lead to contracture or functional impairment or if there is lack of improvement after 1 year of therapy, because scars may take 1 to 2 years to fully mature. As an important reminder, surveillance for signs of abuse-related burn injuries is encouraged.[6]

Contraindications/Cautions/Risks

Intralesional Corticosteroids

- Contraindications include active skin infection and history of triamcinolone hypersensitivity.
- Adverse effects include lipoatrophy, hypopigmentation (higher risk in darker skin), telangiectasia, pain, bleeding, bruising, infection, contact allergic dermatitis, impaired wound healing, and, rarely, systemic side effects including rare reports of Cushing's syndrome.

Laser Therapy

- Contraindications for laser therapy include photosensitivity, recent history of sun tanning, seizure disorder triggered by light, and prior/current gold therapy if using a Q-switched laser. If the patient is currently on a photosensitizing medication such as isotretinoin or has a history of hypertrophic scars, consider treating less aggressively with lower fluences. Relative contraindications also include Fitzpatrick skin types IV and above because laser treatments can lead to dyspigmentation.
- Adverse effects include mild to moderate pain, erythema, perifollicular edema, temporary dyspigmentation (often 2-3 months), blistering, crusting, infection, and scarring.

Equipment Needed

Intralesional Corticosteroids
- Triamcinolone acetonide (TAC) 10 or 40 mg/mL
- Sterile saline or 1% or 2% lidocaine without epinephrine
- 27- to 30-gauge needles
- 1- or 3-mL syringe(s)

Laser Therapy
- Appropriately sized eye protection with coverage of appropriate laser wavelengths
- Laser with smoke evacuator system
- Cooling method (eg, ice, cooled gel, cryogen spray, solid air flow)
- Topical anesthesia
- Gauze (to wipe off the topical anesthetic)

Surgery
- Sterile gloves and mask
- Chlorhexidine or Betadine antiseptic
- 4 × 4 gauze
- Cotton-tipped applicators
- 1-, 3-, 5-mL syringes
- 25- and 30-gauge needles
- Local anesthetic (eg, 1% lidocaine with epinephrine)
- Fenestrated disposable drape
- Small-tipped hemostats
- Scalpel, No. 11 blade
- Needle holder
- Sutures
- Iris scissors
- Adson forceps
- Suture needles
- Electrocautery

Preprocedural Approach

- Transfer appropriate patients to a burn center, per the American Burn Association guidelines (eg, partial-thickness burns affecting >10% of the total body surface area; burns affecting the face, hands, feet, genitalia, or joints; third-degree burns; electrical or chemical burns; inhalation injury; patients with medical disorders complicating management; patients at underequipped hospitals; and patients requiring special intervention).
- Obtain a thorough history to assess the patient's candidacy for the procedure, current medications, prior treatments and associated adverse effects, and patient/family goals.
- Extensive sun protection before laser therapy should be advised.

Procedural Approach (See Table 65.2)

Silicone-Based Therapy

- Often a first-line conservative option, silicone gel sheets may help flatten hypertrophic scars through occlusion, hydration, and tension reduction.
- The sheets may be stretched and applied over the hypertrophic scar and worn for ≥12 hours daily for ≥1 month (Figure 65.1).
- Therapy should not be initiated until after the wound has reepithelialized.[3]
- Counsel parents to wash the covered area twice daily.[4]
- For large, high-mobility areas or for scars located on the face, patients may prefer the cream or ointment over the silicone sheet.[3] (Level of evidence [LOE]-1b in adults, LOE-4 in children.)

Intralesional Triamcinolone Acetonide

- IL steroids are commonly utilized and are often the first-line treatment for hypertrophic scars and keloids, with reported recurrence rates of 9% to 50% when used as monotherapy.[2]
- Prepare no more than 1 to 2 mL of TAC solution at, typically, 10 to 20 mg/mL (diluted in sterile saline or lidocaine without epinephrine) in a 27- or 30- gauge needle. If there is no improvement with two to three treatment sessions, consider increasing the concentration; thick keloids may require up to a concentration of 40 mg/mL. Exercise caution not to exceed the maximal dose.
- Some authors recommend pretreating hypertrophic scars with liquid nitrogen for 5 to 20 seconds to soften scars, particularly thick keloids, and also for the slight anesthetic effect.
- Inject about 0.1 mL/cm² of the prepared solution of TAC intradermally.
- Exercise caution not to inject too deeply into the subcutaneous layer or too superficially in the epidermal layer so as to prevent lipoatrophy and hypopigmentation, respectively. Multiple treatments at 4- to 6-week intervals may be indicated until significant flattening and acceptable improvement of the scar or until therapy becomes limited by adverse effects.
- If the procedure is poorly tolerated, dilution of corticosteroid with 2% lidocaine may provide some relief.
- A helpful technique for highly fibrotic keloids with difficult infiltration of steroid includes first inserting the needle and subsequently injecting while withdrawing.
- Laser-assisted delivery of IL TAC has been reported[6-8] (LOE-4 in adults, LOE-5 in pediatric patients), whereby TAC is placed topically to the scar after AFL or NAFL treatment.

TABLE 65.2 : Treatment Recommendations by Scar Type

SCAR	DESCRIPTION	RECOMMENDED THERAPY
Immature scar	Erythematous, slightly elevated, sometimes symptomatic (eg, itchy, painful); may take 1-2 y for maturation	Conservative therapy. Silicone gel is often first line (LOE-1b in adults; LOE-4 in children). May also consider hypoallergenic paper tape and onion extract containing formulations. If persistent for >1 mo despite initial therapy, consider another month of silicone gel with or without monthly intralesional corticosteroid injection (if hypertrophic or keloidal). May also proceed with pulsed-dye laser (PDL) or fractional laser therapy.
Linear hypertrophic scar	Erythematous, raised, sometimes symptomatic, confined to borders; develops within weeks of injury. May grow for 3-6 mo, become stable, and subsequently begin to regress	First-line therapy includes silicone gel or sheet. If no improvement after 2 mo or scar is severe[a] or symptomatic, consider monthly intralesional corticosteroid (LOE-4 in children). In adults, monthly 5-FU[b] has been recommended but has not been well established in children. PDL or fractional laser may also be considered. If persistent despite 1 y of conservative management, consider surgical excision combined with postoperative silicone gel or sheeting. It is generally recommended to wait a year before surgical excision, given the scars may mature and regress over the course of a year. Experts also believe that earlier surgical excision may lead to less favorable outcomes. However, earlier surgical treatment is warranted if scarring results in functional impairment.
Widespread hypertrophic burn scar	Widespread, erythematous, raised, sometimes symptomatic, confined to borders	Options include silicone gel, PDL, and fractional lasers (ablative preferred by some over nonablative). Depending on the unique features of the burn scar, combination therapy involving silicone gel sheets, pressure therapy, massage, physical therapy, corticosteroid therapy, and surgical procedures may be considered.
Minor keloid	Focally raised scar extending over borders of wound into normal skin; does not resolve on own	Silicone gel sheeting with monthly intralesional corticosteroid injections. If persistent despite conservative therapy for 8-12 wk, may consider lasers or surgical excision. Surgical excision is best accompanied with adjunctive therapies, such as silicone gel and intralesional corticosteroids. Other adjunctive treatments of bleomycin, mitomycin C, and imiquimod 5% cream have not been well studied in children. In adults, combination intralesional corticosteroids with 5-FU[b] have also been recommended. Radiation therapy has also been reported to be used for refractory keloids in adults; however, it should be avoided in children because of severe side effects on bone growth and other long-term risks.[2]
Major keloid	Large, raised scar (>0.5 cm), sometimes symptomatic; does not regress on own	Monthly intralesional corticosteroid with or without adjuvant cryotherapy. If no improvement in 3-4 mo, consider laser or surgical excision with adjuvant therapy (LOE-4 in children). (In adults, monthly 5-FU[b] is also recommended.)

[a]Risk factors include personal or family history of hypertrophic scars/keloids, location on high-tension sites such as the neck, presternum, thorax, shoulder, and ankle.
[b]Although an increasing body of literature has supported the benefit of intralesional 5-FU in adults, the efficacy and safety of intralesional 5-FU is not well established in children and considered "off-label" (LOE-5).
5-FU, 5-fluorouracil; LOE, level of evidence; mo, month; y, year; wk, week.
Adapted from Gold MH, McGuire M, Mustoe TA, et al. Updated international clinical recommendations on scar management: part 2—algorithms for scar prevention and treatment. *Dermatol Surg*. 2014;40(8):825–831 and Mustoe TA, Cooter RD, Gold MH, et al. International clinical recommendations on scar management. *Plast Reconstr Surg*. 2002;110(2):560–571.

Laser Therapy

- *Setting Up Equipment and Eye Safety*
  - Ensure all equipment is the appropriate size, particularly the eye protection gear.
  - Make sure the child does not remove eye safety gear during the procedure.
  - Use metal corneal shields if treatment site is near the eyes.
  - Before the procedure, ensure that all personnel are wearing eye safety equipment with the appropriately labeled optical density.
  - Prepare and test the cooling method and the evacuator system.
- *Anesthesia*
  - Clean the treatment site with a mild cleanser and water or an alcohol pad, ensuring all alcohol is allowed to dry completely, typically for at least 3 minutes.

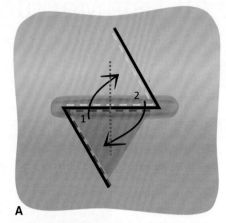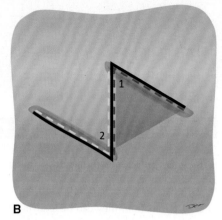

FIGURE 65.2. A, Z-plasty before flap rotation. B, Z-plasty after flap rotation with reoriented scar line.

○ Commonly used topical anesthesia include lidocaine 2.5% and prilocaine 2.5% (EMLA™ [AB Astra Pharmaceuticals, L.P.]) and 4% or 5% liposomal lidocaine cream (LMX.4™ or LMX.5™ [Ferndale Laboratories]). Using a gloved finger, apply a layer about ⅛-in thick and allow it to sit for about 30 minutes and no longer than 1 hour to avoid systemic absorption. Exercise caution that EMLA should not to exceed the maximal dose, because systemic absorption may lead to symptomatic methemoglobinemia in children owing to incomplete maturation of the nicotinamide adenine dinucleotide (NADH)-methemoglobin reductase system.

○ Completely remove topical anesthetic with a gauze to prevent further systemic absorption, and because products may contain flammable ingredients.

○ A more invasive alternative for patients who require more extensive anesthesia is the local injection of 1% lidocaine solution with epinephrine.[9]

• *Selecting and Using Lasers*

○ The 585- or 595-nm PDL has had reported success in reducing erythema and pruritus, whereas the 10 600-nm ablative fractional CO_2 laser has had reported success with improving the thickness and texture of hypertrophic scars. One study on pediatric burn scars suggested that combination therapy with 595-nm PDL and ablative fractional CO_2 laser may be safe and efficacious (significant improvement in pigmentation, vascularity, pliability, height, and the total Vancouver Scar Scale scores).[5]

Surgery

• For large scars with excessive tension or development of contractures, surgical relief may be provided with a Z-plasty or W-plasty, surgical excision, or tissue expansion (Figure 65.2).[2,6]

• Surgical excision of keloids as monotherapy is not recommended given the high recurrence (up to 100%). However, there has been some success with the combination of surgery with intraoperative and postoperative IL steroids, with one study reporting recurrence of keloids and hypertrophic scars in 14.3% and 16.7% of cases, respectively.[6]

• For optimal outcomes, monofilamentous sutures are preferable to braided sutures, which may induce a more inflammatory reaction.

• Sutures should also be left in place for up to a total of 10 to 14 days to prevent wound dehiscence, because corticosteroids may delay wound healing.[2]

POSTOPERATIVE APPROACH

• Following laser therapy, cooling with an ice pack and a mild topical steroid cream may help reduce erythema, swelling, and postoperative pain.

• Educate the patient and family on the importance of extensive sun protection for at least 1 month after the procedure.

• If there are signs of epidermal injury such as blistering, consider topical antibiotics to prevent infections.

• Reassure patients that mild erythema and edema are to be expected, although severe symptoms or those lasting for more than several hours should prompt them to notify their physician.[9]

• Patients with complicated scars may benefit from a multidisciplinary team.

• If the patient received a skin graft, they generally require a bolster dressing for 3 to 5 days to ensure optimal wound healing. Smaller scar revisions may only require small dressings postoperatively.

• Follow-up generally occurs at 1 to 2 weeks.

• For large complex scars, physical therapy may be required over the long term for complete recovery of function particularly in high-tension anatomic sites.

REFERENCES

1. Palmieri TL, Greenhalgh DG. Topical treatment of pediatric patients with burns: a practical guide. *Am J Clin Dermatol.* 2002;3(8):529–534.

2. Berman B, Viera MH, Amini S, Huo R, Jones IS. Prevention and management of hypertrophic scars and keloids after burns in children. *J Craniofac Surg.* 2008;19(4):989–1006.

3. Gold MH, McGuire M, Mustoe TA, et al. Updated international clinical recommendations on scar management: part 2—algorithms for scar prevention and treatment. *Dermatol Surg.* 2014;40(8):825–831.

4. Van den Kerckhove E, Stappaerts K, Boeckx W, et al. Silicones in the rehabilitation of burns: a review and overview. *Burns.* 2001; 27(3):205–214.

5. Zuccaro J, Muser I, Singh M, Yu J, Kelly C, Fish J. Laser therapy for pediatric burn scars: focusing on a combined treatment approach. *J Burn Care Res.* 2018;39(3):457–462.

6. Krakowski AC, Totri CR, Donelan MB, Shumaker PR. Scar management in the pediatric and adolescent populations. *Pediatrics.* 2016;137:e20142065.

7. Waibel JS, Wulkan AJ, Shumaker PR. Treatment of hypertrophic scars using laser and laser assisted corticosteroid delivery. *Lasers Surg Med.* 2013;45(3):135–140.

8. Sklar LR, Burnett CT, Waibel JS, Moy RL, Ozog DM. Laser assisted drug delivery: a review of an evolving technology. *Lasers Surg Med.* 2014;46(4):249–262.

9. Nouri K. *Handbook of Lasers in Dermatology.* London, England: Springer; 2014.

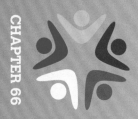
Café au Lait Macules

Dawn Z. Eichenfield and Lawrence F. Eichenfield

Introduction

Café au lait macules (CALMs) are well-circumscribed, uniformly pigmented brown macules or patches noted during infancy or early childhood, which may increase in number and size with age. Although they are present in 10% to 20% of the normal population, they can be associated with genodermatoses such as neurofibromatosis and McCune-Albright syndrome. The CALMs seen in McCune-Albright syndrome are often fewer in number, larger, and have a midline demarcation. Descriptively, they have been classically referred to as the "coast of Maine" (Figure 66.1) subtype given their jagged or ill-defined borders, whereas CALMs in neurofibromatosis are referred to as the "coast of California" subtype (Figure 66.2), because of their smooth and well-defined borders.

To date, CALMs have been treated with topical bleaching agents such as hydroquinone, which has no therapeutic benefit, as well as laser therapy. The response to laser therapy is highly variable, with uneven lesion clearance and high recurrence rates. Multiple lasers have been utilized with variable results, including the Q-switched Ruby laser, Q-switched Alexandrite laser, Q-switched 1064-nm Nd:YAG laser, frequency-doubled Q-switched Nd:YAG laser, 755-nm Alexandrite and 532-nm Nd:YAG picosecond lasers, pulsed dye lasers, copper vapor laser, KTP laser, and Erbium:YAG laser. Recently, a prospective trial utilizing Q-switched 1064-nm Nd:YAG laser showed a

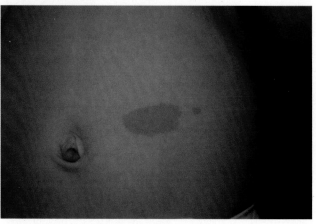

FIGURE 66.2. In neurofibromatosis, café au lait macules are referred to as the *coast of California subtype* because of their typically smooth and well-defined borders.

greater than 50% clinical clearance in 74.4% of lesions. Another study found that CALMs of the "coast of Maine" subtype tend to respond better to treatment than do CALMs of the "coast of California" subtype. Although these studies report favorable outcomes, further studies are needed to better delineate the ideal laser and laser settings for treatment of CALMs.

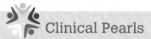 Clinical Pearls

- **Guidelines:** No specific guidelines or expert consensus papers exist for this condition.
- **Age-Specific Considerations:** Patients who are of the age of consent or assent may be treated. Larger lesions and young patients may be considered for general anesthesia to minimize pain and anxiety, and allow for technically appropriate laser surgery.
- **Skin of Color Considerations:** Q-switched Nd:YAG (1064-nm) laser could be utilized for darker skin types with caution given the greater likelihood of posttreatment side effects and complications.

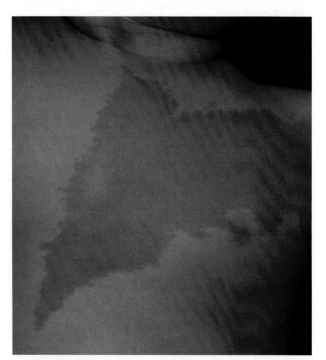

FIGURE 66.1. Café au lait macules typically seen in McCune-Albright syndrome have been referred to as the *coast of Maine subtype* given their jagged or ill-defined borders. This subtype appears to respond more favorably to laser treatment.

Contraindications/Cautions/Risks

Contraindications

- The presence of an active skin infection
- Patients with a history of keloids
- The inability to perform posttreatment wound care

Cautions

- The presence of a suntan or prior history of melasma as well as other pigmentary disorders (postinflammatory hyperpigmentation) may result in increased skin dyspigmentation and other complications post the procedure.

Risks

- Erythema after the laser procedure, transient hypopigmentation or hyperpigmentation, texture changes, light scarring, permanent hyperpigmentation or hypopigmentation, incomplete clearance, repigmentation or recurrence, infection, complications of general anesthesia

---

Equipment Needed

- Wavelength-specific eye shields, glasses, or goggles; metal eye shields for periocular lesions; opaque eye patches
- Laser
- Smoke evacuator
- Gauze
- Normal saline
- Ice or cooling system
- Petrolatum-based ointment
- Nonadherent topical dressing

Preprocedural Approach

- Several months before treatment, we ask patients to minimize sun exposure and maximize sun protection to allow greater contrast between the treatment area and surrounding skin. The purpose is to reduce melanin in the nonlesional skin.
- We ask patients to avoid taking aspirin-containing products for 2 weeks before treatment.
- Patients are asked to bathe the treatment area either the evening or morning before laser surgery.
- Topical anesthetic cream, for example, liposomal lidocaine 4% or a mixture of lidocaine 2.5% and prilocaine 2.5%, is applied under occlusion for 1 hour before the procedure.
- General anesthesia may be required for larger or multiple lesions and/or younger patients.

Procedural Approach

- Informed consent is obtained from the patient. If the patient is a minor, informed consent should be obtained from the parent/guardian and assent obtained from the minor.
- All personnel in the procedure room should wear wavelength-specific appropriate eyeware. Patients may wear correctly fitted metal eye shields, wavelength-specific glasses or goggles, or opaque eye patches.
- Treatment should be initiated at the threshold fluence (a test spot should be used on each patient to determine the threshold fluence to achieve the treatment endpoint, which is variable depending on the laser utilized, ie, the appearance of an ashen gray color to mild nonpetechial erythema immediately after treatment with the Q-switched Nd:YAG laser or immediate epidermal whitening using the Q-switched Alexandrite laser). Higher fluences (eg, fluences above the threshold fluence) can result in overt erythema, edema, blisters, crusting, skin sloughing, and punctuate bleeding. These complications can occur seconds to minutes, and sometimes hours after treatment.

- The frequency of treatments varies from 2 weeks to months. The number of treatments is dependent on lesion response and patient satisfaction.
- Postoperative care can utilize cool compresses or gauze frozen with normal saline.
- Petrolatum-based ointment is liberally applied followed by a nonadherent topical dressing. Any crusting is left on the skin as a biologic dressing.
- Sunscreen (SPF 30 or higher should be regularly applied) and diligent sun protection should be restarted.

Postprocedural Approach

- Any postoperative swelling and pain should quickly decrease with time. For postoperative pain, patients can be asked to take acetaminophen or ibuprofen. Continued intermittent ice compression can be applied to reduce swelling.
- Postoperatively, patients should be informed that bruising and swelling could develop.
- Patients should be monitored for symptoms and signs of infection.
- Postoperative downtime is minimal and the skin heals within several days, usually with basic wound care (continued application of petrolatum-based ointment and diligent sun protection). Patients should be cautioned to remove facial products very gently because the treatment area is fragile during the healing process.
- Patients should be cautioned that there may be lightening or darkening of the treated area for several months after laser treatment that can be covered easily with cosmetics.
- Patients should be encouraged to contact the physician directly for any questions or concerns.
- A follow-up appointment can be made for postoperative care issues in the immediate postoperative phase, or weeks to months post the laser for repeat treatments or to evaluate whether further treatments are needed.

SUGGESTED READINGS

Baek JO, Park IJ, Lee KR, et al. High-fluence 1064-nm Q-Switched Nd:YAG laser: safe and effective treatment of café-au-lait macules in Asian patients. *J Cosmet Dermatol.* 2018;17:380–384.

Belkin DA, Neckman JP, Jeon H, Friedman P, Geronemus RG. Response to laser treatment of Café au lait macules based on morphologic features. *JAMA Dermatol.* 2017;153(11):1158–1161.

Grossman MC, Anderson RR, Farinelli W, Flotte TJ, Grevelink JM. Treatment of café au lait macules with lasers. A clinicopathologic correlation. *Arch Dermatol.* 1995;131(12):1416–1420.

Kim HR, Ha JM, Park MS, et al. A low-fluence 1064-nm Q-switched neodymium-doped yttrium aluminum garnet laser for the treatment of café-au lait macules. *J Am Acad Dermatol.* 2015;73:477–483.

Kim J, Hur H, Kim YR, Cho SB. Treatment of café-au-lait macules with a high-fluenced 1064-nm Q-switched neodymium:yttrium aluminum garnet laser. *J Cosmet Laser Ther.* 2018;20:17–20.

Wanner M, Sakamoto FH, Avram MM, Anderson RR. Immediate skin responses to laser and light treatments: warning endpoints: how to avoid side effects. *J Am Acad Dermatol.* 2016;74(5):807–819.

Wanner M, Sakamoto FH, Avram MM, et al. Immediate skin responses to laser and light treatments: therapeutic endpoints: how to obtain efficacy. *J Am Acad Dermatol.* 2016;74(5):821–833.

CHAPTER 67

Calcinosis Cutis

Jonathan A. Dyer

Introduction

Calcinosis cutis, the deposition of calcium salts within the skin and subcutaneous tissues, may occur in children because of a variety of causes. It is often divided into five categories based on etiology: dystrophic calcification due to trauma; metastatic calcification due to disordered calcium regulatory systems; and idiopathic, iatrogenic, and mixed (an underlying metabolic cause increases the likelihood of dystrophic calcification after trauma). A common form of pediatric calcinosis cutis is the small calcified heel nodules that can develop at sites of heel stick blood draws in the newborn period. Calcinosis cutis frequently favors sites of trauma (such as extensor extremities and over joints), manifesting as hard, white papules that occasionally drain chalklike material. They can be painful and are also prone to ulceration and resultant secondary infection, which leads to significant morbidity.

Several autoimmune connective tissue diseases (ACTDs) are associated with skin calcinosis, most commonly juvenile dermatomyositis, where it occurs in 50% to 70% of patients and the incidence parallels disease severity. It can also be seen in other autoimmune disorders such as systemic sclerosis (especially the CREST [calcinosis, Raynaud phenomenon, esophageal dysmotility, sclerodactyly, and telangiectasia] variant), morphea, cutaneous lupus erythematosus, and lupus panniculitis. Genetic disorders associated with calcinosis cutis include pseudoxanthoma elasticum (PXE), Ehlers–Danlos syndrome, porphyria cutanea tarda, Werner syndrome, and Rothmund–Thomson syndrome. A specific form termed milia-like calcinosis cutis (MICC) has been reported primarily in patients with Down syndrome.

Benign and malignant growths may periodically exhibit calcification, such as pilomatricomas, which develop calcification in over 75% of cases (see Chapter 114. Pilomatricoma [Pilomatrixoma]). These cyst-like tumors are much more common in children than in adults and are associated with β-catenin mutations. With time, the entire cystic tumor may calcify, forming a white nodule under the skin. Surgical removal is typical. Idiopathic calcified nodules of the scrotum, another common form of calcinosis cutis, do not typically develop until adulthood; however, surgical removal of problematic lesions is the current recommended treatment if intervention is desired. Extravasation of intravenous fluids containing calcium can also lead to calcinosis cutis, and treatment immediately with intralesional triamcinolone has been helpful in decreasing inflammation and ulceration in animal models.[1]

No well-documented medical therapy exists for calcinosis cutis, although there are anecdotal reports of promising interventions. Sodium thiosulfate has been reported to be effective. It has been administered intravenously, intralesionally (12.5 mg/mL; 0.1-1 mL every 3-6 weeks), and topically (variable concentrations reported: 12.5 mg/mL compounded 1:1 with petrolatum applied daily; 10% topical sodium thiosulfate in a water-in-oil emulsion cold cream are two examples) with improvement in anecdotal case reports.[2]

A review of calcinosis cases from the Mayo Clinic suggested an approach to managing calcinosis cutis in patients with ACTD.[3] For cases associated with an underlying condition, achieving as much control as possible over the underlying autoimmune process is critical. Surgical excision should be considered in patients with discreet problematic lesions. Sodium thiosulfate could be considered as initial treatment or for inoperable or diffuse lesions. If not effective, other medications to consider include diltiazem (extremely prolonged therapy is often required for notable benefit), colchicine, minocycline, or warfarin. However, reports are quite mixed as to the efficacy of these interventions.

Surgical removal of problematic calcium deposits is a frequently utilized intervention (often considered the treatment of choice when possible), although recurrence does occur. Excision of the calcified area with standard linear closure is most typical. Some lesions may be removed with a snip technique. Alternatively, smaller lesions can occasionally be treated with incision and expression of the calcified material, occasionally with curettage to ensure complete removal of the calcium.

Extracorporeal shock wave lithotripsy improved the involved area of calcinosis and associated pain in nine patients in one small study. Carbon dioxide laser has also been beneficial in treating small superficial lesions in a few small reports. Telangiectasias associated with calcinosis cutis can be treated with pulsed-dye laser, as noted elsewhere in this text (see Chapter 125. Telangiectasia).

Clinical Pearls

- **Guidelines:** No specific treatment guidelines exist for the treatment of calcinosis cutis. Lesions are typically treated on a case-by-case basis, focusing on symptomatic lesions or those developing secondary complications.
- **Anatomy-Specific Considerations:** Calcinosis cutis often occurs over the extensor surfaces of joints, which are less ideal locations for surgical excisions. Care must be taken to consider the resulting scar and any potential complications that could result, whether functional or cosmetic.
- **Age-Specific Considerations:** Ideally, patients should be old enough to speak for themselves when noting pain or functional limitations caused by their calcinosis and requesting treatment for these lesions.
- **Technique Tips:** Complete removal of the local calcium deposit at the site of surgery is advised. There is no extant data on any impact of pre- or postoperative thiosulfate treatment, either topical or intralesional. Severely infected areas may be less than ideal candidates for surgical wound closure upon removal of the calcium deposits.
- **Skin of Color Considerations:** The risk of dyspigmentation from resulting inflammation or scarring increases with darker skin types. There are no data on relative frequency of calcinosis in different ethnicities. Consideration of any genetic tendency toward hypertrophic scar or keloid formation must be taken into consideration.

Contraindications/Cautions/Risks

Contraindications

- Inability to care for postoperative wounds
- Poorly controlled underlying ACTD
- Immunocompromised (relative)

Cautions

- Minimizing movement or trauma at/on the surgical site, especially when operating over a joint, in the postoperative period is very important.

Risks

- Death (infection or anesthesia), scarring (avoid cuticular sutures on the trunk or extremities in children wherever possible), pain, bleeding, recurrence

Equipment Needed

- Procedure dependent
- Sterile syringe and 30-G ½-in needles if intralesional therapy
- Standard curette and simple tray if performing incision and curettage
- Standard surgical tray if traditional excision with layered closure

Preprocedural Approach

- Standard in-office procedural setup
- Cleanse area to be treated.
- Assess landmarks for incision orientation if excising the area.

Procedural Approach

- Informed consent from the parent/guardian and, when possible, assent from the minor are obtained.
- Typically, local anesthesia is utilized because of pain associated with the procedure.
- An appropriate amount of 0.5% to 1% lidocaine (typically with 1:100 000-200 000 units epinephrine) is used to anesthetize the appropriate skin area.
- The site is prepped and draped in a standard manner.
- **Incision and Curettage**
  - The skin overlying the calcinosis is incised with a scalpel blade.
  - An appropriately sized curette is then used to remove the visible calcium. Care should be taken to remove all calcium visible at the surgical site.
  - If necessary, the wound may be flushed with sterile saline to facilitate particulate calcium removal.
  - Once clear, the skin edges may be approximated with sutures.
  - If it is not possible to close the area, then petrolatum-based ointment and a sterile wound dressing is applied and maintained daily until reepithelialization has occurred. The timing of this varies depending on the size of the wound. This method does not work well on idiopathic scrotal calcinosis.
- **Excision**
  - Excision of calcinosis cutis is performed in a typical elliptical manner to remove the calcinosis deposit.
  - Hemostasis is achieved utilizing cautery in a standard manner.
  - Wound edges are then reapproximated, typically using absorbable sutures in a buried manner (subcuticular sutures) and then cuticular sutures are placed if necessary for the best final result.
  - Cuticular sutures should be avoided in children except for facial or scalp excisions because of the risk of "track mark" scarring. Subcuticular sutures should be used instead. If subcuticular sutures are well placed, often the external skin edges may be simply secured with Steri-Strips or DERMABOND™ Topical Skin Adhesive (Ethicon, Somerville, NJ) depending on surgeon preference.

Postprocedural Approach

- Generally, swelling and pain decrease quickly with time.
- Wounds should be cleansed gently once daily. A simple mild cleanser is reasonable. Then, a petrolatum-based ointment is immediately reapplied and maintained until reepithelialization has occurred—typically 5 to 7 days after laser surgery.
- Patients should be monitored for signs and symptoms of infection.
- Patients are encouraged to contact the physician directly for concerns and are often provided with cell phone numbers for direct contact and reassurance.

REFERENCES

1. Reiter N, El-Shabrawi L, Leinweber B, Berghold A, Aberer E. Calcinosis cutis: part II. Treatment options. *J Am Acad Dermatol.* 2011;65(1):15–22; quiz 3–4.
2. Garcia-Garcia E, Lopez-Lopez R, Alvarez-Del-Vayo C, Bernabeu-Wittel J. Iatrogenic calcinosis cutis successfully treated with topical sodium thiosulfate. *Pediatr Dermatol.* 2017;34(3):356–358.
3. Balin SJ, Wetter DA, Andersen LK, Bernabeu-Wittel J. Calcinosis cutis occurring in association with autoimmune connective tissue disease: the Mayo Clinic experience with 78 patients, 1996-2009. *Arch Dermatol.* 2012;148(4):455–462.

CHAPTER 68

Callus

Brian Z. Rayala and Howard Kashefsky

Introduction

Callus or hyperkeratotic skin is defined as skin thickening, usually over a bony prominence or joint, in response to repetitive pressure or friction. Callus commonly occurs in the feet or lower extremities, but can present in any weight-bearing area. It usually precedes or is concurrent with pressure ulcers. At-risk populations include children and adolescents with neurologic problems such as spina bifida, musculoskeletal deformities, immobility, gait abnormalities, and in highly active populations such as athletes.

Paring or scalpel debridement is the most common procedure used to manage pediatric callus. The goal is to trim down or remove hyperkeratotic skin to decrease the pain or foreign body sensation to the area. A nonsurgical alternative to paring callus involves optimizing pressure relief to affected areas using offloading methods (eg, proper-fitting shoes and orthoses, braces, cushions, and mattresses). Paring is effective in removing thickened skin, but calluses usually recur if pressure relief is not adequately addressed.

Performed correctly, paring is safe, relatively painless, and inexpensive; requires minimal time; entails no postoperative recovery; and has minimal complications. Children who may be fearful of seeing a sharp surgical instrument may forgo paring for nonsurgical offloading methods with or without in-home use of pumice stone or similar less invasive skin removal techniques.

Clinical Pearls

- **Guidelines:** Despite the absence of randomized trials, experts recommend nonsurgical offloading techniques before considering surgical interventions for symptomatic callus (Level 5).
- **Age-Specific Considerations:**
  - Paring should only be considered if it can be performed safely. In children who cannot sit still or follow instructions, it is best to use nonsurgical pressure-relief techniques (Level 5).
  - To decrease patient-related fear and anxiety while paring plantar callus, position the patient supine, with the sole perpendicular to the table, and use the child's foot to hide the scalpel from his/her sight (Level 5).
- **Technique Tips:**
  - Short-term paring or scalpel debridement among adults (18 years and older) appears more effective in relieving pain than do topical keratolytics such as potassium hydroxide, trichloroacetic acid, and salicylic acid[1,2] (Level 2b). No data exist for children.
  - In older adults (65 years and older), scalpel debridement appears no better than sham debridement in relieving pain[3] (Level 2b). Data are not available for the pediatric population.
  - Debridement of callus surrounding ulcers may help with wound healing by decreasing the amount of hyperkeratotic skin at the edge and allowing more efficient epithelial migration from the ulcer base to the edge (Level 5).

Contraindications/Cautions/Risks

- There are no absolute contraindications to paring or scalpel debridement as long as patient selection is done correctly.
- Relative contraindications include uncooperative patients and severe pain or dysesthesia in the area of the callus.
- Common adverse events include minor bleeding and formation of superficial wound or abrasion. Serious but rare adverse events include deep laceration; skin and soft-tissue infections; bone infection; and damage to surrounding tendons, ligaments, and joints.

Equipment Needed

- Clean, nonsterile gloves
- Disposable underpad (Chux)
- Alcohol or chlorhexidine swab, or moist gauze
- #10 surgical blade with handle
- 4 × 4 gauze
- Silver nitrate sticks (as needed for hemostasis)

Preprocedural Approach

- Preoperative labs and tests are not necessary for paring a callus.
- Remove shoes, socks, or clothing and fully expose the callus and perilesional skin. Perform careful inspection, always comparing both sides, looking for skin and soft-tissue changes and musculoskeletal deformities that are associated with and contribute to callus formation.
- Before paring, feel the contour and thickness of the callus and compare to perilesional skin. If the callus is on the foot, assess the extremity's neurovascular status.
- Then turn attention to patient's footwear, looking at areas of accelerated wear on the insoles and shoes and evaluating how they relate to the callus.

Procedural Approach

- Whenever possible, place patient in a supine position on the examination table.
- Remove shoes and socks and fully expose the surgical site. The foot should be positioned perpendicular to the table.
- Slide disposable underpad beneath the surgical site.
- Clean the surgical site with alcohol wipes or chlorhexidine swab. An alternative is to wipe the area with gauze moistened with tap water. Because sterility is not required for this procedure, either technique is acceptable. Either method will also work to soften the callus for easier paring. For an excessively thick callus, it may be necessary to perform this step intermittently throughout the procedure as a way to soften the callus at different depths.
- Pare the callus down using a #10 surgical blade (with handle) applied parallel to the skin using a shaving motion and utilizing the middle of the blade to sculpt the callus until its

thickness is close to that of the perilesional skin. Ideally, start at the periphery and work toward the center, which is often the thickest portion.

- Avoid removing thick layers of skin initially. Start with thin slices, getting a feel for how firm the callus is.
- During paring, use the nondominant hand to stabilize the patient's foot or digit. Likewise, use the nondominant hand or digits to continually gauge how much skin has been pared and how much more needs to be removed.
- Discontinue paring once callus thickness is similar to perilesional skin and even throughout.
- If bleeding inadvertently occurs, apply pressure using gauze for a few minutes. If bleeding persists, wipe blood with gauze and apply silver nitrate stick to bleeding surface using a rolling motion. Repeat until bleeding ceases.

Postprocedural Approach

- Because paring is performed without sedation or anesthesia, postoperative recovery is negligible.
- Remind the child's parent or guardian that the callus is likely to recur, usually within a few weeks, if proper offloading is not addressed.
- For calluses due to mild orthopedic issues, the use of proper-fitting off-the-shelf shoes and insoles may be all that is necessary to offload involved area.
- For calluses resulting from significant neurologic or musculoskeletal deformities, referral to an orthotist and consultation

with a physiatrist, occupational therapist, and prosthetist may be necessary to address questions about pressure-relief surfaces (eg, mattresses, cushions) and ambulation-assistive devices (eg, braces, prosthesis, wheelchairs). A referral to a podiatrist or orthopedic foot specialist should also be considered to evaluate the need for surgical correction of the foot deformity.

- If patient sustains a wound or skin injury during the procedure, provide return precautions for infection, such as monitoring for erythema, warmth, swelling, pain, or purulence.
- Schedule a return visit for the patient in about a month to reevaluate the callus and to review progress with offloading strategies.

REFERENCES

1. Hashmi F, Nester CJ, Wright CR, Lam S. The evaluation of three treatments for plantar callus: a three-armed randomised, comparative trial using biophysical outcome measures. *Trials.* 2016;17(1):251.
2. Gijón-Noguerón G, García-Paya I, Morales-Asencio JM, Jiménez-Cebrián A, Ortega-Ávila AB, Cervera-Marín JA. Short-term effect of scalpel debridement of plantar callosities versus treatment with salicylic acid patches: the EMEDESCA randomized controlled trial. *J Dermatol.* 2017;44(6):706–709.
3. Landorf KB, Morrow A, Spink MJ, et al. Effectiveness of scalpel debridement for painful plantar calluses in older people: a randomized trial. *Trials.* 2013;14:243.

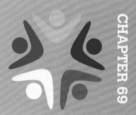

Chalazion

Austin Carter Smith and John C. Browning

Introduction

Chalazia, or meibomian cysts, are common, benign lesions that arise in the eyelid. They are sterile inflammatory collections caused by blockage of the meibomian gland duct (Figure 69.1A and B). Chalazion may present in children of any age and are commonly idiopathic in nature but can be related to blepharitis, acne rosacea, and seborrheic dermatitis. Chalazia appear at similar rates among children regardless of age, gender, or ethnicity. They are most commonly seen in conjunction with blepharitis, or infection of the eyelid, but it is important to note that chalazia are sterile and the cysts do not contain bacteria. If blepharitis is also present, the patient should be treated for that condition as well to prevent recurrence.

The primary approach to chalazia is conservative management with a warm compress four times per day for 15 minutes at a time. If conservative management fails, the lesion may be treated with a steroid injection or surgical removal of the chalazion by an ophthalmologist. One study showed 46% of chalazia resolved when treated with conservative management compared to 84% treated with steroid injections and 87% treated surgically.[1] In the same study, patients were also shown to have

higher satisfaction in the treatment groups compared to the conservative management group.

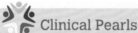

Clinical Pearls

- **Guidelines:** Although no specific treatment guidelines are known to exist for this condition, less invasive techniques should be pursued because of the sensitivity of the anatomically involved area.
- **Age-Specific Considerations:** Patient age should be taken into consideration when attempting steroid injection. Although teens might be able to hold still for an injection so close to the eye, younger patients might be more difficult to restrain when working near such a sensitive area with low room for errors.
- **Technique Tips:**
  - Patients might prefer conservative management because of simple at-home treatment, no out-of-pocket cost, low risk of other complications, and avoidance of injection or surgery near the eye.
  - Steroid injection might be preferred because of one-time treatment rather than daily compresses and is less invasive than is surgery.

- Referral to ophthalmology for surgical removal should be considered when unresponsive to treatment or when steroid injections are contraindicated.
- **Skin of Color Considerations:** Patients should be counseled on postinflammatory hyper- and hypopigmentation, but risk should be low with small-bore steroid injections and internal approach for incision/excision.

WARM COMPRESS TREATMENT

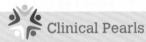

Clinical Pearls

- **Guidelines:** Preferred initial treatment
- **Age-Specific Considerations:** Great for young children because of ease of treatment
- **Technique Tips:** Test warmth with each use to prevent burns.

Contraindications/Cautions/Risks

Cautions

- Rice packs or other heating packs can become too hot, and uneven heating can allow them to be hotter than anticipated in different areas.
- To reduce chance of burns, warm compresses in children should be clean, gentle washcloths or rags or other fabric soaked in warm water to allow the temperature to be more easily regulated and monitored.
- Counsel patients to use a clean fabric with each use to prevent infection.

Risks

- Burns, recurrence of lesion

Equipment Needed

- Clean fabric (gentle washcloth or rag)
- Warm water

Preprocedural Approach

- Parents/guardians should be counseled to check the temperature of the compress on a sensitive area of their own skin such as the back of their hand.
- Temperature of the compress should be tolerable for a 15-minute use without causing significant discomfort.

Procedural Approach

- Warm compress should be applied with light pressure to the affected area three to four times per day for 10 to 15 minutes at a time.
- The lesion can also be softly massaged after use of the warm compress to promote clearance of the material contained behind the blocked duct.

Postprocedural Approach

- Improvement with conservative management may take 3 to 4 weeks.
- If the chalazion fails to decrease in size after 3 to 4 weeks, alternative treatment should be considered.

INTRALESIONAL INJECTION

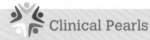

Clinical Pearls

- **Guidelines:** Second-line treatment should be considered after conservative management has failed to produce results
- **Age-Specific Considerations:** Injections near the eye can be difficult at any age, but especially so in young children.
- **Technique Tips:** A chalazion clamp can also be a useful tool in isolating and stabilizing the area.
- **Skin of Color Considerations:** None

Contraindications/Cautions/Risks

- *Contraindications*
  - Do not inject through overlying skin infection.

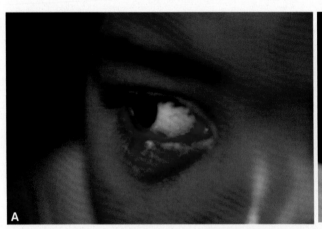
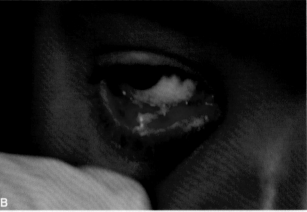

FIGURE 69.1. A, Outward appearance of chalazion with outward bulging of the eyelid. Reprinted with permission from Salimpour RR, Salimpour P. *Photographic Atlas of Pediatric Disorders and Diagnosis.* Philadelphia, PA: Wolters Kluwer Health/Lippincott Williams & Wilkins; 2013. Figure 00C-Unimage 011a. B, Mucosal appearance of the chalazion along the inner eyelid. Reprinted with permission from Salimpour RR, Salimpour P. *Photographic Atlas of Pediatric Disorders and Diagnosis.* Philadelphia, PA: Wolters Kluwer Health/Lippincott Williams & Wilkins; 2013. Figure 00C-Unimage 011b.

- *Cautions*
  - Injecting a drug into the thin skin of the eyelid comes with the risk of moving the needle too far in or, especially in the pediatric population, the patient moving or jerking while the needle is being inserted in this sensitive area.
  - Risk of puncturing the eye can be mitigated by restraining the patient and, if the patient is old enough, explaining what will be done and what they can expect to feel during the injection.
  - There have not been studies as to the relation of chalazion injections and steroid-induced glaucoma specifically, but the risk must still be addressed. The patient and/or parent/guardian should, at least, be aware of the signs and symptoms related to developing this condition. If the patient is at an increased risk, surgical treatment or treatment with a steroid that has been shown to have a lesser effect on intraocular pressure, such as fluorometholone, rimexolone, or loteprednol, should be considered.[2]
  - The steroid injection can also lead to localized skin depigmentation and fat atrophy if administered subcutaneously via the external eyelid. This is a self-limiting process that will usually resolve in 6 to 12 months. The risk can be decreased if the injection is done transconjunctivally or into the inside layer of the eyelid.
- *Risks*
  - Perforation of the globe
  - Steroid-induced glaucoma
  - Localized skin depigmentation and fat atrophy

Equipment Needed

- Corticosteroid (triamcinolone 0.2 mL at 10 mg/mL)
- A 27-gauge short needle
- A 3-mL syringe
- Gloves
- Iodine or alcohol swabs
- Chalazion clamp

Preprocedural Approach

- Fill the syringe with the desired amount of steroid solution to be injected.
- Begin the procedure by sterilizing the chalazion clamp.
- Use the chalazion clamp by inserting the open-circle side of the clamp under the lifted eyelid.
- Carefully expose the inside surface of the eye.
- Apply aqueous povidone-iodine 5% preparation to the eye and lids if injecting transconjunctivally. Alcohol can be used if injecting through external lid.

Procedural Approach

- Carefully inject steroid solution into the middle of the chalazion (Figure 69.2).
- Instruct the patient to look away from the chalazion while performing this procedure.
- It is possible to perform the injection subcutaneously through the external eyelid in some patients, but caution should be used because the area is not as secure as it would be when held with a chalazion clamp when injecting transconjunctivally.

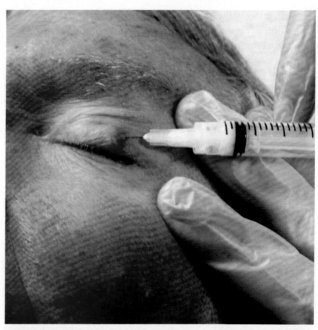

FIGURE 69.2. Demonstrating intralesional injections. Reprinted with permission from McNabb JW. *Practical Guide to Joint and Soft tissue Injections.* 3rd ed. Philadelphia, PA: Lippincott Williams & Wilkins; 2014. Figure 4.2.

Postprocedural Approach

- Patients should be prescribed an antibiotic ointment to apply daily for 5 days to prevent infection.
- Return appointments may be warranted to determine treatment outcomes within 2 to 3 weeks.
- Patients can expect to see decrease in size over 1 to 2 weeks. If no improvement is seen, further injections or referral to ophthalmology may be required.

INCISION AND DRAINAGE OR EXCISION

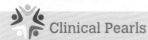 Clinical Pearls

- **Guidelines**
  - Third-line treatment for recurrent or persistent lesions
  - These procedures should be referred to an ophthalmologist if one is available.

Contraindications/Cautions/Risks

Contraindications
- Active skin infection or conjunctivitis

Cautions
- Extra caution should be exercised in sensitive areas.
- Medial chalazia are closely related to the punctum, which can be damaged when using a chalazion clamp.

Risks
- Infection, hemorrhage

○ Infection will be prevented with aqueous povidone-iodine solution applied to the eye before the procedure. Postoperative hemorrhage will be controlled with direct pressure or cautery, if needed. The procedure can be performed under local anesthetic or general anesthetic.

Equipment Needed

- Topical anesthetic
- Local anesthetic
- A 27-gauge needle
- A 3-mL syringe
- Sterile gloves
- Aqueous povidone-iodine
- Chalazion clamp
- A #11 blade
- Small curette
- Fine-toothed forceps
- Fine scissors
- Cautery
- Eye pads

Preprocedural Approach

- Begin the procedure by anesthetizing the external area of the eyelid with topical anesthetic.

- Wipe the area with alcohol to sterilize.
- Inject the surrounding tissue with local anesthetic. Instruct the patient look away from the syringe to minimize any risks related to patient movement or reflexes (Figure 69.2).
- It may also be helpful to mark the area with a waterproof marker.
- Ensure that the area is fully anesthetized before proceeding.
- Apply aqueous povidone-iodine to the eye and eyelid.
- Insert the chalazion clamp under the lifted eyelid with the open-circle end internal to the eyelid, paying close attention to the eye to avoid any external damage to the eye itself.
- Once the clamp is in place, carefully expose the conjunctival aspect of the chalazion (Figure 69.3A).
- Tightening the clamp can also help restrict bleeding.

Procedural Approach

- The chalazion will be identified and a vertical incision will be made with a #11 blade.
- The incision should not involve the lid margin or the external eyelid skin (Figure 69.3B).
- Using the small curette, remove the contents of the chalazion (Figure 69.3C).
- The contents may be collected and sent to pathology if the chalazion is recurrent or has other unusual characteristics (Figure 69.4).

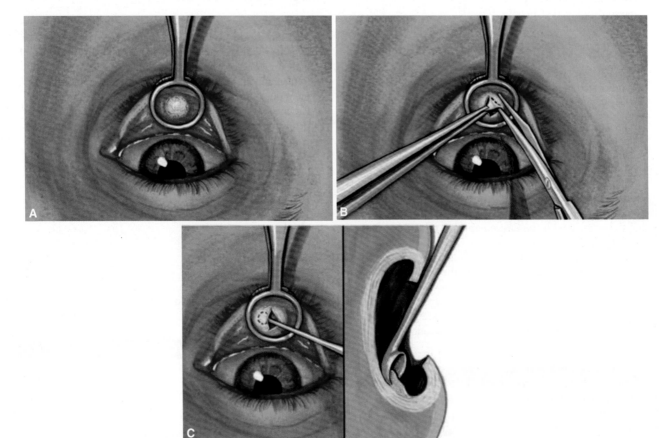

FIGURE 69.3. A, Tighten a chalazion clamp over the eyelid margin with the open plate centered over the pointing lesion on the conjunctival surface. Evert the eyelid to expose the lesion. B, Make a vertical incision through the conjunctiva and the posterior tarsal abscess wall. If possible, the incision should not extend closer than 2 to 3 mm to the eyelid margin. Grasp one edge of the wound and cut a small triangular flap of tarsus and conjunctiva from one side of the posterior cyst wall to allow for drainage. C, Remove the cyst contents completely with a chalazion curette. Explore for loculated pockets toward the eyelid margin, being careful not to injure the eyelash follicles. Scrape the walls of the entire inner surface to remove any epithelium. Using a spreading maneuver with Westcott scissors, carefully explore the interior of the cyst cavity for any remaining loculated pockets. Open these and curette the cavities to the level of the normal tarsus. Reprinted with permission from Dutton JJ. *Atlas of Oculoplastic and Orbital Surgery.* 2nd ed. Philadelphia, PA: Wolters Kluwer; 2018. Figures 4.1, 4.2, 4.3.

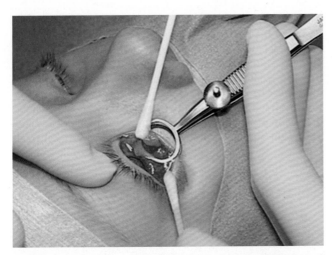

FIGURE 69.4. Chalazion incision and drainage transconjunctival approach. Intraoperative photograph reveals a lipogranulomatous material characteristic of chalazion. Reprinted with permission from Tasman W, Jaeger EA, Augsburger JJ, et al. *Wills Eye Hospital Atlas of Clinical Ophthalmology*. 2nd ed. Philadelphia, PA: Wolters Kluwer; 2018. Figure 10.65.

- Using the fine-toothed forceps, apply traction to the surrounding tissue to excise the chalazion.
- The scissor may be used to release any fibrous tissue or pseudocapsule present.
- Use care to prevent the removal of any normal tissue to preserve normal architecture.
- Once complete, release the clamp.

- Control any bleeding with direct pressure.
- If bleeding is excessive or continual, use of the cautery may be warranted.

Postprocedural Approach

- Topical antibiotic ointment should be used for 5 days.[3]
- Instruct the patient/parent to follow up if there is persistent swelling, redness, or recurrence.
- After resolution of chalazia through any of the avenues discussed, instruct the patient on actions they may perform to prevent recurrence and additional chalazia.
- Patient/parent should be instructed on methods of eyelid cleaning to prevent predisposing conditions such as blepharitis.
- Proper lid hygiene will help prevent gland obstruction as well as blepharitis.
- Patient/parent should be educated on the conservative management methods of warm compress and massaging, which can help resolve future early chalazia as well as prevent recurrence.

REFERENCES

1. Goawalla A, Lee V. A prospective randomized treatment study comparing three treatment options for chalazia: triamcinolone acetonide injections, incision and curettage and treatment with hot compresses: response. *Clin Exp Ophthalmol*. 2008;36(4):395–395. doi:10.1111/j.1442-9071.2008.001744.x.
2. Nuyen B, Weinreb RN, Robbins SL. Steroid-induced glaucoma in the pediatric population. *J AAPOS*. 2017;21(1):1–6. doi:10.1016/j.jaapos.2016.09.026.
3. Gilchrist H, Lee G. Management of chalazia in general practice. *Aust Fam Physician*. 2009;38(5):311–314.

Circumcision Adhesions

Austin Carter Smith and John C. Browning

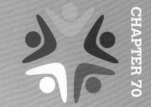

Introduction

Circumcision adhesions are a common occurrence in infants. Circumcisions are most commonly performed within 48 hours of birth. Boys younger than age 3 who have undergone circumcision are at highest risk for adhesions.[1] These adhesions are caused when the skin of the shaft of a circumcised penis adheres to the glans (Figure 70.1). These can be painful and cause discomfort, especially if they persist into adolescence. Adhesions are best treated conservatively, but other options such as steroid injections and lysing have been used, although their effectiveness has been questioned.[1] After adhesions have resolved, it is important to continue care to prevent readhesion. When adhesions are severe, they are referred to as "skin bridges" and must be treated surgically.

Penile adhesions are thought to occur because at the time of circumcision, the epithelium covering the glans has not fully developed and has not keratinized.[2] This immature skin has not fully

formed the barrier it needs. The skin is like an open wound, and as it is healing (ie, keratinizing), it can attach itself to other skin. These unwanted attachments can limit the retraction of the foreskin and cause bacteria to become trapped within the skin folds. These can create issues with development, urination, and erections.

Most adhesions are best treated conservatively by the parents/guardians at home. Many adhesions will require no treatment at all and will resolve on their own.[1] Others that cause significant discomfort or are persistent can be treated with gentle traction. Topical steroid creams have been shown to be useful for the treatment of phimosis in older boys when used in conjunction with manual traction, but their use in circumcision adhesions is unclear.[2]

If adhesions are severe, they can become skin bridges (Figure 70.2). Skin bridges are dense adhesions that can cause tethering of the penis. These skin bridges are band-like connections from the shaft to the glans. Skin bridges will appear as tissue connections that are visible while the skin covering the glans is retracted. After they have fully developed, they

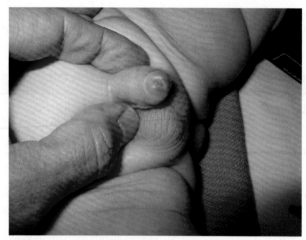

FIGURE 70.1. Circumcision adhesion. Whitish yellow mucosal attachments are noted between the prepuce and shaft of the penis. From Docimo SG, Canning D, Khoury A, et al. *The Kelalis King Belman Textbook of Clinical Pediatric Urology.* 6th ed. Boca Raton, FL: CRC Press; 2019. Copyright © 2019 by Taylor & Francis Group, LLC. Reproduced by permission of Taylor and Francis, a division of Informa plc.

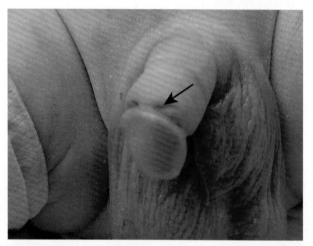

FIGURE 70.2. Penile skin bridge 1 week after newborn circumcision (see arrow). Reprinted with permission from MacDonald MG, Seshia MMK. *Avery's Neonatology.* 7th ed. Philadelphia, PA: Wolters Kluwer; 2015. Figure 40.35b.

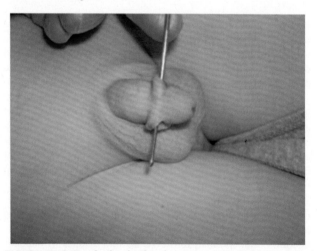

FIGURE 70.3. Penile skin bridge showing extent of space underlying adhesion.

will be attached at the glans and the shaft but will not be connected to the penis skin between those two points. The term "skin bridge" is literal in the sense that a tool can be passed underneath the connecting skin (Figure 70.3). They are believed to be caused by improper healing of the circumcision wound. They must be removed surgically and will not be responsive to the retraction treatment that is used for minor adhesions. Treatment of skin bridges is important because they can cause great pain and curvature during an erection. Surgical treatment can be performed when treating severe adhesions or skin bridges.

APPROACH #1: GENTLE TRACTION

 Clinical Pearls

- **Guidelines:** No specific treatment guidelines are known to exist for this condition.
- **Age-Specific Considerations:** This treatment is appropriate at any age, but the degree of pain and discomfort can be more closely monitored when a child or adolescent is performing it on themselves. The gentle retraction technique for a newly circumcised penis can begin 1 or 2 days after circumcision.
- **Technique Tips:** The best time to perform this is after a bath while the skin is soft and moisturized.
- **Skin of Color Considerations:** None

Contraindications/Cautions/Risks

Contraindications
- None

Cautions
- It is important not to use excessive force because that can tear the adhesion, leading to bleeding and/or infection.

Risks
- Mild bleeding from skin tear, and risk of infection is present with any breakage in skin.

Equipment Needed
- No tools or equipment are required.

Procedural Approach

- This action is very simple and can be demonstrated or explained to the caregiver during a visit to the clinic.
- Instruct the caregiver to gently grip the patient's penis between the thumb and index finger, with the fingers on one hand being on the glans above the adhesion and the fingers of the other hand on the shaft below the adhesion. Carefully slide fingers apart stretching the adhesion.
- The goal of this treatment is to slowly release the adhesion without causing pain or discomfort to the child.

Postprocedural Approach

- The caregiver should be aware that this treatment may take a significant amount of time to see improvement.

- After the adhesion has been released, it is important to regularly pull back and clean any skin covering the glans. This will help prevent future adhesions.[3]
- It is important to educate new parents on retraction and cleaning practices.
- Adhesions after circumcisions can be prevented by periodic retraction, as instructed earlier.
- Periodic preventative retractions will be easier, cause less discomfort to the child, and cause less distress to the parent by preventing future adhesions.
- If the adhesion is persistent, severe, or otherwise causing a great amount of discomfort to the child, the child should be referred to urology for assessment.
- Likewise, if the adhesion has shown no improvement using the traction technique after 6 to 8 weeks, the patient should be referred to urology, where more invasive procedures to resolve the adhesion can be performed.

APPROACH #2: LYSIS

 Clinical Pearls

- **Guidelines:** No specific treatment guidelines are known to exist for this condition.
- **Age-Specific Considerations:** None, skin bridges will require surgical treatment at any age.
- **Technique Tips:** String or suture can also be tied around the skin bridge to allow a point of contact to lift the open section of the bridge. This procedure can be done under either local or general anesthesia, but local anesthetic will be sufficient in most cases.
- **Skin of Color Considerations:** None

Contraindications/Cautions/Risks

Contraindications
- Active skin infection on penis

Cautions
- Lysis of skin bridges can be done quickly and easily but should be done by someone with proper training, such as a urologist.
- Small skin bridges are usually avascular and, therefore, will have a lower chance of bleeding.
- Large bridges can contain blood vessels, so the use of electrocautery may be warranted.

Risks
- Bleeding, infection, scarring, pain, recurrence of adhesions

Equipment Needed
- Lidocaine
- Electrocautery
- Aluminum chloride with applicators
- Scalpel with #15 blade
- Gauze
- Cotton-tipped applicator
- String or suture
- Alcohol or iodine

Preprocedural Approach

- Informed consent from the parent/guardian and, when possible, assent from the minor are obtained.
- Patients should bathe before the procedure.

Procedural Approach

- The provider will start by sterilizing the area with alcohol or iodine.
- The area will then be anesthetized using lidocaine injections, paying special attention to the bases of the skin bridges.
- The small cotton applicator can be passed under the skin bridge allowing it to be propped up and isolated.
- The string or suture can be passed under the skin bridge and tied for easy leverage.
- Once numb, the skin bridges can be carefully cut from their bases using the scalpel.
- The gauze may be used to apply pressure to stop any bleeding, and the aluminum chloride or electrocautery can be used if bleeding is sufficient and persistent.

Postprocedural Approach

- Patients should be prescribed an antibiotic ointment to apply twice daily to prevent infection.
- Follow-up should be scheduled within 2 to 3 weeks to assess healing of the wound.
- Patient and guardian should be educated on signs of a developing infection in the postoperative state.
- The parents should know that there may be slight residual bleeding present in the diaper when changing. If the bleeding is persistent, they should be instructed to apply pressure with a clean cloth. If the bleeding continues to persist for more than 5 minutes, they should seek medical attention.
- Parents should perform sponge baths until the wound has closed.
- It is important to educate the parents on the importance of retracting and cleaning the foreskin regularly to reduce the risk of infection and prevent the development of future adhesions.
- The patient should be scheduled for regular follow-up appointments to ensure that no adhesions have developed.

REFERENCES
1. Ponsky LE, Ross JH, Knipper N, Kay R. Penile adhesions after neonatal circumcision. *J Urol.* 2000;164(2):495–496. doi:10.1016/s0022-5347(05)67410-1.
2. Palmer LS, Palmer JS. The efficacy of topical betamethasone for treating phimosis: a comparison of two treatment regimens. *Urology.* 2008;72(1):68–71. doi:10.1016/j.urology.2008.02.030.
3. Gracely-Kilgore KA. Penile adhesion. *Nurse Pract.* 1984;9(5):22–24. doi:10.1097/00006205-198405000-00005.

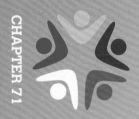

CHAPTER 71

Condyloma Acuminatum

Kevin Yarbrough

Introduction

Also known as "genital warts" or "anogenital warts," condyloma acuminatum refers to an epidermal manifestation of infection with human papillomavirus (HPV), most often with types HPV-6, HPV-10, and HPV-11. Other HPV types including HPV-16, HPV-18, HPV-30, HPV-2, and HPV-4 have also been isolated from condyloma in children. In situ hybridization for HPV or immunohistochemical studies for papillomavirus common antigen can help confirm the presence of HPV, and polymerase chain reaction (PCR) may be used to help identify the specific HPV type.

Lesions may be few or many (Figure 71.1). Modes of HPV transmission are well established and include vertical and perinatal transmission, benign horizontal, autoinoculation or heteroinoculation, and transmission by sexual contact or abuse. The source of infection is often unclear, leading to anxiety for both parents and physicians. The possibility of sexual abuse should be considered when condyloma is found, especially in older children, as the risk of abuse is highest in children older than 3 to 4 years.

The treatment of condyloma is often difficult, given the nature of the lesions and the options available for treatment. One approach, especially in younger children, is watchful waiting, because condyloma may resolve spontaneously in up to 50% of patients over time. Most parents, however, prefer to treat given symptoms associated with the lesions as well as desire for prompt resolution. When choosing a treatment, practitioners should strive to avoid overly aggressive, painful, or scarring treatments. As no single modality stands out as superior to others, many factors are considered to select the right treatment for each patient. These factors include patient and parent preference, cost, patient symptoms, resources available to the practitioner, physician experience, lesion number, location, and morphology. Most physicians and families select topical treatments such as chemovesicants (podophyllin, podophyllotoxin, trichloroacetic acid) or imiquimod as a first-line treatment. Surgical options are most often used in extensive or refractory cases. These include cryotherapy, laser treatment with either carbon dioxide (CO_2) or pulsed dye laser (PDL), and surgical removal by tangential scissors excision, tangential shave excision, or electrosurgery. Prevention of anogenital HPV infection is now possible with the development of HPV vaccines.

Chemovesicants-Topical Immunotherapy

Topical treatments are typically used as first line for pediatric condyloma. Options include in-office treatments such as podophyllin and trichloroacetic acid (TCA) as well as imiquimod and podophyllotoxin (podofilox) applied at home. The authors preferred initial treatment is home treatment with imiquimod or podofilox.[1] In adults, home treatment with podofilox was shown to be cheaper and more effective than in-office treatment with podophyllin.[2] Podophyllin resin contains mutagenic and toxic compounds not present in podophyllotoxin-based products and is generally not recommended.[3] TCA 80% to 90% solution is applied in office. This modality can be used for small acuminate or papular lesions. Optimal use results in a small erosion that heals without scaring. It can be used safely during pregnancy.[4]

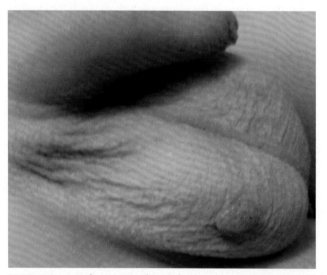

FIGURE 71.1. A discrete papule was slowly enlarging on a 6-year-old male's scrotum. The boy's mother had a history of genital warts that were present during his vaginal birth. Biopsy and subsequent typing by polymerase chain reaction showed both the boy's lesion and his mother's lesions were the same human papillomavirus type. An investigation by Child Protective Services revealed no concerns for sexual abuse. Photo courtesy of Andrew C. Krakowski, MD.

Clinical Pearls: Chemovesicants-Topical Immunotherapy

- **Guidelines:** No formal management guidelines exist for the treatment of pediatric condyloma.
- **Age-Specific Considerations:** These chemical treatment options may be preferable to other more painful options for symptomatic condyloma.
- **Technique Tips:**
  - White petrolatum or other skin protectant applied to surrounding skin can reduce pain and injury to normal skin.
  - TCA is likely most effective for moist nonkeratinized lesions but can be used on keratinized lesions as well.
  - Have sodium bicarbonate or talc available as neutralizing agent for any inadvertent application or spills.
- **Skin of Color Considerations:** Darker skin types are at increased risk for pigmentation changes following treatment and should be counseled appropriately.

Contraindications/Cautions/Risks: Chemovesicants-Topical Immunotherapy

Contraindications

- Very large lesions, hypersensitivity, or allergy to TCA. TCA should not be used for warts of the urethra, vagina, cervix, or rectum.

Cautions

- Potential result of scarring with overtreatment

Risks

- Scarring, infection, pain, and hypopigmentation

Equipment Needed

- TCA 80% to 90%; often 85% is used.
- Cotton-tipped applicators
- White petrolatum
- Sodium bicarbonate or talc as a neutralizing agent

Preprocedural Approach: Chemovesicants-Topical Immunotherapy

- The procedure is explained to the patient and parents, and informed consent is obtained.
- White petrolatum, paraffin, or other skin protectant is applied to surrounding normal skin to avoid inadvertent contact with unaffected skin.

Procedural Approach: Chemovesicants-Topical Immunotherapy

- In all, 80% to 90% TCA is applied with a cotton-tipped applicator (either wooden end or cotton end).
- A small amount is applied to the surface of the lesion and allowed to dry. A white frosting should develop.
- Treatment is repeated every 5 to 7 days for 6 to 10 weeks as needed until clearance.
- If pain is intense or an excess amount of acid is applied cover the area with sodium bicarbonate (ie, baking soda), wash with liquid soap, or cover with talc to neutralize the acid and remove unreacted acid.

Postprocedural Approach: Chemovesicants-Topical Immunotherapy

- Lesions should dry completely before patient sits or stands to avoid spreading.
- Patients can wash the area following treatment or use sitz baths for discomfort. Pain can also be managed with nonsteroidal anti-inflammatory drugs (NSAIDs) or acetaminophen.

Cryosurgery of Genital Warts

Cryotherapy is an effective and frequently used treatment for adults and adolescents with condyloma. Condyloma is treated in a similar manner to common warts. Each lesion undergoes one or two freeze–thaw cycles with a 2-mm zone of frosting surrounding the lesion. Treatments are done at a frequency of 1 to 3 weeks. Clearance rates of 79% to 88% have been reported within three treatments.[5,6] Pretreatment with topical lidocaine can be used to reduce pain.

 Clinical Pearls

- **Guidelines:** No formal management guidelines exist for the treatment of pediatric condyloma.
- **Age-Specific Considerations:** These treatment options work best for older, motivated children able to tolerate painful treatments in a very sensitive location.
- **Technique Tips:**
  - Application of liquid nitrogen with a cotton-tipped applicator allows more precise freezing with less pain and often less anxiety for the patient.
  - Portions of a cotton ball can be added to the cotton-tipped applicator to ensure a larger base for freezing larger/wider lesions.
  - Topical lidocaine applied 1 hour prior to treatment reduces the pain of cryotherapy.
- **Skin of Color Considerations:** Darker skin types are at increased risk for pigmentation changes following cryotherapy and should be counseled appropriately.

Contraindications/Cautions/Risks

Contraindications: Treating areas with compromised circulation, previous adverse reaction to cryotherapy, undiagnosed lesion, lesion requiring pathologic examination

Cautions: Potential result of hypopigmentation/dyschromia in skin of color

Risks: Blistering, scarring, infection, pain, and hypopigmentation

Equipment Needed

- Liquid nitrogen
- Cotton-tipped applicators
- Cotton balls (optional)
- Liquid nitrogen spray equipment (spray gun/canister), if preferred

Preprocedural Approach

- The procedure is explained to the patient and parents, and informed consent is obtained.
- Topical lidocaine is applied 1 hour prior to the procedure and held in place with plastic food wrap.

Procedural Approach

- Liquid nitrogen is applied with either a cotton-tipped applicator or a spray apparatus to each lesion until an ice field encompasses the lesion and the desired margin.
- A second freeze–thaw cycle can be used depending on patient tolerance, location, and previous response.
- Treatment is repeated in 1 to 3 weeks.

Postprocedural Approach

- Side effects are normally mild and resolve quickly.
- Patients monitor for any blistering.

Laser Treatments of Genital Warts

CO_2 laser and PDL have both been used in the treatment of pediatric condyloma.[7-9] An important consideration with laser treatment is the potential for transmission of HPV to the surgeon and medical staff. Treatments that generate a smoke plume are potentially infectious to any bystanders. HPV DNA is found in the smoke generated from destructive treatments, such as laser and electrofulguration/coagulation. Correct appropriately fitting masks and effective smoke evacuator should be used. Viral DNA has been found in the plume generated by CO_2 and electrocoagulation; however, no studies exist evaluating the presence of viral DNA in plumes generated with PDL. PDL typically generates minimal smoke unless used over hair-bearing skin. Regardless, it would be prudent to wear personal protective equipment for any treatment of warts where a smoke plume is generated. Clearance with as few as one treatment and on average 1.59 treatments has been reported with PDL.[8-10]

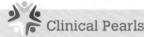

Clinical Pearls

- **Guidelines:** No specific guidelines exist.
- **Age-Specific Considerations:** Most younger patients will likely need general anesthesia for laser treatments in sensitive areas.
- **Technique Tips:** PDL has less potential for scaring and infection as the skin surface is typically maintained.

Contraindications/Cautions/Risks

Caution is recommended when using PDL and CO_2 lasers in skin types III-VI, as dyspigmentation may result.

Risks: Pain, bruising, bleeding, blistering, scaring, infection, pigment change, and recurrence.

Equipment Needed

- PDL or CO_2 laser
- Mechanical smoke evacuation system with a high-efficiency filter to manage the generation of large amounts of laser plume
- Appropriately fitted N95 or N100 respirators to minimize exposure to laser plumes
- White petrolatum to apply postprocedure
- Topical lidocaine cream if needed for local anesthesia

Procedural Approach

- For PDL: Settings of 7-mm spot size, 1.5 ms pulse duration, and 7.5 mJ were used in one pediatric report, and a case series of adults reported the use of 7-mm spot size, 0.45 ms pulse duration, and 6 to 7 mJ for fluence. The tissue reaction end point is purpura of the condyloma histologically corresponding with selective thermolysis of the dilated dermal capillary network supplying the condyloma. Some authors advocate for stacked pulses to achieve this clinical end point.
- For CO_2: This technique will vary by manufacturer's device. One reported method uses a device set at a power of 2 W in the continuous focused mode with a 1-mm spot size.[7-9] One

to four passes are made with the CO_2 laser, until the condyloma can be manually cleared to the level of the papillary dermis with moistened gauze. After clearance, each lesion is treated with one pass in a defocused mode.

Postprocedural Approach

- Acetaminophen or ibuprofen can be given for postprocedural pain.
- Lesions are covered with white petrolatum or topical antibiotics twice daily, and light crusting is expected.
- For CO_2 postoperative care, twice-daily sitz baths for 2 weeks can be helpful.

Surgical Removal-Tangential Scissors Excision, Tangential Shave Excision, or Electrosurgery

Surgical removal has the potential advantage of rendering a patient free of visible warts after one treatment. This can be especially appealing when the warts are numerous, interfering with function, and multiple office visits are not possible. However, the potential for scarring and need for general anesthesia make this method not a great first-line treatment. In adults, electrosurgery is initially more effective than cryotherapy, imiquimod, or podophyllin with clearance during therapy up to 94%. However, at 3 months, efficacy is similar to cryosurgery and podophyllin, with continued clearance around 70%.[6] In a study of 213 patients with extensive genital warts treated with electrosurgery, 83% were able to be cleared with a single procedure, with recurrence rates around 20% over a 5-year period. Various methods of electrosurgical treatment of condyloma have been used, including electrocoagulation, electrofulguration, electrodesiccation, and electrocautery. These terms are sometimes used interchangeably in the literature, making it difficult to accurately describe the techniques used. Regardless of the exact technique used, the goal of treatment is destruction of the condyloma with minimal damage to surrounding tissues. This is accomplished using a fine-tip electrode and starting with a low-power setting, gradually increasing for the desired effect.[11,12] Electrosurgery can also be used in conjunction with tangential excision, especially for larger lesions. Smaller lesions can be treated with tangential scissor/shave excision with or without electrocoagulation of the base to aid with hemostasis and treat any remaining wart tissue remaining after excision.

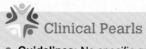

Clinical Pearls

- **Guidelines:** No specific guidelines exist.
- **Age-Specific Considerations:** Most younger patients will likely need general anesthesia as well as local anesthesia.
- **Technique Tips:**
  - Larger lesions have higher potential to leave noticeable scars when treated with this method.
  - Large lesions may need to be debulked with excision, then treated at the base with electrocautery.
  - Electrofulguration tends to generate larger smoke plumes, and appropriate protective measures should be taken during the procedure (as discussed with laser treatment and plume above).

Contraindications/Cautions/Risks

Caution
In darker skin types

Risks
Include pain, bruising, bleeding, blistering, scaring, infection, pigment change, and recurrence.

Equipment Needed
- Electrosurgical unit with fine tip
- Mechanical smoke evacuation system with a high-efficiency filter to manage the generation of smoke plume
- Appropriately fitted N95 or N100 respirators to minimize exposure to smoke plumes
- White petrolatum to apply postprocedure
- One percent lidocaine with epinephrine for local anesthesia
- Sharp iris scissors if performing snip excision
- Forceps

Procedural Approach

- Using a fine-tip and low-power setting, first, coagulate the wart base; then, the exophytic portion may be treated.
- Coagulum can be left in place to minimize open areas.
- Very large lesions can be surgically debulked, then treated by electrosurgery.
- Tangential excision is accomplished by grasping the lesion with forceps and tangentially cutting across the base of the lesion using either a scalpel or scissors.
- Hemostasis can be achieved using aluminum chloride or electrocautery of the base.

Postprocedural Approach

- Acetaminophen and ibuprofen can be given for postprocedural pain.

- The lesions are covered with white petrolatum or topical antibiotics twice daily until healed.
- Sitz baths can also be used.

REFERENCES

1. Moresi JM, Herbert CR, Cohen BA. Treatment of anogenital warts in children with topical 0.05% podofilox gel and 5% imiquimod cream. *Pediatr Dermatol.* 2001;18(5):448–450.
2. Lacey CJN, Goodall RL, Tennvall GR, et al. Randomised controlled trial and economic evaluation of podophyllotoxin solution, podophyllotoxin cream, and podophyllin in the treatment of genital warts. *Sex Transm Infect.* 2003;79(4):270–275.
3. von Krogh G, Longstaff E. Podophyllin office therapy against condyloma should be abandoned. *Sex Transm Infect.* 2001;77(6): 409–412.
4. Lacey CJN, Woodhall SC, Wikstrom A, Ross J. 2012 European guideline for the management of anogenital warts. *J Eur Acad Dermatol Venereol.* 2013;27(3):e263–e270.
5. Yanofsky VR, Patel RV, Goldenberg G. Genital warts. *J Clin Aesthet Dermatol.* 2012;5(6):25–36.
6. Stone KM, Becker TM, Hadgu A, Kraus SJ. Treatment of external genital warts: a randomised clinical trial comparing podophyllin, cryotherapy, and electrodesiccation. *Genitourin Med.* 1990;66(1):16–19.
7. Johnson PJ, Mirzai TH, Bentz ML. Carbon dioxide laser ablation of anogenital condyloma acuminata in pediatric patients. *Ann Plast Surg.* 1997;39(6):578–582.
8. Komericki P, Akkilic M, Kopera D. Pulsed dye laser treatment of genital warts. *Lasers Surg Med.* 2006;38(4):273–276.
9. Tuncel A, Görgü M, Ayhan M, Deren O, Erdogan B. Treatment of anogenital warts by pulsed dye laser. *Dermatol Surg.* 2002;28(4):350–352.
10. Sethuraman G, Richards KA, Hiremagalore RN, Wagner A. Effectiveness of pulsed dye laser in the treatment of recalcitrant in children. *Dermatol Surg.* 2010;36(1):58–65.
11. Challenor R, Alexander I. A five-year audit of the treatment of extensive anogenital warts by day case electrosurgery under general anaesthesia. *Int J STD AIDS.* 2002;13(11):786–789.
12. Taheri A, Mansoori P, Sandoval LF, Feldman SR, Pearce D, Williford PM. Electrosurgery—Part I. Basics and principles. *J Am Acad Dermatol.* 2014;70(4):591.e1–591.e14.

Cutaneous Larva Migrans (Creeping Eruption)

Caroline Stovall and Craig N. Burkhart

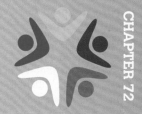

CHAPTER 72

Introduction

Cutaneous larva migrans (creeping eruption) is a pruritic rash caused by a localized infection of the skin with hookworm larva. Humans are accidental hosts, and inoculation occurs when animal hookworm larva directly infect the skin. Hookworm larva is unable to penetrate the basement membrane, so the infection is limited to the epidermis. *Ancylostoma caninum*, *Ancylostoma braziliense*, and *Uncinaria stenocephala* are the most common causative organisms.

The classic eruption typically involves the distal lower extremities, buttocks, or, more rarely, the hands. Presentation is variable, but typically, an infected individual will present with erythematous and edematous serpiginous tracts created by larval migration. Other, more atypical presentations include vesicles, papules, or folliculitis (Figures 72.1 and 72.2).

Individuals who travel to or reside in warmer climates and those who walk barefoot on soil or sand contaminated by animal feces are at highest risk of infection. However, infection can be prevented by prohibiting domesticated animals from beaches and wearing protective footwear.

Cutaneous larva migrans is diagnosed on the basis of history and physical examination. If untreated, the cutaneous eruption will wax and wane for weeks to months until spontaneously

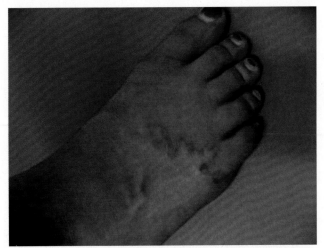

FIGURE 72.1. Cutaneous larva migrans infection after playing beach volleyball in Puerto Rico. Reprinted with permission from Altchek DW, DiGiovanni CW, Dines JS, et al. *Foot and Ankle Sports Medicine*. Philadelphia, PA: Wolters Kluwer Health/Lippincott Williams & Wilkins; 2012. Figure 32.5.

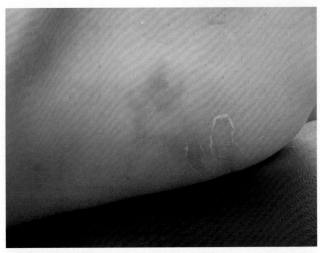

FIGURE 72.2. Cutaneous larva migrans infection on the sole of the foot after walking on a beach in Mexico. Photo courtesy of Andrew C. Krakowski, MD.

self-resolving. However, treatment is usually necessary because the pruritus can be quite severe. Systemic manifestations are rare, but if they occur, can include peripheral eosinophilia or self-limited, mild upper respiratory symptoms. The goal of treatment is to kill the larva, which results in resolution of the eruption and pruritus.

Although medical treatment with antiparasitic medication is the gold standard, some procedural interventions can be helpful. For nonpregnant individuals weighing >15 kg, the first-line medical treatment is systemic ivermectin 200 µg/kg for a single dose. This treatment is 80% to 100% effective in eliminating pruritus and killing larva. If a patient does not demonstrate clinical improvement, a repeat dose 10 days later is recommended. For children weighing <15 kg or individuals with localized disease (single tract), topical albendazole 10% applied to the area of involvement, three times a day, for 7 to 10 days is a suitable alternative therapy. Topical corticosteroids are helpful for symptomatic treatment of inflammation and itching and the recommended treatment for pregnant patients. Another alternative treatment is systemic albendazole 15 mg/kg/d for 3 to 5 days in children >2 years (for a maximum dose of 800 mg/d) or 400 to 800 mg/d for 3 to 5 days in adults. For limited disease, or for patients who cannot tolerate side effects from systemic medications, treatment with 10% to 15% thiabendazole solution/ointment, three times a day, for 15 days is an effective alternative topical treatment.

Cryotherapy can be helpful as an adjunct to systemic therapy, or primary treatment for pregnant patients, those with localized disease, or in patients who cannot tolerate the side effects of systemic medications. Recently, a small case report of 10 cases in the Philippines demonstrates efficacy of treatment of the eruption of cutaneous larva migrans with fractional CO_2 laser.

Clinical Pearls

- Systemic treatment is preferred.
- Treatment of cutaneous larva migrans with cryotherapy with liquid nitrogen has Level 4 evidence of efficacy.

- Cryotherapy with liquid nitrogen can be particularly helpful in treatment of cutaneous larva migrans in pregnant patients, in individuals who cannot tolerate side effects of systemic medications, in patients with isolated disease limited to one to two small tracts, or as adjunctive treatment.
- Patient maturity and pain tolerance must be evaluated when considering cryotherapy as a treatment because of the discomfort associated with the procedure.
- Patients with skin of color are at higher risk of postinflammatory pigmentary changes; this risk must be discussed with the patient before pursuing treatment with liquid nitrogen.

Contraindications/Cautions/Risks

Contraindications

- Very young children, darkly skinned patients concerned for pigmentary changes, several discrete tracts, and patients unable to tolerate side effects of cryotherapy
- No absolute contraindications

Risks

- Pain, swelling, vesicle development, pigmentary changes, recurrence, and infection

Equipment Needed

- Cryospray device (preferred) or cotton-tipped applicator and nonpermeable container for liquid nitrogen
- Spray tips for cryospray device
- Appropriate storage tanks (Dewar flasks) for liquid nitrogen

Preprocedural Approach

- If using cryospray device, select appropriate spray tip for diameter and apparent depth of tract.
- If using cotton-tipped applicator, fill container with liquid nitrogen and position patient.

Procedural Approach

- Apply liquid nitrogen to the leading edge of the tract and, as tolerated by patient, 1 to 2 cm peripherally around the end of the tract, for a freeze–thaw cycle of 5 seconds.
- Two freeze–thaw cycles may be more effective if tolerated by the patient.

Postprocedural Approach

- Counsel patient that the area may blister, bruise, scab, swell, bleed, or be tender for the next few days; instructions for appropriate wound care after cryotherapy should be provided.

- Discuss with patient that pigment changes after cryotherapy may occur and are more common in darkly pigmented individuals.
- More uncommon adverse effects include local hair loss, hypertrophic scarring, and infection.

SUGGESTED READINGS

Davies HD, Sakuls P, Keystone JS. Creeping eruption. *Arch Dermatol.* 1993;129(5):588–591.

Soriano LF, Piansay-Soriano ME. Treatment of cutaneous larva migrans with a single session of carbon dioxide laser: a study of ten cases in the Philippines. *J Cosmet Dermatol.* 2017;16(1):91–94.

Sunderkötter C, Stebut E, Schöfer H, et al. S1 guideline diagnosis and therapy of cutaneous larva migrans (creeping disease). *J Dtsch Dermatol Ges.* 2014;12(1):86–91.

Depigmentation

Nisrine Kawa, Julia Roma May, Morgan Albert, and Thanh-Nga T. Tran[*]

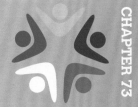

CHAPTER 73

INTRODUCTION

Depigmentation is the total loss of pigment and subsequent localized lightening of the skin that can occur in all ages. Piebaldism is a congenital form of depigmentation that remains stable throughout life. Vitiligo is typically an acquired condition that presents between the ages of 10 and 30 and may be associated with other autoimmune conditions. Some rare cases of congenital forms have also been described and usually exhibit an unpredictable course. Vitiligo is classified as segmental (asymmetric, unilateral, and stable) or nonsegmental (symmetric and often evolving).

The psychosocial aspect of depigmentation disorders is most often the cause of patients' distress, because they often report social rejection and stigmatization, especially at young ages. Although depigmentation may occur in all skin types, it is most disfiguring in those with darker skin because of marked contrast. As a result, not all patients with depigmentation need treatment. Moreover, the progressive nature of vitiligo may lead to relapses, even following treatment success.

In case of piebaldism, repopulation of affected tissue with donor melanocytes is the only treatment option. In vitiligo, selection of the treatment modality depends on subtype, location, and extent of depigmentation, response to treatment, and stability of the lesions. Although some lesions may benefit from topical or systemic regimens, others may require phototherapy or procedures related to melanocyte transfer. These are summarized in Table 73.1. New drugs such as Janus kinase (JAK) inhibitors are promising; however, these are not included in this procedural focus.

Clinical Pearls

- **Guidelines:**
  - No specific treatment guidelines are known to exist for this condition.

- Before proceeding with treatment procedures detailed later, further training and expertise are required.
- Not all patients will require procedural intervention. Adequate initial assessment will guide which patients will benefit from each treatment (Table 73.1).
- **Stability-Based Considerations:**
  - Vitiligo may be considered stable when the patient has no new lesions, progression of existing lesions, and no Koebnerization in the previous year.
  - Active and progressive vitiligo requires *stabilization*. This typically entails oral or topical steroids, with or without calcineurin inhibitors and/or light therapy. No repigmentation procedures are suggested at this stage.
  - Stable lesions can undergo attempts at *repigmentation*. This may require topical treatments or procedural intervention.
- **Subtype-Specific Considerations:**
  - Segmental vitiligo appears to respond better to treatment than does the nonsegmental subtype.
  - Segmental vitiligo often requires melanocyte or epidermal grafting.
- **Considerations for Extent of Vitiligo Spread:**
  - *In severe cases affecting* >40% of total body surface area, patients may prefer depigmentation therapy with topical monobenzene.
- **Location-Specific Considerations:**
  - Facial and truncal lesions respond better than do those on the extremities.
- **Age-Specific Considerations:**
  - Treating younger children is more difficult given the need for cooperation for many of these techniques.
  - In general, rates of treatment success for melanocyte transfer are higher in patients aged 20 and younger.
- **Skin of Color Considerations:**
  - Individuals with fair skin may opt for no treatment and rely on sun avoidance to prevent tanning of normal skin.
  - In general, rates of treatment success are higher in patients with darker skin types (Fitzpatrick IV-VI).

---

[*]Latanya T. Benjamin provided additional editorial review of this chapter.

TABLE 73.1 ⋮ **Summary of Treatment Options for Vitiligo**

TREATMENT MODALITY FOR REPIGMENTATION	INDICATIONS AND RECOMMENDATIONS	OUTCOMES
Medication		
• Steroids	Oral—5-10 mg prednisone for children. Instead of continuous dosing, mini-pulse therapy can be used as a safe option. Topical—to be used when lesions occupy <10% TBSA, applied daily with scheduled interruptions to prevent side effects May be used alone when disease is stable and localized or combined with phototherapy if disseminated[a]	Oral treatment for stabilization of rapidly progressive vitiligo Topical steroids—optimal duration of treatment for topical therapy has not been established yet. Possible steroid-related side effects Response may take up to 12 wk to appear.
• Calcineurin inhibitors	Can be applied daily when lesions <10% TBSA	Preferred over steroids when high risk of skin atrophy (such as face) Similar outcomes to those for steroids for children with facial vitiligo; slight inferiority to steroids for children with nonfacial vitiligo Uncertain link to possible later malignancies—*FDA box warning*
Light Based		
• Psoralen and ultra-violet A	No longer recommended as first line Was considered gold standard in the past	Similar or inferior outcome to those of other phototherapy modalities High side effect profile with phototoxicity, GI disturbance, and risk of skin cancer
• NB-UVB (311 nm)	First-line therapy in case of disseminated disease or when >10% TBSA is involved May be used as combination with steroids when <10%TBSA is involved May be used for stabilization Home devices exist if patient cannot come to office regularly.	Requires multiple sessions a week (2-3) over at least 9 mo 36% success rate at 12 mo defined as >75% repigmentation In case of good response, maintenance sessions every other week can be considered. Response may not occur until after 15-20 sessions. Variable overall long-term success
• Excimer laser or lamp (308 nm)	Indications similar to those of NB-UVB with less need for UV exposure	Session frequency, duration of treatment, and long-term outcome similar to those of NB-UVB 60%-70% response rate after 9 wk of biweekly treatment Overall treatment success at 12 mo is similar or slightly superior to that of NB-UVB.
Melanocyte/epidermis/skin transfer	To be used when localized stable vitiligo is unresponsive to topical and phototherapy treatments May be done using various modalities: • Split-thickness skin grafts (STSG) • Epidermal suction blister grafts • Punch grafts • Cultured and noncultured epidermal cell suspensions: Melanocyte keratinocyte transplant procedure • Hair transplant	In case of grafts involving dermis, donor site morbidity may be considered in keloid forming patients. Potential risk for Koebner phenomenon Highest success rates for STSG and blister grafts: 90% repigmentation Suspensions contain melanocytes and keratinocytes; 80% success rate in repigmenting >90% of treated area Hair transplant may be considered for hairy areas of the body, with around 61% success rate.
TREATMENT MODALITIES FOR DEPIGMENTATION	**INDICATION AND RECOMMENDATIONS**	**OUTCOME**
Depigmentation with monobenzene	Indicated for patients with extensive and recalcitrant vitiligo (generally affecting >40% of body surface area) Apply topical monobenzene to areas of residual pigmentation one to two times a day. Start with 10% for first month then move to 20%.	Irritant contact dermatitis and severe xerosis are possible side effects of treatment.

[a]Disseminated disease refers to spread over body and not based on percentage of involvement.
FDA, U.S. Food and Drug Administration; GI, gastrointestinal; NB-UVB; narrow-band ultraviolet B; TBSA, total body surface area.

Contraindications/Cautions/Risks

Contraindications

- Active local skin infections or sunburn is a contraindication.

Cautions

- Given the time commitment and potential financial expense (ie, multiple copays) patients may prefer to consider "at-home" narrow-band ultraviolet B (NB-UVB) lamp treatments.

Risks

- Light-based treatments such as NB-UVB and excimer laser are generally rapid, relatively painless, and safe with low short-term side effect potential, but variable effectiveness. With frequent treatments over years, photoaging and skin cancer may increase.
- Epidermal grafting procedures are fairly safe as well with low risk of donor or recipient scarring or infection. Possible risks include Koebner phenomenon with onset of a vitiligo lesion at the donor site because of injury. At the recipient site, grafting may lead to unevenness in color, with islands of pigment surrounded by a depigmented base.
- Suction blister grafting can painlessly harvest pure epidermis from a pigmented donor site, but suction often fails to obtain a graft in children younger than age 3.
- Even though it is an approved treatment option, split-thickness grafting should be avoided because of donor site morbidity.

Equipment Needed

Equipment needed varies with treatment choice:
- Generally required equipment
  - Local anesthesia
  - Petrolatum-based ointment
- Phototherapy
  - NB-UVB source, excimer laser, or excimer lamp
  - UV dosimeter
  - Protective eyewear
- Grafting procedures—options for donor site preparation
  - Traditional epidermal blister grafting
    - Two syringes: 10 and 50 mL
    - Three-way connector
    - Curved scissors
    - Glass slide
  - Semiautomated epidermal blister grafting
    - A suction-harvesting system such as the CelluTome (CelluTome® Epidermal Harvesting System; Kinetic Concepts, San Antonio, TX)
    - Adhesive dressing
  - Cultured melanocyte cell suspensions
    - A dermatome
    - A skilled laboratory is needed to prepare cultured melanocyte cell suspensions.
    - Autologous noncultured skin cell suspensions can be made with the RECELL Autologous Skin Cell Harvesting System (RECELL®, Avita Medical, Valencia, CA).
- Grafting procedures—options for removal of recipient site epidermis
  - Laser-assisted removal of epidermis
    - Ablative laser such as CO_2 or erbium lasers
  - Superficial dermabrasion
    - Sterile (autoclave or gas) #120 emery cloth

Preprocedural Approach

Proper diagnosis, procedure planning, and a detailed discussion with the patient and parents is necessary to establish realistic goals, understand the long course of response, the typical need for repeated treatments, and risks involved. Standardized photographic documentation before and after treatment, and during subsequent responses is essential. Equipment should be well maintained, sterile (for grafting procedures), and familiar. For children, fear and even minor pain can make treatment impossible because of lack of cooperation. Painless ways of reducing pain and anxiety are key, including topical anesthesia, local skin cooling, hypnosis, and inhaled or oral sedation. General anesthesia, which carries a potential risk of cognitive development changes in young children, should be used only when warranted.

SPECIFIC PROCEDURAL APPROACHES

Phototherapy

Phototherapy Preprocedural Approach

- Many physicians start topical therapy about 1 month before deciding to begin phototherapy; the two are often synergistic.
- It is convenient to perform minimal erythema dose (MED) exposures the day before treatment.
  - The patient's MED is usually determined on the buttock or other non–sun-exposed skin by exposing small (1-2 cm) patches of skin to a range of exposure doses with about 30% increments.
  - The MED is defined as the lowest exposure dose that causes erythema 1 day later.
- Instruct patients to avoid application of any topical products including sunscreen within 4 hours of treatment.
- Patients may apply mineral oil over dry areas before phototherapy.
- No additional preparatory measures are necessary.

Procedural Approach

I. Narrow-Band Ultraviolet B

- Children older than age 7 can generally stand in the phototherapy cabinet alone, following required instructions.
- An adult can remain in the phototherapy cabinet with younger children as long as they are adequately photoprotected. However, this may lead to unnecessary exposure to the adult or inadvertent shielding of the child.
- UV-blocking goggles should be used, and male genitals should be covered during phototherapy.
- In case of eyelid involvement, exposure while monitoring to be certain the patient's eyes are closed is acceptable. Eyelids are often more sensitive to NB-UVB treatment than is the rest of the body; goggles should be worn after the desired eyelid exposure is achieved.
- Protocols may vary depending on physician experience and light source used (Table 73.2).

II. Excimer Laser (308-nm XeCl Laser)

- Initial treatment dose for excimer laser or excimer lamp treatment is similar to that for NB-UVB.
- Only affected (depigmented) skin lesions are exposed.

TABLE 73.2 Phototherapy Treatment Protocol Considerations

Initial starting dose	About 0.5 minimal erythema dose, which is approximately 200 mJ/cm²
Subsequent dosing	Based on individual response to treatment: • No erythema after last treatment: Increase 50 mJ/cm² • Mild painless erythema: No change in dose • Moderate or painful erythema: Decrease 25 mJ/cm² • Severe, painful erythema: Wait until resolution, then decrease dose by 15%.
Maximal acceptable dosing	• 1500 mJ/cm² for face • 3000 mJ/cm² for body
Dose adjustments for missed sessions	• No change if within 1 wk of last session • Reduce dose by 25% if 8-14 d since last session • Reduce dose by 50% if 15-21 d since last session • Restart at baseline if >21 d since last session

- Eye protection is required.
- Treatment dose should be adjusted depending on response seen in each individual patient.
- If excessive pain, erythema, or blistering occurs, decrease the exposure dose by at least 10%.
- If followed well and done in accordance with guidelines, excimer lamp treatment in the office or at home may be equally effective as excimer laser treatment.

Phototherapy Postprocedural Approach

Sun avoidance and diligent sunscreen application are recommended after phototherapy.

- Phototherapy treatments are typically given two to three times per week.
- Following phototherapy procedures, patients may experience tingling or burning of their skin, which may be erythematous.
- Clinical response will help guide the choice of exposure dose for further treatments, as described.
- Significant pain or blistering are signs of UV injury, and it is best to take a break before resuming treatment at lower doses.
- Improvement may be expected after 15 to 20 sessions, seen as perifollicular outgrowth of pigmentation.
- Outcomes will vary from one patient to another but also at different sites within the same patient, with the poorest response occurring in hairless thick skin such as over the knuckles.
- Maintenance sessions may be continued every other week depending on patient preference.
- Phototherapy failure usually warrants consideration of more invasive procedures.

MELANOCYTE TRANSFER PROCEDURES

Disclaimer: For completion, basic descriptions are provided for the following procedures; however, more extensive training is required before being able to attempt them.

I. Epidermal Grafting by Suction Blister

Preprocedural Approach

- Epidermal grafting should be performed only when the vitiligo lesion is stable and small enough to be treated.
- Donor site must be healthy, normally pigmented skin in an inconspicuous area (usually thigh or buttock) to reduce the risk of disfigurement if Koebnerization (vitiligo in the donor site) should occur.
- If necessary, shave or clip hair on donor and recipient areas, then clean with rubbing alcohol or chlorhexidine solution.

Procedural Approach

- If using the automated CelluTome system, place the epidermal suction blister device on the selected donor site and secure the device ensuring that there is complete contact of the skin with all the microblister holes. Attach the vacuum head and power on to begin the process. An array of 2-mm blisters will have formed after approximately 45 minutes. The patient is required to stay still during this time. Distraction techniques are encouraged for younger patients.
- Epidermal blisters can also be formed without automated systems, but this technique may take longer. This requires attaching a 50-mL syringe to a 10-mL syringe, connected by a three-way connector. The plunger is removed from the 50-mL syringe that is placed against the donor site. Suction is then applied from the 10-mL side and the pressure gradient can then be sealed by closure of the three-way connector. This generally is more time consuming and may require multiple reapplications because syringes easily detach.
- While waiting for the blisters to form, the recipient area can be prepared. Start by anesthetizing the recipient treatment area by local injection or topical numbing cream. Next, remove the depigmented epidermis 1 to 2 mm beyond the border. This can be done using laser ablation (CO_2 or Er:YAG) or dermabrasion with sterilized (autoclave or gas) #120 emery cloth sandpaper to the point of brisk pinpoint bleeding.
- When the blister formation is complete, the epidermis can be harvested and placed onto the prepared recipient site. If using the CelluTome, unlatch the vacuum head and place adhesive film such as Tegaderm® (3M, US) onto the harvesting plate, making sure to press firmly against the raised blisters. Next, pull on the blue cutting latch to separate the epidermal blisters from the donor site, leaving the epidermis attached to the adhesive dressing. This is nearly painless and does not need anesthesia, even in children. This dressing is then removed from the harvesting device and several holes are punctured through the dressing to allow for drainage, and the dressing is then applied to the preprepared recipient site.
- If nonautomated systems are used, the blister can be cut using scissors. Placing a glass slide against the surface of the pierced blister can help collect the epidermal tissue in preparation for placement on recipient site. Once in place, surgical glue may be used to help attach the graft if recipient site is mobile.
- After placement of epidermal grafts, adhesive dressing and gauze are applied and taped down to provide a stable pressure dressing for at least 24 to 48 hours. This applies to both methods of epidermal grafting. Usually, the dressing is taken down after 2 to 3 days in the office.

Postprocedural Approach

- The donor site is a minor (epidermal) wound that can be treated simply with petrolatum ointment and a nonadherent dressing. Pain medication is generally not needed.
- At the recipient site, the array of epidermal blisters adheres within an hour, but takes about 2 days to integrate into the recipient skin.
- Three days after grafting, an array of pigmented macules with surrounding outgrowth of epidermis should be visible through the transparent dressing, and the dressing can be gently removed.
- Abrasion or wiping at this stage should be avoided.
- Both the donor and recipient sites should be treated with standard wound care, such as application of sterile petrolatum and nonadhesive dressings, which can be removed around day 5.
- Patients are asked to avoid swimming, shaving, light exposure, or use of topical medications to the graft site.
- A fully formed new epidermis should be present at about 1 week. Pigmentation, however, requires longer because melanocytes migrate much more slowly than do keratinocytes, as illustrated in Figure 73.1.
- Unlike punch grafting or split-thickness skin grafting, epidermal suction blister grafting does not leave an abnormal texture or pattern.

II. Melanocyte Keratinocyte Transfer Procedures

Preprocedural Approach

- To use this treatment method, vitiligo must be stable.
- This approach refers to any cellular graft, cultured or uncultured. Although cultured graft preparation requires collaboration with a skilled laboratory, uncultured grafts can be prepared in office; however, this requires adequate training.

- For uncultured cell grafts, cells may be provided from epidermis (noncultured epidermal suspension [NCES]) or anagen hairs (outer root sheath hair follicle suspension [ORSHFS]).
- Determine the required amount of donor tissue by estimating a 1:3 to 1:5 donor-to-recipient ratio.

Procedural Approach

- For NCES, epidermal blisters are used as the cell source and may be harvested as mentioned earlier.
- Tissue from the blister is digested using trypsin and incubated until cells separate from the stratum corneum. Trypsin inhibitor is then added to terminate enzymatic degradation. Cells can then be collected and dissolved in Ringer lactate solution.
- Alternatively, the commercially available disposable RECELL system can be used. It includes degradation enzyme and buffer solution. This results in the production of a regenerative epidermal suspension containing fibroblasts, keratinocytes, and melanocytes.
- Prepare the recipient site by removing overlying epidermis, as described in the epidermal blister section.
- The dermabraded recipient site can then be treated with prepared solution that should be evenly spread over the area. If the suspension consistency is too fluid, it can be mixed into hyaluronic acid gels.
- The treated area is then covered with a first layer of collagen dressing, followed by petrolatum-impregnated gauze and covered with a layer of absorbent cotton pads.

Postprocedural Approach

- The donor site is a minor (epidermal) wound that can be treated simply with petrolatum ointment and a nonadherent dressing. Pain medication is generally not needed.
- Recipient site should remain dry and covered with dressing for 4 to 7 days after the procedure.

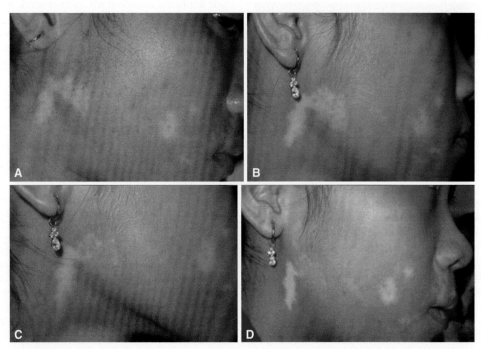

FIGURE 73.1. A 16-year-old Asian girl with segmental vitiligo. A, Pretreatment, just before epidermal blister grafting of one lesion on the lateral face. B, One month post treatment shows transfer of pigmented blister array. C, Two months post treatment shows outgrowth of pigmentation from grafts. D, Six months post treatment shows repigmentation of treated site. Untreated sites remain unchanged.

- Patients are informed that greenish discharge can be expected.
- Patients are asked to avoid swimming, shaving, light exposure, or use of topical medications to graft site.

III. Punch Grafts

Preprocedural Approach

- Full-thickness skin tissue repopulation of vitiliginous lesions can allow transfer of adnexal structures including hair follicles and associated melanocytes.
- This technique is laborious and notorious for having the highest rate of adverse effects. "Polka-dot" or "cobblestone" appearance, scarring, and keloid formation are all possible outcomes associated with such procedures. For this reason, this procedure is generally not recommended.
- Donor site must consist of healthy, normally pigmented tissue, free from injury or infection. Vitiligo at recipient site must be stable.
- Donor and recipient site are cleaned with alcohol before procedure and then anesthetized with local infiltration.

Procedural Approach

- Small 1- to 2-mm grafts are collected from a healthy inconspicuous donor site. Similar caliber grafts are removed from recipient site, spaced 5 to 10 mm apart.
- Collected donor grafts are relocated into the recipient site with the dermal portion of the graft in direct contact with the dermis.
- The ART System is a new harvesting device that is able to collect over 300 microscopic full-thickness tissue columns without the associated side effects of larger biopsies at donor sites. Its utility for treating vitiligo has yet to be assessed; however, it could possibly be a useful tool for tissue collection from the donor site in the future.

Postprocedural Approach

- The donor site can be covered in antibiotic cream and overlying nonadhesive dressing and is left to heal by secondary intention. This should take 1 week.
- The recipient site is covered with gauze and surgical tape to form a pressure dressing, preventing mobility of grafts for 2 weeks. This dressing may be changed 4 to 7 days after the procedure.
- Dressing area for both donor and recipient site must be kept clean, dry and unexposed to sun.

IV. Split-Thickness Skin Grafts

Preprocedural Approach

- A thorough discussion of risks versus benefits should be made. It is difficult to achieve excellent results with this procedure because the texture, pigmentation, and pattern of the donor site are transferred; in contrast, epidermal suction blister and cell suspension grafts take on the texture and pattern of recipient skin.
- Split-thickness grafting is associated with more donor site morbidity. Although suction blister donor sites typically heal to normal skin, split-thickness donor sites typically cause permanent scarring.
- Prepare both donor and recipient sites by cleaning area with antiseptic cleaning product of choice and anesthetizing with local infiltration.
- One week before the procedure, daily application of topical antibiotic may be suggested.

Procedural Approach

- For this procedure, ultrathin grafts of uniform thickness must be used (~0.1 mm). This can be harvested using a dermatome.
- Recipient site is dermabraded as mentioned in the epidermal blister section. Once again, this procedure must go beyond the margins to avoid formation of a hypopigmented halo around the graft.
- Harvested tissue is then relocated to the recipient site while avoiding wrinkling or curling of the graft at the margins. Surgical glue can be used to help adherence at the recipient site. Graft is covered using a pressure dressing.

Postprocedural Approach

- The donor site is covered with Xeroform™ (Covidien/Medtronic) or similar petrolatum-embedded dressing followed by gauze, and can be reinforced with a mild compression dressing. Dressing can be removed around day 3 to 5 and Xeroform can be left to peel off on its own.
- At the recipient site, the sterile gauze is used to dress the wound, which is then covered with pads or combine dressings followed by a soft gauze wrap with equal pressure throughout the wound. The dressing can be changed around day 7, at which time graft will be assessed for adequate adhesion. The area may be gently cleaned one to two times a day, avoiding direct impact of water on to the graft site. The wound must be properly dried with surgical gauze and covered in petrolatum or antibiotic ointment for another week with daily dressing changes.
- Both donor and recipient sites should be kept clean and dry, minimizing sun exposure, and sunscreen should be used. Sun exposure can lead to postinflammatory hyper and hypopigmentation, which is not desirable.
- Patients are asked to avoid swimming, shaving, light exposure, or use of topical medications to graft site.

SUGGESTED READINGS

Bassiouny D, Esmat S. Autologous non-cultured melanocyte–keratinocyte transplantation in the treatment of vitiligo: patient selection and perspectives. *Clin Cosmet Investig Dermatol.* 2018;11:521–540.

Dellatorre G, Bertolini W, Castro CCS. Optimizing suction blister epidermal graft technique in the surgical treatment of vitiligo. *An Bras Dermatol.* 2017;92(6):888–890. doi:10.1590/abd1806-4841.20176332.

Majid I. Grafting in vitiligo: how to get better results and how to avoid complications. *J Cutan Aesthet Surg.* 2013;6(2):83–89.

Shi Q, Li K, Fu J, et al. Comparison of the 308-nm excimer laser with the 308-nm excimer lamp in the treatment of vitiligo—a randomized bilateral comparison study. *Photodermatol Photoimmunol Photomed.* 2013;29(1):27–33. doi:10.1111/phpp.12015.

Vachiramon V. A concise approach to childhood hypopigmentation. *J Cutan Aesthet Surg.* 2013;6(2):73–74.

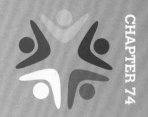
Dermal Melanocytosis (Mongolian Spot)

Dawn Z. Eichenfield and Lawrence F. Eichenfield

Introduction

Dermal melanocytosis usually presents sporadically at birth as blue to blue-gray or blue-brown unilateral or bilateral macules and patches, sometimes coalescing into near-confluent sheets. Because they typically resolve spontaneously in childhood, these lesions almost never require treatment (Figures 74.1 and 74.2). In addition to sporadic dermal melanocytosis, multiple genetic conditions present with extensive dermal melanocytosis, including GM1 gangliosidosis, lysosomal storage diseases (Hunter and Hurler syndrome), and phakomatosis pigmentovascularis.

Phakomatosis pigmentovascularis is a group of congenital skin conditions, which phenotypically manifests as a collision of a vascular and melanocytic lesion (often dermal melanocytosis) and is thought to be due to a postzygotic mutation in the *GNA11* or *GNAQ* gene. Dermal melanocytoses are present in three types of phakomatosis pigmentovascularis, type II (phakomatosis cesioflammea consisting of port wine stain + dermal melanocytosis +/− nevus), type IV (port wine stain + dermal melanocytosis + nevus spilus +/− nevus anemicus), and type V (phakomatosis cesiomarmorata consisting of cutis marmorata telangiectatica congenita + dermal melanocytosis) phakomatosis pigmentovascularis. Oftentimes, these dermal melanocytosis can be persistent and may be a source of anxiety for the patient. For that reason, remnant dermal melanocytosis may be treated with laser therapy.

Here, we discuss the treatment of dermal melanocytosis with Q-switched ruby, Q-switched alexandrite, Q-switched Nd:YAG lasers, and picosecond alexandrite lasers. There are reports of other lasers being utilized (eg, fractionated 1440-nm Nd:YAG laser). Multiple treatments are usually needed and the response to treatment ranges from lesion lightening to complete clearance.

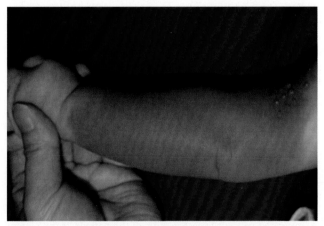

FIGURE 74.1. Dermal melanocytosis on a 3-month-old boy prior to treatment. Photo courtesy of Hyunchang Ko, MD, PhD.

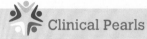

Clinical Pearls

- **Guidelines:** No specific guidelines or expert consensus papers exist for this condition.
- **Age-Specific Considerations:** Patients who are of the age of consent or assent may be treated. Larger lesions and young patients may be managed utilizing general anesthesia to minimize pain and anxiety, and allow for technically appropriate laser surgery.
- **Skin of Color Considerations:** Q-switched ruby laser and Q-switched alexandrite laser can be utilized for skin types I to III. Picosecond alexandrite laser can be utilized for skin types I to IV. Q-switched Nd:YAG laser can be utilized for darker skin types, with caution given the greater likelihood of posttreatment side effects and complications.

Contraindications/Cautions/Risks

Contraindications

- The presence of an active skin infection
- Patients with a history of keloids
- The inability to perform posttreatment wound care

Cautions

- The presence of a suntan or prior history of melasma as well as other pigmentary disorders (postinflammatory hyperpigmentation) may result in increased skin dyspigmentation and other complications after the procedure.

Risks

- Edema and erythema after the laser procedure, transient hypopigmentation or hyperpigmentation, texture changes, slight scarring, permanent hyperpigmentation or hypopigmentation, incomplete clearance, repigmentation or recurrence, infection, and complications of general anesthesia

Equipment Needed

- Wavelength-specific eye shields, glasses, or goggles; metal eye shields for periocular lesions; opaque eye patches
- Q-switched ruby (694-nm) laser
- Q-switched alexandrite (755-nm) laser
- Q-switched Nd:YAG (1064-nm) laser
- Picosecond alexandrite (755-nm) laser
- Smoke evacuator
- Marking pen (white, "gelly roll" gel-ink pens preferred)
- Ice or cooling system
- Petrolatum-based ointment

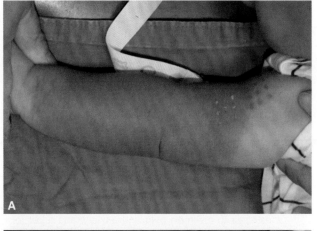

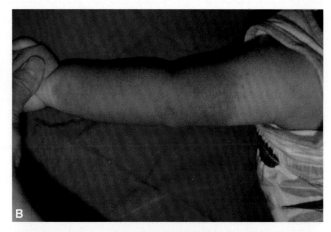

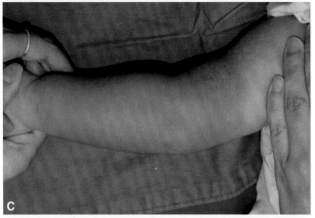

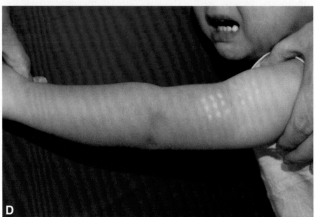

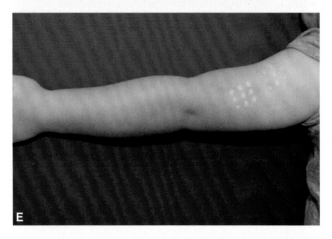

FIGURE 74.2. Dermal melanocytosis treated with Q-switched Nd:YAG (1064-nm) laser after two (A), four (B), six (C), twelve (D), and eighteen sessions (E). The lighter spots on the proximal arm are hypopigmented scars from stamp-type BCG vaccination, which were covered by pigmentation from the dermal melanocytosis and became more visible after laser treatment. Photo courtesy of Hyunchang Ko, MD, PhD.

Preprocedural Approach

- Several months before treatment, we ask patients to minimize sun exposure and maximize sun protection to allow greater contrast between the treatment area and surrounding skin. The purpose is to reduce melanin in the nonlesional skin.
- If there is a history of herpes simplex, prophylaxis for herpes simplex is started 1 to 2 days before laser surgery and continued for 1 week after surgery.
- Patients are asked to bathe the treatment area either the previous evening or in the morning before laser surgery.
- Topical anesthetic cream, for example, liposomal lidocaine 4% or a mixture of lidocaine 2.5%/prilocaine 2.5%, is applied under occlusion for 1 hour before the procedure.

- Oral analgesics (eg, acetaminophen) may be utilized for non–general anesthesia procedures, 30 minutes before the procedure.
- General anesthesia may be required for larger lesions and/or younger patients.

Procedural Approach

- Informed consent is obtained from the patient. If the patient is a minor, informed consent should be obtained from the parent/guardian and assent obtained from the minor.
- All personnel in the procedure room should wear wavelength-specific appropriate eyewear. Correctly fitted metal eye shields should be worn by the patient for periocular nevus of Ota. Wavelength-specific eye shields (glasses or goggles) or opaque eye patches may be utilized otherwise.

- Treatment should be initiated at the threshold fluence (eg, the minimum fluence to produce the laser endpoint of immediate tissue whitening). Higher fluences can result in erythema, edema, and punctuate bleeding.
- There is great variability in laser settings and output, and laser settings should be determined by the clinical endpoint.
- The clinical endpoint is immediate tissue whitening. There should be no overlapping of pulses in general. Treatments should be performed at 2- to 4-month intervals until patient satisfaction.
- Immediately after surgery, intermittent ice compression can be applied for 20 minutes to reduce pain and swelling.
- Petrolatum-based ointment is liberally applied. Any crusting is left on the skin as a biologic dressing.
- Sunscreen and diligent sun protection should be restarted.

Postprocedural Approach

- Postoperative swelling and pain should quickly decrease with time. For postoperative pain, patients can use acetaminophen or ibuprofen with standard dosing. Continued intermittent ice compression can be applied to reduce swelling.
- For patients with a history of herpes simplex, they should continue herpes prophylaxis for a total of 7 to 10 days.
- Postoperatively, patients should be informed that bruising may develop in areas with more pigment. Over the next several days, shallow blisters or crusting may develop.
- Patient should be monitored for symptoms and signs of infection.
- Postoperative downtime is minimal and the skin heals within 7 to 10 days, usually with basic wound care (continued application of petrolatum-based ointment and diligent sun protection). Any crusted dark spots should peel off within

10 to 14 days of treatment. Cosmetics and sunscreen can be applied to the treatment area. Patients should be cautioned to remove facial products very gently because the treatment area is fragile during the healing process.

- Patient should be cautioned that there may be lightening or darkening of the treated area for several months after laser treatment that can be covered easily with cosmetics if desired.
- Patients should be encouraged to contact the physician directly for any questions or concerns.
- Postoperative appointments at 2 weeks and several months after the laser treatment may be offered to evaluate healing and the need for further treatments.

SUGGESTED READINGS

Chan JC, Shek SY, Kono T, Yeung CK, Chan, HH. A retrospective analysis on the management of pigmented lesions using a picosecond 755-nm alexandrite laser in Asians. *Lasers Surg Med.* 2016;48(1):23.

Levin MK, Ng E, Bae YS, Brauer JA, Geronemus RG. Treatment of pigmentary disorders in patients with skin of color with a novel 755 nm picosecond, Q-switched ruby, and Q-switched Nd:YAG nanosecond lasers: a retrospective photographic review. *Lasers Surg Med.* 2016;48(2):181–187.

Ohshiro T, Ohshiro T, Sasaki K, Kishi K. Picosecond pulse duration laser treatment for dermal melanocytosis in Asians: a retrospective review. *Laser Ther.* 2016;25(2):99–104.

Shah VV, Bray FN, Aldahan AS, Mlacker S, Nouri K. Lasers and nevus of Ota: a comprehensive review. *Lasers Med Sci.* 2006;31:179–185.

Tay YK, Chan YC, eds. *Textbook of Laser and Light Dermatology in the Asian Skin.* Hackensack, NJ: World Scientific Publishing; 2011.

Wanner M, Sakamoto FH, Avram MM, et al. Immediate skin responses to laser and light treatments: therapeutic endpoints: how to obtain efficacy. *J Am Acad Dermatol.* 2016;74(5):821–833.

Wanner M, Sakamoto FH, Avram MM, Anderson RR. Immediate skin responses to laser and light treatments: warning endpoints: how to avoid side effects. *J Am Acad Dermatol.* 2016;74(5):807–819.

Dermatofibrosarcoma Protuberans

Guilherme Canho Bittner and Nelise Ritter Hans-Bittner

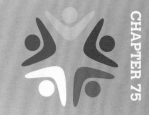

CHAPTER 75

INTRODUCTION

Dermatofibrosarcoma protuberans (DFSP) is an infiltrative low-grade malignancy expressing CD34. Its annual incidence per million inhabitants is 4.2 in the United States. Soft-tissue sarcomas represent less than 1% of malignant tumors overall, and the prevalence of DFSP before 20 years of age is very rare: 1.0 per million.[1,2]

It does not coexist with other dermatologic conditions. Because of the rarity of the tumor, diagnosis of DFSP in children is quite difficult (Figure 75.1).

Histologically, DFSP exhibits small, elongated cells arranged in a storiform pattern extending into the subcutaneous fat. It is usually seen in adults but can occur in infancy and childhood.[1]

Herein we offer our step-by-step instructions to treat this tumor. Excision is with wide margins (3 cm) or, our preferred option, Mohs micrographic surgery (MMS). Both carry an excellent prognosis, but Mohs surgery tends to save more tumor-free tissue and has less chance of recurrence.[1-3]

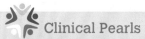
Clinical Pearls

- **Guidelines:** MMS is a 2A recommendation, although a wide excision (3 cm) can be performed.[3]
- **Age-Specific Considerations:** Some patients are old enough to be aware of the procedure and cooperate with the surgeon. In these patients, the MMS procedure can be performed with local anesthesia.
- **Technique Tips:**
  - Bupivacaine 0.5% with epinephrine 1:200 000 is a long-lasting anesthetic and is well tolerated after lidocaine. It acts as an adjunct in decreasing the patient's pain during the procedure.
  - Usually because of the recurrence rate (~6% without MMS and 2% with MMS), a flap is not the recommended first option for reconstruction.
- **Skin of Color Considerations:** The technique can be performed in any skin color.

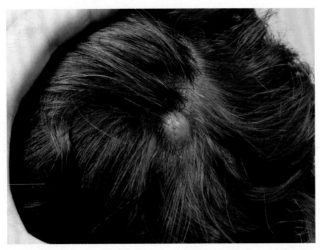

FIGURE 75.1. A 7-year-old boy who was misdiagnosed with a pilar cyst and ended up needing Mohs surgery for this myxoid dermatofibrosarcoma protuberans. Photo courtesy of Andrew C. Krakowski, MD.

Contraindications/Cautions/Risks

Contraindications
- Active skin infection on surgical site
- Inability to care for postoperative wounds

Cautions
- History of bleeding and allergic reactions (check family history)

Risks
- Death (infection or anesthesia), scarring, pain, bleeding, recurrence of lesions. The parents must be aware that permanent scarring sometimes resulting in poor cosmesis can occur, especially with skin grafts.

Equipment Needed
- Lidocaine 1% with epinephrine 1:100 000
- Saline
- Bupivacaine 0.5% with epinephrine 1:200 000
- Scalpel
- Scissors
- Clamps
- Hooks
- Hemostatic clamps
- Electrocautery
- Smoke evacuator
- Gauze
- Surgical marker pen
- Tissue stain
- Mohs laboratory (cryostat, hematoxylin and eosin stain)
- Suture
- Petrolatum-based ointment
- Micropore Surgical Tape™ (3M, US)

Preoperative Approach

- Bring all medications to show the doctor. Continue taking all regular medicines except those that affect bleeding.
- Prophylaxis for herpes simplex is not necessary.
- Patients should bathe either the evening before or on the morning of their surgery.

- Patients should be advised not to take supplements such as ginkgo, vitamin E, niacin, fish oil tablets, or nonsteroidal anti-inflammatory medicines (ibuprofen, naproxen, etc) for 1 week before surgery because they can increase bleeding.

Procedural Approach

- Informed consent from the parent/guardian and, when possible, assent from the minor are obtained.
- Typically, general anesthesia (sometimes with concurrent local anesthesia) is utilized in young children.
- During the laboratory period, depending on the size of the tumor, the patient remains under general anesthesia (usually for no more than 4 hours at a time).
- If the laboratory work will take more than 4 hours, we wake up the patient and he or she waits for the result in a hospital room with his or her family.
- The area of the tumor is marked with a permanent pen. The first margin is 1 to 1.3 cm from the visible tumor edge.
- The surgery site must be cleansed, usually with alcohol 70%, chlorhexidine 2%, or a combination of both, such as Chlora-Prep (BD).
- We recommend lidocaine 1% with epinephrine 1:100 000 for local anesthesia. To reduce pain during anesthesia infiltration, inject slowly. A repetitive movement with the finger tips around the needle can reduce the pain of injection. Also, good conversation and ambient music can help distract the patient and keep him or her relaxed during the procedure.
- When the patient is sufficiently anesthetized, bupivacaine 0.5% with epinephrine 1:200 000 is then infiltrated around the area. Sometimes laboratory work can take several hours depending on the tumor size; this long-acting anesthetic will keep the area numb.
- The surgical site is cleansed again with another antiseptic, either with alcohol 70%, chlorhexidine 2%, or a combination of both, such as ChloraPrep™ (Becton, Dickinson and Company, US).
- The tumor is then cut to the subcutaneous layer with a number 15 scalpel.
- A Mohs layer is taken after that, with a second scalpel (preventing tumor contamination) and the tissue is marked with proper tissue stains.
- Good hemostasis is then made with electrocauterization, using clamps if necessary.
- A dressing with saline and gauze should cover the surgical defect until the closure or a new Mohs surgery stage.
- The procedure continues for as many stages as needed until all surgical margins are cleared.
- Next, after clear margins are obtained, reconstruction is performed.
  - Usually, because of the recurrence rate (~6% without MMS and 2% with MMS), a flap is not the recommended first option.
  - For some areas, depending on the tumor size and dimension (oval, circle, or another shape), a primary closure is an option.
  - A full-thickness graft is often required.
    - We typically harvest from the supraclavicular site because of the thickness of this skin area (it is thinner than other areas) and because it closes fairly easily.
    - The donor site is then closed, first, with deep sutures, such as Monocryl™, Vicryl™, or PDS™ (Ethicon US, LLC). External suturing is performed with Prolene™ (Ethicon US, LLC) or plain gut fast absorbable.

- The graft is sutured in the wound's edge with Prolene or another nonabsorbable suture.
- Clean the surgical site with saline and dry well.
- Afterward, a petrolatum-based ointment is applied over the graft with overlying nonabsorbable gauze.
- A second layer of the dressing is made with another layer of gauze and Micropore Surgical Tape to keep pressure on the wound and prevent bleeding.

- In some places, where MMS is not an option to treat patients with DFSP, a similar approach is made; however, the margin from the tumor edges is wider (3 cm). Personally, we recommend marking the edge of the specimen, after the excision with a suture (eg, "12 o'clock" with one suture and "3 o'clock" with two sutures) and two small cuts at "6 o'clock" and "9 o'clock" to have an idea where the further approach should be made if a margin is positive for additional tumor.

Postprocedural Approach

- Generally, pain increases the night after the excision. Pain medications such as Tylenol are usually enough to control it. After the second day, pain should decrease.
- It is normal to have swelling and bruising around the surgical site. The bruising will fade in approximately 10 to 14 days. Elevate the area to reduce swelling.
- The outer bandage remains in place for 24 hours. Remove it carefully after this time.
- The inner bandage is left in place for 1 week. Keep it dry.
- For skin grafts, avoid prolonged exposure to extremely cold temperatures for 3 weeks.

- Patients should be vigilantly monitored for signs and symptoms of infection, especially for symptoms of pain, fever, or increasing redness in the area.
- Postoperative downtime is significant, and patients should expect to be absent from school or work for at least 1 week.
- After a follow-up appointment to directly assess the graft about 7 to 10 days after surgery, the sutures should be removed (absorbable sutures often work better for children).
- One week after surgery, patients should be instructed to gently cleanse the area with soapy water using a Q-tip or gauze pad (shower/bathe normally). Dry the wound and apply Vaseline™ (Conopco, Inc., US), Polysporin™ (Johnson & Johnson, US), or bacitracin ointment (do *not* use Neosporin™ [Johnson & Johnson, US]).
- Cover the wound with a nonstick gauze pad and paper tape.
- Repeat wound care once a day for another week.
- After 1 week, continue to apply ointment until fully healed.
- Patients are encouraged to contact the physician directly for concerns, and our surgeons often provide their cell phone numbers for direct contact and reassurance.

REFERENCES

1. Buteau AH, Keeling BH, Diaz LZ, et al. Dermatofibrosarcoma protuberans in pediatric patients: a diagnostic and management challenge. *JAAD Case Rep.* 2018;4:155–158. doi:10.1016/j.jdcr.2017.09.022.
2. Wollina U. Dermatofibrosarcoma protuberans in a 10-year-old child. *J Dermatol Case Rep.* 2013;7:121–124. doi:10.3315/jdcr.2013.1160.
3. Saiag P, Grob JJ, Lebbe C, et al., Diagnosis and treatment of dermatofibrosarcoma protuberans. European consensus-based interdisciplinary guideline. *Eur J Cancer.* 2015;51:2604–2608. doi:10.1016/j.ejca.2015.06.108.

Dermoid Cysts

John C. Browning and Folawiyo Babalola

CHAPTER 76

Introduction

A dermoid cyst (DC) can be clinically described as an epithelium-lined cavity in the body containing differentiated structures such as sebaceous glands, hair follicles, or sweat glands that form subcutaneously as a result of entrapment of tissue at fusion lines during development. These cysts are usually asymptomatic and may go unnoticed until early childhood when they begin to enlarge. They normally present within the first decade of life and at equal rates among males and females, regardless of race or ethnicity.[1,2] They usually appear as bluish or skin-colored subcutaneous nodules, and because they are usually so clinically evident, they comprise the most frequently diagnosed benign orbital lesions in children.

DCs most commonly develop on the head and neck, particularly around the eyebrows, forehead, scalp, or below the chin. DCs seen in children can be categorized into four groups based on their location (Figure 76.1):

- Group 1 cysts develop in the periorbital region and appear along the naso-optic groove between the maxillary and mandibular processes during embryonal closure.

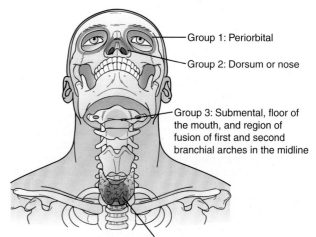

Group 1: Periorbital

Group 2: Dorsum or nose

Group 3: Submental, floor of the mouth, and region of fusion of first and second branchial arches in the midline

Group 4: Midventral and middorsal fusion in suprasternal, thyroidal, and suboccipital regions

FIGURE 76.1. Common dermoid cyst locations on the head and neck.

- Group 2 cysts develop over the dorsum of the nose and are thought to develop during ossification of the frontonasal plate.
- Group 3 cysts are found in the submental region, the floor of the mouth, and the region of fusion of the first and second branchial arches in the midline.
- Group 4 cysts are formed at the midventral and middorsal fusion in the suprasternal, thyroidal, and suboccipital regions, where they are typically confused with thyroglossal duct cysts or thyroid neoplasms, suprasternal masses and enlarged lymph nodes, or meningoencephaloceles.[3]

DCs tend to be located superficially, making definitive management of the lesion usually quick and relatively straightforward. However, some DCs can develop with a sinus tract that allows communication between the skin surface and the cystic components, leading to a high risk of infection. Prior to definitive procedural management, DCs may be investigated using ultrasound or computed tomography (CT) scan to better delineate involvement of the surrounding tissues. If a sinus is found to be present, it should be explored using a sinogram at the surgeon's discretion.

Currently, there are two main approaches for the treatment of DCs, which include open, direct excision and endoscopic removal. Both approaches require complete resection of the DC to prevent recurrence and are both equally effective. Patients typically prefer the endoscopic approach because of better cosmetic outcomes and minimal scarring compared to direct excision.

Cost-effectiveness and the potential for hair loss are factors that may influence physicians to prefer direct excision, and this is the focus of this chapter.

Clinical Pearls

- **Guidelines:** No specific treatment guidelines are known to exist for this condition.
- **Age-Specific Considerations:** The age of the child and the child's ability to cooperate with the surgical team typically guide the decision to perform this procedure under general anesthesia.
- **Technique Tips:** Direct excision has been noted and widely supported by dermatologists as an appropriate measure for the removal of DCs. In the rare instance that a child presents with an ovarian cyst, laparoscopic surgery is the preferred approach.
  - Different DC locations have particularly preferred incision sites. For example, in the case that the DC is endophytic (inside the orbital rim), superficial lesions should be approached through crease incision. If the DC is exophytic (extending outside the orbital rim), lesions should be approached through infrabrow incision. If the DC is a deep orbital lesion with a defective wall, the approach should be through exposure, intended evacuation, dissection, and excision of the remaining cyst wall.[1,2] In endophytic and deep orbital lesion excisions, oculoplastics or ophthalmology consults should be considered.
  - DC presenting in the *midline* can have intracranial extensions. If CT and magnetic resonance imaging (MRI) demonstrate intracranial extension, the standard approach is the anterior bifrontal craniotomy.

This consists of a bicoronal incision with subpericranial scalp elevation. A neurosurgery consult should be considered.
- **Skin of Color Considerations:** No specific considerations

Contraindications/Cautions/Risks

Contraindications
- Active skin infection in the surgical area
- Inability to care for postoperative wounds

Cautions: Consider possibility of intracranial extensions for midline lesions

Risks: Risks associated with direct excision are generally minimal. The primary risk is that of recurrence with failure of complete removal of the DC. During the procedure, caution should be taken to prevent cyst rupture, which increases the risk of recurrence. There may also be localized inflammatory reactions to retained cyst material, seroma and hematoma formation, infection, and edema at the site of the incision. Additionally, patients and their families should be made aware of the potential for scar and/or bruising.

Equipment Needed
- Blade
- Marking pen
- Suture
- Fine forceps
- Skin hooks
- Scissors
- Saline
- Cauterizer
- Antiseptic wipe

Preprocedural Approach

- Prior to surgery, different imaging techniques should be used to gauge the status of the child. For instance, when a nasal midline DC is suspected, ultrasound, followed by CT or MRI, can be employed to rule out intracranial involvement.[4] In children under 2 years of age, CT and MRI sometimes require general anesthesia to be properly performed. General anesthesia should also be provided prior to the procedure in children who have exceptional fear of needles or other parts of the procedure.
- Methylene blue has recently been indicated as a valuable tool to facilitate appropriate, morbidity-sparing management of midline DCs.[4] Methylene blue is used as a dye and can demonstrate the extent of the cyst. This technique is most useful in cases of equivocal imaging or to confirm the absence of intracranial extension.[4]

Procedural Approach

- The child should be locally anesthetized with lidocaine in addition to general anesthesia.

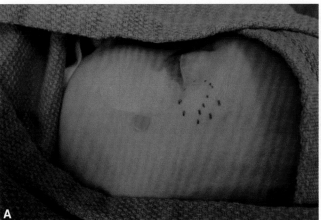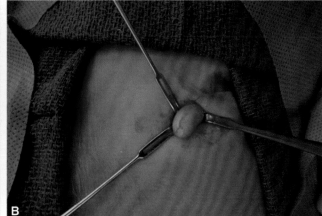

FIGURE 76.2. A, Preoperative photo with periorbital dermoid cyst delineated with blue surgical marker; the child is under general anesthesia. B, Intraoperative photo with periorbital dermoid cyst fully exposed in preparation for complete dissection.

- A fenestrated drape can be placed on the patient with the fenestrated portion bordering the DC.
- Once the child is appropriately anesthetized, pomade should be added to the eye prior to surgery to protect the eyeball, particularly if the cyst is periorbital.
- The DC area should be wiped with an antiseptic such as alcohol.
- Borders of the cyst and the incision site should be marked with the marking pen (Figure 76.2A).
- Different DC locations have particularly preferred incision sites. For example, in the case that the DC is endophytic (inside the orbital rim), superficial lesions should be approached through crease incision. If the DC is exophytic (extending outside the orbital rim), lesions should be approached through infrabrow incision. If the DC is a deep orbital lesion with a defective wall, the approach should be through exposure, intended evacuation, dissection, and excision of the remaining cyst wall.[1,2] In the occasion that the DC is located nasofrontally, a vertical or horizontal incision should be made parallel to the relaxed skin tension lines directly over the mass.
- After selecting the correct incision site, an incision should be made 1 cm in size with the blade, making sure not to expose the contents of the cyst.
- Sharp dissection with scissors should be made to expose the cyst.
- Once exposed, skin hooks should be placed at the site of incision to assist with the feasibility of dissection (Figure 76.2B).
- The DC should be lightly grasped using forceps.
- At this point, the DC should then be bluntly dissected from fascial attachments for complete evacuation.
- In the instance that the contents of the DC are exposed, irrigation of the site with a saline solution should be done to ensure complete removal of the cyst to prevent recurrence.
- Once the cyst is completely resected, the incision site should be cauterized.
- Lastly, a suture should be placed at the site.
- In group 1 cysts, a suture of the orbicularis oculi muscle must be fixed prior to suturing of the skin.

Postprocedural Approach

- Recovery is typically uneventful. A follow-up appointment should be made for wound evaluation 2 weeks after the procedure.
- Parents are instructed to gently clean the incision site with soap and warm water and to monitor the wound for excessive redness or pus formation, in which case parent needs to return before the 2-week follow-up.
- Recurrence is also common when the cyst is not completely removed and should be monitored by the parent.
- At the 2-week follow-up, the wound is evaluated for infection and rupture and removal of nondissolvable sutures.
- If a craniotomy was performed, the patient must be prescribed intravenous (IV) steroids to prevent serious complication of meningitis.

REFERENCES

1. Eldesouky MA, Elbakary MA. Orbital dermoid cyst: classification and its impact on surgical management. *Semin Ophthalmol.* 2018;33:170–174. doi:10.1080/08820538.2016.1182636.
2. Khanna G, Sato Y, Smith RJH, Bauman NM, Nerad J. Causes of facial swelling in pediatric patients: correlation of clinical and radiologic findings. *Radiographics.* 2006;26(1):157–171. doi:10.1148/rg.261055050.
3. Pryor SG, Lewis JE, Weaver AL, Orvidas LJ. Pediatric dermoid cysts of the head and neck. *Otolaryngol Head Neck Surg.* 2005;132(6):938–942. doi:10.1016/j.otohns.2005.03.005
4. Phelan AL, Jones CM, Ceschini AS, Henry CR, Mackay DR, Samson TD. Sparing a craniotomy. *Plast Reconstr Surg.* 2017;139(6):1445–1451. doi:10.1097/prs.0000000000003369

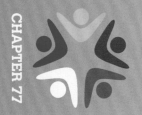

Epidermal Inclusion Cysts and Pilar Cysts

Austin Carter Smith and John C. Browning

CHAPTER 77

Introduction

Cysts of all types are a common occurrence in any patient population, including pediatrics. Epidermal inclusion cysts and pilar cysts are among the most common cutaneous cysts in pediatric populations. These cysts are easily treatable with excision and have positive treatment outcomes. Cutaneous cysts in children are commonly found when they become infected. Infections in cysts should be resolved before they are excised to decrease the risk of spreading the infection. The basic outline for cyst treatment is addressed and specific directions for treating each cyst are explained.[1]

EPIDERMAL INCLUSION CYSTS

Epidermal inclusion cysts, also known as epidermoid cysts, are derived from epidermal cells that proliferate within the dermis. The cells proliferate within an enclosed space, and a growth comprising squamous cell debris develops. They can be caused by invagination of epidermal cells owing to trauma or surgery. They present as skin-colored dermal nodules and regularly have a visible central punctum. Epidermal inclusion cysts are among the most common cysts in adults, but they can also found in children. If a pediatric patient has recurrent or excessive epidermoid cysts, this can be suggestive of an underlying disorder such as Gardner syndrome. These cysts are found in the same rates among boys and girls regardless of race or ethnicity. Epidermoid cysts do not always cause discomfort or pain. They do occasionally become infected but can also become inflamed because of external irritation.

These cysts do not usually need to be imaged with ultrasound or computed tomography (CT) because these do not typically penetrate underlying tissues in the way, for example, that dermoid cysts may do. Epidermal inclusion cysts can break apart easily during extraction, so additional care must be exercised to ensure total removal. It is helpful to examine and flush the defect with sterile saline once the cyst has been removed to ensure no remnants have been left behind. If completely removed, these cysts do not typically recur.

There are a few ways to approach the procedural treatment of an epidermoid cyst.

APPROACH #1: INTRALESIONAL CORTICOSTEROID

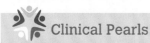 Clinical Pearls

- **Guidelines:** If the cyst is only transiently irritated and the patient does not want to undergo an excision, then the cyst can be injected with corticosteroids.
- **Age-Specific Considerations:** None
- **Technique Tips:** Inject small volumes around the cyst while avoiding injecting into the cyst itself. When injecting, it is important to inject only small amounts of the solution into the cyst.
- **Skin of Color Considerations:** Steroid injections can cause hypopigmentation in darker skin; use with caution.

Contraindications/Cautions/Risks

Contraindications
- None

Cautions
- If excessive solution is injected into the cyst, there is a risk that it will rupture and cause scarring.

Risks
- Hypopigmentation, atrophy, infection

Equipment Needed
- Corticosteroid (triamcinolone 0.2 mL at 10 mg/mL)
- 27-gauge short needle × 2
- 3-mL syringe × 2
- Gloves
- Alcohol swabs
- Lidocaine

Preprocedural Approach
- Informed consent from the parent/guardian and, when possible, assent from the minor are obtained.

Procedural Approach
- Begin by sanitizing the area with alcohol.
- Inject lidocaine to numb the area.
- Inject corticosteroid into the dermis surrounding the cyst, trying to inject as closely as possible to the cyst without puncturing the cyst wall.
- Move the needle in the skin to inject in a wider area without requiring excessive needlesticks for the patient.

Postprocedural Approach
- The patient should be instructed to keep the area clean and watch for any signs of infection.
- The inflammation should decrease within 3 to 5 days.
- The patient should be instructed to return if the cyst becomes inflamed or infected in the future.
- Further treatment with excision might be required.

APPROACH #2: SURGICAL EXCISION

 Clinical Pearls

- **Guidelines:** Excision is a definitive treatment for cysts.
- **Age-Specific Considerations:** This treatment is appropriate at any age but might require general anesthesia in younger pediatric patients.
- **Technique Tips:** It is important to remove the entire intact cyst if possible. There is a risk of recurrence if the

cyst wall is ruptured or if the cyst is incompletely removed. Remove any remnants of the cyst wall if it is not intact. It can be helpful to grasp the cyst between index finger and thumb to provide outward force and elevate cyst.
- **Skin of Color Considerations:** None

Contraindications/Cautions/Risks

Contraindications
- None

Cautions
- Avoid excisions while the cyst is actively inflamed because it will be more difficult to remove intact. Cyst remnants that are left behind will regularly lead to recurrence.

Risks
- Minimal. Bleeding, infection, recurrence

Equipment Needed
- Scalpel and blade
- Local anesthetic
- Aqueous povidone-iodine or alcohol
- Operating scissors
- Forceps
- Electrocautery
- Sutures

Preprocedural Approach

- Informed consent from the parent/guardian and, when possible, assent from the minor are obtained.

Procedural Approach

- Begin with sanitizing the area with iodine or alcohol and administering the local anesthetic.
- When injecting the anesthetic, it must be injected around the cyst rather than into it to get the full effect of the anesthesia as well as to prevent puncture and rupture of the cyst upon removal.
- After the area is sufficiently numb, the cyst will be removed using a direct approach.
- The physician will mark an ellipse that is equal to the diameter of the cyst (Figure 77.1).
- Make a superficial incision over the midline of the cyst, paying special attention not to cut or rupture the cyst (Figure 77.2).
- The initial incision should be made in a direction that will allow the sutures and future scar to be placed in a position for optimal cosmetic and functional outcomes (Figure 77.3).
- The cyst should be dissected out using the operating scissors (Figure 77.4).
- The cyst should be freed on every surface as well as the underside and released from the base.
- Forceps can be used to grip the cyst and manipulate it to reach all angles.
- The cyst should be carefully removed from the opening and the area should be visually inspected for any remnants.
- If the cyst does rupture on removal or dissection, the remnants should be removed using curettage and liberal irrigation.
- The wound should then be closed using sutures (Figure 77.4).

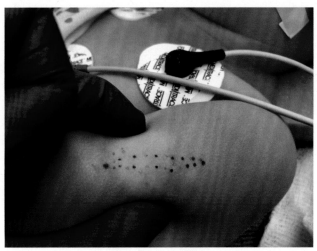

FIGURE 77.1. Photograph of cyst excision prep on upper arm. Note the ellipse outlining the planned excision. Blanching is due to local anesthetic. Photo courtesy of John C. Browning, MD.

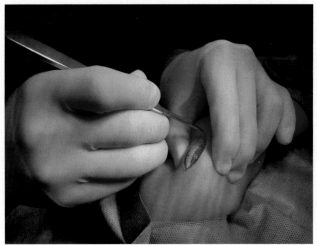

FIGURE 77.2. Excision of cyst. Note grasping technique. Photo courtesy of John C. Browning, MD.

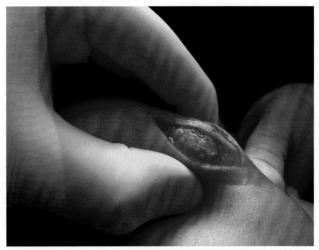

FIGURE 77.3. Close-up of cyst. Note elevation by grasping technique. Photo courtesy of John C. Browning, MD.

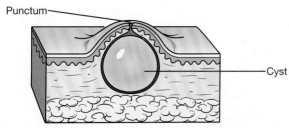

1. Cross section

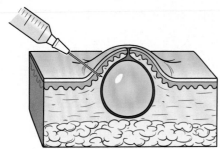

2. Injection of local anesthetic

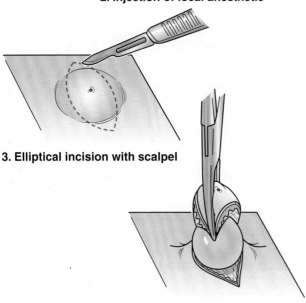

3. Elliptical incision with scalpel

4. Removal of cyst

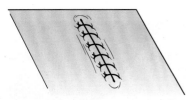

5. Final suture line

FIGURE 77.4. Cyst excision steps.

Postprocedural Approach

- Standard wound care practices should be followed.
- The patient/guardians should be informed of what to expect during the recovery process.
- There may be bruising and redness.

- The area should be kept dry for 24 hours and kept clean until suture removal.
- The sutures can be removed after 1 week.
- The parents should monitor the excision site for any signs of infection or recurrence of the cyst.
- Follow-up can be scheduled as needed.

APPROACH #3: MINIMAL INCISION TECHNIQUE

Another variation to the standard excision is the "punch incision" or "minimal incision" technique (Figure 77.5). These techniques require a smaller incision and, therefore, will leave a smaller scar. The punch incision technique uses a 4-mm punch biopsy instrument to create a hole over the center of the cyst without piercing the capsule. The minimal incision technique uses a small incision over the center of the cyst. This incision is small enough to carefully eject the cyst through and is usually equal to or slightly smaller than the diameter of the cyst itself. For both techniques, lateral pressure helps release the cyst and eject it through the opening. These methods are preferred for cosmetic purposes in areas such as the face. The recurrence rate of these techniques has been reported to be between 4% and 8%.[2]

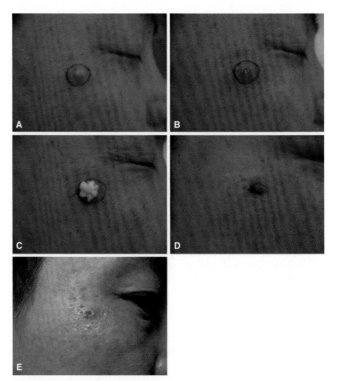

FIGURE 77.5. Minimal incision technique. A, Cyst before procedure. B, Incision into center of skin overlying cyst with a small punch tool. C, Extrusion of cyst. D, Appearance immediately after procedure. E, Appearance 1 week following procedure. Reprinted by permission from Springer: Wu H, Wang S, Wu L, Zheng S. A new procedure for treating a sebaceous cyst: removal of the cyst content with a laser punch and the cyst wall with a minimal postponed excision. *Aesthetic Plast Surg.* 2009;33(4):597–599. Copyright © 2009 Springer Nature.

PILAR CYSTS

Pilar cysts, or trichilemmal cysts, are derived from the root of hair follicles. They are most commonly found on the head and present similarly to epidermal inclusion cysts as firm subcutaneous nodules.[3]

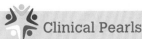 Clinical Pearls

- **Guidelines:** The treatment approach is identical to that for epidermal inclusion cysts. The cyst may be injected with steroids if inflamed or excised.
- **Age-Specific Considerations:** Identical to those listed for epidermoid cysts
- **Technique Tips:** These cysts have a firm capsule and can be extruded through a small opening with lateral pressure. Pilar cysts are found on hair-bearing areas. Surrounding hair may be shaved, but shaving is usually not necessary.
- **Skin of Color Considerations:** None

Contraindications/Cautions/Risks

- Same as listed earlier for epidermal inclusion cyst

Equipment Needed

- Same as listed earlier for epidermal inclusion cyst

Preprocedural Approach

- Same as listed earlier for epidermal inclusion cyst

Procedural Approach

- Begin with sanitizing the area with iodine or alcohol and administering the local anesthetic.
- When injecting the anesthetic, it must be injected around the cyst rather than into it to get the full effect of the anesthesia as well as to prevent puncture and rupture of the cyst upon removal.

- After the patient is sufficiently numb, the cyst will be removed using a direct approach.
- The physician will mark an ellipse that is equal to the diameter of the cyst.
- Make a superficial incision over the midline of the cyst, paying special attention not to cut or rupture the cyst.
- The orientation of the incision is not as important because of the low visibility of scarring under the hair.
- Lateral pressure should be applied to the cyst to extrude the contents.
- If the cyst is not completely expelled, it should be dissected out using the operating scissors and forceps.
- The cyst should be freed on every surface as well as the underside and released from the base.
- The cyst should be carefully removed from the opening and the area should be visually inspected for any remnants.
- The cotton-tipped applicator can be used to clean the area that contained the cyst.
- The wound should then be closed using sutures.
- Special attention should be paid to the hair when closing the wound. Hairs that become trapped under or within the wound can produce a foreign body reaction and create another cyst.

Postprocedural Approach

- The postoperative course is also identical to that of epidermal inclusion cysts.

REFERENCES

1. Orozco-Covarrubias L, Lara-Carpio R, Saez-De-Ocariz M, Duran-Mckinster C, Palacios-Lopez C, Ruiz-Maldonado R. Dermoid cysts: a report of 75 pediatric patients. *Pediatr Dermatol.* 2013;30(6):706–711. doi:10.1111/pde.12080.
2. Mehrabi D, Leonhardt JM, Brodell RT. Removal of keratinous and pilar cysts with the punch incision technique. *Dermatol Surg.* 2002;28(8):673–677. doi:10.1097/00042728-200208000-00005.
3. Al-Khateeb TH, Al-Masri NM, Al-Zoubi F. Cutaneous cysts of the head and neck. *J Oral Maxillofac Surg.* 2009;67(1):52–57. doi:10.1016/j.joms.2007.05.023.

Epidermal Nevi

Allison Zarbo and Marla N. Jahnke

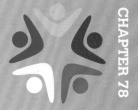

CHAPTER 78

Introduction

Epidermal nevi (ENs) are a heterogeneous group of hamartomatous lesions distributed in the lines of Blaschko (Figure 78.1). These benign, yet sometimes cosmetically disfiguring, lesions, can be unilateral or widespread, localized or extensive. The majority arise at birth or are noticed in early childhood and, although generally stable once present, may appear to extend over time. Lesions are generally asymptomatic, although pruritus is sometimes noted. Extracutaneous abnormalities can rarely be associated with large EN. An appropriate workup to rule out EN syndromes in concerning cases should be pursued prior to treatment.

Owing to the benign course, the treatment of EN is generally considered cosmetic; in some cases, however, the pruritus is severe enough to warrant treatment. Electrodesiccation and curettage, surgical excision, and carbon dioxide (CO_2) laser ablation are discussed in this chapter. Nonsurgical treatment options are often unsatisfactory and limited by significant irritation; they may include topical retinoids, chemotherapeutics (5-fluorouracil), or keratolytics (lactic acid, salicylic acid, urea). Destruction is favored for more immediate and effective treatment, regardless of the lesion thickness. Surgical excision is reserved for smaller lesions where definitive treatment is required, because other destructive methods have a risk of recurrence and

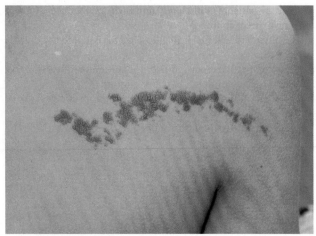

FIGURE 78.1. Photo illustrating the Blaschkolinear nature of a typical epidermal nevus.

may need multiple treatment sessions to maintain the appearance. The authors favor electrodesiccation and curettage because it is a relatively quick, well-tolerated and effective in-office procedure that may be utilized even in young children with the use of local anesthesia.

PROCEDURE: ELECTRODESICCATION AND CURETTAGE

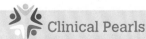 **Clinical Pearls**

- **Guidelines:** No guidelines exist for the treatment of EN.
- **Age-Specific Considerations:** The patient should be old enough to request treatment and willing to sit comfortably for treatment under local anesthesia.
- **Technique Tips:**
  - Histologically, ENs are superficial lesions. The surgeon does not need to curette past the superficial dermis in order to achieve a nice result.
  - In very thick lesions, cautery and curettage do not penetrate well. It can be helpful to initially shave or trim the exophytic portion of the EN with a blade or tissue scissor and then desiccate and curettage the base of the lesion to decrease the risk of recurrence.
- **Skin of Color Considerations:** All skin types are at risk for postinflammatory dyschromia, but darker skin types have an increased likelihood. Those with a predilection to keloid should be made aware that this may be a complication.

Contraindications/Cautions/Risks

Contraindications
- Extensive involvement
- Skin infection
- Inability to care for the wound

Cautions
- Cosmetically sensitive areas
- Skin of color

Risks
- Pain
- Bleeding
- Infection
- Scarring
- Keloids/hypertrophic scars
- Postinflammatory hyperpigmentation or hypopigmentation
- Recurrence is high.

Equipment Needed
- Camera for preoperative documentation
- Masks with eye protection
- Chlorhexidine
- Topical anesthesia
- Local anesthesia
- Sterile curette
- Electrodesiccation device
- For thick lesions, iris scissor or #15 blade or Dermablade™ (Accutec Blades Inc., US)
- Sterile gauze
- Sterile petrolatum–based ointment
- Nonadherent dressing and tape

Preprocedural Approach
- Preprocedural photographs
- Informed consent from the parent/guardian and, when possible, assent from the minor are obtained.
- Application of topical anesthesia approximately 60 minutes prior to procedure

Procedural Approach
- Thoroughly clean with chlorhexidine.
- Inject local anesthesia into the targeted area.
- Trim thick lesions, if applicable, with scissor or blade.
- Desiccate the EN using the lowest setting possible for destruction of tissue.
- Debride charred tissue using curette.
- Repeat electrodesiccation and curettage of tissue until the EN is level with normal surrounding skin.
- Dress with sterile petroleum jelly and occlusive nonadherent dressing.

Postprocedural Approach
- Patients should wash once to twice daily with gentle, unscented soap, apply sterile petroleum jelly, and bandage until wound is epithelialized.
- Minor swelling, erythema, and pain are normal during the first 2 to 3 days postoperatively.
- Pain should be managed as needed with acetaminophen every 4 to 6 hours without exceeding maximum doses per day.
- Return to activity should be expected within a few days, depending on patient's age, lesion size, and complications. Many children do not require downtime.
- *Red flags:* Significant increase in pain and signs and symptoms of infection should prompt immediate evaluation and corresponding treatment.

PROCEDURE: SURGICAL EXCISION

Clinical Pearls

- **Guidelines:** No guidelines exist for the treatment of EN.
- **Age-Specific Considerations**: With regard to local anesthesia, assessment of the ability to tolerate injections, listen to commands, and stay still for at least an hour should be performed. Generally, patients over the age of 12 may be considered for excision in the ambulatory procedure setting, whereas younger children require treatment in the operating room. There is, however, high variability as to which patients can tolerate this.
- **Technique Tips:** Dermoscopy can help identify the borders of the lesion. Surgical excision is most amenable to small lesions in noncosmetically sensitive areas. For large lesions, serial staged excisions with primary closure, tissue expansion, flaps, or grafts may be required and should be performed by dermatologists with advanced surgical skills or plastic surgeons. From herein, we address surgical excision with local anesthesia and primary closure.
- **Skin of Color Considerations:** Those with a predilection to keloid should be made aware that this may be a complication.

Contraindications/Cautions/Risks

Contraindications: Extensive lesions

Cautions
- Cosmetically sensitive sites
- Inadequate resection and partial-thickness excision will lead to high risk of recurrence.

Risks
- Pain
- Bleeding
- Infection
- Scarring
- Keloids
- Hypertrophic scars
- Contractures if located over joints
- Postinflammatory dyschromia
- Recurrence

Equipment Needed
- Camera for preoperative documentation
- Masks with eye shields
- Chlorhexidine
- Sterile surgical tools (blade, needle driver, forceps, skin hooks, undermining scissor)
- Dissolvable deep sutures
- Epidermal sutures: dissolvable or nondissolvable
- Electrocautery device
- Sterile gauze
- Sterile petrolatum–based ointment
- Topical anesthesia
- Local anesthesia
- Nonadherent dressing
- Tape for dressing

Preprocedural Approach

- Preprocedural photographs
- Measure lesion size
- Informed consent with a thorough review of side effects, discussion of expectations, and potential of recurrence should be obtained from patient (if applicable) and guardian.
- Application of topical anesthesia approximately 60 minutes prior to procedure

Procedural Approach

- Mark the site of the EN, clean and inject local anesthesia.
- Thoroughly clean with chlorhexidine.
- Full-thickness excision to the level of the subcutaneous fat.
- Primary closure may be obtained with deep dissolvable sutures to remove tension and top sutures with either dissolvable or nondissolvable sutures.
- Dress with sterile petroleum jelly and occlusive nonadherent dressing.

Postprocedural Approach

- Patients should wash once to twice daily with antibacterial unscented soap, apply sterile petroleum jelly, and cover with bandage until suture removal.
- If nondissolvable sutures employed, patient should return for suture removal with timing depending on the surgical site.
- Swelling, erythema, and pain are normal during the first 2 to 3 days postoperatively.
- Pain should be managed as needed with alternating acetaminophen every 4 to 6 hours without exceeding maximum doses per day.
- Return to school should be expected within a few days, depending on patient's age, lesion size, and complications. Activity should be minimized as much as possible for as long as possible with return to rigorous activity only once sutures are removed, at the earliest.
- *Red flags:* Significant increase in pain and signs and symptoms of infection should prompt immediate evaluation and treatment.

PROCEDURE: CO$_2$ LASER ABLATION

Clinical Pearls

- **Age-Specific Considerations:** CO$_2$ laser ablation is performed under local anesthesia in older children, typically a consideration in patients over 12 years of age. Patients should be able to obey commands and stay still for at least 30 minutes. Otherwise, the procedure should be performed in the operating room or delayed until the patient can tolerate.
- **Technique Tips:**
  - CO$_2$ laser ablation should be performed with a pulsed technique as opposed to continuous owing to greater control over thermal damage to minimize scarring.
  - Avoid treating the reticular dermis owing to greater scar risk.

- Best response can be seen in smaller EN with surface area <20 cm² or EN of the face/neck.[2]
- Repeat sessions, typically up to 8 to 10 treatments,[1,2] may be performed every 4 weeks.
- **Skin of Color Considerations:** Appropriate discussion of postinflammatory dyspigmentation and keloid scarring is necessary.

Contraindications/Cautions/Risks

Contraindications
- Predilection for keloid or hypertrophic scars

Cautions
- Bleeding disorders
- Poor efficacy in widespread, extensive[3] EN >100 cm²
- Poor efficacy in hyperkeratotic nevi, which may result in hypertrophic scars[4]

Risks
- Bleeding
- Infection
- Atrophic scars
- Keloid or hypertrophic scars
- Postinflammatory dyschromia
- Recurrence (20%-30%)[2,3]

Equipment Needed
- Camera for preoperative documentation
- CO_2 laser
- Smoke evacuator
- Wavelength-specific eye shields
- One set of metal eye shields
- Masks
- Chlorhexidine
- Sterile saline
- Sterile gauze
- Sterile petrolatum–based ointment
- Topical anesthesia
- Local anesthesia
- Nonadherent dressing and tape

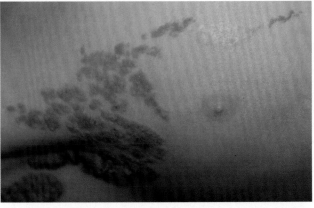

FIGURE 78.2. Extensive hypertrophic epidermal nevus with "test spot" (directly superior to nipple) showing excellent response to laser ablation. Photo courtesy of Andrew C. Krakowski, MD.

Preprocedural Approach

- Preoperative photographs
- A *test spot* of a representative area to evaluate efficacy and monitor for side effects (Figure 78.2)
- Prophylaxis for herpes simplex virus in affected patients 1 to 2 days prior
- Informed consent with a thorough review of side effects, discussion of expectations, and potential need for further sessions should be obtained from patient (if applicable) and guardian.

Procedural Approach

- Apply topical anesthesia to the targeted area 60 minutes prior (Figure 78.3A).
- Protective eyewear and masks for everyone in the procedure room, metal eye shields for the patient
- Clean with chlorhexidine.
- Inject local anesthesia.
- CO_2 laser in unfocused mode for a beam diameter of 2 mm, power of 4 to 15 W
  - Power may be adjusted to target lesion thickness.[2]
- Smoke evacuator employed by a second operator

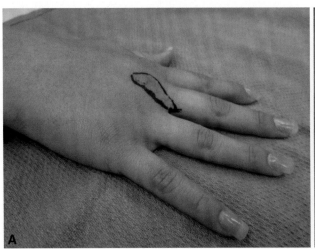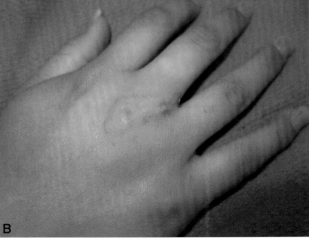

FIGURE 78.3. A, Preoperative photo with flesh-colored epidermal nevus delineated by surgical marker. B, Intraoperative photo demonstrating near full-field ablation. The white areas are the superior portion of the papillary dermis; deeper ablation increases the risk for scarring, so a "less is more" approach is recommended. Photos courtesy of Andrew C. Krakowski, MD.

- Apply a paintbrush pattern until exposure of white dermis is visible to establish an acceptable level of tissue destruction aimed at destruction of the papillary dermis with preservation of the reticular dermis[3] (Figure 78.3B).
  - Take care not to destroy the reticular dermis, which increases the risk of scarring.[2]
- Clean charred surface after each ablation with gauze soaked in sterile saline[2,3] and apply pressure for bleeding as needed.[2]
- Anywhere from one to four passes may be required for complete destruction.[2]
- A final pass should be performed to coagulate surface vessels.[2]
- Dress with sterile petroleum jelly and occlusive nonadherent dressing.

Postprocedural Approach

- Apply petroleum jelly with or without occlusion with a nonadherent dressing until erosions/ulcerations are healed within approximately 10 to 15 days.[2,3]
- Within the first 2 postoperative days, expect erythema and pain.
  - Erythema should improve within 4 weeks after procedure.[2]

- Pain should be managed with acetaminophen every 4 to 6 hours without exceeding maximum doses per day.
- Return to school should be expected within 2 to 3 days.
- *Red flags:* Significant increase in pain and signs and symptoms of infection should prompt immediate evaluation and treatment.
- Evaluate postoperative healing and response at 2 months or sooner.

REFERENCES

1. Lee BJ, Mancini AJ, Renucci J, Paller AS, Bauer BS. Full-thickness surgical excision for the treatment of inflammatory linear verrucous epidermal nevus. *Ann Plast Surg.* 2001;47(3):285–292.
2. Alonso-Castro L, Boixeda P, Reig I, de Daniel-Rodriguez C, Fleta-Asin B, Jaen-Olasolo P. Carbon dioxide laser treatment of epidermal nevi: response and long-term follow-up. *Actas Dermosifiliogr.* 2012;103(10):910–918.
3. Bhat YJ, Hassan I, Sajad P, et al. Evaluation of carbon dioxide laser in the treatment of epidermal nevi. *J Cutan Aesthet Surg.* 2016;9(3):183–187.
4. Paradela S, Del Pozo J, Fernandez-Jorge B, Lozano J, Martinez-Gonzalez C, Fonseca E. Epidermal nevi treated by carbon dioxide laser vaporization: a series of 25 patients. *J Dermatolog Treat.* 2007;18(3):169–174.

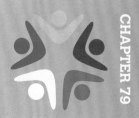

Epidermolysis Bullosa

Madeline L. Gore and Kristen P. Hook

CHAPTER 79

Introduction

Epidermolysis bullosa (EB) describes a subset of genetic skin conditions in which a mutation of a structural protein in the skin and/or mucous membranes leads to fragility and blistering. Typically, these diseases are present from birth, with an incidence of about 19 per 1 million live births. There are four major types of EB, with several subtypes: epidermolysis bullosa simplex (EBS; intraepidermal), junctional epidermolysis bullosa (JEB; intraepidermal through the lamina lucida, Figure 79.1), dystrophic epidermolysis bullosa (DEB; subdermal through the lamina densa, Figures 79.2 and 79.3), and Kindler's syndrome (mixed). EB acquisita is an autoimmune acquired blistering disorder that often presents with a phenotype similar to that of dystrophic EB, although it is not classified as an EB subtype. Owing to chronic open wounds and blisters, it is imperative to use proper blister care, wound dressings, and gentle skin care to aid the healing process, reduce pain and itch, and prevent infection.

The subtype of EB will often determine the severity and amount of blistering that occurs. It is recommended that blisters be lanced with a sterile needle to prevent enlargement of blisters and, subsequently, painful wounds. This is the standard blister care for all subtypes. Patients with EBS will often need their blisters drained and sometimes covered with nonadhesive bandages. However, many patients with EBS, especially with age, will rely less on complex wound dressings. Blistering is often exacerbated by minimal friction, sweating, and heat. Patients with JEB or DEB often have chronic, more severe wounds and erosions that will need adequate cleansing and dressings that are changed every day or every other day depending on the severity of the wound and whether infection is present. It is often recommended for patients of all subtypes to use emollients (often bland ointments such as petrolatum jelly) under or spread on the contact layer of bandages as well as dilute vinegar, salt, or dilute bleach soaks for cleansing after bandage removal. Wound care and dressing changes can be very painful and overwhelming to patients and caregivers. Herein we describe brief procedures that optimize healing and comfort.

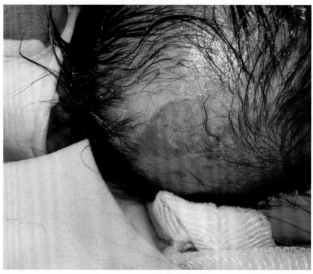

FIGURE 79.1. Junctional epidermolysis bullosa in an infant.

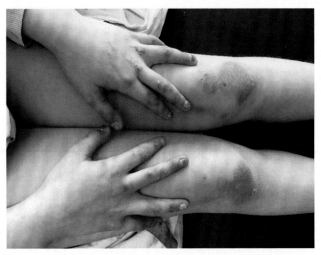

FIGURE 79.2. Dominant dystrophic epidermolysis bullosa in a child.

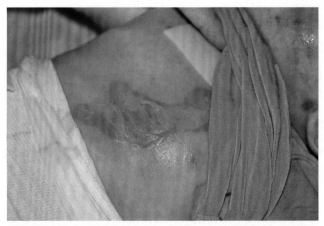

FIGURE 79.3. Recessive dystrophic epidermolysis bullosa in an infant.

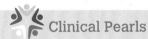

Clinical Pearls

- **Guidelines:** Published clinical guidelines by *Pope et al.* (*J Am Acad Dermatol 2012*) described consensus recommendations for wound care in patients with EB.
- **Anatomic-Specific Considerations:** Patients with JEB or DEB may have digit fusion (pseudosyndactly) or be at risk for digit fusion, thus it is important to dress properly between the fingers and toes.
- **Age-Specific Considerations:** Infants may need more care and protection from blistering:
  - Lay infants on egg-crate mattress (before the baby is able to roll) or on sheepskin (after baby can roll) to reduce skin trauma.
  - Remove elastic in diapers or line with nonadhesive dressings such as foam dressings.
  - Dress infants with clothes inside out to reduce trauma from seams; remove external tags.
  - Extra bandaging/padding on bony prominences (knees, dorsal feet) or use Glidewear™ (Tamarack Habilitation Technologies Inc., US) or other special garments for crawling.
  - Do not lift infants/toddlers from their axillae. It is recommended to lift from behind the head and under the buttocks.
  - Breastfeeding and bottle-feeding may cause oral mucosal blisters and erosions. Lubricating the nipple or the mouthpiece of the bottle with Vaseline™ (Conopco, Inc., US) or Aquaphor® (Beiersdorf AG, US) may lessen lesions. Some patients use the Haberman Feeder that requires less suckling.
  - Nutrition must be monitored closely. Consult a nutritionist or seek referral to pediatric gastroenterology as indicated.
- **Skin of Color Considerations:** Patients with darker skin types may have more dyspigmentation with time.
- **Subtype Considerations:** Dressings vary with subtype and patient/caregiver preference, because patients with milder subtypes (EBS or dominant dystrophic epidermolysis bullosa [DDEB]) may not regularly prefer to dress wounds or even require this regularly. Patients with more severe subtypes have greater systemic associations and often require more complex wound care and dressings.

Contraindications/Cautions/Risks

Contraindications

- *If EB is suspected or diagnosed, strict avoidance of adhesive materials on the skin should be followed, whether inpatient or in the home setting. Avoid friction and significant pressure on skin, depending on the EB subtype.*

Cautions

- Confirm diagnosis to ensure adequate resources, care, and counseling.

Risk

- Neonates: beware of increased infection risk, increased transepidermal water loss, increased caloric needs due to skin turnover, and in some forms of EB, significant risk of early demise.
- Monitor temperature of patients, particularly if a large portion of their body surface is bandaged. This is especially important in infants because patients may have a decreased ability to sweat and are therefore at increased risk for higher body temperatures.

Equipment Needed

- Small-gauge lancet (30G, ½ in for infants and smaller blisters; 22 G, 1 in for larger blisters and adolescents/adults)
- Sterile gauze
- Gentle would cleanser
  - Sterile saline, sterile water, Dremol 500 (available only in the United Kingdom), and others
  - Dilute bleach solution, dilute vinegar solution, salt bath
- Scissors
  - Clean, bandage scissors are ideal to cut dressings to size.
  - Wound scissors to remove dressings and reduce risk of injury
  - Scissors that are used for soiled dressings should never be used for cutting clean dressings.
- Topical preparations (examples)
  - Nonprescription brand emollients: Aquaphor, petrolatum jelly, Restore (Hollister) DimethiCreme (contains lavender, a possible contact irritant), Dimethicone Skin Protectant, Curefini ointment, allantoin cream, and others

- Prescription topical antimicrobial preparations (mupirocin, gentamicin, silver sulfadiazine)
  - Medical-grade honey preparations
- Dressing supplies (examples)
  - **First layer or contact layer:** serves as a non-adherent protective layer, fluid permeable, that is in direct contact with the wound/skin surface; examples include impregnated gauze (eg, petrolatum impregnated gauze) and foam dressings (eg, Mepitel®, Restore Foam)
  - **Second layer:** provides a cushion and absorbency, especially for wounds with excessive drainage beyond the first layer
    - Examples: foam dressings (eg, Mepilex® Lite [2019 Mölnlycke Health Care AB], Mepilex, Restore Foam, Polymem® [Ferris Corp, US], Telfa)
  - **Third layer:** provides structural support and slight pressure
    - Examples: Kerlix™ (Covidien/Medtronic, US) or Conform Rolled Gauze
  - **Fourth layer:** outer layer used to gently hold layers in place
    - Retention dressings (eg, Coban, Surgilast® [Derma Sciences Inc.], Tubifast® [2019 Mölnlycke Health Care AB])
    - Utilize a clean surface for preparing and laying out clean dressing supplies.
    - Provide a clean, safe and padded surface for dressing change.

Preprocedural Approach

- Assess the blister: size, depth, pain level, and infection status.
- If the dressing is adherent to the wound or blister, soaking the dressed wound in a bath or using sterile saline or water to remove dressing will help limit further trauma and may reduce pain.
- Cleanse wounds with mild cleansers as tolerated (saline, water, Dermol 500, dilute bleach solution, dilute vinegar solution, among others).
- Pain control: oral medication such as acetaminophen or ibuprofen may be given if the anticipated procedure is deemed to be painful (not for daily/chronic use, in general). Topical anesthetics, such as lidocaine, per patient need (although in the author's experience, this is rarely needed). Opioid analgesics may be utilized for severe pain associated with wound care, dressing changes, and blister care but are not generally recommended for chronic use and chronic pain (see Chapter 134. Pain Management). Patients requiring frequent opioid and nonopioid pain medications should be evaluated by a pain management team or expert provider.

Procedural Approach

- Hold clean gauze gently against outer edge of blister.
- With a sterile needle, puncture the blister surface in the most highly filled area.
- It is helpful to puncture more than once depending on the size of the blister.
- Do not pull the needle to tear the overlaying skin, because this may cause severe pain. Keeping overlaying skin intact also allows for a natural biologic "dressing" for the wound.

- Gently press on the blister, if tolerated by the patient, to remove the fluid. Gauze can also be pulled taut and gently pressed against the blister to remove fluid.
- Bacteria culture may be done at this time.
- Try to drain blister fully to allow scab formation. If not drained fully, the punctures can close and the blister can reform.
- Care after blister puncture depends both on the subtype and patient preference.
- Here are some helpful guidelines for general wound care for EB patients and commonly used supplies (Figure 79.4):
  - EBS: If blister is infected or inflamed, medication can be applied either directly to the wound if tolerated or to the contact layer bandage, if being covered (often preferred).
    - Older patients may not prefer not to bandage.
  - JEB, DEB, and Kindler's syndrome:
    - Wrapping the fingers and hands require careful technique that should be demonstrated to families; helpful videos and resources can often be found on the internet at the websites of EB centers and support groups (Figures 79.5 and 79.6).

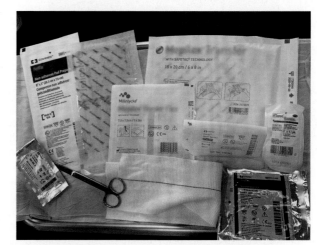

FIGURE 79.4. Commonly used wound care supplies.

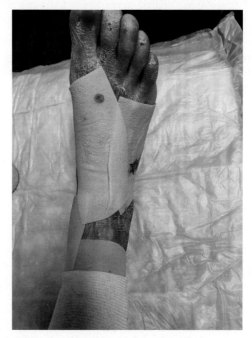

FIGURE 79.5. Absorbent dressing layer (Mepilex).

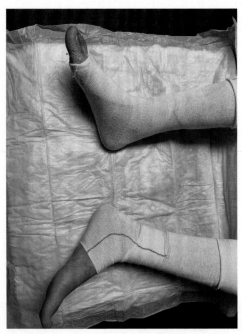

FIGURE 79.6. Secure dressing layer (Tubifast).

- Soft gloves made especially by wound care companies can also be useful and may help prevent scarring and fusion along the digits. It is helpful to have the family consult with an occupational therapist about dressing between the digits.
- There are many choices for dressings, including those containing silver for antimicrobial effects, medical-grade honey for its anti-inflammatory effects, iodine, or polyhexamethylene biguanide. However, ionized silver has been found in the circulation of patients with EB, so use should be limited to a small surface area. Medical-grade honey has been noted to increase pain and exudate with long-term use, so use may only be helpful temporarily.

Postprocedural Approach

- The patient may be in great pain following the wound care, especially those patients with more severe forms of EB.
- Some wounds in EB may not reach full healing, and therefore require pain-reducing and infection-preventing care with regular dressing changes.
- If the patient presents with fever, spreading redness from the wound, or an acute increase in blistering, these may be signs of a deep or systemic infection that should be treated with systemic antimicrobials.
- It is of utmost importance to consider the patient's opinions, feelings, and preferences throughout care because there is a great amount of variability among types of EB and wound care options.
- Bathing with dilute salt, bleach, and vinegar have various antimicrobial and wound healing effects for EB patients.
  - **Salt:** Reduces pain during bath time, especially with open wounds
    - Babies/infants: Add 2.5 to 5 teaspoons of salt to each gallon of bathwater
    - Teens/adults: Add 1 to 2 lb of salt to a half-filled bathtub (~40 gallons of bathwater)
    - Optional to rinse after salt bath. It has not been shown that salt baths cause itching without rinsing.
    - Salt can be table salt or pool salt purchased at pool supply stores, hardware stores, and bulk supply stores. Aquarium salt may also be used, which can be found at pet supply stores.
  - **Bleach:** fights infection, anti-inflammatory
    - ¼ cup standard bleach (not ultraconcentrated) per half-tub (40 gallons)
    - Typically, 1-2 teaspoons bleach per gallon of water; may increase up to 3 teaspoons (1 tablespoon) if indicated clinically
  - **Vinegar:** Fights infection
    - 3% vinegar: 1 part 3% vinegar to 12 parts bathwater
    - 5% vinegar (Heinz): 1 part 5% vinegar to 20 parts bathwater
  - In our experience, four cups of 5% vinegar per half-tub yields a similar molality and effect, and is easier to use for families.

SUGGESTED READINGS

Centers for Medicare and Medicaid Services. Billing and coding guidelines for wound care (L34587). https://downloads.cms.gov/medicare-coverage-database/lcd_attachments/34587_21/L34587_GSURG051_BCG.pdf. Accessed June 20, 2020.

Centers for Medicare and Medicaid Services. Local coverage determination (LCD): debridement services (L34032). https://www.cms.gov/medicare-coverage-database/details/lcd-details.aspx?LCDId=34032. Published September 12, 2019. Accessed February 18, 2020.

Debra of America. Dystrophic Epidermolysis Bullosa Research Association. http://www.debra.org/. Accessed June 13, 2018.

Fine J-D, Eady RA, Bauer EA, et al. The classification of inherited epidermolysis bullosa (EB): Report of the Third International Consensus Meeting on Diagnosis of Classification of EB. *J Am Acad Dermatol.* 2008;58(6):931–950. doi:10.1016/j.jaad.2008.02.004.

Pope E, Lara-Corrales I, Mellerio J, et al. A consensus approach to wound care in epidermolysis bullosa. *J Am Acad Dermatol.* 2012;67(5):904–917. doi:10.1016/j.jaad.2012.01.016.

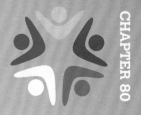
Epstein's Pearl

Emily M. Becker and Jessica Parappuram

Introduction

Discovered in 1880 by Alois Epstein, a Czech pediatrician, Epstein's pearls are a type of intraoral retention cyst found in newborns, which are made up of accumulations of keratin. Initially, the classification of various nodules/cysts in the oral cavities of newborns was broad and the term "Epstein's disease" was used to encompass any newborn oral cyst. In 1967, Alfred Fromm undertook an extensive evaluation of oral cysts in 1367 infants, which allowed him to further classify these oral cysts on the basis of location and composition. In recognizing that these intraoral cysts were distinctly different on the basis of clinical presentation and histologic characteristics, Fromm created the terminology we use today: Epstein's pearls, Bohn's nodules, and dental lamina cysts.[1] Unfortunately, many sources incorrectly use these terms interchangeably. "Palatal cysts of the newborn" is the proposed preferred terminology that more appropriately encompasses them. For the purposes of this chapter, we are limiting the discussion of oral cysts in the newborn to that of Epstein's pearls alone, because these are the most commonly encountered.

Bohn's nodules and dental lamina cysts occur on the buccal/lingual ridges and crest of the alveolar mucosa, respectively. In contrast, Epstein's pearls appear in the mouth along the midline of the hard palate, specifically in the location of the median palatine raphe (Figure 80.1). Most commonly, they can be seen at the junction of the hard and soft palate. The lining of these cysts consists of stratified squamous epithelium surrounding a keratin-filled center. Either solitary or multiple, Epstein's pearls can range in size from 1 to 3 mm and appear as yellowish-white, fluid-filled vesicles. They are thought to originate from the epithelium trapped along the line of fusion during the development of the palate, which occurs during the first trimester of pregnancy. This palatal fusion is completed by the end of the fourth month of gestation. Other less common theories include that

Epstein's pearls are actually epithelial remnants arising from the formation of the minor salivary glands.[2]

Epstein's pearls are a frequent neonatal condition and can be seen in approximately 60% to 80% of newborns. Gender does not seem to play a role in the development of Epstein's pearls, but they are seen more commonly in Japanese newborns, followed by Caucasian, and then African-American newborns. Maternal factors during pregnancy and at the time of delivery have been shown to play only a minor role. A greater rate has been shown in term babies, those with higher birth weight, and infants born to multigravida mothers, although this is not entirely reproducible throughout the literature.[1,2]

Crucially, this is a case of where "less is more" because Epstein's pearls are harmless and disappear roughly from 2 weeks to 3 months of age of life. They are thought to involute or express their keratin material into the mouth over time. Despite the widely held recommendations against surgical intervention/removal as mentioned earlier, limited case reports in the literature demonstrate rare instances of procedural intervention for dental lamina cysts (although not for Epstein's pearls).

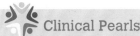 **Clinical Pearls**

- **Guidelines:**
  - There are no consensus guidelines or treatment parameters to date.
  - To the contrary, the dental literature stresses that management of palatal cysts of the newborn (Epstein's pearls, Bohn's nodules, and dental lamina cysts) should not include surgical intervention because of the self-limiting nature. Instead, treatment should entail parental counseling and reassurance.[1-3]
- **Age-Specific Considerations:**
  - Epstein's pearls typically resolve spontaneously by 2 weeks to 3 months of age.
- **Technique Tips:**
  - The differential diagnosis for cystic lesions in the mouth of a neonate includes Epstein's pearls, Bohn's nodules, dental lamina cysts, natal/neonatal teeth, congenital epulis, congenital ranula, and alveolar lymphangioma.
  - A key distinction in diagnosing these self-limiting lesions is that they do not progressively increase in size.
  - These lesions do not typically interfere with feeding or tooth appearance or development.
  - Epstein's pearls do not necessitate medical intervention or removal; however, benign removal for cosmetic purposes can be considered with discretion.
  - Multiple cysts that appear larger in nature at atypical locations should be referred to a dental surgeon for proper diagnostic evaluation and monitoring.
- **Skin of Color Considerations:**
  - These lesions are seen more commonly in Japanese newborns, followed by Caucasian and then African-American newborns.
  - Otherwise, no special considerations

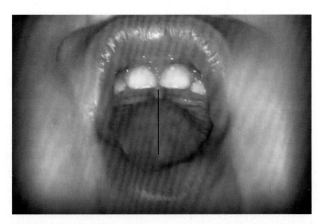

FIGURE 80.1. Epstein's pearls appear in the mouth along the midline of the hard palate, specifically in the location of the median palatine raphe (indicated by black line).

Contraindications/Cautions/Risks

Contraindications

- Active infection intraorally
- Inability to care for postoperative wounds

Cautions

- All interventions should be avoided in newborns with craniofacial anomalies such as cleft/lip palate because of the anatomic changes seen with such conditions.
- Care should be taken regarding avoidance of bleeding or excessive amount of time that the infant is crying.
- Bleeding or excessive secretions in the oral cavity in newborns can be problematic because the infants are at risk for aspiration of liquid contents because they are unable to protect the airway in the same manner as do older children and adults.

Risks

- Death (infection or anesthesia), scarring, pain, bleeding, recurrence of lesions

Equipment Needed

- 11 blade
- Cotton-tipped applicators (CTAs)
- Comedone extractor (optional)
- Hyfrecator 2000™ (Conmed, Utica, NY) (optional)

Preprocedural Approach

- Ice may be applied directly to the area for purposes of numbing the area locally.
- Local anesthesia is generally not necessary.

Procedural Approach—Incision and Drainage

- Surgical intervention, if absolutely necessary, may be undertaken by a simple incision and drainage procedure.
  - A tiny nick is made very superficially into the cyst wall.
  - Gentle pressure is applied using either a comedone extractor or CTAs to extract the keratinaceous material.

Procedural Approach—Electrodesiccation

- Alternatively, benign destruction with electrodesiccation at a low setting can be considered.
  - The Hyfrecator should be placed at a relatively low setting (no more than 2) so that local/topical anesthesia is typically not required.
  - The cyst wall is then gently cauterized in an attempt to extrude the contents.

Postprocedural Approach

- Ice or a cold drink such as a milkshake may help alleviate pain and local edema.

REFERENCES

1. Marini R, Chipaila N, Monaco A, Vitolo D, Sfasciotti GL. Unusual symptomatic inclusion cysts in a newborn: a case report. *J Med Case Rep.* 2014;8:314.
2. Singh RK, Kumar R, Pandey RK, et al. Reminder of important clinic lesson: dental lamina cysts in a newborn infant. *BMJ Case Rep.* 2012;2012:bcr2012007061.
3. Nazif MM, Martin BS, McKibben DH, et al. In Zitelli BJ, Davis HW, ed. Oral Disorders. *Atlas of Pediatric Physical Diagnosis.* 5th ed. Philadelphia, PA: Mosby Elsevier; 2007:755–779.

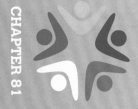

CHAPTER 81

Fibroma (Subungal or Periungal)

Mimi R. Borrelli, Ruth Tevlin, and H. Peter Lorenz

Introduction

Ungual fibromas are rare benign fibrous lesions of the fingers or toes. They are described as "periungual" when they arise under the proximal nail fold and "subungual" when they originate from under the nail plate (Figure 81.1). Ungual fibromas most commonly originate from the proximal border of the nail and more rarely from the matrix region.

The term *acral fibrokeratomas* refers to both acquired garlic clove–shaped fibromas and the congenital fibromas associated with conditions such as tuberous sclerosis, where they can present in multiple clusters. Periungual and subungual fibromas may be the only clinical abnormality of tuberous sclerosis, and in this context are called "Koenen's tumor."[1,2] The pathophysiology of acquired *acral fibrokeratomas* is unknown, and trauma may be a predisposing factor.

Generally, ungual fibromas are small (3-5 mm), dome-shaped popular lesions that are firm on palpation and are well demarcated. They may be flesh-colored or range in color from pink-to-red. Ungual tumors are often symptomatic; fibroma growth can significantly distort the nail plate and even eventually destroy the nail, or, alternatively, place excessive pressure on the nail matrix, making them tender to touch. There are no U.S. Food and Drug Administration (FDA)-approved topical or systemic treatment options. Multiple procedural techniques have been described favorably in the literature, including CO_2 ablation or shave excision with nail matrix phenolization. Surgical excision is indicated for ungual fibromas that are cosmetically disturbing, catch on clothing, or are painful. Surgical excision can be executed with ease, is reproducible, and does not require special or expensive equipment. Complete surgical excision is recommended because of the risk of recurrence following partial excision or curettage. There are various surgical techniques for the surgical excision of ungual fibromas, which depend on whether the tumor arises from above or below the nail plate. Surgical excision of acral fibrokeratomas is challenged by the

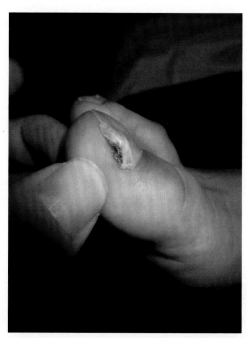

FIGURE 81.1. Right toe subungal fibroma. Photo courtesy of Andrew C. Krakowski, MD.

possibility of irreversible nail dystrophy. Conservation of the proximal nail fold and the integrity of the nail plate are not always possible. Herein, we describe a technique for the excision of *acral fibrokeratomas* based on our experience.

 Clinical Pearls

- **Guidelines:** There are no specific treatment guidelines for ungual fibroma treatment.
- **Age-Specific Considerations:**
  - Fibroma may be associated with tuberous sclerosis; patients should be comprehensively examined (ie, with a Wood's lamp, if possible) for other signs of systemic disease.
  - Periungual fibromas usually develop around puberty and are less frequent in young children.
  - In young children, acquired digital fibrokeratomas occur most commonly on rudimentary supernumerary digits.
  - General anesthesia or intravenous sedation is usually required for younger children.
- **Technique Tips:**
  - Surgical excision should aim to eliminate the entire tumor and preserve the germinal cells of the nail matrix.
  - One author describes the use of Monsel solution, a ferric sulfate solution that has a high hemostatic potential and can be applied with a cotton bud or gauze swab after suturing.[3]
- **Skin of Color Considerations:** There are no specific skin of color considerations.

Contraindications/Cautions/Risks

Contraindications
- Local infection
- Inability to care for the postoperative wound
- If significant patient comorbidities exist, then shave and phenolization or CO_2 laser vaporization may be preferred.

Cautions
- The nail matrix is very sensitive to compression or trauma, which can result in permanent deformities. Defects in the nail matrix greater than 3 mm in diameter generally lead to permanent nail dystrophy.
- Although complete surgical excision can create a cosmetic defect, this may be preferable to the possibility of a tumor involving the nail.
- Differential diagnoses include pyogenic granuloma, supernumerary digit, cutaneous horn, neurofibroma, and amelanotic melanoma, so always send the specimen for histopathologic examination.

Risks
- Bleeding: Ungual fibromas tend to bleed despite suturing.
- Nail dystrophy including abnormal nail growth, nail striations
- Scarring; however, the cosmetic outcome is usually very good.
- Recurrence
- Infection

Equipment Needed
- Nerve block local anesthetic (1% or 2% lidocaine is generally used)
- Digit tourniquet
- Monsel solution
- No. 15 scalpel
- Scissors
- Hemostat
- Needle holder
- Forceps
- 4-0 or 5-0 nylon sutures

Preprocedural Approach

- Preoperative diagnosis of subungual or periungual lesions can be made on clinical history examination alone.
- Imaging modalities can help rule out other inflammatory or infectious conditions.
- Imaging may also be helpful in elucidating the exact origin of the fibroma in relation to the nail bed; this allows for the optimal choice for the surgical excision and may result in the least trauma.

Procedural Approach

- Surgical excision is usually performed under digital nerve block anesthesia.
- Digital tourniquets provide a bloodless surgical field.
- Two oblique incisions can be made at either end of the eponychium.
- The nail fold can be lifted to expose the lesion.
- The tumor should be excised proximal to its base to ensure complete excision and to reduce the risk of recurrence.
- Lesions arising from above the nail plate can be excised after lifting the proximal nail fold as a banner flap. Lesions arising from below the nail plate require partial or total removal of the nail.
- The wound site should be irrigated, and the skin reapproximated.
- Adequate hemostasis is essential given the risk of bleeding. Monsel solution is a ferric sulfate solution that has a high

hemostatic potential and can be applied with a cotton bud or gauze swab after suturing.[3]

- The skin can be closed under minimal tension with 4-0 or 5-0 nylon sutures.

Postprocedural Approach

- The wound should heal in 1 to 2 weeks, after which the patient can return to full activities.
- A histopathologic examination should be performed in all cases because the diagnosis of abnormal growths can be a challenge. Ungual fibromas have distinct histopathologic features; they are nonencapsulated and have dense hyalinization and irregular collagen bundles, suggesting proliferation of the connective tissue.

- Follow-up is important to assess for recurrence. Ultrasonography can be used to monitor for recurrence.
- If the lesion recurs, excision should be repeated.
- Excellent functional recovery is expected, although nail regrowth may be unpredictable.

REFERENCES

1. Vinson R, Angeloni V. Acquired digital fibrokeratoma. *Am Fam Physician.* 1995;52:1365–1367.
2. Baran R, Perrin C, Baudet J, Requena L. Clinical and histological patterns of dermatofibromas of the nail apparatus. *Clin Exp Dermatol.* 1994;19:31–35.
3. Yélamos O, Alegre M, Garcés J, Puig L. Periungual acral fibrokeratoma: surgical excision using a banner flap. *Actas Dermosifiliogr* [in English, Spanish]. 2013;104:830–832.

CHAPTER 82

Deep Fungal Infection

Talia Noorily, Joan Fernandez, Christopher Rizk, Renata S. Maricevich, and Audrey Chan

Introduction

There are a variety of organisms responsible for deep fungal infections, and many of these infections manifest clinically with cutaneous pathology. Pediatric patients most susceptible to infection include immunocompromised individuals, premature infants, low-birth-weight neonates, and those with other comorbid medical conditions including hematologic disorders, diabetes with recurrent diabetic ketoacidosis, and severe burn injuries[1] (Figure 82.1).

There are many therapeutic modalities used for the treatment of deep fungal infections, including both medical and surgical interventions. Mortality may be improved in certain fungal infections, such as invasive mucormycosis when surgical interventions are combined with medical therapy.[2] It is hypothesized that in angioinvasive infections, surgery may improve outcome by limiting dissemination and reducing overall burden of disease to improve response to medical therapy.[2] Subcutaneous mycoses such as eumycetoma, phaeohyphomycosis, and chromoblastomycosis are often challenging to manage, usually requiring surgical management in addition to systemic and local therapies.[3]

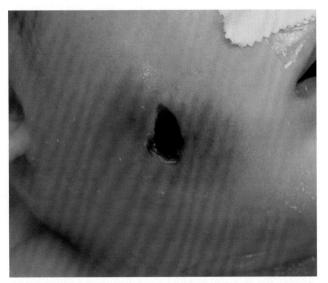

FIGURE 82.1. Former premature infant with erythematous nodule with central eschar concerning for deep fungal infection. Photo courtesy of Renata S. Maricevich, MD.

Clinical Pearls

- **Guidelines:** No specific treatment guidelines are known to exist for this condition in pediatric patients. We recommend working closely with the infectious disease experts to most appropriately select patients who would benefit from surgical management.
- **Age-Specific Considerations:** Although successful treatment using Mohs surgery to clear fungal infections has been reported in an adult population, its utility has not been reported in children.
- **Technique Tips:**
  - Recommend working in concert with infectious disease experts whenever possible
  - Aggressive soft-tissue infections require wide local excision, with the goal of achieving negative margins (Figures 82.2 and 82.3). An average of six debridements are usually required for aggressive disease, whereas indolent fungal infections require an average of two debridements.
- **Skin of Color Considerations:** None

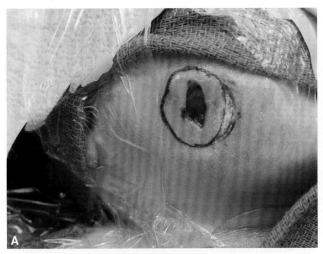

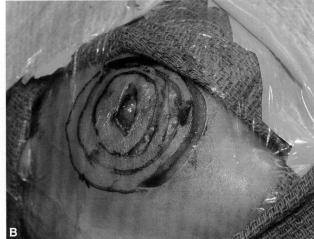

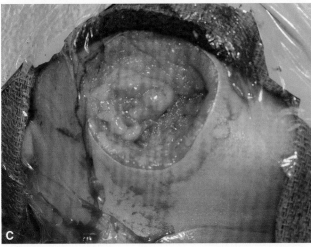

FIGURE 82.2. Marking of initial planned excision, with 1-cm margin circumferentially, notable for gross involvement and persistent deep fungal infection (A), followed by sequential markings at 1-cm intervals (B). Final resection with negative margins at 3 cm down through the level of superficial fascia (C). Photos courtesy of Renata S. Maricevich, MD.

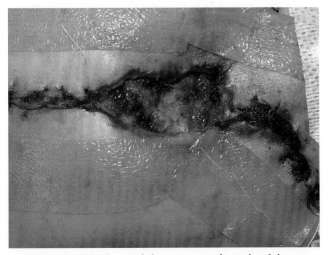

FIGURE 82.3. Partial wound closure was performed and the center portion was allowed to heal by secondary intention. Photo courtesy of Renata S. Maricevich, MD.

Contraindications/Cautions/Risks

Contraindications

○ Hemodynamically unstable patient or other criteria that would make the patient unsuitable for surgery such as active cardiopulmonary disease; excessive bleeding risk (platelets <50 000-100 000, or known bleeding disorder); risk factors for thromboembolism; or severe heart disease, kidney disease, and liver disease

○ For lesions arising within or near critical vascular and/or nervous structures, systemic antifungal therapy alone may be considered on a case-by-case basis depending on the severity of infection.

○ Patient selection regarding appropriate size and location will depend on individual expertise of dermatologic surgeon.

Risks

● Death (iatrogenic spread of infection or anesthesia), pain, bleeding, scarring, recurrence of lesions, damage to surrounding structures (nerves, vessels, tendon, bone)

Equipment Needed

- General surgical equipment (per surgeon preference)
  - Eye protection
  - Antiseptics (chlorhexidine, povidone-iodine)
  - Local anesthesia (injectable 1% lidocaine with 1:100 000 epinephrine) ± general anesthesia
  - Hemostasis equipment for heat cautery, electrocautery, electrodesiccation, or electrofulguration
  - Smoke evacuator
  - Sterile equipment
    - Sterile draping
    - Sterile gauze
    - Sterile curette
    - Scalpel (#10 or #15 blade depending on location)
    - Surgical scissors (eg, Iris, Gradle, Westcott, O'Brien, Metzenbaum)
    - Surgical forceps
    - Sterile suture scissors (eg, Spencer)
    - Suture (based on location and surgeon preference)
  - Petroleum-based ointment
  - Pressure dressing

Preprocedural Approach

- Evaluate need for anesthesia and/or sedation: Age, level of anxiety in relation to procedure, surface area involved
- Recommend evaluation by infectious disease for management of most appropriate systemic antifungal therapy and to determine utility of surgical management.
- Complete blood count (CBC). Other preoperative labs will depend on individual patient risk.
- For immunosuppressed patients, large lesions, or fixed areas of involvement, consider imaging studies (eg, magnetic resonance imaging [MRI]) to rule out deep involvement, which might necessitate referral to general surgery or plastic surgery.

Procedural Approach

- Informed consent from the parent/guardian and, when possible, assent from the minor are obtained before the procedure.
- Appropriate protective eyewear, facemasks, and sterile gloves should be worn. If the patient is on contact precautions, follow outlined procedures on a case-by-case basis.
- The procedure may take place at the bedside or in the operating room depending on patient age, patient disposition, extent of debridement, and expectation of pain.
- Appropriate anesthesia (injectable lidocaine 1% with 1:100 000 epinephrine ± general anesthesia) around the area to be debrided
- Clean the surgical field with antimicrobial detergent (chlorhexidine, povidone-iodine).
- Using sterile towels, drape the surgical field.

- Debridement
  - Using a sharp, sterile curette, debride the wound until healthy, bleeding tissue is encountered around all margins of the lesion.
  - Achieve hemostasis.
  - Immediately after debridement, a petroleum-based ointment should be applied to the bed of the wound.
- Excision
  - Using a sharp, sterile scalpel with a #10 or #15 blade, depending on the location of the lesion, excise the lesion with circumferential, minimum 1 cm margins, down to the superficial fascia (Figure 82.2).
  - Achieve hemostasis.
  - Excision site may be closed primarily, and a purse-string suture may be performed to decrease the wound size. Alternatively, excision site may be allowed to heal by secondary intention with or without the assistance of negative pressure wound therapy (ie, vacuum-assisted closure; Figure 82.3).
  - Specimen should be sent for histopathology to confirm clear margins with fungal stains.

Postprocedural Approach

- Systemic antifungal therapy should be considered if the patient is not already receiving it. Consultation with infectious disease experts may be appropriate.
- Postoperative pain should be managed with appropriate analgesics.
- Typically, patients are instructed to keep postoperative dressing in place for 48 hours.
- Apply petroleum-based ointment to the affected area two to three times daily.
- Patients are instructed to keep physical activity to a minimum for the first 24 hours, with resumption of normal activity in 2 weeks; however, this will depend on size of wound and type of closure.
- Patients should be carefully monitored for signs and symptoms of infection and/or recurrence, including significant erythema, warmth, worsening pain, fevers, and chills.
- Duration of wound healing and recovery will depend on the size of the wound and whether the site was closed primarily or left to heal by secondary intention.
- Patient should be followed up closely by infectious disease and/or dermatology for signs of recurrent fungal infection. Frequency of monitoring will depend on fungal organism.

REFERENCES

1. Marcoux D, Jafarian F, Joncas V. Deep cutaneous fungal infections in immunocompromised children. *J Am Acad Dermatol.* 2009;61:857–864.
2. Pana ZD, Seidel D, Skiada A, et al. Invasive mucormycosis in children: an epidemiologic study in European and non-European countries based on two registries. *BMC Infect Dis.* 2016;16:667.
3. Garnica M, Nucci M, Queiroz-Telles F. Difficult mycoses of the skin: advances in the epidemiology and management of eumycetoma, phaeohyphomycosis and chromoblastomycosis. *Curr Opin Infect Dis.* 2009;22(6):559–563.

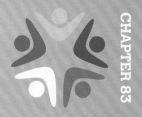

CHAPTER 83

Granuloma Annulare

Jennifer Ornelas and Smita Awasthi

Brief Introduction of Condition

Granuloma annulare (GA) is characterized by smooth papules and nodules arranged in an annular configuration without overlying scale. GA typically involves the hands, feet, wrists, and ankles, but can occur anywhere on the body. Lesions can be solitary or involve multiple sites, such as in the generalized form. The classic pink to purplish lesions can range in size from 5 mm to several centimeters (Figure 83.1). GA may also present as subcutaneous nodules typically on the scalp and distal extremities. The cause of GA remains unknown. Reported disease associations with GA include dyslipidemia (in adults), thyroid disease, and diabetes, although the latter is controversial. Children of any age can be affected with GA, although school-aged children are the most commonly affected.

Lesions typically resolve within months to 2 years and are often asymptomatic, so treatment is not usually necessary. However, if treatment is desired for symptomatic disease or cosmetic reasons, several options are available. For localized GA, treatment options include high-potency topical steroids, topical tacrolimus, intralesional steroid injections, cryotherapy, shave biopsy, and laser.[1] For diffuse GA, a variety of systemic treatments have been used, including oral steroids, antibiotics (dapsone, doxycycline, rifampin, ofloxacin, minocycline), immunosuppressants (cyclosporine, methotrexate), biologics (infliximab, adalimumab, etanercept, efalizumab), and isotretinoin; however, the risk of these agents often does not outweigh the potential benefits. Narrowband ultraviolet B (NB-UVB) and psoralen plus ultraviolet A therapy (PUVA) have also been described.[1] Here, we review intralesional steroid, cryotherapy, and laser treatment options for localized GA.

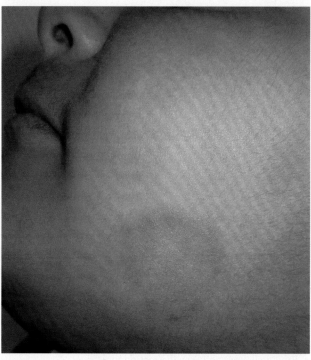

FIGURE 83.1. Granuloma annulare on the face of a young girl. She was misdiagnosed with tinea faciei and nummular eczema and treated with multiple courses of topical and oral antifungals and topical steroids, without improvement. The lesion resolved after two treatments with intralesional corticosteroid. Photo courtesy of Andrew C. Krakowski, MD.

Clinical Pearls

- **Guidelines:** Treatment is not usually required for GA because lesions are typically asymptomatic and self-resolve within months to a few years. However, biopsy may be needed to aid in diagnosis, and other treatment options may be utilized for cosmetic purposes or if symptomatic.
  - Intralesional triamcinolone injection: Strong expert consensus as first-line treatment for localized GA[2]
  - For widespread GA, consider antimalarial medications or phototherapy.
  - Trauma alone has been shown to improve lesions of GA.
  - There is a lack of quality data for other treatment options.
- **Age-Specific Considerations:** Consider age and ability of child to tolerate a specific procedure when selecting a treatment method.
- **Technique Tips:** The use of distraction techniques is recommended to help reduce stress, anxiety, and pain associated with treatments.
- **Skin of Color:** Dyspigmentation secondary to intralesional triamcinolone and cryotherapy is more common in skin of color.

Contraindications/Cautions/Risks

Contraindications
- Active infection
- Allergy to injected anesthesia
- Inability to tolerate procedure or remain sufficiently still for duration of procedure

Cautions
- Carefully weigh risks/benefits of treatment because GA is usually asymptomatic and often self-resolves.

Risks
- Pain, bleeding, infection, reaction to anesthesia, atrophy, telangiectasias, postinflammatory pigmentary changes, especially with skin of color, no improvement, recurrence.

Equipment Needed
- Cryotherapy
  - Liquid nitrogen in either a canister or Styrofoam cup
  - Cotton-tipped applicators
  - Cotton swab
- Intralesional injection of triamcinolone
  - Kenalog 5 to 10 mg/mL, depending on thickness of lesion to be treated

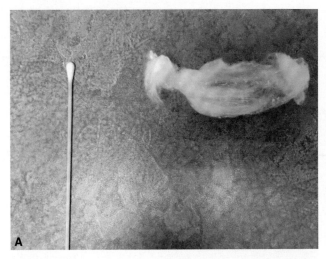

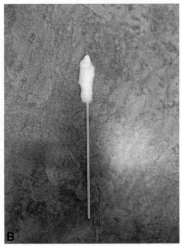

FIGURE 83.2. A, Portion of unwrapped cotton ball and cotton-tipped applicator. B, Cotton swab wrapped at base of cotton-tipped applicator to provide a reservoir of liquid nitrogen to keep the tip cooler when treating each lesion.

- 585- or 595-nm pulsed-dye laser (PDL)
- 308-nm excimer laser
- 1440-nm Nd:YAG laser

Preoperative Approach

- Consider intervention only if needed for symptomatic treatment or for cosmetic purposes.
- Explain procedure to patient in age-appropriate manner.
  - Utilize pictures to demonstrate the procedure to the patient.
  - Allow patients the opportunity to ask any questions.
- Provide patient with any distraction tools.
  - Allow patient to choose video to watch or music to listen to during the procedure.
- We recommend the use of topical anesthetic cream when utilizing laser. Also consider use of anesthetic cream when utilizing intralesional steroid injections for younger children or needle-phobic children.
  - Thirty minutes before treatment, apply topical anesthetic cream to the area(s) to be treated; then, cover with occlusive dressing, such as Tegaderm® (3M, US).

Intraoperative Technique

- Cryotherapy
  - Approach #1: Use a liquid nitrogen canister to apply steady stream of liquid nitrogen to the lesion for 10 to 12 seconds.
  - Approach #2: Loosely wrap cotton swab to base of cotton tip of cotton-tipped applicator and dip into Styrofoam cup filled with liquid nitrogen (Figure 83.2). Press tip of the cotton-tipped applicator to individual lesion for 10 to 12 seconds. Repeat for each individual lesion.
- Intralesional steroid injection
  - Clean area to be treated with alcohol.
  - Use a 30-gauge needle with 5 to 10 mg/mL of intralesional triamcinolone (diluted with sterile saline, if needed) to inject directly to the lesion. Take care to space injections approximately 0.5 cm apart and to avoid pain and other risks from too closely spaced injections.
- 585-nm PDL laser (Candela Corp., Wayland, MA)
  - 6.75 J/cm^2, 5-mm spot size, 36 to 43 pulses per session, three sessions over 13 months[1]

- 595-nm PDL laser
  - Fluence 11 to 15 J/cm^2, spot size not reported, pulse duration 1.5 to 2.0 ms, number of treatments two to three done with Vbeam, Candela or Vstar, Cynosure[3]
  - Fluence 8, spot size 7 mm, pulse duration 1.5, number of treatments one[3]
- 308-nm Excimer laser
  - 300 mJ/cm^2, 5 doses per session, 9 to 15 treatments needed[1]
- 1440-nm Nd:YAG laser (Affirm, Cynosure, Westford, MA)
  - 6 J/cm^2, 3 ms pulse duration, two full passes with 25% overlap, treat every 3 weeks, with two to three treatment sessions per area[1]
- Phototherapy (for generalized GA)
  - For generalized GA, phototherapy is a reliable treatment option examined in a number of different studies.
  - PUVA[1]
    - Oral PUVA: 38 treatments, cumulative dosage 60.4 J/cm^2
    - Bath PUVA: 6 treatments, cumulative dosage 60.4 J/cm^2
  - NB-UVB[2]
    - Median number of treatments: 35, cumulative dosage 47.7 J/cm^2
  - Photodynamic therapy with aminolevulinic acid or methylaminolevulinate acid[1]

Postoperative Approach

- One-hundred percent white petrolatum and ice packs applied after laser treatment
- Sun protection after phototherapy
- Monitor for recurrence.
- Patient should be monitored for signs and symptoms of diabetes mellitus by primary physician. Consider checking serum lipids whether systemic GA is present.

REFERENCES

1. Thornsberry LA, English JC III. Etiology, diagnosis, and therapeutic management of granuloma annulare: an update. *Am J Clin Dermatol.* 2013;14(4):279–290.
2. Piette EW, Rosenbach M. Granuloma annulare: pathogenesis, disease associations and triggers, and therapeutic options. *J Am Acad Dermatol.* 2016;75(3):467–479.
3. Verne SH, Kennedy J, Falto-Aizpurua LA, Griffith RD, Nouri K. Laser treatment of granuloma annulare: a review. *Int J Dermatol.* 2016;55(4):376–381.

Infantile Hemangioma

Ayan Kusari, Allison Han, and Sheila Fallon Friedlander

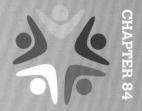

CHAPTER 84

Introduction

Infantile hemangiomas (IHs) are benign, high-flow vascular tumors that present during infancy and are characterized by a relatively programmed life cycle, with rapid growth in the postnatal period, followed by slower involution over a span of years. IH may be superficial, deep, or may contain both deep and superficial components and treatment depends on which components are present. The prevalence of IH is approximately 5% in Western populations.[1] IH is more common in Caucasians, in females, and in preterm neonates. Between 50% and 70% of IHs resolve without treatment, and most involute before age 4. Given this tendency toward spontaneous resolution, watchful waiting has historically been the standard for IH management. Since 2008, however, oral propranolol and, more recently, topical timolol, have become widely used therapies for IH because of their efficacy and relative safety.[2] However, not all patients—particularly those with pulmonary, cardiac, or central nervous system vascular disease (ie, those with PHACES [posterior fossa malformations, hemangiomas of the face, arterial anomalies, aortic coarctation, cardiac anomalies, eye anomalies, sternal anomalies] or LUMBAR [lower body hemangiomas, urogenital anomalies, myelopathy, bone deformities, anorectal malformations, arterial anomalies, renal anomalies] syndrome[3])—are suitable candidates for β-blocker therapy, and not all patients respond fully to medical therapy. Moreover, medical therapy cannot always prevent complications of hemangioma such as ulceration (Figure 84.1) or residua of IH, most commonly parchment-like scars or fibrofatty tissue.[4] As such, laser treatment and surgical excision remain useful tools for the treatment of IH.

Procedural management of IH should be targeted to the needs of each patient, and a "one-size-fits-all" approach is not advisable. For example, patients with superficial telangiectatic residua or ulceration may benefit from pulsed-dye laser (PDL) therapy, whereas those with deeper fibrofatty residua are more likely to benefit from surgical excision. Early surgical excision for active IH is rarely performed because of the efficacy of topical timolol and oral propranolol, but if there is a contraindication to these therapies and the hemangioma is in a functionally disabling or disfiguring location (ie, nasal tip), then early surgical intervention is suitable.

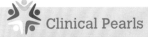

Clinical Pearls

- **Guidelines:** In 2015, the American Academy of Pediatrics issued an executive summary on the diagnosis and management of IH.[1]
- **Age-Specific Considerations:** IHs undergo rapid growth followed by gradual resolution, but for hemangiomas that persist to age 4, complete involution is unlikely and dramatic changes in size are uncommon. Regression is difficult to predict, however, and does not correlate with number or size of lesions.
- **Technique Tips:**
  - A piece of white gauze can be cut to fit the lesion; soaking the gauze and applying it over the lesion before laser surgery can protect surrounding skin from being inadvertently lased.
  - Treatment of IH with propranolol or timolol may leave residua that are resistant to medical therapy.
  - 595-nm PDL is useful for treating superficial vascular residua and ulcerative lesions.
  - Ablative or nonablative fractionated lasers are suitable for more sclerotic lesions and for fibrofatty residua.
  - Surgical excision is suitable for deeper fibrofatty residua and for active lesions in rare circumstances, such as when oral medications cannot be administered or are ineffective. As hemangiomas are often circular in shape and act locally as tissue expanders, the purse-string suture technique is a simple and effective option for closure.
- **Skin of Color Considerations:** PDL settings should be adjusted for darker skin types. Typically, longer pulse durations and lower fluences may help decrease the risk of dyspigmentation and blistering. Epidermal cooling should always be used to decrease the risk of epidermal injury.

Contraindications/Cautions/Risks

Contraindications to Laser Therapy
- Sunburn at treatment site
- Active skin infection at treatment site (ie, herpetic or staph infection)

Cautions
- Presence of a suntan may increase dyspigmentation.
- We do not typically use eutetic mixture of lidocaine and prilocaine, also known as EMLA™ (AB Astra Pharmaceuticals, L.P.) in young infants and children because of the risk of methemoglobinemia. If EMLA must be used, then particular caution should be demonstrated when applying it to large or ulcerated lesions, because absorption may be higher.

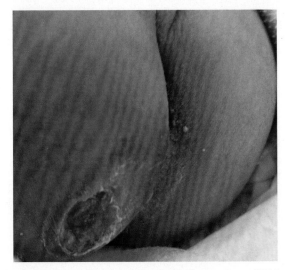

FIGURE 84.1. Deeply ulcerated infantile hemangioma (IH) located on buttock of infant; this lesion was painful and at great risk for superinfection given its anatomic location. Photo courtesy of Andrew C. Krakowski, MD.

Risks

- Blistering, bruising, erythema, peeling, swelling, hypo/hyperpigmentation

Equipment Needed—Laser Therapy

- Wavelength-specific eye shields
- PDL device with epidermal cooling
- Smoke evacuator
- Sterile cotton-tipped applicators
- Sterile water
- Petrolatum-based ointment
- Ice

Equipment Needed—Surgical Excision

- Syringe filled with 1% to 2% Xylocaine ± epinephrine
- Sterile gloves
- No. 15 scalpel blade and handle
- Needle holder
- Scissors
- Adson forceps

Preprocedural Approach

- Before surgery, we ask that patients minimize sun exposure and maximize sun protection so that their skin is as light (ie, untanned) as possible; although this may be somewhat seasonally and geographically dependent, the approach reduces melanin in the skin as a competing chromophore.
- Patients should bathe either the evening before or on the morning of their surgery.

Procedural Approach—Pulsed-Dye Laser Treatment of Ulcerated Infantile Hemangioma

- The risks, benefits, and alternatives of treatment are discussed with the patient and the family. If all parties are agreeable, informed consent from the parent/guardian and assent from the minor are obtained.
- Local anesthetic, particularly lidocaine cream (LMX.4™ or LMX.5™ [Ferndale Laboratories]) is applied to the area to be treated. LMX.4 cream is available over the counter and should be applied to the treatment area 45 minutes to 1 hour before the procedure for maximum effect.
- Appropriate protective eyewear should be worn, and patients should have eye pads (disposable adhesive eye shields offering full eye protection from medical lasers with wavelengths between 190 and 11 000 nm at an optical density greater than 7; OD 7@190-11 000 nm) or correctly fitted metal eye shields in place.
- PDL (595-nm Vbeam Perfecta™ [Candela Corporation, US]) is employed to treat the "proliferating vascular" component of the lesions. A 7- or 10-mm spot size, fluence of approximately 5.5 to 8 J/cm², and 0.45- to 1.5-ms pulse width are typically used, depending on skin type and clinical response. Minimal overlap of pulses is the goal, and the clinical endpoint is mild to moderate purpura. Cryogen cooling spray should always be used for epidermal protection when operating the PDL device.
- Treatment may be repeated as necessary as often as every 1 to 3 weeks.

Procedural Approach—Pulsed-Dye Laser Treatment of Infantile Hemangioma or Associated Telangiectasia

- The risks, benefits, and alternatives of treatment are discussed with the patient and the family. If all parties are agreeable, informed consent from the parent/guardian and assent from the minor are obtained.
- Local anesthetic, particularly lidocaine cream (LMX.4 or LMX.5), is applied to the area to be treated. LMX.4 cream is available over the counter and should be applied to the treatment area 45 minutes to 1 hour before the procedure for maximum effect.
- Appropriate protective eyewear should be worn, and patients should have eye pads (disposable adhesive eye shields offering full eye protection from medical lasers with wavelengths between 190 and 11 000 nm at an optical density greater than 7; OD 7@190-11 000 nm) or correctly fitted metal eye shields in place.
- PDL (595-nm Vbeam Perfecta) is employed to treat the "proliferating vascular" component of the lesions. A 7- or 10-mm spot size, fluence of approximately 7 to 12 J/cm², and 0.45- to 1.5-ms pulse width are typically used, depending on skin type and clinical response. Lower fluences and shorter pulse durations should be used for proliferative lesions because of the risk of ulceration. A 10% to 20% overlap of pulses is the goal, and the clinical endpoint is mild to moderate purpura (Figure 84.2A and B). Cryogen cooling spray should always be used for epidermal protection when operating the PDL device.

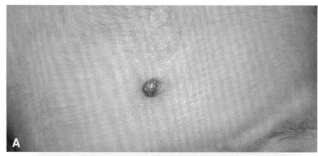
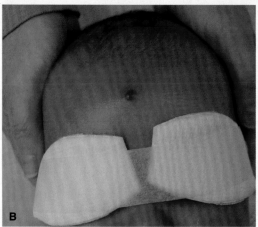

FIGURE 84.2. A, Preop photograph of a young child with a fast-growing IH in the middle of the forehead; the decision was made to treat with pulsed-dye laser (PDL) to help halt rapid expansion. B, Immediate post-op photograph demonstrating mild to moderate purpura. Photo courtesy of Andrew C. Krakowski, MD.

Procedural Approach—Fractional Carbon Dioxide Treatment of Fibrofatty Residua

- The risks, benefits, and alternatives of treatment are discussed with the patient and the family. If all parties are agreeable, informed consent from the parent/guardian and assent from the minor are obtained.
- The treatment site is sterilized with povidone-iodine or chlorhexidine gluconate (Hibiclens; Mölnlycke Health Care, Gothenburg, Sweden), and marked with a sterile surgical marker. Chlorhexidine-containing cleansers should *not* be used for IH near the ears or eyes because of this agent's ototoxicity and oculotoxicity.
- Local anesthetic, particularly lidocaine cream (LMX.4 or LMX.5) is applied to the area to be treated. LMX.4 cream is available over the counter and should be applied to the treatment area 45 minutes to 1 hour before the procedure for maximum effect. Ice applied directly to the to-be-treated area for 5 minutes is also very helpful. Despite best efforts, however, general anesthesia may be required given the painful nature of this procedure.
- Appropriate protective eyewear should be worn, and patients should have eye pads (disposable adhesive eye shields offering full eye protection from medical lasers with wavelengths between 190 and 11 000 nm at an optical density greater than 7; OD 7@190-11 000 nm) or correctly fitted metal eye shields in place.
- A smoke evacuator is necessary to help remove plume smoke, and all present should wear masks.
- Areas of fibrofatty residua are treated using an ablative microfractionated 10 600-nm carbon dioxide laser (FCO_2) (UltraPulse™ [Lumenis, Yokneam, Israel]). Laser settings are individualized depending primarily on the estimated fibrofatty residua thickness and degree of tissue redundancy; a reasonable starting point for most lesions would be 20 mJ and 5% to 10% density. The entire area is treated as a single "sheet" with a single pulse, nonoverlapping stamping technique. With subsequent treatments, remember that treatment density is typically decreased with increasing pulse energies to prevent excessive thermal injury. Depending on the anatomic location of the area being treated, it may be necessary to treat the entire cosmetic unit and/or the contralateral (ie, unaffected) cosmetic unit so that the skin "matches" post the laser.
- Adjunctive laser-assisted delivery of triamcinolone acetonide (40 mg/mL) may be attempted when residua is thick and indurated, although this application remains largely untested. In this technique, intralesional-grade triamcinolone acetonide suspension is "dripped" over the treatment site and rubbed gently over the ablated columns within 2 minutes of laser treatment to facilitate dermal delivery through capillary action. Atrophy is a concern with this technique, so avoid triamcinolone in lesions where atrophy is already present.
- Immediately after laser surgery, a petrolatum-based ointment is applied (Aquaphor® [Beiersdorf AG, US] ointment, Beiersdorf, Inc., Wilton, CT) and continued two to three times a day until complete reepithelialization occurs within approximately 5 to 7 days.
- Ice may be applied to help decrease discomfort and limit local edema.

Procedural Approach—Surgical Excision of Infantile Hemangioma or Fibrofatty Residua

- Surgical excision of active IH should be performed if (1) there are small, active IH in potentially disfiguring sites *and* (2) β-blocker therapy (either oral propranolol or topical timolol)

is contraindicated or has failed after an adequate trial. As of 2018, β-blockers are first-line therapy for active IH. At our institution, surgical excision of active IH is often performed by plastic surgeons, because, in most cases, these lesions are being excised as a result of their location in a cosmetically sensitive and anatomically complex area (ie, nasal tip, philtrum, eyelid).
- Fibrofatty residua may be surgically excised if there is a significant quantity following medical or laser therapy, and the patient's family desires such removal.
- The risks, benefits, and alternatives of treatment are discussed with the patient and the family. If all parties are agreeable, informed consent from the parent/guardian and assent from the minor are obtained.
- The treatment site is sterilized with povidone-iodine or chlorhexidine gluconate (Hibiclens; Mölnlycke Health Care), and marked with a sterile surgical marker. Chlorhexidine-containing cleansers should NOT be used for IH near the ears or eyes because of this agent's ototoxicity and oculotoxicity.
- Local anesthesia is utilized for this procedure, typically 1% to 2% lidocaine with epinephrine. Despite conventional teaching that epinephrine should be avoided at the fingertip, penis, and nasal tip, current evidence indicates that epinephrine improves hemostasis and does not increase risk of necrosis, particularly in young patients without cardiac or vascular disease.
- Depending on anatomic considerations and operator preference, either a lenticular/elliptical excision or circular excision may be performed (Figure 84.3).
- Here, we detail the lenticular/elliptical technique. Using a no. 15 scalpel blade, a fusiform incision should be made parallel to the lines of least tension (Langer lines), with the blade held perpendicular to the skin surface. Once the fusiform incision has been completed, the scalpel should be turned parallel to the skin surface and used to separate the central island of skin from underlying fat.
- If significant bleeding is noted, then electrocautery (Bovie Aaron 940 [Bovie Medical Corporation, Purchase, NY] *or* Hyfrecator 2000™ [Conmed, Utica, NY]) may be used to stanch the flow of blood (see Chapter 17. Electrosurgery/Hyfrecation).
- Interrupted deep sutures should be placed, at an interval of approximately one per centimeter of wound, to eradicate any space at the bottom of the wound and promote healing. Simple interrupted, continuous, or running subcuticular sutures may be placed to close the wound superficially, taking care not to crush skin with forceps and being sure to evert the wound edges. Smaller, circular lesions may be closed using the purse-string technique, as discussed earlier.

Postprocedural Approach

- Generally swelling and pain should decrease quickly with time.
- Patients may remove bandages when bathing. Petrolatum-based ointment is immediately reapplied and maintained until reepithelialization has occurred—typically 5 to 7 days after treatment.
- Families should self-monitor for signs and symptoms of infection.
- The authors do not perform any laboratory evaluation as routine monitoring. Retreatment may be required. Patients are encouraged to contact the physician directly for concerns.

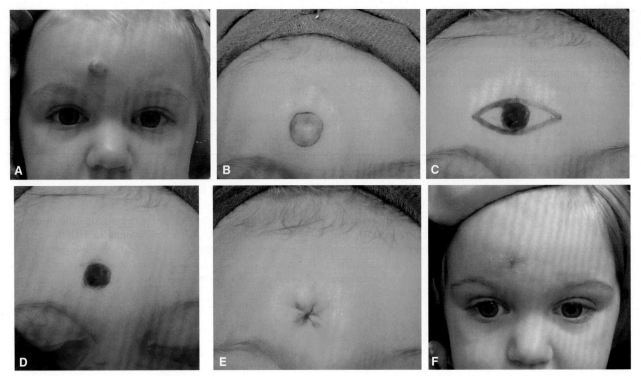

FIGURE 84.3. A, B, A 2.5-year-old female child with frontal IH and fibrofatty residuum. C, Lenticular excision would result in a scar approximately three times the diameter of the tumor. D, E, Circular excision/purse-string closure. F, A small scar 3 months postoperatively that itself could be treated with PDL and/or fractional CO$_2$ laser. Reprinted with permission from Fischer J. *Fischer's Mastery of Surgery*. 7th ed. Philadelphia, PA: Wolters Kluwer; 2018. Figure 27.4.

- Serial photography (ie, "selfies") may be used if the photos are sent through a secure system.
- Ulcerated hemangiomas should be monitored and treated for signs and symptoms of superinfection and pain.

REFERENCES

1. Darrow DH, Greene AK, Mancini AJ, Nopper AJ; Section on Dermatology, Section on Otolaryngology–Head and Neck Surgery, and Section on Plastic Surgery. Diagnosis and management of infantile hemangioma. *Pediatrics*. 2015;136(4):e1060–e1104.
2. Moehrle M, Léauté-Labrèze C, Schmidt V, et al. Topical timolol for small hemangiomas of infancy. *Pediatric dermatology*. 2013;30(2):245–249.
3. Metry Denise W., et al. PHACE syndrome: current knowledge, future directions. *Pediatric dermatology*. 2009;26(4):381–398.
4. Léaute-Labrèze, Christine, et al. Safety of oral propranolol for the treatment of infantile hemangioma: a systematic review. *Pediatrics*. 2016;138(4):e20160353.

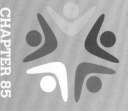

CHAPTER 85

Hematoma

Mimi R. Borrelli, Ruth Tevlin, and H. Peter Lorenz

Introduction

Hematomas are large collections of blood outside the vasculature that can become painful as they swell and enlarge. They can throb, give rise to a pressure sensation, and fluctuate the tissues. They may be named after the body cavity within which they form (eg, subdural hematoma) and give rise to symptoms specific to that cavity. Hematomas may present with ecchymoses, which are small losses of blood into the interstitial space. Ecchymoses occur first in the soft tissues, and they migrate in the direction of gravity and turn from a purple color to a blue/black and then yellow.

Most often, hematomas arise from an injury to a blood vessel. They may form slowly because of continuous bleeding from smaller blood vessels or may expand rapidly if larger vessels are involved. Surgery is a situation where blood vessels may be damaged, and minor postoperative bleeding into a cavity created by surgery is the most common complication of dermatologic surgery. Hemorrhages mostly occur in the first 6 hours following surgery. They are largely due to insufficient surgical hemostasis, leading some to question the use of vasoconstrictors, which may conceal the need for more extensive hemostasis. Hematomas usually occur within the first 24 to 72 hours of surgery.

Postoperative bleeding is most effectively reduced when potential causes of coagulopathy are identified, both preoperatively and postoperatively.[1] A multidisciplinary team involving nurses, physicians, and surgical technicians can work together to provide optimal preoperative, intraoperative, and postoperative care, helping to prevent hemorrhage or hematoma. Prevention can be facilitated by a preoperative workup to assess bleeding risk, a meticulous surgical technique with thorough hemostasis, and the use of compressive bandages or drains. Of note, cutaneous surgeons often operate on patients taking Aspirin, Plavix, and/or warfarin if the risk is too high to withhold these medications.

It is important to recognize the presence of a hematoma early, because hematomas further increase the risk of wound infection and delay wound healing. Hematomas can usually be diagnosed clinically as an expansile fluctuant mass under a recent surgical site, associated with ecchymoses at the skin surface (see Figure 85.1). For patients with suspected or confirmed hematomas, serial clinical examinations with or without the need for additional imaging can be used to monitor progression. Patients may be encouraged to rest, elevate, and apply ice and pressure to the area. For large hematomas that give rise to symptoms, a surgical evacuation may be required. There are a number of techniques and hemostatic agents. We describe our approach for postoperative hematomas.

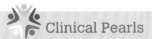

Clinical Pearls

- **Guidelines:** Most hospitals publish guidelines for hematomas within certain cavities—such as epidural, subdural, and for optimizing prescribed medications and anticoagulant or antiplatelet agents before undergoing surgery.

- **Age-Specific Considerations:** Signs of blood loss, such as tachycardia, are better compensated for in children and younger healthy patients in the early phases.
- **Technique Tips:** The amount of collateral tissue damage with coagulation devices can be reduced by applying electrocoagulation to tissue forceps or, instead, through the routine use of bipolar cautery.
- **Skin of Color Considerations:** Bleeding and hematomas may be easier to detect in patients with Fitzpatrick types I and II. Additional clinical suspicion may be required in those with darker skin tones.

Contraindications/Cautions/Risks

Contraindications

- Antiplatelet/anticoagulant medications including Aspirin (acetylsalicylic acid, ASA), Coumadin (warfarin) Plavix (clopidogrel), or Persantine (dipyridamole) can increase the chances of developing a hematoma. The risk of holding the medication preoperatively must be weighed against the benefits of operating without these agents and the potential to reduce the risk of intraoperative hemorrhage or postoperative hematoma. The clinician must be aware of why the medication is being prescribed and discuss a plan with the patient regarding these medications at the preoperative visit because this will allow discussion with specialist teams, if required. This may involve consultation with a hematologist.
- Many herbal remedies such as St. John's wart, Ginkgo biloba, and garlic supplements can also increase bleeding risk. Our practice is to ask patients to hold herbal remedies for at least 1 week before surgery.

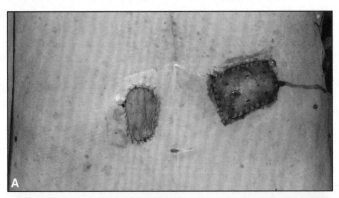

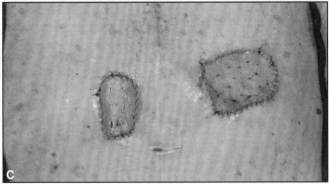

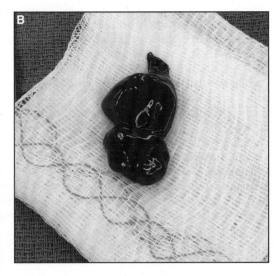

FIGURE 85.1. A, A hematoma under a skin graft. B, The hematoma itself. C, The skin graft laid back down after hematoma removal.

- Other conditions such as chronic renal or liver disease, excessive alcohol use, blood cancers, thrombocytopenia, or bleeding disorders such as hemophilia and von Willebrand disease can also increase the chance that a patient develops a hematoma.
- Cautery selection is affected by the presence of implantable cardioverter defibrillators and pacemakers. In general, bipolar diathermy is safer in such patients.

Cautions

- A hematoma may indicate the presence of another, yet unknown, bleeding disorder.
- If using electrocautery, care must be taken with preparatory agents. For example, if using alcohol, one must allow the alcohol to fully dry before placing drapes. Chlorhexidine/alcohol ChloraPrep™ (Becton, Dickinson and Company, US), a commonly used preparative agent, must be allowed to dry for 3 minutes before applying surgical drapes.

Risks

- Recurrence or inadequate hemostasis
- Would healing complications: necrosis, infection

Equipment Needed

- Hemostat
- Electrocautery Bovie pen
- Vicryl™ (Ethicon US, LLC) 3-0 and 4-0 sutures for the deep planes
- Chalazion clamp

Preprocedural Approach

- A drug history should include the use of ASA, which reversibly inhibits platelets and should be stopped 5 to 7 days before surgery and started again at least 7 days after surgery, depending on the risk of a stroke or myocardial infarction. Warfarin may also be stopped 2 to 4 days before surgery based on consideration of the patient's circumstances and the international normalized ratio (INR). Warfarin can be replaced with heparin subcutaneously until the day after surgery, when warfarin can be restarted. However, there are no hard and fast rules, because the risk of stopping the medication may be greater than is the benefit.
- Blood tests can be used to identify quantitative deficiencies, including the platelet count. The prothrombin time can assess the function of the coagulation cascade, and the partial thromboplastin time detects abnormalities in the intrinsic pathway.
- A complete blood count (CBC), coagulation, and metabolic and chemistry panel can help in the workup to assess for the presence of any underlying conditions. This is low yield and rarely done for outpatient surgery preoperatively, unless the patient is known to be thrombocytopenic. A patient's INR level may also be checked in the setting of anticoagulation.
- Imaging using computed tomography (CT) or magnetic resonance imaging (MRI) can help visualize within certain cavities, like the head or abdomen.
- Correction of any underlying disorders is essential to treating the hematoma.

Procedural Approach

- Clinical suspected hematomas should be reopened to localize bleeding blood vessels and to evacuate the hematoma.
- Most anesthetic agents can cause vasodilation and increase blood loss. Vasoconstrictive agents such as epinephrine and norepinephrine can help control blood loss and can prolong the anesthetic effect postoperatively. Alternatively, tumescent anesthesia can be used where dilute lidocaine (0.1%) and epinephrine concentrations (1:1 000 000) can be subcutaneously injected into the surrounding tissue to provide anesthesia. The anesthetic effect can last for 48 hours.
- The site can then be prepped for surgery using chlorhexidine and avoiding alcohol-based products if electrocautery is to be used.[2]
- Tourniquets can help decrease blood flow to a procedural area in extremity surgery.
- The site should be inspected for the affected vessels. Sterile gauze pads can be inserted into a body cavity to soak up excess blood and improve visualization of the surgical field, or cotton applications if the cavity is small. In addition, they can help compress bleeding sites to enhance coagulation.
- Hemostasis may be achieved using electrocautery or suture ligation.
- Instruments such as the chalazion clamp or hemostat can provide hemostasis by being placed around a vessel to tamponade the bleeding, at least momentarily until sutures can be placed in a clear space.
- If bleeding continues despite attempts at coagulation, a drain can be placed, or other topical hemostatic agents can be tried, for example, Monsel's solution or aluminum chloride.
- Acrylates can be applied to the skin, such as octyl-2-cyanoacrylate (DERMABOND™ Topical Skin Adhesive [Ethicon US, LLC]).
- Full debridement of the clotted tissue is necessary to eliminate material that increases the chances for infection, reduces the inflammation, and creates a cleaner space for closing.
- Hematomas that present late may be gelatinous and firm (Figure 85.1B). They can be evacuated or left to heal by secondary intension.
- Hematomas eventually undergo resorption and liquefactive necrosis. At this point, they can be either aspirated or drained with a 16- to 18-gauge needle.
- Once hemostasis is achieved, the cavity layers should be closed, and resutured, from deep to superficial. Surgical techniques that can help decrease bleeding and close areas in large defects are mattress sutures (Figure 85.1C).
- A clean pressure dressing can be applied.
- If the cavity is large or vascular and the risk of bleeding is high, drains can be inserted and monitored for daily output.

Postprocedural Approach

- The highest risk of bleeding is in the first 24 hours after surgery.
- Place a dressing immediately postoperatively and keep it in place for at least 24 hours to reduce the risk of a recurrent hematoma.
- In the immediate postoperative period, the clinical team is responsible for looking for early warning signs of bleeding, to track the recovery, and to escalate care where needed.

Common signs of hemorrhage include mental status change, obvious bruising or ecchymoses, tachycardia, drop in venous pressure, diminished cardiac output, reduced urine output, and swelling of the extremities.[1]

- Hematomas are a nidus for infection and prophylactic antibiotics should be prescribed for 5 to 7 postoperative days.
- Drains ideally should be removed after 24 hours, dependent on the blood loss, because of the increased risk of infection if they are left longer.

- Patients should be encouraged to be only minimally active for the first 24 hours, and to refrain from strenuous exercise for at least 1 month. Alcohol is a vasodilatant and should be discouraged until 1 week postoperatively.

REFERENCES

1. Dagi TF. The management of postoperative bleeding. *Surg Clin North Am.* 2005;85:1191–1213, x.
2. Hemani ML, Lepor H. Skin preparation for the prevention of surgical site infection: which agent is best? *Rev Urol.* 2009;11:190.

Hidradenitis Suppurativa (Acne Inversa)

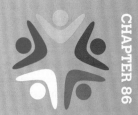

Christopher J. Sayed and Karina M. Paci

CHAPTER 86

Introduction

Hidradenitis suppurativa (HS), or acne inversa, is a debilitating chronic follicular disease, usually arising after puberty, that causes painful inflammation and scarring with a predilection for intertriginous areas. Ninety-six percent of pediatric patients present after age 10 years, and, similarly to adults, prevalence is increased in female and African-American patients. Early-onset disease is particularly likely to be linked to a family history of disease. Medical management is often helpful in reducing symptoms and inflammation, but the presence of cutaneous sinuses often requires surgery for the best results. Procedural management techniques include unroofing, incision and drainage (I&D), lasers for follicular destruction (see Chapters 18. Laser Surgery and 89. Hypertrichosis), and excision (limited, wide, or regional). Other treatment options, including botulinum toxin and cryosurgery, have limited utility with some mention in case reports in the medical literature. Surgical excision of affected areas shows the lowest recurrence rates, although other treatment methods, such as laser therapy, are emerging as successful.

We propose a brief procedural manual for treatment of HS in the outpatient setting with a focus on unroofing, intralesional triamcinolone, I&D, excisional procedures, and Nd:YAG/other follicular lasers. Dermatologists have the skillset necessary to play a central role in the surgical management of HS and have the knowledge needed to medically manage the patient before and after procedures to prevent recurrences.

Clinical Pearls

- **Guidelines:** No standard treatment guidelines exist for acne inversa.
- **Age-Specific Considerations:** Assessing willingness to undergo and tolerate procedures is important. Many procedures can be performed with local anesthesia; alternatively, an operating room setting with general anesthesia can be considered when treatment is medically indicated and patients cannot tolerate the discomfort associated with injecting local anesthesia or other aspects of a procedure.
- **Technique Tips:**
  - Consider anxiolytic therapy for anxious patients (eg, *appropriately dosed diazepam*).
  - Staging procedures can help keep wound sizes small to allow for wound suturing, mitigating patient fear, and simplifying wound management and recovery.
  - Local Anesthesia: Use 5- to 20-mL syringes, up to 100 mL for larger cases. Buffer and dilute to 0.5% to avoid lidocaine toxicity for larger volumes. Use a 0.5-in, 30-gauge needle for the first injection, then switch to 1.5-in 25-gauge needles to avoid hand fatigue and allow more rapid coverage in subcutaneous and dermal planes with fanning technique. Consider tumescent anesthesia for large areas.

Contraindications/Cautions/Risks

	UNROOFING AND MARSUPIALIZATION	INCISION AND DRAINAGE	EXCISIONAL PROCEDURES	LASERS (ND:YAG AND FOLLICULAR LASERS)
Contraindications	Inability to care for postoperative wounds	No absolute contraindications	Inability to care for postoperative wounds	No absolute contraindications
Cautions	Indication limited to mild to moderate severity of disease (Hurley stage I and II)	Indicated for relief of acute pain	Consider severity of disease to decide between local, wide, and radical excision	Requires minimum of three to four sessions for best results
Risks	Bleeding, hypertrophic scar, neuralgia (including axillary intercostobrachial neuralgia) at wound site	Recurrence is typical for chronic lesions.	Bleeding, infection, scarring, recurrence, rare risk of squamous cell carcinoma	Postlaser hyper- or hypopigmentation; minimal risk with appropriate device

Equipment Needed

UNROOFING AND MARSUPIALIZATION	INCISION AND DRAINAGE	EXCISIONAL PROCEDURES	LASERS (ND:YAG AND FOLLICULAR LASERS)
• Fistula probe • Scissors • Scalpel (usually #10 blade) • CO_2 laser • Sterile gauze • Electrosurgical loop • Nonstick dressing • 20% aluminum chloride	• Ice packs • Local anesthesia • 4- to 8-mm punch • Sterile gauze • Normal saline • Nonstick wound dressing/pad • 20% aluminum chloride solution	• Fistula probe • Scalpel (usually #10 blade) • CO_2 laser • Sterile gauze • Suture (*larger closures:* 2.0 absorbable for subcutaneous plicating; *superficial:* fast-absorbing gut or skin adhesive) • Petrolatum-based ointment • Nonstick wound dressing/pad	• Wavelength-specific eye shields • Appropriate laser device

Preprocedural Approach

For All Procedures: Consider severity of disease in assessing candidacy for treatment. Areas with extensive active and recurrent painful lesions make operative interventions more appropriate (Figure 86.1).

Procedural Approach

- Informed consent from the parent/guardian and assent from the minor are obtained.

INTRALESIONAL TRIAMCINOLONE

- The smallest possible gauge needle (27-30 G) should be used to inject 0.1 to 0.5 mL of solution into acute or chronically inflamed painful lesions (see Chapters 14. Injectables and 15. Injectable Corticosteroids [Intralesional Kenalog, Intramuscular]).
- Concentrations of 5 to 40 mg/mL can be considered with caution to avoid the superficial dermis when possible to avoid steroid-induced hypopigmentation.

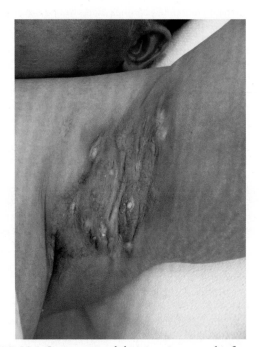

FIGURE 86.1. Interconnected draining sinuses and inflammatory nodules in a female with Hurley stage 3 disease.

- When possible, keep total injected dose below 40 mg to minimize systemic steroid effects.
- Placebo-controlled trials are currently lacking, but uncontrolled prospective data suggest improvement of pain in the days following treatment.

UNROOFING AND MARSUPIALIZATION

- Anesthesia is infiltrated from treatment area border and worked into the center.
- Probe is used to determine extent of disease tunnels, during and throughout the procedure, looking for additional extensions (Figure 86.2A).
- Scissors, scalpel, or CO_2 laser is used to incise and expose bases of tunneled areas and further bevel overlying tissue (Figure 86.2B). This can be done with the probe in place to help guide depth and direction of cutting. This procedure mostly involves the dermis, with little subcutaneous exposure.
- Beveling free edges to remove the "roof" of the opened sinus and prevent the wound from healing together at the free edges is essential (Figure 86.2B and C).
- For small chronic lesions, an 8-mm punch tool used for a single punch or a few contiguous punches may be adequate for unroofing.
- Roof excision with electrosurgical loop is an option, leading to quick hemostasis and helping to maintain the lining of the sinus floor.
- Probing along wound edges for communicating side passages is crucial for unroofing success.
- Often 20% aluminum chloride is adequate for hemostasis. Electrocautery can also be used once the aluminum chloride solution has fully dried.
- Wounds are dressed with petrolatum and nonstick bandaging and left to heal by secondary intention with daily changes. Wet-to-dry dressings and wound packing are typically not necessary and add to discomfort.

INCISION AND DRAINAGE

- Given the intense pain often present, an ice pack applied for 20 seconds immediately before injection of small amounts of local anesthesia is helpful.
- Using a punch tool, the site is quickly accessed, drained, and cleaned with sterile gauze and saline. Larger punches allow for more rapid drainage, less pressure, and discomfort; and continued drainage in the following days prevents abscesses from quickly reforming, as is often encountered with small scalpel or needle incisions.

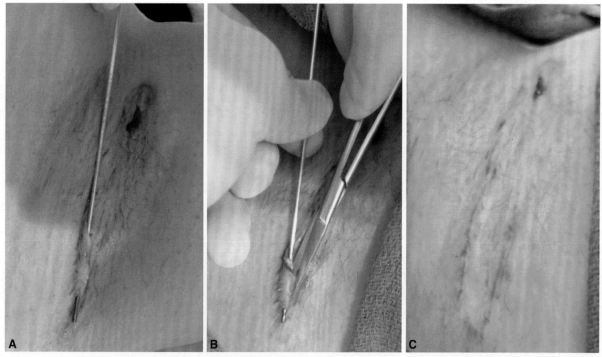

FIGURE 86.2. A, Probing to delineate areas of involvement. B, Opening sinus with scissors. C, Partial-thickness wound after unroofing.

- Wounds are dressed with petrolatum and nonstick bandaging and left to heal by secondary intention. Packing with gauze is typically not necessary given its limited benefit and the discomfort experienced with changes.

EXCISION

- Anesthesia is injected and probing occurs before excision to verify planned borders (Figure 86.3A).
- Excision, via a scalpel (#10 blade) or CO_2 laser, is performed in a superficial subcutaneous plane. If disease visibly extends into fat, deeper excision targeting specific areas can occur, but removal of large fat pads is usually not necessary (Figure 86.3B).
- Visual inspection and probing of borders is needed with extension of the excision when appropriate.
- Healing by secondary intention or suturing when confident that the disease is cleared is acceptable (Figure 86.3C). For large closures, a subcutaneous plicating suture (the author uses 2.0 Vicryl™ [Ethicon US, LLC]) is helpful in reducing tension on dermal sutures. Buried dermal sutures are selected depending on surgeon preference. For the superficial layer, a fast-absorbing gut suture or skin adhesive may reduce skin tearing around sutures.
- Open wounds are dressed with copious petrolatum and nonstick dressings changed daily.

LASER

- Regions frequently developing new nodules and abscesses tend to have the best response. Established sinuses do not typically resolve with lasers used for follicular destruction. Surgical intervention is typically still necessary in these cases in addition to laser.
- Protective eyewear should be worn.

- Typical treatment plans encompass three to four sessions spaced every 4 to 6 weeks, although additional treatments for maximal hair reduction may be beneficial.
- Local cooling can be used, but additional anesthesia is typically not necessary.
- Settings are based on skin type and individual laser devices (see Chapter 18. Laser Surgery).
- Delayed perifollicular erythema and edema are the primary clinical endpoints.

Postprocedural Approach

FOR ALL PROCEDURES

- Worsening pain and drainage should trigger patients to contact their physicians; infection rates are very low.
- Adequate concurrent medical management is key for reducing recurrence rates.
- Exuberant granulation tissue interfering with healing often responds to triamcinolone ointment applied daily for 1 week.

UNROOFING AND MARSUPIALIZATION

- Healing time varies from 3 to 4 weeks for narrow wounds to 6 to 8 weeks for larger areas. For small procedures, patients can return to work in 1 to 2 days, but it may take up to 2 to 3 weeks for very large cases.

INCISION AND DRAINAGE

- Wounds will continue to drain freely for up to 7 days following the procedure.
- Considering indication for acute pain relief, I&D is not a definitive management for most chronic lesions, with exceptions for small completely unroofed or excised lesions. Patients will likely need further management with unroofing, excision, or lasers.

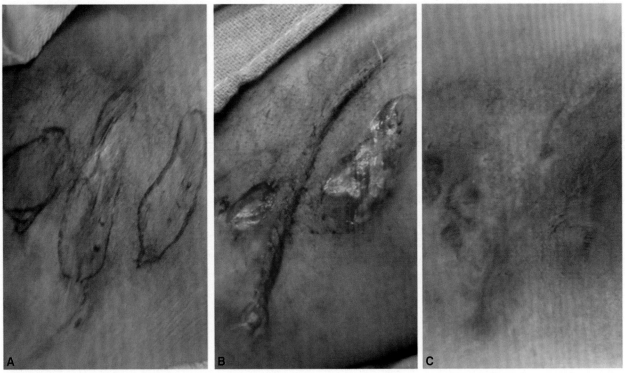

FIGURE 86.3. A, Preoperative lesions. B, Central excision with primary closure, with two unroofing wounds on either side. C, Scars following complete healing.

EXCISION

- Healing time spans 2 to 4 weeks for small, sutured wounds; and 8 to 12 weeks for larger wounds.
- Recurrence rates are lowest with complete excisions of affected areas.

LASER

- Ice packs can be used for analgesia.
- Sun avoidance for 2 weeks before and after each procedure is recommended.

SUGGESTED READINGS

Garg A, Wertenteil S, Baltz R, Strunk A, Finelt N. Prevalence estimates for hidradenitis suppurativa among children and adolescents in the United States: a gender-and age-adjusted population analysis. *J Invest Dermatol.* 2018;138(10):2152–2156.

Liy-Wong C, Pope E, Lara-Corrales I. Hidradenitis suppurativa in the pediatric population. *J Am Acad Dermatol.* 2015;73(5, suppl 1):S36–S41.

Ritz JP, Runkel N, Haier J, Buhr HJ. Extent of surgery and recurrence rate of hidradenitis suppurativa. *Int J Colorectal Dis.* 1998;13(4):164–168.

Saunte DML, Jemec GBE. Hidradenitis suppurativa: advances in diagnosis and treatment. *JAMA.* 2017;318(20):2019–2032.

Van hattem S, Spoo JR, Horváth B, Jonkman MF, Leeman FW. Surgical treatment of sinuses by deroofing in hidradenitis suppurativa. *Dermatol Surg.* 2012;38(3):494–497.

CHAPTER 87

Hyperhidrosis
Jane Sanders Bellet

OVERVIEW

Primary focal hyperhidrosis is excessive sweating due to no known underlying cause. Frequently beginning in adolescence, it also can begin in very early childhood. The axillae, palms, and soles are most commonly affected. Other locations such as the craniofacial and groin areas may also be involved. Many treatment options exist including topical medications, systemic medications, iontophoresis, microwave destruction, and, for severe cases, sympathectomy. Botulinum toxin A injections work particularly well for the axillae, but they can also be used for palmar, plantar, groin, and craniofacial hyperhidrosis. Results are variable, but many patients will have significant improvement of symptoms for 6 to 12 months before retreatment is required.

Clinical Pearls

- **Guidelines:** No specific treatment guidelines exist for hyperhidrosis.
- **Age-Specific Considerations:** Botulinum toxin A injections for hyperhidrosis are used off-label for those younger than 18 years of age. OnabotulinumtoxinA BOTOX®, [©2020 Allergan, Irvine, CA] is currently the only form of botulinum toxin A approved by the U.S. Food and Drug Administration (FDA) for use in patients with axillary hyperhidrosis older than 18 years of age. Injections are approved for children as young as 12 for blepharospasm and strabismus and for those with cervical dystonia older than 16 years. AbobotulinumtoxinA (Dysport® [Galderma Laboratories ©2020 US]) is approved for treatment of cervical dystonia and glabellar lines in adults, although it is used in other parts of the world for hyperhidrosis. Axillary injections can be well tolerated in the office with the use of topical anesthetic. Palmar and plantar injections are not well tolerated in young patients and require either general anesthesia or ulnar/radial nerve blocks for those younger than 18 years of age.
- **Technique Tips:** Use an easy-to-remove marking pen (white or green, WhiteEZ® Removable Ink or GreenEZ® Removable Ink [Viscot Medical, LLC, East Hanover, NJ]), not Gentian violet because that will take a few days to wash off.
  - Apply topical anesthetic to the axillae for at least 60 minutes (preferably 75 minutes) because this allows for both decreased pain and superior vasoconstriction, which decreases the amount of leakage of the botulinum toxin.
  - After the injection, push slightly in and then pull out; this also helps reduce leakage of the botulinum toxin.
  - Do not "flick" or tap the syringe. You do not want to lose any of the botulinum toxin A.

Contraindications/Cautions/Risks

Cautions
An FDA black box warning has been issued because of the risk of generalized muscle weakness and respiratory difficulty secondary to distant spread of the toxin. This can occur hours to weeks after injection; however, this has not been reported when used for hyperhidrosis. Informed consent is essential before botulinum toxin A usage.

Contraindications
- Active skin infection at injection site
- Hypersensitivity
- Neuromuscular conditions: Amyotrophic lateral sclerosis (ALS), myasthenia gravis, motor neuropathy, and Guillain-Barré.

Risks
- Pain
- Swelling
- Ecchymosis
- "Flulike" syndrome
- Botulism
- For palmar injections, transient weakness can occur with diffusion into the hand muscles. With repeated treatments, permanent weakness can result. This risk should be discussed before the first treatment as well as before every subsequent treatment.

Equipment Needed
- Topical anesthetic (lidocaine 4% cream, LMX.4™ [Ferndale Laboratories])
- Plastic wrap (Glad Press' N Seal® [Glad Products Company, Oakland, CA] works best)
- Botulinum toxin A (brand and number of units determined by physician)
- Preservative-free 0.9% NaCl (normal saline)
- 1-mm Luer-Lok® Disposable Syringes (Becton, Dickinson and Company, Franklin Lakes, NJ)
- 30-gauge needles
- Marking pen (white or green, WhiteEZ Removable Ink or GreenEZ Removable Ink)
- Gauze
- Alcohol wipes
- Optional: Betadine, cornstarch

Preoperative Approach

- No special preparation is required before treatment.
- If the patient wishes to exercise on the day of treatment, recommend that it be done before the treatment.
- If the patient removes axillary hair via shaving, depilatory, or waxing, then the procedure is easier to perform; however, this is not required.
- Be sure that the tamper-evident seal of the vial is intact before opening. Be sure the vial is legitimate, because there have been counterfeit vials sold. If using BOTOX, a holographic film on the vial label that contains the name "Allergan" within horizontal lines of rainbow color will be seen for BOTOX products; in addition, U.S. license number 1145 will be on the carton and vial label.
- Reconstitute the botulinum toxin A with preservative-free 0.9% sodium chloride injection to the dilution desired. Some options include the following: If injecting 100 units total, dilute with 4.4 mL of sodium chloride per 100 unit vial, and if injecting 200 units total, dilute with 2.2 mL of sodium chloride per 100 unit vial.

Intraoperative Technique

- Informed consent is obtained from the patient and parent.
- Minor's starch iodine test can be performed before injections and can be helpful to visualize the affected areas. Betadine is swabbed onto the area(s) of interest. Allow it to thoroughly dry. Dust a small amount of cornstarch over the dry Betadine. Wait 10 minutes. The ambient temperature of the room can be increased to facilitate sweating. Wherever deep purple color is visible, this indicates that sweating has occurred. This area can be delineated with a marking pen.
- For axillary injections, treatment is usually well tolerated in the office setting with the use of a topical anesthetic such as lidocaine 4% cream (LMX.4). Allow at least 60 minutes for adequate penetration. More time decreases pain and increases vasoconstriction. For palm and sole injections, these are not usually well tolerated by children or adolescents and require either general anesthesia or ulnar and radial nerve blocks. Median and ulnar nerve blocks have their own risks; consequently, general anesthesia would be employed by this author.
- Have the patient lie down on the examination table and raise the arm over the head and rest it on the pillow. Mark injection sites approximately 1.5 to 2 cm apart in a "diamond grid" pattern with a marking pen so that the diffusion areas overlap

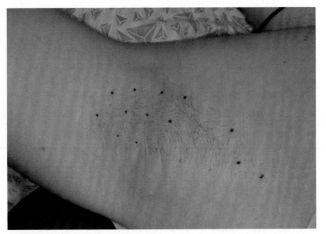

FIGURE 87.1. Mark injection sites approximately 1.5 to 2 cm apart in a "diamond grid" pattern with overlapping diffusion.

(Figure 87.1). Give the patient a "stress squeezy ball" because this gives them a focal point for any pain they may experience. Make sure that you have adequate visualization of the entire axilla. With the skin stretched, a 30-gauge needle on a 1-mL Luer-Lok syringe is used and should be inserted into the dermis to a depth of approximately 2 mm and at a 45° angle with the bevel up (Figure 87.2). Inject just below each pen mark, so as to avoid any potential for tattooing. The entire volume is divided into 0.1 to 0.2 mL aliquots and distributed among 15 to 30 sites, which are 1 to 2 cm apart. Fifty units per axilla is a standard starting point; however, efficacious dosages range up to 200 units per axilla. Change the needle frequently (approximately every six to seven injections), as a dull needle hurts more. When finished with each axilla, wipe the pen marks off with an alcohol wipe and put the patient's arm down on the examination table (patients do not need to keep their arms above their head).

- For palmar or plantar injections, a similar grid pattern is marked, being sure to include the fingers or toes. A higher dose is usually required, often at least 100 units per palm or sole.

Postoperative Approach

- No special care is required of the treated site.
- Mild bruising and swelling as well as discomfort may occur. Acetaminophen or ibuprofen can be given if needed.

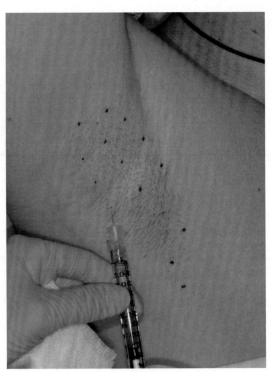

FIGURE 87.2. Injections given at 45° angle with the bevel up.

- No exercise for 24 hours. This is more precautionary than an absolute.
- Improvement should be noted within 4 to 5 days. Maximum improvement is usually seen by 14 days postoperative.
- Subsequent treatments are performed when the effect wears off. Ideally, this is at least 6 months and hopefully longer.

SUGGESTED READINGS

Bohaty BR, Hebert AA. Special considerations for children with hyperhidrosis. *Dermatol Clin.* 2014;32(4):477–484.

Coutinho dos Santos LH, Gomes AM, Giraldi S, Abagge KT, Marinoni LP. Palmar hyperhidrosis: long-term follow-up of nine children and adolescents treated with botulinum toxin type A. *Pediatr Dermatol.* 2009;26(4):439–444.

Glaser DA, Pariser DM, Hebert AA, et al. A prospective, nonrandomized, open-label study of the efficacy and safety of onabotulinumtoxinA in adolescents with primary axillary hyperhidrosis. *Pediatr Dermatol.* 2015;32(5):609–617.

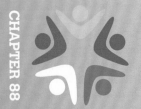

CHAPTER 88

Hyperpigmentation

Nicholas Ryan Lowe, Nisma Mujahid, Tara L. Rosenberg, Denise W. Metry, and Audrey Chan

Introduction

Hyperpigmentation is a frequently encountered condition with a myriad of underlying etiologies with varying characteristics. Most pigmented lesions contain melanin and have epidermal, dermal, or mixed components. Certain conditions with primarily superficial pigmentation may be targeted with topical retinoids, corticosteroids, and/or bleaching agents; however, these are usually ineffective for melanocytic lesions. With the advent of laser therapy, management of hyperpigmented lesions due to either melanin or other nonmelanin pigments has become feasible, especially in locations unfavorable to excision or in lesions with a pigment that is situated at levels not adequately managed with topical therapies (Figure 88.1).

Melanin has a wide absorption spectrum, meaning that many different lasers can be used to target melanin; however, different wavelengths have variable ability to penetrate to deeper layers of the skin instead of dissipating energy in more superficial lesions. On the basis of these principles, knowledge of the histologic depth of lesions is important in the selection of the wavelength used. Pulse duration is also important, because pulse durations limited to less than half of the thermal relaxation time of the target chromophore minimizes destruction to the surrounding tissue. Longer pulse durations can be used in specific scenarios where adjacent damage is desired, such as in elimination of nested melanocytes. Unfortunately, there is limited published literature on use of laser therapy in the treatment of pigmented lesions in children.[1,2]

 Clinical Pearls

- **Skin of Color Considerations:** Patients with darker skin phenotypes are at greater risk of dyspigmentation. When treating lesions with dermal or mixed components, wavelengths with greater melanin absorption will be absorbed by nonlesional melanin, which may lead to dyschromia.
  - To minimize risk of dyschromia
    - Use lasers with longer wavelengths (such as 1064 nm) to allow penetration with minimal absorbance by more superficial melanin; however, lower fluences should be employed.
    - Maximize cooling mechanisms for that particular laser.
    - Perform conservative "test spots" before treating larger areas.
- **Technique Tips:** Lasers that have a wavelength close to absorption peaks of hemoglobin are also effective on melanin; using simultaneous compression with a compression handpiece or other compression medium minimizes intravascular red blood cells, and thus minimizes absorption by off-target chromophores.

Contraindications/Cautions/Risks

Contraindications
- Active skin infection
- Inability to care for postoperative wounds

Risks
- Death (infection or anesthesia), scarring, bleeding, pain, dyspigmentation, recurrence of lesion
- There are often residual melanocytes left in the deeper reticular dermis after treatment of melanocytic lesions, which may mask future malignant transformation; treatment sites must be closely monitored.

Cautions
- Presence of a suntan may increase risk of dyspigmentation.

Equipment Needed
- Wavelength-specific eye shields, optical density (OD) 5+ rated
- Laser (see Table 88.1 for laser selection and settings published in the literature)
- Cooling equipment
- Topical anesthetic or coordination for general anesthesia
- Petrolatum-based ointment

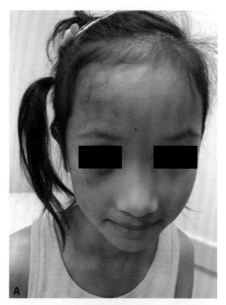

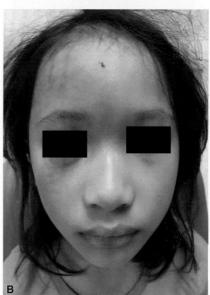

FIGURE 88.1. A, Right facial nevus of ota 3 years s/p alexandrite laser and q-switched Nd:YAG laser treatments. B, Same patient 2 months s/p 3 more alexandrite laser treatments with improved appearance of hyperpigmentation.

Preprocedural Approach

- Evaluate for anesthesia and/or sedation: age, level of anxiety in relation to procedure, surface area involved
- For laser treatment on face, in patients with history of herpes simplex infections: prophylaxis for herpes simplex started 1 to 2 days before laser surgery
- Patients should bathe before their surgery.
- Strict sun protection and sun avoidance is advised 4 to 6 weeks before treatment.

Procedural Approach

- Informed consent from the parent/guardian and, when possible, assent from the minor are obtained.
- Typically, general anesthesia is used because of pain associated with the procedure.

TABLE 88.1 ⋮ Conditions Associated With Hyperpigmentation With Published Laser Selection and Parameters

LESION	AUTHOR	LASER (WAVELENGTH)	SETTINGS	PATIENT CHARACTERISTICS	REPORTED RESULTS
Nevus of Ota (see Chapter 110. Nevus of Ota and Nevus of Ito)	Belkin et al. (2018)[3]	Q-switched ruby (694 nm) Q-switched Nd:YAG (1064 nm)	No settings available	N = 23 children Age: range 3 mo-12.4 y; mean age 3.9 y Skin types: 4 receiving Q-switched ruby (71%) 5-6 receiving Q-switched Nd:YAG (29%)	86% saw at least 50% improvement; Improvement was better in lower Fitzpatrick types.
Nevus of Ota	Felton et al. (2014)[4]	Q-switched alexandrite (755 nm) Q-switched Nd:YAG (532 nm)	Q-switched alexandrite: (4.2-18 J/cm², 2-4 mm) Q-switched Nd:YAG: (0.5-5 J/cm², 2-5 mm)	N = 21 patients (of which 4 were children) Q-switched alexandrite: N = 2 Age and skin types: 15 y with skin type 5 Q-switched Nd:YAG N = 2 Age and skin types: 18 y with skin type 4 16 y with skin type 5	Q-switched alexandrite: One patient noted 50% improvement after seven treatments, the other noted 90% improvement after eight treatments. Q-switched Nd:YAG: 18-y-old patient with 90% improvement after 13 treatments; 16-y-old patient with 100% improvement after eight treatments
Dermal melanocytosis (see Chapter 74. Dermal Melanocytosis [Mongolian Spot])	Kagami et al. (2012)[5]	Q-switched alexandrite (755 nm)	Fluence: 4-5 J/cm² Pulse duration: 50 ns Spot size: 4 mm	N = 16 patients (of which 3 were children) Age, skin type, location: 14-y-old patient with skin type 3 with buttock involvement 18-y-old patient with skin type 3 with facial involvement 18-y-old patient with skin type 3 with trunk and extremity involvement	14-y-old patient with "good" results after nine treatments 18-y-old patient with facial involvement, noted "good" results after eight treatments 18-y-old patient with trunk/extremity involvement, noted "good" results after 12 treatments, but complicated by hypopigmentation
Lentigines (facial and labial in Peutz–Jeghers)	Li et al. (2012)[6]	Q-switched alexandrite (755 nm)	Fluence: 5-7 J/cm² Pulse duration: 75 ns Spot size: 2.4 mm	N = 43 patients Age: range 5-43 y (data on individual patients not available) Skin type: 3-5	Three treatments 55.8% with more than 75% clearance
Lentigines (labial in Peutz–Jeghers)	Kato et al. (1997)[7]	Normal-mode ruby (694 nm)	Fluence: 20 J/cm² Pulse duration: 450 µs Spot size: 6 mm	N = 2 Age: 10 and 12 y Skin types: not available	10-y-old patient with four treatments at 1- or 2-mo intervals with nearly complete resolution, no recurrence at 3-y follow-up 12-y-old patient with two treatments at 2-mo intervals with complete resolution, no recurrence at 2-y follow-up
Café-au-lait macules (see Chapter 66. Café au Lait Macules)	Artzi et al. (2018)[8]	Picosecond frequency-doubled Nd:YAG (532 nm)	Fluence: 0.8-1.6 J/cm² Spot size: 4-5 mm	N = 16 patients (of which 4 were children) Age, skin type, location: 18 y, skin type 3, eye corner 8 y, skin type 2, nose 17 y, skin type 2, abdomen 14 y, Fitz II, face	18-y-old patient: nearly complete resolution after one treatment 8-y-old patient: nearly complete resolution after one treatment 17-y-old patient: 50%-75% clearance after two treatments 14-y-old patient: nearly complete resolution after one treatment

TABLE 88.1 : Conditions Associated With Hyperpigmentation With Published Laser Selection and Parameters (*continued*)

LESION	AUTHOR	LASER (WAVELENGTH)	SETTINGS	PATIENT CHARACTERISTICS	REPORTED RESULTS
Café-au-lait macules (see Chapter 66. Café au Lait Macules)	Kim et al. (2015)[9]	Q-switched Nd:YAG (1064 nm) Q-switched frequency-doubled Nd:YAG (532 nm)	1064-nm settings: Fluence: 2.6 -3 J/cm^2 Spot size: 7 mm 10 Hz 3 passes 532-nm settings: Fluence: 1.0-1.2 J/cm^2 Spot size: 2.6 mm 2 Hz 1 pass	$N = 32$ patients Age: range 2-36 y (data on individual patients are not available) Skin type: 4	100% patients in 1064-nm group had "good" or "better" clinical response, but only 67% of the patients in the 532-nm group had any clinical response.
Congenital melanocytic nevus	Funayama et al. (2012)[10]	Q-switched ruby (694 nm) PLUS PDL (595 nm)	Ruby Fluence: 6-10 J/cm^2 PDL Fluence: 6-10 J/cm^2 Spot size: 7 mm	$N = 6$ (of which 3 were children) Age, %BSA, location: 12-y-old patient with 10% BSA on abdomen and leg 12-y-old patient with 2% BSA on nape 4-y-old patient with 5% BSA on arm Skin types: not available	Average number of treatments was 7. All three patients had nearly completely response. The 4-y-old patient developed hypopigmentation.
Congenital melanocytic nevus	Minakawa et al. (2012)[11]	Q-switched ruby (694 nm)	Settings not available	$N = 18$ Age: range 4 mo-14 y (mean 5.5 y) Skin types: 3 and 4	Patient underwent 2-44 treatments with poor results to slight improvement. After 3+ y of follow-up: 11 continued to have slight improvement, 5 were repigmented within 1 mo
Congenital melanocytic nevus	Kono et al. (2005)[12]	Normal-mode ruby (694 nm) vs. normal-mode ruby + Q-switched ruby	Normal-mode ruby (694 nm): Fluence: 20-30 J/cm^2 Pulse duration: 1 ms Spot size: 10 mm Q-switched ruby (694 nm): Fluence: 7 J/cm^2 Pulse duration: 30 ns Spot size: 4 mm	$N = 15$ (data on individual patients not available) Ages: range 5 mo-55 y (data on individual patients not available) Skin types: 3-5	Average of six treatment sessions at 1-3 mo intervals. Combination resulted in better outcomes (64%-72% significantly lightened) vs. NMRL alone. None of the treated lesions were cleared histologically, regardless of treatment cohort.
Congenital melanocytic nevus of the ala	Zeng et al. (2016)[13]	CO_2 laser alone or with Q-switched Nd:YAG (1064 nm)	CO_2: Power: 1-3 W Spot size: 0.2-0.4 mm Nd:YAG Fluence: 5-8 J/cm^2 Pulse duration: 8 ns Spot size: 2-3 mm	$N = 8$ (of which 7 were children) Age: range 9-18 y	Patients underwent one to six treatments. CO_2 laser found to be more effective, because Nd:YAG alone lightened some of the nevi but left hyperplastic tissue requiring follow-up treatment with CO_2 laser. One patient had moderate response, three patients had good response, and two patients had excellent response. Scarring noted in two out of six children. Pigmentation noted in two out of six children. Dyspigmentation noted in three out of six children

BSA, body surface area; NMRL, normal-mode ruby laser; PDL, pulsed-dye laser.

- Confirm that protective eyewear is OD 5 or higher for the wavelength of the laser being used. Patients should be provided with eye protection as well: adhesive eye pads or metal eye shields may be used.
- Use the selected laser on lesional skin. Cooling with cryogen sprays, cool air blower, or a cooling handpiece (if available) may be used to mitigate thermal damage to nontarget structures (Table 88.1).
- After session, petrolatum-based ointment is applied liberally to area.
- Ice may be applied to area to decrease discomfort and limit edema.

Postprocedural Approach

- For laser treatment on face, in patients with history of herpes simplex infections: continue herpes prophylaxis for 7 to 10 days.
- Patients are instructed to gently wash treated areas with warm soap and water three times daily.
- Patients are instructed to keep laser-treated area covered with generous amounts of Vaseline.
- Patients should make every effort to keep areas treated elevated, including while sleeping.
- Patient/parents advised to watch for signs and symptoms of infection.
- Strict sun protection and sun avoidance is advised 4 to 6 weeks after treatment.
- Depending on lesion and clinical response, patient may require multiple treatment sessions with adjustments in laser settings as needed.

REFERENCES

Introduction
1. Carpo BG, Grevelink JM, Grevelink SV. Laser treatment of pigmented lesions in children. *Semin Cutan Med Surg.* 1999;18(3):233–243.
2. Shahriari M, Makkar H, Finch J. Laser therapy in dermatology: Kids are not just little people. *Clin Dermatol.* 2015;33(6):681–686.

Nevus of Ota
3. Belkin DA, Jeon H, Weiss E, Brauer JA, Geronemus RG. Successful and safe use of Q-switched lasers in the treatment of nevus of Ota in children with phototypes IV-VI. *Lasers Surg Med.* 2018;50(1):56–60.
4. Felton SJ, Al-Niami F, Ferguson JE, Madan V. Our perspective of the treatment of nevus of Ota with 1,064-, 755-and 532-nm wavelength lasers. *Lasers Med Sci.* 2014;29(5):1745–1749.

Dermal Melanocytosis (Mongolian Spot)
5. Kagami S, Asahina A, Uwajima Y, et al. Treatment of persistent Mongolian spots with Q-switched alexandrite laser. *Lasers Med Sci.* 2012;27(6):1229–1232.

Lentigines Associated With Peutz-Jeghers Syndromes
6. Li Y, Tong X, Yang J, Yang L, Tao J, Tu Y. Q-switched alexandrite laser treatment of facial and labial lentigines associated with Peutz-Jeghers syndrome. *Photodermatol Photoimmunol Photomed.* 2012;28(4):196–199.
7. Kato S, Takeyama J, Tanita Y, Ebina K. Ruby laser therapy for labial lentigines in Peutz-Jeghers syndrome. *Eur J Pediatr.* 1998;157(8):622–624.

Café-au-Lait Macules
8. Artzi O, Mehrabi JN, Koren A, Niv R, Lapidoth M, Levi A. Picosecond 532-nm neodymium-doped yttrium aluminium garnet laser—a novel and promising modality for the treatment of cafe-au-lait macules. *Lasers Med Sci.* 2018;33(4):693–697.
9. Kim HR, Ha JM, Park MS, et al. A low-fluence 1064-nm Q-switched neodymium-doped yttrium aluminium garnet laser for the treatment of cafeau-lait macules. *J Am Acad Dermatol.* 2015;73(3):477–483.

Congenital Melanocytic Nevi
10. Funayama E, Sasaki S, Furukawa H, et al. Effectiveness of combined pulsed dye and Q-switched ruby laser treatment for large to giant congenital melanocytic naevi. *Br J Dermatol.* 2012;167(5):1085–1091.
11. Kono T, Ercocen AR, Nozaki M. Treatment of congenital melanocytic nevi using the combined (normal-mode plus Q-switched) ruby laser in Asians: clinical response in relation to histological type. *Ann Plast Surg.* 2005;54(5):494–501.
12. Minakawa S, Takeda H, Korekawa A, Kaneko T, Urushidate S, Sawamura D. Q-switched ruby laser therapy and long-term follow-up evaluation of small to medium-sized congenital melanocytic naevi. *Clin Exp Dermatol.* 2012;37(4):438–440.
13. Zeng Y, Ji C, Zhan K, Weng W. Treatment of nasal ala nodular congenital melanocytic naevus with carbon dioxide laser and Q-switched Nd:YAG laser. *Lasers Med Sci.* 2016;31(8):1627–1632.

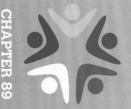

CHAPTER 89

Hypertrichosis

Deborah Moon, Shauna Higgins, and Ashley Wysong[*]

INTRODUCTION

Hypertrichosis refers to excessive hair growth in nonandrogen dependent areas. This is in contrast to *hirsutism*, which specifically describes excessive hair growth in androgen-dependent areas (eg, upper lip, chin, anterior chest, linea alba, upper inner thighs, legs), in women or prepubertal children.[1] Hypertrichosis can generally be classified as *primary* versus *secondary*, congenital versus acquired, and localized versus generalized. It may occur as part of a larger congenital syndrome or secondary to neurologic conditions (such as encephalitis and traumatic brain injury), medications (notably phenytoin and cyclosporine), hypothyroidism, anorexia nervosa and malnutrition, porphyria, dermatomyositis, and acrodynia (Tables 89.1 and 89.2).[2]

Early and appropriate treatment is crucial given the psychosocial impact hypertrichosis may have on children. If hypertrichosis is secondary to an underlying condition or part of a

*Latanya T. Benjamin provided additional editorial review of this chapter.

TABLE 89.1 : Localized/Circumscribed Hypertrichosis

TYPES OF LOCALIZED HYPERTRICHOSIS	CLINICAL PRESENTATION AND COURSE	ASSOCIATED SYMPTOMS/ CONDITIONS	WORKUP
Congenital nevocellular nevus (congenital)	May have hair within lesion	—	Consider serial excisions if >20 cm or increased risk of malignant degeneration (see Chapter 109. Nevi).
Nevoid hypertrichosis (congenital)	Patch of terminal hair, often solitary	No associated abnormalities. Consider spinal abnormalities if presents in a faun tail distribution (see "Spinal hypertrichosis (congenital)")	—
Spinal hypertrichosis (congenital)	Patch of terminal hair over the sacrum ("faun-tail"), or midline vellus hair ("silky down")	Spinal abnormalities, including dermal cyst or sinus, myelomeningocele, diastematomyelia, vertebral abnormalities, or subdural or extradural lipoma	Obtaining magnetic resonance imaging is critical, as early surgical intervention may be necessary.
Smooth muscle hamartoma (congenital)	Skin colored to hyperpigmented slightly elevated plaque often with vellus hypertrichosis. Can be distinguished from Becker nevus by rubbing the lesion, which induces a "pseudo-Darier" sign (surfaces changes and a transient piloerection) in smooth muscle hamartoma.	May be isolated or seen within a Becker nevus	—
Hypertrichosis cubiti (congenital)	Symmetric hair growth on elbows. Often appears in infancy, progresses in childhood, and improves or resolves during adolescence.	May be isolated or associated with Wiedemann-Steiner syndrome (rare autosomal dominant condition characterized by distinct facial features, short stature, intellectual disability, and hypertrichosis cubiti).	If patient with concerning features, may consider genetic testing
Hairy cutaneous malformation of palms and soles (congenital)	Rare, autosomal dominant. Women and children have vellus hairs on bilateral palms and/or soles. Vellus hairs become terminal for males at puberty.	—	—
Hypertrichosis associated with neurofibroma (congenital)	Hyperpigmentation, hypertrichosis overlying neurofibroma	Neurofibroma; may occur in isolation or in association with neurofibromatosis	Begin with thorough examination for possible signs of neurofibromatosis, including café-au-lait macules, freckling in axillary or inguinal regions, neurofibromas, or Lisch nodules.
Hemihypertrophy (congenital)	Patients may have terminal hypertrichosis on hypertrophic side	May be isolated or associated with Beckwith-Wiedemann syndrome, neurofibromatosis, Klippel-Trenaunay-Weber syndrome, and Proteus syndrome. May also be associated with Wilms' tumor, hepatoblastomas, brain tumors, adrenocortic neoplasms, internal hemangiomas, and genitourinary malformations	Requires thorough initial workup. Subsequent serial abdominal ultrasounds are recommended by some.
Anterior cervical hypertrichosis (congenital)	Patch of terminal hair superior to the laryngeal prominence	Sometimes associated with peripheral neuropathy	—
Becker nevus (typically acquired)	Often solitary, hypermelanotic patch with increased hair growth at puberty; more common in males and on the torso	Often isolated but may occur as part of a Becker nevus syndrome (unilateral breast and areolar hypoplasia, focal acne, pectus carinatum, limb asymmetry, and spina bifida)	Treatment is generally discouraged, although hypertrichosis may be treated with laser depilation, if desired.

(continued)

TABLE 89.1 ⋮ Localized/Circumscribed Hypertrichosis (*continued*)

TYPES OF LOCALIZED HYPERTRICHOSIS	CLINICAL PRESENTATION AND COURSE	ASSOCIATED SYMPTOMS/ CONDITIONS	WORKUP
Hypertrichosis associated with local inflammation (acquired)	May arise from chemically induced dermatitis (psoralen, iodine), orthopedic casts, friction, other inflammatory causes	—	—
Hypertrichosis of the pinna (acquired)	Often older men but also seen with diabetes, in babies with diabetic mothers, babies with XYY syndrome, and AIDS	See "Clinical Presentation and Course"	Depending on clinical presentation, consider working up for a possible underlying condition.
Trichomegaly (acquired)	Acquired hypertrichosis of the eyelashes	Trichomegaly has been reported in HIV, systemic lupus erythematosus, and with use of medications, such as latanoprost.	Depending on clinical presentation, consider working up for a possible underlying condition.

Adapted from Wendelin DS, Pope DN, Mallory SB. Hypertrichosis. *J Am Acad Dermatol*. 2003;48(2):161-181. Copyright © 2003 American Academy of Dermatology, Inc. With permission.

TABLE 89.2 ⋮ Generalized Hypertrichosis

TYPES OF GENERALIZED	CLINICAL PRESENTATION AND COURSE	ASSOCIATED SYMPTOMS/CONDITIONS	WORKUP
Primary			
Congenital hypertrichosis lanuginosa (congenital)	Lanugo hairs retained diffusely; often decrease in hair over trunk and limbs in late childhood; autosomal dominant and sporadic cases	Case reports of dental anomalies	—
Acquired hypertrichosis lanuginosa (acquired)	Conversion of normal hair to lanugo hair often in craniocaudal spread, signs of internal malignancy	May see other cutaneous manifestations of internal malignancy	Internal malignancy workup
Congenital generalized hypertrichosis (congenital)	Extremely rare; diffuse terminal hair hypertrichosis; X-linked	—	—
Gingival fibromatosis with hypertrichosis (congenital)	Dark terminal hairs on peripheral face, central back and extremities, with gingival hyperplasia; autosomal dominant	Gingival hyperplasia, ~50% cases with mental retardation, seizures	Rule out medications (eg, antiepileptic, cyclosporine), which may cause hypertrichosis and gingival hyperplasia.
Secondary			
Medication (eg, phenytoin, cyclosporine, minoxidil, diazoxide, acetazolamide, latanoprost, psoralen, valproic acid, streptomycin) (acquired)	Distribution of hair growth may vary by medication.	—	May resolve with discontinuation
Thyroid abnormalities (acquired)	Generalized hypertrichosis more common in children; resolves with thyroid hormone replacement	Cold intolerance, weight gain, dry skin, constipation, fatigue, pretibial myxedema, poor growth, coarse and brittle scalp hair	Thyroid function panel
Porphyrias (Porphyria cutanea tarda, erythropoietic porphyria, erythropoietic protoporphyria, hereditary coprophyria, variegate porphyria, acquired porphyrias) (congenital or acquired)	Blistering photosensitivity with scarring, pigmentary changes, and hypertrichosis in sun-exposed areas (esp. the face and limbs). Porphyria cutanea tarda can have isolated findings of hypertrichosis over the face and upper torso.	Often elevated liver transaminase	**Initial workup:** Total plasma, serum, or spot urine porphyrins

TABLE 89.2 Generalized Hypertrichosis (*continued*)

TYPES OF GENERALIZED	CLINICAL PRESENTATION AND COURSE	ASSOCIATED SYMPTOMS/CONDITIONS	WORKUP
Anorexia/malnutrition (acquired)	Generalized vellus hypertrichosis	Multisystem complications depending on severity	Complete blood count (CBC), comprehensive chemistry panel, thyroid-stimulating hormone, vitamin D, and electrocardiogram. Rule out organic causes.
Cerebral disturbances (acquired)	May be seen in encephalitis, traumatic head injury, or other cerebral disturbances	Variety of neurologic symptoms	—
Paraneoplastic (eg, polymyositis) (acquired)	More common in adults	Proximal muscle weakness	Creatine kinase, aldolase, antinuclear **antibody** and myositis-specific Ab, chest imaging
Dermatomyositis (acquired)	Hypertrichosis on face and limbs, more in males	Gottron's papules, heliotrope rash, proximal muscle weakness	As above
Acrodynia (acquired)	From chronic mercury exposure	Increased salivation and perspiration, painful hands and feet	Mercury levels in serum or 24 h urine collection
Teratogenic (fetal hydantoin syndrome, fetal alcohol syndrome) (congenital)	**Fetal hydantoin syndrome** (from phenytoin, carbamazepine exposure): Hypertrichosis, cleft lip, midfacial hypoplasia, nail hypoplasia, low birth weight. **Fetal alcohol syndrome:** growth deficiency, developmental delay, mental retardation, distinct facial features	(See left)	—
Infection (eg, tuberculosis, AIDS) (acquired)	Transient hypertrichosis	Variable depending clinical presentation, subacute/chronic constitutional symptoms, immunosuppression	Chest imaging, sputum specimen, tuberculin skin test (for latency)
POEMS (Crow-Fukase) syndrome (acquired)	Generalized hypertrichosis (especially more over lower extremities), hyperpigmentation, cutaneous angiomas, edema, digital clubbing	Polyneuropathy, organomegaly, endocrinopathy, M protein, skin changes; plasma cell dyscrasias	Eye examination for papilledema, serum vascular endothelial growth factor, CBC with differential, peripheral blood smear, serum protein electrophoresis, urine protein electrophoresis, metastatic bone survey, endocrine evaluation
Osteochondrodysplasia with hypertrichosis (Cantú syndrome) (congenital)	Autosomal recessive skeletal dysplasia	Often short stature; may have macrosomia and cardiomegaly	Refer for thorough workup involving skeletal radiographs and chromosomal analysis; severe forms may be diagnosed in utero via ultrasound
Other syndromes (Brachmann-de Lange, Berardinelli-Seip, Lawrence-Seip, Donohue, Hurler, Hunter, Sanfilippo, Stiff-skin, Winchester, Rubinstein-Taybi, Schinzel-Giedion, Barber-Say, Coffin-Siris, MELAS, Hemimaxillofacial dysplasia, craniofacial dysostosis, hypomelanosis of Ito) (congenital)	Various congenital syndromes that may present with hypertrichosis	May have facial and skeletal abnormalities, mental retardation, and other multisystem abnormalities (cardiac, lung gastrointestinal/ genitourinary, metabolic, hyperinsulinemia)	Requires thorough workup and multidisciplinary approach

Adapted from Wendelin DS, Pope DN, Mallory SB. Hypertrichosis. *J Am Acad Dermatol.* 2003;48(2):161-181. Copyright © 2003 American Academy of Dermatology, Inc. With permission.

larger congenital syndrome, a multidisciplinary team should be employed to evaluate and treat the underlying cause and address associated conditions. Additional treatments to areas of excess hair growth include concealment, depilation (removal of hair along the shaft), epilation (the removal of the *entire* hair shaft), and eflornithine cream (not approved for use by those younger than 12 years), which prevents new hair growth (Tables 89.3 and 89.4).[2] Factors to consider in selecting treatment include patient and family convenience, the patient's pain tolerance, the patient's Fitzpatrick skin type, the anatomic location of the excess hair growth, and the cost of treatment.

Clinical Pearls

- *Safety and efficacy of laser hair removal in the pediatric population*—Although laser hair removal has been reported as a common nonsurgical cosmetic procedure among minors, its evidence in those under the age of 18 is not robust (Oxford Level of Evidence 4). Despite this, the long-pulsed ruby, alexandrite, and Nd:YAG have been proven to have some utility in small case studies.
- Some recommend waiting until puberty for laser hair removal, as hair growth patterns (and style preferences) may change.

- *Managing expectations about laser treatment*—Laser therapy is an effective long-lasting, though not always permanent, means of hair removal. It requires multiple sessions and is optimal for dark hair on light skin (the laser selectivity optimizes in high contrast).[3]
- **Age-Specific Considerations:**
  - Before and after photos of laser treatments in children may be reassuring for both patients and their parents.[2]
  - If older children are anxious, it may be helpful to describe what the laser will feel like (eg, a band snapped against skin) so they are aware of what to expect.[4]
  - Ensure thorough preprocedure preparation to minimize the time the child must remain still and cooperative. The child may become anxious after donning eye protection equipment and it may be reassuring for the provider or the parent to talk to the patient so that they know they are not alone.
- **Skin of Color Considerations:**
  - The long-pulsed Nd:YAG (1064 nm) is the wavelength of choice for darker skin types (Fitzpatrick IV-VI), given the lower risk of epidermal melanin absorption and damage with this longer wavelength.
  - The diode may also be used for some darker skin types, although the Nd:YAG may have an improved safety profile in Fitzpatrick IV skin types and above.[4]

TABLE 89.3 : Treatment Options for Hypertrichosis

TREATMENT OPTIONS	PROS	CONS	LONGEVITY	OTHER COMMENTS
Concealing Methods				
Cover, make-up	Easy, painless	Variable effect	Daily	—
Bleaching	Quick, easy, painless	Skin irritation; may be undesirable for darker skin, as dark hair will be discolored yellow causing hair to be more noticeable	Up to 4 wk	—
Depilation (hair removal along any part of the hair shaft)				
Mechanical • Shaving • Trimming	Easy, inexpensive	Need to shave daily, otherwise blunt hair ends may worsen cosmetic appearance. It may be considered psychosocially unacceptable for females to have "stubble" on the face.	Up to 4 wk, but typically 1-2 wk per reported expert experience	Shaving does not increase growth rate, pigmentation, or thickness. May appear thicker, given hair ends are blunted rather than tapered.
Chemical depilation • Sulfides • Thioglycates	Easy home treatment	Allergic contact dermatitis; irritation; unpleasant odor (sulfides); not recommended for extensive areas, given possible risk of systemic absorption and toxicity	About a week	Consider a test site first. **Sulfides:** More effective but have an unpleasant odor and more irritating **Thioglycates:** Less effective with slower action but less irritating and without odor
Enzymatic	Less irritating	Less effective than chemical depilation	About a week	Consider for localized areas; Caution against toxic reactions from systemic absorption for larger surface areas
Epilation (removal of entire hair shaft)				
Mechanical • Plucking • Waxing	Lasts longer than depilation	May be more painful for prepubertal children; hair needs to be at least 2-3 mm for effective waxing. **Adverse effects:** hyperpigmentation, folliculitis, scarring, ingrown hairs	Regrowth 4-6 wk	—

TABLE 89.3 ⋮ Treatment Options for Hypertrichosis (*continued*)

TREATMENT OPTIONS	PROS	CONS	LONGEVITY	OTHER COMMENTS
Electrolysis	Permanent hair removal	Most painful; poorly tolerated in children even with topical anesthetic; long process; operator dependent **Adverse effects**: transient erythema, edema, and bruising; postinflammatory hyperpigmentation in darker skin	Permanent	Performed by an electrologist
Laser	Less painful than electrolysis, rapid, effective	Pain may be uncomfortable for children. **Adverse effects**: pigmentary changes, erythema, edema, discomfort, (rarely) scarring	Total suppression of hair growth may last 3-6 mo; hair may take up to 2 wk to fall out	Consider topical anesthesia. **Goal:** Highest tolerable fluence that gives the desired endpoints of perifollicular erythema and edema without epidermal damage (eg, blistering). Most effective on dark hairs
Intense pulsed light (IPL) (570-1200 nm)	Greatest safety when using appropriate cooling, cheaper than laser	May not be as effective as laser. There are reports of greater efficacy and few side effects with the Nd:YAG laser compared to the IPL for darker skin types.	About 6-8 wk; hair falls out in 1-3 wk	Shorter pulse durations for finer hair; Longer pulse durations for thicker hair.
Eflornithine cream 13.9% BID at least 8 h apart (not approved for use by those <12 y old)	Rather than removing hair, this treatment prevents hair regrowth.	Hair growth returns after discontinuing.	Onset of improvement around 4-8 wk	Do not use over widespread areas given risk of toxicity from systemic absorption (myelosuppression).

Adapted from Olsen EA. Methods of hair removal. *J Am Acad Dermatol*. 1999;40(2):143–155 and Nouri K. *Handbook of Lasers in Dermatology*. London, UK: Springer; 2014.

TABLE 89.4 ⋮ Lasers for Hair Removal

LASER	PROS	CONS	LONGEVITY	OTHER COMMENTS
Long-pulsed ruby (694 nm)	Long history of use, effective for Fitzpatrick skin types I-III	Not recommended for darker skin types.	Total suppression of hair growth may last 3-6 mo.	Less commonly used today. Caution: pulsing >3-4 ms can be problematic. A study with 28 cases of hair removal using the Ruby laser in children <16 y old showed efficacy and tolerability.[7]
Long-pulsed alexandrite (755 nm)	Effective for lighter skin types (I-III) with less risk of adverse effects compared to the Ruby laser given its longer wavelength.	Not recommended for darker skin types.	3-6 mo	Use appropriate cooling or may have postinflammatory pigmentary changes even in skin type II or suntanned type II. A study of 24 children under 16 years reported successful hair removal with the alexandrite and Nd:YAG.[8]
Diode (800-810 nm)	Effective for darker skin types (I-IV, and up to VI in some cases). More efficacious than the long pulsed Nd:YAG but with increased risk of adverse effects. Small, portable, user friendly	Narrower margin of safety compared to the long-pulsed Nd:YAG	3-6 mo	Relatively safer for darker skin types, but should still be used with caution given increased risk of adverse effects compared to the Nd:YAG Pulse durations >100 ms may be used to improve safety in darker skin. For even darker skin types (eg, type VI), pulse durations >400 ms have been reported; aggressive skin cooling is essential.
Long pulsed Nd:YAG (1064 nm)	Safest for darker skin types (IV-VI).	Less effective than the above lasers.	3-6 mo	Safest for darker skin when pulse durations are ≥30 ms with aggressive skin cooling, but may be less effective.

Adapted from Nouri K. *Handbook of Lasers in Dermatology*. London, UK: Springer; 2014; Alexis AF, Barbosa VH. *Skin of Color: A Practical Guide to Dermatologic Diagnosis and Treatment*. New York, NY: Springer; 2013; Bolognia J, Jorizzo JL, Schaffer JV. *Dermatology*. Philadelphia, PA: Elsevier Saunders; 2012; and Paller AS, Mancini AJ. *Hurwitz Clinical Pediatric Dermatology E-Book: A Textbook of Skin Disorders of Childhood and Adolescence*. London, UK: Elsevier Health Sciences; 2015.

Contraindications/Cautions/Risks

Contraindications

- Contraindications for laser therapy include: Photosensitivity, recent sun tanning, seizure disorder triggered by light, and prior/current gold therapy.

Cautions

- Consider using lower fluences for those with a higher risk of adverse effects (eg, darker skin type, propensity for keloid formation, and/or use of photosensitizing medications such as isotretinoin).

Risks

- Mild to moderate pain, erythema, perifollicular edema, temporary dyspigmentation, blistering, crusting, infection, scarring, and paradoxical hypertrichosis (occurring in 0.6%-10% of patients and more commonly on the face and neck and in darker skin types). This phenomena is proposed to be related to subtherapeutic fluences during treatment.[3]

Equipment Needed

- Consent form
- Camera
- Appropriately sized eye protection with the appropriate optical density for all individuals in the room (occasionally, overlapping gauze is applied to fit the contour of the periorbital region, as standard gear may not provide adequate protection for small children)
- Metal corneal shields for periorbital laser treatments, including anesthetic eye drops and protective eye ointment
- Laser with smoke evacuator system, as surgical smoke may be carcinogenic
- Cooling method (eg, ice, cooled gel, cryogen spray, solid air flow)
- Topical anesthetic (eg, EMLA™ [AB Astra Pharmaceuticals, L.P.], LMX.4™ or LMX.5™ [Ferndale Laboratories])
- Gauze (to remove topical anesthetic)
- Mild topical corticosteroid

Preprocedural Approach

- Obtain a thorough history to assess the patient's candidacy for the procedure (see Contraindications), symptoms of endocrinopathies (irregular menstruation, acne), current medications, and prior treatments and associated outcomes and adverse effects.
- If the patient has a history of herpes simplex at the treatment site, provide prophylactic therapy.
- Refer concerning patients for workup of underlying conditions.[3]
- Counsel patients to sun protect 6 weeks prior to and after treatment, to stop any epilatory treatments 2 to 4 weeks prior, to shave the night before, and to not apply skin care products on the day of procedure.[3]

Procedural Approach

- *Equipment and eye safety*
  - Ensure all individuals are wearing appropriate eye safety equipment prior to and throughout the procedure.
  - Prepare the cooling method, and activate the evacuator system during laser treatment, as surgical smoke may be carcinogenic.
  - Exercise caution to clear any flammable substances from the laser.[3]
- *Anesthesia*
  - Clean the treatment site with a mild cleanser and water or an alcohol pad, ensuring the alcohol is allowed to dry completely (at least 3 minutes).
  - Commonly utilized topical anesthesia includes lidocaine 2.5% and prilocaine 2.5% (EMLA) and 4% or 5% liposomal lidocaine cream (LMX.4). Exercise caution to adhere strictly to the recommended safe dosages and administration of EMLA, as overdose from systemic absorption may result in symptomatic methemoglobinemia. Some have discouraged use for premature infants and those under 1 month of age, while others recommend extra caution up to 3 months of age, given immature enzyme systems.[5]
  - Using a gloved finger, apply a layer and allow it to sit for about 30 minutes and no longer than 1 hour to avoid systemic absorption (Figure 89.1).
  - Completely remove topical anesthetic with a gauze to prevent further systemic absorption and to remove any residual flammable substances.[3]
  - Topical anesthetics should only be applied in the clinic where the patient can be monitored and should not be given for the patient to apply at home.
  - Additional anesthetic options include local injectable 1% lidocaine solution with epinephrine or general anesthesia. Although general anesthesia is considered to be a reasonable option for treating children with functionally

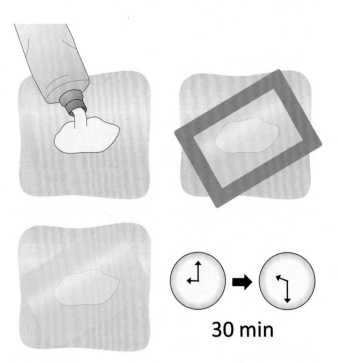

FIGURE 89.1. Topical anesthetic applied to skin and allowed to sit for about 30 minutes and no longer than 1 hour to avoid systemic absorption.

significant or cosmetically disfiguring lesions, the risks of general anesthesia for those under 3 years are poorly understood. Recent literature has suggested that children exposed to greater than one general anesthesia episode by age 4 may be at increased risk of learning disabilities and cognitive dysfunction.[6] The Food and Drug Administration has also issued a recent warning to consider avoiding serial general anesthesia in children younger than 3 years or in pregnant women during their third trimester because it may affect the development of children's brains. Consequently, for elective cosmetic procedures it may be best to delay exposure to general anesthesia until the child is over 4 years.

- *Selecting and using lasers*
  - Consult the manual for specific instrument operating instructions and setting recommendations.
  - Prior to starting treatment, the laser should be test fired away from the patient to ensure that it is working properly and that cooling spray (if on the device) is firing.
  - Depending on the laser hand piece, it may be placed approximately 1 to 2 cm from the surface of the skin (typically with a spacer) or applied directly to the skin.
  - The laser is activated by pressing the appropriate button on the hand piece or foot pedal. The hand piece should be moved along a deliberate path and passes made with an approximate 10% overlap of the treatment area.
  - A reasonable goal is to treat with the highest tolerable fluence that gives the desired endpoints of perifollicular erythema and edema. During the first treatment, it is prudent to perform "test spots" with several fluences to find the ideal settings, waiting approximately 10 to 15 minutes for the desired endpoints.
  - Signs that the fluence is too high include epidermal changes such as graying, crusting, or blistering.
  - Fluence in future treatments should also be lowered if patient reports excessive pain, erythema, and edema lasting for several hours.
  - Darker skin types are at increased risk of epidermal injury. Appropriate and increased cooling compared to lower Fitzpatrick skin types reduces risk of adverse effects. The long-pulsed Nd:YAG (1064 nm) has been most widely recommended for darker skin types (Fitzpatrick IV-VI), as there is less absorption of energy by epidermal melanin with longer wavelengths. The diode (800-810 nm) has been used for skin types I to IV and up to VI by some, although the risk of adverse effects is higher as the shorter wavelength is not ideal for darker skin types. For lighter skin types (Fitzpatrick type I-III), the long-pulsed ruby (694 nm) and the alexandrite (755 nm) lasers are also safe and effective choices (Table 89.4).[3,4]

- *Laser tolerability*
  - If concerned about laser tolerability in certain patients (eg, darker skin type, history of hypertrophic scars, anxious patients/parents, location on a cosmetically sensitive area in a new patient), a test spot may be performed (four spots overlapping by 10%) in a less cosmetically sensitive area with similar skin color, hair density, and sun exposure.
  - Signs of cutaneous side effects in patients with darker skin may not be visible until 2 days post-treatment, and therefore, skin evaluations should be performed at least 48 hours after the laser test spot was performed to determine appropriate parameters.[4]

Postprocedural Approach

  - Cooling with an ice pack and a mild topical steroid cream may help reduce erythema, swelling, and postoperative pain.
  - Educate patients and families on the importance of extensive sun protection for at least 1 month after the procedure.
  - If a folliculitis-type reaction occurs, it should be treated with antibiotics and/or corticosteroids.
  - Reassure patients that they should expect shedding of the hair within 1 to 2 weeks of their laser treatment.
  - Reassure patients that mild erythema and perifollicular edema are to be expected, although symptoms lasting for more than several hours should prompt them to notify their physician.[3]

REFERENCES

1. Paller AS, Mancini AJ. *Hurwitz Clinical Pediatric Dermatology E-Book: A Textbook of Skin Disorders of Childhood and Adolescence.* London, UK: Elsevier Health Sciences; 2015.
2. Wendelin DS, Pope DN, Mallory SB. Hypertrichosis. *J Am Acad Dermatol.* 2003;48(2):161–179; quiz 180–181.
3. Nouri K. *Handbook of Lasers in Dermatology.* London, UK: Springer; 2014.
4. Alexis AF, Barbosa VH. *Skin of Color: A Practical Guide to Dermatologic Diagnosis and Treatment.* New York, NY: Springer; 2013.
5. Lillieborg S, Otterbom I, Ahlen K. Topical anaesthesia in neonates, infants and children. *Br J Anaesth.* 2004;92(3):450–451.
6. Backeljauw, Barynia, et al. Cognition and brain structure following early childhood surgery with anesthesia. *Pediatrics.* 2015;136(1):e1–e12.
7. Morley S, Gault D. Hair removal using the long-pulsed ruby laser in children. *J Clin Laser Med Surg.* 2000;18(6):277–280.
8. Rajpar S, Hague JS, Abdullah A, Lanigan SW. Hair removal with the long-pulse alexandrite and long-pulse Nd: YAG lasers is safe and well tolerated in children. *Clin Exp Dermatol.* 2009;34(6):684–687.

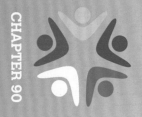

CHAPTER 90

Hypertrophic Scars and Contractures

James J. Contestable and Peter R. Shumaker*

Introduction

Hypertrophic scars (HTSs) are pathologic fibrotic skin responses that can arise in any phase of childhood in response to dermal injury from a variety of inciting events, such as surgery, trauma (eg, lacerations and burns), and inflammation (eg, acne and infections). Keloids are associated with overlapping stimuli and treatment modalities, but demonstrate a range of differences, including histopathologic basis, more aggressive tumor-like growth, and greater resistance to treatment. This chapter focuses on the management of HTS and contractures, especially following trauma.

Multiple variables contribute to HTS formation, including body location, depth of injury, degree of tension, patient age, and individual predisposition. Contractures arise from a progressive shortening of the scar tissue across a joint, resulting in loss of range of motion and related functional sequelae. In addition to functional disability and disfigurement, HTSs and contractures can be associated with symptoms such as pain and itch and psychosocial impairment. This constellation of issues is compounded during the active growth and development of children. Current management and mitigation strategies include conservative measures such as silicone gels and sheets, injectables such as corticosteroids, massage, and physical and occupational therapy. Lasers such as the 595-nm pulsed-dye laser (PDL), 1064-nm neodymium-doped yttrium-aluminum-garnet (Nd:YAG), nonablative fractional lasers (NAFLs), and ablative fractional lasers (AFLs) are increasingly working their way into institutional paradigms.[1] The latter in particular has revolutionized the treatment of HTSs and contractures over the past decade. This chapter emphasizes minimally invasive procedures such as lasers and injectables that can be added to standard management. Repeated interventions and observation over months and years are expected.

Clinical Pearls

- **Guidelines:** A lack of randomized controlled trials limits the available level of evidence for the management of traumatic scars and contractures, though the preponderance of current literature supports the efficacy of laser treatment.
- **Age-Specific Considerations:** Younger patients with more extensive involvement are more likely to require general anesthesia. Longitudinal management must accommodate ongoing growth and development.
- **Anatomic-Specific Considerations:** Scars in virtually any anatomic location will respond to treatment. Fractional lasers, offering tunable depth of penetration and density, are flexible platforms for the treatment of scars of variable thickness and reduced healing potential.
- **Technique Tips:** Since early evidence suggests scars may respond better to early intervention, and to mitigate the impact of HTSs and contractures on growth and development, proactive management should be considered

in the first weeks and months after the inciting event when feasible (Figure 90.1A and B). Adjuncts to anesthesia including cold packs, vibratory stimuli, and distraction techniques (eg, movies, video games, virtual reality) may be helpful in selected patients.
- **Skin of Color Considerations:** AFL and NAFL are options suitable for all skin types because the target is tissue water. Consideration should be given to reducing settings by about 30% in darker skin types, as well as increasing intervals between treatments. Millisecond 1064-nm lasers are more suitable than PDL for darker skin types because of decreased melanin absorption. Topical bleaching agents (eg, hydroquinone) are not frequently used by the authors in the setting of HTSs and contractures.

Contraindications/Cautions/Risks

Contraindications
- Active skin infection (eg, herpes labialis and impetigo)
- Inability to care for postoperative wounds

Cautions
- Baseline pigmentation and postprocedural sun exposure may exacerbate dyspigmentation.
- Treatment options include potential triggers for post-traumatic stress reactions (ie, anxiety, pain, sounds, odors). Mitigation of these stimuli (ie, earplugs, masks, distraction techniques, suitable transparent eye protection, etc) should be considered where feasible.
- Oxygen delivered by cannula or mask may accumulate in layered towels around the head and neck and become a fire hazard.
- Avoid excessive surface area of topical anesthetics; special caution with compounded anesthetics in children owing to enhanced and unpredictable absorption; anesthetics containing prilocaine in very young children (methemoglobinemia)[2,3]
- Though commonly used, medications such as triamcinolone acetonide suspension (TAC) applied after ablative fractional resurfacing (laser-assisted delivery or LAD) have not yet been formulated or approved for this mode of delivery.

---

*Disclaimer: The views expressed in this article are those of the authors and do not reflect the official policy or position of the Department of the Navy, Department of Defense, Department of Veterans Affairs, or the U.S. government. Dr. Contestable is a military service member. This work was prepared as a part of his official duties. Title 17, U.S.C. §105 provides that copyright protection under this title is not available for any work of the U.S. Government. Title 17, U.S.C., §101 defines a U.S. Government work as a work prepared by a military service member or employee of the U.S. Government as part of that person's official duties.

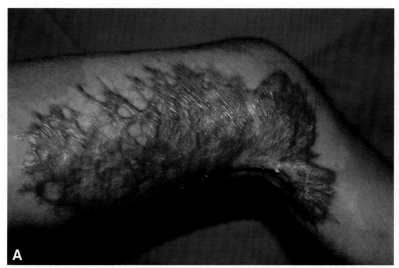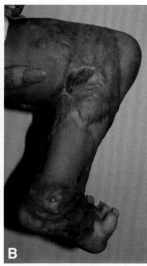

FIGURE 90.1. A, Hypertrophic scar with a developing contracture in a 9-year-old child approximately 4 months following a thermal injury. Intervention with minimally invasive techniques such as vascular and fractional lasers at early stages of recovery (ie, within weeks and months of injury) can help prevent or mitigate hypertrophic scar and contracture formation and occupy a paradigm-shifting position between conservative techniques (eg, pressure garments, therapy) and surgical intervention. In this patient with significant hypertrophy and an incipient contracture, ablative fractional laser resurfacing with laser-assisted delivery of corticosteroids would be a good initial choice in combination with other standard measures, such as massage, pressure garments, and physical therapy. The peripheral hypopigmentation without hypertrophic scarring demonstrates the importance of injury depth on hypertrophic scar formation. Vascular-specific devices can be incorporated for same-day or alternating treatments. B, Inadequate posthospital care and ongoing anticipatory scar management can result in catastrophic contractures that are debilitating for both the patient and family.

- Fractional lasers should be used at a low-density setting to minimize the risk of worsening scarring.
- Caution should be used when contemplating anesthetic blocks in traumatized digits; lower volumes of lidocaine without epinephrine should be considered.

Risks
- Procedural pain; bleeding; dyspigmentation; infection; atrophy; persistent, recurrent, or worsening scarring; death (infection or anesthesia)

Equipment Needed
- Appropriately sized laser-safe, internal/external eye shields, or appropriate wavelength-specific goggles for patients
- Wavelength-specific goggles for laser operators and supporting personnel
- Laser signage, window coverings, door locks, fire extinguishers, and other safety equipment as dictated by national and institutional requirements
- Laser-safe endotracheal tube and moist towels, especially when working around the face in anesthetized patients
- Topical (eg, 4% lidocaine cream) and injectable (eg, 1% lidocaine with and without epinephrine) anesthetics
- Cold pack/forced air chiller
- Distraction techniques such as electronics and vibratory stimuli
- Smoke evacuator (specifically HEPA filtration, 25-35 CFM, 2-3 cm from operative site)
- Masks suitable for particulates for operators and support staff (eg, N95)
- Sterile gauze
- Petrolatum or petrolatum-based ointment

- Nonstick dressings
- Triamcinolone acetonide suspension (TAC) 10 and 40 mg/mL
- High-potency steroid ointment and steroid tapes
- 5-fluorouracil (5-FU) 50 mg/mL
- 1-mL Luer-Lok® syringe (Becton-Dickinson and Company, Franklin Lakes, NJ) and 30-gauge ½ in needle
- 595-nm PDL
- Fractional CO_2 laser (10 600-nm) or Er:YAG laser (2940-nm)
- Fractional nonablative laser (eg, 1540-, 1550-, 1565-nm)
- Short- (nanosecond/picosecond) and long-pulsed (millisecond) 755- and 1064-nm lasers
- Fillers such as hyaluronic acid and poly-L-lactic acid

Preprocedural Approach

- For at least 4 weeks before and after laser surgery, patients with darker skin types should maximize sun protection and avoidance to reduce the risk of dyspigmentation.
- Prophylaxis for herpes simplex may be considered beginning the day of or 1 day prior to laser procedures, particularly in the context of perioral treatment locations and a strong history of recurrent outbreaks.
- Patients should bathe either the evening before or the morning of their ablative laser procedure.
- For relatively small treatment areas or prior to treatments associated with modest discomfort, topical anesthetics may be adequate alone or prior to injections of lidocaine solution. It is prudent to apply the cream in clinic, particularly if using compounded high-potency topical anesthetics to avoid excessive areas of application. Appropriate dosing (including concentrations and area of application) will vary depending

on the age and weight of the patient.[2,3] It should be noted that vascular blanching associated with topical anesthetics may impact the efficacy of vascular laser treatments.

- Cold packs, forced chilled air, vibrating devices, and other distraction techniques including electronics can also be utilized during local anesthetic injection, or during the procedure for added pain management. However, given that the efficacy of these adjuncts can vary and most of these procedures are associated with limited postoperative pain, it may be better on balance to simply proceed.
- Younger children with larger areas of involvement, relatively painful procedures such as AFL, or body locations associated with increased pain (ie, palms, face) may require a referral for general anesthesia.
- Patients with functional deficits should receive physical/occupational therapy consultation to assess baseline status and augment rehabilitation during the course of treatment and beyond.
- Mental health issues are common in traumatically injured patients, and a referral should be considered if there is any suspicion of undiagnosed or untreated disorders such as post-traumatic stress and depression.
- Prior to laser procedures, all topical anesthetic and makeup residue (if present) should be removed with moist gauze, cleansing wipes, or soap and water. Aside from general cleansing and simple alcohol wipes, sterile skin preparation (eg, chlorhexidine, iodine-based cleansers) is not commonly used by the authors before laser procedures.
- Informed consent from the parent/guardian (and assent for older children) should be obtained for each distinct procedure.
- A surgical timeout should be performed to verify items such as patient identification and treatment site, allergies, eye protection for patient and providers, appropriate safety equipment (eg, fire extinguisher and smoke evacuator), treatment settings, medication dose, and locked treatment room doors.

Procedural Approach ▶

Traumatically injured areas may display a variety of findings concurrently, such as erythema, hypertrophy, atrophy, hyperpigmentation, hypopigmentation, and contracture; each finding merits a tailored approach. Although a variety of techniques are often combined, fractional lasers fill a unique niche as they do offer a degree of efficacy for each of these components. With experience, it is possible to safely combine different techniques in the same area in the same treatment session. However, scars have reduced healing potential compared to uninjured skin, and excessive cumulative injury should be avoided. When less experienced, it may be safer to perform interventions in alternating treatment sessions at several week intervals; this is especially true for younger scars associated with more profound erythema.

RED PORTIONS OF SCAR

- Other interventions may impact the degree of swelling and erythema of the scar, so erythematous areas should often be addressed first.
- PDL is well tolerated and can be effective for scar-associated pain and itch, such as following burns.
- The 595-nm PDL is the best studied of the vascular-specific lasers and light devices. For lighter skin types, the scar is frequently treated with a 7- or 10-mm spot size, a pulse width of

1.5 ms, moderate cooling settings, and fluence depending on the selected spot size. The clinical end point is light purpura; for a 7-mm spot, the fluence is frequently in the range of 7 to 9 J/cm² (595-nm Vbeam Perfecta™ [Candela Corporation, US]). For a 10-mm spot, the fluence is frequently in the range of 4 to 6 J/cm². Pulses are delivered in a single pass with approximately 10% overlap.

- PDL should be used with caution in skin types III and IV because of increased epidermal melanin. Lower fluences, a longer pulse width, and greater attention to cooling may be considered for these skin types.
- PDL is generally not appropriate for skin types V and VI. Millisecond 1064-nm lasers are often overlooked and may be beneficial in all skin types. The authors use settings of 6 mm, 40 to 65 J/cm² (depending on skin type), 20 to 30 ms pulse width, and 30/20/0 ms cooling (Gentle Max; Syneron-Candela Corporation).
- PDL may be the only intervention for flat red scars.
- Other vascular-specific devices such as intense pulsed light and 532-nm lasers may also be applied for erythematous scars. Fluences used for scars should generally be lower than those used for vascular destruction (by ~30%) because the overall goal is the induction of a remodeling response.
- Prolonged erythema is a sign of ongoing inflammation and may be a harbinger of incipient hypertrophy.

CHANGES IN TEXTURE/ELEVATION OF THE SCAR

Hypertrophy and atrophy result from an imbalance in extracellular matrix deposition and degradation in response to injury and inflammatory processes. Both AFL and NAFL alone may have some benefit for both hypertrophic and atrophic scars.

SELECTING ABLATIVE FRACTIONAL LASER PARAMETERS

- The important parameters pertaining to AFL resurfacing include the microbeam diameter, pulse width, treatment depth, and microcolumn density. Microbeam diameter and pulse width are generally fixed depending on the laser platform, whereas treatment depth (pulse energy) and density can be adjusted by the operator. Selection of a platform with a relatively narrow beam diameter (up to a few hundred microns) and pulse width (<1 ms) are key to safe scar treatments.
- Likewise, a low treatment density will help minimize the risk of worsening scarring. Density should be inversely proportional to the treatment depth to minimize thermal injury and may frequently be at the lowest setting (1%-10%).
- Treatment depth should be proportional to the estimated scar thickness. Approximately 3.5 mm is the greatest treatment depth available with current technology. Thick, contracted scars may be treated with the highest pulse energy and the lowest density, whereas atrophic scars may be treated with low or moderate pulse energy and density settings.

HYPERTROPHY

- Hypertrophy may be managed in part with corticosteroids and antimetabolites, most commonly TAC and 5-FU solution, respectively.

- TAC is commonly used in a range of concentrations from 10 to 40 mg/mL, proportional to the degree of hypertrophy in a particular area. It may be injected intralesionally, applied topically after ablative fractional resurfacing (LAD), or both. TAC can be associated with prolonged cutaneous atrophy, so judicious injections into the scar tissue avoiding adjacent normal skin are necessary. Injections are performed by the authors with a 30-gauge ½ in needle attached to a Luer-Lok syringe. Injections are performed in a retrograde manner after advancing the needle, above the level of adjacent normal skin. Appropriate injection pressure is associated with subtle vascular blanching of the scar tissue. A lack of resistance may indicate excessive depth of injection. Consideration must be paid to the overall quantity of corticosteroid as the body surface area-to-weight ratio of a pediatric patient is considerably higher than adults. Hypothalamic–pituitary axis suppression is a concern when excessive doses are used. When injected, a maximum single dose of 1 to 1.5 mg/kg is reasonable. The maximum safe amount of TAC applied through LAD is more difficult to decipher as most applied product will end up on the gauze after application. TAC is frequently delivered by the authors at 3- to 4-week intervals.
- Similar to TAC, 5-FU may be injected intralesionally or applied topically using LAD. To our knowledge, there are no published articles on the use of 5-FU via LAD for pediatric scars. However, extrapolating from successful use in adults indicates it is worth additional study. It may be used alone in a concentration of 50 mg/mL, but most commonly in adults, it is combined with TAC in ratio of 3:1 or 9:1 (5-FU:TAC). Efficacy appears to be similar between the two medications in adults, but 5-FU may be associated with less risk of atrophy.
- Pretreatment of larger scars with an AFL may facilitate intralesional injection.
- When performing LAD, treat elevated areas with the fractional laser first. The medication is squirted onto the treatment area and rubbed over top of the laser channels within a few minutes of treatment. The excess is simply wiped away with gauze. Once the medication has been applied to elevated areas, the remainder of the scar can be treated with the laser.

ATROPHY

- Cutaneous fillers may be combined with fractional laser treatment to manage scars associated with atrophy.
- A course of AFL or NAFL resurfacing prior to filler injection may facilitate contour restoration by improving scar pliability and tethering.
- Cutaneous fillers such as poly-L-lactic acid (Sculptra; Galderma Laboratories, LP; Fort Worth, TX) can be applied through LAD as well as injection.
- Autologous fat grafting can improve contour as well as facilitate scar remodeling through the action of adipose-derived stem cells (see Chapter 23. Autologous Fat Transfer).

CONTRACTURES

- AFL can be categorized as *micro*-fractional (narrow columns in the micron range with deeper penetration) and *macro*-fractional (column diameter in the millimeter range with shallower penetration and greater surface coverage).
- For areas of tethering, restricted movement, or scar-associated erosions and ulcers, micro-fractional AFL should be considered as a primary intervention. The entire scar sheet should

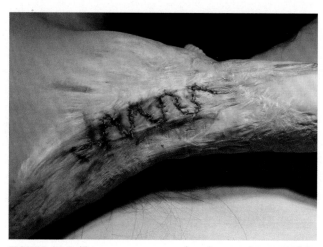

FIGURE 90.2. Tissue rearrangement for a large contracture of the axilla of a child followed by same-session ablative fractional CO_2 laser resurfacing. The ablative columns are visible as small gray dots approaching the suture line. A combined approach can offer the best results for large and severe traumatic scars.

be treated, though density and pulse energy (depth) settings may be adjusted as appropriate for the scar thickness. Contractures should be treated with a relatively high pulse energy (proportional to the thickness of the scar) and a low density (often the lowest setting).

- Surgical and laser scar revision may be combined in the same treatment session for patients with severe contractures and large areas of involvement. In the authors' experience, surgical revision (flaps, grafts, etc) is performed first and then laser treatment performed over the remaining scarred areas. If top stitches are placed, the laser treatment area can proceed close to, but not including, the sutured area to avoid suture ligation (Figure 90.2). Splinting and therapy can proceed in the typical manner after surgery.
- Procedures such as focal follicular unit transplantation and autologous fat grafting may be beneficial in areas of alopecia and contour deficit, respectively, especially once laser treatment has been initiated.
- If PDL and AFL are combined in the same session, PDL should be performed first.

TEXTURAL ABNORMALITIES AND DYSCHROMIA

- Macro-fractional and nonfractional ("full-field") ablative lasers may have a limited role after micro-fractional treatment for smoothing areas of elevation and blending dyspigmentation. The operator should avoid denuding large confluent areas of epidermis because of the decreased healing potential of scar tissue. A small single-spot (ie, 1 mm) handpiece or a small spot on the pattern generator is selected. The elevations are ablated to the desired level in nonfractional mode with periodic wiping with sterile saline-soaked gauze or cotton-tipped applicators to remove char and assess the level of ablation.
- NAFL appears to have a role in the mitigation of developing HTS, or treating scars with mild or moderate textural irregularity and dyspigmentation (eg, split-thickness skin grafts).

In patients prone to HTS, NAFL may be considered in the first week(s) after surgery or laceration repair (ie, suture removal or soon thereafter) at monthly intervals to help reduce the risk of pathologic scarring. The use of NAFL for thick existing HTS and contractures is less clear because of reduced depths of penetration compared to AFL. However, NAFL may be initiated after a course of AFL and other adjuncts has reduced scar tension and elevation to treat persistent texture and color issues.

- Short-pulsed (nanosecond and picosecond) lasers may be helpful focally in areas with hyperpigmentation.

Postprocedural Approach

AFTER AFLS

- Immediately after surgery, a petrolatum-based ointment is applied to the treatment area. A high-potency steroid ointment such as clobetasol may be mixed with petrolatum in hypertrophic areas. Nonstick dressings may be used for convenience, though uncovered areas may be left open. Ointment should be continued for approximately 2 to 3 days until the epidermal barrier is reconstituted.
- Pain and swelling generally decrease rapidly after treatment, and pain medication is rarely required.
- Patients should continue herpes simplex virus prophylaxis for a total of 5 to 7 days, if indicated.
- Bacterial infections appear to be very rare after AFL. However, they are a theoretical concern with temporary disruption of the epidermal barrier. The authors very rarely use prophylactic topical or oral antibiotics after a treatment. Patients are advised to avoid hot tubs and swimming in untreated water for several days. Mycobacteria can be found in municipal water, though the incidence of infection appears to be quite low. Judgment is warranted, but showering and bathing are generally permitted within the first 1 to 2 days without scrubbing or prolonged submersion.
- Postoperative downtime (absence from school, sports, etc) is more an issue of convenience and perception than necessity. Pain is not generally an issue. Modest serous discharge may merit nonstick dressings for approximately 2 days after a treatment. Treatment areas will be apparent to others for approximately 2 weeks after an ablative fractional treatment, starting with significant erythema and mild oozing on day 1 followed by decreasing daily degrees of erythema. One to 2 days of the absence from school and normal sports activities is, therefore, a conservative estimate.
- In the experience of the authors, a course of three to five treatments at 8- to 12-week intervals will produce the majority of the functional gains. However, additional improvements in function, texture, pliability, and color may be associated with continuing AFL and NAFL and other treatments.

- Patients with HTSs and contractures may be treated with an alternating regimen of AFL and LAD/injection of TAC/5-FU, followed in approximately 1 to 2 months by PDL/NAFL/1064-nm laser treatments and intralesional TAC/5-FU.

AFTER PDL, NAFLS, AND 1064-NM LASER TREATMENTS

- Generally, swelling and pain should decrease quickly with time, typically within 48 hours.
- Petrolatum or antibiotic ointment can be used focally for any crusting or blistering.
- Treatments are performed at 4- to 8-week intervals.

BETWEEN TREATMENTS

- Conservative management such as pressure garments, silicone, massage, and physical therapy may continue between treatments. From a practical standpoint, it is probably best to initiate these after a few days when epidermal continuity is restored in the treatment area.
- Topical steroids creams, ointments, and tapes may be applied focally for hypertrophic areas associated with itch in between treatment sessions. To help reduce the risk of atrophy, dosing 2 to 4 days/week should be considered.
- Dosing of intralesional/LAD TAC and 5-FU is at approximately 4-week intervals.

Case Example

Figure 90.3A and B demonstrates the foot of a 2-year-old male approximately 4 months after a scald injury that resulted in second- and third-degree burns requiring escharotomy and skin grafting during reconstruction. Focal areas of erythema, hypertrophy, and contracture are noted on the sole and medial portion of the foot. The parent noted increasing impact on his developing ambulation. The presence of these clinical findings indicates that AFL, intralesional and LAD TAC, and vascular lasers could all be beneficial in his treatment course. He received a series of combined treatments at approximately 3-month intervals. Owing to the patient's young age, injury location, and potential procedural pain associated with AFL and injection, treatments were performed under anesthesia. Erythematous areas were treated first with a 10-mm spot, pulse width of 1.5 ms, and fluence 5 to 6.5 J/cm^2 (595-nm Vbeam Perfecta). AFL was performed over contracted bands at pulse energies of 40 to 50 mJ and density of 5% (UltraPulse™ [Lumenis, Yokneam, Israel]). Triamcinolone suspension at a concentration of 40 mg/mL was applied over fractional-treated hypertrophic areas, and supplemented with intralesional injections into thicker scar bands in earlier treatment sessions. He received a total of three combination treatment sessions over 10 months (Figure 90.3C and D). Additional improvements in texture and color could be achieved with NAFL performed in the clinic after topical anesthesia.

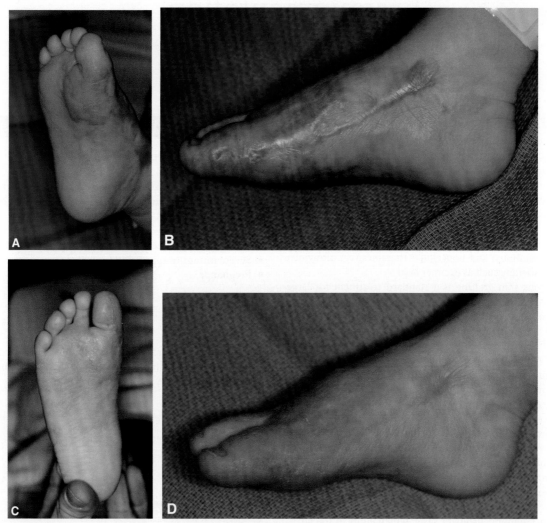

FIGURE 90.3. A, B, Preoperative photos approximately 4 months after a scald injury to the foot of a 2-year-old male. Progressive hypertrophy, pain, and itch were interfering with developing ambulation. C, D, Approximately 10 months after initiating a course of ablative fractional CO_2 laser resurfacing (UltraPulse) at settings of 40 to 50 mJ and 5% density, with laser-assisted delivery of triamcinolone acetonide at 40 mg/mL supplemented by intralesional triamcinolone acetonide suspension to the most hypertrophic areas during the initial treatment. During each treatment session, erythematous areas were treated first with a pulsed-dye laser (595-nm Vbeam Perfecta) with a 10-mm spot, 5 to 6.5 J/cm², 1.5 ms, and 30/20 ms cooling. The patient received a total of three treatment sessions at approximately 3-month intervals. Additional improvements could be obtained with nonablative fractional laser for residual minor color and textural irregularities.

REFERENCES

1. Krakowski A, Shumaker PR, eds. *The Scar Book*. Philadelphia, PA: Wolters Kluwer; 2017.
2. Young, KD. What's new in topical anesthesia. *Clin Ped Emerg Med.* 2007;8:232–239.
3. Kouba DJ, LoPiccolo MC, Alam M, et al. Guidelines for the use of local anesthesia in office-based dermatologic surgery. *J Am Acad Dermatol.* 2016;74:1201–1219.

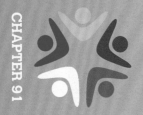

CHAPTER 91

Hypopigmentation

Mohammed D. Saleem and Jennifer J. Schoch

INTRODUCTION

Hypopigmentation of the skin is a common problem encountered by pediatric dermatologists and may be associated with social stigmatization. Treatment may reduce disease progression and improve a patient's quality of life. Treatment of global hypopigmented conditions focuses on photoprotection and management of associated systemic symptoms. In contrast, localized hypopigmentation may be amenable to procedural interventions, which include cellular therapies (eg, tissue or cell transplantations) and noncellular therapies (eg, ultraviolet light-based therapy such as excimer laser).

Autologous skin grafting is a standard treatment for large burn injuries, but has the potential to produce severe scarring, achromic fissuring, and graft contracture. Melanocyte-keratinocyte transplantation and tiny epidermal particles grafts may be more effective and less traumatic than autologous skin grafting. Other techniques include cultured cell suspensions, tissue-engineered grafts, and noncellular therapies such as micropigmentation, excimer laser, and fractional resurfacing plus topical latanoprost or bimpatoprost. Tissue engineering has evolved over the past decade and may be applicable to a variety of hypopigmented conditions in the future.

Here we focus on the use of the excimer laser, which has shown to be effective in the treatment of nevus depigmentosus, postinflammatory hypopigmentation, progressive macular hypomelanosis, idiopathic guttate hypomelanosis, pityriasis alba, hypopigmented scars, and striae alba. The excimer laser is a xenon chloride monochromatic laser, which emits in the ultraviolet range at 308 nm. With a few exceptions, the efficacy and safety of the excimer laser in the treatment of hypopigmented pediatric skin disease is limited to case series and low-quality trials. Treatment of hypopigmented scars that result from burn injuries has been more extensively studied.

Clinical Pearls

- **Guidelines:** No general guidelines that specifically address hypopigmentation exist.
- **Age-Specific Considerations:** Infants with neurologic abnormalities and hypopigmented macules should be evaluated for tuberous sclerosis complex.
- **Technique Tips:**
  - Perilesional hyperpigmentation may be reduced by applying sunscreen to unaffected skin that flanks the margins of the to-be-treated areas.
  - Adjuvant therapy with topical corticosteroids, calcineurin inhibitors, calcipotriene, khellin, tetrahydrocurcuminoid, and bimatoprost may produce a better response, although the evidence is limited.
- **Skin of Color Considerations:** The maximum rate of repigmentation is achieved with two to three treatment sessions per week, with skin types III or higher responding more rapidly than do lighter skin types.

Contraindications/Cautions/Risks

Relative or Absolute Contraindications

- Active skin infections
- Known photosensitivity disorder (eg, xeroderma pigmentosum, Cockayne syndrome, Bloom syndrome, lupus erythematosus)
- Previous or current diagnosis of melanoma
- Actively treated with known phototoxic medications (eg, amiodarone, quinine, voriconazole, tetracyclines, sulfonamides)
- Severe immunosuppression (eg, renal transplant patients)
- Pregnancy

Cautions

- History of koebnerization or keloid formation

Risks

- Persistent erythema, bullae formation, burning sensation, dyspigmentation, increased risk of cutaneous malignancy, herpes reactivation

Equipment Needed

- Ultraviolet eye protection for all personnel and patients
- Narrow-band ultraviolet light device (excimer laser)
- Sunscreen

Preprocedural Approach

- A brief medical history and examination should be performed, and the presence or absence of contraindications documented.
- Pre- and post-treatment photographs are recommended to assist in evaluating efficacy.
- Topical agents (eg, sunscreen) should not be applied to the treated skin before treatment; however, perilesional hyperpigmentation may be reduced by applying sunscreen to unaffected skin that flanks the margins of the to-be-treated areas (Figure 91.1).
- Treatment sites should be cleaned before device use to reduce the risk of infection.

Procedural Approach

- Adverse effects and treatment expectations should be discussed before therapy and informed consent obtained, with assent from the patient if appropriate. Review concomitant medications and adverse events before each session.
- All personnel should wear ultraviolet eye protection.
- Set up and calibrate the excimer laser per manufacturer's guidelines.
- Minimal erythema dose (MED) testing may be considered to determine initial treatment settings. The MED is the lowest exposure required to induce an area of erythema to sun-protected skin 24 hours after exposure.

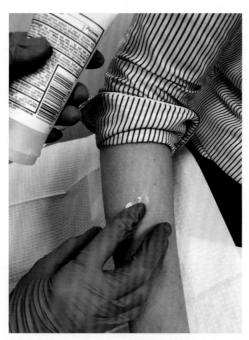

FIGURE 91.1. Sunscreen is applied to unaffected skin around the treatment area.

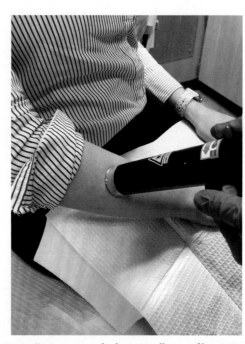

FIGURE 91.2. Excimer is applied to a small area of hypopigmentation.

- The dose applied to affected skin depends on the documented MED, body region, and the clinical response to previous sessions. Excimer is applied to affected areas two to three times a week on nonconsecutive days (Figure 91.2). Response is noted, on average, after 10 to 12 sessions.
- Retreatment of affected areas should be skipped if blistered, eroded, or painful areas develop. Therapy, at a reduced dose (per manufacturer recommendation), can be resumed once any such lesions resolve.
- In the absence of blisters, erosions, or tenderness, the administered dose of narrow-band ultraviolet B (NB-UVB) can be increased per the manufacturer's recommendation (often 20%-25% per session).
- The treatment dose and number of sessions required to achieve a satisfactory cosmetic response (often defined as >50%-75% of repigmentation) varies by condition and between subjects.

Postprocedural Approach

- Treated areas should be protected from excessive sun exposure or physical trauma.
- A moderate amount of emollient (ie, Vaseline™ [Conopco, Inc., US]; Aquaphor® [Beiersdorf AG, US] or similar) should be applied regularly to the treated areas.
- If burning is noted, the patient should report this at the next session to adjust settings.

SUGGESTED READINGS

Alexiades-Armenakas MR, Bernstein LJ, Friedman PM, Geronemus RG. The safety and efficacy of the 308-nm excimer laser for pigment correction of hypopigmented scars and striae alba. *Arch Dermatol.* 2004;140(8):955–960.

Beggs S, Short J, Rengifo-Pardo M, Ehrlich A. Applications of the excimer laser. *Dermatol Surg.* 2015;41(11):1201–1211.

Gordon JRS, Reed KE, Sebastian KR, Ahmed AM. Excimer light treatment for idiopathic guttate hypomelanosis. *Dermatol Surg.* 2017;43(4):553–557.

Onychocryptosis (Ingrown Nail)

Jane Sanders Bellet

Introduction

Onychocryptosis (ingrown nail) is the embedding of a spicule of the nail plate into the lateral nail fold, often leading to a very painful toe, with drainage, swelling, and bleeding (Figure 92.1). The goals of treatment are to relieve pain and prevent further complications with ongoing granulation tissue, drainage, and bleeding. Many different approaches to onychocryptosis exist: conservative measures with warm soaks, cotton or dental floss under the free edge of the nail, and taping, as well as softening and chemical avulsion with topical urea (gel or ointment under occlusion). These treatments are frequently efficacious and therefore help to avoid a procedure. For severe, recalcitrant ingrown nails, permanent ablation of the nail matrix may

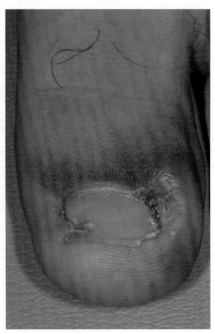

FIGURE 92.1. Onychocryptosis.

be undertaken. Phenol ablation is the most frequently used method. Other methods include surgical excision with electrocautery, destruction with carbon dioxide laser, or radiofrequency ablation.

Clinical Pearls

- **Guidelines:** There are currently no specific guidelines regarding management of onychocryptosis.
- **Age-Specific Considerations**:
  - Consider whether the procedure can be avoided using conservative measures.
  - Local versus general anesthesia. As a general rule, children younger than age 12 will require general anesthesia and, in certain circumstances, even older adolescents may require general anesthesia. Some physicians do these procedures on young children with the initial use of topical anesthetic under occlusion for 2 hours.
- **Technique Tips**:
  - To decrease risk of ischemia, use minimal anesthetic volume.
  - A bloodless field is crucial to success with phenol ablation; phenol is inactivated by blood.
  - Bandage in a longitudinal manner to avoid ischemia.
  - Removal of tourniquet should be done only by the operating surgeon to ensure proper removal.

Contraindications/Cautions/Risks

Cautions
- With phenol ablation, the nail plate is permanently diminished in width.
- Spicules can form if the lateral matrical horns are not adequately ablated.
- Recurrence of ingrown nail can occur.

Risks
- Phenol is an organic compound that can cause severe chemical burns when in contact with skin, eye, or mucosal surfaces. Care must be taken so that no inadvertent application or splash occurs.
- Pain, dysesthesia, bleeding, ischemia that leads to gangrene and possible amputation, infection, drainage, septic arthritis or osteomyelitis if the joint space is violated, flexor or extensor tendon injury (should not be encountered in usual phenol ablation), scarring, nail dystrophy

Equipment Needed
- Protective eyewear for everyone in the room
- Local anesthetic (ropivacaine or lidocaine)
- Ethyl chloride spray and/or vibrating massager
- Sterile scrub, such as chlorhexidine (surgical scrub brush is easy to use)
- Tourniquet (T-ring tourniquet or Penrose drain and hemostat)
- Sterile drapes
- Freer nail elevator (Figure 92.2)
- English anvil action nail splitter (Figure 92.3)
- #15 blade scalpel (preferably Teflon coated)

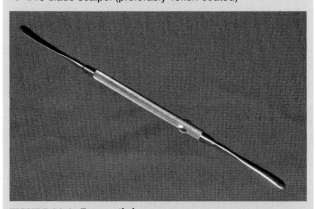

FIGURE 92.2. Freer nail elevator.

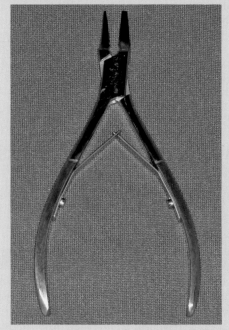

FIGURE 92.3. English anvil action nail splitter.

- Metal curette
- Forceps (Adson or Castro-Viejo)
- Hemostat
- Phenol 88% (preferably in individually wrapped swabs [Phenol EZ swabs, Pedinol, a division of Valeant Pharmaceuticals, North America LLC]).
- Normal saline (for flush)
- 50-mL syringe
- Sterile bowl
- Chucks
- Vaseline™ (Conopco, Inc., US)
- Scissors to cut T-ring tourniquet
- Cotton-tipped swabs
- 4 × 4 gauze
- Gel foam (potentially)
- Electrocautery
- Hypafix tape (or other strong tape)
- 2 × 2 gauze
- Mastisol (or other skin adhesive)
- Stockinette (small sizes)
- Splint/orthopedic shoe (potentially)

Preoperative Approach

- Photographs before the procedure to document the onychocryptosis and the appearance of the entire nail unit are useful.
- Soaking the entire foot in warm water and chlorhexidine for 10 to 30 minutes before the procedure helps soften the nails, as well as start the cleansing process.

Procedural Approach

- Informed consent should be obtained from the parent/guardian before any nail procedure.
- Often, both a digital and wing block are placed, although for most procedures, a wing block is sufficient. These blocks are placed using local anesthetic. Some providers prefer plain 1% lidocaine; some prefer 1% lidocaine with epinephrine or ropivacaine 0.2% to 1%. Still others prefer a mixture of short- and long-acting local anesthetics such as 0.5% lidocaine and 0.25% bupivacaine, which provides for further anesthesia after the procedure.
- The actual volume of local anesthetic injected must be monitored carefully because there is a risk of ischemia due to pressure of the volume itself, especially if the anesthetic is inadvertently infiltrated as a total ring block. The smallest volume possible should be used. Most digital and wing blocks are fully functional with 1 mL or less of local anesthetic; however, if the ingrown nail is very inflamed, then it can be difficult to achieve adequate anesthesia because of local tissue acidosis. If more anesthesia is needed, very careful attention should be paid to the total volume.
- For awake patients, the injections of a digital and wing block are much better tolerated with the use of ethyl chloride spray before each injection, as well as the use of a vibrating massager, which uses the gate theory in reducing pain perception.
- There are multiple techniques for digital blocks. One of the simplest and safest is to use a 30-gauge needle on a 3-mL syringe, with the first injection of the digital block placed in the interdigital web space into the subcutaneous fat in the middle of the proximal phalanx (Figure 92.4A and B). This then is repeated on the other side of the digit, sometimes with extension across the top of the base of the digit.

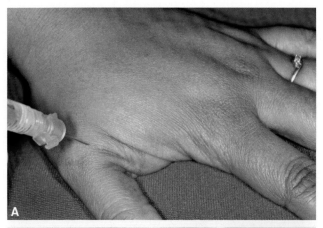

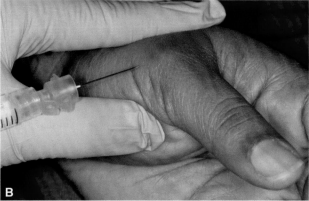

FIGURE 92.4. A, B, Digital block.

- A wing block can be placed in addition to a digital block or as a stand-alone block. A wing block is placed with the first injection 2 to 3 mm proximal to the lateral proximal nail fold; this is then repeated on the opposite side. Then, a point 1 to 2 mm proximal to the center of the proximal nail fold is infiltrated. Each side of the lateral nail fold more distally is injected and then finally the eponychium in three separate sites (Figure 92.5). At this point, the functionality of the block should be checked in an awake patient.
- Once the digit is fully anesthetized, the entire hand or foot is cleansed with surgical scrub. A chlorhexidine surgical scrub brush works well.
- The hand or foot is then draped sterilely. In an older child or adolescent, a sterile glove can be pulled over the entire hand; however, this technique does not work well in smaller patients, nor very well for toenails. A fenestrated drape is often useful, to isolate the single digit on which the procedure will be done.
- A tourniquet is usually needed because phenol application must be performed in a bloodless field. There are a number of different ways in which to apply a tourniquet. One method is to snip the tip of the sterile glove that is already in place on the patient's hand and roll back the finger of the glove to the base of the digit. The residual material of the glove finger can then be clamped with a hemostat. Alternatively, the flat side of a small Penrose drain can be wrapped from the most distal aspect of the digit to the base of the digit and then clamped using a mosquito or Halsted hemostat. The more distal portion is then unwrapped, effectively exsanguinating the digit. Even more effective is the proprietary "T-ring" tourniquet (Figure 92.6) (Precision Medical Devices, LLC, Thousand

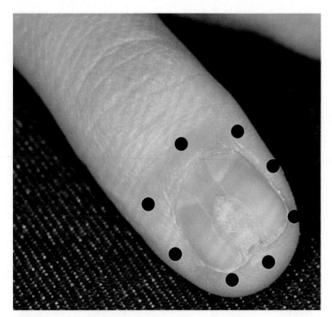

FIGURE 92.5. Wing block.

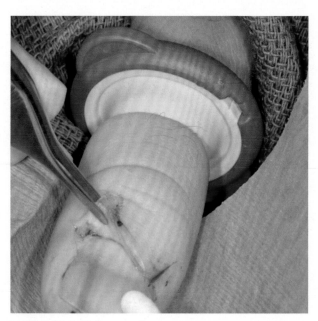

FIGURE 92.6. T-ring tourniquet.

Oaks, CA), which provides equal pressure circumferentially, as well as a more predictably bloodless field.

The biggest risk with tourniquet use is ischemia due to lack of oxygen delivery, leading to acidosis. The shortest amount of time a tourniquet is in place, the better. Monitoring the exact amount of time a tourniquet is in place is very important; therefore, an assistant should mark the starting and ending time. In general, 20 minutes should be sufficient for phenol ablation and clinically important ischemia is unlikely at times less than this, as long as a small volume of local anesthetic was used.

- **Phenol ablation (chemical matricectomy)**

  There are many techniques for phenol ablation. One approach is presented here. Granulation tissue is debrided either with a sharp metal curette or 15 blade scalpel. Partial nail avulsion is then performed. A Freer nail elevator is used to free the proximal nail fold and distal nail plate. An English anvil action nail splitter is used to cut the nail plate longitudinally distal to proximal. A Halsted hemostat is secured to the nail plate distally and then the nail plate is rolled laterally. The partial nail plate is then removed. Care should be taken to be sure that all parts of the nail, spicule, and matrix are removed. A curette can be used in the lateral sulcus. At this point, all persons in the room, including the patient, must wear protective eyewear. Vaseline is applied to the proximal and lateral nail folds. Phenol 88% is placed in the nail cul-de-sac using small prepprepared swabs. Swabs are placed for 1 minute ×3 applications for a total of 3 minutes on each side. The tissue should turn gray-white indicating cell death (Figure 92.7). Some providers flush the area with 50 mL of normal saline, with gauze held around the digit, to prevent splash. Others do not do this step.

- Once the ablation is complete, the tourniquet is released and the time noted for "tourniquet time." There is often not much bleeding at all with phenol ablation. Even with active bleeding, the digit can usually be bandaged. This is in contrast to

cutaneous excisional surgery. If the bleeding seems excessive, pressure can be held for 10 minutes before bandaging and then a piece of Gelfoam (Pharmacia and Upjohn Company, Kalamazoo, MI) can be placed over the site after which bandaging can proceed. Pressure should be held by compressing the distal interphalangeal (DIP) joint laterally on both sides, so that the digital arteries are occluded.

- Many different bandaging methods exist. One method includes application of a small piece of petrolatum gauze or bismuth tribromophenate-impregnated gauze (Xeroform™ [Covidien/Medtronic]), followed by regular gauze, and then

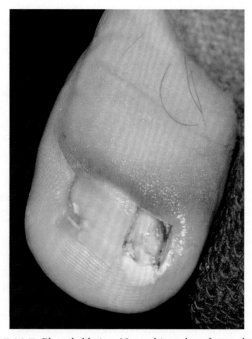

FIGURE 92.7. Phenol ablation. Note white color of treated tissue.

tape. Another technique includes application of plain petro-latum, then a nonstick pad such as Telfa (Covidien LP, Mansfield, MA), followed by regular gauze, and then tape. Tape application often requires an adhesive such as Mastisol and should only be done in a longitudinal manner to prevent postoperative ischemia of the digit (Figure 92.8A and B). Because the patient is either under general anesthesia or cannot sense how much pressure is being applied owing to a block, circumferential bandaging is not advisable. Tubular gauze or stockinette can provide a snug cohesive final layer (Figure 92.8C).

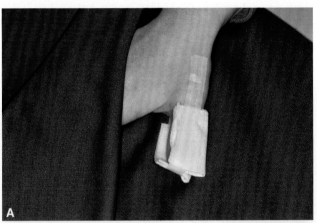
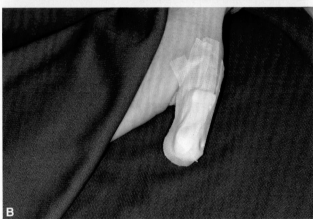
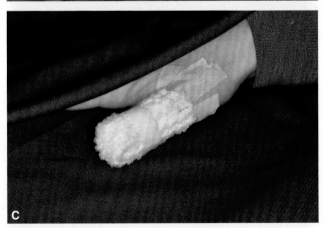

FIGURE 92.8. A and B, Longitudinal bandaging with Mastisol, gauze, and tape. C, Final appearance of bandage with stockinette.

The patient is then monitored for approximately 15 to 20 minutes to ensure there is no bleeding through the bandage. Patients undergoing general anesthesia should be reassessed in recovery before discharge. If there is excessive bleeding through the bandage at this point, a new bandage should be applied. If there is just a small area of bleeding, that part of the bandage can be reinforced with more gauze.

- A toe splint or an orthopedic shoe can be used to prevent inadvertent trauma while the digit heals.

Postoperative Approach

- Patients should keep their foot elevated on the way home. For those older adolescents who may be able to drive, it is important that someone else drives them home.
- Sometimes there is already bleeding through the bandage on the day of the procedure, in which case the patient should either reinforce that portion of the bandage if possible or reapply the entire bandage.
- Postoperative pain management is very important. Phenol nail ablations are usually not that painful postoperatively, because the phenol acts as a topical anesthetic. Acetaminophen should be given on arrival at home, and may be all that is required. Ibuprofen alternating with acetaminophen can be used and is often quite effective. Narcotic pain medications such as oxycodone may be required for 1 to 3 days, because there can be significant throbbing for the first 36 hours postoperatively. Alternating these two agents often works well. If pain is not under good control and continues to be significant, the patient should be evaluated to assess for causes of pain. For 1 to 3 weeks postoperatively, there can be dull pain at the surgical site. Most patients are able to walk well within 5 to 7 days, with return to full function in 3 to 4 weeks, depending on individual recovery. Wearing clean, nonrestrictive footwear is advisable.
- Daily wound care is required, usually starting 48 hours after the phenol nail ablation. Soaking the bandage off in a bath or bowl of warm water facilitates the process. Epsom salts or regular table salt can be added to the water if desired. Bleach or vinegar soaks are not needed. The finger or toe should be gently dried and Vaseline applied to the nail unit. The entire nail unit should then be rebandaged. At this point, this can be done circumferentially because the patient has full sensation and can sense whether the bandage is too tight and potentially causing ischemia. Bandaging daily is done for a number of reasons: to prevent infection; collect drainage; and to provide protection from inadvertent trauma and subsequent pain. More padding will be required in the first week because there usually is more drainage; this diminishes with time. Often, bandaging is necessary for 3 to 4 weeks, because of drainage, especially of the great toe.

SUGGESTED READINGS

de Berker DA. Phenolic ablation of the nail matrix. *Australas J Dermatol.* 2001;42(1):59–61.

Haricharan RN, Masquijo J, Bettolli M. Nail-fold excision for the treatment of ingrown toenail in children. *J Pediatr.* 2013;162(2):398–402.

Yang G, Yanchar NL, Lo AY, Jones SA. Treatment of ingrown toenails in the pediatric population. *J Pediatr Surg.* 2008;43(5):931–935.

CHAPTER 93

Juvenile Xanthogranuloma

Jennifer Ornelas and Smita Awasthi

INTRODUCTION

Juvenile xanthogranuloma (JXG) is a type of non–Langerhans cell histiocytosis that typically presents in infants, younger children, and, less frequently, in adults. Cutaneous JXG present as pink to tan papules that become more yellow over time, most often affecting the head, neck, and trunk (Figure 93.1). The typical size is ≤2 cm, but giant forms that are larger (up to 10 cm) exist. JXG can present with extracutaneous involvement, affecting the eye, the skeletal muscles of the trunk, as well as the lungs, liver, spleen, central nervous system (CNS), bone, and kidney.[1,2] JXGs are typically benign, with the exception of those that involve the liver, CNS, or impede vital functions. Multiple JXGs are associated with intraocular JXG (especially in the setting of café au lait macules and neurofibromatosis [NF] type 1) and with a higher risk of childhood leukemia (particularly in children 2 years of age and younger). Those patients with both JXG and NF need monitoring for leukemia. Ocular lesions often require intervention, such as topical or intralesional corticosteroids, excision, or radiation. Complications from ocular JXG include glaucoma, hyphema, and blindness; therefore, early referral to ophthalmology is important. Other sites of systemic involvement are typically monitored with treatment considered only if there is risk of functional impairment.

JXGs typically regress over 1 to 5 years, although there can be residual hyperpigmentation, atrophy, or anetoderma. Treatment of cutaneous lesions is therefore not necessary unless pathology is needed to aid in diagnosis or for cosmetic reasons. Management options for cutaneous JXG include observation, shave removal, punch excision, or conventional surgical excision. Intralesional corticosteroid injections, which may be less invasive and less traumatic to the patient than is conventional

surgery, have also been utilized to help spur regression; herein, we describe our approach to this technique. Once regression has occurred, the carbon dioxide laser has been utilized to improve any residual anetoderma.[3,4] For any surgical approach, we recommend employing the use of distraction techniques before and during these procedures to help minimize the stress, anxiety, and pain felt by the child during the procedure. We also recommend deferring any surgical treatment that would require general anesthesia until after the age of 3, if possible, to avoid any potential side effects of general anesthesia on learning and behavior.

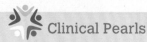
Clinical Pearls

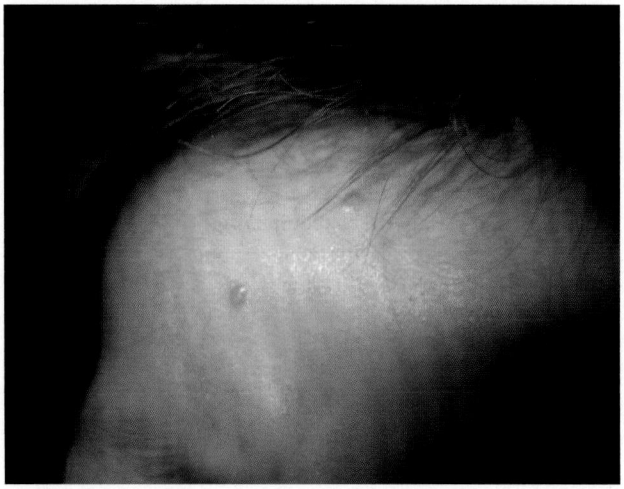

- **General Guidelines:**
  - No specific consensus guidelines exist for the treatment of primary JXG.
  - A full skin examination should be performed to assess for the presence of multiple JXG and other lesions such as café au lait spots and neurofibromas.
- **Age-Specific Considerations:**
  - For children 2 years of age and younger or with multiple JXGs, evaluation by ophthalmology for intraocular JXG is recommended. If no intraocular JXGs are detected, continue screening every 6 months until 2 years of age.[5]

Contraindications/Cautions/Risks

Contraindications
- Active skin infection overlying the lesion
- Allergy to injected anesthesia
- Inability to remain sufficiently still for the procedure

Cautions
- If the differential diagnosis includes a Spitz nevus or amelanotic melanoma, care should be taken to remove the whole lesion.

Risks
- Reaction to anesthesia, pain, bleeding, infection, dyspigmentation, certainty of scar, hypertrophic or keloid scar, recurrence

TREATMENT OF PRIMARY LESION: INTRALESIONAL CORTICOSTEROID

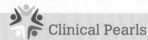
Clinical Pearls

- **Guidelines:**
  - No specific consensus guidelines exist for the treatment of primary JXG lesions.
  - Treatment of primary JXGs is often not needed because they typically spontaneously regress, but may be considered to help incite regression due to cosmetic concerns.

FIGURE 93.1. Multiple juvenile xanthogranulomas on the forehead of a young child with skin type III. He had several other lesions on his back and lower extremities; thankfully, ophthalmologic examination did not reveal any intraocular lesions. Photo courtesy of Andrew C. Krakowski, MD.

- **Age-Specific Considerations:** Ideally, patients should be old enough to ask for treatment, understand the risks and benefits of the procedure, and be able to cooperate with an injection.
- **Technique Tips:**
  - Although the diagnosis of JXG is usually clinical, pathology may be needed in atypical cases and a standard approach to biopsy or removal applies.
  - Various corticosteroids have been used for intralesional injection, although the most commonly used and published is triamcinolone acetonide.
  - The use of distraction techniques is recommended to help reduce stress, anxiety, and pain associated with the procedure.
- **Skin of Color Considerations:** The risk of hypopigmentation with intralesional corticosteroid is greater in darker skin types.

Contraindications/Cautions/Risks

Contraindications
- Allergy to corticosteroids
- Inability to sit still for injection or assent to injection

Cautions
- Smaller lesions have an increased risk of atrophy after injection.
- Darker skin types are at higher risk for dyspigmentation.

Risks
- Death (anaphylaxis to corticosteroids), systemic absorption of corticosteroids and adrenal suppression, local atrophy, hypopigmentation

Equipment Needed
- Syringe
- 30 G ½ in needle
- 18 G needle
- Triamcinolone acetonide 10 mg/mL injectable suspension
- Normal saline
- Alcohol wipe
- Sterile gauze

Preprocedural Approach

- Draw up the desired strength of triamcinolone acetonide by diluting it with normal saline for injection. Alternatively, the dilution can be performed with lidocaine if desired. Typically, a concentration of between 2.5 and 10 mg/mL is utilized.
- The resulting solution should be manually mixed by gently rolling or shaking the syringe.
- Replace the 18 G needle with a 30 G needle before proceeding with the injection.

Procedural Approach

- Informed consent from the parent/guardian and assent from the minor are obtained. For this minor procedure, this is usually in the form of verbal consent, although some practitioners may opt for written consent.

- Typically, anesthesia is not utilized given that the pain of the procedure is minimal. However, should the patient be apprehensive about any discomfort, a topical numbing agent can be applied before the procedure. Alternatively, ice or a forced air-cooling device could be utilized to anesthetize the area just before injection.
- It is recommended that the practitioner wear protective eyewear during the injection.
- Gently cleanse the area to be treated with ethyl alcohol.
- Next, insert the needle so that the tip is in the middle of the JXG lesion. Pressure is applied slowly and steadily to the syringe to inject enough corticosteroid into the lesion until it slightly fills and blanches.
- Upon blanching of the lesion, the needle is withdrawn, and firm pressure is applied with a gauze. Pressure is usually adequate to stop minimal bleeding and a small bandage can be placed if needed, but is often not necessary.
- During injection, the patient will experience a burning sensation. Given that solution (corticosteroid) is injected into the JXG lesion, the patient may have an increased sense of pressure in the area just after injection as well.

Postprocedural Approach

- A BAND-AID™ (Johnson & Johnson, US) can be placed if necessary or is requested.
- It is expected that the lesion will be smaller and softer within 4 weeks.

TREATMENT OF RESIDUAL ANETODERMA: CARBON DIOXIDE LASER

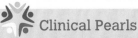 Clinical Pearls

- **Guidelines:** No specific consensus guidelines exist for management of anetoderma secondary to JXG regression. Treatment is not usually needed, but may be considered for cosmetic concerns.
- **Age-Specific Considerations:** Ideally, patients should be old enough to ask for treatment, understand the risks and benefits of the procedure, and be able to cooperate.
- **Technique Tips:**
  - Fractional carbon dioxide would be a reasonable approach as well.
  - The use of distraction techniques is recommended to help reduce stress, anxiety, and pain associated with the procedure.
- **Skin of Color Considerations:** There is a greater risk of dyspigmentation in darker skin types compared to lighter skin types.

Contraindications/Cautions/Risks

Contraindications
- Active infection in the to-be-treated area
- Inability to sit still for injection or assent to procedure

Cautions
- Consider prophylaxis against herpes simplex virus in the appropriate clinical setting.

Risks
- Pain, erythema, scarçring, bleeding, infection, postinflammatory hyper- or hypopigmentation, no change

Equipment Needed

- Carbon dioxide laser
  - Ultra-pulse CO_2 laser (SNJ-1000 U; SNJ Co., Ltd; South Korea)
  - Continuous-wave CO_2 laser (Sharplan 1020, 10 W)[4]
- Topical anesthetic (if needed)
- Syringe
- 30 G ½ in needle
- 18 G needle
- Lidocaine with or without epinephrine
- Chlorhexidine
- Alcohol wipes
- Sterile gauze
- Vaseline™ (Conopco, Inc., US)
- Ice pack(s)

Preprocedural Approach

- Consider necessity of intervention.
- Explain procedure to patient in age-appropriate manner.
  - Utilize pictures to demonstrate the procedure to the patient.
  - Allow patients the opportunity to ask any questions.
- Provide patient with any distraction tools.
  - Allow patient to choose video to watch or music to listen to during procedure.
- Utilize ice, topical anesthesia, and/or local anesthesia depending on location and size of the JXG(s) and tolerance of the child.
  - For younger children, or needle phobic children, consider utilization of topical anesthetic cream before local anesthetic.
- Apply topical anesthetic cream to the area(s) to be treated 30 minutes before treatment, and then cover with occlusive dressing, such as Tegaderm® (3M, US).

Procedural Approach

- Informed consent from the parent/guardian and assent from the minor are obtained.
- The practitioner and all those present in the room, including the patient, must wear protective eyewear during laser treatment.
- Broadly cleanse area with ethyl alcohol and/or chlorhexidine.
- Lee et al. described treatment of anetoderma secondary to JXG using a pinhole method with an Ultra-pulse CO_2 laser

(SNJ-1000 U). They performed treatment in ultra-pulse wave mode with the following settings:

- Spot diameter: 1 mm
- Pulse duration: 0.2 ms
- Peak power: 800 W
- Multiple, small holes were made 1 to 2 mm in diameter and to the depth of the papillary dermis, which were spaced 3 mm apart over the area of anetoderma.
- Two treatment sessions 4 weeks apart led to improvement in the treated patient.
- Klemke et al.[4] treated multiple JXGs with a continuous-wave CO_2 laser (Sharplan 1020). The authors describe the treatment as being well tolerated with no recurrence, but unfortunately did not list their settings.

Postprocedural Approach

- Apply ice to the treated site to reduce pain and swelling.
- Apply 100% white petrolatum ointment to the treated site followed by a wound dressing.
- Advise patient to avoid direct sunlight to the area and to keep the area clean and dry for 24 to 48 hours, after which warm soapy water can be used, followed by 100% white petrolatum ointment and a bandage until healed.
- Schedule follow-up to determine whether more treatment is needed.

REFERENCES

1. Dehner LP. Juvenile xanthogranulomas in the first two decades of life: a clinicopathologic study of 174 cases with cutaneous and extracutaneous manifestations. *Am J Surg Pathol.* 2003;27(5):579–593.
2. Freyer DR, Kennedy R, Bostrom BC, Kohut G, Dehner LP. Juvenile xanthogranuloma: forms of systemic disease and their clinical implications. *J Pediatr.* 1996;129(2):227–237.
3. Lee SM, Kim YJ, Chang SE. Pinhole carbon dioxide laser treatment of secondary anetoderma associated with juvenile xanthogranuloma. *Dermatol Surg.* 2012;38(10):1741–1743.
4. Klemke CD, Held B, Dippel E, Goerdt S. Multiple juvenile xanthogranulomas successfully treated with CO laser. *J Dtsch Dermatol Ges.* 2007;5(1):30–33.
5. Hernandez-Martin A, Baselga E, Drolet BA, Esterly NB. Juvenile xanthogranuloma. *J Am Acad Dermatol.* 1997;36(3 pt 1):355–367; quiz 368–359.

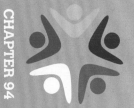

CHAPTER 94

Keratosis Pilaris

Manisha Notay, Jennifer Ornelas, and Smita Awasthi

Introduction

Keratosis pilaris (KP) is a common, hereditary skin condition of follicular plugging affecting both children and adults. The characteristic rough, keratotic follicular papules often accompanied by erythema typically affect the cheeks and proximal extremities (Figure 94.1). Children with KP often have xerosis and, occasionally, atopy. The severity of KP is highly variable and, though usually asymptomatic, can be cosmetically bothersome depending on the degree of erythema present.

Treatment of KP is frequently disappointing but includes the use of topical emollients including those containing topical keratolytics, such as lactic acid, salicylic acid, glycolic acid, or urea. Topical retinoids and gentle mechanical exfoliation

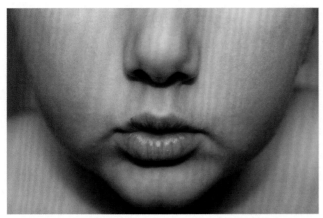

FIGURE 94.1. Keratosis pilaris with concurrent erythema on the cheeks of a young child. Photo courtesy of Andrew C. Krakowski, MD.

are also used. For patients with significant erythema, topical anti-inflammatory agents such as low-potency topical steroids or topical calcineurin inhibitors can be useful. Pulsed dye laser (PDL) can also be used for cosmetically bothersome erythema, such as in the setting of keratosis pilaris rubra (KPR). A combined laser treatment and microdermabrasion has also been reported with some reduction in roughness and erythema. For maintenance of results, treatment must be continued or lesions will recur. In this chapter, we provide details on treatment of KP with topicals and with laser, with or without microdermabrasion.

Clinical Pearls

- **Guidelines:** No specific treatment guidelines are known to exist for KP.
  - All patients with KP will benefit from dry skin care measures such as avoiding long hot showers or baths, using gentle, unscented soaps or soap-free cleansers, and applying thick, fragrance-free emollients after bathing.
  - First-line treatment: Emollients and topical keratolytics. For example, CeraVe® SA (L'Oreal), Amlactin 12% lotion (Sandoz), Gold Bond® Rough and Bumpy Daily Therapy Cream, Glytone® KP Kit
  - Second-line treatment: Low-potency topical steroids, topical calcineurin inhibitors, and topical retinoids
  - Third-line treatment: Laser therapy (PDL, long-pulsed 755 nm alexandrite laser, 810 nm long-pulsed diode laser, long-pulsed 1064 nm Nd:YAG laser) and microdermabrasion
  - Patients with cosmetically bothersome erythema are typically those who seek both second- and third-line treatment options.
- **Age-Specific Considerations:**
  - Consider the age of child and the ability of child to tolerate a specific procedure when selecting a treatment method.
  - Trial emollients alone first in younger patients and, if nonresponsive, select emollients containing mild topical keratolytics (e.g., CeraVe SA).
- **Technique Tips:**
  - The use of distraction techniques is recommended to help reduce stress, anxiety, and pain associated with treatments.
  - Start a strict regimen of sunscreen use and sun avoidance several weeks prior to planned laser treatment to help ensure the to-be-treated skin is as little "tanned" as possible.

- **Skin of Color Considerations:**
  - Erythema may be more difficult to notice, and postinflammatory pigmentary changes may be more notable in patients with darker skin tones.

Contraindications/Cautions/Risks

Contraindications
- Sunburn, open ulcers to treatment area, or infection at any skin site prior to laser treatment
- Use of topical or oral photosensitizing medications prior to laser treatment
- Inability to tolerate procedure or remain sufficiently still for duration of procedure
- Inability to wear protective eye-gear during laser treatment

Cautions
- Caution using topical keratolytics, steroids, or calcineurin inhibitors over a large body-surface area in infants and children, especially in those with impaired skin barrier
- Caution with selection of laser and laser settings in patients with tan present or darker skin types

Risks
- Pain; bleeding; infection; reaction to topical anesthetic cream; postinflammatory pigmentary changes, especially with darker skin types; blistering; bruising; no improvement or only temporary improvement; and recurrence

Equipment Needed
- Topical anesthetic cream: EMLA™ (AB Astra Pharmaceuticals, L.P.) (lidocaine 2.5% and prilocaine 2.5%) or LMX.4™ (Ferndale Laboratories) (lidocaine 4%)
- Protective eye shields for patient
- Wavelength-specific goggles for selected laser
- Ice packs
- Topical petrolatum
- Laser
  - 532-nm potassium titanyl phosphate laser
  - 585-nm PDL
  - 595-nm PDL
  - PDL for KPR
  - Long-pulsed 1064-nm Nd:YAG
  - 810-nm diode laser
  - Long-pulsed 755-nm alexandrite
- Microdermabrasion

Preprocedural Approach

- Consider intervention with laser only in highly motivated patients for which their KP is very cosmetically bothersome because treatment results are modest and usually only temporary.
- Several weeks prior to laser treatment, patients should increase sun protection as they should have no tan to decrease risk of dyspigmentation from the laser treatment.
- Explain procedure to patient in age-appropriate manner.
  - Utilize pictures to demonstrate the procedure to the patient.
  - Allow patients the opportunity to ask any questions.
- Provide patient with any distraction tools.
  - Allow patient to choose music to listen to during procedure.

TABLE 94.1 :: Laser Therapy and Supporting Case Studies for Keratosis Pilaris

WAVELENGTH	595 nm[1,2]	810 nm Diode[3]	Long-Pulsed 1064 nm[4]	QS 1064 nm[5]	532 nm[6]	595/755 nm + Microdermabrasion[7]
Spot size (mm)	7 or 10		15	4-6	7	595 nm: 7 755 nm: 18
Fluence (J/cm^2)	5-9 4.5-11.5	45-60	34	5.9-8	12-14	595 nm: 8 755 nm: 10
Pulse duration (ms)	0.5-1.5 1.5-10	30-100	30	Pulse rate: 10 Hz	5-10	595 nm: 10 755 nm: 3
Cooling	Continuous airflow cooling		20/20			595 nm: 30/30 755 nm: 50/30
Number of treatments	1-7 1-4	3	3	5	7	2.5
Interval	8 wk	4-5 wk	4 wk	Weekly	6-8 wk	1 mo
Number of patients	8 (8-35 y) 8 teens	18 (18-65 y)	17 (15-42 y)	10	1	26 (19-45 y)
Type of study	Case series	RCT	RCT	Case series	Case report	Retrospective
Follow-up time period	1 y 1-19 mo	12-15 wk	12 wk	2 mo	18 mo	3 mo
Outcome	Lasting improvement in erythema, few cases with recurrence	Improved roughness, no change in erythema	Improved erythema and keratotic papules. Satisfaction in half of patients	Fair to excellent clinical improvement of hyperpigmentation in all 10 patients	Improved papules and erythema	Improvement in texture, redness, and dyschromia in half of patients
Additional comments		Lidocaine/prilocaine-based cream applied prior to treatment Two non-overlapping passes separated by a 1-min delay			4% amethocaine gel applied prior to treatment	Start with 595 nm, then 2 wk later 755 nm, 1 wk later microdermabrasion.[a] EMLA prior to treatment, ice pack after

[a]2B Bio Peeling was used according to manufacturer's instructions and rubbed on upper arms and lower legs for 7 minutes each, then gently wiped away with wet gauze. Main ingredients of 2B Bio Peeling powder include Havnejordit lava, Badiaga halichondria spongia coelente rata, Acacia gum, crystallized Quartz, Equisetum arvensis, Calendula officinalis, and arrow root.

RCT, randomized controlled trial.

- Recommend the use of topical anesthetic cream when utilizing laser.
  - Apply topical anesthetic cream to the to-be-treated area(s) 30 to 60 minutes before treatment, then cover with occlusive dressing, such as Tegaderm® (3M, US).

Procedural Approach

- PDL appears to be the most widely used; thus, recommendations for the use of PDL in KP are described herein. See Table 94.1 for additional laser settings for other wavelengths.
- PDL for KPR is based on two case series of eight adolescent patients[1] and eight patients aged 8 to 35 years.[2]
- Initiate treatment at low settings and use test spots to titrate settings to the development of purpura. Mild purpura at the time of treatment was associated with efficacy. Test spots were used in three patients; for the others, treatment was initiated at a low setting and titrated to the development of purpura (Table 94.1).
- Spot size 7 to 10 mm
- Laser settings varied markedly with fluence, ranging from 4.5 to 11.5 J/cm² (most patients were treated with fluence of 8-11.5 J/m²).
- Pulse duration range: 0.5 to 10 ms (most patients were treated with a pulse duration of 1.5-3 ms)

Postprocedural Approach

- Apply petrolatum ointment over the treated area.
- Consider ice packs for analgesia and to reduce any potential swelling.
- Can advise the use of over-the-counter oral analgesic, such as ibuprofen or acetaminophen.

- Monitor signs or symptoms of infection.
- Follow-up at specified treatment intervals or sooner as needed. For the abovementioned PDL study, the number of treatments needed for improvement was "1 to 4." Over follow-up of "1 to 19 months," patients were satisfied with results, though some patients had recurrence.

REFERENCES

1. Schoch JJ, Tollefson MM, Witman P, Davis DM. Successful treatment of keratosis pilaris rubra with pulsed dye laser. *Pediatr Dermatol.* 2016;33(4):443–446.
2. Alcantara Gonzalez J, Boixeda P, Truchuelo Diez MT, Fleta Asin B. Keratosis pilaris rubra and keratosis pilaris atrophicans faciei treated with pulsed dye laser: report of 10 cases. *J Eur Acad Dermatol Venereol.* 2011;25(6):710–714.
3. Ibrahim O, Khan M, Bolotin D, et al. Treatment of keratosis pilaris with 810-nm diode laser: a randomized clinical trial. *JAMA Dermatol.* 2015;151(2):187–191.
4. Saelim P, Pongprutthipan M, Pootongkam S, Jariyasethavong V, Asawanonda P. Long-pulsed 1064-nm Nd:YAG laser significantly improves keratosis pilaris: a randomized, evaluator-blind study. *J Dermatolog Treat.* 2013;24(4):318–322.
5. Park J, Kim BJ, Kim MN, Lee CK. A pilot study of Q-switched 1064-nm Nd:YAG laser treatment in the keratosis pilaris. *Ann Dermatol.* 2011;23(3):293–298.
6. Dawn G, Urcelay M, Patel M, Strong AM. Keratosis rubra pilaris responding to potassium titanyl phosphate laser. *Br J Dermatol.* 2002;147(4):822–824.
7. Lee SJ, Choi MJ, Zheng Z, Chung WS, Kim YK, Cho SB. Combination of 595-nm pulsed dye laser, long-pulsed 755-nm alexandrite laser, and microdermabrasion treatment for keratosis pilaris: retrospective analysis of 26 Korean patients. *J Cosmet Laser Ther.* 2013;15(3):150–154.

Labial Adhesion

John C. Browning and Giselle Castillo

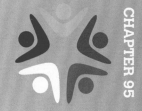

CHAPTER 95

Introduction

Labial adhesion is the fusion of the labia minora or majora (Figure 95.1). This fusion often occurs near the clitoris and can go by other names including synechia vulvae or labial agglutination. This is a common gynecologic problem that often presents in childhood between the ages of 3 months to 6 years of age and affects around 2% of prepubertal girls.

The exact cause of labial adhesions still remains unknown, although it is believed that low levels of estrogen may be an important contributing factor. This had led to treatment options centering around estrogen cream and achieving positive results. Other less common causes are believed to be centered around vulvar irritation. These irritants can come in many forms, some common ones being harsh soaps, wet diapers, infections, or even trauma.

The diagnosis of labial adhesion is made clinically and does not require any labs or imaging.

For the majority of cases, the adhesion is an incidental finding because of lack of symptoms. There is rarely a need to send the patient to a gynecologist for evaluation because the majority of cases resolve without any therapy within 18 months. It is reported that up to 80% will resolve without treatment. If the patient is clinically asymptomatic, the clinician's primary role will be to provide reassurance. Clinical manifestations, if present, usually consist of dysuria, postvoid dripping, hematuria, and local inflammation around the labial area. One of the major indications of treatment is the presence of a urinary tract infection (UTI). If the labial adhesion resolves successfully, the risk of infection decreases.

Treatment options for labial adhesions often come in the form of estrogen and/or steroid creams or ointments. The most effective treatment consists of an estrogen cream. Other treatment options include topical betamethasone and surgical removal. Surgical management should be considered if topical management has failed.

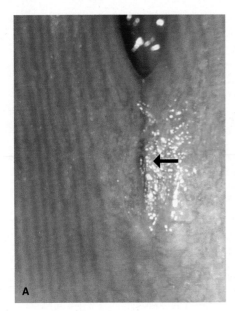
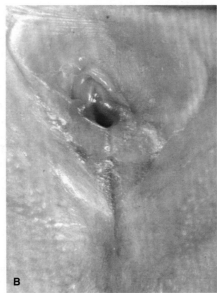

FIGURE 95.1. Labial/vulvar adhesions. Posterior adhesions (A) and nearly complete adhesion (B) with small opening below the clitoris. Reprinted with permission from Emans SJ, Laufer MR, DiVasta A. *Goldstein's Pediatric and Adolescent Gynecology*. 7th ed. Philadelphia, PA: Wolters Kluwer; 2019. Figure 14.13.

Clinical Pearls

- **Guidelines:** No specific treatment guidelines are known to exist for this condition.
- **Age-Specific Considerations:** Adhesions may keep reforming until the patient goes through puberty (around 10% of patients will report a recurrence); recurrences are managed the same way that a primary labial adhesion would be treated.
- **Technique Tips:**
  - Surgical separation is generally only needed in cases of pain, impaired urination, or where other treatment options have failed.
  - Treatment usually depends on the size and severity of the adhesion.
  - Small adhesions that do not cover the vaginal introitus are more likely to separate by themselves.
  - Adhesions that cover the urethral meatus or larger portions of the vaginal introitus may require more aggressive intervention.
  - Complicated adhesions that involve the area around the urethra or clitoral hood should be referred to a pediatric gynecologist or urologist.
- **Skin of Color Considerations:** None specifically

Contraindications/Cautions/Risks

- The majority of patients who present with labial adhesions are asymptomatic, leading to treatment often being nonsurgical. This leads to few, if any, contraindications or risks. For individuals who are symptomatic, drug allergies should be discussed before treatment with topical estrogen or steroids.
- Side effects of estrogen cream include breast tenderness and pigmentation to the area applied.
- Risks associated with high-potency topical steroids include thinning of the skin, increased risk for infection of the hair follicle, redness, thinning of hair growth, and itchiness on the area applied.
- If topical management fails, surgical treatment should be considered.
  - Contraindications to surgery include undiagnosed vaginal bleeding, atypical anatomy, or problems with healing.

Forceful separation is always contraindicated because of the trauma that may result and the increased chance of recurrence.
- When surgery is required, it is important to discuss the risks (bleeding, infection, scar, recurrence) as well as benefits (reduction in pain, urinary problems, etc) and alternatives (waiting, estrogen cream, topical corticosteroid).

Equipment Needed

- General anesthesia is often required.
- Local anesthetic with 1% lidocaine with epinephrine or 0.25% bupivacaine with epinephrine (local anesthetic is required when not using general anesthesia, but it is also recommended during general anesthesia to reduce postoperative pain; epinephrine helps reduce bleeding and is not contraindicated on this part of the body)
- #15 blade
- Curved hemostats
- Iris scissors
- Needle holder
- Suture scissors
- Bovie or Hyfrecator 2000™ (Conmed, Utica, NY) to control bleeding

Preprocedural Approach

- Around 80% of labial adhesions resolve within 18 months without treatment. This makes the preoperative, or pretreatment approach, the most common.
- If the patient is asymptomatic, no treatment is necessary.
- It is important for the clinician to reassure the patient and their family that the adhesion will likely resolve once puberty begins.

Topical Estrogen

- For adhesions that require treatment, the most effective first-line option has proved to be topical estrogen cream.
- This cream should be applied twice a day for a period of time until the adhesions resolve.
- It is important to note that once the adhesions begin to separate, the estrogen cream should not be placed inside the vaginal opening.

- After the estrogen cream is no longer used, it may be beneficial for the patient to switch to a nonprescription lubricating ointment such as petroleum jelly or zinc oxide cream. This may reduce the chances of recurrence of the adhesion.

Topical Corticosteroid

- A high-potency topical steroid such as topical betamethasone or clobetasol is another management option.
- The same method of application as that for topical estrogen should be used.
- It is important to note that there is no precise length of treatment that is currently recommended, so the clinical picture should dictate duration of therapy, balancing benefits against side effects.

Procedural Approach: Surgical Separation

- This type of procedure may require general anesthesia.
- The adhesions should be clearly identified and then injected with local anesthetic with epinephrine.
- Next, the adhesions should be removed from the normal tissue using a #15 blade.
- For larger adhesions, a curved hemostat can help secure the adhesion during this process.
- One might also find that an absorbent suture such 4-0 plain gut can be used to tie off each end of the adhesion before removal with the #15 blade or iris scissors.
- When not using a suture, the Bovie or Hydrecator can be used to control bleeding.

Postprocedural Approach

- Once the labial adhesions have been separated, whether by topical treatment or surgery, a generous amount of petrolatum should be used for 6 to 12 months to keep the labia open. This helps prevent or lessen irritation of the area and decreases the chances of recurrence.
- Zinc oxide may also be considered because some patients find petroleum jelly to be greasier and less adherent in the groin area.
- Other ways to decrease irritation include the avoidance of harsh soaps, bubble bath products, tight clothing, and scrubbing the vulva.
- Recurrences are common in labial adhesions regardless of the treatment method that is used. This is due to the fact that the adhesions may keep reforming until the patient goes through puberty. It is estimated that around 10% of cases will report a recurrence. Recurrences may be managed the same way that an original labial adhesion would present.

SUGGESTED READINGS

Bacon, JL, Romano ME, Quint, EH. Clinical recommendation: labial adhesions. *J Pediatr Adolesc Gynecol.* 2015;28:405.

Kumar GK. Labial adhesion: an office problem in pediatric urology. *Pediatr Urol Case Rep.* 2017;4(1):248. doi:10.14534/pucr.2017124186.

Mayoglou L, Dulabon L, Martin-Alguacil N, Pfaff D, Schober J. Success of treatment modalities for labial fusion: a retrospective evaluation of topical and surgical treatments. *J Pediatr Adolesc Gynecol.* 2009;22(4):247–250. doi:10.1016/j.jpag.2008.09.003.

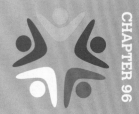

Laceration Repair

Samuel H. Lance and Amanda A. Gosman

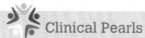

INTRODUCTION

Traumatic lacerations remain one of the most common surgical procedures performed in the urgent or emergent setting. Early intervention and closure of traumatic lacerations can improve long-term scarring and functional outcomes. Timely and appropriate treatment further decreases morbidity by reducing the risk of subsequent wound infection.

Although timely management of traumatic injuries is critical to optimizing outcomes, closure should still be considered even in the setting of delayed presentation. Delayed closure is most important in areas of significant aesthetic importance, most notably the face, nose, and ears.

Assessment of associated injuries to the aesthetic and neurovascular structures with subsequent restoration of anatomic landmarks and neurovascular repair, if indicated, is critical to obtaining optimal outcomes following laceration repair. Practitioners should assess the extent and location of the wound and seek the assistance of additional specialists should the complexity of the wound warrant additional evaluation.

Clinical Pearls

- **Guidelines:** No specific treatment guidelines are known to exist for this condition.
- **Technique Tips:**
  - Traumatic lacerations require meticulous irrigation and debridement of the wound to reduce the risk of infection.[1]
  - Periprocedural antibiotics should be considered for lacerations that present with gross contamination or that are due to bite injuries.[2]
  - The patient's tetanus status should be assessed and additional administration of tetanus prophylaxis provided if required.
  - Appropriate setup with the arrangement of all necessary equipment and materials before initiation of the procedure is critical to operative success and building patient confidence. Multiple breaks in sterility to access needed instrumentation and supplies increase the risk of infection and lengthen procedural time.

- Care should be taken to avoid overexcision of damaged tissue during the initial closure. This principle is of paramount importance when addressing the facial and extremity tissues. Ultimate viability of traumatized tissues at these aesthetically sensitive areas is difficult to assess immediately following injury. Overresection can result in loss of otherwise viable tissue and distortion of critical structures with resultant poor aesthetic outcomes.
- Multilayered closure with precise approximation of each anatomic sublayer is critical to obtaining optimal tissue approximation, minimizing scarring, and decreasing distortion of the surrounding structures. Closure of deep layers with deep sutures also allows for early removal of the more superficial epithelial sutures.
- Early removal of superficial sutures before epithelialization along the suture track can further optimize tissue scarring and minimize scar visibility.

Contraindications and Risks

- Active infection and the presence of retained foreign bodies are clear contraindications to closure of traumatic lacerations.
- If closure would jeopardize already injured vital structures surrounding the laceration, the surgeon may consider stabilizing the injured vital structures before proceeding with closure.
- Realistic expectations of aesthetic outcomes following scarring as well as potential future functional limitations are critical to achieving patient satisfaction following repair.
- It serves to be noted that following infiltration of local anesthetic, nerve injuries may be difficult to precisely assess. Thus, potential nerve injury without clear diagnosis remains a relative contraindication to repair. Once clear diagnosis of the nerve injury is achieved, closure can be safely performed.

Equipment Needed

- 1% lidocaine with epinephrine 1:100 000
- Normal saline irrigation; 1 L/2 cm^2 of injury
- Betadine prep solution
- Fine-toothed forceps
- Tenotomy/iris scissors
- Needle driver
- Sutures
  - Deep 5-0 Monocryl™ (Ethicon US, LLC) to 3-0 Monocryl
  - Superficial 5-0 or 6-0 fast gut suture
  - 5-0 or 6-0 Nylon
- Bacitracin ointment

Preprocedural Approach

- Complete workup including history, mechanism of injury, and evaluation for additional traumatic injuries should be completed before intervention.
- Should the presence of a foreign body be suspected, imaging with plain film x-ray or computed tomography (CT) scan can be utilized to identify radiopaque foreign bodies. Nonradiopaque foreign bodies are best visualized with ultrasound or magnetic resonance imaging (MRI) modalities.
- Specialist consultation should be obtained as directed by the nature of each traumatic injury.

- Patient maturity and the extent of the traumatic laceration should be assessed to determine whether local anesthesia alone is adequate for the procedure. If local anesthesia alone is deemed insufficient to obtain adequate patient comfort and a safe surgical environment, the use of sedation or general anesthesia should be arranged.

Procedural Approach

- Local anesthesia is achieved with infiltration as a field block versus nerve block. Local anesthetic containing epinephrine solution should be used to improve visualization and examination of the traumatized tissue.
- After achieving appropriate anesthesia, the wound is prepped with Betadine solution. Alcohol-based prep solutions should be avoided in the setting of open wounds given the risk of tissue damage associated with alcohol-based preps.
- The tissues are examined with the use of loupe magnification as necessary. Exploration of the deep structures should be performed in the setting of a penetrating injury. The anatomic layers of involved tissue should be identified and marked as needed.
- The area is then irrigated extensively with normal saline solution. All visible debris and foreign bodies should be removed. Confirmatory imaging can be obtained to verify foreign body removal if a foreign body is noted preoperatively.
- Tissue that appears clearly devitalized should be judiciously removed with sharp excision.
- Hemostasis is achieved with electrocautery, as needed, taking care to avoid damage to any vital structures previously identified. Layers are then closed, beginning with monofilament absorbable suture to the deep muscular or fascial layers extending up to the level of the deep dermis. It is recommended that these layers be closed with interrupted suture. The dermis should be well approximated following completion of the deep layers to avoid excessive tension to the epidermal and dermal closure (Figures 96.1 to 96.3).
- The authors recommend proceeding with epidermal closure utilizing nonabsorbable monofilament permanent suture in aesthetically sensitive areas to minimize the inflammatory response at that level of the epidermis. If the area is not considered aesthetically sensitive or patient factors are unfavorable

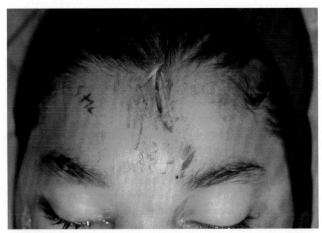

FIGURE 96.1. Preoperative photograph demonstrates a complex and deep laceration to forehead.

for the future removal of sutures, then rapidly absorbable plain gut suture may be used.

- After antibiotic ointment is used, a light dressing is then applied.

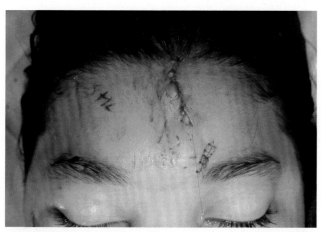

FIGURE 96.2. Intraoperative photograph demonstrates complex closure.

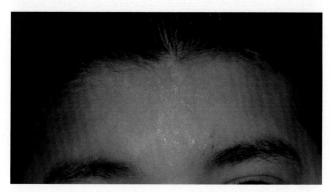

FIGURE 96.3. Well-healed laceration 6 months after the procedure.

Postprocedural Approach

- Wound care overlying incisions can be performed with light daily washing using soap and water, followed by patting the area dry and application of antibiotic ointment.
- Patients should be reevaluated at 1 week after the procedure for assessment of appropriate wound healing.
- Nonabsorbable sutures should be removed at 5 to 7 days following the procedure, thus avoiding epithelialization along the monofilament suture.
- After suture removal, patients may be transitioned to daily incision care with washing and drying, followed by application of nonallergenic, petroleum-based, moisturizing ointments.
- Strict sun protection is recommended starting immediately after the intervention.
- Scar reduction techniques such as silicone application and scar massage may be initiated around 2 weeks after the intervention.

REFERENCES

1. Collins S, White J, Ramsay M, Amirthalingam G. The importance of tetanus risk assessment during wound management. *IDCases.* 2015;2(1):3–5.
2. Ghafouri HB, Bagheri-Behzad B, Yasinzadeh MR, Modirian E, Divsalar D, Farahmand S. prophylactic antibiotic therapy in contaminated traumatic wounds: two days versus five days treatment. *Bioimpacts.* 2012;2(1):33–37.

Lichen Planus

Alexandra Zeitany and Craig N. Burkhart

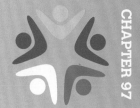

Introduction

Lichen planus (LP) is a condition characterized by small, discrete, polygonal, flat-topped, pruritic, violaceous-to-purple papules, caused when autoreactive T lymphocytes attack basal keratinocytes located in the skin (Figures 97.1 and 97.2), mucous membranes, hair follicles, and/or nails (Figure 97.3). The etiology is still unclear, but various viruses, including hepatitis C, and medications have been implicated. LP is most common in the fourth to sixth decades of life, but it can occur at any age. There is no known predilection for sex or ethnicity; however, there are geographic clusters (eg, in the Mediterranean and Japan) that may be related to the high incidence of certain viruses in these regions. The condition can spontaneously resolve, typically after 1 year, or it can follow a chronic, relapsing course. The therapeutic goals are 2-fold: resolution of cutaneous lesions and resolution or symptomatology, most notably pruritus.

Although data on its efficacy are limited and placebo-controlled randomized trials have not been performed, phototherapy has proved useful as a treatment for this condition. Although psoralen plus ultraviolet A (PUVA) can be utilized, narrow band ultraviolet B (nb-UVB) is the most common modality used. nb-UVB is relatively inexpensive and may be a good treatment option for patients with widespread disease, especially those who prefer to avoid systemic therapy or have a contraindication to such. It is typically given three times per week and then downtitrated once a response is demonstrated. If no response is observed after 3 to 4 months, therapy should be discontinued.

One major disadvantages of nb-UVB is that it is quite time intensive, requiring multiple visits to a provider several days a week. This may not be feasible for some families and time away from work and travel expenses are often not calculated in the total costs of this intervention. In addition, it is absolutely contraindicated in conditions such as xeroderma pigmentosum and lupus erythematosus and is relatively contraindicated in anyone with a history of a photosensitivity disease, history of melanoma, history of ionizing radiation, and immunosuppression for organ transplant. Most

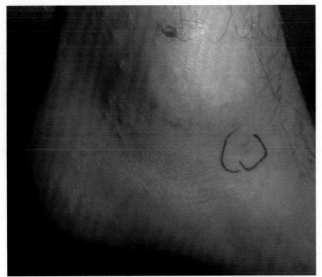

FIGURE 97.1. Purple, flat-topped papules are the classic morphology of lichen planus. The circled lesion was singled out for punch biopsy to confirm the diagnosis. Photo courtesy of Andrew C. Krakowski, MD.

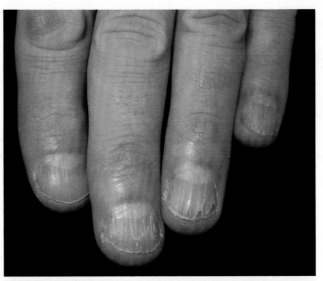

FIGURE 97.3. Lichen planus of the nails, demonstrating thinning and ridging.

notable side effects are primarily cutaneous including erythema, dryness, pruritus, blistering, and reactivation of herpes simplex. Long-term adverse effects include photoaging and the possibility of photocarcinogensis (a systemic review suggests that nb-UVB does not increase the risk of skin cancer; however, larger studies are needed[1]).

Emerging treatments also include laser and photodynamic therapy (PDT). There are several case reports that have attempted Q-switched Nd:YAG laser and PDT in the treatment of oral LP. Fractionated laser has also been attempted for delivery of corticosteroids. In one case report, a single patient was treated with fractionated CO_2 laser (fluence of 60 J/cm^2 and a treatment density of 100 microthermal zones/cm^2) followed by triamcinolone 10 mg/mL solution, and the authors reported "near-complete" clearance after four sessions. Results with these novel modalities are

promising, but further research is required to characterize their efficacy in cutaneous disease. Moreover, these techniques may not be feasible in pediatric patients given the associated pain.[2] The main focus of this procedural chapter is on the use of intralesional corticosteroids, which is detailed herein.

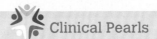

Clinical Pearls

- **Guidelines:**
  - Treatment of LP with intralesional corticosteroids has level 4 evidence of efficacy.
  - Often considered first line for both cutaneous and nail disease (especially if there are three nails or less involved)
  - Data on efficacy are limited and placebo-controlled randomized trials have not been performed.
- **Age-Specific Considerations:**
  - Although there are no gender- or age-specific considerations, patient maturity and pain tolerance must be evaluated and considered given the discomfort associated with the procedure.
  - Tips for younger patients
    - Avoid allowing the patients to see the needle before the procedure.
    - Cold packs or vibration can be used to minimize pain and distract the patient.
  - Those patients unable to tolerate intralesional corticosteroids or those with widespread lesions may consider phototherapy.
- **Technique Tips:**
  - Relatively inexpensive and often covered by insurance
  - Set appropriate expectations and counsel patients that multiple treatments may be required.
    - Injection itself is somewhat painful, but discomfort is short lived.
    - No downtime required
    - Often requires numerous treatments spaced 4 to 6 weeks apart
  - Corticosteroids should never be injected into sites where there is a concern for infection.
  - Caution must be exercised when injecting into the nasal tip or perinasally to avoid the angular artery

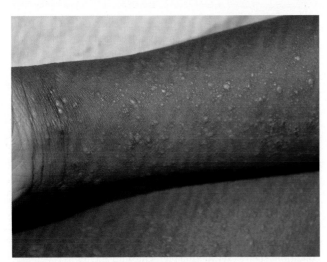

FIGURE 97.2. Involvement of the volar wrists is quite classic for lichen planus. This photograph also demonstrates evidence of excoriation, a prototypical secondary change noted in lichen planus. Photo courtesy of Andrew C. Krakowski, MD.

(see further details in Chapter 9. Anatomy and Superficial Landmarks of the Head and Neck).

- For nail involvement, intralesional corticosteroid can be injected into both the proximal and lateral nail folds.
  - The injection is placed intradermally and then diffuses into the underlying matrix. Injection directly into the nail matrix is exquisitely painful.
  - Injections are typically continued at monthly intervals until the proximal half of the nail normalizes.
- There are several techniques that can minimize the risk of hypopigmentation and atrophy.
  - Use the lowest concentration and smallest quantity of triamcinolone needed. Even if this requires repeat injection, this is preferable to overestimating the dosage.
  - Placement too deeply into the subcutaneous layer may produce more atrophy.
  - Injecting too superficially in the upper dermis and epidermis may cause hyperpigmentation and desquamation.
- **Skin of Color Considerations:**
  - Skin of color is more susceptible to hypo- and depigmentation. Caution must be used when injecting these patients and they must be counseled about this potential complication.

Contraindications/Cautions/Risks

Contraindications
- There are no absolute contraindications to intralesional corticosteroids. Attention must be paid to anatomic site, particularly the head and neck, to avoid important neurovascular structures.
- Relative contraindications include localized infection.

Cautions
- Caution must be taken in skin of color because the risk of hypopigmentation is higher.

Risks
- Side effects primarily cosmetic in nature
  - Most common: localized pain (from injection), atrophy and hypopigmentation. Usually self-limited and resolves over several weeks; however, it can occasionally persist longer or be permanent. Fitzpatrick skin types III or greater are most susceptible.
- Systemic side effects are rare.
  - Repeated frequent injections producing a cumulative dose greater than 40 mg/month have anecdotally been reported to cause adrenal suppression and menstrual irregularities, but strong data are lacking.
- Adverse events: Studies estimating the frequency of these events are lacking.
  - Hypo- or depigmentation
  - Atrophy
  - Sterile abscess formation (rare)
  - Exacerbation of localized infection (rare)
  - Systemic absorption leading to menstrual abnormalities and adrenal abnormalities. This is exceedingly rare, especially if the cumulative dose of triamcinolone is less than 40 mg/month.

Equipment Needed
- Triamcinolone acetonide 5 to 20 mg/mL
- Sterile saline
- 1- to 3-cc Luer-Lok® syringe (Becton-Dickinson and Company, Franklin Lakes, NJ)

- An 18-gauge needle
- A 30-gauge needle
- Alcohol swabs
- 2 × 2 gauze pads
- Nonsterile gloves
- Eye protection

Preprocedural Approach

- The primary preoperative consideration is the patient's pain tolerance and maturity because this affects the patient's ability to tolerate the procedure. This is not always directly correlated with the patient's chronologic age. Even with avoidance of the nail matrix, injections into the nail bed are quite painful.
- It is critical to evaluate the extent of disease.
  - If lesions are widespread and involve a large body surface area, intralesional triamcinolone may not be feasible. Phototherapy or systemic medications may prove more efficacious.
  - This also applies to nail involvement. If the patient has more than three nails involved, consider systemic therapy.
  - It may be prudent to target the most symptomatic or hypertrophic lesions.
- Hypertrophic lesions may be more recalcitrant to therapy and patients should be counseled that multiple treatments may be required to achieve a response.
- Again, caution should be taken in skin of color given the increased risk of dyspigmentation.
- Providers may choose to treat a limited number of lesions on body surfaces that are not highly visible (eg, the torso) to evaluate the patient's response before treating numerous lesions or lesions in cosmetically sensitive areas.
- If injecting lesions on the face, familiarize yourself with facial anatomy to avoid important neurovascular structures.
- There are no medications required before the procedure.

Procedural Approach

- Prioritize symptomatic or hypertrophic lesions.
- Draw up the triamcinolone acetonide with an 18-gauge needle.
- Dilute to the appropriate concentration using sterile saline.
- Clean the lesion with an alcohol swab.
- Using a 30-gauge needle, slowly inject the triamcinolone at a 45° angle into the dermis.
- When the lesion blanches, stop injecting and remove the needle carefully.
- Minimize the amount of triamcinolone introduced to the normal surrounding skin; this will minimize the risk of atrophy and hypopigmentation.
- Hold pressure with 2 × 2 gauze pads to achieve hemostasis.
- Repeat this process until all lesions are treated or you reach a maximum triamcinolone dosage of 40 mg.

Postprocedural Approach

- Pain during the procedure is expected and burning from the triamcinolone can last 3 to 5 minutes after injection.
- Although some bleeding is expected, this is minimal and hemostasis is quickly achieved with pressure alone.
- There is no downtime required.

- *Red flags* include worsening erythema, edema, and pain at the site of injection, which may indicate infection. Neurologic dysfunction, particularly involving the cranial nerves when injecting the head, is also concerning for introduction of corticosteroids into neurovascular structures.
- Results are apparent within 4 to 6 weeks. Follow-up at this time is appropriate and the need for repeat injection can be established at that time.

REFERENCES

1. Archier E, Devaux S, Castela E, et al. Carcinogenic risks of psoralen UV-A therapy and narrowband UV-B therapy in chronic plaque psoriasis: a systematic literature review. *J Eur Acad Dermatol Venereol.* 2012;26(3):22–31.
2. Majid I. Fractional carbon dioxide laser in combination with topical corticosteroid: an innovative treatment for hypertrophic lichen planus. *J Am Acad Dermatol.* 2017;77(3):e67–e68.

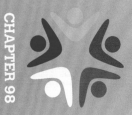

CHAPTER 98

Lipoma

Mimi R. Borrelli, Ruth Tevlin, and H. Peter Lorenz

INTRODUCTION

Lipomas are benign soft-tissue tumors composed of mature white adipocytes with uniform nuclei arranged in lobules. Many lipomas are encapsulated within a thin fibrous capsule. The exact etiology of lipomas is uncertain but involves the proliferation of mature adipocytes.

Lipomas occur in any part of the body where fat normally exists, usually in the subcutaneous tissue, and most frequently over extensor surfaces or on the neck and trunk. Lipomas occur in 1% of the population and are the most common soft-tissue tumors of adulthood; however, they rarely occur in children; the WHO reported that 6% of lipoma occur in children and 94% were benign. Lipomas are slow growing and have benign characteristics. Typically, lipomas are round, mobile, and have a soft-to-firm texture. They involve no change in color to the overlying skin. They are painless but may cause discomfort with direct pressure. The size of lipomas varies depending on their localization and time.

The diagnosis of superficial lipomas can usually be made clinically where they are visible or are detected on palpation. Lipomas deep to the investing fascia are more difficult to assess on clinical examination and may warrant additional imaging. Occasionally, lipomas grow rapidly and result in cosmetic and functional disabilities because of compressive symptoms.[1] Nonencapsulated lipomas may become "infiltrating lipomas" and infiltrate nearby muscle. Although it has been hypothesized that large lipomas may occasionally undergo malignant transformation, this pathogenesis has never been convincingly demonstrated.

Nonexcisional treatment of lipomas is common and involves regular observation, medical treatment with steroid injections to induce fat atrophy, or liposuction. Liposuction is U.S. Food and Drug Administration (FDA) approved and can help avoid scarring, but requires additional training and equipment. Surgical excision of lipomas often results in a cure and is indicated for large lipomas (>5 cm), compressive symptoms (pain or discomfort), lipomas growing rapidly, when the diagnosis is uncertain, or for cosmetic indications.[2] Lipomas can also be cauterized or removed by lasers, but laser removal involves larger incisions.

 Clinical Pearls

- **Guidelines:** No specific treatment guidelines exist for lipoma excision.
- **Age-Specific Considerations:** Children are generally treated only if the lipoma is causing issues and is especially large.
- **Technique Tips:** Great care should be taken to appreciate the lipoma from surrounding subcutaneous fat by recognizing the different consistency of the lipoma fat (more dense) from that of the subcutaneous fat, or indeed by developing your plane of excision along the investing fascia of the lipoma.
- **Skin of Color Considerations:** Lipomas involve no changes to the color of overlying skin.

Contraindications/Cautions/Risks

Contraindications

- No contraindications for surgical excision of lipomas exist unless the location of the lipoma makes excision infeasible or there are other contraindications to surgery.

Cautions

- Rarely, liposarcomas can be confused for lipomas because they present in a similar manner. Preoperative magnetic resonance imaging (MRI) can be used if there is any concern for sarcomatous features (pain, large, rapid growth, less mobile). We recommend sending excised specimens for histology to confirm the tumor is benign. Complete surgical excision of lipomas is recommended by some to exclude the possibility of a liposarcoma.
- Lipomas are associated with a number of diseases including Gardner's syndrome, Cowden syndrome, Dercum's disease, adiposis dolorosa, and Madelung disease. Preteen children with multiple lipomas are more likely to have syndromic and genetic causes.
- Differential diagnoses include neurofibromas, sebaceous cysts, vascular lesions, and fibroadenomas.
- Lipomas involving the fascial nerve and tendons may require specialist referral.

Risks

- Infections: Cellulitis, fasciitis, periostitis
- Bleeding: Ecchymoses, hematoma
- Seroma
- Scarring, permanent contour deformity
- Fat embolus
- Injury to nearby structures: Nerves → paresthesia, vessels → vascular compromise, muscle
- Recurrence

Equipment Needed

- Local anesthetic (1% or 2% lidocaine with or without epinephrine)
- Skin marker pen
- 3-mm curette
- No. 15 scalpel (larger lipomas may require a No. 10)
- Metzenbaum scissors
- Hemostat
- Needle holder
- Forceps
- 3-0 or 4-0 Vicryl™ (Ethicon US, LLC) sutures
- 4-0 or 5-0 Nylon sutures

Preprocedural Approach

- Radiography can support the clinical diagnosis of lipoma.
- Ultrasonography is often the first-line modality because it is easily accessible, inexpensive, noninvasive, relatively sensitive, and specific. The majority of lipomas appear hyperechoic, although some may be hypoechoic or isoechoic.[3]
- Computed tomography (CT) scans often observe lipomas as an encapsulated, low-density homogeneous mass. A low density is the definitive diagnostic for the lipoma.
- MRI is the most frequently used method because it has high soft-tissue resolution and can show the distribution and depth.
- Histopathology examination of large lipomas is recommended in all specimens to rule out malignancy.

Procedural Approach

- First, a marker can be used to draw around the border of the lipoma to delineate its margins, which may otherwise become easily obscured after administration of local anesthetic. Palpation can be used to help define the edges of the lipoma.
- The skin is then thoroughly cleaned with povidone-iodine (Betadine) or chlorhexidine.
- The sterile area is created by draping sterile towels.
- Local anesthetic (1%-2% lidocaine with or without epinephrine) can be administered in the subcutaneous area surrounding the operative field. Larger lipomas involving the deeper fascia may require general anesthesia.

Enucleation

- Enucleation can be used to remove small lipomas. This involves the creation of a small linear incision over the lipoma, half to one-third of its diameter, directly on the skin overlying the lipoma along Langer's lines, and down to the lipoma capsule.
- A curette or Metzenbaum scissors can be placed into the incision and used to create space between the lipoma and surrounding tissue, thus freeing the tumor from the fibrous bands connecting the fat lobules to the surrounding tissue. Great care must be taken to not pierce the lipoma and thus leak its contents.
- The tumor is then enucleated through the incision using the curette.
- Very little dissection may be required in some cases and the lipoma can be squeezed out with direct pressure.

Elliptical Excision

- Larger lipomas (>3-4 mm) are best removed by incisions that include a small ellipse of skin. This helps reduce any redundancy at closure and maximizes the visualization of the surgical field (Figure 98.1A).
- The incision should be made in a fusiform shape.
- The central island of skin can be removed first; a hemostat can be used to grasp the skin and provide tension to facilitate the removal of the lipoma.

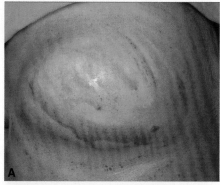

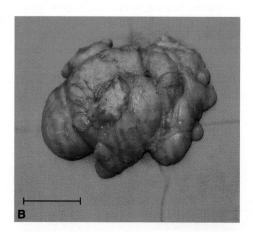

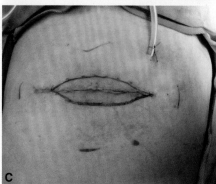

FIGURE 98.1. A, A large lipoma on the chest prior to surgical removal. B, The lipoma itself, *scale bar: 5 cm.* C, Chest skin closed after lipoma removal. Skin closed with running subcuticular 4-0 Monocryl suture with knots buried.

- Dissection is then performed beneath the subcutaneous fat to the tumor. Any tissue cutting is performed under direct visualization.
- Once the lipoma is freed, it can be removed whole, or in segments (Figure 98.1B).
- Take care to avoid nerves and blood vessels in the tissue surrounding the lipoma.

Closure

- After the lipoma is removed, the resultant cavity can be explored to ensure adequate hemostasis.
- The dead space beneath the skin can be closed using buried interrupted 3-0 or 4-0 Vicryl sutures. When large lipomas are removed, the remaining cavity can be significant and should be carefully closed to obliterate dead space.
- Drains can be placed to help the drainage of fluid and collapse dead space for lipomas greater than 5 cm in diameter.
- The skin is then closed per surgeon's preference (Figure 98.1C).

Postprocedural Approach

- The patient is given standard wound care instructions.
- The wound is checked in 1 to 2 weeks, earlier for larger lesions.
- The sutures are removed after 7 to 32 days depending on the body location: shorter times on the head and neck and longest times on the extremities.
- Specimens may be sent for histopathologic analysis.
- There is a risk of recurrence after a variable period, especially with large lipomas, and long-term follow-up is recommended in such patients.

REFERENCES

1. Patel S, Jindal S, Singh M. Giant lipoma of the posterior neck—a rare entity. *JIMSA*. 2012;25:245.
2. Usatine RP, Pfenninger JL, Stulberg DL, Small R. *Dermatologic and Cosmetic Procedures in Office Practice E-Book*. Philadelphia, PA: Elsevier Health Sciences; 2011.
3. Inampudi P, Jacobson JA, Fessell DP, et al. Soft-tissue lipomas: accuracy of sonography in diagnosis with pathologic correlation. *Radiology*. 2004;233:763–767.

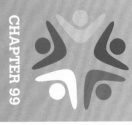

CHAPTER 99

Lymphatic Malformations

Shehla Admani and Joyce M. C. Teng

Introduction

Lymphatic malformations (LMs) are congenital vascular anomalies composed of dilated and disorganized lymphatic networks. LMs can be classified as macrocystic, microcystic, or a combination. LMs tend to increase in size over time and complications can include infection, pain, swelling, disfigurement, and functional impairment. Macrocystic LMs are often amenable to sclerotherapy and consultation with an interventional radiologist should be considered. Microcystic lesions can be more difficult to target with sclerotherapy, and additional management options include observation, surgical excision/debulking, laser treatment, and medical therapy (eg, rapamycin, sildenafil).

Although LM can be a challenging lifetime disorder, long-term condition control is possible even for complex LMs. However, a multidisciplinary approach is often required. Laser treatment can be effective for the superficial component of LM. Similar to venous malformations, LMs are "low-flow" vascular malformations; therefore, the treatment algorithms for these two disorders overlap (refer to treatment protocol in Chapter 127. Venous Malformations) with a few exceptions detailed later.

Clinical Pearls

- **Guidelines:** There are no published laser treatment guidelines for this condition.
- **Age-Specific Considerations:**
  - Because these lesions tend to progress over time, early intervention could be beneficial; however, in cases that require general anesthesia, it is reasonable to postpone the elective procedure until general anesthesia is considered to be safe.

  - Laser surgery can be coordinated with other procedures to minimize the overall number of general anesthesia needed for these treatments.
- **Technique Tips:**
  - In select cases, the authors consider pre- or concurrent use of mammalian target of rapamycin (mTOR) inhibitors such as rapamycin or the use of systemic sildenafil. Rapamycin is typically started at 0.8 mg/m^2 twice daily and titrated to a trough level of 10 to 15 ng/mL. Sildenafil dosing is weight based. Patients weighing 8 to 20 kg are treated with 10 mg sildenafil three times a day (30 mg/d) and those weighing greater than 20 kg are treated with 20 mg three times daily (60 mg/d). In cases where three-time daily dosing is not feasible, oral tadalafil can also be used, for children under 20 kg, a dose of 1 mg/kg/d is well tolerated.
  - Coordinated sclerotherapy with interventional radiology should be considered especially for macrocystic lesions.
  - Some experts will consider the use of intralesional bleomycin injection; this can be done in isolation or intraoperatively to an open wound bed during a partial resection.
- **Skin of Color Considerations:** Laser settings should be adjusted to minimize epidermal pigment damage and strict sun protection is always advised for darker skin patients.

Contraindications/Cautions/Risks

Contraindications

- Active skin infection
- Inability to care for postoperative wounds (eg, upcoming sporting events, vacations)

Cautions

- Presence of a suntan may increase dyspigmentation after laser surgery.

Risks

- Possible complications: Pain, bleeding, blistering, infection, dyspigmentation, and scarring
- Use of adjunctive medications such as rapamycin carries additional potential risks that are beyond the scope of this brief procedure description.

Equipment Needed

- Wavelength-specific protective eyewear (ie, goggles)
- Age-appropriate, laser-safe eye protection for patients if the periorbital area is to be treated (laser eye pads, correctly fitting metal eye shields, etc)
- Long-pulsed alexandrite laser
- Long-pulsed Nd:YAG laser
- Sterile water
- Gauze (wet and dry)
- Petrolatum-based ointment
- Ice
- Anesthetic: Choice of anesthetic can vary from case to case and generally consists of either topical or general anesthesia followed by injectable local anesthetic. For further details, see Chapter 127. Venous Malformations.
- Surgical prep (isopropyl alcohol, chlorhexidine, Betadine, followed by sterile water)
- Dressing (will vary depending on treatment site)

Preprocedural Approach

- Sun protection is recommended before the procedure to reduce the risk of epidermal damage and to assure optimal treatment.

- Antiviral prophylaxis should be considered when treating patients with facial venous malformations and history of herpes labialis.
- Although controlled studies are needed, there is anecdotal experience suggesting that the use of antiangiogenic therapy such as mTOR inhibitors can be beneficial before and/or concurrent with laser treatments.

Procedural Approach

- Appropriate protective eyewear should be worn by both care providers and patients during the entire procedure.
- To decrease fire risk in the operating room, wet towels should be placed around the treatment area. When a facial lesion is being treated, patient safety and protection of the airway should be paramount, and an appropriate laser-safe protocol should be implemented. For short procedures, nasal cannula oxygenation can be a safer alternative. For intraoral procedures, room air ventilation may be used to decrease percentage of oxygen in the surgical field and thereby reduce the fire risk. Airway fires are lethal and appropriate precautions should be taken when treating facial/oral lesions.
- A combination of alexandrite (755 nm) and Nd:YAG lasers may be used for treatment of LMs depending on the epidermal, dermal, and subcutaneous involvement of the malformations (Figure 99.1).
- For LMs with obvious epidermal involvement, long-pulsed alexandrite laser is the best choice. For LMs involving subcutaneous tissue, long-pulsed Nd:YAG may be more effective. For details on baseline settings and treatment endpoints, see Chapter 127. Venous Malformations. It is important to note that patients treated with Nd:YAG do get some fibrosis and hypertrophic changes may occur when there is epidermal ulceration post treatment.
- Unlike venous malformations, LM does not often benefit from pulsed-dye laser treatment.

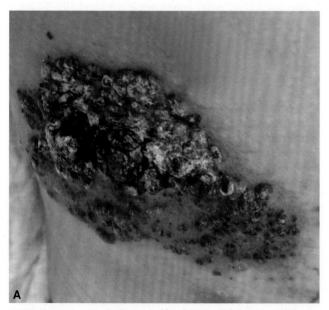
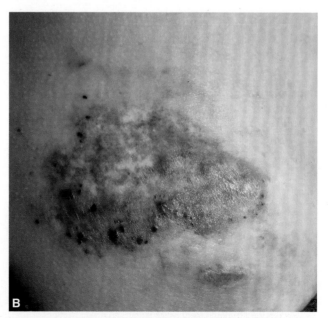

FIGURE 99.1. A, Lymphatic malformation with hypertrophic change that was treated with a combination of alexandrite (755 nm, 3-mm spot size, fluence of 44 J/cm^2, microsecond pulse width) and long-pulsed Nd:YAG laser (1064 nm, 4-mm spot size, pulse duration of 30 μs, fluence of 60 mJ/cm^2). B, Lymphatic malformation after multiple treatment sessions. The foci of hypopigmentation are areas of prior hypertrophic lymphatic malformation that have responded excellently to treatment.

- In the authors' experience, LMs have a tendency to bleed or ooze immediately after laser treatment; in such cases, electrocautery or silver nitrate sticks can be used.
- Immediately after surgery, a petrolatum-based ointment should be applied liberally.
- Application of intra- and postoperative cooling is very important to help decrease discomfort and minimize edema.
- Combined sclerotherapy and laser treatment should be used cautiously because excessive tissue destruction can result in localized skin ulceration.
- Combined treatment with intralesional bleomycin carries an increased risk of hyperpigmentation. Therefore, special attention should be paid to prevent skin friction, pressure, or trauma at the treatment and surrounding sites.

Postprocedural Approach

- The postoperative approach is similar to that of venous malformations; for further details, see Chapter 127. Venous Malformations.

SUGGESTED READINGS

García-Montero P, Del Boz J, Sanchez-Martínez M, Escudero Santos IM, Baselga E. Microcystic lymphatic malformation successfully treated with topical rapamycin. *Pediatrics*. 2017;139(5):e20162105.

Lee HJ, Kim TW, Kim JM, et al. Percutaneous sclerotherapy using bleomycin for the treatment of vascular malformations. *Int J Dermatol*. 2017;56(11):1186–1191.

Tu JH, Tafoya E, Jeng M, Teng JM. Long-term follow-up of lymphatic malformations in children treated with sildenafil. *Pediatr Dermatol*. 2017;34(5):559–565.

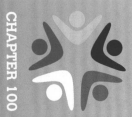

CHAPTER 100

Mastocytoma

Allison Truong, Latanya T. Benjamin, Carol E. Cheng, and Marcia Hogeling

INTRODUCTION

Mastocytosis describes a group of disorders characterized by excessive mast cell accumulation in one or multiple tissues. Mastocytosis is subdivided into cutaneous mastocytosis (CM) and systemic mastocytosis (SM). Patients with CM should have skin-limited involvement and should not fulfill diagnostic criteria for SM (Table 100.1). According to the World Health Organization,

there are three forms of CM: maculopapular cutaneous mastocytosis (MPCM) or urticarial pigmentosa (UP), diffuse cutaneous mastocytosis (DCM), and solitary cutaneous mastocytoma. Telangiectasia macularis eruptive perstans (TMEP) and nodular mastocytosis are sometimes classified as CM.

Mastocytosis is a rare disorder with an estimated prevalence of 1 in 10 000 people. Males and females are equally affected, although there is a slight male predominance in childhood and slight female predominance in adulthood. Fifty-five to 80% of mastocytosis cases occur before age 2 years and 10% between ages 2 and 15 years. A majority of these cases are skin limited and eventually improve or resolve by adolescence. In contrast, only 5% of adult-onset mastocytosis are cutaneous only, with most adults having systemic involvement. Children also have a lower risk of anaphylaxis at 6% to 9% compared to that in adults (49%). On physical examination, the Darier's sign (ie, the eliciting of erythema and an urticarial wheal with brisk stroking or rubbing the lesion) is helpful for diagnosis (Figure 100.1). Annual laboratory studies including complete blood count and serum chemistries including liver function test and tryptase are recommended to evaluate for SM. In addition, serum tryptase level reflects mast cell burden, and its determination is recommended in the diagnosis and follow-up. When tryptase levels are >6 ng/mL, children are more likely to require treatment to manage symptoms and prevent severe episodes. When levels are >15.5 ng/mL, they are at higher risk for hospitalization because of severe symptoms. Additional studies can be considered such as peripheral blood and/or bone marrow, which can be evaluated for c-KIT mutation at codon D816V and bone marrow aspirate and biopsy for foci of ≥15 mass cells, morphology of mast cells, and expression of CD2 and/or CD25 by bone marrow mast cells.

TABLE 100.1 : Diagnostic Criteria for Systemic Mastocytosis; 2016 Update from the World Health Organization

If the Major Criterion and one Minor Criterion or at least three Minor Criteria are fulfilled, then the diagnosis of systemic mastocytosis can be established.

Major Criterion:
- Multifocal dense infiltrates of mast cells (≥15 mast cells in aggregates) in bone marrow (BM) biopsies and/or in sections of other extracutaneous organ(s)

Minor Criteria:
- In biopsy sections of BM or extracutaneous organs, >25% of the mast cells in the infiltrate are spindle shaped or have atypical morphology or, of all mast cells in BM aspirate smears, >25% are immature or atypical.
- KIT point mutation at codon 816 in the BM or another extracutaneous organ
- Mast cells in BM or blood or another extracutaneous organ express CD25 with/without CD2 in addition to normal mast cell markers.
- Serum total tryptase level persistently >20 ng/mL (unless there is an associated myeloid neoplasm).

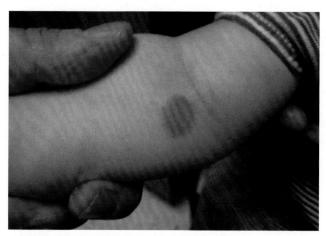

FIGURE 100.1. Solitary mastocytoma in a young boy in the antecubital fossa region of the right arm. Because of its location it was "almost always" inflamed secondary to mechanical irritation. Photo courtesy of Andrew C. Krakowski, MD.

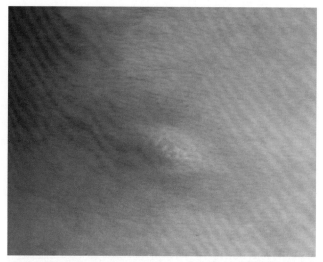

FIGURE 100.2. The waistband of this patient's diapers mechanically irritated this solitary mastocytoma on the lower abdomen. The patient's age (ie, not potty trained), anatomic location, and inherent elliptical shape make surgical excision a consideration. Photo courtesy of Andrew C. Krakowski, MD.

There are no current therapies to change the natural course of disease, although the prognosis is generally favorable in children. Initial management includes practical measures such as the use of lukewarm water for bathing instead of hot water, air-conditioning during hot weather, and avoidance of triggers for mast cell degranulation. Parents and caretakers should recognize anaphylaxis and carry at least 2 doses of epinephrine in self-injectable form at all times. Hypotension is the most common presentation in anaphylaxis in patients with mastocytosis. Additional symptomatic treatment with topical and/or oral steroids and antihistamines is helpful. Phototherapy can be used in UP and DCM, with reported improvement of pruritus, leathery skin thickening, and dermatographism but with persistent cutaneous lesions. Treatment with biologics, chemotherapy, combination therapy, and surgical therapy are typically reserved for SM. Omalizumab (humanized murine monoclonal antibody conjugates free serum immunoglobulin [Ig] E and reduces binding to high-affinity IgE receptor FCεRI on mast cells and basophils), imatinib (KIT-targeting tyrosine kinase inhibitor), and cladribine (a chemotherapy agent) have been used with reported success in cases report or case series. Allogeneic hematopoietic stem cell transplant (Allo-HCT) is often used as salvage therapy for systemic disease.

In most cases, mastocytoma lesions gradually increase in size for several months before stabilizing. Symptoms associated with solitary mastocytoma may include pruritus or discomfort, urtication, and, rarely, blister formation. Treatment is for symptomatic management. It is reasonable to observe residual, biopsy-confirmed mastocytoma in patients who are asymptomatic and who do not have systemic disease. A recent study found that complete resolution rate for mastocytoma was 10% per year compared to 1.9% per year for UP. Intralesional triamcinolone acetonide injections have been used to treat solitary mastocytomas with various efficacies in infants and adults. Negative Darier's sign and flattened lesions following three injections given at monthly intervals have been reported. However, others reported decreased itching but neither change in size or cessation of urtication with intralesional injections.

The definitive treatment of a solitary mastocytoma includes excision, which can be done as an excisional biopsy during initial evaluation or subsequently on histologic confirmation of the pathology. Of note, degranulation secondary to trauma or urtication has been reported in biopsy specimens, leading to poor demonstration of granules and possible precipitation of severe symptoms. Avoidance of trauma during biopsies can help retain granules and aid in an accurate diagnosis. Surgical excision offers a rapid, relatively simple, and effective mode of treatment. In the case of a single or a few symptomatic lesions, surgical excision can be tried as first-line therapy (Figure 100.2). However, the surgeon should take care to entirely remove the lesion or the scar that forms may develop symptoms such as urtication. It is also important to counsel families about spontaneous resolution of mastocytomas, whereas surgery will leave a permanent scar. If the lesion is large, with minimal symptoms, then total excision would likely be unnecessary because the lesion tends to involute.

Clinical Pearls

- **Guidelines:**
  - Level 4 evidence for intralesional triamcinolone of solitary mastocytomas
  - Level 4 evidence for surgical excision of solitary mastocytomas: B
- **Technique Tips:**
  - Consider using lower doses of triamcinolone in areas of the face, groin, and axillae.
  - Avoid vibratory devices used for preoperative pain management because they may lead to urtication.
  - Be careful while gently cleaning with alcohol preoperatively because it may lead to urtication.
- **Age-Specific Considerations:** Consider the anatomic location of the lesion because it relates to the specific age of the patient; some lesions may be more problematic at different ages (eg, a small lesion on the back of a mostly supine 4-month-old and the same lesion on the back of an adolescent wearing sports equipment).
- **Skin of Color Considerations:** Urtication may be more difficult to appreciate in darker skin tones.

PROCEDURAL APPROACH #1: INTRALESIONAL INJECTION

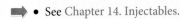 • See Chapter 14. Injectables.

Equipment Needed

- Intralesional triamcinolone
- Normal saline (for dilution if needed)
- 30G needle
- 16G needle (or other needle for drawing up medication)
- 1-cc Luer-Lok® syringe (Becton-Dickinson and Company, Franklin Lakes, NJ)
- Gauze
- Alcohol pad

Preprocedural Approach

- Complete blood count, serum chemistries including liver function test, and tryptase
- Consideration for peripheral blood and/or bone marrow and bone marrow aspirate and biopsy

Procedural Approach

- Avoid massaging or scratching the skin because of risk of urtication.
- Gently wipe area of skin clean with alcohol pad, being careful not to mechanically urticate the lesion.
- Insert 30-gauge needle at 30° to 45°.
- Slowly infiltrate desired amount of medication depending on location on body starting at 2.5 to 5 mg/mL for face and 10 to 20 mg/mL for trunk and extremities.

Postprocedural Approach

- Injections should be spaced at 4- to 6-week intervals.
- Usually takes two to three injections to see improvement in pruritus and discomfort

PROCEDURAL APPROACH #2: SURGICAL EXCISION

Contraindications/Cautions/Risks

Contraindications
- Because patients have higher risk of anaphylaxis with general anesthesia, local anesthetics are preferred.

Cautions
- See Table 100.2.

Risks
- Atrophy, dyspigmentation, and scar
- Recurrence or incomplete treatment with subsequent urtication within scar

TABLE 100.2 : Potential Irritants for Children With Mast Cell Disease

PHYSICAL STIMULI	Exercise, skin friction, hot baths, cold exposure (especially swimming), ingestion of hot beverages, spicy foods, or ethanol
MEDICATIONS	Aspirin, alcohol, morphine, codeine, polymyxin B, thiamine, quinine, D-tubocurarine, radiographic dyes, scopolamine, procaine, opiates, nonsteroidal anti-inflammatory agents, gallamine, decamethonium
OTHERS	Intravenous high-molecular-weight polymers (dextran), cheese, crayfish and lobsters, emotional stress, temperature extremes, bacterial toxins, envenomation by insects, snake venoms, polypeptides released by *Ascaris*, jellyfish

- Rarely, at higher doses and regular intervals, risk of adrenal insufficiency can occur.

Equipment Needed

- Lidocaine with epinephrine
- Excision tray
- Suture

Preprocedural Approach

Same as above

Procedural Approach

- Gently wipe area of skin clean with alcohol pad or other antiseptic agent.
- Apply local anesthetic to skin.
- Perform elliptical excision of skin lesion based on clinical margins.

Postprocedural Approach

- Suture removal in 7 to 14 days depending on location of surgery

SUGGESTED READINGS

Brockow K, Jofer C, Behrendt H, Ring J. Anaphylaxis in patients with mastocytosis: a study on history, clinical features and risk factors in 120 patients. *Allergy.* 2008;63(2):226–232.

Cohen PR. Solitary mastocytoma presenting in an adult: report and literature review of adult-onset solitary cutaneous mastocytoma with recommendations for evaluation and treatment. *Dermatol Pract Concept.* 2016;6(3):31–38.

Valent P, Akin C, Metcalfe D. Mastocytosis: 2016 updated WHO classification and novel emerging treatment concepts. *Blood.* 2017;129(11):1420–1427.

CHAPTER 101

Median Raphe Cyst

Paul A. Mittermiller, Clifford C. Sheckter, and H. Peter Lorenz

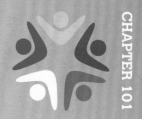

INTRODUCTION

Median raphe cysts occur on the midline ventral surface of the penis, scrotum, or perineum. One example of the presentation on the ventral surface of the penis is shown in Figure 101.1. There are two theories regarding the formation of these cysts. One posits that tissue is trapped as the urethral or genital folds close during development, and the other suggests that these form as outgrowths after the primary closure of the folds.[1] The cysts rarely communicate with the urethra.

These cysts are usually present at birth but are sometimes detected later in life. They commonly present as painless, subcutaneous cysts or canals. However, patients can also present with localized infections or pain with intercourse.[2] Diagnosis is suggested on the basis of history and physical examination. Differential diagnosis should include other benign cysts and masses of the skin. Surgeons should also consider urethral diverticula given the greater complexity in management.[2]

There are three different histologic types that demonstrate epithelial linings composed of columnar stratified, pseudostratified, or squamous cells, and pathology confirms the diagnosis.[3,4] Surgical excision is the treatment of choice for providing definitive management of the lesion. A description for excision of median raphe cysts is included later.

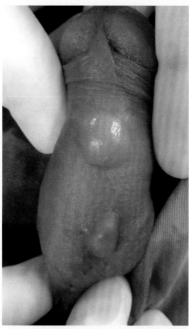

FIGURE 101.1. Two median raphe cysts on the ventral surface of the penis. Reprinted by permission from Springer: Shao IH, Chen TD, Shao HT, et al. Male median raphe cysts: serial retrospective analysis and histopathological classification. *Diagn Pathol.* 2012;7:121. Copyright © 2012 Springer Nature.

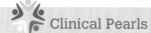
Clinical Pearls

- **Guidelines:** There are no specific treatment guidelines for treatment of median raphe cysts.
- **Age-Specific Considerations:** General anesthesia or intravenous sedation should be considered for children given the sensitive location of the cysts.
- **Technique Tips:** Surgical excision should aim to remove the entire lesion without damaging any neighboring structures (eg, the urethra).
- **Skin of Color Considerations:** As with all surgical procedures, there is a risk of scarring postoperatively. The degree of scarring may vary depending on skin tone and type.

Contraindications/Cautions/Risks

Contraindications

- No specific contraindications for surgical removal of median raphe cysts
- If the surgeon believes the cyst may represent a urethral diverticulum, consultation with urology is recommended.
- If significant patient comorbidities exist, excision can potentially be performed under local anesthesia to avoid the risks of general anesthesia.

Cautions

- The surgeon should take care to not damage the nearby urethra.

Risks

- Bleeding
- Infection
- Damage to the urethra

Equipment Needed

- Local anesthetic (1% or 2% lidocaine or 0.25% bupivacaine)
- #15 scalpel
- Scissors
- Electric cautery
- Needle holder
- Forceps
- Suture

Preprocedural Approach

- Urology should be consulted if there is concern for communication with the urethra.

Procedural Approach

- A sterile field is created using antiseptic prep safe for the urethra (eg, Betadine).
- The borders of the lesion are identified and a wedge-shaped excision is designed around the cyst or canal to remove the entire lesion and overlying skin.
- Local anesthesia is injected around the lesion.
- A scalpel is used to incise the skin.
- Dissection should be carried around the lesion using either sharp dissection with the scalpel or scissors or by blunt spreading.
- The lesion should be excised in its entirety without violating the cyst contents to prevent local recurrence.
- Adequate hemostasis is obtained using electric cautery.
- The wound site is irrigated and the skin reapproximated.
- The skin is closed in two layers. Deeper penile tissues are approximated with absorbable monofilament suture. The skin is approximated with absorbable sutures (particularly in children) to prevent the need for removal in clinic.

Postprocedural Approach

- The incision should be well healed within 3 weeks.
- After the incision has healed, the patient can return to full activities, including intercourse for sexually active patients.
- A histopathologic examination should be performed in all cases to confirm the diagnosis.
- If the lesion recurs, this likely resulted from inadequate primary excision. Additional excision may be repeated to remove all contents.

REFERENCES

1. Krauel L, Tarrado X, Garcia-Aparicio L, et al., Median raphe cysts of the perineum in children. *Urology.* 2008;71:830–831.
2. Little JS, Keating MA, Rink RC. Median raphe cysts of the genitalia. *J Urol.* 1992;148:1872–1873.
3. Romaní J, Barnadas MA, Miralles J, Curell R, de Moragas JM. Median raphe cyst of the penis with ciliated cells. *J Cutan Pathol.* 1995;22:378–381.
4. Shao IH, Chen TD, Shao HT, Chen HW. Male median raphe cysts: serial retrospective analysis and histopathological classification. *Diagn Pathol.* 2012;7:121.

CHAPTER 102

Melanoma

Mimi R. Borrelli, Ruth Tevlin, and H. Peter Lorenz

INTRODUCTION

Cutaneous malignant melanomas are the most sinister of skin cancers. In the pediatric population, melanomas are rare; however, diagnoses in those 15 to 19 years of age are increasing in the United States by 2% each year, and melanomas are the second leading cause of cancer in adolescents and young adults aged 15 to 29 years.[1]

The majority of pediatric melanoma cases are sporadic and related to ultraviolet (UV) radiation exposure. Other risk factors include fair skin, sunbed use, family history of melanoma, the presence of multiple atypical nevi, congenital melanocytic nevi, xeroderma pigmentosum, and germline mutations involving cell-cycle mediators.

Early recognition is important to prevent melanoma progression. At least one cohort study suggested that the conventionally taught ABCDE detection criteria (ie, *A*symmetry, *B*order irregularity, *C*olor variegation, *D*iameter >6 mm, and *E*volution) may not represent the most common presentations of pediatric melanoma; consequently, the criteria of *A*melanotic; *B*leeding, *B*ump; *C*olor uniformity; *D*e novo development, any *D*iameter—used together with conventional criteria—may aid in the earlier detection and treatment of melanoma in children.[2]

Surgical excision is the treatment of choice for all localized cutaneous lesions suspected of being a melanoma. Punch or shave biopsies may be performed but are suboptimal because tumor thickness may be underestimated. Management of malignant melanomas requires a multidisciplinary team including medical oncologists, radiation oncologists, dermatologists, oncology nurses, as well as surgeons to ensure the best staging, therapy, and prognosis. We discuss our surgical approach to the excision of malignant melanomas.

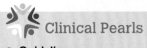

Clinical Pearls

- **Guidelines:**
  - Adolescents and young adults have not benefited from clinical trials as much as their older or younger counterparts.
  - There are no optimum excision margins specific to minors, and standard adult guidelines may be recommended: 1-cm margins for ≤1-mm lesions, or where morbidity precludes wider margins in 1- to 2-mm depth, and 2-cm margins for thicker lesions.
  - Younger children may not require as large margins even for thicker melanomas.
- **Age-Specific Considerations:**
  - In young adults, melanomas are more likely to arise from dysplastic nevi that have evolved rather than from congenital nevi.
  - At the time of presentation, children are more likely than are adults to have localized disease, to be Caucasian with fair skin, and to have been exposed to UV radiation and sunbeds.
  - A high degree of suspicion is needed for children because they may present atypically: 60% of children aged younger than 10 years and 40% of adolescents did not meet the traditional ABCDE criteria, and,

resultantly, it took longer than 6 months to diagnose 82% of cases.[2] Cordoro et al.,[2] therefore, propose the following criteria to detect characteristics more specific to melanomas in children: A, amelanotic; B, bleeding, bump; C, color uniformity; D, de novo, any diameter; and E, evolution of mole.

- **Technique Tips:**
  - Whenever possible, diagnostic biopsies should include complete excision with narrow margin of normal skin as follow-up sentinel lymph node biopsy results can be skewed by initial wide excision.
  - For extremity lesions, surgical biopsy incisions should always be oriented vertically so as to not interfere with or complicate subsequent definitive excision and reconstruction. Planned elliptical excision can facilitate closure.
- **Skin of Color Considerations:**
  - Acral lentiginous melanomas are more common in black than in white individuals.
  - Melanomas in white individuals are more likely to be localized at diagnosis.

Contraindications/Cautions/Risks

Contraindications

- Surgical excision is unlikely to cure those with metastatic disease, and if surgery is used in these cases, it is to control, as opposed to cure, the disease.
- The patient must be medically fit to withstand the planned surgery.

Cautions

- The main caution with melanoma surgery is the choice of margin width for in situ melanomas, because there are currently no known randomized studies. Case series evidence suggests that 5-mm margins are often adequate in most cases, but does not completely diminish the risk of disease recurrence.[3]

Risks

- Lymphedema or lymphocele
- Pain
- Swelling, bruising, bleeding
- Nerve damage, paresthesia
- Infection
- Seroma
- Wound dehiscence
- Poor functional/cosmetic outcome with scarring and disfigurement
- Recurrence, at site or at distant site

Equipment Needed

- No special equipment is needed.
- 4-0 or 5-0 Nylon sutures for superficial closure
- 3-0 or 5-0 Vicryl™ (Ethicon US, LLC) sutures for deep closure
- No. 15 scalpel
- Local or general anesthesia
- Ruler
- Needle holder
- Forceps

Preprocedural Approach

- Clinical evaluation includes asking about family history and a history of precursor lesions in the area including congenital melanocytic nevi.
- The area should be photographed, and its color and size adequately documented.
- Extensive imaging and laboratory tests are not generally recommended for the asymptomatic patient with a new diagnosis of a primary melanoma.
- Histologic confirmation of metastatic disease is critical and can be performed using fine-needle aspiration biopsy under radiologic (computed tomography [CT] or ultrasound) guidance of any lymph nodes felt to be enlarged on physical examination.
- A full review of the histologic findings should be undertaken before planning the local excision.

Procedural Approach

- Informed consent from the parent/guardian and, when possible, assent from the minor are obtained.
- General anesthesia is typically used for children because of the pain associated with the procedure and need to excise adequate depth of tissue. Local anesthesia is sufficient for the older patient. Mohs resection is generally not performed in the pediatric patient who requires general anesthesia.
- The area can be thoroughly cleaned with Betadine or chlorhexidine and a sterile field created with drapes.
- If local anesthesia is used, 1% Xylocaine without epinephrine, or 1% Xylocaine and 0.25% to 0.5% bupivacaine in a 50:50 mixture can be used to infiltrate the region of the proposed incision without directly injecting into the lesion.
- Marginal biopsy is first indicated, followed by a wide local excision.
- For a wide local excision, a marker pen can be used to demarcate the planned excision. The primary goal of excision is to achieve negative margins. First, using a ruler and a marker pen, a circle can be drawn around the lesion to include the appropriate margin depending on the depth of the melanoma (Breslow thickness) (see Guidelines in "Clinical Pearl" box for children). In general, the following margins may serve to guide the clinician:
  - In situ lesions require at least a 0.5-cm margin.
  - Invasive melanomas <1 mm require a 1-cm margin.
  - Melanomas >2 mm in depth require a 2-cm margin.
- The circle can be reshaped to an ellipse to improve the closure. The long axis should be orientated along the lymphatic drainage to the ipsilateral lymph node.
- Excise down to, but not including, the fascia, and maintain the perpendicular angle of the scalpel while determining the excision margins.
- Orient the specimen for pathology with clips or a suture.
- Gloves and surgical instruments should be changed after excision of the melanoma to avoid wound contamination.
- Ensure hemostasis and close the skin in layers. Excision sites are most often closed primarily with interrupted sutures. Deep closure can be achieved with interrupted or running 3-0 Vicryl sutures. Subcuticular monofilament closure (if there is minimal skin tension) or nylon mattress sutures can be used for the skin closure (Figure 102.1).
- Larger defects may require use of a split- or full-thickness skin graft, or a flap such as a rotational or advancement flap.

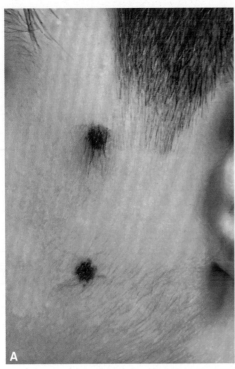
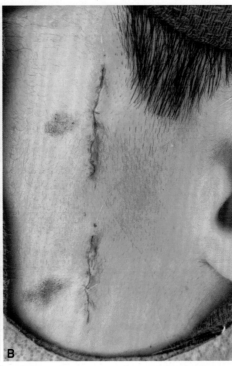

FIGURE 102.1. A, Two facial nevi lesions preoperatively. B, Following skin closure by buried running subcuticular suture technique. The pathology report for both lesions read "compound melanocytic nevus."

- If there is any lymph node involvement, the lymph node biopsy or dissection can be performed within the same procedure. Sentinel node biopsy is typically performed in conjunction with melanoma excision for melanomas ≥1 mm in depth and for those presenting with malignant features (ulceration, angiolymphatic invasion, high mitotic rate). If performed, the sentinel node biopsy is usually performed before lesion excision.

Postprocedural Approach

- Sutures should remain in place for 7 to 14 days depending on anatomic location.
- Melanomas have a propensity to recur. There are clear guidelines regarding follow-up intervals, for example, those published by the American Academy of Dermatology and the British Association of Dermatology.
- Clinicians should have a low threshold for detecting metastatic disease with a comprehensive review of systems and thorough physical exam. Laboratory tests and imaging studies may also be indicated; however, the clinician should be aware of the possibility of false positive and false negative results.

REFERENCES

1. Barr RD, Ries LA, Lewis DR, et al. Incidence and incidence trends of the most frequent cancers in adolescent and young adult Americans, including "nonmalignant/noninvasive" tumors. *Cancer.* 2016;122:1000–1008.
2. Cordoro KM, Gupta D, Frieden IJ, McCalmont T, Kashani-Sabet M. Pediatric melanoma: results of a large cohort study and proposal for modified ABCD detection criteria for children. *J Am Acad Dermatol.* 2013;68:913–925.
3. Links S. What are the recommended definitive margins for excision of primary melanoma? [Version URL: https://wiki.cancer.org.au/australiawiki/index.php?oldid=199874, cited 2020 Jan 4]. Available from https://wiki.cancer.org.au/australia/Clinical_question:What_are_the_recommended_safety_margins_for_radical_excision_of_primary_melanoma%3F/In_situ. In: Cancer Council Australia Melanoma Guidelines Working Party. Clinical practice guidelines for the diagnosis and management of melanoma. Sydney: Cancer Council Australia. Available from: https://wiki.cancer.org.au/australia/Guidelines:Melanoma.

CHAPTER 103

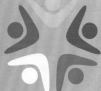

Milium

Allison Truong, Latanya T. Benjamin, Carol E. Cheng, and Marcia Hogeling

INTRODUCTION

Milia (the plural of "milium") are small, benign, subepidermal keratin cysts arising from the pilosebaceous units or eccrine sweat ducts. They usually have a wall of several layers of stratified squamous epithelium with a central keratinous material, similar to an epidermal inclusion cyst. They present as 1- to 2-mm firm, white papules usually on the face. They can occur at all ages and are a common finding in newborns (40%-50% of babies). In newborns, they are frequently found on the nose and cheeks and usually self-resolve within the first few weeks of life, although they may persist into the second or third month.

The development of milia can be spontaneous or may result as part of the healing process of second-degree burns, blistering diseases (ie, porphyria cutanea tarda, epidermolysis bullosa), dermabrasion, or ablative laser resurfacing. Some autoimmune skin disorders, genetic syndromes (eg, Loeys–Dietz, Bazex–Dupre–Christol, Rombo, Rasmussen, orofacial digital syndrome type 1, and atrichia with papular lesions), systemic drugs (eg, tyrosine kinase inhibitors such as dovitinib and sorafenib), photodynamic therapy, electron beam therapy (for mycosis fungoides), topical creams (eg, imiquimod, clobetasol), and allergic contact dermatitis (eg, poison ivy) have also been reported to be associated with the development of milia.

There is currently no standardized treatment for this condition. Given its benign nature, watchful waiting is a reasonable consideration. Milia can be treated for cosmetic reasons with topical or oral retinoids. Case reports of milia en plaque have been successfully treated with oral minocycline. Further, surgical treatments such as curettage, incision, electrodesiccation, and manual extraction methods have also been tried with success but can be labor intensive depending on the number of lesions. Herein we describe one approach to manual extraction.

MANUAL EXTRACTION

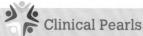

Clinical Pearls

- **Guidelines:** Level 1 evidence for manual extraction of milia
- **Technique Tips:** Children can be distracted with video on phone or Buzzy® Mini Healthcare (MMJ Labs, Atlanta, GA).
- **Age-Specific Considerations:** Age 5+ or ability to stay still during procedure
- **Skin of Color Considerations:** In all skin types, dyspigmentation due to skin inflammation should be discussed before the procedure.

Contraindications/Cautions/Risks

Contraindications
- Active infection, bleeding disorder, poor healing

Cautions
- Considerations for anatomic location such as periorbital areas given increased risk of pain and purpura

Risks
- Risk of adverse events includes recurrence, pitted scarring, bleeding, and infection.

Equipment Needed
- Alcohol pad
- 18-gauge needle or 11 blade scalpel
- Two cotton-tipped applicators
- Comedone extractor
- Paper clip

Preprocedural Approach

- Verbal and/or written consent may be obtained before procedure.
- Proper stabilization and positioning of patient will help to ensure a pleasant procedural experience

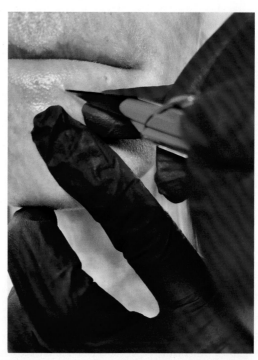

FIGURE 103.1. Inverted 11 blade used to nick the skin surface overlying the milium.

Procedural Approach

- Wipe area of skin clean with alcohol pad.
- Nick surface of milium using an 18-gauge needle or inverted (ie, "blade up") 11 blade scalpel (Figure 103.1).
- Using cotton swab portion of two cotton-tipped applicators, place lateral pressure in different directions on the individual milium to express keratin debris (Figure 103.2). Nicking may need to be repeated if initial hole is too small.

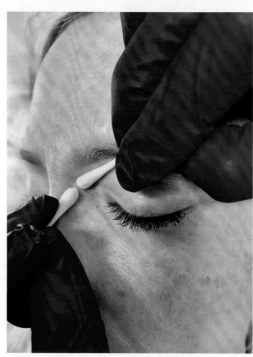

FIGURE 103.2. Manual extraction of keratinaceous debris from milia using two cotton-tipped applicators.

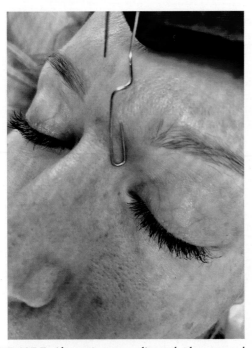

FIGURE 103.3. Alternative paper clip method to extract keratinaceous debris from milia.

- Alternatively, a comedone extractor can be used to express the contents of the individual milium. A paper clip bent such that the two looped ends are opposite one another can also be used if no comedone extractor is available and cost is a concern (Figure 103.3). This should be sterilized before use to minimize infection.

Postprocedural Approach

- Apply Vaseline™ (Conopco, Inc., US).
- Bandage daily until resolution.
- Consider prescribing topical retinoid nightly to decrease risk of recurrence.

SUGGESTED READINGS

Bridges AG, Lucky AW, Haney G, Mutasim DF. Milia en plaque of the eyelids in childhood: case report and review of the literature. *Pediatr Dermatol.* 1998;15(4):282–284.

George DE, Wasko CA, Hsu S. Surgical pearl: evacuation of milia with a paper clip. *J Am Acad Dermatol.* 2006;54(2):326.

George DE, Wasko CA, Hsu S, Connelly T. Eruptive milia and rapid response to topical tretinoin. *Arch Dermatol.* 2008;144(6):816–817.

Hinen HB, Gathings RM, Shuler M, Wine Lee L. Successful treatment of facial milia in an infant with orofaciodigital syndrome type 1. *Pediatr Dermatol.* 2018;35(1):e88–e89.

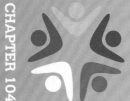

CHAPTER 104

Miliaria

Allison Truong, Latanya T. Benjamin, Carol E. Cheng, and Marcia Hogeling

Introduction

Miliaria is a common, benign, transient condition caused by blockage of the eccrine sweat ducts. It is colloquially known commonly as "heat rash," "sweat rash," or "prickly heat." Miliaria is divided into crystallina, rubra, and profunda depending on the level of blockage of the duct. Crystallina blocks the duct within the stratum corneum; rubra blocks the duct within the stratum malpighi; and profunda blocks the duct at the dermal–epidermal junction or dermis. Miliaria crystallina (sudamina) is commonly seen in neonates, peaking at 1 week of age with a reported frequency of 4% to 9%. Miliaria rubra is the most common subtype of miliaria and reported in 4% of neonates and up to 30% of all ages. Miliaria profunda (tropical anhidrosis or mammillaria) is a less common subtype more frequently seen in adult males in more tropical climates. Because this is a disorder of the sweat glands, anything that causes sweating can lead to miliaria in patients of all ages including fever, exercise, skin occlusion, and hot and humid climates. Other associations include medications (ie, isotretinoin), hypernatremia, ultraviolet or ionizing radiation, bacteria, and rare genetic diseases such as type I pseudohypoaldosteronism and Morvan syndrome.

The distinction between these subtypes can be seen during the physical examination. Crystallina presents as fragile, asymptomatic, 1- to 2-mm clear vesicles on the head, neck, and upper trunk, resembling water droplets, easily subject to rupture (Figure 104.1). It tends to not cause a significant inflammatory

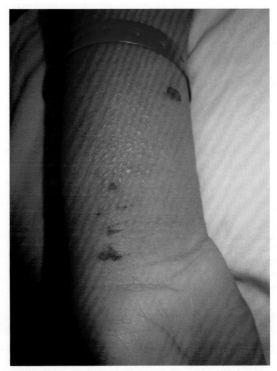

FIGURE 104.1. Miliaria crystallina in a hospitalized pediatric patient. Photo courtesy of Andrew C. Krakowski, MD.

response. Rubra is characterized by leakage of sweat into the periductal tissue resulting in inflammation. It generally presents as 2- to 4-mm, nonfollicular, erythematous papules on the head, neck, axillae, or groin in children and scalp, trunk, back, neck, and flexural areas in adults and may be papulovesicular or pustular. When pustular, miliaria rubra is called miliaria pustulosa. These lesions tend to be symptomatic and patients may describe itching or stinging. Miliaria profunda presents as 1- to 4-mm nonfollicular, skin-colored or erythematous papules. The process occurs deep in the skin; therefore, the affected areas show little or no sweating and the lesions themselves are generally asymptomatic. Miliaria lesions appear within days to weeks and resolve within hours to days. Miliaria profunda is usually a benign entity, but it can also rarely present with systemic symptoms associated such as hyperthermia, heat exhaustion, weakness, malaise, dyspnea, tachycardia, and cardiovascular collapse.

Clinical Pearls

- **Guidelines:** There are no published treatment guidelines for this condition. There is no strong evidence for any one specific treatment option.
- **Age-Specific Considerations:** Monitor younger children to ensure they do not become hypothermic during treatment or, conversely, they do not overheat from lack of being able to sweat.
- **Technique Tips:**
  - These lesions typically will self-resolve, so aggressive procedural treatment is NOT indicated.
  - Treatment centers on minimizing sweating and obstruction of eccrine sweat ducts.
  - Identifying the etiology of the miliaria and finding ways to alleviate the patient's overheating are keys to expediting resolution and prevent recurrence.
    - For symptomatic treatment of miliaria rubra, mild to mid-potency steroids such as hydrocortisone or triamcinolone cream twice daily for 1 to 2 weeks may decrease pruritus and inflammation. Avoidance of ointments is important to decrease risk of exacerbations.
    - Topical antibiotics such as clindamycin or erythromycin solution are generally reserved for patients with miliaria pustulosa.
    - There is little information in the literature for treatment of miliaria profunda. Oral isotretinoin 40 mg daily for 2 months and topical anhydrous lanolin before exercise were reported to be helpful. Of note, anhidrosis may occur in affected areas and may persist for 3 weeks or longer, putting patients at risk for systemic symptoms of overheating.
  - Gradual exposure to hot and humid environments can help with acclimation.
  - Cooling the patient down via cooling devices (ie, cold packs, fans, air-conditioners), taking cool showers, changing clothes into breathable fabrics or exposing involved skin, removing occlusive bandages, and treating fever with antipyretics have all proved useful.
  - Daily gentle exfoliation can help remove debris that may be occluding eccrine duct, improving miliaria.
- **Skin of Color Considerations:** None

Contraindications/Cautions/Risks

Contraindications
- Active skin infection

Cautions
- Monitor young children for hypothermia.

Risks
- Discomfort during cooling process

Equipment Needed
- Clean, gentle washcloth or gauze material
- Fan
- Ice
- Water
- Basin or bucket

Preprocedural Approach

- Move to an air-conditioned room at approximately 69°F to 72°F (20°C-22°C)
- Remove any occlusive clothing or bandages or medicaments (eg, thick ointments).

Procedural Approach

- Mix water and ice to make cold water.
- Soak the washcloth or compress material in ice water mixture.
- Wring out the majority of ice water.
- Apply cool compress to affected areas.
- Use fan to evaporate cool water mixture off skin and to increase air flow over skin.
- Consider applying mild cortisone lotion or cream (avoid ointment), if necessary.

Postprocedural Approach

- Encourage light activity that helps motivate the patient to get out of bed.
- Consider providing an antipyretic such as acetaminophen.
- Avoid skin-to-skin contact by placing a gentle, clean, cotton washcloth or gauze between skin folds.
- Wear light, breathable cotton clothing.
- Ensure good water intake for overall hydration.

SUGGESTED READINGS
Carter R, Garcia AM, Souhan BE. Patients presenting with miliaria while wearing flame resistant clothing in high ambient temperatures: a case series. *J Med Case Reports.* 2011;5:474.

Lyons RE, Levine R, Auld D. Miliaria rubra, a manifestation of staphylococcal disease. *Arch Dermatol.* 1962;86:282–286.

Wenzel FG, Horn TD. Nonneoplastic disorders of the eccrine glands. *J Am Acad Dermatol.* 1998;38:1–7.

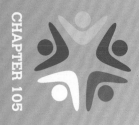

CHAPTER 105

Molluscum Contagiosum

Allison Truong, Latanya T. Benjamin, Carol E. Cheng, and Marcia Hogeling

Molluscum contagiosum is a viral disorder of the skin and mucous membranes characterized by single or multiple (sometimes demonstrating the phenomenon of koebnerization), pink or skin-colored, dome-shaped smooth papules with central umbilication or indentation, usually on the trunk, axillae, antecubital and popliteal fossa, and crural folds (Figure 105.1). They are caused by the poxvirus *Molluscipoxvirus*, and they may trigger a local eczematous dermatitis or generalized autoeczematization reaction, also known as id reaction. It is estimated that 5% of children have clinical evidence of molluscum contagiousum in the United States, whereas the number of cases in adults are more varied.

Molluscum is a common disease of childhood with transmission occurring via skin-to-skin contact or by scratching or touching. Infection can also be spread via fomites on bath sponges or towels and within swimming pools, leading to the nickname "water bumps." When seen in healthy adolescents and adults, it often presents in relation to contact sports or as a sexually transmitted infection. It is also associated with immunocompromised or deficient states such as inherited or acquired immunodeficient states (eg, transplant patients, immunosuppression by medication, human immunodeficiency virus infections, etc). Patients with atopic dermatitis may have a higher risk of having molluscum. Berger et al. showed that 18% to 45% of patients with molluscum have atopic dermatitis, which is higher than the 10% to 20% of general pediatric population with atopic dermatitis.

Symptoms tend to be minimal and can be associated with pruritus. The lesions themselves can become inflamed. Before resolution of the viral infection, the molluscum lesions may become tender, crusted, and erythematous, suggesting a positive host response, which has been described in the literature as the "BOTE" ("beginning of the end") sign. Given the self-limited nature of the condition, treatment is usually for symptomatic or cosmetically sensitive lesions. Molluscum typically self-resolves in 6 to 18 months, but can persist upwards of 2 to 3 years.

There is currently no specific antiviral therapy for molluscum. A Cochrane systematic review performed in 2009 and an update in 2017 found insufficient evidence to conclude that any particular treatment for molluscum was definitively effective, but the review was limited in its number of studies and randomized controlled trials. Thus, the choice of therapy depends on the patient's age, number and location of lesions, and immune status and comorbidities. Because lesions do tend to self-resolve, watchful waiting is an acceptable consideration in healthy patients. It is recommended to treat secondary infections with topical antibiotics and local eczematous or autoeczematization reactions with topical steroids and emollients to prevent scarring and further spreading of the molluscum virus. Interventions can be justified for patients with cosmetic concerns, underlying immunodeficiencies, or parental desires to hasten resolution, prevent further autoinoculation, or transmission to close contacts.

Treatment options of physical destructive methods include manual extrusion of individual lesions with cotton-tipped applicators, an 18-gauge needle, or fine forceps, cryotherapy, curettage, and, less commonly, pulsed-dye laser and photodynamic therapy. Studies have found that manual extrusion was more effective than was cryotherapy. Cryotherapy is a rapid procedure still commonly used in adult populations, however, it may be painful for children and may lead to unnecessary dyspigmentation and/or scarring.

A common chemical destructive approach is the in-office use of topical cantharidin 0.7%, an extract of the blister beetle and a non–U.S. Food and Drug Administration (FDA)-approved vessicant. It is not widely available and must be ordered from a compounding pharmacy. A retrospective review of 300 children with topical cantharidin application applied by a clinician for 4 to 6 hours found a 90% clearance rate after a mean of 2.1 treatments.

Other chemical destructive therapies that have been reported include topical retinoids (especially for molluscum located on the face or neck), 0.3% to 0.5% podophyllotoxin (antimitotic agent), 5% acidified nitrite applied with 5% salicylic acid, topical 12% salicylic acid gel, 10% povidone-iodine and 50% salicylic acid plaster, 40% silver nitrate paste, 0.0001% diphencyprone, Australian lemon myrtle (*Backhousia citriodora*), topical 3% cidovfovir, 0.05% tretinoin, 10% benzoyl peroxide cream, 0.1% adapalene, tea tree oil (*Melaleuca alternifolia*) and iodine, 0.015% ingenol mebutate, 10% sinecatachins ointment, and homeopathic calcarea carbonica.

Significant scarring has been reported from potassium hydroxide and phenol and thus is not recommended. Imiquimod cream 1% to 5% has also been used; consider caution in the use of this topical medication in the pediatric population because severe application site reactions have been reported. Systemic therapies that have also been utilized include intralesional Candida antigen, cimetidine, and subcutaneous interferon-α injections.

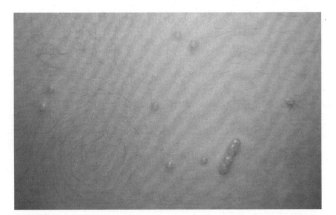

FIGURE 105.1. Typical clinical presentation of molluscum contagiosum. Note Koebnerization phenomenon as the molluscum virus "tracks" in a linear array subsequent to trauma (ie, scratching).

PROCEDURAL APPROACH #1: MANUAL EXTRUSION

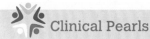 Clinical Pearls

- Level 1 evidence for manual extrusion with gloves or forceps for molluscum
- It is recommended that a topical anesthetic, frozen ice pack, or other numbing technique be applied to decrease pain 1 hour before the procedure.

Contraindications/Cautions/Risks

- Contraindications include a child unable to tolerate the procedure or if the lesion to be treated exists within an area of local infection.
- Risk of adverse events includes pain, bleeding, infection, and scarring.

Equipment Needed

- Gloves or forceps
- Alcohol pad
- Cotton-tipped applicator
- Aluminum chloride (if needed)
- Bandage

Preprocedural Approach

- Apply topical anesthetic such as eutectic mixture of local anesthetics (lidocaine and prilocaine cream) 1 hour before the procedure.

Procedural Approach

- Wipe area of skin clean with alcohol pad.
- Use gloved fingers or forceps tips to squeeze individual lesions expressing contents (Figure 105.2).

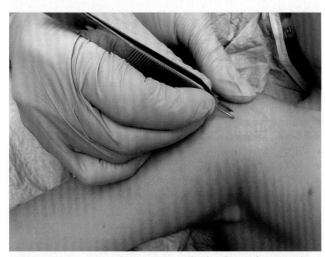

FIGURE 105.2. Manual extrusion method utilizing forceps. Photo courtesy of Andrew C. Krakowski, MD.

- Wet cotton end of cotton swab with aluminum chloride and apply to lesion as needed for hemostasis.

Postprocedural Approach

- Apply Vaseline™ (Conopco, Inc., US) petrolatum to treated area.
- Bandage daily until resolution.
- Counsel patient that there should be limited pain after the procedure and that it can take 1 to 2 weeks for lesions to resolve.

PROCEDURAL APPROACH #2: CRYOTHERAPY

 Clinical Pearls

- Level 1 evidence for cryotherapy for molluscum
- Cryotherapy is considered a relatively fast procedure.
- We recommend applying a topical anesthetic or other numbing technique when possible to decrease pain 1 hour before the procedure, especially if a cluster of lesions is being treated.

Contraindications/Cautions/Risks

- Risk of adverse events includes dyspigmentation, infection, scarring, bleeding, blistering, and pain.

Equipment Needed

- Liquid nitrogen in cup with cotton-tipped applicator or liquid nitrogen sprayer can
- Cut gauze to protect unaffected (ie, "normal") skin.

Preprocedural Approach

- Apply topical anesthetic such as eutectic mixture of local anesthetics (lidocaine and prilocaine cream) 1 hour before the procedure.

Procedural Approach

- Use cotton swab in cup of liquid nitrogen or liquid nitrogen sprayer can to treat each individual lesion for 5 to 10 seconds (Figure 105.3).
- Repeat once for total of two-step freeze–thaw cycle.
- Ensure complete thawing (no residual frost overlying lesion) before second freezing cycle.
- Repeat every 2 to 6 weeks until lesion is gone.

Postprocedural Approach

- Apply Vaseline petrolatum and a bandage postprocedurally.
- Counsel the patient that there is usually burning or stinging pain that occurs after the procedure, and it can take as little as 1 week for the lesion to resolve.
- The treated areas may blister if aggressive cryotherapy is performed.
- Dyspigmentation can also occur after healing in patients with skin of color.

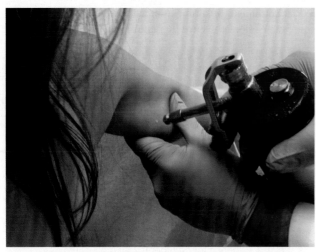

FIGURE 105.3. Cryotherapy method utilizing liquid nitrogen delivered from a liquid nitrogen spray dispenser. Photo courtesy of Andrew C. Krakowski, MD.

PROCEDURAL APPROACH #3: CURETTAGE AND ELECTRODESICCATION

 Clinical Pearls

- Level 2 evidence for curettage and desiccation for molluscum
- This technique is often associated with pain and fear in young children.
- It is recommended that a topical anesthetic or other numbing technique be applied to decrease pain 1 hour before the procedure. Intralesional lidocaine with epinephrine can be considered on a case-by-case basis depending on the number of lesions and the child's aversion to needles.

Contraindications/Cautions/Risks

- Risk of adverse events includes significant scarring, bleeding, infection, and pain.

Equipment Needed

- Alcohol pad
- Hebra curette
- Cautery tip
- Aluminum chloride (if needed)

Preprocedural Approach

- Apply topical anesthetic such as eutectic mixture of local anesthetics (lidocaine and prilocaine cream) 1 hour before the procedure.

Procedural Approach

- Wipe area clean with alcohol pad.
- Use curette to scrape lesions away removing their central core.

- Electrodesiccation can be used for hemostasis.
- Repeat again in 4 to 6 weeks if necessary.

Postprocedural Approach

- Apply Vaseline petrolatum and bandage daily until resolution.
- There should be limited pain after the procedure.

PROCEDURAL APPROACH #4: CANTHARIDIN APPLICATION

 Clinical Pearls

- Level 2 evidence for topical cantharidin for molluscum
- This technique is preferred in the clinical setting given the rapid application and lack of pain upon initial application.
- Have families set their smartphones as a physical reminder to clean the area with soap and water within 4 to 6 hours of application (or as soon as any pain develops at a site of treatment) to remove the cantharidin because of its potential for development of severe blistering or significant inflammatory reaction with prolonged skin contact.
- Avoid application in areas near mucosal surfaces or in occluded areas.
- With time and use, the cantharidin supply tends to become "tacky" toward the bottom of the container and may be more concentrated than is a fresh supply.

Contraindications/Cautions/Risks

- Risk of adverse events includes blistering (expected), burning, pain, erythema, pruritus, scarring, dyspigmentation, inflammatory reaction, or toxicity of agent if ingested.

Equipment Needed

- Alcohol pad
- Cantharidin
- Cotton-tipped applicators with wooden blunted end

Preprocedural Approach

- Counsel patient that the procedure is quick and essentially painless.
- Ensure that the opened container of cantharidin is kept in a secure area and out of contact with the patient or staff.
- Apply protective eye wear if necessary.
- Gently mix the contents of the cantharidin bottle to get a more even concentration of product.

Procedural Approach

- Wipe area clean with alcohol pad.
- Use blunt wooden end of cotton-tipped applicator to dip superficially into cantharidin bottle.
- Apply a small amount of cantharidin to slightly wet the surface of an individual lesion but without excess. If there is excess, use the "cotton end" of the cotton-tipped applicator to remove the product from the skin, taking care not to spread it beyond the lesion.
- Discard individual cotton swabs with each use (ie, avoid "double dipping").

Postprocedural Approach

- Have the patient remain in the examination room for about 5 minutes before putting on clothes so that the cantharidin may completely dry.
- Have the family set an alarm on a smartphone as a physical reminder to wash all treated areas in no more than 4 to 6 hours (or sooner if the patient notes any pain in the treated areas); a shower is preferable to a bath to decrease the chance that any cantharidin could contact a mucosal or ocular surface.
- Some proceduralists will apply a bandage over each lesion to avoid spreading of cantharidin to unaffected sites, whereas others purposefully avoid this step out of concern for causing a more robust skin reaction.
- There should be limited pain immediately after the procedure.
- Counsel families to expect that blisters may develop within the next few days. Likewise, patients may develop a local eczematous dermatitis reaction around the treated area; this should not be confused with cellulitis.
- Have families repeat treatments every 2 to 4 weeks until fully resolved.

SUGGESTED READINGS

Berger EM, Orlow SJ, Patel RR, Schaffer JV. Experience with molluscum contagiosum and associated inflammatory reactions in a pediatric dermatology practice: the bump that rashes. *Arch Dermatol.* 2012;148(11):1257.

Dohil MA, Lin P, Lee J, Lucky AW, Paller AS, Eichenfield LF. The epidemiology of molluscum contagiosum in children. *J Am Acad Dermatol.* 2006;54(1):47.

van der Wouden JC, van der Sande R, Kruithof EJ, Sollie A, van Suijlekom-Smit LW, Koning S. Interventions for cutaneous molluscum contagiosum. *Cochrane Database Syst Rev.* 2017;5:CD004767.

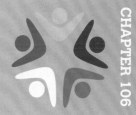

Mycosis Fungoides

Laura Huang and Andrew C. Krakowski*

CHAPTER 106

INTRODUCTION

Mycosis fungoides (MF) is the most common type of cutaneous T-cell lymphoma. Although it is more common in adults, it has been increasing in frequency in the adolescent population. The cancer registries from 1973 to 2002 in the United States report 14 cases in those younger than 9 years of age and 33 cases in those between 10 and 19 years of age; the calculated incidence for that time period is 0.1/1 000 000 person-years for the younger cohort and 0.3/1 000 000 person-years for the older cohort.

The clinical presentation of MF is more variable in adolescents compared to that of adults, with a greater proportion of children having nonclassic features. One of the more common variants seen in children is the hypopigmented type. This typically presents as slightly scaly, hypopigmented macules and patches (Figure 106. 1). Involvement of sun-protected areas (eg, the buttocks) may be an important clinical clue.

Because MF is rare in children and mimics benign dermatologic conditions, it is often misdiagnosed. Multiple biopsies of clinically "affected" versus "unaffected" skin—especially tissue sampled from sun-protected skin—are often helpful in histopathologic diagnosis. Although the presence of T-cell clonality supports the diagnosis of MF, the absence of clonality should never rule it out; clinical hypervigilance and serial biopsies are often necessary to confirm the evolving diagnosis when there is strong suspicion.

Once diagnosed, it is important to determine the disease stage to guide treatment and management. In early-stage MF,

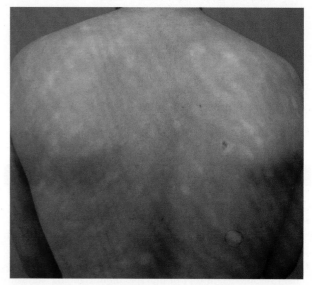

FIGURE 106.1. Hypopigmented mycosis fungoides presenting in an adolescent male. The patient had previously been diagnosed with tinea versicolor and presented only after multiple treatment failures with oral antifungals. Photo courtesy of Andrew C. Krakowski, MD.

---

*Latanya T. Benjamin provided additional editorial review of this chapter.

skin-directed treatments are first line. This includes topical corticosteroids, phototherapy (narrowband ultraviolet B [nbUVB]), and photochemotherapy (psoralen plus ultraviolet A [PUVA]). Advanced-stage disease treatment usually includes systemic therapies in conjunction with the skin-directed treatments. Systemic therapies include oral retinoids, interferon, methotrexate, extracorporeal photopheresis, and, at times, chemotherapy. This chapter focuses on the use of nbUVB (311-313 nm), which is efficacious, has a low side effect profile, and is relatively available (see Chapter 20. Phototherapy and Photodynamic Therapy).

Clinical Pearls

- **Guidelines:** In 2016, JAAD published the United States Cutaneous Lymphoma Consortium's guidelines for phototherapy of mycosis fungoides and Sezary syndrome; while not "pediatric" specific, it is a helpful guide to therapy. The National Comprehensive Cancer Network also publishes regularly updated guidelines.
- **Age-Specific Considerations:** Consider setting up the phototherapy "process" to be as child-oriented as possible by offering the following:
  - Hours before and after school/extracurricular activities
  - Pediatric-friendly environment physically separated from adult patients
  - Illustrated pamphlet or video that helps demonstrate the process to the child
  - Headphones and music/video to entertain child while occupying phototherapy booth
  - A platform for child to stand on while inside the phototherapy booth
- **Technique Tips:**
  - Physical examination should include sun-protected areas and lymph nodes, with further testing (imaging, biopsy) as directed by clinical suspicion.
  - Important laboratory testing includes T-cell receptor (TCR) gene analysis, lactate dehydrogenase (LDH), complete blood count (CBC), Sezary cell count, peripheral blood flow cytometry, and human T-cell leukemia virus type 1 (HTLV-1) serology.
  - Depending on disease extent, a multidisciplinary team with a dermatologist, oncologist, dermatopathologist familiar with cutaneous lymphoma, and radiation oncologist should be considered.
- **Skin of Color Considerations:** Hypopigmented variant may be more readily apparent in darker skin types and can easily be missed in lighter skin tones.

Contraindications/Cautions/Risks

Contraindications
- Absolute contraindications include xeroderma pigmentosum, Gorlin's syndrome, and photosensitive conditions (such as lupus erythematosus).
- Relative contraindications include porphyria, history of malignant melanoma, history of multiple nonmelanoma skin cancers, claustrophobia, and inability to follow safety instructions.

Cautions
- Avoid additional ultraviolet light exposure (sun, tanning booths, etc) in conjunction with phototherapy.

- If possible, discontinue any photosensitizing medications.
- Consider other treatment options in patients with a history of nonmelanoma skin cancers, atypical nevi, multiple common nevi, aphakia, and immunosuppression.

Risks
- Burning
- Erythema
- Xerosis
- Blistering
- Photodamage
- Pruritus
- Exacerbation of preexisting dermatoses (eg, herpes simplex and acne)
- Photosensitivity reactions to medications
- Idiopathic guttate hypomelanosis–like reaction
- Light-induced lentigines
- Effect on serum levels of vitamins (eg, folate and Vitamin D)
- Photocarcinogenicity (theoretical)
- Ocular effects (eg, cataracts)

Equipment Needed
- Phototherapy unit (eg, 311-313 nm)
- UV-blocking eye protection
- If face is not involved, protect face with sunscreen or a cloth barrier.
- Genital shields
- Mineral oil (optional)

Preprocedural Approach

- Preliminary evaluations and discussions:
  - Clinicians should discuss any financial constraints, transportation issues, and medical limitations (eg, inability to tolerate heat, inability to stand for long periods in the phototherapy booth, claustrophobia, and anxiety) around the use of in-office phototherapy.
  - Impact of routine phototherapy sessions (ie, two to three times a week) on school and extracurricular activities should be addressed.
  - A detailed history that includes a patient's history of immunosuppression; previous ionizing radiation to treatment area; history of nonmelanoma skin cancer; history of UV light exposure (including any related skin eruptions and "burn" history); history of known photosensitivity disorders (eg, xeroderma pigmentosum, lupus erythematosus, porphyria, ad vitiligo); history of photosensitizing medication use (eg, doxycycline); and unwillingness to forego sunbathing or sun tanning beds should be obtained.
  - A full skin examination (including eyes, nails, and genitalia) with particular reference to the body surface area involved, patient's Fitzpatrick skin type, lymphadenopathy exam, presence of any organomegaly, and the presence of aphakia, lentigines, actinic keratoses, atypical pigmented or multiple common nevi, and suspected nonmelanoma or melanoma skin cancers should be performed.
  - Biopsy of any suspicious lesions found on baseline physical exam should be performed prior to initiation of phototherapy.

○ Lab evaluation prior to phototherapy should be guided by clinical indication or suspicion (eg, screening labs for lupus erythematosus or porphyria).

○ Women of child-bearing age receiving nbUVB should take folate supplementation to decrease the risk of neural tube defects resulting from unplanned pregnancies.

○ Informed consent discussion around the most common potential side effects including acute reaction (skin erythema, discomfort, feeling faint in the phototherapy booth, etc), skin pigmentation (ie, "tanning"), repetitive exposure to UV radiation associated with accelerated skin aging (ie, wrinkling), and increased risk of skin cancer

- Phototherapy treatment considerations:
  ○ Patients with stages IA, IB, and IIA MF are candidates for monotherapy with nbUVB; UVA may be a better option for thick plaques or folliculotropic involvement because of superior skin penetration.

  ○ nbUVB may be helpful for erythrodermic MF; however, the preexisting cutaneous erythema may make assessment of nbUVB treatment-related erythema difficult, which may jeopardize the process of safely increasing the UV dose.

  ○ Failure to clear with nbUVB as monotherapy in patients with stage IA to IIA MF should prompt consideration for the addition of a systemic agent.

  ○ Patients with poor prognostic factors and/or who have stage IIB, IVA, and IVB MF should be considered for phototherapy in conjunction with a systemic agent.

  ○ Consider application of a thin layer of emollient such as petrolatum or mineral oil (ie, photochemotherapy) to increase the effectiveness of phototherapy and reduce UV-induced erythema.
    - Reimbursement is usually higher for photochemotherapy than phototherapy alone.
    - It is recommended to always include a contemporaneous note stating that the photochemotherapeutic agent was applied with the direct involvement of a clinical staff member; this documentation may help in the event of an audit.

  ○ The primary goal of phototherapy for MF—a malignant condition—is to induce a long-lasting remission off therapy (ie, goal of 100% clearance).
    - Clinical clearing of disease may occur without and sooner than histologic clearing; persistence of MF at time of discontinuation of nbUVB may account for a short remission.
    - Phototherapy treatment for MF may take longer than that seen in nonmalignant conditions such as psoriasis.
    - Patient adherence is critical to the success of the treatment.
      • Patients should be instructed that on the day of phototherapy they should not apply sunscreen prior to their phototherapy session—either as part of their normal skin care regimen or with the intent of protecting areas that demonstrated a photoreaction at the prior visit.
      • Patients should be instructed on proper anatomic positioning while in the phototherapy booth so as to properly expose as much of the body (especially the axillae, flanks, medial thighs, dorsal feet, and under breasts) to the nbUVB light source as possible.

○ Patients may need to stand on a short platform to better treat the lower legs and feet.

○ The use of alternate therapies (topical adjuvants or combination therapy with a systemic agent) should be considered to aid in the treatment of any areas where light does not reach.

- Patients should be instructed on how to maintain proper and consistent distance from the light source so that unwanted photoreactions (ie, burning of an area held too close) do not occur.

- Certain areas of skin should be protected as much as possible.
  ○ In early-stage disease, when the face is not clinically involved, patients may elect to shield their face during phototherapy with a towel or sunscreen.
  ○ Men should shield their genitals by either wearing an athletic supporter or a sock or some other suitable covering.
  ○ Nipples may be shielded with a broad-spectrum SPF ≥50 sunscreen or a physical blocker (eg, zinc oxide paste).
  ○ Areas of recent skin cancer or new surgical scars should be shielded.
  ○ Appropriate protective eyewear should be provided and worn during treatment.
  ○ Any parent accompanying the child into the booth should remain clothed and should wear appropriate eye protection.

Procedural Approach

- Induction/Clearing phase: The time from when nbUVB is started to the time of 100% clearing (a documented response should be present for ≥1 month). During this period, the dose is incrementally increased while the treatment frequency remains fixed.

  ○ Frequency of treatments in this phase is, typically, three times a week on nonconsecutive days. Two times a week will work (if cost and transportation are limiting factors) but will require more time.

  ○ Initial dosing (and incremental increase) is determined using one of two methods:
    - Method #1: By assessing the patient's Fitzpatrick skin type (skin phototype)
      • See Table 106.1 for a guide to help assess patient's Fitzpatrick skin type by skin color and burn/tan characteristics.
      • Estimated initial dose and incremental increase in dose by skin type are as follows:
        ○ Skin type I: Initial dose of 130 mJ/cm²; increase incrementally by 15 mJ/cm²
        ○ Skin type II: Initial dose of 220 mJ/cm²; increase incrementally by 25 mJ/cm²
        ○ Skin type III: Initial dose of 260 mJ/cm²; increase incrementally by 40 mJ/cm²
        ○ Skin type IV: Initial dose of 330 mJ/cm²; increase incrementally by 45 mJ/cm²
        ○ Skin type V: Initial dose of 350 mJ/cm²; increase incrementally by 60 mJ/cm²
        ○ Skin type VI: Initial dose of 400 mJ/cm²; increase incrementally by 65 mJ/cm²

TABLE 106.1 : Assessment of Skin Type by Skin Color and Burn/Tan Characteristics

SKIN TYPE	SKIN COLOR	CHARACTERISTICS
I	White, very fair, red or blond hair, blue eyes, freckles	Always burns, never tans
II	White; fair; red or blond hair; blue, hazel, or green eyes	Usually burns, tans with difficulty
III	Cream-white, fair with any eye or hair color	Sometimes mild burn, gradually tans
IV	Brown, typical Mediterranean white skin	Rarely burns, tans with ease
V	Dark brown, Middle Eastern skin types	Very rarely burns, tans very easily
VI	Black	Never burns, tans very easily

- If no response is noted after approximately 20 treatments, then the dose may be increased by an additional 50-100 mJ/cm^2 above the previous incremental increase.
  - Method #2: By determining the patient's MED (see Chapter 20. Phototherapy and Photodynamic Therapy)
    - It is usually unnecessary to do formal MED testing; in fact, using MED for directing phototherapy has been shown to be associated with a higher cumulative dose of UV light as compared to using Fitzpatrick skin type.
    - Typically, an initial dose equal to "50% to 70% of MED" may be used with incremental increases of 10% to 20% per session (decreasing as appropriate if any photoreaction occurs) for the first 20 treatments.
    - Additional increases after the first 20 treatments are usually left to the discretion of the treating physician.
  - Session-to-session dosing may be adjusted based on several factors:
    - Presence of patient's subjective symptoms of burning (stinging, pain, or itch)
    - Patient's response to phototherapy as assessed by the degree and duration of erythema (ie, photoreaction):
      - Mild photoreaction (ie, pinkness of irradiated skin that blanches on pressure and is not symptomatic) ➜ No increase for next treatment
      - Moderate photoreaction (ie, markedly red skin with discomfort to touch, no blisters) ➜ Hold phototherapy until clear and decrease next incremental increase by 10%

- Missed treatments (ie, gaps between treatments) typically require dose adjustment as follows:
  - If patient missed ≤1 week ➜ Hold previous dose constant
  - If patient missed >1 to ≤2 weeks ➜ Decrease previous dose by 25%
  - If patient missed >2 to ≤3 weeks ➜ Decrease previous dose by 50%
  - If patient missed >3 weeks ➜ Return to initial dose (ie, restart as if patient is completely new to phototherapy)
- A clinical response should typically be observed within 1 month of treatment initiation.
- Clearance of lesions should be determined by a clinician experienced in assessing MF lesions in various Fitzpatrick skin types.
- Obtaining a skin biopsy is not necessary to document clinical clearing; however, it may be helpful in the specific clinical setting of trying to differentiate pigment changes or erythema from residual MF versus postinflammatory pigmentation changes versus phototherapy-related erythema.
- Consolidation phase: The time period after clinical clearance of lesions in which the UV dose and frequency of treatments are both held steady
  - Dosage and frequency are typically held steady, from the last session utilized in Induction/Clearing phase, for 1 to 3 months.
  - This additional exposure to phototherapy after clearance may help to extend resulting remission.
  - Patients deemed "clear" should be reassessed at ≥1 month but ≤3 months later before moving into Maintenance phase of treatment.
- Maintenance phase: The period of gradual decrease of frequency of treatments while in clinical remission before discontinuation of therapy
  - Dosage of nbUVB is typically held constant from Consolidation phase unless erythema occurs or unless the patient has missed enough treatments such that erythema would be expected to occur.
  - The minimal duration of time necessary to reduce phototherapy frequency from two to three times per week to discontinuing altogether has been reported to be approximately 3 months.
  - Special attention should be given to the clinical status of the patient's disease (ie, the patient is still clear of lesions) before the next reduction in frequency.
  - Frequency of treatments is typically reduced every 4 to 8 weeks in the following stepwise order:
    - Three times a week
    - Two times a week
    - Once a week
    - Every 10 days
    - Every 2 weeks (consider decreasing dose by 25% to prevent unwanted photoreactions at this much reduced frequency)
  - Some patients (ie, those with a prior history of relapse after discontinuation of phototherapy) may consider longer periods of maintenance therapy.

Postprocedural Approach

- Sunscreen with an SPF of ≥30 should be applied to all sun-exposed areas of skin on days NOT receiving nbUVB and after phototherapy.
- Document the history of phototherapy in the patient's medical record.
- Follow patient regularly for skin exams and reassessment.

SUGGESTED READINGS

Elmets CA, Lim HW, Stoff B, et al. Joint American Academy of Dermatology-National Psoriasis Foundation guidelines of care for the management and treatment of psoriasis with phototherapy. *J Am Acad Dermatol.* 2019;81(3):775–804

Lebwohl MG, Heymann WR, Berth-Jones J, Coulson IH. Mycosis fungoides and Sezary syndrome. *Treatment of Skin Disease: Comprehensive Therapeutic Strategies.* 5th ed. Philadelphia, PA: Elsevier; 2018:532–537.

Menter A, Korman NJ, Elmets CA, et al. Guidelines of care for the management of psoriasis and psoriatic arthritis: Section 5. Guidelines of care for the treatment of psoriasis with phototherapy and photochemotherapy. *J Am Acad Dermatol.* 2010;62(1):114–135.

Olsen EA, Hodak E, Anderson T, et al. Guidelines for phototherapy of mycosis fungoides and Sezary syndrome: a consensus statement of the United States Cutaneous Lymphoma Consortium. *J Am Acad Dermatol.* 2016;74(1):27–58.

Virmani P, Levin L, Myskowski PL, et al. Clinical outcome and prognosis of young patients with mycosis fungoides. *Pediatr Dermatol.* 2017;34(5):547–553.

Myiasis

Jamie R. Manning and Diana H. Lee[*]

CHAPTER 107

Introduction

Myiasis is an infestation of the skin by the larvae of flies of the order Diptera. It is a common disease of travelers returning from South America and sub-Saharan Africa but does have a worldwide incidence. The most common flies causing human infestation worldwide is *Dermatobia hominis* (human botfly) and *Cordylobia anthropophaga* (tumbu fly).

There are three main clinical cutaneous types of myiasis: furuncular, wound, and migratory, often associated with a pruritic sensation or lancinating pain. In furuncular myiasis, larvae penetrate the skin forming a small pruritic papule that enlarges into a large nodule with central punctum, allowing for larval respiration (Figure 107.1) . The wound form is characterized by deposition of larvae into a suppurative wound or on decomposing flesh and can be accompanied by systemic symptoms including fever, chills, leukocytosis, and eosinophilia. If wound myiasis occurs periorificially, the larvae can burrow into the nasal bones and eyes or brain tissue with serious clinical sequelae. Migratory myiasis is typically found in patients working or living near cattle or horses and present with pruritic serpentine lesions.

Diagnosis is usually made clinically, although dermoscopy, ultrasound, and magnetic resonance imaging (MRI) can assist in difficult cases. Myiasis is self-limited in the majority of

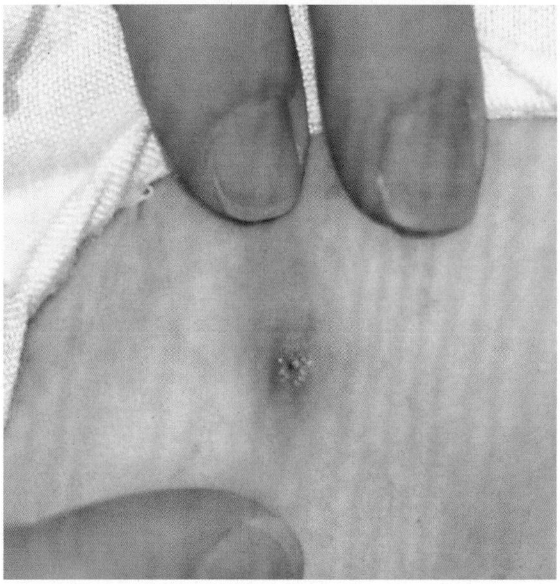

FIGURE 107.1. Typical-appearing papule with central punctum resulting from botfly infection. Reprinted with permission from Fleisher GR, Ludwig S, Baskin MN. *Atlas of Pediatric Emergency Medicine.* Philadelphia, PA: Lippincott Williams & Wilkins; 2004. Figure 3.8.

cases; however, treatment is often indicated for pain reduction. Removal of the larvae is curative in all forms of myiasis (Figure 107.2). Treatment regimens include occlusion, manual extraction of the larvae, and use of larvicides.

---

[*]Latanya T. Benjamin provided additional editorial review of this chapter.

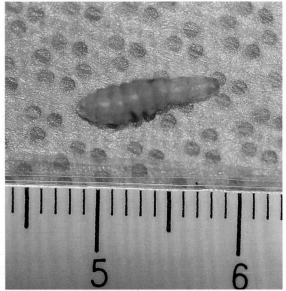

FIGURE 107.2. The human botfly (*Dermatobia hominis*) after manual extraction from a pustular lesion. The flask shape, tapered neck, and encircling spines of the larva are evident. Reprinted with permission from Fleisher GR, Ludwig S, Baskin MN. *Atlas of Pediatric Emergency Medicine.* Philadelphia, PA: Lippincott Williams & Wilkins; 2004. Figure 6.17.

Clinical Pearls

- **Guidelines:** The U.S. Centers for Disease Control and Prevention is a helpful resource for the prevention and treatment of this condition.
- **Age-Specific Considerations:** Less invasive treatment options, such as the occlusion technique or larvicides, may be preferred for patients unable to tolerate or sit still for the procedure within the outpatient setting.
- **Clinical Tips**
  - Treatment options include occlusion (or suffocation) to force the larva to the surface for air (may take several hours), manually squeezing out the larva, debridement with irrigation, or oral ivermectin.
  - Myiasis has been associated with poor hygiene and housing conditions, and thus physicians should inquire about these potential risk factors.
  - Myiasis is commonly related to ulcerated cutaneous malignancies including basal cell and squamous cell carcinoma, and melanoma, but it can also be seen within chronically draining wounds, prolonged infections, malnutrition, as well as mental and physical debilitation. Providers therefore must be aware of potential confounding factors that may complicate infection and wound healing.
  - Myiasis can be a portal of entry for *Clostridium tetani*, and so always consider vaccination of affected individuals.
  - Myiasis of the orbital, nasal, aural, and urogenital systems often requires combination therapy of oral and endoscopic intervention to eradicate the larvae and prevent potentially life-threatening sequelae.
- **Skin of Color Considerations:** None

Contraindications/Cautions/Risks

Contraindications
- Surgical extraction is contraindicated in the setting of active skin infections (ie, active cellulitis).

Cautions
- Caution use of forceful removal of larvae from cutaneous wounds because the tapered shape and rows of spines can prevent simple extraction.
- Retained larvae can elicit an inflammatory response, leading to the development of foreign body granuloma and, eventually, calcification.
- Pyogenic infections can complicate myiasis infestations and thus appropriate antibiotics must be administered if secondary infection is suspected.
- Myiasis lesions have an increased risk of infection with *C. tetani*, so vaccination of affected persons should be considered.

Risks
- As with most procedures, there is risk of bleeding, scarring, and pain.

Equipment Needed
- Chlorhexidine solution
- Petrolatum-based ointment or other occlusive dressing as detailed later (ie, bacon strips, beeswax, paraffin, chewing gum, or cigarette tobacco)
- Ivermectin (1%-10% topical solution or oral tablet)
- Liquid nitrogen
- 1% Lidocaine
- 3 mL syringe
- 30-gauge needle
- A 15 blade with handle, Adson forceps with teeth, 4- to 5-mm punch
- 4 × 4 sterile gauze

Preprocedural Approach

- A thorough history and physical examination should be performed in all patients before the procedure. Myiasis has been associated with poor hygiene and housing conditions, and thus physicians should inquire about these potential risk factors.
- Patients must be warned that with each of these techniques there is risk that dead larvae may be trapped within the skin. The risk of attempted occlusion is that the organism can asphyxiate without emerging, making conventional methods of extraction difficult. Furthermore, the presence of backward- and forward-directed spines on the larvae allows for numerous anchoring points, increasing the risk of retention of larvae fragments and eliciting a severe inflammatory response.

Procedural Approach

Therapeutic objectives include doing no further harm and, if possible, complete removal of the larvae. There are many treatment regimens for the eradication of myiasis infestation. Herein we offer step-by-step instructions for occlusion, manual extraction methods, and topical and oral larvicides.

APPROACH #1: OCCLUSION TECHNIQUE

- Occlusion of the punctum impairs respiratory exchange for the larvae, either suffocating or inducing it to migrate toward the surface and out of the sinus.
  - A variety of readily available materials have been used to occlude the central pore including petrolatum, mineral oil, animal fat (ie, bacon strips), beeswax, paraffin, chewing gum, or cigarette tobacco.
  - Authors have documented the efficacy of injecting 1% lidocaine to paralyze the larvae as well as liquid nitrogen to stiffen the larvae, making extraction easier.
  - Application of a topical toxic substance, such as 1% ivermectin, has also proved to be a successful larvicide.
- The central pore is occluded for around 24 hours to achieve the desired effect and after migrating toward the skin, the larvae is grasped with forceps.

APPROACH #2: MANUAL EXTRACTION

- There are a variety of surgical methods described for extraction of larvae. Given that myiasis is a self-limited disease, manual or surgical extraction of larvae is usually not necessary, unless causing significant distress to the patient.
- If surgical removal is preferred, the skin lesion is locally anesthetized with lidocaine, a cruciate incision is made lateral to the central punctum, and the larva is removed with forceps.
- Care must be taken to prevent laceration of the larvae, leading to incomplete extraction and a foreign body response.
- A probe and forceps can be helpful after the procedure to ensure all larval parts are removed.
- The use of an inexpensive, commercially available snake venom extractor has proved effective and useful in patients with concurrent superimposed bacterial infections where surgery is contraindicated.
- Furthermore, larvae can be extracted by digital manipulation or use of instruments to expel the organisms from the wound.
- Alternatively, lidocaine can be injected forcibly into the base of the lesion in an attempt to create enough fluid pressure to force the larvae out of its pore.
- Another surgical approach involves performing a punch excision of the overlying punctum to manually extract the larva.
  - In this case, an orifice is created using a 4- to 5-mm punch biopsy tool.
  - Light compression is used to manually extract the larvae.
  - The pedicle of the skin fragment cut by the punch biopsy tool is kept intact and then relocated for good aesthetic result.
  - The wound is covered with an occlusive dressing to permit proper wound healing.
- Depending on the size of the cruciform incision, wounds can be allowed to heal by secondary intention or can be sutured if deemed necessary.

APPROACH #3: LARVICIDES

- Ivermectin is a broad-spectrum antiparasitic agent that has been successful in the treatment of myiasis. It acts by causing paralysis of the nematodes, arthropods, and insects by blocking chemical transmission across nerve synapses. As mentioned earlier, application of 1% ivermectin in propylene glycol solution (400 µg/kg) for 2 hours leads to decreased pain and death of all larvae within 24 hours.
- Other cases have documented similar use with topical 1% to 10% ivermectin solution.
- Ivermectin, in a single oral dose of 200 µg/kg, also appears to be effective.

Postprocedural Approach

- Postoperative wounds typically heal without complication.
- Wounds should be monitored for signs and symptoms of infection, watching for warmth, erythema, discharge, and significant postoperative pain.
- Open wounds should be irrigated and cleaned and covered with protective dressings, and standard hygiene and sanitation methods should be employed to reduce infestations.
- Supplemental treatments can be used including isopropyl alcohol, hydrogen peroxide, or Dakin's solution to keep the wound clean.
- Postoperative antibiotics are usually not warranted if adequate hygiene is ensured.
- Patients should be monitored on an ongoing basis until the wound is fully reepithelialized.
- Patients should be extensively counseled on prevention techniques because most infestations can be avoided if proper precautions are taken. Most important is to wear protective clothing and utilize mosquito nets, insect repellents, and proper footwear to prevent the responsible larvae vectors from reaching the skin. All damp clothing and linens should be properly dried and hot ironed to prevent transmission of residual eggs to travelers.
- Myiasis can be a portal of entry for *C. tetani*, and so always consider vaccination of affected individuals.

SUGGESTED READINGS

Chen C, Phelps RG. Myiasis. In: Lebwohl MG, Heyman WR, Berth-Jones J, Coulson I, eds. *Treatment of Skin Disease, Comprehensive Therapeutic Strategies*. 5th ed. New York, NY: Elsevier, 2018:538–540.

McGraw TA, Turiansky GW. Cutaneous myiasis. *J Am Acad Dermatol*. 2008;58(6):907–926.

Pascoal G, de Oliveira FQ, Siqueira RR, Lopes MGA, Martins Neto MP, Gamonal ACC. Treatment of furuncular myiasis using a punch: a simple, practical and aesthetic method. *An Bras Dermatol*. 2016;91(3):358–361.

CHAPTER 108

Neurofibromas

Laura Huang*

Introduction

Neurofibromas are benign tumors of neural origin, composed mainly of Schwann cells, endoneurial fibroblasts, perineurial cells, and mast cells. They are present in males and females equally and can vary greatly clinically. Neurofibromas can appear as soft or rubbery, skin-colored to pink-tan papules that range from 0.5 to 3 cm (Figure 108.1) and sometimes invaginate with gentle pressure in the center, oftentimes called the "buttonhole sign." Generally, if there is just one lesion, it appears on the trunk or head. Multiple neurofibromas (<10 to >1000) may be indicative of neurofibromatosis 1 (NF1), a systemic autosomal dominant genetic disorder caused by mutation of the *neurofibromin* gene on chromosome 17. NF1 is relatively common, found in 1/3000 people. One variant of neurofibroma, the plexiform type, is pathognomonic of NF1. Plexiform neurofibromas present at birth or soon after. These lesions are often described as feeling like a "bag of worms." Plexiform neurofibromas can be associated with overlying pigmentation and hypertrichosis, and they have a higher probability of malignant transformation.

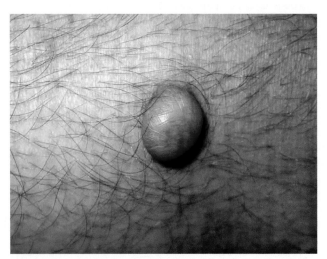

FIGURE 108.1. Solitary neurofibroma. Reprinted with permission from Requena L, Kutzner H. *Cutaneous Soft Tissue Tumors.* Philadelphia, PA: Wolters Kluwer Health; 2014. Figure 114.2.

---

*Latanya T. Benjamin provided additional editorial review of this chapter.

In general, neurofibromas are removed for symptomatic or cosmetic purposes. Current management strategies include surgical excision, electrodesiccation, laser photocoagulation, CO_2 laser, radiofrequency ablation, photodynamic therapy, as well as upcoming pharmacologic therapies. Although large controlled trials are lacking, factors that can help one choose a method include number of lesions, thickness of neurofibromas, and patient skin type. When there are many lesions, two methods that can treat hundreds of lesions per session when used in conjunction with general anesthesia and have high patient satisfaction are electrodesiccation and CO_2 laser. This chapter describes the use of CO_2 laser therapy.

Clinical Pearls

- **Guidelines:** No specific treatment guidelines exist for treating neurofibromas specifically; however, the American Academy of Pediatrics updated its clinical report, "Health Supervision for Children with Neurofibromatosis Type 1," which is a very useful set of established clinical guidelines for anyone taking care of a patient with neurofibromatosis type 1.
- **Anatomic-Specific Considerations:** Use of imaging (magnetic resonance imaging [MRI], positron emission tomography/computed tomography [PET/CT]) to determine extent of plexiform neurofibroma, especially if there are symptoms or neurologic abnormalities
- **Referrals:** Neurology or neurosurgery if there is perineural extension or neurologic compromise
- **Skin of Color Considerations:** There is a higher risk of scarring with hypertrophic scar and/or dyspigmentation in people with darker skin types.
- **Technique Tips:**
  - There is a rare but reported risk of hypertrophic scar formation with CO_2 laser. A test lesion can be performed first under local anesthesia.
  - Pre- and postoperative photographs should be taken to objectively measure treatment outcome.
  - Plan for several sessions. Treatment area for each session can be chosen to optimize postoperative positioning and care.

Contraindications/Cautions/Risks

Contraindications
- Active skin infection
- Appendageal abnormality
- Inability to care for postoperative wounds

Cautions

- History of abnormal scarring or keloid formation
- History of herpes simplex

Risks

- Death, scar, dyspigmentation, pain during and after, bleeding for days to weeks after the procedure, recurrence, infection
- Speak to the patient and the parents/guardians about possibility of scarring and recurrence to set their expectations.

Equipment Needed

- Wavelength-specific eye shields
- Masks
- Smoke evacuator
- CO_2 laser
- Moist gauze
- Forceps
- Sterile water
- Sterile Vaseline™ (Conopco, Inc., US)

Preprocedural Approach

- Avoid sun and maximize sun protection weeks to months before and after the procedure.
- Stop topical retinoids and bleaching creams few days before treatment.
- Antiviral prophylaxis for herpes simplex may be started if clinically indicated 1 to 2 days before laser surgery and continued until reepithelialization has occurred.

Procedural Approach

- Informed consent from the parent/guardian and, when possible, assent from the minor are obtained.
- Typically, general anesthesia is recommended to minimize pain and to allow for treatment of multiple lesions per session.
- Appropriate protective eyewear should be worn, and patients should have eye pads (disposable adhesive eye shields offering full eye protection from medical lasers with wavelengths between 190 and 11 000 nm at an optical density > 7; OD 7@190-11 000 nm) or correctly fitted metal eye shields in place.
- CO_2 laser is used. A smoke evacuator is necessary to help remove plume smoke, and all present should wear masks.
  - Pedunculated lesions: Forceps should be used to grasp the lesion and pull it to the side, on top of wet gauze. Next, 10 to 15 W of power should be focused at the base with a 0.1 to 0.2 mm beam. This specimen can be submitted for histologic examination.
  - Sessile lesions: Use high power, up to 35 to 60 W, slightly defocused to vaporize the superficial portion of the neurofibroma. Then, the subcutaneous portion can be treated by squeezing the sides of the lesion, allowing the deep part of the tumor to protrude through the skin defect.
  - Subcutaneous lesions: Use a focused beam to create an opening superficial to the mass. Pinch and squeeze the tumor through the opening, to allow for direct visualization while treating.
  - Sutures may be placed for any large defects.
- Cleanse areas lightly with moist gauze.
- Apply a petrolatum-based ointment.
- Ice and cold packs can also be applied to minimize edema and pain.

Postprocedural Approach

- Generally, swelling and pain should decrease quickly with time. Mild analgesics can be given for pain and antihistamines for pruritus.
- Patients should continue herpes prophylaxis for a total of 7 to 10 days, or until reepithelialization has occurred.
- At least 2 to 3 times a day, patients should gently cleanse the treated areas using a mixture that consists of one capful of acetic acid (ie, food-grade white distilled vinegar) combined with 1 L of distilled water. Gauze is soaked in this mixture and, with patients lying supine, left in place on the treated areas for 10 minutes. Then, the gauze is removed, and the area is rinsed gently with fresh water. Petrolatum-based ointment is immediately reapplied and maintained until reepithelization has occurred—typically 5 to 7 days after laser surgery.
- Patients should be vigilantly monitored for signs and symptoms of infection, with special consideration paid to viral, fungal, and atypical mycobacterial infections, as well as the more typical bacterial culprits. For example, post-treatment, Candida or fungal infections tend to evolve as bright red eruptions that may be intensely itchy.
- Postoperative downtime is significant, and patients should expect to be absent from school or work for at least 1 week.
- Patients are encouraged to contact the physician directly for concerns.

SUGGESTED READINGS

Becker DW Jr. Use of the carbon dioxide laser in treating multiple cutaneous neurofibromas. *Ann Plast Surg.* 1991;26(6):582–586.

Meni C, Sbidian E, Moreno JC, et al. Treatment of neurofibromas with a carbon dioxide laser: a retrospective cross-sectional study of 106 patients. *Dermatology.* 2015;230(3):263–268.

Miller DT, Freedenberg D, Schorry E, et al. Health supervision for children with neurofibromatosis type 1. *Pediatrics.* 2019;143(5): e20190660. doi:10.1542/peds.2019-0660.

Verma SK, Riccardi VM, Plotkin SR, et al. Considerations for development of therapies for cutaneous neurofibroma. *Neurology.* 2018;91:S21–S30.

CHAPTER 109

Nevi

Shauna Higgins, Deborah Moon, and Ashley Wysong[*]

Introduction

Nevi are benign neoplasms of melanocytes or hamartomatous growths that can be categorized into dermal and epidermal subtypes with varied presentations, workup, and management schema (Table 109.1). Cutaneous growths such as nevi in children can negatively impact school performance, parent–child interactions, social development, and self-esteem. They can lead to feelings of shame and depression, in addition to aversive behavior, causing children to become socially handicapped and to develop both behavioral and emotional problems secondary to their physical appearance. This can ultimately affect psychological health and a child's ability to contribute to society as an adult.[1] Thus, treating disfiguring skin lesions at a younger age has been shown to decrease the psychosocial sequelae of the deformity.[1] Predominant management techniques in the pediatric population include watchful waiting, surgical excision, and laser therapy; however, unique procedural considerations are required in this vulnerable cohort.

Given the increased life expectancy in children relative to adults, the treatment decision should be made considering the risk for progression to melanoma in melanocytic nevi and the "risks" associated with a cosmetically disfiguring appearance.[2] Age, anatomic location (proximity to vital structures), complexity of removal, and potential cosmetic outcome should also be considered.[2]

Clinical Pearls

- **Guidelines:** There are no published treatment guidelines for nevi in children.
- **Age-Specific Considerations**:
  - Unique management considerations in the pediatric cohort include risk of malignant transformation early in life, psychosocial consequences of untreated lesions, potential long-term risks associated with general anesthesia, and the patient's pain tolerance.[1]
  - In the case of disfiguring congenital nevi in cosmetically sensitive areas, clinicians may consider treating the lesion before preschool, when children's awareness of others' comments may impact their self-esteem.[1]
  - Other lesions that may benefit from earlier treatment include the nevus of Ota, which becomes less responsive to therapy in older children, and giant congenital melanocytic nevi, which may have the potential to undergo malignant transformation (2%-15%), with most cases occurring within the first decade of life.[3]
  - It is ideal to remove lesions on the lower extremity before 10 months of age or before walking begins to minimize the tension on the wound. If a procedure must be performed in an older toddler, waiting until the walking becomes much more stable is advised.[4]
  - Regarding the effects of general anesthesia, there may be increased risks in children exposed to general anesthesia at ages younger than 4, although there exist conflicting data in the literature.[5]

- **Technique Tips:** All lesions should be photographed and documented before anesthesia; all specimens should be sent for histopathlogic examination.
- **Skin of Color Considerations:** Some of the treatments for nevi may have a greater risk for skin dyspigmentation in darker skinned patients.

Contraindications/Cautions/Risks

Contraindications
- Active skin infection
- Inability to care for postoperative wounds (eg, upcoming sporting events, vacations)

Cautions
- In the pediatric population, it is essential to communicate the risks of treatment versus surveillance.

Risks
- Risks of cutaneous excisions include bleeding, infection, pain, scarring, recurrence of pigmentation, and reactions to anesthetic.
- Common adverse effects of laser therapy include dyspigmentation, scarring, incomplete removal, and textural changes.
- Exercise caution when using anxiolytics such as midazolam, given the risk of respiratory depression.
- If using eutectic mixture of local anesthetics (EMLA™ [AB Astra Pharmaceuticals, L.P.]), it should be applied to small areas and used with caution in children younger than 3 years because of immature nicotinamide adenine dinucleotide (NADH)-methemoglobin reductase systems and resulting risk of methemoglobinemia. The maximal safety dose should not be exceeded.

Equipment Needed: All Procedures
- Consent form
- Distraction tool for children (eg, portable DVD player, iPad, etc)
- Digital camera
- Alcohol pads
- Topical anesthesia
- Nonadherent dressing for occlusion of topical anesthetic

Equipment Needed: Surgical Excision
- Sterile gloves
- Surgical mask
- Chlorhexidine (or Betadine if near or around the eye or ear)
- Surgical drapes
- 1 or 3 mL syringe
- 25- and 30-gauge needles
- Local anesthetic (eg, 1% lidocaine with epinephrine)
- Scalpel (eg, #15 blade)
- Cotton-tipped applicators
- 4 × 4 gauze
- Needle driver

---

[*]Latanya T. Benjamin provided additional editorial review of this chapter.

TABLE 109.1 ⋮ Nevi: Presentations and Treatment

NEVUS	CLINICAL PRESENTATION	AGE	TREATMENT	OTHER CONSIDERATIONS
Nevus of Ota	Blue-brown unilateral patch on the face; usually follows the first two branches of the trigeminal nerve; involvement of the ipsilateral sclera is possible.	Two peaks at onset: early childhood before 1 y (with the majority present at birth) and at puberty	Treatment with Q-switched lasers (including alexandrite, Nd:YAG, and ruby) has been successful[6] (Grade B). Camouflage with make-up is another favored treatment. Other options include epidermal peeling, cryotherapy, and dermabrasion, some of which may be unfavorable because of hypopigmentation and scarring[7] (Grade C).	Secondary malignancies are rare. Treating these lesions earlier in life when they are more superficial may lead to improved outcomes and fewer required treatment sessions.
Nevus of spilus (also called "speckled lentiginous nevus")	Light brown or tan macule speckled with smaller, darker macules or papules; often on trunk or lower extremities	Common in school-aged children and adolescents. Some believe it is congenital, although it may take several years to develop the speckled appearance.	Removal by Q-switched ruby laser or Q-switched alexandrite (Grade C) may require many sessions for acceptable results.	Malignant melanoma has been reported to be more common in the macular type compared to the papular type, although rare in both
Benign melanocytic nevi	The common mole, hyperpigmented macules, or papules; epidermal, dermal, or junctional	Quantity increases over first three decades of life	Treatment is generally not warranted, although an excision may be considered if there are concerning signs of malignant transformation or if patient complains of irritation (eg, neckline, beltline). May also remove for cosmesis (QS ruby, QS alexandrite, QS Nd:YAG, long-pulsed ruby, diode, Er:YAG, CO_2) (Grade D)	Partially treated melanocytic nevi may recur, and subsequent biopsies may appear distorted ("pseudomelanoma" or "recurrent nevus").
Becker nevus	Hyperpigmented, hypertrichotic patch on the upper trunk or proximal upper extremities	Usually begins before puberty	Not often treated because of asymptomatic nature	Almost all patients are males.
Spindle and epithelioid cell nevus (also known as "Spitz nevus")	Pink, smooth-surfaced, raised, round, firm, papules	Usually occur during the first two decades of life, although they can occur in adulthood in one-third of cases	Dermoscopically asymmetric lesions with spitzoid features should be completely excised whenever possible with tumor-free margins (margins of approximately 1 cm recommended for atypical variants). Management of dermoscopically symmetric spitzoid lesions requires integration of clinical and dermoscopic information[8] (Grade A).	Key is to differentiate from melanoma or atypical Spitz variant.
Pigmented spindle-cell nevus (also known as "Reed nevus")	Pigmented variant of Spitz nevi	Found in children and young adults. Few have been reported at birth, although average age of diagnosis is 25 y.	Complete excision with clear margins to prevent recurrence, because pathology may be difficult to distinguish from melanoma. Wider margins are advised for nevi with atypical features.	—

(continued)

TABLE 109.1 ⋮ Nevi: Presentations and Treatment (*continued*)

NEVUS	CLINICAL PRESENTATION	AGE	TREATMENT	OTHER CONSIDERATIONS
Congenital melanocytic nevus	Large, darkly pigmented hairy patches in which smaller, darker patches may be interspersed	Present at birth and grow proportionally with the body	Routine excision of uniform-appearing small- and medium-sized nevi may no longer be required given the small melanoma risk. Acceptable alternative to surgical excision is baseline photography and yearly follow-up. For larger lesions, serial excision is the method of choice, although some cases may warrant skin grafting or tissue expansion. Alternative approaches include dermabrasion, curettage, CO_2 laser ablation, or use of Q-switched Nd:YAG, ruby, and alexandrite lasers.	Incidence of developing melanoma within a large congenital melanocytic nevus (LCMN) is 2%-15%. Half of all melanomas associated with LCMN occur in deep structures and, thus, prophylactic removal of the upper portions may reduce but does not eliminate risk of melanoma[3,9] (Grade D). Surgical excision of large congenital nevi with distant flap coverage offers a good option for treatment on the extremities.
Dysplastic nevus	Clinically atypical melanocytic nevi with irregular or ill-defined borders, irregular color, and/or a size of >5 mm; histologically graded as mild, moderate, or severe	Usually develop by late adolescence in those with a family history of atypical melanocytic nevi; otherwise, sporadic lesions may occur anytime, even as late as the sixth decade.	Excision of individual atypical nevi should be limited to those suspicious for melanoma (ie, increase in diameter, focal enlargement, radial streaming, peripheral black dots, and clumping in the pigment network). Complete excision with 2-mm margins and margins no more than 5 mm are advised (even with severe atypia). Avoid overly aggressive procedures, surgery, and follow-up. Reexcision of margin-positive mildly and moderately dysplastic nevi is not recommended[10] (Grade C).	Marker for dysplastic nevus syndrome, which is characterized by >50 nevi (many with atypical clinical features), nevi with histologically distinct features, and a family history of melanoma in a first- or second-degree relative
Blue nevus	Blue-gray discoloration **Common type:** Well-circumscribed, dome-shaped papule or nodules, often on dorsa of hands and feet **Cellular type:** Surface is smooth but sometimes uneven, usually on buttocks or sacrococcygeal area.	Usually acquired with onset in childhood or adolescence	Mainstay of treatment is excision. Success has been reported with Q-switched ruby laser. Intratumoral interferon-β has also been reported.	**Other subtypes:** Cellular, epithelioid, deep penetrating nevus, amelanotic, atypical cellular, malignant[3]
Epidermal nevus	Benign hamartomatous lesions often present at birth or early childhood, characterized by hyperplasia of epidermis or adnexal structures. May be classified as keratinocytic (eg, linear verrucous epidermal nevus) or organoid (eg, nevus sebaceous, follicular nevi). May appear flat and slightly pigmented initially but develop into thicker, verrucous lesions. Follows lines of Blaschko (the trail of epidermal cell migration during embryogenesis)	Most commonly first seen at birth or during early childhood	Small lesions can usually be removed by full-thickness surgical excision, because recurrence is common when only the epidermis is removed (ie, by shave or curettage). Topical therapies tried but of limited utility: corticosteroids, retinoic acid, tar, anthralin, 5-fluorouracil, podophyllin. Chronic therapy with oral retinoids has been reported to be helpful in decreasing thickness of systematized epidermal nevi, but does not cause resolution. CO_2 and Er:YAG laser treatment may also be effective.	Epidermal nevus syndrome (ENS) is characterized by extensive epidermal nevi associated with systemic abnormalities often of the central nervous system, eyes, and skeletal system. Syndromes include Schimmelpenning syndrome, nevus comedonicus, pigmented hairy ENS, Proteus syndrome, congenital hemidysplasia with ichthyosiform nevus and limb defects (CHILD) syndrome, phakomatosis pigmentokeratotica.

TABLE 109.1 ⋮ Nevi: Presentations and Treatment (*continued*)

NEVUS	CLINICAL PRESENTATION	AGE	TREATMENT	OTHER CONSIDERATIONS
Keratinocytic	Verrucous, skin-colored, dirty gray brown papules that coalesce to form serpiginous plaques	Onset generally at birth but may develop within first 10 y of life	—	—
Nevus comedonicus	Closely arranged, grouped, often linear, slightly elevated papules that have their center keratinous plugs resembling comedones; most commonly unilateral but can be bilateral	Usually arises before age 10	Often resistant to treatment. Localized lesions can be surgically excised, although excisions of larger lesions may be challenging. Other options include manual comedo extraction, dermabrasion, keratolytic agents (eg, salicylic acid and ammonium lactate). Pore-removing cosmetic strips and comedone expression may improve cosmetic appearance. Treatments for the inflammatory type include surgical excision and oral isotretinoin given chronically at the minimum effective dose (0.5 mg/kg/d or less if possible), which may partially suppress the formation of cysts and inflammatory nodules, although is often unsuccessful.	An "ENS" or "nevus comedonicus syndrome" has been reported with electroencephalogram abnormalities, ipsilateral cataract, corneal changes, and skeletal abnormalities (ie, hemivertebrae, scoliosis, and absence of the fifth ray of the hand).
Inflammatory linear verrucous epidermal nevus	Erythematous papules and plaques with fine scale; may be morphologically nondescript and, if not recognized, could be easily overlooked as an area of dermatitis; usually unilateral, but may be bilateral	Most common type appears by age 5 in 75% of cases with most presenting before 6 mo	Surgical excision is effective. Other treatments: topical steroids, topical retinoids (limited benefit), topical vitamin D (calcipotriol and calcitriol), topical anthralin, and pulsed-dye laser, and CO_2 laser[11]	—
Nevus sebaceous	Sharply circumscribed, yellow-orange hamartoma that may initially appear velvety in childhood but more cerebriform in adulthood. The scalp is the most common location (50%), with other areas being head and neck (45%) and trunk (5%); lesions are usually alopecic.	Often noticed at birth but may be subtle and not noticeable until later in childhood	Clinical monitoring is recommended; monitor for any changes and new growths that may warrant biopsy. Surgical removal of unchanging, nonbothersome lesions remains controversial. Prophylactic excisions are less common, because a majority of growths are benign.	Numerous neoplasms, most of them benign adnexal (eg, trichoblastoma, syringocystadenoma, papilliferum), have been described arising in a nevus sebaceous. Given the small risk of malignancy (basal cell carcinoma, keratoacanthoma, squamous cell carcinoma, apocrine carcinoma, malignant eccrine poroma) that almost always develops after adolescence, surgical removal of a nevus sebaceous may be delayed until adulthood.
Hair follicle nevus	Small papule from which fine hairs protrude evenly from the surface; often on face near the ear	—	No treatment required; conservative complete excision may be considered.	—

- Sutures
- Electrosurgical tools
- Hemostats
- Iris scissors
- Adson forceps

Equipment Needed: Laser Therapy

- Appropriately sized eye protection for all individuals in the room
- Laser with smoke evacuator system
- Cooling method

Preprocedural Approach

- Perform preoperative counseling to accurately and thoroughly describe the impending events to patients and family members, while making an effort to avoid language that may induce anxiety for children (eg, "needle" or "prick").[4]
- Lesion(s) should be photographed and documented before anesthesia.
- Topical anesthetics are preferred in children given their safety profile; however, when more complete anesthesia is required, intradermal injection, conscious sedation, or general anesthesia may be utilized.[1]
- Techniques to decrease injection-related pain include the use of counterstimulatory methods (pinching or tapping an adjacent area), deep infiltration of the local anesthetic, use of small (30-gauge) needles, buffering and warming of lidocaine (1 mL of 8.4% bicarbonate [1 mEq/mL] per 10 mL of 1% lidocaine), and slow infiltration of the anesthetic.
- Nonanesthetic techniques for pain reduction include the use of ethyl chloride, vapocoolant, and oral sucrose.[4]

Procedural Approach ▶

MODALITY: SURGICAL

Approach #1: Standard Surgical Excisions

- Use a sterile marking pen to demarcate an ellipse (3:1 length-to-width ratio with apical angles at 30°) around the lesion in parallel to skin tension lines, taking into account the local anatomy, functional units, and cosmetic units.
- While stabilizing the surrounding skin, make a vertical incision to the depth of the subcutaneous layer using a #15 blade starting distally over the demarcated area.
- Dissect the lesion from the surrounding connective tissue and send the specimen to pathology for confirmation of the diagnosis.
- Undermine the skin to reduce wound tension.
- Ensure hemostasis with electrocautery or direct pressure.
- To minimize risk of dehiscence, close the defect in a layered manner (eg, a deeper layer of absorbable subcutaneous/intradermal sutures with a superficial layer of nonabsorbable percutaneous sutures or adhesive material).
  - Options for buried sutures include variations of vertical and horizontal mattresses (often placed in a manner bisecting the unclosed wound, "rule of halves"), running subcuticular/intradermal sutures, and purse-string sutures.
  - If wounds are at sites of high tension (eg, scalp, back), consider a pulley stitch or vertical mattress stitch (Figure 109.1).

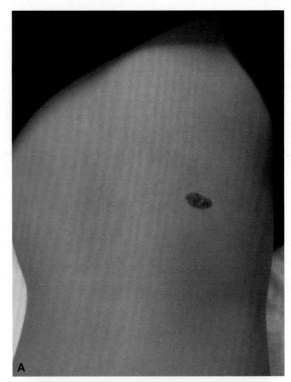

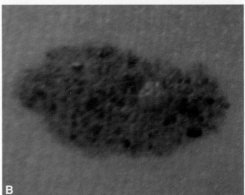

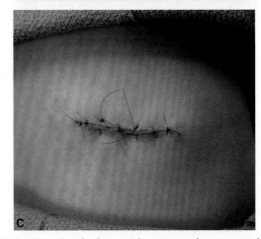

FIGURE 109.1. Standard surgical excision of a congenital melanocytic nevus. A, Preoperative appearance. B, Close-up showing details of the atypical-appearing lesion that caused this adolescent to demonstrate anxiety and social isolation. C, Postoperative photo demonstrating good approximation in a high-tension area (ie, the back) using a combination of simple interrupted sutures (shorter blue stitches) and two vertical mattress sutures (longer blue stitches). Photos courtesy of Andrew C. Krakowski, MD.

Approach #2: Serial Excisions

This approach is particularly useful for removing large congenital melanocytic nevi (LCMN), although there is insufficient evidence to demonstrate that surgery can lower risk of malignant transformation (Grade D).[3] The modified technique offers the advantage of removing larger lesions that would otherwise result in too large a wound defect to close in a single-staged excision.

- Excise as much of the central area of the lesion as possible taking into consideration tissue laxity and wound tension.
- Perform subsequent excisions at intervals of 4 to 6 weeks for smaller lesions or about 3 months for larger lesions, until the entire lesion is excised.
- Send all excised specimens to pathology to evaluate for malignant degeneration, in which case appropriate melanoma treatment should be employed.
- *Large excisions are generally conducted under general anesthesia, although local anesthesia may be appropriate for some patients.*

Approach #3: Skin Grafting

Skin grafting for large nevi such as LCMN is preferable when the surrounding tissue reservoir is inadequate for closure (eg, ear, eyelid), although the resulting depressed and hairless patch may be less cosmetically appealing. Although not always possible, attempts should be made to find a donor site that matches the color, thickness, hair density, and texture of the skin at the recipient site.

- Donor skin is incised and removed by dissection, defatted to improve graft survival, and washed with sterile saline.
- Secure the graft by suturing onto the recipient tissue bed and placing a tie-over "bolster" dressing to ensure adequate contact with the nourishing recipient bed.
- In highly vascular sites (eg, scalp, face, hands), consider creating slits in the skin graft with a No. 11 blade for improved drainage, although this should be balanced with the increased risk of scar formation.

Approach #4: Tissue Expansion

Tissue expansion for LCMN is an alternative method that can offer a more cosmetically pleasing outcome compared to skin grafts, although it is highly operator dependent and may be poorly tolerated in children (pain and possibly difficult cooperation during filling of the expanders, psychosocial morbidity as expanders become visible to peers, and frequent office visits). Complications include infection, malposition, deflation, malfunction, extrusion, tissue necrosis, wound dehiscence, and rupture of the expander. The wound is undermined to accommodate the expander, which is inserted in the subcutaneous fat and expanded over 6 to 8 weeks.

MODALITY: LASERS

Accurate diagnosis as a benign nevus before treatment is critical. Laser therapy would be inappropriate in malignant lesions because the laser surgeon cannot ensure complete removal of the entire lesion. Laser therapy of benign melanocytic nevi is more controversial. The theoretical risk of malignant transformation of nevus cells as a result of laser irradiation is often raised as a counterargument to lasing nevi; there is virtually no evidence to suggest that this is even a real phenomenon (Grade D). More practical is the concern that lasing nevi could disrupt one's ability to monitor a particular nevus over

time, preventing or delaying diagnosis of potential malignant transformation.[12]

- Clean the treatment site with a mild cleanser and water or an alcohol pad, ensuring the area is allowed to completely dry.
- Apply a topical anesthetic (eg, EMLA, LMX.4™ or LMX.5™ [Ferndale Laboratories]) for 30 minutes, after which it should be completely removed with gauze.
- Consider precooling the treatment site with ice, given that the shorter pulses in Q-switched lasers may not provide opportunity for intraoperative cooling.
- See Table 109.1 for selection of lasers for different conditions.

Postprocedural Approach

After any procedure, praising the child and offering rewards such as stickers and lollipops may improve the overall experience of both the child and the present family members.[4] It also may be beneficial to have a "rescue parent" who stays out of the room for the procedure, then "rescues" the child immediately after.

MODALITY: SURGICAL

- A pressure dressing should be placed postoperatively.
- Provide clear verbal and written postoperative wound care instructions.
  - Keep bandages dry to avoid maceration.
  - Keep wound covered with ointment.
  - Return for follow-up for suture removal in 4 to 7 days for the face or in 7 to 14 days for other sites.
  - If the area is under tension, the patient can use Steri-Strips postoperatively and for 1 week or more after suture removal to stabilize the wound.

MODALITY: LASER THERAPY

- Status after laser therapy, cooling with an ice pack and a mild topical steroid cream may help reduce erythema, swelling, and postoperative pain.
- Educate the patient and family on the importance of extensive sun protection for at least 1 month after the procedure.
- If there are signs of epidermal injury such as blistering, consider topical antibiotics to prevent infection.
- Reassure patients that mild erythema initially and a darkening or "coffee grounds" appearance after a few days (for melanocytic nevi) are to be expected, although worsening symptoms or those lasting for more than several days should prompt them to notify their physician.

REFERENCES

1. Shahriari M, Makkar H, Finch J. Laser therapy in dermatology: kids are not just little people. *Clin Dermatol.* 2015;33(6):681–686.
2. Bolognia J, Jorizzo J, Rapini R. *Dermatology.* Vol. 2. New York, NY: Mosby; 2003.
3. James WD, Elston D, Berger T. *Andrew's Diseases of the Skin: Clinical Dermatology.* New York, NY: Elsevier Health Sciences; 2011.
4. Metz BJ. Procedural pediatric dermatology. *Dermatol Clin.* 2013;31(2):337–346.
5. Pride HB, Tollefson M, Silverman R. What's new in pediatric dermatology? Part II. Treatment. *J Am Acad Dermatol.* 2013;68(6):899. e1–899.e11.
6. Watanabe S, Takahashi H. Treatment of nevus of Ota with the Q-switched ruby laser. *N Engl J Med.* 1994;331(26):1745–1750.
7. Chan HH, Kono T. Nevus of Ota: clinical aspects and management. *Skinmed.* 2003;2(2):89–98.
8. Lallas A, Apalla Z, Ioannides D, et al. Update on dermoscopy of Spitz/Reed naevi and management guidelines by the International Dermoscopy Society. *Br J Dermatol.* 2017;177(3):645–655.

9. Krengel S, Hauschild A, Schäfer T. Melanoma risk in congenital melanocytic naevi: a systematic review. *Br J Dermatol.* 2006;155(1):1–8.
10. Strazzula L, Vedak P, Hoang MP, Sober A, Tsao H, Kroshinsky D. The utility of re-excising mildly and moderately dysplastic nevi: a retrospective analysis. *J Am Acad Dermatol.* 2014;71(6):1071–1076.
11. Conti R, Bruscino N, Campolmi P, Bonan P, Cannarozzo G, Moretti S. Inflammatory linear verrucous epidermal nevus: why a combined laser therapy. *J Cosmet Laser Ther.* 2013;15(4):242–245.
12. Rogers T, Krakowski AC, Marino ML, Rossi A, Anderson RR, Marghoob AA. Nevi and lasers: Practical considerations. *Lasers in Surgery and Medicine.* 2018;50(1):7–9.

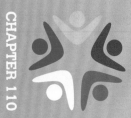

CHAPTER 110

Nevus of Ota and Nevus of Ito

Dawn Z. Eichenfield and Lawrence F. Eichenfield

Introduction

Nevus of Ota and nevus of Ito are types of dermal melanocytosis, predominantly affecting females and common in the Asian population. Although present at birth in about half of patients, the remainder appear around puberty.

Nevus of Ota generally presents as blue to blue-gray or blue-brown unilateral or bilateral facial patches and can involve the eye, ear (and associated structures), nose, palate, or pharynx (Figure 110.1). This melanocytic lesion normally follows the first (ophthalmic) and second (maxillary) branches of the trigeminal nerve. Involvement of the sclera on the ipsilateral side is common and necessitates ophthalmologic evaluation for possible glaucoma. Although melanomas can occur in association with these lesions, less than 20 cases have been reported in the literature. A similar entity, acquired nevus of Ota-like macules (Hori's nevus), commonly presents as blue-gray to gray-brown macules in the zygomatic area, forehead, upper outer eyelids, and nose in Asian women. This entity is commonly misdiagnosed as melasma; treatment is similar to nevus of Ota.

Nevus of Ota has been classified histologically into five types based on the location of the dermal melanocytes, which are superficial, superficial dominant, diffuse, deep dominant, and deep. Generally, more superficial lesions are located on the cheeks, whereas deeper lesions occur on the temple, forehead, and periorbital region. This variability in depth may explain the sometimes inconsistent response to treatment with different lasers. For instance, treatment with shorter wavelengths such as the Q-switched 532-nm Nd:YAG laser may be more effective for superficial lesions. Multiple treatments are usually needed, and the response to treatment ranges from lesion lightening to complete clearance.

Nevus of Ito usually presents along the posterior supraclavicular and lateral cutaneous brachial nerves. Typically, it manifests as a slate-brown or blue/gray colored birth mark. It may infrequently be associated with sensory changes in the involved skin area. Very rarely does nevus of Ito become cancerous, and the exact cause of malignant transformation is unknown.

These lesions are most commonly found in Asian populations and appear more frequently in females. They are very uncommon in Caucasians.

Nevus of Ota and nevus of Ito are manifestations of dermal melanocytosis usually present at birth. Unlike dermal melanocytosis that usually resolves during childhood, Nevus of Ito and Ota tend to be more persistent and may require treatment. Nevus of Ota and nevus of Ito can usually be treated effectively with laser surgery. Here, we discuss the treatment of these lesions with Q-switched ruby, Q-switched alexandrite, Q-switched Nd:YAG (532- and 1064-nm) lasers, and Picosecond alexandrite lasers. There are reports of other lasers being utilized (eg, Fractionated 1440-nm Nd:YAG laser), as well.

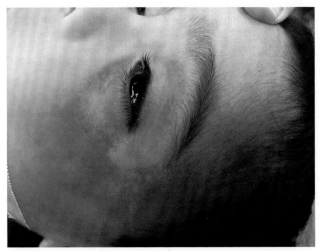

FIGURE 110.1. Preoperative photograph demonstrating nevus of Ota predominantly involving the left eye and temple. Photo courtesy of Harper Price, MD.

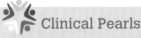 Clinical Pearls

- **Guidelines**
  - Involvement of the sclera on the ipsilateral side is common and necessitates ophthalmologic evaluation for possible glaucoma.
- **Technique Tips:**
  - The primary clinical endpoint is immediate dermal whitening limited to the lesion itself and not occurring when adjacent "normal" skin is lased.
  - Oftentimes, the dermal whitening effect may be less robust (ie, less "crisp") than is epidermal whitening associated with lesions such as lentigines.

- **Age-Specific Considerations:**
  - Patients who are of the age of consent or assent may be treated.
  - Larger lesions and young patients may be managed utilizing general anesthesia to minimize pain and anxiety, as well as to allow for technically appropriate laser surgery and eye protection.
- **Skin of Color Considerations:**
  - Although no formal recommendations are available, laser surgeons typically utilize the Q-switched ruby laser and Q-switched alexandrite lasers for skin types I to III.
  - The Q-switched (532- and 1064-nm) Nd:YAG laser as well as the picosecond alexandrite laser may be used for skin types I to IV.
  - For darker skin types (IV-VI), a test spot should be conducted before initiating treatment given the greater likelihood of post-treatment side effects and complications.
  - With caution, the Q-switched alexandrite has been utilized for skin type IV and the Q-switched 1064-nm Nd:YAG laser for darker skin types (IV-VI). Other lasers may also be utilized in darker skin types with care.

Contraindications/Cautions/Risks

Contraindications
- The presence of an active skin infection
- Patients with a history of keloids
- The inability to perform post-treatment wound care

Cautions
- The presence of a suntan or prior history of melasma, as well as other pigmentary disorders (postinflammatory hyperpigmentation) may result in increased skin dyspigmentation and other complications after the procedure.

Risks
- Edema and erythema after the laser procedure, transient hypopigmentation or hyperpigmentation, texture changes, slight scarring, permanent hyperpigmentation or hypopigmentation, incomplete clearance, repigmentation or recurrence, infection, complications of general anesthesia

Equipment Needed
- Wavelength-specific protective eye wear; the authors recommend metal eye shields for periocular lesions; opaque eye patches may be utilized in the appropriate clinical setting.
- Q-switched ruby (694-nm) laser
- Q-switched alexandrite (755-nm) laser
- Q-switched Nd:YAG (532- and 1064-nm) laser
- Picosecond alexandrite (755-nm) laser
- Smoke evacuator
- Marking pen (white, "Gelly Roll" gel-ink pens preferred)
- Ice or other appropriate cooling system
- Petrolatum-based ointment (for aftercare)

Preprocedural Approach

- Several months before treatment, we ask patients to minimize sun exposure and maximize sun protection to allow greater contrast between the treatment area and surrounding skin. The purpose is to reduce melanin in the nonlesional skin.

- If there is a history of herpes simplex, prophylaxis for herpes simplex is started 1 to 2 days before laser surgery and continued for 1 week after surgery.
- Patients are asked to gently cleanse the treatment area either the evening or morning before laser surgery. The treatment area should be free of other topical products, such as emollients or sunscreen, before laser application.
- Topical anesthetic cream, for example, liposomal lidocaine 4% or lidocaine 2.5%/prilocaine 2.5%, is applied under occlusion for 1 hour before the procedure.
- Oral analgesics (eg, acetaminophen) may be utilized for non–general anesthesia procedures, 30 minutes before to the procedure.
- General anesthesia may be required for larger lesions and/or younger patients.

Procedural Approach

- Informed consent is obtained from the patient. If the patient is a minor, informed consent should be obtained from the parent/guardian and assent obtained from the minor when age appropriate.
- All personnel in the procedure room should wear wavelength-specific appropriate eyewear. Correctly fitted metal corneal eye shields should be worn by the patient for periocular nevus of Ota. Wavelength-specific protective eye wear (goggles or glasses) or opaque eye patches may be utilized in an appropriate clinical setting.
- Treatment should be initiated at the threshold fluence that produces the clinical endpoint (eg, the minimum fluence to produce immediate dermal whitening limited to the lesion itself and not occurring when adjacent "normal" skin is lased). Higher fluences can result in erythema, edema, and punctuate bleeding. Unwanted adverse tissue response includes formation of blisters or epidermal sloughing.
- There is great variability in laser settings and output, and laser settings should be determined by the clinical endpoint.
- Generally, higher fluences are required with multiple treatments spaced at least 6 weeks apart. Some authors have utilized lower fluences with a low incidence of side effects.
- The spot size and energy should be optimized depending on the depth of the lesion.
- Laser settings are highly dependent on the clinical endpoint and should be optimized based on the immediate tissue response. Individual lasers from the same manufacturer can often differ in their output.
- The clinical endpoint is immediate tissue whitening (Figure 110.2).
- There should be no overlapping of pulses in general.

Postprocedural Approach

- Immediately after surgery, intermittent ice compression can be applied for 20 minutes to reduce pain and swelling.
- Petrolatum-based ointment should also be liberally applied. Any crusting is left on the skin as a biological dressing.
- Sunscreen and diligent sun protection should be restarted.
- Treatments are typically performed at 2- to 4-month intervals until patient satisfaction.
- Three or more treatment sessions may be necessary before any clinical improvement can be observed (Figure 110.3).
- Postoperative swelling and pain should quickly decrease with time. For postoperative pain, patients can use acetaminophen

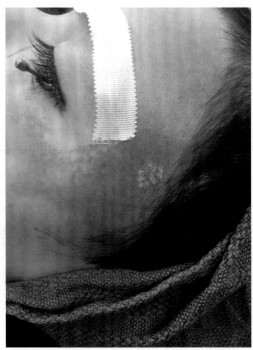

FIGURE 110.2. Intraoperative photograph with metal eye shield and tape to protect the eyebrow in place; a test spot is seen laterally yielding the excellent clinical endpoint of "immediate dermal whitening." Photo courtesy of Harper Price, MD.

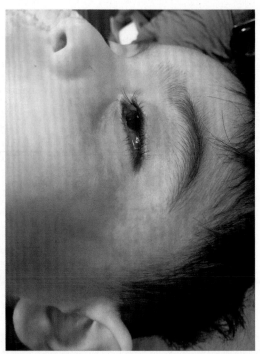

FIGURE 110.3. Postoperative photograph demonstrating significant lightening of treated areas without loss of eyebrow; this patient underwent subsequent treatments for additional lightening of the affected areas. Photo courtesy of Harper Price, MD.

or ibuprofen with standard dosing. Continued intermittent ice compression can be applied to reduce swelling.

- For patients with a history of herpes simplex, herpes prophylaxis should be utilized for a total of 7 to 10 days.
- Postoperatively, patients should be informed that bruising may develop in areas with more pigment. Over the next several days, minimal crusting may develop.
- Patients should be monitored for symptoms and signs of infection; any blistering or erosion formation should prompt urgent examination by the treating physician.
- Postoperative downtime is minimal and the skin heals within 7 to 10 days usually with simple wound care (continued application of petrolatum-based ointment, gentle cleansing daily and diligent sun protection). Any crusted dark spots should peel off within 10 to 14 days of treatment. Cosmetics and sunscreen can be applied to the treatment area. Patients should be cautioned to remove facial products very gently since the treatment area is fragile during the healing process.
- Patients should be cautioned that there may be lightening or darkening of the treated area for several months after laser treatment that can be covered easily with cosmetics if desired.

- Patients should be encouraged to contact the physician directly for any questions or concerns.
- Postoperative appointments at 2 weeks and several months after the laser may be offered to evaluate healing and the need for further treatments.

SUGGESTED READINGS

Belkin DA, Jeon H, Weiss E, Brauer JA, Geronemus RG. Successful and safe use of Q-switched lasers in the treatment of nevus of Ota in children with prototypes IV-VI. *Laser Surg Med.* 2018;50(1):56–60.

Chan JC, Shek SY, Kono T, Yeung CK, Chan HH. A retrospective analysis on the management of pigmented lesions using a picosecond 755-nm alexandrite laser in Asians. *Laser Surg Med.* 2016;48(1):23.

Ge Y, Yang Y, Guo L, et al. Comparison of a picosecond alexandrite laser versus a Q-switched alexandrite laser for the treatment of nevus of Ota: a randomized, split-lesion, controlled trial. *J Am Acad Dermatol.* 2019. doi:10.1016/j.jaad.2019.03.016.

Rani S, Sardana K. Variables that predict response of nevus of Ota to lasers. *J Cosmet Dermatol.* 2019;18:464–468. doi:10.1111/jocd.12875.

Shah VV, Bray FN, Aldahan AS, Mlacker S, Nouri K. Lasers and nevus of Ota: a comprehensive review. *Laser Med Sci.* 2006;31:179–185.

Yan L, Di L, Weihua W, et al. A study on the clinical characteristics of treating nevus of Ota by Q-switched Nd:YAG laser. *Laser Med Sci.* 2018;33(1):89–93.

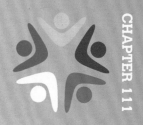
Nevus Sebaceous

Samuel H. Lance and Amanda A. Gosman

Introduction

The nevus sebaceous, first described in 1895, is a congenital lesion presenting in approximately 0.3% of newborns.[1] These lesions are histologically hamartomas with various epithelial elements including sebaceous glands, sweat glands, and hair follicles.[2] Although these lesions remain relatively benign in nature, excision has been advocated as a means of managing the potential secondary neoplasms. These neoplastic transformations include both benign and malignant tumors, with the clear majority of secondary tumors being benign in nature. Of the malignant tumors presenting in the nevus sebaceous, most occur in adults with no malignant secondary tumors identified in the nevus sebaceous at less than 10 years old.[3] Given this information, it is reasonable to delay excision of these lesions until puberty unless otherwise indicated.

The primary site of presentation of the nevus sebaceous is the scalp. It can, however, present at any anatomic location. Aside from the potential of secondary malignancy, these lesions can present with bothersome production of sebaceous material as well as texture and color changes during the pubertal period. These signs and symptoms may be the impetus for excision at an earlier age.[2]

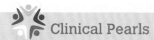

Clinical Pearls

- **Guidelines:** Current recommended margins are 2 to 3 mm, thus mirroring the recommendations for basal cell carcinoma.[2]
- **Age-Specific Considerations:**
  - Excision during the early adolescent period allows for improved tissue laxity, easing soft-tissue closure following excision. Early excision has the added benefit of eliminating the lesions before the structural changes apparent during the pubertal growth phase of the nevus sebaceous.
- **Technique Tips:**
  - Complete excision of the nevus should include skin through the deep dermis as well as the subcutaneous tissue given the presence of adnexal structures within these lesions.
  - Soft-tissue laxity is an important preoperative consideration when planning excision and primary closure versus tissue expansion with secondary excision and closure of large lesions.
  - Serial excision of larger lesions has been described. However, it is the authors' recommendation to proceed with tissue expansion before the excision of large lesions with advancement of the expanded tissue after excision. This staged technique provides ample soft tissue for closure, allowing the surgeon to optimize excisional margins and improve scar outcomes.

Contraindications/Cautions/Risks

Contraindications

- Active infection at the surgical site is considered a strong contraindication to excision.

Cautions

- Lesions overlying complex aesthetic structures of the face, neck, ears, or hands should be evaluated carefully before excision.
- Resultant scars and distortion of adjacent aesthetic structures should be discussed in detail with the family and patient before excision.
- Potential loss of critical structures should be weighed with the risk of secondary malignant transformation.
- Given the depth of the nevus sebaceous into the deep dermis and the adjacent adnexal structures of the superficial subcutaneous tissue, careful attention should be directed to any underlying anatomic structures, most notably facial nerve branches when addressing facial lesions.
- The surgeon should consider referral to appropriate surgical specialists when addressing lesions involving both anatomic areas of high aesthetic priority and potentially vital subcutaneous anatomic structures.

Risks

- Risk of recurrence following inadequate excision should be mitigated by ensuring adequate margins of excision in the depth of excision.

Equipment Needed

- Marking pen
- Local anesthetic with epinephrine
- Scalpel blade #15
- Electrocautery with needle point
- Skin hooks
- Tenotomy scissors
- Needle driver
- Suture
- 3-0 Vicryl™ (Ethicon US, LLC)
- 5-0 Monocryl™ (Ethicon US, LLC)
- 4-0 Monocryl
- 5-0, 6-0 nylon
- 6-0 fast gut
- 3-0 chromic gut
- 3- or 4-in Kerlix™ (Covidien/Medtronic, US) bandage
- 1-in silk bandage tape
- #5 to 8 surgical netting

Preprocedural Approach

- Before excision, critical analysis of the lesion and surrounding tissues should be performed and a clear reconstructive plan outlined.

- Although lesions may appear amenable to primary closure, local tissue rearrangement should be considered as a secondary means of achieving minimal tension closure even in the setting of a planned primary closure.
- Lesions should be identified in conjunction with the patient and parents before surgery and marked accordingly.
- Discussions regarding postoperative scar, resulting alopecia, and distortion of surrounding tissues should be addressed in detail.

Procedural Approach

Operative technique and management of the nevus sebaceous will vary depending on the atomic location and size of the lesion.

Scalp

- Hair surrounding the lesion is trimmed, allowing for clear identification of margins and a sufficient area to allow for rotation of local tissue versus dog ear excisions (Figure 111.1).
- The lesion is then marked at its periphery with 2- to 3-mm margins (Figure 111.2). It is the author's preference to mark the margins of the lesion only at the onset and proceed with marking dog ears for excision versus local tissue rearrangement flaps as needed during closure. Dog ears are well tolerated in the hair-bearing portion of the scalp and will smooth out over time.
- The area is infiltrated with local anesthetic solution that, ideally, contains epinephrine. Local anesthetic containing epinephrine is highly recommended for lesions in the scalp given the extensive vascular network. This will improve surgical visibility during excision and closure.
- Once infiltration of local anesthetic is complete, an incision is made through the skin into subcutaneous tissue of the scalp. Care is taken to incise parallel to the hair follicles, thus minimizing alopecia in the resultant scar. Care should be taken to minimize use of an electrocautery within the scalp, reducing thermal injury to the hair follicles.
- The dense nature of scalp tissue limits mobility during closure. This may require extending the depth of excision below the galea aponeurosis. Subgaleal dissection can then easily be

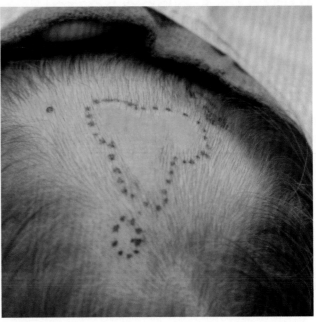

FIGURE 111.2. Intraoperative photograph demonstrating intended margins around lesion.

continued bluntly in a relatively bloodless field circumferentially below the area of excision. Subgaleal dissection should extend approximately two times the width of closure to allow for adequate mobility of the scalp and reduced tension to the overlying skin.
- Closure should begin with the galeal layer using 3-0 Vicryl suture in an interrupted manner. The galeal closure maintains most of the closure tension, allowing for approximation of the skin. Skin closure can then be performed with either interrupted chromic suture versus staples (Figures 111.3 and 111.4).
- Surgical head bandage can be applied with Kerlix wrapped around the occiput to the forehead and secured with surgical netting (Figure 111.5).

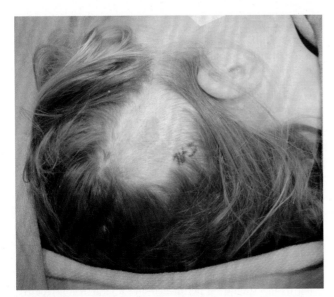

FIGURE 111.1. Preoperative photograph demonstrating nevus sebaceous on the scalp; hair is trimmed appropriately.

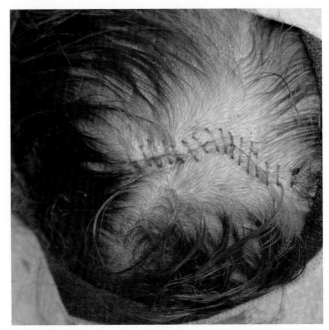

FIGURE 111.3. Intraoperative photograph showing placement of absorbable sutures for scalp closure.

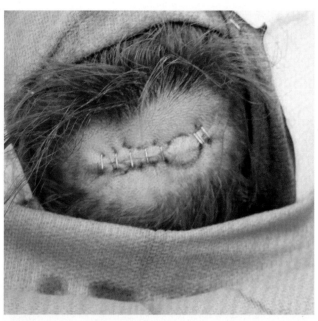

FIGURE 111.4. Alternate scalp closure using staples.

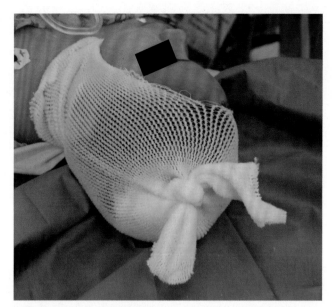

FIGURE 111.5. Surgical head bandage.

Face

- Marking of lesion and margins should be as noted earlier. Attempts should be a made to minimize margin excision in the face, thus approximating a 2-mm margin. Overresection of critical facial tissue can lead to unwanted soft-tissue distortion during closure.
- Care should be taken to clearly identify anticipated pathways of underline facial nerve branches.
- Local infiltration is then injected into the subcutaneous plane.
- Incision is made just through the skin and sharp dissection carried carefully into the subcutaneous tissue just below the dermis. Additional attention is directed to carefully preserving the subcutaneous fat layer in the face, minimizing risk of injury to facial nerve branches.
- Following excision, primary closure versus adjacent tissue transfer should be utilized for closure. Relaxed skin tension lines and animation folds should be used if possible to direct closure. It is the authors' recommendation to proceed with a deep dermal closure utilizing 5-0 Monocryl suture. Closure requiring heavier gauge suture likely represents inadequate mobilization of adjacent tissue and excessive tension to the closure line. Monofilament nylon or other permanent suture is recommended for closure of superficial cutaneous layers of the face.

Trunk and Extremities

- Similar marking of the lesion and margins should be performed as noted earlier.

- Subcutaneous fascial layers can be identified in the trunk and extremities and mobilized as necessary to allow for decreased tension during closure.
- The subcutaneous fascial layers can be approximated with 3-0 Monocryl suture followed by interrupted 4-0 Monocryl suture in a deep dermal manner.
- A subcuticular running 4-0 Monocryl suture is the authors' preference for closure of the final cutaneous layer.

Postprocedural Approach

- Given the variability of location, postoperative management should be directed toward the specific location and closure type.
- Removal of permanent sutures and staples should be performed in a timely manner to minimize scarring.
- Extremities can be protected with splinting or bulky dressings as needed depending on patient maturity and cooperation.

REFERENCES

1. Benjamin LT. Birthmarks of medical significance in the neonate. *Semin Perinatol.* 2013;37(1):16–19.
2. Moody MN, Landau JM, Goldberg LH. Nevus sebaceous revisited. *Pediatr Dermatol.* 2012;29(1):15–23.
3. Idriss MH, Elston DM. Secondary neoplasms associated with nevus sebaceus of Jadassohn: a study of 707 cases. *J Am Acad Dermatol.* 2014;70(2):332–333.

CHAPTER 112

Nevus Simplex

Molly J. Youssef and Megha M. Tollefson

INTRODUCTION

Nevus simplex (salmon patch) is a very common vascular lesion of infancy, occurring in at least 30% to 40% of newborns. It is classified as a capillary malformation but may represent persistent fetal circulation. Nevus simplex appears as pink to red macules and patches in characteristic locations including the scalp, posterior neck, upper eyelids, glabella, and forehead (often in a V-shape: Figure 112.1). They may also occur on the nose, philtrum, nasolabial areas, and lumbosacral back, with involvement of multiple locations sometimes being referred to as "nevus simplex complex." These are typically isolated lesions without associated abnormalities. Terms including "median telangiectatic nevus" or "butterfly nevus" (butterfly-shaped vascular patch on the lumbosacral back) have been used in the literature and represent nevus simplex. However, nevus simplex is the preferred terminology.

TREATMENT RECOMMENDATIONS

No treatment is usually indicated for nevus simplex (in contrast to port-wine birthmark/nevus flammeus, where early and

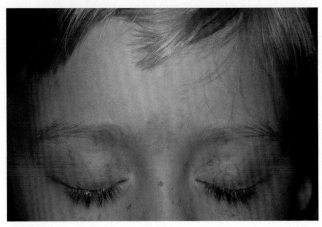

FIGURE 112.2. Persistent nevus simplex on the glabella in a 7-year-old girl. Used with permission of Mayo Foundation for Medical Education and Research. All rights reserved.

aggressive treatment may be indicated). Lesions located on the face almost universally fade within the first 2 years of life. Those on the scalp and neck may fade or persist, but are typically covered with hair and therefore not a cosmetic concern. Nevus simplex occasionally develops an overlying dermatitis, which can be treated with topical steroid.

In some instances, patients may have persistent facial nevus simplex (Figure 112.2). In those cases, treatment with pulsed-dye laser could be considered for cosmetic purposes, akin to treatment for other visible capillary malformations (eg, port-wine birthmark, see Chapter 115. Port-Wine Birthmarks). There is a case report that utilized the following settings for treatment of an inflamed nevus simplex on the nape of the neck: laser wavelength 585 nm, pulse duration 0.45 ms, spot size 5 mm, and fluence of 6 J/cm^2. We suggest similar conservative pulsed-dye laser settings for persistent facial nevus simplex: pulse duration 1.5 ms, spot size 7 mm, and fluence of 7 to 8 J/cm^2. However, pulsed-dye laser settings should be adjusted on a case-by-case basis depending on the location and color of the lesion, the patient's skin type, and response to a test pulse.

SUGGESTED READINGS

Juern AM, Glick ZR, Drolet BA, Frieden IJ. Nevus simplex: a reconsideration of nomenclature, sites of involvement, and disease associations. *J Am Acad Dermatol.* 2010;63(5):805–814.

Leung AKC, Barankin B, Hon KL. Persistent salmon patch on the forehead and glabellum in a Chinese adult. *Case Rep Med.* 2014; 2014:1–3.

Pasyk KA, Wlodarczyk SR, Jakobczak MM, Kurek M, Aughton DJ. Familial medial telangiectatic nevus: variant of nevus flammeus—port-wine stain. *Plast Reconstr Surg.* 1993;91(6):1032–1041.

Tay YK, Morelli J, Weston WL. Inflammatory nuchal-occipital port-wine stains. *J Am Acad Dermatol.* 1996;35(5 pt 2):811–813.

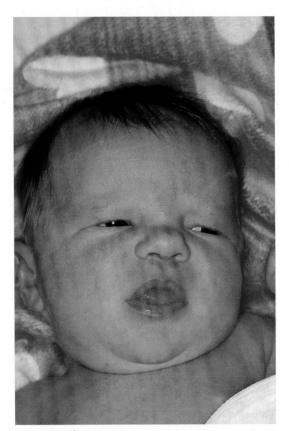

FIGURE 112.1. Nevus simplex on the nose, philtrum, and V-shape on the forehead. Used with permission of Mayo Foundation for Medical Education and Research. All rights reserved.

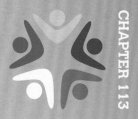

CHAPTER 113

Pigmentary Mosaicism

Nisrine Kawa, Garuna Kositratna, and Thanh-Nga T. Tran*

Introduction

Pigmentary mosaicism is a spectrum of abnormal mosaic-like distribution of skin pigmentation presenting at birth or soon thereafter. These colored patterns run along distinctive arrangements and vary according to affected cell type, timing, and mechanism of mosaicism (Figure 113.1). Skin discoloration ranges from beige or brown, to black. The etiology of pigmentary mosaicism is heterogeneous.

The genetic change may be due to lyonization, mutations, chromosomal aberrations, chimerism, or following an epigenetic mechanism. Examples of mosaic skin conditions are listed in Table 113.1. Uncommonly, these may be accompanied by extracutaneous manifestations, requiring additional surveillance.[1] This entails examination of skin with Wood's light, systematic physical examination, and cytogenetic evaluation of peripheral blood lymphocytes, and skin fibroblasts from both normal and affected skin. Following baseline assessment, longitudinal follow-up of dermatologic, neurologic, musculoskeletal, ophthalmologic, and/or dental examinations are recommended, because the condition may progress over time. Owing to the genetic involvement of these cases, examination of the mother in

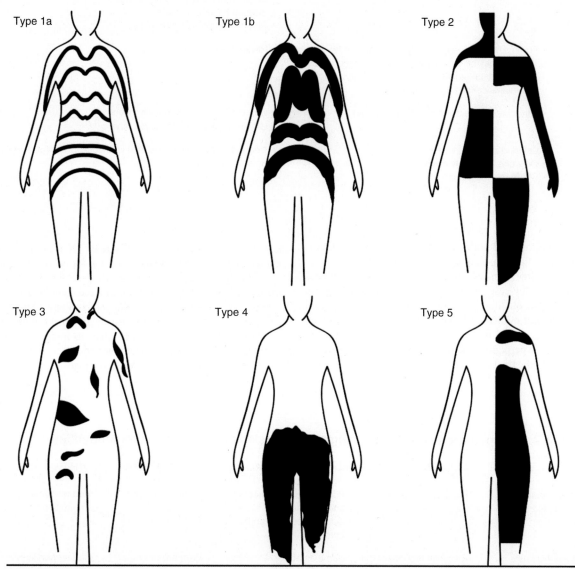

FIGURE 113.1. Patterns of pigmentary mosaicism. Modified from Kromann AB, Ousager LB, Ali IKM, et al. Pigmentary mosaicism: a review of original literature and recommendations for future handling. *Orphanet J Rare Dis.* 2018;13(1):39. http://creativecommons.org/licenses/by/4.0/.

*Latanya T. Benjamin provided additional editorial review of this chapter.

TABLE 113.1 ⋮ Examples of Conditions Following Mosaic Patterns

Type 1	• The most common pattern of cutaneous mosaicism • Narrow (type 1a) and broad (type 1b) bands • Follows Blaschko's lines, representing direction of ectodermal development patterns	• Hypomelanosis of Ito • Incontinentia pigmenti • Linear and whorled neviod hypermelanosis • Inflammatory linear verrucous epidermal nevus • Porokeratotic eccrine ostial and dermal duct nevi • Goltz's syndrome • Speckled lentiginous nevus • McCune-Albright syndrome
Type 2	• Block-like "checkerboard" pattern • Alternating affected areas on either side of the body • Abrupt interruption at the midline	• Nevus spilus • X-linked congenital generalized hypertrichosis • Café-au-lait macules • Becker's nevus/smooth muscle hamartoma • Speckled lentiginous nevus • Port-wine birthmark • Capillary-lymphatic-venous malformation • Venous malformation • Segmental infantile hemangioma • Segmental leiomyomata • Segmental neurofibromatosis
Type 3	• Phylloid "leaf-like" hypo- or hyperpigmented lesions • Typically may be associated with other comorbid conditions (mental, auditory, or visual defects; craniofacial and musculoskeletal abnormalities)	• Phylloid hypomelanosis
Type 4	• Large patches without midline separation	• Congenital nevomelanocytic nevus • Giant congenital melanocytic nevi
Type 5	• Lateralization • Only one hemibody involved • Sharp midline demarcation	• Congenital hemidysplasia with ichthyosiform nevus and limb defects syndrome

X-linked conditions and both parents in autosomal conditions followed by genetic counseling are recommended.

Treatment often focuses on reducing disfigurement and varies on a case-by-case basis. Treatment may also improve functionality and quality of life. Q-switched and long-pulsed (microsecond and millisecond) pigment-specific lasers, as well as fractional lasers, and full resurfacing may be used in treatment of some hyperpigmented lesions (Table 113.2). Surgical excision may be the treatment of choice, or may be considered if laser treatment outcome is inadequate.[2,3] New epidermal grafting techniques are an alternative option for unifying pigment.

Although energy-based and grafting devices are great treatment options, not all lesions can or need to be treated. In fact, cosmetically sensitive areas are the main regions of interest. Expectations must be set preoperatively, because treatment often involves multiple sessions, with intent to improve overall appearance rather than cure. Moreover, the elective nature of the condition may preclude insurance coverage.

TABLE 113.2 ⋮ Responsiveness of Various Pigmented Lesions to Different Laser Modalities

	LENTIGO; FRECKLES	CAFÉ-AU-LAIT MACULES	NEVUS OF OTA	CONGENITAL NEVI
Q-switched lasers (alexandrite; Nd:YAG)	Excellent response	Poor response (smooth border lesions) Good response (rough border lesions)	Excellent response	Good response in combination
Long-pulsed lasers (alexandrite)	Excellent response	Same as above	Dangerous	Good response in combination
Intense pulsed light	Excellent response	Not recommended	Dangerous	Not recommended
Fractional ablative lasers	Good (partial) response	Not recommended	Not recommended	Useful for texture changes
Fractional nonablative	Good (partial) response	Not recommended	Not recommended	Not recommended

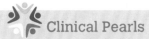
Clinical Pearls

- **Guidelines:** No specific guidelines for this condition have been published.
- **Age-Specific Considerations:**
  - Young children as well as patients with large lesions will likely need to undergo the procedure under general anesthesia, which may be suboptimal for children younger than age 3 because of possible adverse effects on brain development. Older and more mature children may be able to transition back to office treatments.
- **Technique Tips**:
  - Optimal treatment using lasers requires extensive training and understanding of the parameters of the selected device, because under- or overtreatment can be problematic or even harmful.
  - The need for anesthesia is driven by both lesion- and patient-related factors.
    - Although topical anesthetics may suffice for smaller lesions, more extensive ones may require sedation in an operating room setting.
    - If the lesion is small and necessitates only a few laser pulses, infants may be easily restrained by parents and treated in an office setting.
  - There are some known variations in lesion responsiveness to treatment, which will help estimate outcome and set expectations.
    - Café-au-lait macules with smooth borders (coast of California) will respond less to treatment than do those with irregular borders (coast of Maine) (see Chapter 66. Café au Lait Macules).
    - Utility of lasers in the case of giant congenital nevi is controversial given the potential malignant transformation. In these cases, surgical interventions may be more appropriate. Excisions may also be useful for small melanocytic lesions.
    - Hairy lesions may be tricky to treat because melanin in the follicle also comes into play. These have the potential to repopulate melanin locally, and thus should be removed to improve outcomes of the laser treatment on the skin. In this case, laser hair removal may be the best option to improve cosmetic appearance.
    - Hypopigmented and hyperpigmented spots may also be treated with epidermal grafting to normalize the pigment by repopulating the recipient area with skin from the selected normal donor site. This necessitates the use of a dermabrasion device or superficially ablative laser to prepare the recipient site. A suction blister device such as the CelluTome® (Epidermal Harvesting System; Kinetic Concepts, San Antonio, TX) is also needed.
  - Wood's lamp can be used to help localize and determine the depth of abnormal melanin pigment, which in turn will allow better procedural planning.
  - The treated area must be well sun protected before treatment to achieve desired outcome, but also to prevent side effects such as laser burns.
  - When regions close to the eye are treated, adequate eye protection with eye shields is essential.
- **Skin of Color Considerations:** Fitzpatrick skin types 4 to 6 have a higher risk of blister formation and scarring from laser surgery.

Contraindications/Cautions/Risks

Contraindications
- Active skin infection in area being treated
- Refrain from laser treatment in populations at increased risk for melanoma.

Cautions
- As long as it is done in accordance with standard operating procedures, there are no reported contraindications to the use of epidermal grafting devices. It has been noted that inherent pliability of the dermis in children younger than age 3 makes production of suction blisters very difficult, even if the device is used correctly.

Risks
- When performed by trained specialists, laser procedures are relatively safe.
- General laser safety precautions must be taken, such as use of appropriate goggles, adequate cooling, and smoke evacuation.
- Tanned skin may have a higher propensity for side effects, because melanin serves as the main chromophore for certain nonablative pigment-specific lasers.
- Fitzpatrick skin types 4 to 6 have a higher risk of blister formation and scarring.
- Adverse events may include local pain and skin irritation, laser burns, hypopigmentation, or local atrophy.
- Anesthesia-related risks must also be considered.
- Patients with tendencies to develop herpetic lesions may suffer from recurrences and may need appropriate prophylaxis.
- Rarely, skin infections may occur, especially following ablative laser treatments; however, postprocedural care and monitoring will decrease this risk.

Equipment Needed
- Wood's lamp
- Device selection is done according to colors and conditions of lesions, and a variety of lasers will tailor to different lesion types.
  - Pigment-specific devices can be Q-switched or long pulsed and include the ruby, alexandrite, and neodymium-doped yttrium aluminum garnet (Nd:YAG) lasers.
  - Resurfacing devices include CO_2 and erbium lasers. Both full resurfacing and fractional treatment can be used.
- Cooling devices such as the Zimmer may be needed in some procedures, especially in Fitzpatrick skin types 3 to 6 because of the higher amount of melanin absorption of laser.
- Automated epidermal blister devices such as CelluTome
  - In the absence of such a device, traditional epidermal grafting can be done. This would require:
    - Two syringes: 10 and 50 mL
    - Three-way connector
    - Curved scissors
    - Glass slide

Preprocedural Approach: General
- Consideration for patient age, lesion type, size, and location, as well as for predicted cosmetic outcome must be taken into account before initiating the procedure because these will determine the type of treatment and extent of anesthesia that are required.
- Structural concerns to keep in mind include the presence of hypertrichosis and extent of hyperplasia because the excess hair may be clipped and thicker lesions debulked with ablative measures.

- Treatable conditions include localized pigmentary birthmarks in cosmetically sensitive areas such as café-au-lait macules (CALMs) (see Chapter 66. Café au Lait Macules), small congenital nevi (see Chapter 109. Nevi) in cosmetically sensitive areas, and epidermal nevi (see Chapter 78. Epidermal Nevi).
- In the case of epidermal grafting, an adequate donor site must be assessed, because this area must be clean and free from any infection. This is often the thigh or buttock, which must have normal appearing skin in generally good condition.
- Pretreatment photography is worthwhile to monitor improvement over time.

PROCEDURAL APPROACH #1: ENERGY BASED DEVICES

Preprocedural Approach: Energy Based Devices

Modern medicine and technologic advancements have allowed physicians to have a large armamentarium of treatment options for pigmented lesions. It is important to note, however, that treatment modality selection must be tailored to each lesion and that a combination of devices may be needed. It is also imperative to know when not to treat such as in the case of any dysplastic nevi or melanoma. Response to various lasers can be found in Table 113.2 and some treatment results are presented in Figure 113.2.

Many of these techniques will require additional training. The following will serve as a guide but is not sufficient to replace formal training.

GENERAL CONSIDERATIONS FOR ENERGY BASED DEVICES

- Before starting the procedure, a marking pen may be used to demarcate the region of interest, because it may be difficult to see while goggles are on.
- If the area has a lot of hair, clipping or shaving is recommended.
- It is important to ensure that safety measures are taken and that all personnel in the room are wearing the correct eye protection. This may be in the form of external an or extraocular eye shield for the patient.
- Signage outside the treatment room should indicate that a laser procedure is taking place to prevent possible accidental room entry and subsequent eye injury.
- Laser rooms should also be equipped with adequate smoke evacuation and fire extinguishers.

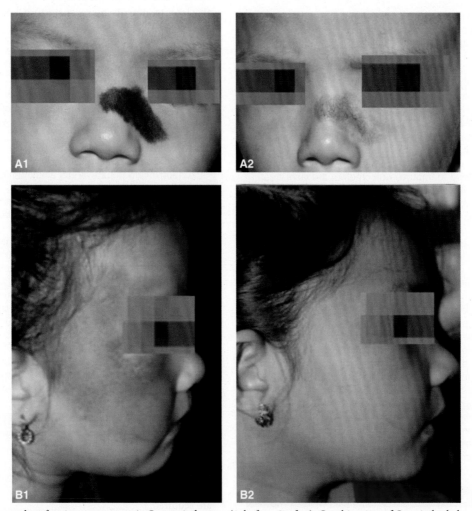

FIGURE 113.2. Examples of patient outcomes. A, Congenital nevus (1: before; 2: after). Combination of Q-switched alexandrite + pulse dye lasers. Result after four treatments. B, Nevus of Ota (1: before; 2: after). Nine treatments of Q-switched alexandrite. Courtesy of Anh Quynh Ngoc Phan, MD and Minh Van Hoang, MD, Vietnam Vascular Anomalies Center, Ho Chi Minh City.

Procedural Approach: Energy Based Devices

- After settings are selected and the device is calibrated, dispense a single pulse directed at the floor to ensure adequate functioning of the laser and cooling system.
- After treating the lesion with a few pulses, stop to ensure that desired immediate endpoints are being met. If that is not the case, reconsider the calibration settings and start again.
- It is noteworthy that in some instances, when treating extremely large areas, the device may heat up and need to be given time to cool down.
- Cumulative splatter onto the laser window may occur after prolonged continuous use, which may necessitate cleaning.
- Correct immediate responses (ie, clinical endpoints) to laser treatments of pigmented lesions are as follows:
  - For Q-switched lasers: immediate whitening
  - For long-pulsed lasers and intense pulsed light (IPL): subtle color change
  - For fractional lasers: very small dots or holes
  - Blisters (Nikolsky's sign) or contraction is never a good sign.

Pigment-Specific Energy-Based Devices

When treating pigmented lesions with these modalities, melanin serves as the target chromophore. Melanin has a wide absorption spectrum, ranging from ultraviolet (UV) to near infrared (IR). As such, wavelengths between 600 and 1100 nm are needed, which can be provided by various devices discussed here.

- *Q-switched alexandrite or Nd:YAG*
  - The use of Q-switching with these pigment-specific lasers allows delivery of high "doses" of energy in very short pulses. This allows targeting of the dendritic cells of melanocytes located deeper in the dermis.
  - These lasers are a great treatment option for conditions with dermal melanocytosis such as nevi of Ota, Ito (see Chapter 110. Nevus of Ota and Nevus of Ito), and blue nevus.
  - Ragged border–type CALMs usually respond well to this laser, whereas the smooth border–type respond more poorly.
  - It is important to treat the area uniformly and avoid pulse stacking, which may create skin indentations.
  - Lesions that immediately show anticipated clearing may have a lower recurrence rate than do those that do not clear as much.
- *Long-pulsed lasers*
  - Devices such as the long-pulsed alexandrite deliver energy more slowly, allowing larger targets to be treated.
  - Oftentimes, it may be necessary to follow a version of Kono's technique, combining both Q-switched and long-pulsed or pulsed-dye laser (PDL) treatments.
    - In this method, the long-pulsed or PDL is used without epidermal cooling to remove the epidermis, which is then wiped off.
    - The Q-switched laser is subsequently used to target the dermal pigment.
    - This applies to congenital nevi or nevi with junctional components such as nevus spilus.
    - Although some may recommend this modality for Becker's nevus (see Chapter 62. Becker's Nevus) to target both the hair and the skin pigment, response is limited and unpredictable.
    - PDL can also be used to treat pigmented lesions as long as the dynamic cooling device (DCD) is turned off.

Intense Pulsed Light

- These devices are flashlamps and not considered to be lasers.
- They provide a wide range of wavelengths and may provide results similar to those seen with long-pulsed lasers.
- This is not a targeted treatment and, therefore, provides general improvement in pigmented and erythematous lesions but is not considered as effective as more selected methods.

Fractional Ablative Laser Resurfacing

- Ablative lasers such as CO_2 and erbium YAG target water in the skin.
- This technique causes full-thickness microscopic destruction of tissue, allowing the physician to eliminate dermal and epidermal melanocytes, and induces more normalized healing of the treated skin.
- As the treatment is done, minor bleeding is to be expected.

Postprocedural Approach: Energy Based Devices

- Immediately following laser treatments, patients may be given an ice pack to help with analgesia. Pain usually resolves relatively quickly and does not necessitate any medication use.
- In case the area around the eye is treated, pupils must always be examined directly after the procedure. Eccentric positioning or distortion of the pupil indicates laser-related injury to the eye.
- In the case of ablative procedures, keep in mind that the barrier function provided by the epidermis is now lost. Physicians should therefore not apply anything *on to* the skin that they are not comfortable injecting *into* the skin.
- Patients are instructed to keep the treated areas protected from the sun to avoid potential postinflammatory pigmentation changes.
- Instructions about detecting signs of skin infections are also to be discussed specifically in the case of ablation to avoid postprocedural growth of harmful organisms.
- The patient should be informed that they will "look worse before they look better," whereby minor redness, local swelling, and possible crusting is to be expected over the next couple of days, but that it should resolve with no intervention. A single dose of fluconazole may be prescribed at day 2 following ablative procedures to prevent fungal overgrowth.
- In the case of epidermal grafts, these take approximately 3 days to adhere, at which point a first follow-up is needed. In the meantime, standard wound care should be done to both the donor and recipient sites, and continued for up to 1 week.

PROCEDURAL APPROACH #2: EPIDERMAL GRAFTING

- This technique can be used in hypopigmented areas to allow creation of a more uniform appearance of the skin.
- Blisters can be generated by automated systems such as the CelluTome device or by means of traditional suction blister techniques.

Preprocedural Approach: Epidermal Grafting

- Healthy, normally pigmented skin in an inconspicuous area should be selected as the donor site. Buttock or thigh skin is usually used.
- The harvesting procedures are nearly painless and will not necessitate anesthesia.
- Clipping or shaving of the donor and/or recipient site may be necessary if hair is present.
- Both donor and recipient sites must be cleaned with rubbing alcohol.

Procedural Approach: Epidermal Grafting

- If using the automated CelluTome device, start by placing the contact surface securely against the selected donor area. Ensure that there is complete contact between skin and microblister array. Attach the vacuum head component of the CelluTome device and power on. Ensure that the patient stays still during the blister formation process. This will take approximately 45 minutes.
- The recipient area must be pretreated with a dermabrasion or superficial ablative technique, which can be achieved with the use of ablative lasers or #120 emery cloth sandpaper. This step can be completed while waiting for blisters to form.
- After the blisters are successfully raised, unlatch the vacuum head and place an adhesive film such as Tegaderm® (3M, US) onto the surface of the harvesting plate. Press adhesive tape down firmly to ensure attachment to blisters.
- Pull on the blue cutting latch to separate raised blisters from the donor site. These will now be attached to the adhesive and are ready for grafting.
- Puncture the adhesive tape a few times before placing against the recipient site to allow for drainage.
- If traditional suction blister formation is desired, start by connecting a 50-mL syringe to a 10-mL syringe using a three-way connector. Remove the plunger from the 50-mL side and place the syringe firmly against the donor site. Suction can then be applied on the 10-mL side and the three-way connector is sealed to maintain pressure.
- This technique may be more time consuming and can require frequent repositioning because the syringes may lose contact with the skin. In the meantime, the same recipient area preparation should be followed.
- When blisters are raised, scissors can be used to collect the skin. A glass slide can then be placed against the pierced blister to collect the epidermal tissue, which can then be placed onto the recipient site. Surgical glue may be used to attach the grafts on to the recipient site.
- Irrespective of the selected harvesting technique, stable pressure is required to secure the grafts after replacement. This can be done by means of adhesive dressing and gauze.
- The dressing can be removed in the office itself after 2 to 3 days.

Postprocedural Approach: Epidermal Grafting

- The donor site can be treated with petrolatum and a nonadherent dressing.
- It will take an hour for the epidermal grafts to adhere and about 2 days to integrate into the recipient site. Patients should be asked to avoid wiping the recipient area during this time and to keep the site clean, dry, and sun protected.
- Patients are also asked to refrain from swimming or shaving during the healing time.
- Sterile petrolatum and nonadherent dressing can then be used on the recipient site till day 5 after the treatment.
- A fully formed epidermis should be seen at around 1 week.

PROCEDURAL APPROACH #3: SURGICAL INTERVENTIONS

- Excision of certain pigmented lesions such as small melanocytic nevi can also be considered.
- Excision is usually considered for giant congenital nevi, because alternative treatments are still controversial. In this case, tissue expansion may be needed to fill the surgical gap.

REFERENCES

1. Kromann AB, Ousager LB, Ali IKM, Aydemir N, Bygum A. Pigmentary mosaicism: a review of original literature and recommendations for future handling. *Orphanet J Rare Dis.* 2018;13(1):39.
2. Rogers T, Krakowski AC, Marino ML, Rossi A, Anderson RR, Marghoob AA. Nevi and lasers: practical considerations. *Lasers Surg Med.* 2018;50(1):7–9.
3. Alster T, Husain Z. The role of lasers and intense pulsed light technology in dermatology. *Clin Cosmet Investig Dermatol.* 2016;9:29. doi:10.2147/ccid.s69106.

CHAPTER 114

Pilomatricoma (Pilomatrixoma)

Ashley M. Rosa and Lucía Z. Díaz

Introduction

Pilomatricoma (or pilomatrixoma) is a benign neoplasm of the skin derived from the hair matrix cells. They are most often seen in children on the head and neck; however, they can be found on any hair-bearing sites and can develop at any age. There is a slight female predominance of 3:2. Lesions usually present as a firm, mobile, single papule or nodule that is skin colored to bluish. Owing to the calcifications and fibrosis within the lesion, an angulated shape can be appreciated when stretching the overlying skin. This is referred to as the "tent" sign. The presence of multiple lesions has been associated with disorders such as myotonic dystrophy, Turner syndrome, and Gardner syndrome.

The differential for pilomatricomas in the pediatric population includes sebaceous and dermoid cysts. Several different techniques to aid in the clinical diagnosis have been described, including fine-needle aspiration, dermoscopy, imaging, and transillumination. The otoscope is a quick and cost-effective way to evaluate the lesion clinically. In a dark room, the otoscope is placed on the lesion to transilluminate it. In the case of a pilomatricoma, a dark shadow is typically cast just distally to where the otoscope superficially touches the skin (Figure 114.1A and B).

Pilomatricomas will not spontaneously regress, so if the patient or parent desires removal, the treatment of choice is enucleation or excision. Additional therapies that have been reported include cryotherapy as well as incision and curettage.

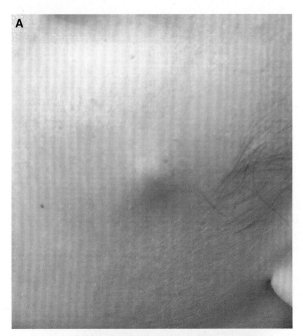

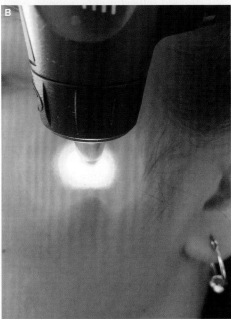

FIGURE 114.1. A, The clinical diagnosis of pilomatricoma is suspected in this female with skin type I. B, Same patient with otoscope placed adjacent to the lesion to transilluminate it; pilomatricomas typically do not allow light to pass through and, instead, cast a dark shadow, as demonstrated here. Photo courtesy of Catalina Matiz, MD.

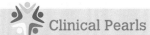

Clinical Pearls

- **Guidelines:**
  - No specific treatment guidelines are known to exist for this condition.
  - Excision is the generally accepted treatment modality.
- **Age-Specific Considerations:**
  - Ideally, patients should be old enough to assent to treatment given this is a benign lesion.
  - If the patient is unable to tolerate an in-office procedure using local anesthesia, then excision may be performed under sedation. However, the parent must be aware of the potential risks.
- **Anatomic-Specific Considerations:**
  - If the lesion is overlying any vital structures, then imaging may be done to evaluate depth of the mass and relation to surrounding tissue (eg, a preauricular pilomatricoma in close proximity to the parotid gland).
- **Technique Tips:**
  - Otoscope can be helpful and cost-effective for prompt "in-clinic" diagnosis.
  - Lesion can be excised with or without the removal of overlying skin. If the skin has been stretched thin by the rapid expansion of the lesion, then excision may help improve cosmesis.
- **Skin of Color Considerations:**
  - Discuss possibility of keloid formation.

Contraindications/Cautions/Risks

Contraindications
- No absolute contraindications

Cautions
- If lesion is deep and overlying vital structures, imaging may be done before excision.

Risks
- Scarring, pain, bleeding, infection, recurrence of lesions, damage to surrounding structures

Equipment Needed
- Otoscope (for diagnosis)
- Antiseptic skin cleansing agent (eg, chlorhexidine)
- Sterile drape
- Scalpel
- Forceps
- Hemostat
- Needle driver
- Cautery
- Suture
- Sterile gauze
- Sterile gloves
- Sterile cotton-tipped applicators
- Petrolatum-based ointment
- Adhesive bandage

Preprocedural Approach

- If the lesion is preauricular or overlying any vital structures, imaging may be done to evaluate depth of the mass and relation to surrounding tissue. It can also be a helpful diagnostic tool if the diagnosis is unclear.
  - Ultrasound is preferred for pediatric patients because it is quick, painless, and cost effective.

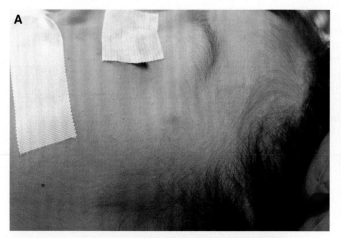

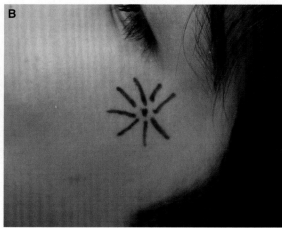

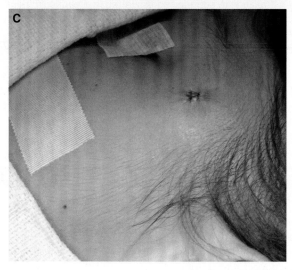

FIGURE 114.2. A, A rock-hard, bluish-hued papule helps clinically define this pilomatricoma, seen here in a young girl with skin type III; she required general anesthesia for the procedure because the lesion was close to her eye. B, A guiding "North star" can be drawn over the lesion using a blue surgical marker; this helps prevent the small pilomatricoma from becoming lost as the surrounding tissue becomes indurated by local anesthetic. C, Patient postoperatively with two small sutures in place. Photo courtesy of Andrew C. Krakowski, MD.

○ Computed tomography (CT) or magnetic resonance imaging (MRI) will give more detailed information about involvement of underlying structures but is costlier and may require sedation.

• Depending on the patient's age and location, topical anesthetic may be applied 30 minutes before the procedure.

Procedural Approach

• Informed consent from the parent/guardian and, when possible, assent from the minor are obtained.

• Typically, local anesthesia is utilized because it is a quick procedure; general anesthesia may be required for procedures on the face or other "at-risk" anatomic areas (Figure 114.2A).

• The site is cleansed, and the area marked (Figure 114.2B).

• A linear incision is made overlying the lesion with an attempt to remove the lesion without excising the overlying skin.

• If the lesion is connected to the overlying dermis, it may be excised along with the tumor in an elliptical manner.

• Ensure the entirety of the lesion is removed to prevent recurrence.

• Internal dissolving deep sutures are placed to approximate the wound edges. Undermining is usually not necessary; however, it can be done if the area is under a significant amount of tension.

• The overlying epidermis is closed with nondissolvable sutures (Figure 114.2C).

• The area is cleansed and petrolatum ointment is applied under an occlusive dressing.

Postprocedural Approach

• There should be limited pain after the procedure. Tylenol may be used if analgesic is required.

• We recommend that the dressing be left in place and kept dry for 24 hours. The patient can then gently cleanse the area and apply petrolatum ointment twice a day.

• Patients should be monitored for signs and symptoms of infection.

• There is no significant postoperative downtime and patients may return to school or work the day of the surgery or the next day. Depending on the area involved, there may be activity restrictions.

• Top sutures are removed in 1 to 2 weeks.

• Patients are encouraged to contact the office with concerns.

SUGGESTED READINGS

Berreto-Chang O, Gorell ES, Yamaguma MA, Lane AT. Diagnosis of pilomatricoma using an otoscope. *Pediatr Dermatol.* 2010;27:554–555.

Danielson-Cohen A, Lin SJ, Hughes CA. Head and neck pilomatrixoma in children. *JAMA Otolaryngol Head Neck Surg.* 2001;27(12):1481–1483.

Young-Hwang J, Wha Lee S. The common ultrasonographic features of pilomatricoma. *J Ultrasound Med.* 2005;24:10.

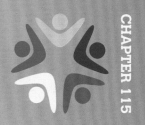
Port-Wine Birthmarks

Hao Feng and Roy G. Geronemus

Introduction

A port-wine birthmark, or nevus flammeus, is a capillary malformation that is typically congenital and affects 0.3% to 0.5% of newborns. The lesions usually present initially as a flat, irregular, pink or light red unilateral patch on the head or neck. Over time without treatment, the lesions grow in proportion to the child's growth, thicken, and become darker in color because of progressive vascular ectasia. They may also develop nodular vascular blebs and pyogenic granulomas. Port-wine birthmarks can be associated with leptomeningeal involvement, occult spinal dysraphism, and soft-tissue and bony overgrowth. Associated syndromes include Sturge–Weber syndrome, Klippel–Trenaunay syndrome, and phakomatosis pigmentovascularis.

The 595-nm pulsed-dye laser (PDL) is the gold standard treatment for port-wine birthmarks. It utilizes the principle of selective photothermolysis to target oxyhemoglobin, resulting in photocoagulation and destruction of vessels, while minimizing thermal injury to the surrounding epidermis and dermis. Studies have shown that multiple treatment sessions are necessary for maximum benefit, and frequent, high-energy PDL before 6 months of age offers the best chance of clearance. Other lasers utilized include 755-nm alexandrite laser and the 1064- and 532-nm neodymium:yttrium-aluminum-garnet lasers (Nd:YAG). Topical agents, such as timolol, rapamycin, and imiquimod, have been investigated, but there is no topical adjuvant to PDL that reliably improves results.

In the authors' experience, early intervention, ideally before 6 months of age, achieves the best response and long-term clearance. Our protocol utilizes frequent PDL treatments without general anesthesia at 2- to 4-week intervals to achieve clinical improvement while minimizing adverse events.

Clinical Pearls

- **Guidelines:**
  - A consensus statement on the dermatologic management and treatment of port wine birthmarks in the setting of Sturge-Weber syndrome is expected to be published in 2020-21.
  - PDL is the gold standard treatment for port-wine birthmarks; other vascular lasers can be utilized in conjunction with PDL.
- **Age-Specific Considerations:**
  - Laser therapy is more effective in infants than in adults because lesions are proportionally smaller, and the thinner skin enables better penetration of laser energy.
  - Ideally, patients begin treatment as soon as possible and before 6 months of age.
- **Technique Tips:**
  - Frequent, relatively high fluence PDL at an early age can induce significant lightening and resolution.
  - Tissue response should be watched closely with initial pulses and throughout treatment; the desired clinical end point is immediate mild-moderate purpura.

- **Skin of Color Considerations:**
  - There is increased risk of dyspigmentation in patients with darker skin types.
  - Appropriate epidermal cooling and laser settings are necessary to minimize risk in patients with skin of color.

Contraindications/Cautions/Risks

Absolute Contraindications
- Active skin infection on areas of treatment (especially herpes labialis or impetigo)

Relative Contraindications
- Photo-aggravated skin diseases

Cautions
- Presence of a suntan and patients of darker phototype may increase chance of post-treatment dyspigmentation.

Risks
- Pain, redness, edema, pruritus, purpura, bleeding, scar, postinflammatory dyspigmentation

Equipment Needed
- Wavelength-specific eye protection
- Pulsed-dye laser (PDL)
- Petrolatum-based ointment
- Ice
- Anesthetic eye drops (if treatment is provided near the eye)
- Eye shields (if treatment is provided near the eye)

Preprocedural Approach

- Encourage early intervention and frequent treatment (Figure 115.1).
- Minimize sun exposure and maximize sun protection as much as possible to reduce competing epidermal melanin content.

Procedural Approach

- Informed consent needs to be obtained from the patient. If patient is a minor, informed consent is obtained from the parent/guardian and, when possible, the minor.
- Typically, no anesthesia is utilized. However, topical anesthesia may be used depending on patient preference. Immobilization of toddlers and school-age children becomes a challenge and may require general anesthesia, especially if treating large lesions. The swaddling technique may be used for infants.
- Appropriate protective eyewear should be worn, and patient and parent(s)/guardian(s) should have appropriate eye protection. If treating close to the eye, the patient should have correctly fitted metal eye shields in place.
- To treat the lesions, 595-nm PDL (595-nm Vbeam Perfecta™ [Candela Corporation, US]) is employed. The port-wine birthmarks are treated with a 10-mm spot size, fluence of

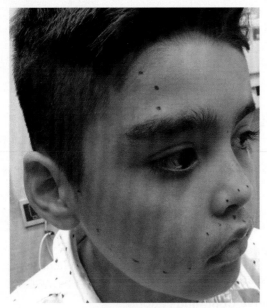

FIGURE 115.1. A Fitzpatrick skin type IV patient with hemifacial port-wine birthmark and associated Sturge–Weber syndrome, before any treatment.

approximately 7 to 9 J/cm^2, and 0.45 to 1.5 ms pulse width, depending on age, skin type, and clinical response. A 10% to 20% overlap of pulses is the goal, and the clinical end point is immediate mild-moderate purpura (Figure 115.2).
- If treating near the eyes, a petrolatum-based ointment can be applied to the eyebrows and eyelashes for protection.
- Ice may be applied to help decrease discomfort and limit edema.

Postprocedural Approach

- Patients should be counseled that the treated area may become purpuric immediately following treatment and the discoloration will become somewhat darker over the next several hours and resolve over the course of 1 to 2 weeks (Figure 115.3).
- Erythema, swelling, and pruritus present in areas surrounding the treated lesion will resolve within several days.

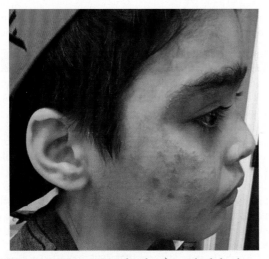

FIGURE 115.2. Patient immediately after pulsed-dye laser treatment with erythema and purpura.

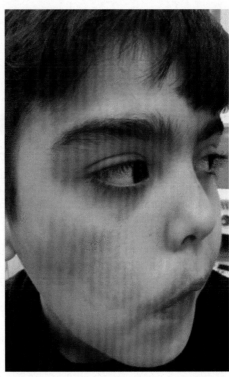

FIGURE 115.3. Patient with clinical improvement after three treatment sessions with pulsed-dye laser.

- Patients should sleep with head elevated and apply ice packs should there be swelling after the treatment, which can occur when the treated area is near the eye or upper cheek.
- If the treated area crusts or blisters, patients are instructed to gently cleanse the area using a gentle cleanser and apply topical petrolatum-based ointment two times daily. It is not necessary to wear a bandage. However, if a bandage is preferred, a nonadhesive bandage should be applied and can be cut to size and secured with paper tape.
- Direct exposure to sunlight should be avoided following PDL treatment. If there is no crusting or blistering, a broad-spectrum sunscreen of SPF-30 or higher should be applied to the treated area for 2 months following the treatment to avoid sun exposure.
- Makeup may be worn if there is no blistering or crusting following the procedure. Particular care must be taken to avoid irritating the skin while removing the makeup. Abrasive or irritating makeup remover should not be used.
- Patients are encouraged to contact the physician directly for concerns and often are provided with cell phone numbers for direct contact and reassurance.
- Serial photography (ie, "selfies") may be used if the photographs are sent securely.

SUGGESTED READINGS

Anolik R, Newlove T, Weiss ET, et al. Investigation into optimal treatment intervals of facial port-wine stains using the pulsed dye laser. *J Am Acad Dermatol.* 2012;67(5):985–990.

Chapas AM, Eickhorst K, Geronemus RG. Efficacy of early treatment of facial port wine stains in newborns: a review of 49 cases. *Lasers Surg Med.* 2007;39(7):563–568.

Chen JK, Ghasri P, Aguilar G, et al. An overview of clinical and experimental treatment modalities for port wine stains. *J Am Acad Dermatol.* 2012;67(2):289–304.

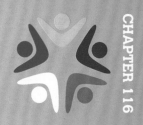

CHAPTER 116

Psoriasis

Kevin Yarbrough and Andrew C. Krakowski

Introduction

Psoriasis is a relatively common chronic inflammatory disease of the skin. The etiology of psoriasis is complex and multifactorial, with many genes conferring an increased risk. In children with an inherited susceptibility, an environmental trigger is thought necessary to induce alterations in the inflammatory pathways, leading to hyperproliferation and inflammation.

Most pediatric psoriasis is managed medically; however, procedural interventions can be very useful as adjunctive treatments and occasionally as stand-alone interventions. Procedures that can be used in treating pediatric psoriasis include narrow-band ultraviolet B (nbUVB) therapy, excimer laser, and intralesional corticosteroid injections.

PHOTOTHERAPY: NARROW BAND ULTRAVIOLET B (311-313 nm)

Ultraviolet therapy has been widely utilized for many years in the treatment of psoriasis. When used appropriately, it presents a useful alterative to systemic therapy in patients not controlled with topical treatments alone. Most studies examining safety and efficacy have been done in adults; however, a systematic review by de Jager et al. identified five studies evaluating ultraviolet B (UVB) treatments in pediatric patients.[1] In those studies, the Psoriasis Area and Severity Index (PASI) 90 ranged from 45% to 60%, with one study reporting complete clearance in all 10 patients treated. Short-term side effects are uncommon and most often related to overexposure. Long-term effects of treatment in pediatric patients remain unclear but could include photoaging and increased risk of skin cancer. Although psoralen plus ultraviolet A (PUVA) has been associated with increased incidence of non–melanoma skin cancer in both children and adults, the long-term risk of nbUVB in pediatric patients is not known, but likely minimal based on safety studies in adults. Studies evaluating long-term effects of nbUVB in pediatric patients are needed. Several challenges are encountered when using nbUVB in this population. Young children can often be nervous and/or uncooperative when standing in an ultraviolet (UV) unit and especially when wearing required eye protection. More information on treating pediatric patients with nbUVB can be found in Chapter 20. Phototherapy and Photodynamic Therapy.

PHOTOTHERAPY: TARGETED EXCIMER LASER (308 nm) PHOTOTHERAPY

Excimer laser therapy is a very useful treatment modality for pediatric psoriasis. Advantages include increased efficacy compared to nbUVB, and targeted treatment resulting in decreased overall UV exposure. Similar to nbUVB, prolonged clearance of psoriatic lesions is possible following treatment. Some barriers to treatment with this modality include increased cost compared to topical treatments, frequent office visits and time commitment, and prolonged time needed to treat widespread disease. Patient cooperation is essential for successful treatment sessions, so very small children are not the best candidates because the appearance and noise of the machine can be intimidating. Few studies that look specifically at safety and efficacy in children are available, but those available for adults are reassuring. Pahlajani et al. compared efficacy and tolerability of excimer for psoriasis in 7 children compared to 18 adults.[2] Side effects were minor and temporary in most patients. The most common side effects encountered were erythema and blistering.

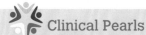

Clinical Pearls

- **Guidelines:** In January 2020, the American Academy of Dermatology and National Psoriasis Foundation published guidelines of care for the management and treatment of psoriasis in pediatric patients.[3]
- **Age-Specific Considerations:** These treatment options work best for older children; however, with some creativity and adult supervision to ensure correct use of protective eyewear, even young children can be treated with phototherapy.
- **Technique Tips:** See Chapter 20. Phototherapy and Photodynamic Therapy, for guidelines in using phototherapy in pediatric patients.
- **Skin of Color Considerations:** Starting dosages of nbUVB and excimer are determined by skin type and minimal erythema dose. Caution should be used in patients with skin types I/II.

Contraindications/Cautions/Risks

Contraindications

- Few absolute contraindications exist for phototherapy, but these include patients with generalized erythroderma or cutaneous cancer syndromes (eg, xeroderma pigmentosum).
- Typically, psoralen use is avoided in children younger than 12 years old.

Cautions

- Photosensitizing medications, history of photosensitizing disorder (must consider the action spectrum of the specific photodermatosis); history of melanoma; multiple atypical nevi; and multiple risk factors for melanoma, multiple non–melanoma skin cancers, and immunosuppression
- The phototherapy booth may be an anxiety-inducing structure for a child so special preparation, education, and assistance may be necessary to ensure a pleasant experience.

Risks

- Short-term side effects are uncommon and most often related to overexposure. They include erythema, pruritus, blistering, and activation of herpes virus.
- Long-term effects of treatment in pediatric patients remain unclear but could include photoaging and increased risk of skin cancer.

379

- Office-based phototherapy may be time consuming, expensive, and inconvenient, especially for school-aged children.

Equipment Needed

- Appropriate eye protection for patient and parents (when in the room during excimer laser treatment or in phototherapy box with child)
- nbUVB booth (311-313 nm) or excimer laser or light (308 nm)
- Mineral oil or thin film of petrolatum (if utilizing photochemotherapy)
- Shielding for genitals
- Shielding or mineral-based sunblock for the face and other nontreated areas, when appropriate

Preprocedural Approach

- Patient and parents are given an orientation to the treatment with either nbUVB unit/excimer laser with a chance to see the booth and protective eyewear before their first treatment so as to reduce anxiety.
- Need for regular treatments and risks/benefits discussed
- Full history and physical examination determining skin type, any risks, contraindications or precautions for phototherapy

Procedural Approach

PROCEDURAL APPROACH: NARROWBAND ULTRAVIOLET B PHOTOTHERAPY[4]

- nbUVB phototherapy is recommended as a treatment option for moderate to severe pediatric plaque and guttate psoriasis.
- Informed consent is obtained from parent or caregiver.
- Appropriate protective eyewear and shielding for face/genitals are provided and worn during treatment.
- Any parent accompanying the child into the booth should remain clothed and should wear appropriate eye protection.
- Women of child-bearing age receiving nbUVB should take folate supplementation; nbUVB is recommended for pregnant women with generalized plaque psoriasis and guttate psoriasis.
- Application of a thin layer of emollient such as petrolatum or mineral oil (ie, photochemotherapy) is recommended before nbUVB treatment sessions because this technique can increase effectiveness of phototherapy and reduce UV-induced erythema.
  - Typically, reimbursement is higher for photochemotherapy than phototherapy alone.
  - It is recommended to always include a contemporaneous note stating the photochemotherapeutic agent was applied with the direct involvement of a clinical staff member; this documentation may help in the event of an audit.
- Initial dosing is determined using one of two methods:
  - Method #1: By assessing the patient's Fitzpatrick skin type (skin phototype)
    - See e-Table 116.1 for a guide to help assess patient's Fitzpatrick skin type by skin color and burn/tan characteristics.
    - Estimated initial dose by Fitzpatrick skin type as follows:
      - Skin types I and II: initial 300 mJ/cm^2
      - Skin types III and IV: initial 500 mJ/cm^2
      - Skin types V and VI: initial 800 mJ/cm^2
  - Method #2: By determining the patient's minimal erythema dose (MED) (see Chapter 20. Phototherapy and Photodynamic Therapy)
    - Select a region of sun-protected area of skin (eg, the hip or buttock) appropriate for MED testing.
      - The total area should be uniform and large enough to accommodate a series of eight test areas approximately 2 × 2 cm in size.
      - Each individual test area should be delineated with a skin pen to help identify the delivered dose.
      - The dosing schedule (mJ/cm^2) for MED testing depends on the individual patient's Fitzpatrick skin type.
        - For skin types I and II: 250, 400, 550, 700, 850, 1000, 1150, 1300
        - For skin types III and IV: 350, 500, 650, 800, 950, 1100, 1250, 1400
        - For skin types V and VI: MED testing should not be performed; instead, these patients should be started at an initial dose of 800 mJ/cm^2 and increased as tolerated according to the protocol described next.
    - With all other areas of skin remaining covered and with appropriate eye protection in place, begin the delivery of UV light.
    - MED testing starts with all testing areas left fully exposed to the UV light source.
    - Each individual testing area is subsequently covered (ie, the dose is stopped) once the specified dose of UV light has been delivered.
    - The entire test region should remain covered for the next 24 hours and exposure to natural or artificial UV light should be avoided.
    - The patient returns 24 hours later and each of the test areas is carefully examined.
    - The patient's MED is the lowest dose with any identifiable erythema within a tested area. Initial dose is typically "50% to 70% of MED" (though some clinicians may use actual MED).
- Subsequent dosing is adjusted based on several factors:
  - Decrease dose by 20% if phototherapy device has been re-calibrated or bulb replacement has occurred between treatments.
  - Decrease dose by 33% if patient is started on tazarotene, isotretinoin, or acitretin.
  - Presence of patient's subjective symptoms of burning (stinging, pain, or itch)
  - Patient's response to phototherapy as assessed by the degree and duration of erythema
    - Minimal erythema lasting <24 hours following treatment → Increase dose by 20%
    - Erythema persistent for >24 hours but <48 hours → Hold dose at previous level until erythema lasting <24 hours
    - Erythema lasting >48 hours → Hold treatment for that visit; when restarting treatment, return to last lower dose that did not cause persistent erythema.
  - Missed treatments (ie, gaps between treatments) as follows:
    - If patient missed ≤1 week or less → Hold previous dose constant

– If patient missed >1 to ≤2 weeks ➔ Decrease previous dose by 25%

– If patient missed >2 to ≤4 weeks ➔ Decrease previous dose by 50%

– If patient missed >4 weeks ➔ Return to initial dose (ie, restart as if patient is completely new to phototherapy)

- Treatments should be two to three times a week (quicker response has been noted with frequency of three times a week).
- Once the patient's psoriasis has cleared, maintenance dosing may begin as follows:
  ○ Maintenance dose = the last dose given prior to clinical clearance
  ○ To taper patient off phototherapy, hold the maintenance dose constant and deliver treatments twice weekly for 4 weeks; then, once weekly for 4 weeks; then, discontinue.
  ○ For prolonged maintenance therapy, the final dose should be decreased by 25% and held constant for all maintenance treatments, which should be delivered every 1 to 2 weeks.
- Maximum dosing
  ○ Facial areas: Regardless of Fitzpatrick skin type, the maximum dose for treatment should not exceed 1 J/cm^2.
  ○ For nonfacial areas, the recommended maximum dose of UV phototherapy is as follows:
    – Skin types I and II ➔ 2000 mJ/cm^2
    – Skin types III and IV ➔ 3000 mJ/cm^2
    – Skin types V and VI ➔ 5000 mJ/cm^2
  ○ Once the maximum dose is reached, the prescribing clinician should be notified.
  ○ Dosing may be increased typically by 5% to 10% at each treatment as tolerated if skin is not clear.
  ○ Higher doses should be prescribed by a physician's order based on individual patient conditions.

PROCEDURAL APPROACH: TARGETED PHOTOTHERAPY WITH EXCIMER LASER (308 nm)[4]

- Use of excimer laser in children with psoriasis may be efficacious and well tolerated but has limited supporting evidence.
- Advantages of targeted phototherapy include sparing of unaffected skin, the ability to deliver high-energy doses, lower cumulative dose, faster clearing, and less risk.
- Targeted UVB phototherapy, including excimer laser (308 nm) and excimer light (308 nm), is recommended for use in adults with localized plaque psoriasis (<10% body surface area), for individual lesions, or in patients with more extensive disease.
  ○ Excimer laser is generally considered more efficacious than excimer light, which is more efficacious than localized nbUVB (311–313 nm) for the treatment of localized plaque psoriasis in adults.
  ○ Excimer laser and excimer light are recommended for use in adults with plaque psoriasis, including palmoplantar psoriasis.
  ○ Excimer laser is recommended in the treatment of scalp psoriasis in adults.
  ○ Excimer laser may be combined with topical corticosteroids in the treatment of plaque psoriasis in adults.
- Informed consent is obtained from parent or caregiver.
- Appropriate protective eyewear is provided to and worn by all people present during treatment.
- Always follow the dosing recommendations and instructions supplied by the specific device's manufacturer.

- Initial dosing is usually determined by one of two methods:
  ○ Method #1: Fixed-dose protocol
    – See e-Table 116.1 for a guide to help assess patient's Fitzpatrick skin type by skin color and burn/tan characteristics.
    – Estimate initial dose by considering plaque thickness and patient's Fitzpatrick skin type (skin phototype) as follows:
      • Skin types I, II, and III:
        ○ Mild plaque psoriasis (induration score = 1) ➔ 300 mJ/cm^2
        ○ Moderate plaque psoriasis (induration score = 2) ➔ 500 mJ/cm^2
        ○ Severe plaque psoriasis (induration score = 3) ➔ 700 mJ/cm^2
      • Skin types IV, V, and VI:
        ○ Mild plaque psoriasis (induration score = 1) ➔ 400 mJ/cm^2
        ○ Moderate plaque psoriasis (induration score = 2) ➔ 600 mJ/cm^2
        ○ Severe plaque psoriasis (induration score = 3) ➔ 900 mJ/cm^2
  ○ Method #2: By determining the patient's MED (see ⬅ Chapter 20. Phototherapy and Photodynamic Therapy)
    – See previous section for MED-determining protocol
    – Typically, a dose of two to four MED may be given as the initial dose.
- Subsequent dosing is adjusted based on several factors:
  ○ Presence of patient's subjective symptoms of burning (stinging, pain, or itch)
  ○ Objective presence of moderate or severe erythema (with or without blistering) ➔ Reduce dose by 25%, avoiding treatment to blistered area until full resolution has occurred.
  ○ Patient's clinical response to targeted phototherapy as assessed by the degree of erythema and clinical response. An example of one approach is as follows:
    – "No effect" (no erythema at 12 to 24 hours and no plaque improvement) ➔ Increase dose by 25%
    – "Minimal effect" (slight erythema at 12 to 24 hours but no significant improvement) ➔ Increase dose by 15%
    – "Notable effect" (mild-to-moderate erythema at 12 to 24 hours with notable improvement) ➔ Maintain dose
    – "Significant effect" (significant plaque thinning, reduced scaliness, or pigmentation) ➔ Maintain dose or reduce dose by 15%
- Treatment frequency should be two to three sessions a week.
- Treatments should be at least 48 hours apart.
- Maximum dosing is similar to nbUVB protocol (see above).
- A total of 10 to 20 treatment sessions are typically anticipated (more or less may be necessary based on clinical response).

Postprocedural Approach

- Side effects are normally mild and resolve quickly.
- Patients monitor for any blistering or signs of overexposure and inform their provider of any concerns or complications.

INTRALESIONAL CORTICOSTEROID INJECTIONS

Painful treatments are not often used in pediatric patients when painless and efficacious alternatives exist; however, intralesional corticosteroid injections may be useful for individual recalcitrant psoriatic plaques in motivated older patients as well as for symptomatic nail disease. Nail involvement in psoriasis can be quite common, affecting up to 50% of patients.[5] One study from Singapore evaluated intralesional triamcinolone injections at 10 mg/mL in four pediatric patients for nail pitting.[6] In this study, it was reported that injections were efficacious and fairly well tolerated in the four patients treated younger than age 12. Studies in adults show good improvement, particularly for nail changes related to nail matrix psoriasis (pitting, ridges, and crumbling). Treatment consists of triamcinolone acetonide, typically in concentrations of 2.5 or 5 mg/mL (but ranging from 1 to 10 mg/mL) injected slowly using a 30-gauge needle into the proximal nail fold (PNF) and lateral nail fold. Injection intervals range from 3 to 8 weeks, decreasing in frequency as clearance is achieved. The volume injected is typically 0.1 mL in up to four areas along the PNF and lateral nail fold or up to 0.3 mL in one injection centrally. Pain is the main limitation of this treatment modality, but in the authors' experience, injections into the PNF are well tolerated with the use of pretreatment topical lidocaine in combination with vapocoolant spray and vibration at the time of injection. Ring blocks can also be used before injections, but injection of lidocaine is quite painful in itself.

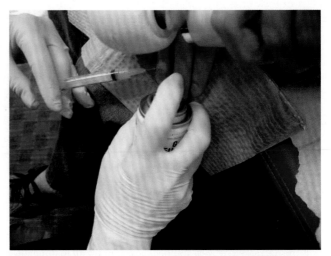

FIGURE 116.1. Intraoperative use of vapocoolant and vibration with intralesional corticosteroid injection of the nail. Photo courtesy of Phoebe Rich, MD.

 Clinical Pearls

- **Guidelines:** In January 2020, the American Academy of Dermatology and National Psoriasis Foundation published guidelines of care for the management and treatment of psoriasis in pediatric patients; however, intralesional injections are not discussed.[3]
- **Age-Specific Considerations:** Patients should be old enough to desire treatment and successfully undergo treatment without forcible restraint or significant distress.
- **Technique Tips:** Pain with nail injections can be reduced by placing injections more superficially and allowing diffusion of triamcinolone down to the matrix and using other techniques such as vibratory analgesia and ethyl chloride spray. Injections directly into the matrix and nail bed are more painful.[7]

Contraindications/Cautions/Risks

Contraindications

- Allergy to triamcinolone, active infection of nail fold

Risks

- Include pain, subungual hematoma, paresthesia, atrophy at injection site, and atrophy of the underlying terminal phalanx with repeated injections
- Theoretical risks not well documented include collagen atrophy and rupture of the extensor tendon.

Equipment Needed

- Syringe with 30-gauge ½-in needle
- Injectable triamcinolone acetonide suspension
- 1% Lidocaine without epinephrine for diluting triamcinolone to desired concentration
- Vapocoolant spray or ice for precooling
- Alcohol wipes
- Vibration source, for example, handheld wand-style massager or Buzzy® Mini Healthcare (MMJ Labs, Atlanta, GA)
- Topical lidocaine cream

Preprocedural Approach

- Topical lidocaine, if used, is applied 60 minutes before the procedure and kept in place using plastic food wrap.
- If using ice for precooling, this can be applied for 20 minutes before the procedure.

Procedural Approach

- The patient is placed in a comfortable reclined position with the hand elevated.
- Vibration is applied proximal to the injection site.
- Injection site is cleaned with alcohol swab.
- Vapocoolant spray is applied in a fine stream from approximately 8 to 18 cm from skin surface for 4 to 10 seconds until the skin just turns white (Figure 116.1).
- Triamcinolone acetonide, diluted in 1% lidocaine without epinephrine or saline, in a concentration of 2.5 to 5 mg/mL is injected slowly using a 30-gauge needle into the PNF and lateral nail fold.
- Inject small amount (0.1 mL or less) initially and then proceed with additional injections when the nail fold is anesthetized.
- The volume injected is typically 0.1 to 0.2 mL in up to four areas along the PNF and lateral nail fold or up to 0.3 mL in one injection centrally.
- Gentle pressure is applied after injection for hemostasis and diffusion of triamcinolone.

Postprocedural Approach

- Acetaminophen can be given for postprocedural pain.
- Injection intervals range from 3 to 8 weeks in decreasing frequency as clearance is achieved.

REFERENCES

1. de Jager MEA, de Jong EMGJ, van de Kerkhof PCM, Seyger MMB. Efficacy and safety of treatments for childhood psoriasis: a systematic literature review. *J Am Acad Dermatol.* 2010;62(6):1013–1030. doi:10.1016/j.jaad.2009.06.048.
2. Pahlajani N, Katz BJ, Lozano AM, Murphy F, Gottlieb A. Comparison of the efficacy and safety of the 308 nm excimer laser for the treatment of localized psoriasis in adults and in children: a pilot study. *Pediatr Dermatol.* 2005;22(2):161–165.

3. Menter A, Cordoro KM, Davis DMR. Joint American Academy of Dermatology–National Psoriasis Foundation guidelines of care for the management and treatment of psoriasis in pediatric patients. *J Am Acad Dermatol.* 2020;82(1):161–201.

4. Elmets CA, Lim HW, Stoff B, et al. Joint American Academy of Dermatology—National Psoriasis Foundation guidelines of care for the management and treatment of psoriasis with phototherapy. *J Am Acad Dermatol.* 2019;81(3):775–804.

5. Jiaravuthisan MM, Sasseville D, Vender RB, Murphy F, Muhn CY. Psoriasis of the nail: anatomy, pathology, clinical presentation, and a review of the literature on therapy. *J Am Acad Dermatol.* 2007;57(1): 1–27. https://www.clinicalkey.com/#!/content/playContent/1-s2.0-S0190962205032287?scrollTo=%23hl0001320. Accessed June 30, 2018.

6. Khoo BP, Giam YC. A pilot study on the role of intralesional triamcinolone acetonide in the treatment of pitted nails in children. *Singapore Med J.* 2000;41(2):66–68.

7. Hare AQ, Jefferson J, Rich P. How to choose my treatment. In: Rigopoulos D, Tosti A, eds. *Nail Psoriasis.* Springer; 2014:149–156.

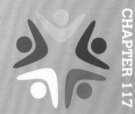

Pyogenic Granuloma

Molly J. Youssef and Megha M. Tollefson

CHAPTER 117

Introduction

Pyogenic granuloma (PG), also known as lobular capillary hemangioma, is an acquired idiopathic vascular neoplasm of the skin and mucous membranes. It presents as a rapidly growing, red, friable papule or polyp (Figure 117.1). PGs are benign and commonly occur in children, most frequently on the head, neck, and extremities. Minimal trauma often leads to profuse bleeding that is difficult to control, leading to the "BAND-AID sign" (Figure 117.2). PGs rarely resolve spontaneously, and therefore treatment is usually warranted. Many different management strategies have been reported including silver nitrate, topical imiquimod, topical and oral β-blockers, cryotherapy, electrocautery, electrodesiccation and curettage, shave removal (± electrodesiccation of base), surgical excision, injection of sclerosing agents, pulsed-dye laser (PDL), and carbon dioxide laser.

Treatment Recommendations

No specific treatment guidelines are known to exist for this condition, but shave removal followed by electrodesiccation is the

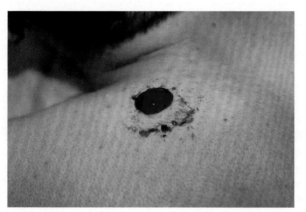

FIGURE 117.1. Pyogenic granuloma typically presents as a red, friable papule that bleeds easily. Photo courtesy of Andrew C. Krakowski, MD.

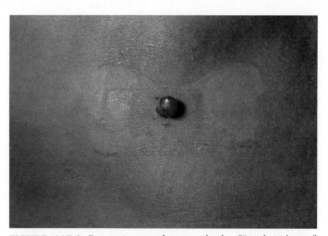

FIGURE 117.2. Pyogenic granuloma with the "Band Aid sign" around the lesion, due to a BAND-AID™ (Johnson & Johnson, US) in place to control bleeding. Used with permission of Mayo Foundation for Medical Education and Research. All rights reserved.

preferred treatment of most experts on the basis of literature review. There is a low risk of recurrence with this method, and the cosmetic outcome is typically satisfactory. Although the procedure is straightforward, we discuss important considerations in the pediatric population.

There are certain situations in which shave removal followed by electrodesiccation may not be the best treatment choice. Some children are unable to tolerate the procedure because of their age, developmental stage, or the presence of significant anxiety. In addition, an alternative treatment may be desired to avoid scar, pain, and/or postinflammatory hyperpigmentation. In these instances, we recommend a trial of topical β-blocker therapy. There are numerous reports of successfully treating PGs with topical timolol 0.5% gel-forming solution applied twice daily, with response seen within 1 to 2 months. There are instances of nonresponse or partial response with use of topical β-blockers. If the PG is not responding to topical β-blocker therapy, we advise removal of the lesion and sending for pathologic diagnosis. There is one report documenting use of oral β-blocker therapy on a recurrent mucosal PG, with resolution of the lesion after 6 months.

Imiquimod is another topical agent that can effectively treat PGs, but local irritation and necrosis can occur. A suggested imiquimod course is three times weekly initially, increasing to daily if tolerated, with treatment duration of up to 2 months. Treatment should be discontinued 1 week after complete disappearance of the lesion.

PDL is an additional option, especially for small PGs with minimal elevation. This procedure is mildly painful but is very quick. A topical anesthetic (eg, LMX.4™ [Ferndale Laboratories]) or eutectic mixture of local anesthetic (EMLA™ [AB Astra Pharmaceuticals, L.P.]) cream can be applied prior if needed. Published laser parameters for PG include laser wavelength 585 nm, pulse duration 0.45 ms, 5-mm spot size, fluence of 6 to 7 J/cm². Individual pulses were minimally overlapped as needed depending on lesion size. Retreatments were administered every 2 weeks until the lesion cleared. It is important to remember that PDL settings must be adjusted on a case-by-case basis, depending on the location and size of the lesion, the patient's skin type, and response to a test pulse.

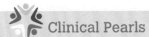

Clinical Pearls

- **Guidelines:** No specific treatment guidelines are known to exist for this condition, but shave removal followed by electrodesiccation is the preferred treatment of most experts on the basis of literature review. There is a low risk of recurrence with this method. We recommend always sending the specimen for pathologic diagnosis (ie, to rule out amelanotic melanoma).
- **Age-Specific Considerations:** Many young patients can tolerate the procedure with appropriate distraction techniques.
- **Pertinent History:** May consider alternative treatment option if the patient has a history of keloid formation
- **Skin of Color Considerations:** There is a greater risk of postinflammatory dyspigmentation with darker skin types.

Contraindications/Cautions/Risks

Contraindications
- Active skin infection near the site
- Inability to care for postoperative wounds

Cautions
- Depending on the location of the pyogenic granuloma, the surgeon should be aware of any critical nearby anatomic structures.
- Lesions around the face, especially the eye, may increase patient anxiety so good distraction and proper patient stabilization techniques should be utilized.

Risks
- Infection, scarring, pain, bleeding, recurrence of lesion, lack of histologic confirmation unless a specimen is sent

Equipment Needed

- Nonflammable cleanser (eg, chlorhexidine or povidone-iodine)
- Local anesthetic (eg, 1% lidocaine with epinephrine)
- Blade (such as Gillette or Dermablade™ [Accutec Blades Inc., US])
- Electrodesiccation device (eg, Hyfrecator 2000™ [Conmed, Utica, NY]), prefer blunt electrode tip (see Chapter 17. Electrosurgery/Hyfrecation)
- Petrolatum-based ointment
- BAND-AID
- ± Surgical curette
- ± Lidocaine-prilocaine cream (EMLA)
- ± Topical anesthetic skin refrigerant (eg, Pain Ease™ Mist Spray [Gebauer Company, US])
- ± Vibration device (eg, Buzzy® Mini Healthcare [MMJ Labs, Atlanta, GA])

Preprocedural Approach

- If the patient is scheduling the procedure for a future date and time, consider prescribing a topical anesthetic to be applied before the visit. We recommend application of 2.5% lidocaine and 2.5% prilocaine in a cream base (eg, EMLA) at home under occlusion for at least 2 hours (maximum 4 hours) before the procedure. Occlusion can be achieved using gauze with tape or adhesive polyurethane film dressing (eg, Tegaderm® [3M, US]).

Procedural Approach

- Informed consent from the parent/guardian and, when possible, assent from the minor are obtained.
- If EMLA was not applied before the procedure, consider application in the office followed by occlusion for 45 to 60 minutes.
- Cleanse the affected area with a nonflammable cleanser.
- Inject local anesthetic slowly. Topical anesthetic skin refrigerant and vibration devices can help reduce pain and provide distraction.
- Using a blade, remove the PG at its base; some proceduralists prefer a slightly scooped shave excision (Figure 117.3).

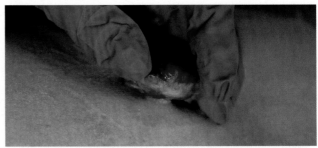

FIGURE 117.3. Intraoperative photograph of pedunculated pyogenic granuloma being grasped firmly and lifted gently to expose the base before shave removal. Photo courtesy of Andrew C. Krakowski, MD.

- At this point, some providers perform curettage of the base, but in our experience it is not necessary to prevent recurrence.
- Place the lesion in the specimen jar to send for pathologic diagnosis.
- Treat the exposed base of the lesion with electrodesiccation (suggest starting on "high" at 8-10 W).

Postprocedural Approach

- Apply petrolatum-based ointment.
- Cover with a BAND-AID.
- Recommend standard wound care instructions.

SUGGESTED READINGS

Lee LW, Goff KL, Lam JM, Low DW, Yan AC, Castelo-Soccio L. Treatment of pediatric pyogenic granulomas using β-adrenergic receptor antagonists. *Pediatr Dermatol.* 2014;31(2):203–207.

Pagliai KA, Cohen BA. Pyogenic granuloma in children. *Pediatr Dermatol.* 2004;21(1):10–13.

Tay Y-K, Weston WL, Morelli JG. Treatment of pyogenic granuloma in children with the flashlamp-pumped pulsed dye laser. *Pediatrics.* 1997;99(3):368–370.

Tritton SM, Smith S, Wong L-C, Wong LC, Zagarella S, Fischer G. Pyogenic granuloma in ten children treated with topical imiquimod. *Pediatr Dermatol.* 2009;26(3):269–272.

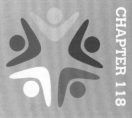

Perianal Pyramidal Protrusions

Kathryn S. Hinchee-Rodriguez

CHAPTER 118

Introduction

Infantile perianal pyramidal protrusions (IPPPs) were first described in the literature in 1989, classified at that time as "skin tags/folds," and it was not until 1996 that the term IPPP was coined (https://pubmed.ncbi.nlm.nih.gov/8961878/). This misidentification highlights the broad differential for IPPP, which includes hemorrhoids, hemangiomas, rectal prolapse, granulomatous perineal lesions of Crohn's disease, sexual abuse, condyloma, molluscum contagiosum, and skin tags. IPPP is a rare, benign condition, which lends itself to being mistaken for more serious lesions. It most commonly presents in infant females[1]; of the over 108 cases in the literature, all but one is in prepubertal females. Age of diagnosis ranges from birth to 13 years; however, the literature suggests that IPPP presents overwhelmingly during infancy.[1]

IPPP lesions tend to be solitary protrusions that predominantly lie perianally along the medial raphe (Figure 118.1). Although they can be found both posterior and anterior to the anus, the anterior location is most common. In coloration, they can be skin-colored, red, or with whitish plaques if associated with lichen sclerosus et atrophicus (LSA). Despite the name, not only do they occur in a pyramidal shape but they also have been described as "leaf-like," "peanut," "hen's nest," and "tongue-tip."[1,2] The protrusions generally do not bleed nor do they show signs of excoriations, helping differentiate them from other diagnoses. Cases have been reported from European, American, Indian, and Korean populations, and ethnic or racial predilection for IPPP has not been shown. Constipation is a comorbidity associated with acquired IPPP[1]; however, IPPP is generally congenital in its presentation.[1]

IPPP is thought to exist in three main subtypes: (1) Congenital/constitutional, (2) acquired/functional, and (3) associated with LSA. In the congenital variety, the protrusion, present at birth, is believed to be a residual tip of the urogenital septum

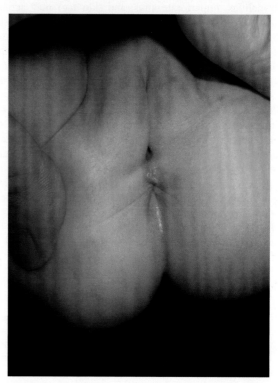

FIGURE 118.1. Example of infantile perianal pyramidal protrusion occurring along the medial raphe in a young female. The lesion resolved spontaneously. It did *not* require procedural intervention. Photo courtesy of Andrew C. Krakowski, MD.

from its embryologic lengthening to form the perineum. In addition, the inherent laxity of the female perineum is believed to contribute to the development of the protrusion, which suggests why the condition is found so predominantly in females. Those with congenital IPP most often have spontaneous regression of the protrusion within weeks of birth; however, some cases have shown that it may persist for years.

Acquired IPPP is believed to be secondary to constipation and straining during defecation, developing as early as 3 weeks of life. Wiping and cleaning, diarrhea, and diaper region inflammation are also thought to contribute. Management strategies involve improving constipation, through dietary or behavioral modification as well as use of stool softeners. Upon improvement of mechanical causative factors, protrusions generally regress.

IPPP associated with LSA can be differentiated by a porcelain white atrophic appearance or recurrent anogenital erythema, and can sometimes clinically herald oncoming LSA that has yet to manifest.[1,3] This form does not tend to spontaneously regress in the same manner as the other two subtypes do, and necessitates topical steroid therapy for resolution.[3] Topical steroids such as clobetasol propionate 0.05% or 0.1% methylprednisolone aceponate[3] resolve the erythema; however, they do not always completely resolve the protruding mass itself.

In addition to coexisting with LSA, IPPP has been found concurrent with infantile hemangiomas.[2] One case report posited that PELVIS syndrome (*p*erineal hemangioma, *e*xternal genitalia malformations, *l*ipomyelomeningocele, *v*esicorenal abnormalities, *i*mperforate anus, and *s*kin tag) may actually include IPPP.[2] Given its rarity, IPPP may be mistaken for skin tags. Hemangiomas, just like IPPP, spontaneously regress over time and generally require no surgical intervention unless they become complicated or persistent, in which case pharmacologic management with topical or oral β-blockers is usually now the first step.

Physical examination and clinical history is generally sufficient for diagnosis; however, biopsy can be done to rule out other potential diagnoses. In histopathology, congenital and acquired IPPP demonstrate epidermal acanthosis and dilated vessels with fibrous tissue; however, normal histopathology has also been reported.[1-3] In LSA-associated IPPP, additional findings include dermal edema, infiltration of inflammatory cells, and dermal vacuolar changes.[1-3]

Overall, IPPP tends to spontaneously regress within a few years in most patients, and requires no specific procedural intervention on behalf of the physician.

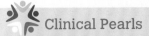

Clinical Pearls

- **Guidelines:** No specific guidelines exist for the procedural treatment of this condition. Unfortunately, given the rarity and common misdiagnosis of IPPP, there is little literature available on the lesion. No meta-analyses, randomized control trials, and cohort or case control studies are available, and what is available is limited to case reports and expert opinion. Because there is no level of evidence of I or II available, only level III and IV, by the GRADE system, IPPP management receives Grade D.
- **Age-Specific Considerations:** The lesion tends to resolve with time.
- **Technique Tips:** Although it does occur almost entirely in females, anatomy does not affect management, because the strategy is to allow the protrusion to resolve on its own.
- **Skin of Color Considerations:** Given that IPPP has no racial or ethnic preference and tends to spontaneously regress, there are no specific considerations in management.

Contraindications/Cautions/Risks

Management involves allowing time for spontaneous regression; there are no known contraindications or risks in IPPP resolution.

Equipment Needed

- Tincture of time

Preoperative Approach

Don't do it. It will likely resolve on its own.

Intraoperative Technique

Seriously, don't do it.

Postoperative Approach

See, we told you it would resolve on its own.

REFERENCES

1. Zavras N, Christianakis E, Tsamoudaki S, Velaorasb K. Infantile perianal pyramidal protrusion: a report of 8 new cases and a review of the literature. *Case Rep Dermatol.* 2012;4(3):202–206.
2. Verma SB, Wollina U. Infantile perianal pyramidal protrusion with coexisting perineal and perianal hemangiomas: a fortuitous association or incomplete PELVIS syndrome? *Indian J Dermatol.* 2014;59(1):71.
3. Kim BJ, Woo SM, Li K, Lee DH, Cho S. Infantile perianal pyramidal protrusion treated by topical steroid application. *J Eur Acad Dermatol Venereol.* 2007;21(2):263–264.

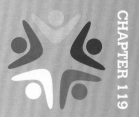
Rosacea

Krystal M. Jones and Lucía Z. Díaz

Introduction

Rosacea is a chronic inflammatory skin disease commonly diagnosed in patients with fair skin, although in skin of color it may be underdiagnosed. It is typically more common in women than in men, and although it classically presents in those older than 30 years, it can present at any age.

Rosacea has been traditionally classified into multiple subtypes depending on morphologic characteristics, namely, erythematotelangiectatic, papulopustular, ocular, and phymatous types. Newer data and clinical experience have shown significant overlap between rosacea's many morphologies, and suggest they may exist on a continuum; that is, flushing and centrofacial erythema may progress to papules and pustules, and in a small number of cases, progress to the development of phymas.[1]

Removing the barriers of subtypes may lead to a more individualized treatment approach for patients. The diagnosis of rosacea is considered with either fixed centrofacial erythema or phymatous change. Phenotypic signs may include papules and pustules, flushing, telangiectasia and ocular manifestations such as blepharitis with or without keratoconjunctivitis. Burning or stinging, edema and a dry appearance are common symptoms. Treatment is based on the presentation of the patient and is often multimodal, with multiple agents simultaneously, because each patient can present with a myriad of phenotypes.

A cornerstone in the treatment of all of rosacea includes sun protection and general skin care, including sunscreen with sun protection factor 30+, frequent moisturizers, gentle cleansers, and known trigger avoidance. Transient erythema can be treated with topical α-adrenergics or oral β-blockers. The most effective therapy for persistent erythema and telangiectasia is laser and light treatment. Mild papulopustular disease can be targeted with topical creams including azelaic acid, ivermectin, and metronidazole, and more moderate to severe cases with oral tetracyclines. Severe papulopustular and/or phymatous disease may require oral isotretinoin, and ocular disease requires lid hygiene and, often, oral tetracyclines.

Although some patients' rosacea may manifest with only persistent erythema and telangiectasia, this may be the only sign remaining following successful medical management of their inflammatory papules and pustules. Thus, laser and light treatment to target the erythema and telangiectasia is key in the overall management of rosacea at some point in the treatment course of many patients.

The pulsed-dye laser (PDL) and intense pulsed light (IPL) are the two most commonly used therapies for persistent erythema and telangiectases seen in rosacea. By emitting a light selectively absorbed by oxyhemoglobin, PDL selectively destroys vessels without surrounding collateral tissue damage. IPL therapy utilizes broadband flash lamps that emit polychromatic incoherent light that ranges from visible to infrared. Optical filters are used to customize the polychromatic light to target multiple chromophores. Although the IPL can be helpful with the many targets seen in facial photoaging, for example, dyspigmentation and erythema, the target of the PDL is more specific to rosacea. Selection of the laser or light therapy is often based on the resources, preferences, and experience of the provider. The discussion in this chapter focuses on PDL, with the caveat that there are many other effective medical, laser, and light modalities used in the treatment of rosacea.

Clinical Pearls

- **Guidelines:** For the treatment of persistent facial erythema and telangiectasia, The Global Rosace Consensus Panel lists IPL and PDL as a first-line therapy, and the American Acne and Rosacea Society encourages laser- and light-based systems for the treatment for persistent erythema and telangiectases as part of the comprehensive approach to the overall management of rosacea.[2]
- **Age-Specific Considerations:** Ideally, patients should be old enough to ask for treatment for themselves and be developed enough to be assist in detecting and reporting postsurgical complications such as increasing pain, redness, warmth, swelling, fever/chills.
- **Technique Tips:**
  - Rosacea-associated facial telangiectases tend to be distributed on the central face. This is in contrast to telangiectases associated with sun damage, which tend to locate on the lateral face and neck, and may be associated with other poikilodermatous change.
  - It is paramount that autoimmune disorders, such as systemic lupus erythematosus and dermatomyositis, which are also characterized by centrofacial erythema, be distinguished from rosacea. These diseases are not only photoaggravated and could be exacerbated with laser- or light-based treatments, but, furthermore, leaving them undiagnosed can result in untreated systemic disease with permanent sequelae.
  - Persistent facial erythema is due to fixed small vessel dilation. Medical management with topical α-adrenergics such as brimonidine is very effective in the treatment of persistent erythema; however, it is limited to the several hours following application, requiring scheduled dosing.
  - Although shorter pulse durations with standard PDL are highly effective, subsequent purpura and the potential for postinflammatory hyperpigmentation at these settings are often intolerable for patients. Longer pulses deliver equivalent energy at a slower rate to heat vessels uniformly and gently, minimizing post-treatment purpura while allowing the treatment of larger vessels. In general, pulse durations longer than 6 ms are nonpurpuric, whereas pulse durations shorter than 3 ms produce purpura. Smaller vessels that contribute to persistent erythema require higher energy delivered in a shorter period of time for destruction. Larger telangiectases can be targeted with longer millisecond pulse durations.

- The absorption spectrum of oxyhemoglobin also shares that of melanin, which can impact treatment of patients with darker skin types or tanned skin. A test spot evaluated in 24 to 48 hours can always be utilized if there is any doubt. Contact cooling can prevent damage from melanin absorption of light.
- **Skin of Color Considerations:** The technique is best suited for skin types I and II, because the risk of dyspigmentation increases with darker skin types.

Contraindications/Cautions/Risks

Contraindications

- Avoid laser treatments in patients with any active skin infection at the treatment location. It is recommended that patients with significant inflammatory papules and pustules be optimally managed medically, likely with oral antibiotics, before treating erythema or telangiectasia with laser.
- Consider the presence of an underlying connective disorder such as lupus or the concurrent/recent use of a photosensitizing medication such as doxycycline.

Cautions

- Eye safety is of utmost importance for both the patient and provider, because blindness occurs rapidly and painlessly. Wrap-around glasses and goggles at an optical density greater than or equal to 4 at the wavelength of the laser or light emitted must be used.

Risks

- Adverse effects of laser and light therapies can include transient erythema and edema, bruising and dyspigmentation.
- Cutaneous burning is a risk, although primarily due to improper device, dosimetry, and/or treatment technique.

Equipment Needed

- Eye protection for patient and provider, staff
- All entrances to procedure room marked with cautionary signage requiring eye protection to enter
- Laser with spot size attachments
- Topical anesthetics
- Cooling roller or cool pack
- Aloe vera
- Broad-spectrum physical sunscreen, such as zinc oxide

Preprocedural Approach

- Although papules, pustules, and ocular rosacea are best managed medically, laser therapy is the treatment of choice for rosacea characterized by persistent facial erythema or telangiectases (Figure 119.1).
- Once the decision has been made to pursue laser treatment with PDL, management of expectations is imperative. One can expect improvements of 50% to 75% in facial telangiectases in one to three treatments, depending on how aggressive the settings. This is a critical discussion to have because the more aggressive the settings, the more efficacious the treatment; however, this comes at the expense of purpura.
- Determining the patient's expectations and wishes for downtime with purpura can help you decide on the treatment settings and number of sessions to break the treatment into.

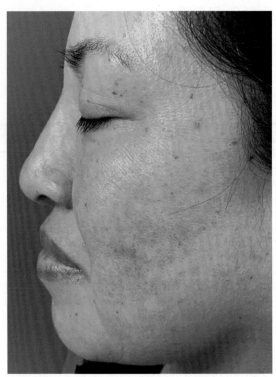

FIGURE 119.1. Rosacea. Persistent erythema and scattered telangiectases on the midface.

- If the patient wishes to apply a topical anesthetic cream such as lidocaine 2.5% and prilocaine 2.5% (EMLA™ [AB Astra Pharmaceuticals, L.P.]) or lidocaine 4% (LMX.4™ [Ferndale Laboratories]), it should be applied to the areas to be treated for 30 to 60 minutes before the procedure.

Procedural Approach

- Consent for the procedure should include a discussion of risks, benefits, and alternatives, as discussed previously. Notable risks include dyspigmentation, bruising, burning, and discomfort.
- Following informed consent of the procedure, place the patient in a position comfortable for them and optimal for the provider to access all treatment areas with the laser hand piece.
- Before starting the procedure, cautionary signage should be hanging from all entrances noting the use of laser devices and the room requires eye protection upon entry. You may hang an extra pair of goggles from the sign, so that anyone needing to enter during the procedure may use them.
- The patient should wear well-fitting metal safety goggles, with instructions to keep the eyes shut, during the procedure (Figure 119.2). The provider, staff, and anyone in the room must also wear wrap-around glasses at an optical density greater than or equal to 4 at the wavelength of the laser or light emitted. If at any point in time the device is not in use for treatment, it should remain in "standby" mode.
- The area to be treated should be cleaned with a gentle cleanser and wiped dry. All makeup including mascara should be removed. If alcohol or acetone was used to clean the skin, this must be allowed to dry completely. All hair should be pinned back and out of the treatment field.

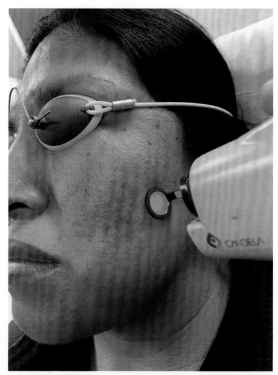

FIGURE 119.2. Rosacea treated with pulsed-dye laser. During the procedure, the patient is wearing well-fitted metal safety goggles and has been instructed to keep her eyes closed.

- For treatment of generalized facial erythema with PDL, use a 7- to 10-mm spot size, and start with a 6 to 10-ms pulse duration and a fluence of 6.5 to 8.5 J/cm². Select a representative test spot location on the lateral face and pulse the laser at your initial settings, paying close attention to the response of the target. The desired end point to assess for is a fleeting black and blue blush. If the target does not reach its clinical end point, you may gradually increase the fluence, or decrease the pulse duration. In general, to avoid purpura, it is recommended to use a pulse duration of 6 ms or longer.
- For the treatment of facial telangiectases, a pulse duration of 10 to 40 ms with fluences from 9 to 15 J/cm² is a reasonable nonpurpuric starting point. After pulsing the laser in a test spot on a desired target, again assess for the desired clinical end point, in this case, transient purpuric change. If you do not see this end point, the fluence can be increased or the pulse duration decreased gradually until the desired end point is reached.
- Overlap between pulses is important to avoid "foot printing." For even and uniform improvement, an overlap of 10% to 15% between pulses is recommended.

Postprocedural Approach

- Once the treatment session has concluded, application of a cooling pack or a cold roller followed by aloe vera can be utilized. A broad physical sunscreen such as zinc oxide should be applied upon leaving the clinic.
- When using nonpurpuric settings, the patient may experience transient edema and erythema for 24 hours. Oral antihistamines and topical application of cool packs can be helpful for this. If the patient did develop purpura, this may last up to 2 weeks to resolve.
- The patient must employ strict sun protection to avoid postinflammatory hyperpigmentation.
- Patients should be counseled on trigger avoidance, because recurrence of flushing can lead to recurrence of disease.
- Follow-up for additional treatments can be scheduled in 4 to 6 weeks. The duration of response is variable; a good estimate is 3 to 5 years.

REFERENCES

1. Gallo RL, Granstein RD, Kang S, et al. Rosacea comorbidities and future research: the 2017 update by the National Rosacea Society Expert Committee. *J Am Acad Dermatol.* 2018;78:167–170.
2. Schaller M, Almeida L, Bewley A, et al. Rosacea treatment update: recommendations from the global ROSacea COnsensus (ROSCO) panel. *Br J Dermatol.* 2017;176:465–471.

Scabies

Craig N. Burkhart

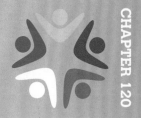

CHAPTER 120

Introduction

Scabies affects all ages, races, and socioeconomic groups. Nodular lesions in the axillae and diaper area are characteristic signs of scabies in young children (see Figures 120.1 and 120.2). It is transmitted by close personal contact and fomites, and incidence increases with overcrowding. Crusted scabies (ie, Norwegian scabies) is a severe infestation with scabies that may occur in immunocompromised individuals or those with decreased sensory functions. Individuals with crusted scabies may have thousands of mites on their skin, and live mites can be found in the sheets, chairs, floors, and other areas of their environment.

Diagnosis of scabies is often confirmed with mineral oil preparations of skin scrapings from clinically infested areas of the skin (crusted nodules or burrows as seen in Figure 120.3). Skin scraping findings are often negative, in which case the diagnosis can be confirmed by response to empirical treatment with an antiscabetic medication.

This chapter reiterates the diagnostic approach to scabies, offering several useful pearls to increase sensitivity and to decrease anxiety in a pediatric population. In addition, this chapter focuses on the "procedural" treatment of scabies from the perspective of how to properly apply topical medications, take oral medications, and environmentally manage scabies in the household.

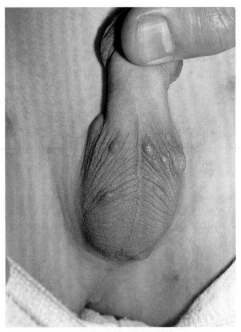

FIGURE 120.1. Papulonodular lesions on the scrotum is not uncommon. Reprinted with permission from Burkhart CN, Morrell D, Goldsmith L, et al. *VisualDx: Essential Pediatric Dermatology.* Philadelphia, PA: Wolters Kluwer Health/Lippincott Williams & Wilkins; 2010. Figure 4-205.

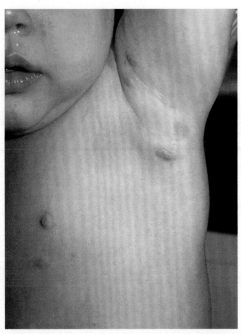

FIGURE 120.2. Papulonodular lesions in the axilla. Reprinted with permission from Burkhart CN, Morrell D, Goldsmith L, et al. *VisualDx: Essential Pediatric Dermatology.* Philadelphia, PA: Wolters Kluwer Health/Lippincott Williams & Wilkins; 2010. Figure 4-202.

Clinical Pearls

- Symptoms can typically take 4 to 8 weeks to develop after infestation; if a person has had scabies before, then symptoms may appear much sooner (1-4 days) after exposure.
- The palms and soles of infants and children may be more likely to yield more positive results than do other anatomic sites.
- A disposable curette may be used instead of a #15 blade to increase acceptability and safety in children.
- The sensitivity of scrapings is low, so it is important to scrape multiple sites and initiate empiric therapy if the patient clinically appears to have scabies.
- The most common reason for treatment failure is reinfestation from untreated family members and other contacts who live in the same household.
- Itching due to hypersensitivity reaction to mites and scybala (their feces) may persist for several weeks after treatment and can be treated with topical steroids if necessary.

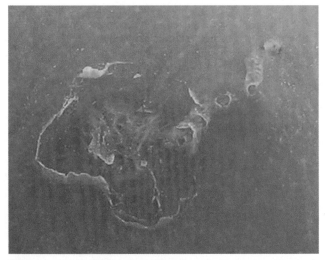

FIGURE 120.3. Scabies burrow (nonpolarized magnification). Photograph by Michael Geary. https://commons.wikimedia.org/w/index.php?curid=1338177.

Equipment Needed

- Mineral oil
- Glass slide
- #10 or #15 blade or disposable curette
- Microscope
- Dermatoscope

PROCEDURAL APPROACH #1: SCABIES PREPARATION FOR MICROSCOPIC EXAMINATION

- Apply mineral oil over the skin lesion to be scraped (preferably a burrow or crusted nodule).
- Firmly scrape the surface of the lesion with a number 15 blade or disposable curette.

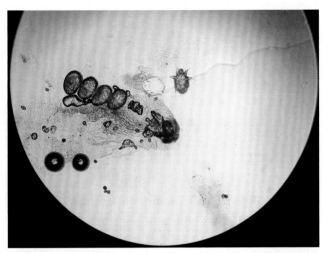

FIGURE 120.4. The "Triple Crown" of scabies preparation for microscopic examination: Scabies mite, four ova, and scybala. Photo courtesy of Andrew C. Krakowski, MD.

- Stop scraping when pin point bleeding or significant scale is removed.
- Apply the mineral oil and scale mixture to a glass slide.
- Repeat scrapings on multiple lesions and add to the glass slide.
- Examine collection of scrapings under a microscope for mites (larvae, nymphs, or adults), eggs, or scybala (feces) (Figure 120.4).
  - Eggs are ovoid shaped and 0.1 to 0.15 mm in length.
  - Larvae emerge from eggs with three pairs of legs and last about 3 to 4 days before molting into nymphs, which have four pairs of legs and look similar to adults, only smaller.
  - Adult females are 0.3 to 0.45 mm long and 0.25 to 0.35 mm wide; males are slightly more than half the size of females.
- Dispose of contaminated slide in appropriate container.

PROCEDURAL APPROACH #2: DERMOSCOPY

- Search for burrows, which may be shaped like an "s" or "z" (Figure 120.3).
- Magnification using dermoscopy can reveal a triangle or "delta wing jet" sign of the scabies head parts along with translucent structures, representing the scabies body and eggs.

PROCEDURAL APPROACH #3: PROPER TREATMENT

- Treating all individuals who live in the same household is important to prevent reinfestation by asymptomatic carriers.
- Apply permethrin 5% cream
  - For infants and young children, apply the cream to the entire body, including the head, neck, and face. For older children and teenagers, apply from scalp down, avoiding the face.
  - Cream should be applied to clean skin and left on 8 to 12 hours (usually overnight) and then completely washed; clean clothing should be worn after treatment.
  - Because permethrin is not 100% ovicidal, it is necessary to repeat in 1 to 2 weeks to kill mites that could potentially hatch from the remaining live eggs.

- Permethrin is not FDA approved for infants younger than age 2 months. However, if it is used in this age group, the medication can be applied to dry skin and washed off in cool water 6 hours later to limit systemic absorption.
  - Permethrin can be used in pregnant and lactating women.
  - A typical 70-kg adult will use approximately 30 g (1/2 tube) of permethrin cream per application. Young children and infants older than 2 months of age should use less than 15 g (1/4 tube) of cream per application.
- Ivermectin 3 mg tablets
  - Dosing is 150 to 200 μg/kg once; repeat in 7 to 14 days (oral ivermectin is not ovicidal, so repeat dosing is required to kill mites that may have hatched from unkilled eggs).
  - In the United States, dosing is weight based, and there is no maximum dose (in low-resource countries without access to scales, ivermectin dosing is based on height).
  - Do not give to pregnant women or children under 15 kg.
- Lindane 1% lotion (rarely used)
  - Lindane 1% lotion has been used to treat scabies, though in limited use due to associated risks.
  - Lindane lotion is contraindicated in premature infants and individuals with known uncontrolled seizure disorders. Seizures and deaths have been reported following application with repeat or prolonged application, but also in rare cases following a single application used according to directions.
  - Lindane lotion is contraindicated for patients with crusted (Norwegian) scabies and other skin conditions (eg, atopic dermatitis, psoriasis) that may increase systemic absorption of the drug.
  - Lindane lotion should be used with caution for infants, children, the elderly, and in those individuals who weigh < 110 lbs (50 kg) as they may be at risk of serious neurotoxicity.
  - Apply from neck down, leave on overnight, and repeat in 1 to 2 weeks (lindane lotion is not 100% ovicidal, so repeat dosing is required to kill mites that may have hatched from unkilled eggs).
- Topical sulfur and benzyl benzoate need to be compounded by a compounding pharmacist and are rarely utilized or available.

Postprocedure Environmental Management

- For regular scabies:
  - It is important to wash and dry (using the dryer's "high heat" setting) any bedding, clothing, and towels used in the household during the previous 3 days before the "day of treatment." Items that cannot be washed (stuffed animals, a favorite blanket, etc) should be dry-cleaned and sealed in a plastic bag for at least 72 hours (the scabies mite does not generally survive more than 2-3 days away from human skin).
  - Insecticide sprays and fumigants are not recommended for regular scabies.
- For *crusted scabies* or for scabies outbreaks in an institutional setting (eg, nursing home, hospital, long-term care facility, prison), follow prevention and control measures as suggested by CDC. gov and any local and/or state health department guidelines.

SUGGESTED READING

Burkhart CN, Burkhart CG, Morrell DS. Infestations. In: Bolognia JL, Schaffer JV, Cerroni L, eds. *Dermatology*. London, England: Elsevier; 2018:1503–1515.

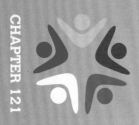

CHAPTER 121

Solitary Fibrous Hamartoma of Infancy

Paul A. Mittermiller, Danielle H. Rochlin, and H. Peter Lorenz

Introduction

Fibrous hamartomas of infancy are benign soft-tissue tumors.[1] The lesions are usually present at birth and are often identified during the first few years of life. They commonly present as painless, mobile, subcutaneous masses without involvement of the overlying skin. Most commonly, they may be found in the upper arm and shoulder regions, but have been described in multiple areas throughout the head, torso, and limbs. An example of a folliculopilosebaceous hamartoma is shown in Figure 121.1. The diagnosis is made through histologic examination of the lesion, which reveals fibrous tissue, adipose tissue, and primitive mesenchyme.[2]

Surgical excision is the preferred treatment because it allows for removal of the mass and for obtaining a diagnosis to differentiate the lesion from other subcutaneous masses. A single surgical excision is often curative,[1] although recurrence is not uncommon and is thought to be due to incomplete excision. An example of the surgical closure following excision of a forehead hamartoma is shown in Figure 121.2. A description for excision of hamartomas is included here.

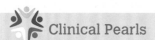

Clinical Pearls

- **Guidelines:** There are no specific treatment guidelines for hamartomas.
- **Age-Specific Considerations:** General anesthesia or intravenous sedation should be considered for young children.
- **Technique Tips:** Surgical excision should aim to remove the entire lesion without damaging any neighboring structures.
- **Skin of Color Considerations:** As with all surgical procedures, there is a risk of scarring postoperatively. The degree of scarring may vary depending on skin tone and type.

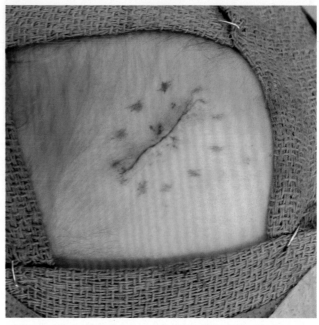

FIGURE 121.2. Photograph of the surgical site following excision of a hamartoma; absorbable suture was used to minimize anxiety at the follow-up visit. Photo courtesy of H. Peter Lorenz, MD.

Contraindications/Cautions/Risks

Contraindications
- There are no specific contraindications for surgical removal of hamartomas. If significant patient comorbidities exist, excision can potentially be performed under local anesthesia to avoid the risks of general anesthesia.

Cautions
- Depending on the location of the hamartoma, the surgeon should be aware of any critical nearby structures.

Risks
- Bleeding
- Infection
- Recurrence

Equipment Needed
- Local anesthetic (1% or 2% lidocaine or 0.25% bupivacaine with or without epinephrine)
- #15 scalpel
- Scissors
- Electric cautery
- Needle holder
- Forceps
- Suture

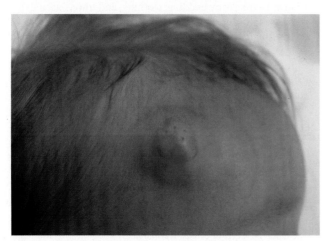

FIGURE 121.1. Photograph of a folliculopilosebaceous hamartoma in a child. Photo courtesy of H. Peter Lorenz, MD.

Preprocedural Approach

- Imaging can help rule out vascular lesions, but it is often inconclusive for differentiating between other subcutaneous soft-tissue tumors.

Procedural Approach

- The lesion is marked before injecting local anesthesia to prevent distortion of the skin and location of the mass.
- Local anesthesia is injected around the lesion for its anesthetic affect and to allow time for vasoconstriction to occur as a result of the epinephrine.
- A sterile field is created using Betadine or chlorhexidine.
- A scalpel is used to create an incision overlying the lesion. If the skin is involved, a skin ellipse should be excised with the lesion.
- Dissection should be carried out around the lesion using either sharp dissection with the scalpel or scissors or by spreading around the lesion bluntly.
- The lesion should be excised in its entirety to prevent local recurrence.
- Adequate hemostasis is obtained using electric cautery.

- The wound site is irrigated and the skin reapproximated.
- The skin is closed using permanent or absorbable sutures. In young children, absorbable suture is preferred because it does not need to be removed in clinic (Figure 121.2).

Postprocedural Approach

- The incision should be well healed within 3 weeks.
- After the incision has healed, the patient can return to full activities.
- A histopathologic examination should be performed in all cases to confirm the diagnosis and to rule out any malignant etiologies.
- If the lesion recurs, excision should be repeated.

REFERENCES

1. Ake Y, Kouameb J, Moh E, et al. Skin hamartoma in children: diagnosis and therapeutic issues. *J Pediatr Surg Case Rep.* 2014;2:319–321.
2. Sotelo-Avila C, Bale PM. Subdermal fibrous hamartoma of infancy: pathology of 40 cases and differential diagnosis. *Pediatr Pathol.* 2009;14:39–52.

Squamous Cell Carcinoma

Guilherme Canho Bittner and Nelise Ritter Hans-Bittner

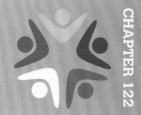

CHAPTER 122

Introduction

Cutaneous squamous cell carcinoma (cSCC) is the second most common form of human cancer and has an increasing annual incidence. Although most cSCC is cured with office-based therapy, advanced cSCC poses a significant risk for morbidity, impact on quality of life, and death.[1]

Cases of cSCC in the pediatric population have been reported in association with xeroderma pigmentosum, oculocutaneous albinism, or as a metastasis of SCC from other sites.[2,3]

Herein we offer our step-by-step instructions for cSCC excisions in children and tips to make the surgery less traumatic. Our protocol is to perform Mohs micrographic surgery (MMS) for high-risk cSCC, but excisions with wide margins (5 mm) can be made in low-risk cSCC (Table 122.1) . We further explain both techniques and how to achieve the best results in both.

Clinical Pearls

- **Guidelines:** MMS is the treatment of choice for most cSCC, especially for the high-risk subtypes. Standard surgery can be performed in low-risk subtypes with a 5-mm margin from the visible tumor.
- **Age-Specific Considerations:**
  - The biopsy experience before surgery is a good indicator of the child's ability to cooperate with surgery under local anesthesia. Consider sedation with an anesthetist if the child does not understand or collaborate.
  - Some patients are old enough to be aware of the procedure and cooperate with the surgeon. In these patients, the MMS can be done with local anesthesia.
- **Technique Tips:**
  - Bupivacaine 0.5% with epinephrine 1:200 000 is a slow-onset local anesthetic that is well tolerated after lidocaine; its extended duration of action can help minimize pain throughout a long procedure and postoperatively.
  - Margins of the tumor can be marked utilizing dermoscopy.
- **Skin of Color Considerations:** The technique can be performed in any skin color.

TABLE 122.1 ⋮ NCCN Clinical Practice Guidelines in Oncology (NCCN Guidelines®) for Squamous Cell Skin Cancer: Risk Factors for Local Recurrence or Metastasis*

PARAMETERS	LOW RISK	HIGH RISK
Clinical		
Location[c]/size[d]	Area L < 20 mm Area M[a] < 10 mm	Area L ≥ 20 mm Area M ≥ 10 mm Area H[b]
Borders	Well defined	Poorly defined
Primary versus recurrent	Primary	Recurrent
Immunosuppression	No	Yes
Site of prior radiation therapy or chronic inflammatory process	No	Yes
Rapidly growing tumor	No	Yes
Neurologic symptoms	No	Yes
Pathologic		
Degree of differentiation	Well to moderately differentiated	Poorly differentiated
High-risk histologic subtype[e]	No	Yes
Depth (thickness or level of invasion)[f]	</=6 and no invasion beyond subcutaneous fat	>6 mm or invasion beyond subcutaneous fat
Perineural, lymphatic, or vascular involvement	No	Yes

*NCCN Guidelines for Squamous Cell Skin Cancer are intended for use in adult patients.
[a]Location independent of size may constitute high risk.
[b]Area H constitutes high risk on the basis of location, independent of size.
[c]Area L consists of the trunk and extremities (excluding hands, feet, nail units, pretibia, and ankles); area M consists of cheeks, forehead, scalp, neck, and pretibia; and area H consists of central face, eyelids, eyebrows, periorbital skin, nose, lips, chin, mandible, preauricular and postauricular skin/sulci, temple, ear, genitalia, hands, and feet.
[d]Greatest tumor diameter; must include peripheral rim or erythema.
[e]Acanthyolytic (adenoid), adenosquamous (showing mucin production), desmoplastic, or metaplastic (carcinosarcomatous) subtypes.
[f]If clinical evaluation of incisional biopsy suggests that microstaging is inadequate, consider narrow-margin excisional biopsy. Deep invasion is defined as invasion beyond the subcutaneous fat OR >6 mm (as measured from the granular layer of adjacent normal epidermis to the bas of the tumor, consistent with AJCC 8th edition).
Adapted with permission from the NCCN Clinical Practice Guidelines in Oncology (NCCN Guidelines®) for Squamous Cell Skin Cancer V.1.2020.

Contraindications/Cautions/Risks

Contraindications
- Active skin infection on surgical site
- Inability to care for postoperative wounds

Cautions
- History of bleeding and allergic reactions (check family history)

Risks
- Death (infection or anesthesia), scarring, pain, bleeding, recurrence of lesions

Equipment Needed
- Lidocaine 1% with epinephrine 1:100 000
- Saline
- Bupivacaine 0.5% with epinephrine 1:200 000
- Scalpel

- Scissors
- Clamps
- Hooks
- Hemostatic clamps
- Electrocautery
- Smoke evacuator
- Gauze
- Surgical marker pen
- Tissue stain
- Mohs laboratory (cryostat, hematoxylin and eosin stain)
- Suture
- Petrolatum-based ointment
- Micropore Surgical Tape™ (3M™, US)

Preprocedural Approach
- Have the family bring all medications to show the doctor. Take all regular medicines except those that can affect bleeding or healing.

- Prophylaxis for herpes simplex is not necessary.
- Patients should bathe either the evening before or on the morning of their surgery.
- Patients must be advised to avoid supplements such as herbs, vitamin E, niacin, fish oil tablets, or nonsteroidal anti-inflammatory medicines (ibuprofen, naproxen, etc) for 1 week before surgery because they can increase bleeding.

Procedural Approach

- Informed consent from the parent/guardian and, when possible, assent from the minor are obtained.
- The surgery site must be cleaned with alcohol 70%.

MOHS MICROGRAPHIC SURGERY

- The area of the tumor is marked with a permanent pen. The first margin is 1 to 2 mm from the dermoscopy tumor edge.
- Lidocaine 1% with epinephrine 1:100 000 is typically used for local anesthesia.
- To reduce anesthesia infiltration pain, infiltrate it slowly. Repetitive movements with the fingertip around the needle can help reduce pain during the injection. Also, conversation and ambient music can help distract the patient and keep him or her relaxed during the procedure.
- After the patient is anesthetized, bupivacaine 0.5% with epinephrine 1:200 000 can be infiltrated around the area. Sometimes laboratory work can take several hours depending on the tumor size. This adjuvant will help keep the area numb.
- The surgical site is cleansed again with another antiseptic, with alcohol 70%, chlorhexidine 2%, or a combination of both as ChloraPrep™ (Becton, Dickinson and Company, US).
- Curettage or a superficial excision of the tumor is now performed.
- A first layer is taken after that, 2 to 3 mm from the curettage or superficial excision with a second scalpel (preventing tumor contamination) and the tissue is marked with proper tissue stain.
- Good hemostasis is then made with electrocauterization using clamps if necessary.
- A dressing with saline and gauze cover the surgical defect until the closure or a new Mohs surgery stage.
- The procedure continues as many stages as needed until clear in all surgical margins.
- After clear margins are obtained, reconstruction is performed. In some areas, depending on the tumor size and dimension (oval, circle, or another shape), primary closure when possible is the best option, but a flap or graft are options for bigger wounds.
- Suture the wound first using absorbable inner stitches as Monocryl™, Vicryl™, or PDS™ (Ethicon US, LLC).
- External suturing is performed with Prolene™ (Ethicon US, LLC) or plain gut fast absorbable.
- The wound sometimes will be left open to heal by second intention. Head, legs, or small defects in the fingers are the usual areas.
- Clean the surgical site with saline and dry well.
- Afterward, a petrolatum-based ointment is applied and a dressing with gauze and Micropore Surgical Tape is placed over the wound.

CONVENTIONAL SURGERY

- In some places, where MMS is not an option to treat their patients, a similar approach is made; however, the margin from the tumor edges is wider (5 mm).
- Conventional surgery can be performed if the tumor is a "low risk" in the stratification (Table 122.1).
- Personally, the authors recommend marking the edge of the specimen with a suture (eg, 12 o'clock one suture and 3 o'clock two sutures) and two small cuts (at 6 o'clock and 9 o'clock) on the specimen when conventional surgery is performed to have an idea where a further approach should be made if a margin is positive to the tumor.

Postprocedural Approach

- Pain often increases during the night after the excision. Pain medications such as Tylenol are usually enough to control it. After the second day, pain should decrease.
- It is normal to have swelling and bruising around the surgical site. The bruising will fade in approximately 10 to 14 days. Elevate the area to reduce swelling.
- The bandage stays in place for 48 hours. Remove after this time, cleaning daily with saline and gauze and closing with a BAND-AID™ (Johnson & Johnson, US) or gauze and tape (Micropore Surgical Tape).
- For skin grafts, avoid prolonged exposure to extremely cold temperatures for 3 weeks.
- Patients should be vigilantly monitored for signs and symptoms of infection, especially if there is pain, fever, or a reddish area.
- Postoperative downtime is significant, and patients should expect to be absent from school or work for 3 days for minor reconstructions and 5 days to a week for the bigger ones.
- When the suture is not absorbable, the stiches must be removed after 7 days.
- One week after surgery, the area should be cleaned with soapy water using a Q-tip or gauze pad (shower/bathe normally). Dry the wound, apply Vaseline™ (Conopco, Inc., US), Polysporin™ (Johnson & Johnson, US), or bacitracin ointment (do *not* use Neosporin™ [Johnson & Johnson, US]).
- Cover the wound with a nonstick gauze pad and paper tape.
- Repeat wound care once a day for another week.
- After 1 week, continue to apply ointment until fully healed.
- Patients are encouraged to contact the physician directly for concerns and physicians often provide their cell phones for direct contact and reassurance.

REFERENCES

1. Kim JYS, Kozlow JH, Mittal B, Moyer J, Olenecki T, Rodgers P; Work Group; Invited Reviewers. Guidelines of care for the management of cutaneous squamous cell carcinoma. *J Am Acad Dermatol.* 2018;78:560–578. doi:10.1016/j.jaad.2017.10.007.
2. Reena S, Reecha S, Kaushal K, Kumar VP, Singh JK. Laryngeal squamous cell carcinoma (SCC) in a 12-year-old boy with cutaneous metastasis: an unusual presentation. *J Clin Diagn Res.* 2014;8:QD01–QD02. doi:10.7860/JCDR/2014/8252.4582.
3. Kauvar AN, Arpey CJ, Hruza G, Olbricht SM, Bennett R, Mahmoud BH. Consensus for nonmelanoma skin cancer treatment, Part II: squamous cell carcinoma, including a cost analysis of treatment methods. *Dermatol Surg.* 2015;41:1214–1240. doi:10.1097/DSS.0000000000000478.

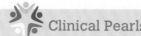

CHAPTER 123

Supernumerary Digits

Samuel H. Lance and Amanda A. Gosman

Introduction

Accessory or supernumerary digits, also referred to as poly-dactyly, can present on both the ulnar and radial aspects of the hand. Although polydactyly may present in all ethnicities, it presents at a rate 10-fold higher among African American ethnicities.[1] Ulnar polydactyly is referred to as "postaxial poly-dactyly" with radial polydactyly described as "preaxial poly-dactyly." Postaxial polydactyly remains the most common form of polydactyly and is often the simplest form to address. Polydactyly is further divided into multiple subtypes with type I being the mildest duplication.[1] Type I polydactyly presents as a small skin redundancy containing no associated bone or nail bed structures (Figure 123.1). Given the complexities of preaxial polydactyly and any polydactyly more significant than type I, it is the authors' recommendation for referral to a pediatric hand surgery specialist for management of these more complex duplications. The subject of this chapter focuses on type I postaxial polydactyly.

Simple ligation of simple polydactyly remains a common practice of treatment for many duplications. However, simple ligation as definitive polydactyly treatment has been shown to result in an increased rate of amputation neuromas and high rates of future revisions.[2] Anatomic studies have also demonstrated the presence of an accessory digital nerve within the duplicated polydactyly tissue. Consequently, managing these duplications via a more precise and anatomically directed approach may be more prudent.

This chapter addresses a directed approach for identification of the accessory digital nerve, protection of the ulnar small finger neurovascular bundle, appropriate ligation of the accessory neurovascular structures, and management of the overlying skin redundancy.

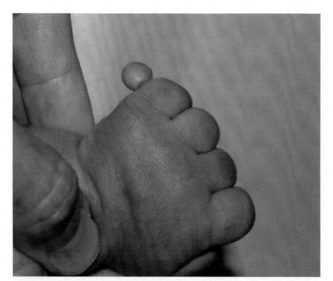

FIGURE 123.1. Preoperative photograph demonstrating type I postaxial (ulnar) polydactyly.

Clinical Pearls

- **Guidelines:** No specific treatment guidelines are known to exist for this condition.
- **Age-Specific Considerations:**
  - Damage to the native neurovascular bundle of the small finger may remain undiagnosed during infancy, presenting later in childhood. Inadvertent injury may lead to loss of protective sensibility, neglect of the digit with function, and delayed fine motor skill development.
  - The procedure can be safely performed on an infant under local anesthesia in the office or procedure room setting without the necessity for general anesthesia. The infant can be held by the parent during infiltration of the local anesthetic. Following infiltration, the infant can be fed and will often fall asleep. Once asleep following appropriate anesthesia, the procedure can be safely performed, with an assistant securely holding the affected extremity during the procedure.
- **Technique Tips:**
  - Loupe magnification should be utilized during this surgical procedure to allow for adequate visualization of the accessory neurovascular bundle and precise differentiation from the ulnar neurovascular bundle of the small finger.
  - Local anesthetic containing epinephrine remains a valuable adjunct allowing for a clear, bloodless surgical field that minimizes the need for electrocautery and, subsequently, reduces the risk of inadvertently damaging the ulnar neurovascular bundle.

Contraindications/Cautions/Risks

- As is true with any pediatric surgical discussion, the concerns for neurologic development following general anesthesia in the very young pediatric patient remain a subject of intense investigation. Type I polydactyly excision can safely be performed under local anesthesia by the experienced surgeon. Thus, it remains our recommendation for treatment of these lesions under local anesthesia when possible.
- Risks of nerve damage or postoperative neuroma formation should also be addressed with parents before surgery.

Equipment Needed

- Loupe magnification
- Local anesthetic, 1% lidocaine with epinephrine 1:100,000 (0.3 mL)
- Betadine or alcohol-containing prep solution
- Blade #15c (preferred) or #15
- Fine-toothed forceps
- Fine-tipped tenotomy scissors
- Fine needle driver
- 5-0 fast absorbing gut suture
- Skin adhesive glue (DERMABOND™ Topical Skin Adhesive [Ethicon US, LLC])

Preprocedural Approach

- A crucial element of success in the management of polydactyly begins with correct diagnosis of the underlying duplication.
  - Plain film X-rays of the affected hand should be obtained before treatment to assess for any underlying bony abnormalities.
  - A complete motor and neurovascular examination of the hand should be performed to identify any additional hand abnormalities.
  - Although the majority of polydactyly remains isolated without syndromic association, appropriate general pediatric follow-up with investigation for any associated syndromes should be recommended before surgical management.

Procedural Approach

- Treatment should begin with achieving adequate anesthesia.
  - Local anesthetic containing 1% lidocaine and 1 to 100 000 epinephrine is infiltrated into the area of the duplicated digit. A maximum of 0.3 mL of local anesthetic should be utilized.
  - Care should be taken to avoid excessive infiltration of local anesthetic, thus preventing increased compartment pressures within the digit and minimizing local tissue distortion.
  - The local anesthetic is allowed to remain in situ for approximately 15 minutes before intervention. This allows for maximal vasoconstriction and improves visualization during the procedure with minimal bleeding.
- As mentioned earlier, in the absence of general anesthesia, the infant should ideally be allowed to fall asleep before proceeding. Once asleep or placed under general anesthesia, the extremity is then firmly held in position by an assistant.
- The affected hand is then sterilely prepped with Betadine solution and draped with a surgical drape.
- It is the author's preference to utilize a #15c scalpel blade for incision because the smaller size of this blade allows for improved precision. In the absence of a #15c blade, a standard #15 blade can be utilized.
- A longitudinal ellipse is incised at the base of the duplicated digits, retaining some redundancy of the surrounding tissue to facilitate closure. Care is taken to only incise through the dermis, leaving the deep structures intact for further dissection.
- Following skin incision, fine-tipped tenotomy scissors are utilized under loupe magnification to bluntly dissect the soft tissues until the accessory digital nerve is identified. This can then be traced to its origin at the ulnar, small finger neurovascular bundle. Gentle traction is applied to the accessory digit, and the accessory digital nerve is incised sharply with a scalpel without damaging the adjacent small finger native neurovascular bundle. If bleeding is noted, gentle pressure should be applied to achieve hemostasis. Use of electrocautery may increase the risk of inadvertent injury to the ulnar nerve vascular bundle and should be avoided except in extreme circumstances.
- Following excision of the digit and adequate hemostasis, closure of the elliptical skin incision is then performed utilizing interrupted simple 5-0 fast absorbing suture (Figure 123.2).
- DERMABOND is then applied directly overlying the suture line to achieve a watertight closure.

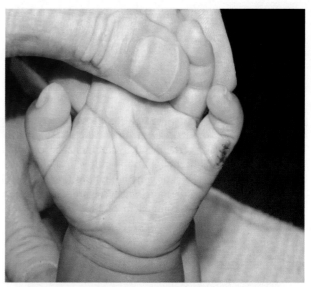

FIGURE 123.2. Intraoperative photograph with sutures and skin glue in place.

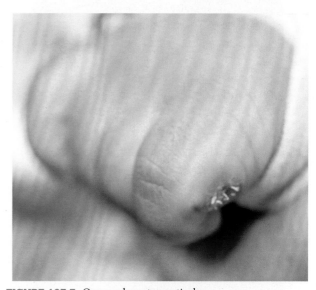

FIGURE 123.3. One week postoperatively.

Postprocedural Approach

- Postoperative antibiotics are not recommended for this procedure.
- Homecare should include normal daily washing with gentle drying of the surgical site.
- The patient should be evaluated in 1 week's time for assessment of appropriate wound healing (Figure 123.3).
- The overlying skin glue will begin to elevate within approximately 10 to 14 days following the procedure.
- Complete absorption of the underlying suture is anticipated by 2 to 3 weeks following intervention.

REFERENCES

1. Delgadillo D, Adams NS, Girotto JA. Supernumerary digits of the hand. *Eplasty*. 2016;16:ic3.
2. Leber GE, Gosain AK. Surgical excision of pedunculated supernumerary digits prevents traumatic amputation neuromas. *Pediatr Dermatol*. 2003;20(2):108–112.

CHAPTER 124

Tattoo Removal

Richard L. Lin, Alexa Beth Steuer, Wesley Andrews Duerson, Sarah Azarchi, and Jeremy A. Brauer

Introduction

Laser tattoo removal is certainly not as common a procedure in the pediatric and adolescent population as it is in adults. In addition to traumatic (carbon or graphite) tattoos (Figure 124.1), the art of tattooing has become widely regarded as a means of self-expression and a component of the identity-forming

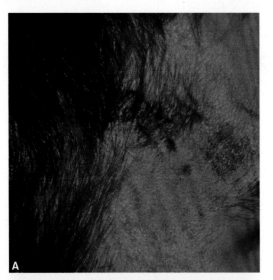

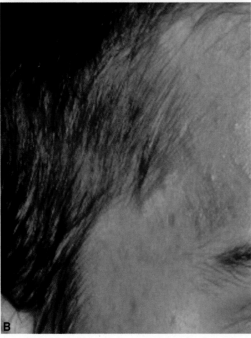

FIGURE 124.1. A, Traumatic "tattooing" with asphalt. B, After three treatments with Q-switched Nd:YAG laser. Reprinted with permission from Krakowski AC, Shumaker PR. *The Scar Book.* Philadelphia, PA: Wolters Kluwer; 2017. Figure 13.16A-B.

experience of adolescence in Western culture, although most parents strongly supported state laws requiring parental consent for tattoos for minors. Many states within the United States allow tattooing in those younger than age 18 with the written consent of a legal guardian.

Although smaller tattoos in certain anatomic locations are amenable to surgical excision, most tattoos are removed by means of laser treatment. Modern laser tattoo removal is largely based on the principle of selective photothermolysis. This principle states that the use of a proper wavelength of light can cause the light energy from that source to be preferentially absorbed by a target chromophore within the skin. This light energy is subsequently converted into heat energy. Different chromophores that can be found in the skin include endogenous (melanin) and exogenous (ink particles) pigments, hemoglobin, and water, which preferentially absorb different wavelengths of light. In this way, lasers can target specific pigments, such as those found in tattoos, while sparing other intradermal structures.

Herein, we discuss the practice and procedure of tattoo removal in the pediatric population that address unique challenges. Our approach seeks to achieve satisfactory clinical results while minimizing adverse events. In the authors' experience, recent innovations have allowed for the successful removal of previously challenging pigments, such as blue and green, with the availability of shorter pulse durations, and the ability to deliver multiple treatments in one session with new tools such as the perfluorodecalin patch.

 Clinical Pearls

- **Guidelines:** No specific treatment guidelines are known to exist for this condition.
- **Age-Specific Considerations:** Ideally, patients should be old enough to ask for treatment for themselves and be developed enough to assist in detecting and reporting postsurgical complications such as increasing pain, redness, warmth, swelling, and fever/chills.
- **Technique Tips:** The authors prefer first anesthetizing the skin with topical and/or injectable anesthetic before laser treatment.
- **Skin of Color Considerations:** The general technique can be used on all skin types; however, the risk of dyspigmentation increases with darker skin types. Threshold responses will normally occur at lower fluences, and longer wavelength devices such as the 1064-nm Nd:YAG laser and use of hydrogel or perfluorodecalin-infused patches should be used to minimize epidermal damage.

Contraindications/Cautions/Risks

Contraindications

- Active skin infection on treated area (especially herpes labialis or impetigo)

- Inability to care for postoperative wounds
- History of gold therapy
- Uncontrolled diabetes
- History of keloid or hypertrophic scar formation

Cautions

- Presence of tanned skin (by sun or artificial means) may increase risk of dyspigmentation; iron oxide–containing tattoos

Risks

- Dyspigmentation, scarring, pain, bleeding, poor cosmesis including paradoxical darkening, and need for multiple treatments, and death (infection or anaphylaxis from anesthesia)

Equipment Needed

- Anesthetics (eg, lidocaine, benzocaine)
- Wavelength-specific goggles
- Eye shields (including intraocular where appropriate)
- Surgical masks
- Gloves
- Smoke evacuator
- Nanosecond, picosecond, and nonablative and ablative fractional lasers
- Perfluorodecalin patch *(optional)*
- Petrolatum-based ointment
- Telfa
- Paper tape
- Ice packs

Preprocedural Approach

- Relevant history includes postinflammatory hyperpigmentation, wound healing disorders, or bleeding disorders.
- A full tattoo history including type (amateur versus professional), age, and location is critical because these factors may influence the number of laser treatments necessary for clearance.
- Fitzpatrick skin type should also be noted, because darker skinned individuals are at a higher risk for complications, and require a more conservative approach in general.
- Counsel patient and parent/guardian that multiple sessions are almost always required for laser tattoo clearance.

TABLE 124.1 : Appropriate Laser Wavelengths and Pulse Durations for Specific Tattoo Pigments

COLOR	WAVELENGTH (nm)	PULSE DURATION
Black	694, 755, 1064	nanosecond; picosecond
Blue	755, 785	picosecond
Green	755, 785	nanosecond; picosecond
Purple	755, 785	picosecond
Red	532	nanosecond; picosecond
Yellow	532	nanosecond; picosecond
Orange	532	nanosecond; picosecond

- Patients should minimize sun exposure and maximize sun protection so that their skin is as light (ie, untanned) as possible. Although there will be seasonal and geographic dependence, the approach reduces melanin in the skin as a competing chromophore.
- Depending on anatomic location and medical history, do consider prophylaxis for herpes simplex.

Procedural Approach ▶

- Informed consent from the parent/guardian and, when possible, assent from the minor, and photographs are obtained.
- Typically, anesthesia is utilized because of pain associated with the procedure. In addition to topical agents, the use of infiltrative anesthesia and, in certain cases, nerve blocks should be employed.
- Surface of tattoo should be meticulously cleaned.
- Appropriate device-specific protective eyewear should be worn, and patients should have eye pads.
- Select the appropriate laser and parameters (Table 124.1).
  - Patients with darker skin types will experience threshold responses at lower fluences; therefore, Q-switched or picosecond devices should be used to minimize epidermal damage.
- A perfluorodecalin patch, which is an optical clearing agent, can be used to facilitate the dissipation of the epidermal whitening due to cavitation effects arising from the laser interaction with the tattoo ink and surrounding tissues. This allows for multiple laser passes to be performed in one treatment setting.
- Initially, a test spot could be done to determine the optimal fluence depending on the tissue response.
  - The ideal response is tissue whitening in the treated area.
  - An undesired response to the laser presents as epidermal disruption or bleeding that may indicate excessive fluence.
  - The physician should adjust the fluence of the laser accordingly when an undesired response occurs.
  - Throughout the treatment course, the parameters (including spot size, pulse duration, and fluence) should be modified accordingly.
- Immediately after surgery, a petrolatum-based ointment is liberally applied with a protective dressing.
- Ice packs may be applied to help decrease discomfort and limit edema.

Postprocedural Approach

- Generally, swelling and pain should decrease quickly with time.
- Patients should continue herpes prophylaxis for a total of 7 to 10 days.
- Whitening of the skin is also expected and this should fade within 20 to 30 minutes of treatment if the perfluorodecalin patch is not utilized.
- Darkening or crusting of the skin in the treated area may also occur, and, if so, the area should be cleaned and covered in occlusive ointments.
- Blistering or vesiculation can occur, and patients should be cautioned to expect this possibility subsequent to laser treatment.
- Emollients, cold compresses, and occlusive dressings may provide relief.

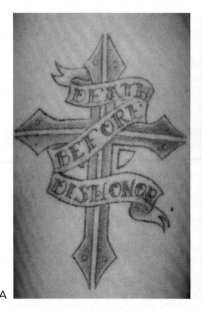
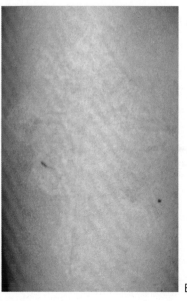

FIGURE 124.2. Black cross tattoo before (A) and after (B) four treatments with a picosecond 755-nm laser. Reprinted from Small R. *A Practical Guide to Laser Procedures.* Philadelphia, PA: Wolters Kluwer; 2015. Figure 14.4A-B. Rebecca Small©, MD.

- It is possible for some patients to experience an urticarial rash, requiring oral antihistamines.
- Minimize long-term complications, namely, hypopigmentation and scarring, by avoiding excess sun exposure.
- Improvement in tattoo pigment should be expected within weeks to months of the treatment, although patients should be extensively counseled on realistic expectations regarding clearance, and that several treatment sessions are almost always required (Figure 124.2).
- Patients are encouraged to contact the physician directly for concerns.

SUGGESTED READINGS

Biesman BS, O'Neil MP, Costner C. Rapid, high-fluence multi-pass q-switched laser treatment of tattoos with a transparent perfluorodecalin-infused patch: a pilot study. *Lasers Surg Med.* 2015;47(8):613–618.

Brauer JA, Reddy KK, Anolik R, et al. Successful and rapid treatment of blue and green tattoo pigment with a novel picosecond laser. *Arch Dermatol.* 2012;148(7):820–823.

Saedi N, Metelitsa A, Petrell K, Arndt KA, Dover JS. Treatment of tattoos with a picosecond alexandrite laser: a prospective trial. *Arch Dermatol.* 2012;148(12):1360–1363.

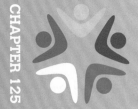

CHAPTER 125

Telangiectasia

Brent C. Martin and Christopher B. Zachary

Introduction

Telangiectasia (interchangeably known as telangiectases) are blood vessels, visible to the naked eye, that are recognized as 0.1- to 1-mm vascular dilatations frequently presenting on the face, especially around the nose, cheeks, and chin. They often appear as a sign of cutaneous photoaging and rosacea. Congenital diseases including hereditary hemorrhagic telangiectasia (HHT) (also known as Osler-Weber-Rendu syndrome) and ataxia-telangiectasia will be diagnosed in part with the development of telangiectases earlier on in life. Current management strategies are largely in the domain of lasers. Treatment is indicated for both medical and cosmetic reasons.

Although telangiectases are the visible component of rosacea, a larger part of this condition is the underlying "blush" of this condition, which is also very amenable to laser treatment. The goal is to achieve optimal clinical improvement while minimizing adverse effects. Using the concept of selective photothermolysis, lasers are the preferred devices for treatment because they can target vessels while avoiding the surrounding tissues.

The workhorse device in the United States has been the pulsed-dye lasers (PDLs) with their 585/595-nm wavelength, variable pulse width, large beam diameter, excellent cooling, and significant speed of delivery. Alternatively, intense pulse light (IPL) can be used to induce a similar response. Individual vessels can be elegantly traced using the potassium titanyl phosphate (KTP; 532 nm) lasers, and, less commonly, the 940-nm wavelength is useful for deeper larger vessels. In this regard, larger vessels on the face or on the trunk and limbs can be eradicated using the more deeply penetrating, longer wavelength devices, namely, the long-pulsed Nd:YAG 1064-nm and alexandrite (755 nm) lasers. Electrocoagulation is still used by some for single telangiectasia, although this modality is less selective and less safe.

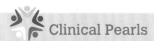 Clinical Pearls

- **Guidelines:**
  - Lasers remain the treatment of choice for telangiectases, although erythematous telangiectatic rosacea can be managed by topical vasoconstrictor agents.
- **Age-Specific Considerations:**
  - The great majority of patients will be older children, adolescents, or young adults with whom a full discussion concerning the optimal treatments, potential complications, and full consent will take place.
  - When pediatric patients are the subject of diagnosis and treatment, they should be brought into the discussion, as appropriate for their age, with their parents or guardians. There should be no surprises; the well-informed child will be more responsive and tolerant than are those who are kept ignorant.
  - In the case of children, they must be positioned to avoid sudden movements, which might induce misplaced laser pulses.
- **Technique Tips:**
  - Wavelength-specific eye protection must always be used. Alternatively, laser-safe adhesive pads or brushed steel eye protectors should be employed.
  - Spider telangiectases can be seen in both children and adults and are best treated with PDLs using short purpuric-inducing 1.5-ms pulses and the dynamic cooling device.
  - PDLs with longer pulse durations (6 ms or greater) can treat telangiectases with minimal purpura. When these longer pulse durations are used, immediate delivery of two to three repeated pulses to the same area (pulse stacking) may be cautiously utilized, but must be delivered with appropriate cooling.
  - Utilization of purpuric settings (pulse durations of 3 ms or shorter) may result in fewer treatment sessions, although some patients may not want purpura.
  - Always examine the laser tissue interaction; a gray tissue response likely indicates epidermal damage. If this occurs, treatment should be stopped or settings adjusted. If gray discoloration is persistent, this may result in scarring. Thus, knowledge of proper treatment end points is critically necessary. The potential for scarring can be minimized by regularly performing test pulses.
- **Skin of Color Considerations:**
  - Tanned skin is never safe to treat.
  - Patients with darker skin tones are at an increased risk for scarring and postinflammatory hyperpigmentation (PIH).
  - Utilization of lower fluences, longer wavelengths, longer pulse durations, and adequate cooling is recommended when treating patients with darker skin types.
  - In addition to proper sun protection, daily applications of a bleaching cream, such as hydroquinone 4% after treatment, can reduce the risk of PIH.

Contraindications/Cautions/Risks

Contraindications

- Active skin infection at the time of procedure, that is, herpes labialis, impetigo, candidiasis

Cautions

- Tanned and darker skin types are at an increased risk for scarring and PIH.

Risks

- Erythema, bruising, swelling, infection, scarring (rare), pain, blistering/erosions, hyper/hypopigmentation, recurrence of telangiectases, eye injury if proper eye protection is not utilized
- Hair loss can occur with millisecond lasers or IPL, particularly in patients with darker hair.

Equipment Needed

- Laser eye protection for all present in room
- 585/595-nm PDL
- 1064-nm Nd:YAG laser
- 532-nm frequency-doubled Nd:YAG laser
- 755-nm alexandrite laser
- 940-nm diode laser
- IPL device
- Hyfrecator 2000 with epilating needle
- Cooling, ice bag
- Petrolatum-based ointment/aloe vera/topical steroid ointment

Preprocedural Approach

- An initial consultation is important to discuss the risks/benefits and treatment options, set expectations, and to determine if additional workup is needed. As with any procedure, it is important to weigh factors such as the patient's budget and availability.
- HHT, ataxia-telangiectasia, and connective tissue diseases need to be considered when evaluating patients with numerous telangiectases involving suspicious areas. Appropriate physical examination, blood work, and imaging should be ordered if suspicions arise.
- Ideally, photographs should be taken before each treatment to track improvement.
- Before treatment, nonsteroidal anti-inflammatory drugs (NSAIDs) should be avoided because they can theoretically inhibit necessary clotting mechanisms and hinder optimal results.

Procedural Approach

- Informed consent should be obtained before the procedure from the parent/guardian.
- Wavelength-specific protective eyewear should be worn at all times by both the patient and all of those present in the room.
- Adequate cooling should be utilized to prevent injury to the epidermis and dermis. Many devices are equipped with cryogen spray or contact cooling devices.
- For superficial/smaller lesions, the 532-nm frequency-doubled Nd:YAG laser is commonly used to treat facial telangiectases with minimal to no purpura. Parameters will vary according to the KTP laser utilized, some being more powerful than others. Moving slowly will allow the operator to trace the individual vessels (Figure 125.1). There is increased melanin absorption at this wavelength and a resultant greater risk in darker skin types.
- Deeper/larger lesions are often resistant to the 532-nm frequency-doubled Nd:YAG laser. The 585/595-nm PDL

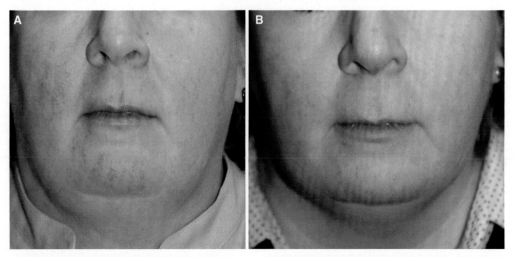

FIGURE 125.1. Preoperative and postoperative results utilizing Excel V (532 nm), 8 J/cm², 10-mm spot size, 10-ms pulse duration. Photos courtesy of Ashish Bhatia, MD and Jeffrey Hsu, MD.

enables the operator to deliver energy somewhat deeper into the skin (fluence varies depending on spot size [7-12 mm] and pulse duration [1.5-20 ms]). Pulses can also be stacked when longer pulse durations are utilized (6 or 10 ms), but associated cooling is imperative. Vessel contraction or transient blue coagulum and/or purpura indicate appropriate end points of therapy.

- PDL Candela Perfecta 595 nm recommended parameters for telangiectasias:
  - Multipulse technique to avoid bruising appearance: 595 nm, 5 to 7 J/cm², 7-mm beam diameter, 6 ms, Dynamic Cooling Device on II or III, multiple pulse technique with three or four pulses until the vessel goes from red to blue to gone
  - Single-pulse technique with bruising: 595 nm, 6 to 7 J/cm², 7-mm beam diameter, 1.5 ms, Dynamic Cooling Device single pulse
- For even larger, more nodular/dark blue lesions, the long-pulsed 1064-nm Nd:YAG laser can be utilized. There is an increased risk of scarring with this wavelength, and this device should be used cautiously by experienced users for treatment of facial lesions.
- For diffuse involvement, IPL can be utilized successfully with a 570-nm cutoff filter. IPL can be less efficacious for the treatment of larger/darker individual vessels.
- If there is an isolated lesion, electrocoagulation by epilating needle is used by some. The epilating needle is attached to a Hyfrecator 2000™ (Conmed, Utica, NY) on the low setting (3-4). The operator should make sure to use the smallest burst of energy possible and move about 5 mm downstream until the vessel blanches and disappears.
- Follow-up treatments are often necessary because telangiectases can recur and new lesions will develop with time.

Postprocedural Approach

- After surgery, ice may be utilized for any discomfort. Some will give a single application of triamcinolone 0.1% ointment to reduce post laser redness and swelling.
- Mild topical emollients, such as petrolatum, can be used if any scabs develop.
- Patients are instructed to wash their face with a mild cleanser daily and to practice sun avoidance and protection as well as limiting trauma to the treated area. This can help decrease future hyperpigmentation and scarring.
- Multiple treatments are often required to achieve the best results for telangiectases and are usually performed at 4- to 6-week intervals until appropriate cosmetic results are obtained. The skin should be evaluated for atrophy, scarring, or dyspigmentation.
- Contact information for the physician is provided to the patient after the procedure. They are encouraged to call with concerns such as blistering, pain, or fever.
- Viral, fungal, and bacterial (including mycobacterial) infections are uncommon after utilization of these minimally invasive lasers, but they do occur. Patients who tend to have herpes simplex virus (HSV) cold sores should be considered for antiviral medications.

SUGGESTED READINGS

Cassuto DA, Ancona DM, Emanuelli G. Treatment of facial telangiectasias with a diode-pumped Nd:YAG laser at 532 nm. *J Cutan Laser Ther*. 2000;2:141–146.

Clementoni MT, Gilardino P, Muti GF, et al. Facial telangiectasias: our experience in treatment with IPL. *Lasers Surg Med*. 2005; 37:9.

Iyer S, Fitzpatrick RE. Long-pulsed dye laser treatment for facial telangiectasias and erythema: evaluation of a single purpuric pass versus multiple subpurpuric passes. *Dermatol Surg*. 2005;31:898.

Umbilical Granuloma

Venkata Anisha Guda and John C. Browning

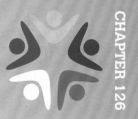

CHAPTER 126

Introduction

Approximately 1 of 500 newborn babies has an umbilical granuloma (umbilical pyogenic granuloma). An umbilical granuloma is an overgrowth of tissue that forms during the healing process of the belly button, after the umbilical cord is cut. It has the appearance of a soft pink or red nodule and can be wet or leak small amounts of clear or yellow fluid. Umbilical granulomas are 3 to 10 mm in size and made up of overgrowth of tissue containing fibroblasts and capillaries (Figure 126.1). They appear during the first few weeks of a baby's life. The granuloma can become infected and result in other symptoms, such as skin irritation around the belly button and fever. The granuloma often appears pedunculated. These can also form in adults because of navel piercings. Normally, after the umbilical cord is cut, a small "stump" is left in the belly button. In most cases, it desiccates and falls off. However, in some cases, when the stump falls off, a granuloma can form. The delay in time for the umbilical cord to fall off can result in the granuloma formation. It can also be due to how the tissue heals as the umbilical cord separates from the baby. Another possibility is due to a subclinical infection in the umbilical stump. Inflammation can result in the presence of an overgrowth of endothelial cells and inadequate epithelialization. As a result, umbilical granuloma formation is due to an inflammatory process and delay in umbilical cord separation. Symptoms and signs of local infection or sepsis such as edema and hyperemia in surrounding skin, fever, drainage, and purulence may accompany an umbilical granuloma; these complications require systemic treatment and hospitalization in the appropriate setting.

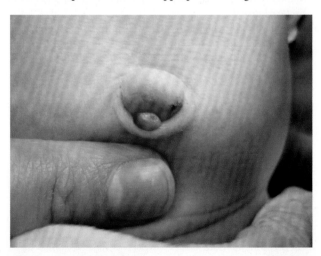

FIGURE 126.1. Umbilical granulomas appear as a soft pink or red nodule, can be wet or leak small amounts of clear or yellow fluid, 3 to 10 mm in size, and are made up of overgrowth of tissue containing fibroblasts and capillaries. Reprinted with permission from Goodheart HP. *Goodheart's Same-Site Differential Diagnosis: A Rapid Method of Diagnosing and Treating Common Skin Disorders.* Philadelphia, PA: Wolters Kluwer Health/Lippincott Williams & Wilkins; 2010. Figure 17.3.

Clinical Pearls

- **Technique Tips**: There are several options to treat a complicated umbilical granuloma.
  - Silver nitrate is the most common treatment option in newborns. It is a local chemical cauterizing agent. Applying this solution causes the granuloma to desiccate and heal with resolution. To prevent tissue injury, extra silver nitrate should be wiped off from the skin and allowed to dry after being put on.
  - Cryosurgery with liquid nitrogen is another treatment option and may offer rapid healing compared to the usage of electrocautery.
  - Excision and the subsequent application of absorbable hemostatic materials is another approach that helps avoid chemical burns. This technique is simple, safe, and inexpensive. Traditional surgery is favored for treating large umbilical granulomas.
  - A surgical thread can also be used to tie off the base of the granuloma. This cuts off the blood supply to the tissue, and it will eventually fall off. Many umbilical granulomas are located deep within the umbilical region and are difficult to locate. The "double-ligature" technique is able to overcome the difficulty of ligating the granuloma at its base.
  - Topical steroid provides an additional safe and effective treatment option. One study found that topical steroid ointment is as effective as silver nitrate and has a reduced risk of causing chemical burns to form. Another study compared the efficacy of silver nitrate versus clobetasol propionate cream versus ethanol wipes and found that treating umbilical granulomas with topical clobetasol propionate cream at home may be as effective as using topical silver nitrate in the clinic.
  - If there is an umbilical granuloma and no sign of infection, then the twice-daily application of a pinch of table salt to the tissue can be used. This is one of the most effective and safe treatments that can be done at home. After the belly button is cleaned with warm water, a small pinch of salt is applied, and, the area should be covered with a piece of gauze for 30 minutes. The salt should then be rinsed off with a clean gauze dressing soaked in sterile water. An alternative approach consists of, first, cleaning the area. Next, common table salt is applied to the lesion; the granuloma is then occluded with surgical adhesive tape for 24 hours. The tape is removed the next day and the area is reassessed for any complications. Both techniques are inexpensive, easy to perform, and can lead to rapid resolution.
  - The tissue may also be removed by a trained professional with a scalpel or knife.[1]
- **Relative Effectiveness:** There is a lack of evidence regarding the best treatment option for umbilical granulomas.

Contraindications/Cautions/Risks

Contraindications
- Active skin infection

Cautions
- Ultrasonography of the abdomen may be required before the procedure if there is concern that the lesion could be an omphalomesenteric or urachal abnormality.
- Because chemical burns to the periumbilical area can be a complication with silver nitrate treatment, caution is necessary (Figure 126.2). The surrounding normal skin should be protected with petroleum jelly.
- Topical silver nitrate should not be applied to broken skin.
- Topical silver nitrate is not suitable for application to anogenital regions and should not be used on the face or for application to large areas.
- Topical silver nitrate should not be used when there are signs of an allergic reaction to the drug or a very bad irritation where the drug is used.
- Silver nitrate can directly reduce fibroblast proliferation, so it should not be used long term.

Risks
- The side effects associated with silver nitrate include chemical burns to the surrounding skin and staining of the skin.
- There can be irritation where the chemical cautery agent is used.
- During treatment with silver nitrate, some patients report pain or a burning sensation that may need a medication or topical anesthetic to alleviate.

Equipment Needed
- Sterile dressing tray
- Sterile gloves
- Normal saline solution
- Bacteriostatic sterile water
- Silver nitrate sticks
- Barrier ointment (eg, sterile petroleum jelly)
- Occlusive dressing

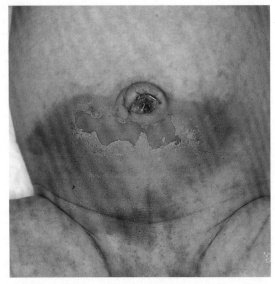

FIGURE 126.2. Chemical burn complication of silver nitrate treatment. Reprinted with permission from Fleisher GR, Ludwig S, Baskin MN. *Atlas of Pediatric Emergency Medicine*. Philadelphia, PA: Lippincott Williams & Wilkins; 2004. Figure 20.1A.

Preprocedural Approach

- In some cases, a topical anesthetic should be applied before the procedure to reduce the pain associated with the silver nitrate.
- Before the procedure, it is important to assess the site for its suitability for applying silver nitrate.
- The site should be cleansed with normal saline (or other appropriate skin cleanser) and dried with sterile dressing or gauze.

Procedural Approach

The intraoperative technique steps for the application of silver nitrate can be found here:
- Wash hands thoroughly using chlorhexidine soap or antibacterial soap.
- Open the dressing tray and add supplies.
- Remove dressing and assess the site for suitability of application of silver nitrate.
- Clean the site thoroughly.
- Apply barrier ointment (eg, sterile petroleum jelly) to the surrounding skin.
- Moisten the tip of the silver nitrate stick with a minimal amount of bacteriostatic sterile water. Make sure that the silver nitrate stick is not so wet that it drips.
- Rub and rotate the tip of the silver nitrate stick along the granuloma tissue beginning at the area proximal to the exit site and moving outward. Two minutes of contact time is usually sufficient. Keep in mind that the degree of caustic action depends on the quantity of silver nitrate delivered, which depends on the length of time the moistened tip is left in contact with the tissue. Avoid touching the silver nitrate stick to the surrounding healthy skin. Repeat with a new silver nitrate stick as required (Figure 126.3).
- For cauterizing purposes, apply pressure during the procedure.
- Stop the treatment procedure if the burning sensation is too much for the patient to endure without any anesthetic.
- Manually remove dead and extra tissue to reduce the risk of bacterial growth.
- Use a damp saline gauze to gently clean the treated area after application. Pat dry to avoid trauma to the surrounding tissue. Do not rub or apply friction to the treated area.

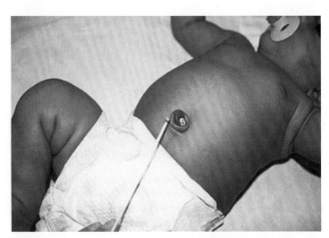

FIGURE 126.3. Umbilical granuloma following treatment with silver nitrate. Reprinted with permission from Chung EK, Atkinson-McEvoy LR, Boom JA, et al. *Visual Diagnosis and Treatment in Pediatrics*. 2nd ed. Philadelphia, PA: Wolters Kluwer Health/Lippincott Williams & Wilkins; 2010. Figure 35.4.

- Apply topical antibacterial solution to the treated area. This can include alcohol, triple dye, bacitracin, silver sulfadiazine, povidone-iodine, chlorhexidine, or hexachlorophene.
- Apply the occlusive dressing to the wound site.

Postprocedural Approach

- It may take more than one treatment to resolve the granuloma. If the granuloma persists after three or four applications that are performed at an interval of 3 to 4 days, then other potential underlying conditions (eg, an omphalomesenteric duct cyst or urachal cyst or other abnormality) and alternative treatments should be considered.
- Follow-up care is very important for umbilical granulomas in neonates.
  - The silver nitrate can cause a dark stain on any skin it touches. The color will go away, but it can take up to a week.
  - In some cases, silver nitrate can cause the skin to burn and become red. There can be a mild skin injury. This will heal with time.
  - The size and quality of the healing granuloma and the nearby skin should be checked daily while the wound heals.
  - An important complication of umbilical granulomas is omphalitis, or umbilical stump infection. Parents should contact their provider if the normal skin around the belly button is open, red, or starts to peel, or if the granuloma does not shrink in size. Providers should also be notified it there is pus draining from the wound area, if the baby develops a fever, if the baby cries when the navel or the skin around it is palpated, if the area bleeds, or if the baby develops a rash, pimples, or blisters around the navel.
  - It is important to clean the area at least once a day and as needed during diaper changes or baths. All drainage should be removed. A cotton swab should be soaked in warm water and mild soap. Excess water should be squeezed out. The sides of the navel should be wiped. The skin around the navel should also be wiped. The area should be patted dry with a soft cloth.
  - The baby's diaper should be folded below the navel until the granuloma is completely healed to prevent mechanical irritation. If that is not practical, then an area should be cut out in front of the diaper to keep the navel exposed to the air.
  - The baby should be bathed with a sponge or a damp wash cloth. The area should be kept above the water level until it heals. The surrounding tissue should be protected with Vaseline™ (Conopco, Inc., US).

SUGGESTED READINGS

Brodsgaard A, Nielsen T, Molgaard U, Pryds O, Pedersen P. Treating umbilical granuloma with topical clobetasol propionate cream at home is as effective as treating it with topical silver nitrate in the clinic. *Acta Paediatr.* 2015;104(2):174–177.

Murrell D. What is umbilical granuloma and how is it treated? Healthline. https://www.healthline.com/health/umbilical-granuloma#-causes. Accessed November 8, 2017.

MyHealth.Alberta. Umbilical granuloma: care instructions. https://myhealth.alberta.ca/Health/aftercareinformation/pages/conditions.aspx?hwid=abp5555. Accessed May 12, 2017.

Venous Malformations

Shehla Admani and Joyce M. C. Teng

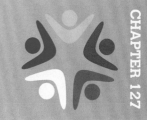

CHAPTER 127

Introduction

Venous malformations (VMs) are congenital vascular anomalies that are present at birth but may not always be immediately recognizable (Figures 127.1 and 127.2). They tend to increase in size over time, and accelerated growth is often noted with hormonal changes (such as during puberty). Larger lesions can be complicated by associated coagulopathy and phleboliths, resulting in pain, swelling, and erythema.

Management options include observation, laser surgery, sclerotherapy, and excision and medical therapy for malformation as well as associated complications. For localized small VMs, surgical excision offers a possible definitive treatment option. For complex and extensive VMs, combined medical and surgical interventions may be beneficial. The superficial components of these large VMs can often be treated with laser surgery to improve cosmesis as well as to reduce intermittent bleeding at the affected sites. However, the intradermal and subcutaneous components can often benefit from sclerotherapy by a skilled interventional radiologist comfortable working with children. Sclerotherapy can also be performed before surgery to decrease the size of the lesion, surgical complexity, and resultant surgical scar. It can also be performed before or concurrent with laser treatment to optimize the overall outcome. A multidisciplinary, multimodal approach should therefore be employed in the management of complex VMs.

The scope of this chapter is to offer step-by-step instruction for the treatment of VMs. Our protocol utilizes long-pulsed alexandrite laser (755 nm), often in combination with long-pulsed Nd:YAG laser (1064 nm), as well as pulsed-dye laser (595 nm) depending on the morphology of the vascular malformation. We aim to achieve lasting clinical improvement while minimizing adverse events. In the authors' experience, long-term (ie, years) disease remission can be achieved, especially when appropriate combination therapies are employed. However, as demonstrated in recent literature, VMs result from somatic mutations of the *Tie2* gene most of the time. Recurrence, therefore, remains a lifelong possibility. Periodic "touch-up" treatments may be needed, especially in areas where residual lesions remain.

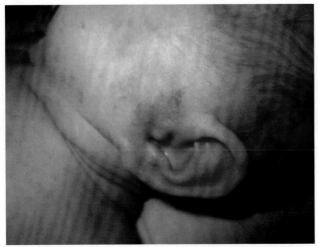

FIGURE 127.1. Young infant with a venous malformation of the left cheek (confirmed by magnetic resonance imaging/magnetic resonance angiography); with the patient's head held in a nondependent position, the lesion is less noticeable clinically. Photo courtesy of Andrew C. Krakowski, MD.

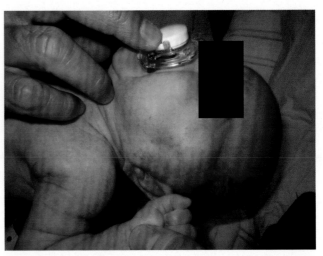

FIGURE 127.2. With the patient's head held in a more dependent position, the lesion fills slowly and becomes more prominent. This technique helps to make the diagnosis of "venous malformation" and may also be utilized to increase the target chromophore during laser surgery. Photo courtesy of Andrew C. Krakowski, MD.

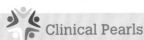
Clinical Pearls

- **Guidelines:** There are no published treatment guidelines for this condition.
- **Age-Specific Considerations:** Because these lesions tend to progress over time, early intervention should be considered. However, in cases that require general anesthesia, it is reasonable to postpone elective laser surgery until general anesthesia is considered to be safe. Laser surgery can also be coordinated with other procedures to minimize the overall number of general anesthesia needed for these treatments.
- **Technique Tips:** Concurrent use of antiangiogenic therapy such as mammalian target of rapamycin (mTOR) inhibitor may reduce disease burden and prevent rebound growth.
- **Skin of Color Considerations:** Laser settings should be adjusted to minimize epidermal pigment damage and strict sun protection is always advised for darker skin patients.

Contraindications/Cautions/Risks

Contraindications
- Active skin infection
- Inability to care for postoperative wounds (eg, upcoming sporting events, vacations)

Cautions
- Presence of a suntan may increase dyspigmentation after laser surgery.

Risks
- Pain, bleeding, blistering, infection, dyspigmentation, and scarring

Equipment Needed
- Wavelength-specific eye shields (metal corneal eye shields if treating periorbital area)
- Pulsed-dye laser
- Long-pulsed alexandrite laser
- Long-pulsed Nd:YAG laser
- Sterile water
- Gauze (wet and dry)
- Petrolatum-based ointment
- Ice
- Anesthetic: can vary from case to case and generally consists of either topical or general anesthesia followed by injectable local anesthetic. Young children (ie, younger than 10 years of age) typically require sedation. Owing to controversial literature on risks and long-term sequelae from general anesthesia in pediatric patients, referral to a tertiary care center is recommended.
  - Because these procedures are associated with significant discomfort when performed in outpatient clinics, higher percentages of topical lidocaine, that is, up to 30% compounded ointment or mixture of lidocaine and tetracaine, are often used. When using higher percentages of lidocaine, it is important to be mindful of the body surface area being treated and limiting application to less than 1% BSA for less than 30 minutes. Before application of topical lidocaine or injection of local lidocaine, risks of potential systemic absorption should be considered. Maximum allowed local anesthetic dosing should be calculated depending on the patient's weight.
- Surgical prep (isopropyl alcohol, chlorhexidine, and Betadine followed by sterile water cleansing to remove residue chemicals on the skin)
- Dressing (will vary depending on treatment site)

Preprocedural Approach

- Sun protection is recommended before the procedure to reduce the risk of epidermal damage and to assure optimal treatment.
- Antiviral prophylaxis should be considered when treating patients with facial VMs and history of herpes labialis.
- Although controlled studies are needed, there is anecdotal experience suggesting the use of antiangiogenic therapy such as mTOR inhibitors can be beneficial before and/or concurrent with laser treatments.

Procedural Approach

- The types of anesthetics used for the laser procedure should be determined depending on age/pain tolerance of the patient, location, and extent of the VM. Although the combined use of topical and local injectable anesthetics may be applicable for adolescents and young adults undergoing these laser procedures, general anesthesia is often needed for young children or those with extensive VMs or VMs involving oral mucosa or genital area. With smaller lesions, it is best to avoid the use of anesthetic with epinephrine because this can cause vasoconstriction and, therefore, reduce the efficacy of the treatment. However, in larger lesions, it can be difficult to obtain adequate analgesia to perform the procedure in office without use of epinephrine. Risks and benefits must be weighed and an appropriate regimen should be determined on an individualized basis.

- Appropriate protective eyewear should be worn by both care providers and patients during the entire procedure. Disposable adhesive eye shields are easy to use on patients and offer full eye protection from medical lasers with wavelengths between 190 and 11 000 nm at an optical density greater than 7 (OD 7@190-11 000 nm). Correctly fitted metal corneal eye shields should be placed when the periorbital area is being treated. Before the insertion of a metal corneal eye shield, it is important to check its integrity and to make sure there are no obvious scratches of the shield that can lead to corneal abrasions. For ease of insertion, it is best to lift the upper eyelid and to start by, first, placing the eye shield inferiorly. After insertion of the shield, it is important to make sure there are no eyelashes caught under the shield that may cause injury to the cornea. The placement of metal corneal eye shields can be challenging for younger children in the outpatient clinic setting.

- To decrease fire risk in the operating room, wet towels should be placed around the treatment area. When a facial lesion is being treated, patient safety and protection of the airway should be paramount, and an appropriate laser-safe protocol should be implemented. For short procedures, nasal cannula oxygenation can be a safer alternative. For intraoral procedures, room air ventilation may be used to decrease percentage of oxygen in the surgical field, and thereby reduce the fire risk. Airway fires are lethal and appropriate precautions should be taken when treating facial/oral lesions.

- A combination of pulsed-dye (595 nm), alexandrite (755 nm), and Nd:YAG (1064 nm) lasers may be used for treatment of VMs depending on the epidermal, dermal, and subcutaneous involvement of the malformations. For malformations with obvious epidermal hypertrophic changes, alexandrite and Nd:YAG lasers are usually the better choices. For example, the use of 3-mm spot size, fluence of 44 J/cm², and microsecond pulse width of alexandrite laser (Candela Gentlelase Pro®) is often effective for VMs with a significant epidermal vascular component and mild hypertrophic changes. It is best to avoid overlap and pulse stacking during initial treatment. Depending on the tissue reaction, a second pass to areas with epidermal hypertrophy is generally well tolerated as long as no blistering is noted during first pass. The clinical endpoint is dark purpura with minimal whitening. To avoid blistering and excessive epidermal damage, cooling should be used during the entire procedure. Concurrent cooling built into the laser device or a separate cold air cooling unit (Zimmer Medizin Systems, Irvine, CA) can be used. When concurrent cooling is not available, ice should be used, with frequent pauses at 10- to 20-second intervals during the procedure.

- For VMs involving subcutaneous tissue, a long-pulsed Nd:YAG laser (1064 nm) may be more effective. Spot size and energy (J/cm²) need to be adjusted depending on patient response as well as the specific laser model being used. In general, laser setting using a 4- to 6-mm spot size, pulse duration of 25 to 40 ms, and fluence of 35 to 70 mJ/cm² may be used. Lower energy settings are recommended for the initial treatment, which can be increased gradually at subsequent treatments. The Nd:YAG laser does not cause significant purpura and the endpoint is often subtle visually, with only minimal edema and tissue contraction being seen. Therefore, it is important not to overlap pulses and inform patients of the possibility of significant postoperative edema. For patients with VMs affecting the oral mucosa and lip, it is important to note that the swelling may affect speech as well as the patient's ability to drink from a cup. A short course of systemic steroid may be needed if there is concern for oral edema leading to airway obstruction.

- Of note, if Nd:YAG laser treatment is performed intraoperatively to an open wound bed, much lower fluences should be used.

- Immediately after surgery, a petrolatum-based ointment should be applied liberally.

- Application of intra- and postoperative cooling is very important to help decrease discomfort and minimize edema as well as risk of blistering.

- Combined sclerotherapy and laser treatment should be used cautiously because excessive tissue destruction can result in localized skin ulceration.

Postprocedural Approach

- Cold compress/ice can be applied as tolerated for the first 24 hours.

- Alternating over-the-counter acetaminophen and ibuprofen are generally sufficient for pain control. However, some patients may also benefit from schedule III narcotic pain medication for breakthrough pain during the first 2 to 3 days.

- Dressing should be applied after the treatment and left in place for the first 24 hours. The treated area can then be cleansed with gentle soap and water daily. If the treated areas are at risk for infection, dilute vinegar or dilute bleach soaks can also be used daily.

- Petrolatum-based ointment is recommended in the immediate postoperative period and also for continued use until the treatment area is fully healed.

- It is important to protect the treatment sites from trauma and friction during the healing process. Protective dressings can be used for 1 to 2 weeks postoperatively. Compression garments can also be helpful to decrease postoperative edema and reduce risks of recurrence with continued use.

- Patients can typically return to school or daily activities within 2 to 3 days.

- Clinic follow-up is recommended 6 to 8 weeks after the treatment to assess response and determine additional management plans. Longer treatment intervals are often preferred for school-aged children to minimize school absences and to reduce the frequency of general anesthesia (if it is being used).

- Although additional evidence is needed, early initiation of treatment for extensive VMs may be beneficial because of the lower disease burden overall at younger ages. Once the disease progression is controlled, additional treatments may be offered as in-office procedures later in life.

- Serial photography to document treatment response is always helpful.

OTHER ASSOCIATED COMPLEX DISORDERS

Multiple VMs in the setting of somatic *Tie2* mutations can be seen in blue rubber bleb nevus syndrome (BRBNS) (see Chapter 64. Blue Rubber Bleb Syndrome). This is a rare disorder characterized by VMs of the skin as well as the gastrointestinal (GI) tract, and, less often, in other organ systems. Morbidity and mortality of BRBNS are mostly attributed to the severity of GI disease. Cutaneous lesions do not need to be treated unless they are symptomatic or in cosmetically sensitive areas, and in such cases, a similar treatment algorithm as outlined earlier can be used.

It is also important to note that VMs can present in isolation or can have an associated lymphatic component. Mixed venolymphatic malformations can be managed with the treatment algorithm described in this chapter as well.

SUGGESTED READINGS

Castillo SD, Tzouanacou E, Zaw-Thin M, et al. Somatic activating mutations in Pik3ca cause sporadic venous malformations in mice and humans. *Sci Transl Med.* 2016;30;8(332):332ra43.

Goldenberg DC, Carvas M, Adams D, Giannotti M, Gemperli R. Successful treatment of a complex vascular malformation with Sirolimus and surgical resection. *J Pediatr Hematol Oncol.* 2017;39(4):e191–e195.

Ünlüsoy Aksu A, Sari S, Eğritaş Gürkan Ö, et al. Favorable response to sirolimus in a child with blue rubber bleb nevus syndrome in the gastrointestinal tract. *J Pediatr Hematol Oncol.* 2017;39(2):147–149.

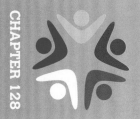

CHAPTER 128

Human Papillomavirus Wart (Verruca)

Jennifer Ornelas and Smita Awasthi

INTRODUCTION

Warts, or verruca, are benign intraepidermal tumors caused by the human papillomavirus (HPV). There are four main types of warts: verruca vulgaris (the common wart), verruca plana (flat warts), verruca plantaris (plantar warts), and condyloma acuminatum (anogenital warts). Warts are typically spread via direct skin-to-skin contact or via fomites that allow the virus to survive by providing a warm and moist environment. Different treatment approaches depend on the age of the patient and type, location, severity, and number of warts, as well as the distress the warts cause the patient and family.

Treatment options include watchful waiting, topicals (salicylic acid, cantharidin, 5-fluorouracil), destructive methods (cryotherapy, paring, and laser), immunotherapy (imiquimod, squaric acid dibutyl ester, and diphencyclopropenone), and injections (*Candida, Trichophyton,* or mumps antigens, bleomycin) among others, though injections are rarely used in young children. Treatment of recalcitrant or numerous warts often requires multiple treatments and more than one treatment modality. For young children, given that warts are usually harmless, asymptomatic, and self-resolve over the course of a few years, watchful waiting is often an appropriate choice. Moreover, treatment methods can be painful and carry risks including postinflammatory pigmentary alteration, scarring, or worsening with the dreaded ring wart.

I. TOPICAL APPROACHES

Approach #1: Salicylic Acid

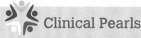 Clinical Pearls

- Ideal for at-home treatment of warts
- Can be used in conjunction with cryotherapy and paring
- Found to be one of the most effective treatments in Cochrane review[1]

Contraindications/Cautions/Risks

- Irritation, blistering, scaling, peeling, pain, stinging, worsening of warts, recurrence of warts, no improvement
- Use is not contraindicated in women who are pregnant or may become pregnant.

Equipment Needed

- OTC salicylic acid preparation with 15% to 17% salicylic acid (or 40% for plantar warts)
- Occlusive tape such as duct tape or surgical cloth tape
- Nail file or pumice stone for paring

Preprocedural Approach

- Begin 1 week after any in-office treatment.
- For thicker warts, soften warts by soaking in warm water for at least 10 minutes, then file gently using a pumice stone or nail file.

Procedural Approach

- Apply salicylic acid preparation directly to each wart nightly. Take care not to apply to unaffected surrounding skin.
- Cover warts with surgical cloth tape or duct tape.

Postprocedural Approach

- Continue daily, including in between in-office treatments, until wart is resolved.
- Stop if surrounding skin appears macerated. Resume when healed.
- Stop and switch treatment modalities if symptoms are not tolerable or if there is worsening.

Approach #2: Cantharidin

Clinical Pearls

- Ideal for younger patients with multiple warts in whom pain associated with other treatment modalities is not tolerable
- A recent systematic review found substantial clearance rates with cantharidin monotherapy for warts and of cantharidin in combination with podophyllotoxin and salicylic acid for plantar warts.[2]

Contraindications/Cautions/Risks

- Ring warts, blistering, burning, erythema, pain, pruritus, postinflammatory pigmentary alteration, recurrence, no improvement
- Use with caution in women who are pregnant or who may become pregnant as it is not known whether or not exposure can cause fetal harm.
- Use of cantharidin for warts confers a greater risk of ring warts compared to other modalities as the blisters caused by it can cause the wart to spread.[3] Counsel family regarding risk.

Equipment Needed

- Cantharidin 0.7% or Cantharadin "PLUS" (30% salicylic acid, 2% podophyllin BP, 1% cantharidin)
- Cotton-tipped applicators
- Occlusive tape

Preprocedural Approach

- Select warts for treatment
  - Avoid facial warts and warts on thin skinned, occluded, or intertriginous areas such as the neck, axilla, genitalia, inguinal creases, and intergluteal crease.
- Discuss increased risk of ring wart compared to other treatment modalities.

Procedural Approach

- Use the wooden end of the cotton-tipped applicator to dip into the cantharadin solution.
- Apply a drop to each individual wart and let air dry for 2 to 3 minutes until completely dry.
- Take care not to apply to unaffected surrounding skin.
- Cover with occlusive tape.
- Remove tape and rinse completely off in 4 to 6 hours for cantharidin 0.7% solution and in 30 minutes to 1-hour for cantharidin PLUS.

Postprocedural Approach

- If vigorous blistering reaction occurs, decrease dwell time; if no blistering reaction or erythema occurs, increase dwell time.
- Repeat treatment every 4 to 6 weeks until wart is resolved.
- Stop and switch treatment modalities if ring wart develops, symptoms are not tolerable, or if there is worsening.

Approach #3: 5-Fluorouracil (Efudex)

Clinical Pearls

- Can be used for treatment of genital and periungal warts

Contraindications/Cautions/Risks

- Erythema, edema, pigmentary alteration, pain, erosions, ulceration, onycholysis, scarring, recurrence of wart(s), no improvement
- Contraindicated in pregnant women or women who intend to become pregnant as exposure may cause fetal harm

Equipment Needed

- 5% fluorouracil cream
- Occlusive tape

Preprocedural Approach

- Begin 1 to 2 weeks after any in-office treatment.

Procedural Approach

- Advise patient to use pumice stone or nail file to pare down hyperkeratotic warts.
- Apply 5-fluorouracil cream directly to each wart. Take care not to apply to unaffected surrounding skin.
- Cover warts with occlusive tape if needed.
  - Not necessary in treatment of genital warts

Postprocedural Approach

- Continue daily for 4 to 12 weeks (until wart[s] resolve).
- Stop and switch treatment modalities if symptoms are not tolerable or if there is worsening.

Approach #4: Imiquimod

Clinical Pearls

- Ideal for treatment of genital warts

Contraindications/Cautions/Risks

- Erythema, erosions, burning, pain, pruritus, psoriasiform eruptions, mucosal ulcerations, hyperpigmentation, flu-like reaction, recurrence, no improvement
- Use with caution in women who are pregnant or who may become pregnant as it is not known whether or not exposure can cause fetal harm.

Equipment Needed

- Imiquimod 5% topical cream

Preprocedural Approach

- Select warts for treatment.
- Pare hyperkeratotic warts prior to treatment.

Procedural Approach

- Instruct patient (or caretaker) to apply to each individual wart at bedtime and leave on overnight 3 times a week for a maximum of 16 weeks.[4]
  - ○ Can alternate every other night with salicylic acid
- Wash hands thoroughly.
- Wash area in the morning.

Postprocedural Approach

- Continue for a total of 12 to 16 weeks.
- Reduce frequency of application if skin reactions occur.
- Stop and switch treatment modalities if symptoms are not tolerable or if there is worsening.

II. DESTRUCTIVE METHODS

Approach #1: Cryotherapy

 Clinical Pearls

- Ideal for treatment of solitary warts and in children old enough to tolerate associated discomfort
- Can be used in conjunction with paring, salicylic acid, and other home treatments
- Use distraction techniques (such as virtual reality headsets, music, short videos, and blowing bubbles) to reduce pain with treatment.

Contraindications/Cautions/Risks

- Burning, pain, erythema, blistering, crusting, ring warts or worsening of wart(s), postinflammatory hyperpigmentation, scarring, recurrence of wart(s), no improvement

Equipment Needed

- Liquid nitrogen in either a canister or Styrofoam cup
- Alcohol swab
- Cotton-tipped applicators
- Cotton swab

Preprocedural Approach

- Select warts for treatment.
- Set up distraction technique.

Procedural Approach

- Use a filled liquid nitrogen dispenser to apply a steady stream of liquid nitrogen to allow for a 10 to 12 second thaw cycle. Repeat once (Figure 128.1).

Or

- Wrap cotton swab around two-thirds of the cotton tip of cotton-tipped applicator (making sure to leave the smaller cotton tip somewhat exposed), then dip the wrapped applicator

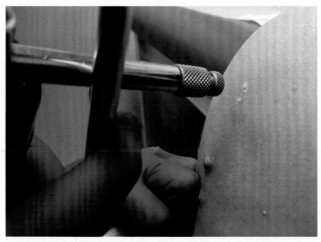

FIGURE 128.1. Cryotherapy using a liquid nitrogen dispenser. The tip of the dispenser is held approximately 1 cm away from wart. Only a small portion of "normal" skin is involved. Photo courtesy of Andrew C. Krakowski, MD.

into the liquid nitrogen in the Styrofoam cup (Figure 128.2A and B). Press tip onto individual lesion for a 10 to 12 second thaw cycle. Repeat for each individual lesion.
  - ○ This technique is ideal for treatment of warts in cosmetically sensitive areas including flat warts on the face or in young children wary of the liquid nitrogen canister.
  - ○ The cotton swab allows for a reservoir of liquid nitrogen to keep the cotton tip of the cotton-tipped applicator colder during treatment.
  - ○ Allows for treatment of multiple warts before having to place applicator back into the liquid nitrogen

Postprocedural Approach

- Apply white petrolatum ointment as needed to warts that have bullae or crusting.
- Repeat treatment every 4 to 6 weeks until wart is resolved. Can treat more frequently for recalcitrant warts (ie, every 2-3 weeks)
- Stop and switch treatment modalities if symptoms are not tolerable or if there is worsening.

Approach #2: Paring

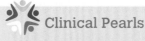 Clinical Pearls

- Ideal for treatment in conjunction with topical salicylic acid, cryotherapy, and laser, as well as other treatment modalities

Contraindications/Cautions/Risks

- Pain, pressure, bleeding

Equipment Needed

- Alcohol swab
- 2 × 2-in gauze
- Sterile #15 blade or curette
- Aluminum chloride

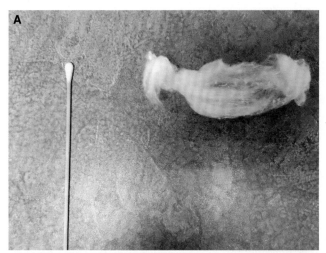

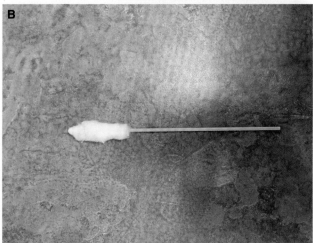

FIGURE 128.2. A, Unrolled cotton ball. B, Unrolled cotton ball rolled onto tip of cotton-tipped applicator allowing finer tip to remain visible for more precise application of the liquid nitrogen.

Preprocedural Approach

- Clean lesions to be treated with alcohol.

Procedural Approach

- Use a sterile #15 blade or curette to gently remove the hyperkeratotic portion of the wart.
- Aluminum chloride can be applied with a cotton-tipped applicator for hemostasis if needed.

Postprocedural Approach

- Repeat treatment once every 4 to 6 weeks as needed.

Approach #3: Laser

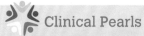 Clinical Pearls

- Ideal for treatment of recalcitrant warts
- Warts should be pared prior to treatment.
- Multiple treatments usually required

Contraindications/Cautions/Risks

- Pain, bleeding, crusting, blistering, postinflammatory pigmentary alteration, scarring, recurrence of wart(s), no improvement

Equipment Needed

- 1064 nm Nd:YAG laser
- 595 nm PDL laser
- 30-gauge needle
- Topical anesthetic
    - Lidocaine 2.5%/prilocaine 2.5% cream
    - Local anesthesia
    - 0.5% to 2% lidocaine with 1:200 000 epinephrine.
- Laser specific eye protective equipment
- Smoke aspiration system
- Cooling system
- Micropore laser mask

Preprocedural Approach

- Clean areas to be treated with alcohol.
- Optional anesthesia:
    - 30 minutes before treatment apply topical anesthetic cream to the area(s) to be treated.
    and/or
    - 10 to 20 minutes before treatment use 30-gauge needle to infiltrate area(s) to be treated with 0.5% to 2% lidocaine with epinephrine.

Procedural Approach

- Laser-specific protective eyewear must be used.
- Recommend also using micropore laser masks and a smoke evacuator to decrease risk of inhaling aerosolized HPV.
- Pare lesions prior to laser treatment.
- Recommend use of cold air device for cooling to minimize pain and thermal burning while applying laser pulses.
- 1064 nm Nd:YAG laser (Table 128.1):
    - Apply laser pulses with overlap to cover the entire wart surface and a 1 mm margin of normal surrounding skin.[5]

TABLE 128.1 : Laser Settings for Wart Treatment

LASER	SPOT SIZE (mm)	PULSE DURATION (ms)	FLUENCE (J/cm²)	ENDPOINT
1064 nm Nd:YAG[5]	4-6	20	200-250	Graying or hemorrhagic bullae[5]
1064 nm Nd:YAG[6]	3	23	180-200	
1064 nm Nd:YAG[7]	5	20	240-300	
595 nm PDL[7]	5 or 7	0.5-1.5	9-14	Intense purpuric response

ND:YAG, neodymium-doped yttrium aluminum garnet; PDL, pulsed dye laser.

○ Endpoint: graying or hemorrhagic bulla forming over the lesion
- PDL-595 nm wavelength (Table 128.1):
  ○ Complete one pass with pulses overlapping 1 to 2 mm. Make sure to include a 2 mm border of normal surrounding skin. Wait 1 minute, then repeat up to two times more for a total of one to three passes.[7]
  ○ Treatment endpoint: Intense purpuric response as clinical endpoint

Postprocedural Approach

- 1064 nm Nd:YAG
  ○ Repeat treatments at 4-week intervals.
  ○ Apply white petrolatum ointment to the treated lesion once daily and cover with a BAND-AID™ (Johnson & Johnson, US) until healed.
- PDL
  ○ Repeat treatments at 3 to 4 weeks intervals as needed until resolved.
  ○ Apply white petrolatum ointment to the treated lesion once daily and cover with a BAND-AID.
  ○ Counsel that purpura is expected to remain for 1 to 2 weeks post-treatment.
- Stop and switch treatment modalities if symptoms are not tolerable or if there is worsening.

III. IMMUNOTHERAPY

Approach #1: Intralesional Immunotherapy

Clinical Pearls

- The authors use *Candida* antigen due to its efficacy, favorable side effect profile, ease of use, and availability. The authors do not use BCG due to inferior efficacy and less favorable side effect profile.
  - In a recent review, *Candida* antigen and MMR were found to have comparable complete response rates (39%-88% vs. 26.5%-92%, respectively), while BCG had inferior clearance rates (33.3%-39.7%).[8]
  - Distant wart resolution rates were noted to be 55.9% to 57.4% with *Candida* antigen and 24.5% to 69.5% with MMR.[8]
- Ideal treatment when multiple warts present
  - Thought to increase HPV recognition by stimulating cell-mediated immunity
- Can be more tolerable than cryotherapy of multiple warts if patient is not needle phobic
- Use distraction techniques (such as virtual reality headsets, music, short videos, and blowing bubbles) to reduce pain with treatment.

Contraindications/Cautions/Risks

- Pain, erythema, edema, pruritus, blistering, rarely fever, myalgia, flu-like symptoms, recurrence of wart, no improvement. Additional risks of BCG injection include papule formation and ulceration at injection site.
- Caution with use of *Candida* and *Trichophyton* antigen and MMR vaccine in women who are pregnant or who may become pregnant as it is not known whether or not exposure can cause fetal harm.

- Caution with use of BCG vaccine in pregnant women as it has only been used in a small number of pregnant women though with no observed direct or indirect fetal harm

Equipment Needed

- Commercially available antigens
  - *Candida* antigen (Candin manurfactured by Nielson BioSciences)
  - *Trichophyton* antigen (Alk-Abello, Round Rock, Texas)
  - BCG vaccine (manufactured by Merk, Dianon systems, and Evans Vaccines)
  - MMR vaccine (manufactured by Merk)
- Alcohol swab
- 1-mL tuberculin syringe
- 30-gauge needle
- 2 × 2-in gauze
- BAND-AID(s)

Preprocedural Approach

- Set up distraction method.
- Clean areas to be injected with alcohol.
- Wear protective eye-gear.

Procedural Approach

- Use 30-gauge needle on a 1-mL tuberculin syringe to inject 0.1 to 0.3 mL of *Candida* antigen or MMR vaccine, or 0.1 mL of BCG vaccine as superficially as possible into the largest wart.[8-10] Readjust tip of needle if solution begins leaking out of wart (Figure 128.3).
- In the case of multiple warts, inject into the largest lesion or split the dose into two different locations (eg, 0.1 mL into one wart on the left hand and one wart on the right hand).[9]

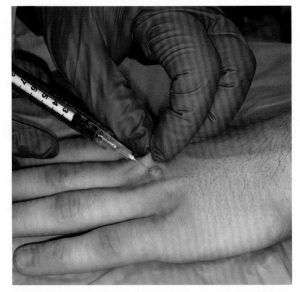

FIGURE 128.3. *Candida* injection using a 1-mL syringe and 30-gauge needle. Note "pinching" used as a nerve distraction technique. Photo courtesy of Andrew C. Krakowski, MD.

Postprocedural Approach

- Repeat treatments:
  - BCG vaccine: every 2 to 4 weeks until lesions are resolved
  - *Candida* antigen: every 3 to 4 weeks until lesions are resolved
  - MMR vaccine: every 2 to 3 weeks until lesions are resolved
- Number of treatments typically needed:
  - BCG vaccine: four to six treatments to see a benefit and/or resolution
  - Candida antigen: three to four treatments to see a benefit and may treat to about six treatments total
  - MMR vaccine: three to six treatments for benefit and/or resolution
- Stop and switch treatment modalities if symptoms are not tolerable or if there is worsening.

Approach #2: Squaric Acid Dibutylester

 Clinical Pearls

- Ideal for younger patients with multiple recalcitrant warts in whom pain associated with other treatment modalities is not tolerable
- Can be done in the office or prescribed to a compounding pharmacy for home treatment
- Ideal for the treatment of multiple warts
- Not recommended for treatment of facial warts

Contraindications/Cautions/Risks

- Erythema, edema, scaling, pruritus, burning, discomfort, dyspigmentation, recurrence of wart(s), no improvement
- Do not use in women who are pregnant or who may become pregnant as it is not known whether or not exposure can cause fetal harm.

Equipment Needed

- Squaric acid dibutylester (SADBE) solution in 0.02% to 2% concentration
  - Typically prepared by a compounding pharmacist who generally purchases SADBE from a chemical distributor

Preprocedural Approach

- Sensitize with 1% to 2% SADBE[11-13]
  - Apply over 2 cm^2 area to the inner forearm and place occlusive dressing (eg, non-stick gauze followed by Tegaderm® [3M, US]).
  - Instruct patient to leave on overnight, then wash off.
  - If rash develops within 1 to 2 weeks, this indicates sensitization and patient may proceed with treatment. If no rash, repeat sensitization in 1-week. If there is still no reaction, consider another treatment modality.

Procedural Approach

- Two weeks after sensitization, start by applying 0.02% to 0.4% SADBE to individual lesions.[11-13]
  - 0.02% for lesions in sensitive areas (eg, perianal lesions) or in those patients with exuberant contact dermatitis with sensitization

- For home use[14]:
  - Parents are instructed to handle the solution using gloves and cotton-tipped swabs to minimize their sensitization.
  - Patients' parents are instructed to apply 0.4% SADBE three times a week to the warts. They then slowly increase the frequency (an additional day per week) to daily application until a mild dermatitis is noted. If no dermatitis is seen at the next clinic visit (by the time the patient is applying the solution daily), the concentration of SADBE is increased by the physician.
- For in-office use:
  - Can start at a slightly higher concentration (1%)
  - Increase to 2% to 5% for lesions that have no change after several applications.

Postprocedural Approach

- May take several months to resolve depending on size and number of warts present. Can continue treatment while there is improvement
- Home use: In-office follow-up monthly to evaluate for the proper reaction and to make changes in the concentration of solution or frequency of use
- Office use: Repeat application once to twice a week to individual lesions until resolved.
- Stop and switch treatment modalities if symptoms are not tolerable or if there is worsening.

Approach #3: Diphencyclopropenone

 Clinical Pearls

- Ideal for younger patients with multiple warts in whom pain associated with other treatment modalities is not tolerable
- Can be used for the treatment of multiple warts
- Not recommended for treatment of facial warts

Contraindications/Cautions/Risks

- Erythema, edema, scaling, pruritus, burning, discomfort, recurrence of wart(s), no improvement
- Do not use in women who are pregnant or who may become pregnant as it is not known whether or not exposure can cause fetal harm.

Equipment Needed

- Diphencyclopropenone (DPCP) 0.05% to 2% in acetone
  - Typically prepared by a compounding pharmacist who generally purchases DPCP from a chemical distributor

Preprocedural Approach

- Sensitize with 1% to 3% DPCP[15-17]
  - Apply to the inner forearm, cover with occlusive dressing
  - Wash off after 8 to 24 hours.
- If rash develops, this indicates sensitization and may proceed with treatment. If no rash, repeat sensitization in 1 week. If there is still no reaction, consider another treatment modality.

Procedural Approach

- During office visit, apply 0.1% DPCP to individual lesions, allow to air-dry, then occlude.[15-17]
  - Instruct patients to wash off after 8 hours.
- Increase concentration gradually to 2% DPCP with each application if needed until mild eczematous reaction occurs.[15-17]
  - Can increase by 0.1% to 0.5% in concentration weekly to every few weeks depending on presence of a reaction and/or whether any improvement of warts is seen

Postprocedural Approach

- Repeat application every 1 to 3 weeks until lesions resolve.
- May take several months to resolve depending on size and number of warts present. Can continue treatment if improvement is noted
- Stop and switch treatment modalities if symptoms are not tolerable or if there is worsening.

REFERENCES

1. Kwok CS, Gibbs S, Bennett C, Holland R, Abbott R. Topical treatments for cutaneous warts. *Cochrane Database Syst Rev.* 2012;(9):CD001781.
2. Vakharia PP, Chopra R, Silverberg NB, Silverberg JI. Efficacy and safety of topical cantharidin treatment for molluscum contagiosum and warts: a systematic review. *Am J Clin Dermatol.* 2018;19(6):791–803.
3. Mathes EF, Frieden IJ. Treatment of molluscum contagiosum with cantharidin: a practical approach. *Pediatr Ann.* 2010;39(3):124–128, 130.
4. Fife KH, Ferenczy A, Douglas JM, Jr, Brown D, Smith M, Owens M. Treatment of external genital warts in men using 5% imiquimod cream applied three times a week, once daily, twice daily, or three times a day. *Sex Transm Dis.* 2001;28(4):226–231.
5. Alshami MA, Mohana MJ. Novel treatment approach for deep palmoplantar warts using long-pulsed 1064-nm Nd:YAG laser and a moisturizing cream without prior paring of the wart surface. *Photomed Laser Surg.* 2016;34(10):448–455.
6. Bingol UA, Comert A, Cinar C. The overlapped triple circle pulse technique with Nd:YAG laser for refractory hand warts. *Photomed Laser Surg.* 2015;33(6):338–342.
7. Shin YS, Cho EB, Park EJ, Kim KH, Kim KJ. A comparative study of pulsed dye laser versus long pulsed Nd:YAG laser treatment in recalcitrant viral warts. *J Dermatolog Treat.* 2017;28(5):411–416.
8. Fields JR, Saikaly SK, Schoch JJ. Intralesional immunotherapy for pediatric warts: a review. *Pediatr Dermatol.* 2020;37:265–271.
9. Khozeimeh F, Jabbari Azad F, Mahboubi Oskouei Y, et al. Intralesional immunotherapy compared to cryotherapy in the treatment of warts. *Int J Dermatol.* 2017;56(4):474–478.
10. Munoz Garza FZ, Roe Crespo E, Torres Pradilla M, et al. Intralesional *Candida* antigen immunotherapy for the treatment of recalcitrant and multiple warts in children. *Pediatr Dermatol.* 2015;32(6):797–801.
11. Lee AN, Mallory SB. Contact immunotherapy with squaric acid dibutylester for the treatment of recalcitrant warts. *J Am Acad Dermatol.* 1999;41(4):595–599.
12. Micali G, Dall'Oglio F, Tedeschi A, Pulvirenti N, Nasca MR. Treatment of cutaneous warts with squaric acid dibutylester: a decade of experience. *Arch Dermatol.* 2000;136(4):557–558.
13. Micali G, Nasca MR, Tedeschi A, Dall'Oglio F, Pulvirenti N. Use of squaric acid dibutylester (SADBE) for cutaneous warts in children. *Pediatr Dermatol.* 2000;17(4):315–318.
14. Pandey S, Wilmer EN, Morrell DS. Examining the efficacy and safety of squaric acid therapy for treatment of recalcitrant warts in children. *Pediatr Dermatol.* 2015;32(1):85–90.
15. Choi Y, Kim DH, Jin SY, Lee AY, Lee SH. Topical immunotherapy with diphenylcyclopropenone is effective and preferred in the treatment of periungual warts. *Ann Dermatol.* 2013;25(4):434–439.
16. Park JY, Park BW, Cho EB, Park EJ, Kim KH, Kim KJ. Clinical efficacy of diphenylcyclopropenone immunotherapy as monotherapy for multiple viral warts. *J Cutan Med Surg.* 2018;22(3):285–289.
17. Suh DW, Lew BL, Sim WY. Investigations of the efficacy of diphenylcyclopropenone immunotherapy for the treatment of warts. *Int J Dermatol.* 2014;53(12):e567–e571.

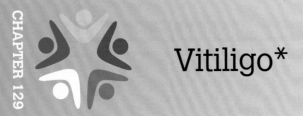

CHAPTER 129

Vitiligo*

Part I: Overview and Phototherapy and Excimer Laser Procedures

Sheena Nguyen, John E. Harris, and Deepti Gupta

INTRODUCTION

Vitiligo is an acquired, autoimmune loss of pigmentation resulting from melanocyte destruction. It affects approximately 1% of the worldwide population, with its onset before the age of 20 years in about half of affected patients and before 8 years of age in one-quarter of patients. In the pediatric population, there is a higher incidence of disease in females versus males, the segmental type of vitiligo is more common, and there is a less frequent association with other systemic autoimmune and endocrine disorders differing from the adult population. Other autoimmune disorders such as hypothyroidism and alopecia areata do occur in pediatric patients with vitiligo, with thyroid autoantibodies described in 11% of patients.[1]

---

*Latanya T. Benjamin provided additional editorial review of this chapter.

Therapy for vitiligo of childhood is almost entirely all "off-label," despite an abundance of articles in the literature describing various treatment regimens. The aim of treatment is to initiate and promote repigmentation of affected lesions. The goal of treatment in childhood is 2-fold, with stabilization of disease being the first endpoint and repigmentation being the secondary endpoint for children with generalized vitiligo.

Phototherapy is traditionally reserved for children with more generalized disease, whereas excimer laser is useful for more localized (ie, segmental) disease. In a recent study of 77 children aged 16 years and younger treated with narrowband ultraviolet (NB-UVB) for vitiligo, 47% demonstrated good response with minimal side effects.

Although the response to **excimer laser** in the childhood population is sparsely reported, a case series of pimecrolimus and excimer laser demonstrated that at 30 weeks, 71% of patients experienced 51% to 100% of repigmentation with the caveat that these patients had used pimecrolimus in conjunction with the excimer laser.[2] As the side effect profile is both limited and localized, combined with the commonality of the segmental type of vitiligo in childhood, excimer would be the light source of choice if available.[3]

Very few reports of **grafting** for childhood vitiligo have been reported; albeit successful in these rare reports, the grafting procedure in its various forms may be painful, may potentially cause scarring, and/or may produce mottled pigmentation in the donor or the recipient sites. In addition, these reports also required the use of either phototherapy or excimer laser to promote more even repigmentation. Grafting is typically reserved for patients with "clinically stable" vitiligo.[2]

Emerging options include melanocyte transfer techniques, in which skin grafts are separated into their cellular components, which are then selectively applied onto recipient skin. The melanocyte keratinocyte transplantation procedure (MKTP) is one such technique that is proving to be a precise, fast, and safe surgical option for treating large areas of depigmentation refractory to medical treatment. This highly-specialized procedure is covered in greater detail below (Part II. Surgical Transplantation).[2]

Regardless of the treatment of choice, it is crucial to involve the parents and/or caretakers of the child, as well as the child, in the decision because it requires coordination with their school schedules and activities, which may be a limiting factor.

Clinical Pearls: Phototherapy and Excimer Laser

- **Guidelines:**
  - **Phototherapy:** Level of Evidence: II and Strength of Recommendation: B
  - **Excimer Laser:** Level of Evidence: II and Strength of Recommendation: B
- **Age-Specific Considerations:**
  - Both phototherapy and excimer laser are therapies that are limited to children who are able to comply with being able to stand or hold still for the treatment to be performed; usually, children age 6 and older have the best success with being able to complete treatments.
- **Technique Tips:**
  - It is critically important to meter the ultraviolet (UV) B machine once weekly.
    - UVB lamps steadily lose power.
    - If UV output is not accurately measured and actual output calibrated into the machine, the clinician may have a false impression that the patient may be treated with higher doses when, in fact, the machine is actually delivering a much lower dose than the dosage entered.
  - Segmental vitiligo of the face has excellent response if treated early in the course with topical tacrolimus with or without NB-UVB.
  - Institution of excimer laser within 5 months of disease activity for facial vitiligo produces best results.
  - Because children are more commonly affected by the segmental type of vitiligo, the excimer laser may prove to be more beneficial in treating limited areas, especially during times when the child may suffer from claustrophobia from the phototherapy booth; this limited risk and the presence of any anxiety should be documented to improve likelihood of insurance coverage.
  - It typically requires at least a 3-month trial before being able to accurately predict/assess true lesional response to any modality.
- **Skin of Color Considerations:**
  - Fitzpatrick skin type I patients may use avoidance of darkening or tanning of their skin as a therapeutic/cosmetic plan because of potential intolerance of other treatment modalities and the minimal appearance of the lesions in this skin type.

Contraindications/Cautions/Risks

Contraindications

- There are no absolute contraindications for phototherapy or excimer laser; however, caution should be exercised in patients with Fitzpatrick skin types I and II who tend to burn easily, those with history of arsenic intake or previous treatment with ionizing radiation therapy, those with history of melanoma or multiple nonmelanoma skin cancers and any medical condition that is severe enough that the patient cannot tolerate heat or prolonged standing in the phototherapy unit.
- A detailed history for photosensitizing medications should be performed.

Cautions

- Long-term data on outcomes and sequelae for pediatric patients a lacking.
- It is crucial to perform a full-body skin examination before initiating therapy and routinely monitor for signs of photoaging, pigmentation, and cutaneous malignancies.
- When used in conjunction with systemic retinoids, dose of both retinoids and UVB may need to be lowered.
- Noncompliance is a real concern given the need for treatments two to three times a week and required copays.

Risks

- There is evidence that adult patients with vitiligo who have received phototherapy have a higher risk of skin cancer than do vitiligo patients who have not received phototherapy. Other studies have shown UVB does not increase skin cancer risk. Putting this concern in context, the risk of skin cancer in vitiligo patients is very low and this treatment modality appears to be very safe.
- The most common side effect of this therapy is UVB-induced sunburn or blistering. This may occur at any time during therapy.
- Increased pigmentation may occur, especially after a blistering sunburn-type reaction, but typically resolves with time.
- UV treatments may cause dryness and itching.

- UV treatments age the skin over time and may increase freckles and pigmentation of the skin.
- UV rays may damage the eyes and increase risk of cataracts. This is preventable with protective eye goggles worn during treatment.
- For phototherapy booth units, specifically, clinicians should discuss possible discomfort, especially if claustrophobia may be an issue.
- For excimer laser, more specific risks include erythema, blistering, and occurrence of erosions at treated sites, but the risk is generally low and limited to the site treated.

Equipment Needed

- Protective eyewear (protective against UVB range from 280 to 315 nm)
- Phototherapy unit (UVB)—properly calibrated on a weekly basis
- Excimer laser device (308 nm)

Preprocedural Approach

- Regardless of the treatment of choice, it is crucial to involve the parents and/or caretakers of the child, as well as the child, in the decision because it requires coordination with their school schedules and activities, which may be a limiting factor.
- A thorough review of systems for conditions that may be associated with vitiligo (and any exam-guided subsequent workup) is recommended.
- Antinuclear antibody testing should be performed when autoimmune photosensitivity is suspected or when a clinically unexpected response to phototherapy is observed.
- Discuss scheduling of sessions in advance. Most effective treatment regimens occur at a frequency of "three times weekly," although benefit may also be seen at "two times weekly" and may be maintained on a "once-weekly" schedule at minimum.

Procedural Approach

Phototherapy using NB-UVB[4]

- Ensure the patient has properly consented for treatment and has signed the consent form (see Chapter 20. Phototherapy and Photodynamic Therapy).
- Have the patient undress and expose the areas of vitiligo to be treated.
  - Male patients should wear an athletic supporter or other appropriate shielding for the genitals.
  - All patients should cover nipples with zinc paste or other protective barrier.
- Eye protection in the form of UV goggles must be worn by all patients and caretakers when inside the phototherapy unit.
- The initial NB-UVB dose (mJ/cm^2) should be the same for all patients with vitiligo: 200 mJ/cm^2. This is derived from calculating 50% of the average MED for Type 1 skin, which is approximately 400 mJ/cm^2.
- There is a manual method for calculating the time (in seconds) to set the NB-UVB control panel to deliver the initial dose:

$$\text{Time (seconds)} = \text{Dose (mJ/cm}^2)/\text{Irradiance (mW/cm}^2)$$

- The measurement of the irradiance can be obtained from a log book that should be kept on a monthly basis.
- The duration of a treatment or total dose of NB-UVB to be delivered can often be calculated by the UV light unit itself, following the manufacturer's instructions in the operation manual that came with the device via inputting the correct information on the control panel before the delivery of the treatment.
- Set the time (dose) on the UV light unit. In some phototherapy units, the session duration is dependent on the dose measured by an internal photometer, and the time must be calculated by the technician.
- Verify that the UV light unit is set on NB-UVB (ie, "narrowband").
- Turn on the fan and have the patient stand in the center of the UV light unit with arms at rest or in the best position to expose the areas being treated.
- Double-check that patients and caretakers are wearing eye protection.
- Instruct patients to exit the UV light box when the lights go out or if they become uncomfortable during the treatment either from burning or stinging of the skin. Inform the patient that the unit doors are not locked.
- Initiate the treatment.
- The frequency of NB-UVB light treatments is two to three times weekly. "Three times a week" dosing tends to produce faster results; however, efficacy is ultimately equivalent. If the patient's schedule permits, it is recommended to start "three times a week" for 3 months and then decrease to "two times a week" thereafter.
- At each subsequent visit, ask the patient about pinkness/tenderness of the skin following the previous dose and document the response in the phototherapy record. A slight erythema persisting less than 24 hours is the optimal response.
  - If the patient notes no pinkness following the previous dose of NB-UVB (and none is noted on exam), then increase the dose by 50 mJ/cm^2.
  - If the patient reports pinkness following the previous dose (or if there is mild pinkness present on exam), then maintain the dose (ie, do not increase dose at that encounter).
  - If the patient reports that pinkness persisted for more than 24 hours (or if there is moderate erythema or any tenderness on exam), then decrease the subsequent dose by 25 mJ/cm^2.
  - If there is severe erythema or pain on exam, the physician should fully evaluate the patient. Further treatments should be delayed until all erythema and pain have resolved. Treatments may then be restarted at a "15% decreased dose" from the previous dose.
  - A typical "holding dose" is 800 mJ/cm^2, though this may vary or be increased over the course of treatment. Once the ordered holding dose is reached, hold at that dose until the patient is next evaluated by the ordering physician, which will generally be 6-12 weeks after starting therapy. The holding dose may be increased at that time.
  - If a significant time lapse between treatments sessions has occurred, then the current treatment dose should be adjusted based on the recommendations in Table 129.1.

Excimer Laser

Using a similar principle as NB-UVB, excimer laser is a highly effective modality that delivers a single wavelength of UVB light (308 nm) through a handheld device. It is typically best-suited

TABLE 129.1 ⋮ Dose Adjustments for Significant Time Lapses Between Treatment Sessions

TIME LAPSE	DOSE ADJUSTMENT
Up to 1 wk	Maintain dose
>1 to 2 wk	Decrease dose by 25%
>2 to 3 wk	Decrease dose by 50%
>3 to 4 wk	Decrease dose by 75%
>4 wk	Restart at 200 mJ/cm²

TABLE 129.2 ⋮ Dose Modifications of Excimer Laser

POST-TREATMENT RESPONSE	DOSE MODIFICATION
No erythema	Increase dose by 50 mJ/cm²
Transient asymptomatic erythema within 24 h	Maintain dose
Persistent asymptomatic erythema over 24 h	Decrease dose by 50 mJ/cm²
Persistent symptomatic erythema with pain or blister	Hold treatment until resolved, then reduce dose by 100 mJ/cm²

for more localized lesions or after NB-UVB has been utilized to treat larger areas of affected skin. Typically, 200 mJ/cm² may be used as the starting dose regardless of anatomic site, though some experts recommend decreasing to 150 mJ/cm² when starting on the face or neck and increasing to 300 mJ/cm² when starting on the hands or feet. Table 129.2 offers practical dose modifications based on the patient's post-treatment clinical response. Because a number of brands of this laser device are available clinicians should follow the instructions specific to their own device.

Postprocedural Approach

- Usually, no recovery time is needed.
- Treated areas may remain pink for a number of days and then self-resolve.
- Counsel on avoidance of excessive sun exposure following procedure.

- Follow-up depends on prearranged schedule, but should ideally be no longer than 1 week for retreatment for best results and no sooner than 48 hours between treatments.

REFERENCES

1. Paller AS, Mancini AJ. *Clinical Pediatric Dermatology*. 5th ed. Edinburgh, Scotland: Elsevier; 2016:245–248.
2. Driessche FV, Silverberg N. Current management of pediatric vitiligo. *Pediatr Drugs*. 2015;17:303–313.
3. Ezzedine K, Silverberg N. A practical approach to the diagnosis and treatment of vitiligo in children. *Pediatrics*. 2016;138:e20154126.
4. Harris JE, Scharf M. Vitiligo nbUVB Treatment Protocol. https://www.umassmed.edu/globalassets/vitiligo/umass-uvb-phototherapy-guidelines.pdf. Accessed July 4, 2020.

Part II: Surgical Transplantation

Maggi Ahmed, Dori Goldberg, and Bassel H. Mahmoud

INTRODUCTION

Vitiligo lesions can fail conventional medical and light treatment options. This treatment resistance is usually related to a complete loss of the melanocyte reservoir in the affected area. Moreover, some vitiligo patches are recalcitrant, especially if they are located on glabrous skin or if leucotrichia is present. In such circumstances, the follicular melanocyte stem cells are absent; therefore, repigmentation will not be achieved unless melanocytes are harvested from normally pigmented skin and then introduced surgically into the affected white area.

Surgical transplantation techniques in vitiligo are divided into two main groups: tissue transplantation and cellular transplantation procedures. The former group entails transferring skin grafts as a whole tissue to the recipient skin. The latter involves further separation of these skin grafts into cellular components. These cellular components are then applied onto denuded recipient skin. Among different techniques, melanocyte keratinocyte transplantation procedure (MKTP) is a cellular transplantation technique that is emerging as an important solution for stable white patches refractory to medical treatment. MKTP is a precise, fast, and safe surgical technique for transplantation that enables treatment of large depigmented lesions during a single surgical operation (Figure 129.1).

Since its debut in 1992, MKTP has proved to be an effective and well-tolerated therapeutic option for the repigmentation of stable vitiligo resistant to other treatments. In contrast to older procedures for treatment of vitiligo, MKTP uses a relatively smaller size of self-donor skin to repopulate a larger recipient area. This allows for better color match and fewer postoperative complications. Despite its proven efficacy, MKTP is an underperformed treatment in the United States. There are currently only a few centers offering MKTP in the United States, likely due

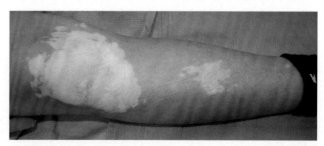

FIGURE 129.1. Vitiligo in an adolescent with skin type 4. Note the islands of repigmentation that are forming at the inferior portion of the knee lesion and within the more distal anterior shin lesion. Photo courtesy of Andrew C. Krakowski, MD.

to both a lack of awareness and availability of trained physician and staff.

Clinical Pearls

- **Guidelines:** No specific guidelines for the use or performance of the MKTP procedure exist.
- **Technique Tips:**
  - MKTP is usually performed in the outpatient dermatology clinic under local anesthesia.
  - It is an autologous transplantation procedure, in which the donor skin comes from the patient.
  - Normal pigment-producing cells (melanocytes) are harvested from unaffected skin of the same patient to be grafted onto vitiligo areas.
  - The skin is processed to make a single-cell suspension that contains healthy melanocytes.
  - Preparing the recipient area for the transplant can be done either by laser ablation or mechanical motorized dermabrasion.
    - Manual dermabrasion costs less compared with other techniques such as erbium yttrium aluminum garnet (Er:YAG) or carbon dioxide (CO_2) lasers but is both time and labor intensive, and it is difficult for large or concave surfaces (eg, eyelids, neck, axilla, and glans penis).
    - Laser resurfacing is faster and yields more uniform deepithelization, but it requires costly equipment and may increase the risk of unwanted color changes.
- **Age-Specific Considerations:**
  - We limit the procedure to children who are old enough to be able to tolerate the intralesional injection of anesthesia and to those who are developmentally mature enough to be able to hold still and to follow the instructions during the procedure.
  - Usually, children aged 8 and older have the best success with being able to comply with the treatment.
- **Skin of Color Considerations:**
  - MKTP is suited for all Fitzpatrick skin phototypes I through VI, with excellent color match among all phototypes.
    - Darker skinned patients experience earlier repigmentation within 1 to 2 months following the procedure.
    - The risk of dyspigmentation in the donor area, however, increases with darker skin types.

Contraindications/Cautions/Risks

Contraindications

- Active vitiligo disease, defined by the appearance of new spots, expansion of the size of current spots, or koebnerization (disease spreading to sites of skin trauma such as scrapes, burns, or scratches) within preceding 12 months
- Active skin infection, particularly herpes labialis or impetigo, at the donor or the recipient areas
- Previous diagnosis of impaired wound healing or history of keloid formation
- History of bleeding tendencies

Risks

- Bleeding
- Infections
- Color mismatch: postinflammatory hyperpigmentation or hypopigmentation
- Scarring: atrophic scar, hypertrophic scar, or keloids

Equipment Needed

Obtaining the Donor Graft

- Sterile marker pen
- Sterile towel packs
- Lidocaine with no epinephrine for intralesional injection
- Silver's skin graft knife, or Dermablade™ (Accutec Blades Inc., US) if skin graft knife is not available
- Petrolatum-based ointment
- Bishop forceps
- Sterile gauze
- DuoDerm® (Convatec/McKesson)
- Sterile adhesive dressing

Preparing the Recipient Site

- Ablative resurfacing laser machine (Er:YAG or CO_2 laser) or motorized dermabrasion
- Lidocaine with no epinephrine for intralesional injection or lidocaine 23% + tetracaine 7% cream
- Vaseline-impregnated gauze (Xeroform™ [Covidien/Medtronic, US])
- Collagen wound dressing (Puracol Microscaffold)
- Transparent occlusive dressing (Tegaderm® [3M, US])
- If laser resurfacing is used:
  - Wavelength-specific eye shields
  - Smoke evacuator
  - Zimmer Cryo Cooler

Preparation of the Suspension

- Tabletop tissue incubator adjusted at 37°C
- Tabletop centrifugation
- One bottle of 0.25% trypsin solution with EDTA tetrasodium
- One bottle of Ringer's lactate
- Two Petri dishes
- Two Bishop forceps
- Plastic pipette
- One 15-mL conical tube
- 1-mL syringe
- 30-gauge 1-in needle

Preprocedural Approach

- Four weeks before surgery, we ask that patients begin to apply tacrolimus ointment; in our experience, this approach improves the repigmentation.
- Prophylaxis for herpes simplex is not needed before laser or mechanical resurfacing, because the ablation depth is superficial (limited to the epidermis).
- Patients are recommended to bathe the morning of their surgery.

Procedural Approach

Donor Area

1. Pick uninvolved skin area to harvest the healthy skin, usually upper lateral aspect of the thigh or gluteal region.
2. Draw the borders of the donor area, which is calculated approximately as one-fifth the size of the recipient area.
3. Disinfect the donor area using chlorhexidine, povidone-iodine, or 70% ethanol.
4. Inject the lidocaine into the borders as well as into the center of the marked area to be harvested.
5. Obtain a thin split-thickness shaved skin sample using either a Silver's skin grafting knife (Figure 129.2A) or a Dermablade (Figure 129.2B).

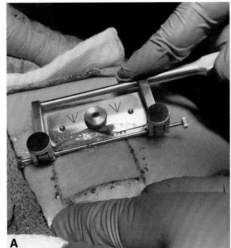
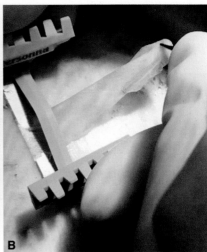

FIGURE 129.2. Obtaining a superficial split-thickness shave skin from a healthy donor site of the patient with a Silver's skin graft knife (A) or surgical Dermablade (B).

6. Obtain the shaved donor skin piece with a Bishop forceps and place it in a Petri dish containing 5 mL of lactate Ringer's solution.

7. Compress the resultant wound with gauze to stop the superficial bleeding. After the bleeding stops, dress the resultant wound with 4 × 4 DuoDerm hydrocolloid dressing, sterile gauze, and adhesive dressing that are removed after 1 week.

Suspension Preparation

1. Wash the obtained shaved donor skin thoroughly with Ringer's lactate in a Petri dish, preferably two to three times for 1 minute.

2. Transfer the donor skin to a new Petri dish containing 5 mL of 0.25% trypsin solution with ethylenediaminetetraacetic acid (EDTA) tetrasodium and incubate it in a tissue incubator for 30 to 60 minutes at 37°C.

3. After incubation, remove the trypsin with a plastic pipette, and wash the skin sample with Ringer's lactate solution to remove residual trypsin.

4. Use two pairs of forceps to separate the dermis (white and thicker part) from the epidermis (skin colored and thinner part) mechanically.

5. Discard the dermis.

6. Break down the epidermis in the Petri dish to multiple small pieces using the forceps. Mince the small epidermal pieces well using the same forceps.

7. Add 1- to 15-mL Ringer's lactate and transfer the minced epidermis using a plastic pipette into a 15-mL conical tube.

8. Centrifuge the conical tube for 5 to 10 minutes, at 2000 rpm to separate the cell pellet (Figure 129.3A).

9. After centrifugation, discard the floating pieces. Do not alter the pigmented pellet that forms because it contains the epidermal cells (mainly melanocytes and keratinocytes).

10. Resuspend the pellet in Ringer's lactate to facilitate the preparation of cell suspension; the final volume will be 1 mL/100 cm^2 (Figure 129.3B).

11. Use a 1-mL syringe to obtain the suspension.

Recipient Area

1. Mark down the area to be treated (ie, the vitiligo lesion) with a sterile marker pen.

2. Measure the marked area to be treated in cm^2. It is ideal that you do not treat more than 100 cm^2 per one treatment session.

3. Disinfect the area to be treated with chlorhexidine and povidone-iodine. Avoid using alcohol if laser is planned for dermabrasion.

4. Anesthetize the area to be treated using 1% Xylocaine, or topically with cream (lidocaine 23% + tetracaine 7%), for 1 hour.

5. Ablate the epidermis of the selected spot using ablative resurfacing laser Er:YAG or CO_2; the depth of ablation is confined to the epidermis 100 to 300 μm (Figure 129.4A).

6. An alternative ablative method is via motorized dermabrasion using a diamond fraise wheel. The operator passes the wheel back and forth on the white patch until achieving homogeneous pinpoint bleeding (Figure 129.4B).

7. Apply cell suspension to the recipient area, using a 1-mL insulin syringe after detaching the needle (Figure 129.5).

8. Cover the transplanted suspension directly with dry, thin collagen wound dressing.

9. Cover the collagen dressing with Vaseline-impregnated gauze that is subsequently covered with sterile gauze pieces and, then, by a transparent film dressing.

10. Finally, cover the wound with gauze; this acts as a pressure dressing to keep the transplanted cells in adherence with the treated area.

11. The donor site and the treated area covering dressing are removed after 1 week.

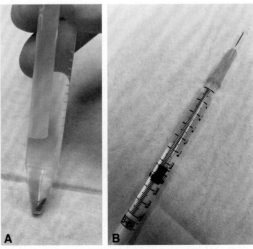

FIGURE 129.3. The epidermal pellet rich in melanocytes after centrifugation (A), resuspended into a single cell suspension (B).

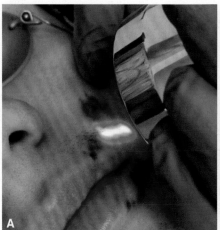 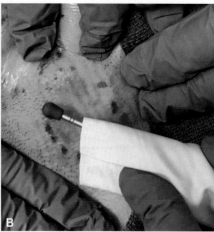

FIGURE 129.4. Preparing the recipient skin by Er:YAG ablative laser (A) or mechanical motorized dermabrasion (B).

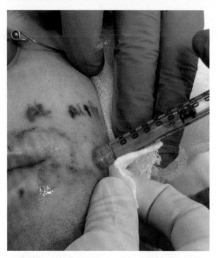

FIGURE 129.5. The cell suspension is applied directly to the dermabraded recipient site.

Postprocedural Approach

- The patient gets discharged home on the same day, an hour after the procedure, remaining still during this time to allow the transplanted cells to settle.

- The patient should avoid showering or swimming or doing any activity that could result in shifting of the dressing until it is removed in the dermatology clinic 1 week postoperatively.
- The treated area will initially appear red; however, early signs of skin repigmentation will be noticed within 4 to 8 weeks, and this will progress up to 4 to 6 months after the procedure.
- The patient can resume usual activities 2 weeks following the procedure.
- Patients are encouraged to contact the physician directly for concerns and are often provided phone numbers for direct contact and reassurance.

The procedure is not covered by insurance in the United States so far. Current Procedural Terminology (CPT) codes for MKTP are institutional; there is no universal code for MKTP.

SUGGESTED READINGS

Falabella R. Surgical treatment of vitiligo: why, when and how. *J Eur Acad Dermatol Venereol.* 2003;17:518–520.

Mulekar SV. Long-term follow-up study of segmental and focal vitiligo treated by autologous, noncultured melanocyte-keratinocyte cell transplantation. *Arch Dermatol.* 2004;140(10):1211–1215.

Parsad D, Gupta S; IADVL Dermatosurgery Task Force. Standard guidelines of care for vitiligo surgery. *Indian J Dermatol Venereol Leprol.* 2008;74(suppl):S37–S45.

CHAPTER 130

Xeroderma Pigmentosum

Nelise Ritter Hans-Bittner, Luciana Paula Samorano,
Maria Cecília Rivitti Machado, Zilda Najjar Prado de Oliveira, and
Eugênio Raul de Almeida Pimentel

Introduction

Xeroderma pigmentosum (XP) is a rare, autosomally recessive inherited disease characterized by extreme sensitivity to sunlight, resulting in sunburn, pigment changes in the skin, and a greatly elevated incidence of skin cancers on the sun-exposed body sites. XP has been found in all continents and across all racial groups. Males and females are similarly affected.

All of the changes seen in photoaging, with the notable exception of solar elastosis, are visible at a very early age, often in early childhood. Later, sun-induced neoplasms appear, including actinic keratoses, keratoacanthomas, squamous cell carcinomas, basal cell carcinomas, and melanomas, often in large numbers (Figures 130.1 to 130.3).

Early diagnosis is crucial for XP. As an inherited condition, a cure cannot be expected. Current management strategy includes

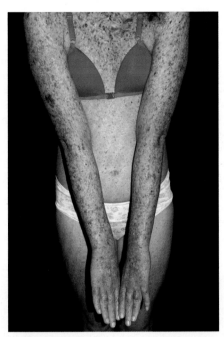

FIGURE 130.1. Teenage female with xeroderma pigmentosum. Presence of suspicious melanocytic skin lesion on the right proximal arm, and postoperative scar on the upper trunk.

careful avoidance of sun exposure, combined with treatment of precancerous and cancerous lesions as they arise. Treatment options for skin cancer in XP include surgery, electrocoagulation, topical 5-fluorouracil, or imiquimod 5% cream.

Herein, we offer our instructions for the management of patients with XP. Our multimodal approach seeks to improve the quality of life and life expectancy of affected individuals. Our protocol utilizes cryotherapy, electrocoagulation and curettage, and surgical resection for the treatment of precancerous lesions and skin cancer, besides recommendations for strict and complete protection from ultraviolet (UV), imiquimod 5% cream, regular follow-up, total body photography and dermoscopy three times a year, and confocal microscopy if necessary. Mohs micrographic

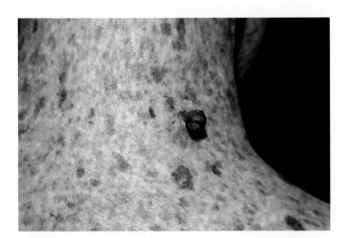

FIGURE 130.2. Presence of suspicious skin lesion (amelanotic melanoma versus squamous cell carcinoma versus basal cell carcinoma) on the posterior neck of a patient with xeroderma pigmentosum. Pigment changes on sun-exposed skin.

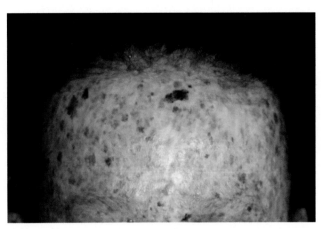

FIGURE 130.3. Presence of several suspicious melanocytic skin lesions on the forehead of a female with xeroderma pigmentosum.

surgery is performed in the case of recurrence of all nonmelanoma skin cancers. In the authors' experience, the use of systemic retinoids in children has failed to prevent skin cancer.

 Clinical Pearls

- **Guidelines:** No specific treatment guidelines are known to exist for this condition.
- **Age-Specific Considerations:** The treatment of premalignant lesions and skin cancer should start very soon after diagnosis. However, most children with XP dislike procedures such as cryotherapy and surgery. In such patients, general anesthesia once or twice a year, depending on the number of lesions to be treated, should be considered to maintain an effective and less painful treatment.
- **Technique Tips:** Skin biopsy and/or confocal microscopy must be done before surgical procedures.
- **Skin of Color Considerations:** Cryotherapy and electrocoagulation may cause dyspigmentation; however, so does XP. Because patients with XP undergo many surgical interventions throughout their lives, we prefer these techniques whenever indicated, instead of conventional surgery.

Contraindications/Cautions/Risks

Contraindications

- **Cryotherapy:** skin tumor without well-defined borders, melanoma, lesions on the angle of the mouth
- **Electrocoagulation:** same as cryotherapy, and periorificial lesions, because of the risk of skin retraction
- **Surgery:** active skin infection on surgical site, inability to care for postoperative wounds

Cautions

- **Electrocoagulation:** patients with cardiac devices; avoid alcohol as an antiseptic agent or allow it to dry completely because it may ignite.
- **Surgery:** history of bleeding and allergic reactions

Risks

- Death (infection or anesthesia), scarring, pain, bleeding, recurrence of lesions

Equipment Needed

- **Cryotherapy**
  - Cryosurgical unit: CRY-AC® (Brymill Cryogenic Systems)
  - Liquid nitrogen
  - Spray-tip size C
- **Electrocoagulation and curettage**
  - Electrosurgical device
  - Disposable electrode tips
  - Smoke evacuator
  - Antiseptic agent (chlorhexidine or povidone-iodine)
  - Curette/scoop
  - Local anesthetics
- **Surgery**
  - Lidocaine 1% with epinephrine 1:100 000
  - Bupivacaine 0.5% with epinephrine 1:200 000
  - Saline
  - Scissors
  - Clamps
  - Hooks
  - Electrocautery
  - Smoke evacuator
  - Gauze
  - Surgical marker pen, tissue stain
  - Mohs laboratory (cryostat, hematoxylin and eosin stain)—if Mohs surgery is necessary
  - Suture
  - Petrolatum-based ointment
  - Micropore Surgical Tape™ (3M™, US)

Preprocedural Approach

- **Cryotherapy**
  - Topical anesthetics 1 hour before the procedure to help reduce the pain associated with freezing
- **Electrocoagulation and curettage and surgery**
  - Special attention to medications that may affect bleeding
  - Prophylaxis for herpes simplex is not routinely indicated.
  - Patients should bathe either the evening before or on the morning of their surgery.

Procedural Approach

Informed consent from the parent/guardian and, when possible, assent from the minor should be obtained.

- **Cryotherapy**—for premalignant lesions
  - Antiseptics are not typically indicated.
  - Open spray technique:
    - Spray liquid nitrogen through a cryospray (CRY-AC, Brymill) directly over the lesion, using spray-tip size C held close to the lesion (approximately 1 cm distance) and perpendicular to the skin surface.
    - Goal: single freeze-thaw cycle, 15 seconds of freezing-time
- **Electrocoagulation and curettage**—for skin cancer (non-melanoma)
  - Smoke evacuator is necessary to help remove plume smoke, and all present should wear masks.
  - The dispersive plate should make good contact with the bare skin of a well-vascularized part of the patients' body.
  - Local anesthetics before the procedure
  - Tumor curettage:
    - Use a large curette (4-6 mm) to debulk all friable tissue.
    - Next, use a small curette (2 mm) to scrape across the surface of the treatment site in every direction.

- Electrosurgical treatment: electrocoagulation current to stop bleeding and potentially remove further tumor
- Repeat this process for a total of three cycles of curettage and electrosurgery, until all friable tissue has been removed.
- **Surgery**—Conventional surgery is our treatment option for all operable melanoma in patients with XP. It is also performed in most of the primary skin cancers in patients with XP. Mohs micrographic surgery is our treatment option in the case of recurrence of all non-melanoma skin cancers.
  - Typically, general anesthesia is utilized in children because of the pain associated with the procedure. However, some older patients might tolerate the procedure under local anesthesia only.
  - The surgical site must be cleaned with alcohol 70%.
  - The tumor area is marked with a permanent pen.
  - Then, the margin is defined depending on the type and location of the tumor, as well as on the type of the surgery (Mohs or conventional excision).
  - Good hemostasis is made with electrocauterization using the clamps if necessary.
  - After tumor removal, reconstruction is made; in some areas, depending on the tumor size and dimension (oval, circle or another shape), a primary closure is an option.
  - Surgical site must be cleaned with saline and adequately dried.
  - Finally, a petrolatum-based ointment is applied and a dressing with gauze and Micropore Surgical Tape is then made.

Postprocedural Approach

- **Cryotherapy**
  - Erythema, local edema, vesicle formation, exudation, crusting, and shallow eschar development are expected after the procedure, and should disappear within 2 to 4 weeks
  - Most lesions require basic wound aftercare, including washing the treated area three times a day with gentle soap and water or with hydrogen peroxide solution 3%. Petrolatum-based ointment is immediately reapplied and maintained until reepithelialization has occurred.
  - Patients are instructed to maintain strict sunlight protection, especially in the treatment area.
  - Patients should be vigilantly monitored for signs and symptoms of infection.
  - Patients are encouraged to contact the physician directly for concerns.
- **Electrocoagulation and curettage**
  - An eschar forms within a few days and separates in about 10 days; deeper wounds should take 2 to 4 weeks to heal (or longer on the lower extremities).
  - Generally, pain medications such as Tylenol are sufficient to prevent discomfort after the procedure.
  - The original bandages should be removed within 24 hours.
  - The exposed wound area should be cleaned with saline using a gauze pad after showering normally.
  - Then, petrolatum-based, Polysporin™ (Johnson & Johnson, US) or bacitracin ointment should be applied (do *not* use Neosporin™ [Johnson & Johnson, US]) with a clean Q-tip being careful not to contaminate the supply of ointment.
  - The wound should be covered with a nonstick gauze pad and Micropore Surgical Tape.
  - Wound care should be repeated once a day until the wound is completely healed.
  - The wound should heal faster with a better cosmetic result if kept moist with ointment and covered with a bandage.

○ Patients should be vigilantly monitored for signs and symptoms of infection.

○ Patients are encouraged to contact the physician directly for concerns.

- **Surgery**
  ○ Generally, pain should increase during the night of the excision. Pain medications as Tylenol are usually enough to control it. After the second day, pain should not be increasing and is generally tolerable by this point.

  ○ Swelling and bruising are normal around the surgical site. The bruising will fade in approximately 10 to 14 days.

  ○ The bandage should remain in place for 48 hours. After this time, it should be removed and cleaned daily with saline and gauze, and then covered with a BAND-AID™ (Johnson & Johnson, US) or gauze and Micropore Surgical Tape.

  ○ For skin grafts, prolonged exposure to extremely cold temperatures should be avoided for 3 weeks.

  ○ Patients should be vigilantly monitored for signs and symptoms of infection, especially symptoms of pain, fever, or reddish area.

  ○ Postoperative downtime is significant, and patients should expect to be absent from school or work for 3 days to the minor reconstructions and 5 days to a week for the bigger ones.

○ When the suture is not absorbable, the stiches should be removed after 7 days.

○ As soon as the stitches have been removed, the wound should be gently cleaned with soapy water using a Q-tip or gauze pad (shower/bathe normally). Then the wound should be adequately dried, followed by application of petrolatum, Polysporin, or bacitracin ointment (do *not* use Neosporin), and then covered with a nonstick gauze pad and Micropore Surgical Tape.

○ Petrolatum, Polysporin, or bacitracin ointment (do *not* use Neosporin) should be applied until the wound is fully healed.

○ Patients are encouraged to contact the physician directly for concerns.

SUGGESTED READINGS

Lambert WC, Lambert MW. Development of effective skin cancer treatment and prevention in xeroderma pigmentosum. *Photochem Photobiol.* 2015;91(2):475–483.

Latour I, Hernández-Martín A, Ged C, Knöpfel N, Taïeb A, Torrelo A. Reversed actinic damage in two children with xeroderma pigmentosum treated with topical imiquimod. *J Eur Acad Dermatol Venereol.* 2018;32(7):e282–e284.

Lehmann AR, McGibbon D, Stefanini M. Xeroderma pigmentosum. *Orphanet J Rare Dis.* 2011;6:70.

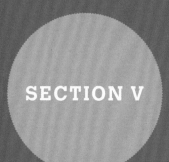

SECTION V

Postprocedural Approach

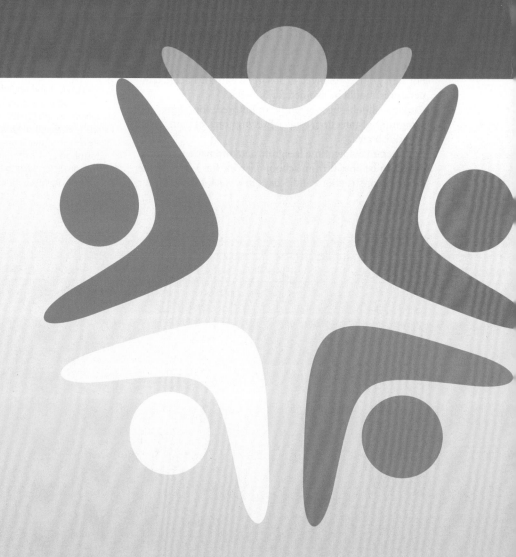

131 Wound Dressings

132 Wound Care and Optimizing Healing

133 Postprocedure Antibiotics

134 Pain Management

135 Photoprotection

136 Surgical Complications

137 Wet Wrap Therapy

138 Bleach Baths

139 Patient and Family Resources

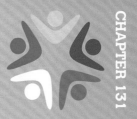
Wound Dressings

Kellie Badger and Harper N. Price

HISTORY OF WOUND CARE

Wound dressings are the basis for wound care and the mainstay treatment to facilitate wound healing. With the vast selection of wound care dressings and topical preparations available today, it easily becomes overwhelming for practitioners to discern the most fitting types of dressings and topical products for wounds in their patients. To date, there are over 5000 different wound care products available and over 1000 wound care centers in the United States. Wound healing has become a medical specialty, with some academic centers even offering fellowship programs.[1] A brief history regarding the initial development and utilization of dressings prefaces this discussion.

Wound care dates back to 2200 BC when the first "plaster" was developed.[1] During this time, the ancients and early moderns developed plasters from mixtures of available substances, including mud or clay, plants, and herbs. The plasters were then applied directly to wounds for protection and to absorb any exudate.[1] Honey grease and lint made from vegetables were the main components of plaster used by the Egyptians. Lint was used for absorption of drainage, whereas grease and honey may have offered protection from infection. The Greeks, too, had great insight on the cleanliness of wounds. They often used boiled water, vinegar, and wine to cleanse wounds. During the 18th century, surgery became an important part of medicine. In the 19th century, the antiseptic technique was introduced, and antibiotics followed in the early half of the 20th century. These breakthroughs significantly reduced infection rates and decreased mortality related to wound infections.

To date, thousands of wound care products, therapies, and methods have been developed and still hold true to many of the historically held beliefs. For example, emollients are often applied to wound dressings to help prevent them from adhering to the wound bed. Likewise, medical grade honey preparations and silver-based products are utilized in wound care for their broad antimicrobial effects, and vinegar is used to control the bacterial load of specific organisms, such as *Staphylococcus aureus* and *Pseudomonas*.

The modern approach to wound dressings starts with a detailed assessment of the wound itself (see Chapter 132. Wound Care and Optimizing Healing) and a clear comprehension of the different categories of dressings and their properties. Table 131.1 illustrates the various categories of wound care products available and their primary function, and brief descriptions of these products follow.

WOUND DRESSINGS AND PROPERTIES

Dressings can be classified depending on their physical properties and material as well as on their function. Various dressing types are available, and these are broadly categorized into *occlusive/moisture retentive dressings*, such as films, foams, hydrogels, alginates, and hydrocolloids, and *open dressings*, such as gauze (Figure 131.1). By definition, occlusive dressings

prevent less water vapor transmission from the wound. Occlusive dressings are ideal, especially in nonsuture wounds, in that they can increase reepithelialization rates and collagen synthesis as compared to wounds left exposed to air.[2] More modern occlusive, nonbiologic dressings include hydrofiber and collagen dressings. Biologic, occlusive dressings include split-thickness, full-thickness, and composite skin grafts (not discussed here), as well as skin substitutes (such as cultured epidermal grafts). Lastly, there are antimicrobial dressings that are occlusive/moisture retentive and offer additional antibacterial effects.

Dressings can also be categorized depending on their properties of adherence, although most dressings, if used improperly, can become adherent. Typical nonadherent dressings include foams (examples include Mepitel, Adaptic® [Johnson & Johnson, US]), gauzes (such as Vaseline™ Petrolatum Gauze [Cardinal Health]), and alginates, which also serve the function of absorption. Nonadherent fabric dressings are often impregnated with components to increase their occlusion potential and prevent adherence; some may contain antimicrobial components, as well. Wound dressings classified as *occlusive/moisture-retentive* as well as *absorptive* include the alginate and foam dressings.

The overall goal of utilization of wound dressings should always be to facilitate wound healing in the least traumatic and most time-efficient way. Several ideal properties of modern wound dressings help in this regard, including the ability to maintain a moist environment, enable gas exchange, prevent infection/contamination, and avoid trauma to the repairing tissues (Table 131.2). Patient compliance to prescribed wound care regimens must also be considered; consequently, bandages should be easy to apply and maintain and should be cost permissive, among other considerations.

Dressing wounds commonly involves up to three layers of products: a contact layer, an absorbent layer, and a secondary or outer layer. The contact layer is placed directly on the wound; oftentimes, a nonadhesive or nontraumatic contact layer is chosen to minimize pain or tissue damage when removed. A plain sterile gauze applied as a contact layer can absorb drainage but will tend to stick to a wound, whether sutured or open; for this reason, a bland ointment such as petrolatum should be applied to prevent adherence to the wound bed. Ointments are also often utilized on nonadherent, occlusive dressings such as foams, to prevent sticking and desiccation of wounds. The absorbent layer of the dressing is designed to absorb exudate away from the wound and provide mechanical cushioning. When a contact layer and absorbent layer are combined in a single product, this is termed the *primary dressing* (eg, Telfa dressing). Lastly, the outer layer or secondary dressing, if needed, is often a gauze wrap or cotton wadding, added for further mechanical protection or to apply pressure on the wound (eg, a pressure dressing for a postsurgical wound); this layer often requires a retention dressing or tape to secure it in place. Secondary dressings can function to help immobilize a wound and apply pressure to prevent bleeding and hematoma formation when applicable. Retention dressings such as rolled gauze or surgical netting can be used to nontraumatically secure a layered dressing in place.

TABLE 131.1 ⦙ Common Wound Dressings and Primary Characteristics and Products

PRODUCT TYPE	APPEARANCE	ABSORPTION	INFECTION PREVENTION OR TREATMENT	NONADHERENT	PROTECTION	RETENTION	EXAMPLE PRODUCTS
NonBiologic Occlusive/Moisture-Retentive Dressings							
Alginates	Woven, fibrous	X	X				Algisite™Ag (Smith & Nephew, Ireland), Melgisorb®Ag (Wound Source)
Hydrocolloid	Soft, opaque pads				X		DuoDerm® (Convatec/McKesson), Restore (Hollister)
Foams	Soft pad	X	X	X	X		Mepilex® Transfer Ag (Molnlycke), Mepilex® Lite (Molnlycke), Polymem® (Ferris Corp, USA), Hydrofera Blue® (Hydrofera, USA)
Films	Transparent film		X		X		Tegaderm® (3M, USA)
Hydrogels	Semitransparent		X	X			Restore® (Hollister), Hydrogel, KeragelT® (Keraplast Technologies LLC)
Antimicrobial							
Honey	Thick liquid in tube or jar, sheet		X				Medihoney® (©2009 Derma Sciences, Inc)
Gauze							
Impregnated gauze	Sheets of moist gauze			X	X		Adaptic® (Johnson & Johnson, US), Vaseline Petrolatum Gauze
Retention Dressings							
Retention dressings	Thin roll					X	Tubifast® (Molnlycke), X-Span® Dressing (Alba Health, Surgilast® (Derma Sciences Inc)

Specific branded products may vary according to the manufacturer's formulary.

Reprinted with permission from Ebnurse.org presented by AdaptHealth Patient Care Solutions. Wound care. http://ebnurse.org/wound-care. Accessed February 4, 2019.

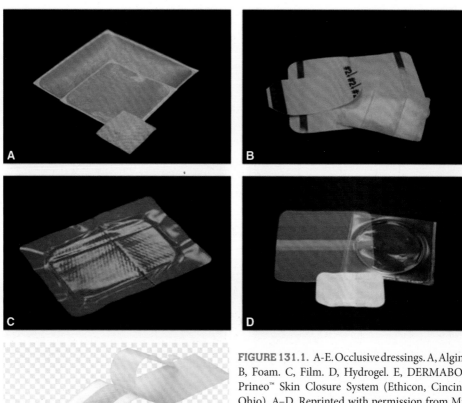

FIGURE 131.1. A-E. Occlusive dressings. A, Alginate. B, Foam. C, Film. D, Hydrogel. E, DERMABOND Prineo™ Skin Closure System (Ethicon, Cincinatti, Ohio). A–D, Reprinted with permission from Miller MG, Berry DC. *Emergency Response Management for Athletic Trainers.* 2nd ed. Philadelphia, PA: Wolters Kluwer; 2016. Figure 14.4. E, DERMABOND Prineo™ Skin Closure System used with permisison from Ethicon, Cincinatti, Ohio 2020.

Alginate Dressings

Alginate dressings are derived from calcium and sodium salts of alginic acid, a seaweed/kelp-based polysaccharide (Figure 131.2A). They create a gel in the wound bed by exchanging calcium ions from the alginate for sodium ions in the wound bed and are used for wounds with a moderate to heavy amount of exudate. They are capable of absorbing 15 to 20 times their own weight in water.[3] These dressings are an excellent choice when infection is present, because infected wounds often have an increased amount of exudate. Silver-impregnated alginate dressings donate additional antimicrobial properties to the wound.

Alginate dressings are soft, nonwoven fibers that become gellike when saturated with exudate. The gel provides a moist environment and promotes wound healing. The gel-forming ability of these dressings prevents the dressing from adhering to the wound bed, allowing for regular removal with water or saline (ie, for wound inspection and cleansing purposes) without damaging the wound bed and with less discomfort to the patient. The alginate sheets or pads should be cut or folded to the shape of the wound and applied directly to the wound surface and then secured with gauze (rolled or sheet) and a retention dressing. These dressings are typically changed on a daily basis. When necessary, they can be left on for several days at a time; however, doing so increases the risk that the dressing will dry and adhere to the wound.

Alginate dressings are best used for chronic or refractory ulcers, wounds with moderate to heavy exudate, and bleeding wounds (due to their hemostatic properties). Specific wound examples include venous insufficiency ulcers, diabetic ulcers, pressure ulcers, surgical wounds, and first- and second-degree burns. They should not be used for minimally draining wounds or third-degree burns. A disadvantage to these dressings is that they may actually dehydrate a wound, impede healing, and adhere to the wound base if desiccated. Thus, they should not be used on wounds with dry crust or eschar. The gel formed in the wound may also be mistaken for purulence, which may be confusing to patients.

TABLE 131.2 ⋮ Ideal Properties in a Wound Dressing

POSITIVE PATIENT FACTORS	PROMOTES HEALING	REDUCES INFECTION RISK
Materials easily obtained and stored	Maintains moisture	Debrides necrotic tissue
Easily applied and maintained	Minimizes trauma/ maceration to wound edges	Absorbs excess exudate
Aesthetically acceptable	Minimizes fluid/ heat loss	Minimizes external contamination
Financially tolerable	Facilitates gas exchange	Removes odor
Nonallergenic	Compression: min- imizes edema, hemostasis	
Pain reducing		

Reprinted with permission from Ebnurse.org presented by AdaptHealth Patient Care Solutions. Wound care. http://ebnurse.org/wound-care. Accessed February 4, 2019.

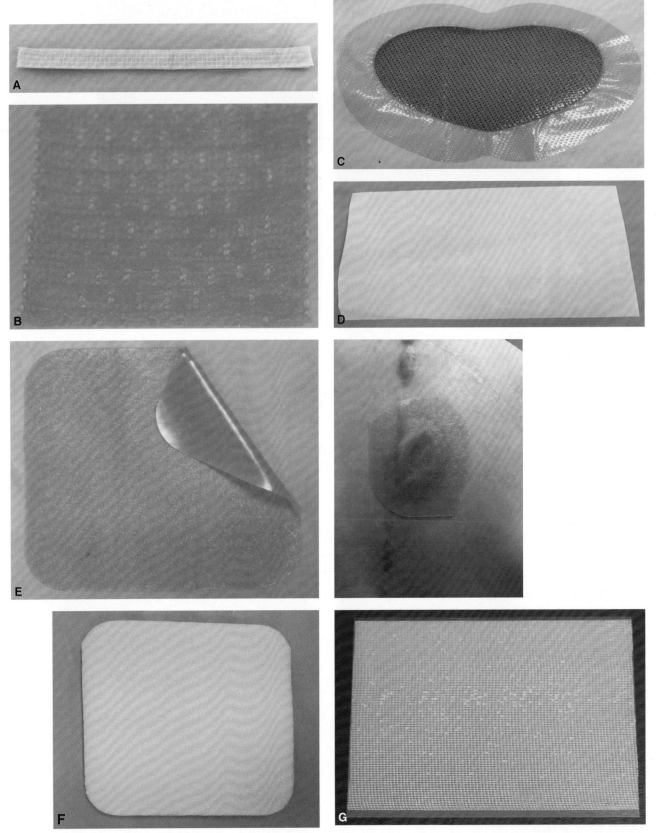

FIGURE 131.2. A-J. Examples of various dressings used in wound care. A, Alginate. B, Antibacterial honey dressing. C, Antibacterial silver dressing; note darker center of dressing is silver. D, Collagen dressing. E, Hydrocolloid dressing (left), dressing applied to wound (right). F, Foam dressing. G, Hydrogel dressing.

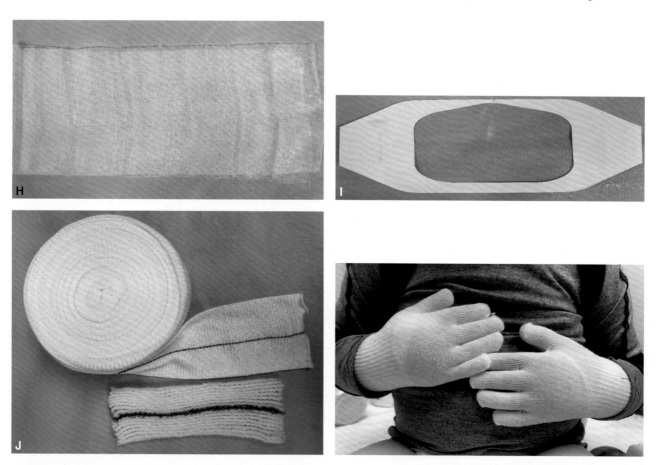

FIGURE 131.2. (*continued*) H, Impregnated gauze dressing. I, Film dressing. J (left), Retention dressings. J (right), Retention dressings (gloves).

Antimicrobial Dressings

Antimicrobial dressings are impregnated with antimicrobial elements that aid in reducing the bacterial load of colonized wounds, prevent infection and the spread of bacteria to surrounding tissues, and keep the wound moist (Figure 131.2B and C). In doing so, overall wound healing time can be reduced. These dressings are typically applied directly to the wound bed and secured in the same manner as are other contact dressings (ie, with rolled gauze and retention dressing). These dressings should be changed depending on the level of exudate and saturation, but they can be left in place for several days when appropriate.

Antimicrobial dressings come in various forms, and the specific dressing type should be carefully considered depending on wound assessment. Silver-containing dressings are common antimicrobial offerings that are purported to work because silver cations disrupt bacterial cell walls, deactivate cellular enzymes and attachment to DNA, and prevent bacterial transcription.[4] Silver-impregnated dressings are bactericidal, with no documented resistance to date, and have a broad spectrum of activity; they also have activity against yeast and fungi. Odors may also be improved with silver dressings.

Silver dressings should be used for short durations because of the potential for systemic absorption; if improvement in the wound is not seen within 2 weeks of use, then other dressings should be considered. These products also have the potential to discolor the skin with a grayish hue if used for any extended length of time; if the skin is noted to have a change in color, then discontinue silver dressings and replace them with a different antimicrobial dressing if still indicated. Lastly, ensure these dressings are removed before magnetic resonance imaging (MRI), electrocardiogram (ECG), or electroencephalogram (EEG) procedures.

There is an increasing interest from patients and providers in the use of honey in wound care as a broad antibacterial agent with no microbial resistance noted to date. Honey-impregnated dressings (gauze and sheets) are also available and have long been thought to have antibacterial benefits (Figure 131.2B). Medical grade honey products can also help promote autolytic debridement.[5] However, solid evidence regarding their efficacy as compared to other dressings is lacking. These types of dressings are helpful to maintain a moist wound bed environment and are best for partial- to full-thickness wounds that have moderate to heavy levels of drainage. These dressings can sometimes be adherent and they may not be suitable for those with fragile skin. Medical grade honey products also come as cream formulations (such as Medihoney) and have the ability to be used underneath dressings or applied onto dressings such as foam. Care should be taken to instruct patients and families that the use of nonmedical grade honey products is not recommended because these may contain microorganisms that could contaminate the wound.

Collagen and Hydrofiber Dressings

Derived from cowhide, collagen dressings contain type 1 bovine collagen and are, accordingly, a relatively newer form of a nonbiologic dressing (Figure 131.2D). Collagen dressings come in sheets, foams, and gels and can be applied directly to the wound bed and moistened with saline to allow better adherence. These dressings provide a collagen matrix for cellular migration into the wound. Collagen dressings may be used for wounds with moderate to exuberant drainage and recalcitrant ulcers, and they can be cut to the size and shape of the wound. These dressings are then secured with rolled gauze and a retention dressing. Uncommonly, these dressings may cause irritation or an initial increase in wound drainage.

Hydrofiber dressings are best for moderate to heavy exudative wounds, especially those that are prone to bleeding, because they are even more absorbent than are alginates. They consist of soft, carboxymethyl cellulose fibers that form a soft gel when in contact with exudate. Hydrofiber dressings are supplied as nonwoven pads or ribbons (which can be used in wound cavities as packing). Because these dressings are nonadherent, they require a secondary dressing. Sterile saline irrigation may be needed to remove the dressing and prevent damage to the underlying granulation tissue.

Hydrocolloid Dressings

Hydrocolloid dressings are manufactured in the form of amorphous sheets, gels, pastes, and powders from substances such as cellulose, gelatin pectin, and guar and come in varying sizes and thicknesses (Figure 131.2E).[5] Hydrocolloids can be used to fill cavities and once absorption of water occurs, they can prevent bacterial proliferation.[6] When the hydrocolloid is placed on a wound with exudate, it absorbs the drainage and forms a gel. These dressing sheets are opaque, self-adhesive, and waterproof, so there is typically no need for a secondary or retention dressing. Hydrocolloids are ideal for wounds over joints, because they can provide some cushion and protection as well. They are an ideal choice for self- (or autolytic) debridement and enhance angiogenesis and granulation tissue formation. Infected wounds should be treated before use. If a large amount of exudate is present, the dressing should be changed daily and may not be the ideal choice in the absence of the need for debridement (eg, consider a more absorptive contact layer); otherwise, this dressing can be changed every 2 to 3 days, depending on saturation. These dressing, when absorbing exudate, may develop an unpleasant odor, and the gel under the dressing can become thick and yellow, creating undue anxiety and concern for a potential infection. The dressings can also leak when heavy exudate is present and may cause local tissue maceration. Figure 131.2E illustrates an example of a common hydrocolloid dressing, Duo-Derm, used in the dermatologic setting.

Because of their autolytic activity, hydrocolloid dressings may cause wounds to slightly enlarge initially. However, their protective and waterproof nature offer distinct advantages. The sheets of hydrocolloid can be cut to more appropriately fit the specific wound size and may be adjusted as the wound evolves. The dressing should extend about 1 cm (or more) from the wound edge so that the dressing will properly adhere to the normal adjacent skin and remain in place. Removal is done when the dressing starts to lift and liquefy; this is often done easily and nontraumatically if adequately timed. Any remaining colloid in the wound bed should be rinsed with sterile saline, and adhesive can be removed gently with mineral oil.

Foam Dressings

Foams are hydrophobic, soft, adsorptive, semiocclusive, and semipermeable polyurethane dressings with an absorbent, gas-permeable inner layer and a nonabsorbent semipermeable outer layer

(Figure 131.2F). The inner layer acts to absorb exudate away from the wound while still keeping the wound bed moist, whereas the outer layer permits release of water vapor and prevents bacterial contamination. These dressings can be adhesive or nonadhesive and can come in varying thicknesses but do not stick to wounds. Foam dressings are often used for wounds with a moderate to large amount of exudate or infected wounds. They provide good protection and comfort to the wound bed. Foam dressings can also be used for wound-prone areas (such as in patients with epidermolysis bullosa) to protect intact skin and/or areas that are frequently prone to mechanical trauma. In addition, they are helpful for pressure relief, such as over bony prominences. Foam can also be used as a secondary dressing for more absorption, if needed. Chronic wounds, burns, and wounds with a moderate amount of exudate are ideal candidates for foams. Foams are also soft and malleable to various sized wounds and anatomic locations.

Foam dressings can be applied directly to the wound bed with the addition of an emollient such as petrolatum ointment or Aquaphor® (Beiersdorf AG, US) ointment. The emollient is applied directly to the dressing before application on the skin. Using a prepackaged wooden tongue depressor to spread the emollient on the contact side of the new, sterile dressings can aid in preparation. The dressing is then secured with a secondary and retention dressing. There are different types and thicknesses of foam dressings depending on the amount of exudate in the wound. There are foam dressings with an adhesive (but nontraumatic) border as well, which do not require a secondary or retention dressing. These types of dressings are quite favorable with patients who have fragile skin conditions such as epidermolysis bullosa and Ehlers-Danlos syndrome.

Foam dressings should not be used on dry wounds or wounds with little exudate because of their absorptive nature. It is also difficult to visualize the underlying wound bed given the opaque nature of these products. If foam dressings desiccate and stick to a wound, patiently soaking with sterile saline is recommended to prevent pain and removal of underlying epidermis.

Hydrogel Dressings

Hydrogel dressings are ideally used for wounds that are dry or contain a thick crust, because they are primarily moisture-donating dressings. These products are semitransparent and semipermeable, and they are made up of hydrophilic polymers with high water content. Hydrogels come in various states such as gel, sheets, and gauzes (Figure 131.2G). These dressings are applied directly to the wound, help keep the wound moist, and serve to actively hydrate the wound. Hydrogels can serve to debride necrotic tissue via autolytic debridement. They are nonadherent unless left in place for multiple days (shorter for necrotic wounds and longer for granulating wounds) and require a secondary dressing to keep them in place. Hydrogels are often reported to be helpful in reducing pain and inflammation at the wound site given their moisture donating properties and also have a cooling effect on application, which can help alleviate pain. Disadvantages to hydrogels include their low absorptive properties, need for a secondary dressing to secure in place, and little antibacterial effect.

Gauze/Impregnated Gauze

Gauze is a widely used fabric dressing in wound care and one with which most practitioners are experienced. Typical plain gauze is absorptive and functions to draw fluids away from the wound, although the absorptive properties of gauze are diminished as it becomes fully saturated with exudate. Using plain, dry gauze against a wound will often result in this dressing sticking to the wound, causing pain and tissue disruption at the time of removal. Gauze can serve many functions in a layered dressing—it can be used to cover a nonocclusive, nonadherent dressing to absorb drainage or over an occlusive dressing as a secondary dressing to keep the primary dressing in place.

To prevent adherence to the wound bed, gauze can be coated (ie, impregnated) with a substance that assists in keeping the wound moist. The most well-known of these products is Vaseline gauze or petrolatum-impregnated gauze (Figure 131.2H). Such impregnated gauze is best utilized with an additional coating of emollient such as petrolatum jelly that further prevents desiccation of the dressing and limits adherence to the wound bed. Other substances that can be impregnated within these dressings include antibacterial agents such as povidone-iodine and bismuth tribromophenate (Xeroform™ [Covidien/Medtronic]). Impregnated gauze dressings should be changed "daily" to "every other day" to help prevent trauma to the wound bed during removal. These products are best used on wounds with little to no drainage because they can cause tissue maceration in otherwise moist wounds. They must be secured with a secondary and retention dressing.

Film Dressings

Transparent film dressings are thin sheets of polyurethane or other synthetic material, with a self-adhesive side (Figure 131.2I). They are nonabsorbent and semipermeable, allowing for moisture retention and gas exchange and preventing accumulation of water. Their transparent nature allows for continued visualization of the wound, and they also serve as a mechanical barrier to microbes, making them ideal candidates to cover intravenous (IV) sites in surgical and hospitalized patients. They can also be utilized in superficial burns, wounds, and ulcers as well as in donor sites for skin grafts. An additional advantage to these dressings is that they are flexible and do not significantly limit range of motion. They can also be utilized for simple wounds, such as postsurgical wounds, overtop a sterile gauze dressing or absorbent pad for sites with mild exudate. To facilitate removal, it is recommended to use slight pressure to stretch the film laterally to help disrupt the adhesive.

Film dressings should not be used on patients with skin fragility owing to their adhesive nature, nor in exudative wounds because these dressings are nonabsorptive. If used in a wound with high fluid content, the dressing seal will eventually be compromised, resulting in the need for more frequent dressing changes.

Placement of film dressings also demands some attention to detail and manual dexterity to prevent the adhesive side from folding onto itself and, thus, rendering the dressing unusable. These dressings also require intact skin around the wound to serve as an anchoring point.

Retention Dressings

Retention dressings are primarily used to hold contact and secondary dressings in place (Figure 131.2J). For patients who have fragile skin such as a patient with epidermolysis bullosa, these types of dressings are helpful because any kind of tape used to secure dressings is likely to cause significant mechanical injury. Retention dressings are also useful for securing bandages around the trunk and axilla because dressings in these anatomic areas are often relatively more difficult to hold in place. Various brands of surgical netting or retention dressings are available

- Wound requires protection from further trauma or contact and friction from clothes.
- Wound is draining or bleeding.
- Wound requires topical treatment for infection.
- Wound is painful and a dressing applied will provide comfort.
- Wound is dry and requires moisture.

FIGURE 131.3. Characteristics of a wound, blister, or erosion that require a bandage. Adapted with permission from Ebnurse.org presented by AdaptHealth Patient Care Solutions. Wound care. http://ebnurse.org/wound-care. Accessed February 4, 2019.

depending on the anatomic location. They are also available as tight woven shirts, gloves, and leggings.

WHEN TO BANDAGE A WOUND

Owing to the variability of wounds and medical conditions seen in pediatric dermatology, it is necessary to understand when wound dressings should ideally be utilized (Figure 131.3).

Dressings are generally indicated in wounds that are infected, bleeding, draining, and causing pain, and those that need protection from trauma, friction, and other external factors. Dressings may also be used when topical preparations are applied to the wound bed or when moisture is needed in the wound bed. Although the hallmark of some medical conditions is skin fragility and frequent wounds, some patients, such as those with mild types of epidermolysis bullosa simplex, prefer to not cover most wounds and do well with this approach. Thus, bandaging recommendations should be individualized depending on the patient, including careful consideration of any underlying diagnoses, adherence to the wound care treatment plan, financial cost, and access and availability.

SELECTING A DRESSING

Choosing the most appropriate dressing for a particular wound depends on multiple factors. An adequate understanding of the physical properties of dressings, and the size, type (ie, infection/exudate), and depth of the wound determine which dressing may best optimize wound healing (Figure 131.4). Selecting the most appropriate type of dressing will primarily be based on this initial wound assessment and, when relevant, the patient's underlying condition (eg, adherent dressings should not be utilized in patients with epidermolysis bullosa). See details in Chapter 132. Wound Care and Optimizing Healing.

Evaluation of the tissue type in the wound is critical. If the tissue appears to be healthy and reepithelialization is occurring, then antibacterial or debriding wound dressings would likely not be warranted; instead, selection of a nontraumatic, moisture-retentive, and nonadhesive dressing would be appropriate. The presence (or likelihood) of infection or necrosis

- Tissue type
- Infection
- Exudate
- Size/depth of wound

FIGURE 131.4. Factors affecting dressing choice.

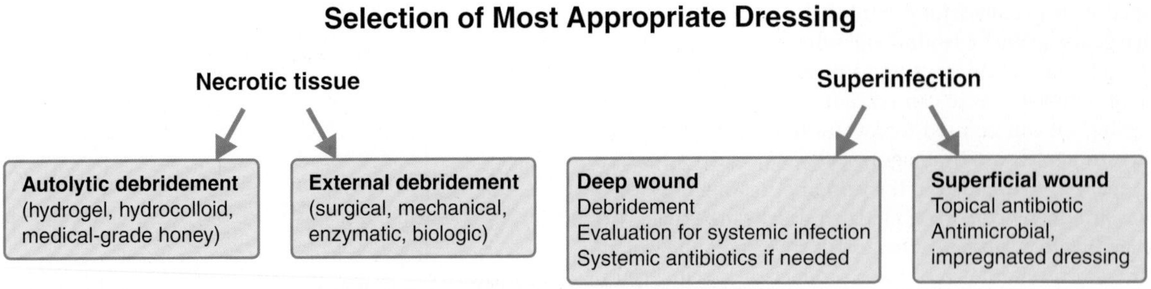

Selection of Most Appropriate Dressing

Necrotic tissue   **Superinfection**

| **Autolytic debridement**
(hydrogel, hydrocolloid,
medical-grade honey) | **External debridement**
(surgical, mechanical,
enzymatic, biologic) | **Deep wound**
Debridement
Evaluation for systemic infection
Systemic antibiotics if needed | **Superficial wound**
Topical antibiotic
Antimicrobial,
impregnated dressing |

FIGURE 131.5. Treatment and dressing choice when necrosis or infection is noted in the wound. Adapted with permission from Ebnurse. org presented by AdaptHealth Patient Care Solutions. Wound care. http://ebnurse.org/wound-care. Accessed February 4, 2019.

Dry wounds
Superficial: hydrocolloid, transparent film,
   gauze + cover (film, foam, tape)
Deep: hydrogel

Wet wounds
Superficial: foam, alginate, hydrofiber
Deep: alginate, hydrofiber

FIGURE 131.6. Recommended dressings based on presence or absence of exudate (moisture level) and depth. Adapted with permission from Ebnurse.org presented by AdaptHealth Patient Care Solutions. Wound care. http://ebnurse.org/wound-care. Accessed February 4, 2019.

must also be assessed and considered when selecting dressings (Figure 131.5). If necrotic tissue is present, external debridement by means of physical disruption (surgical debridement) or enzymatic biologic debridement may be necessary. Autolytic debridement in the form of hydrogel or hydrocolloid dressings or medical grade honey could also be considered. Evaluation of the wound bed for the presence of infection, whether superficial or deep, and if the patient has systemic signs and symptoms of infection, is critical. If a superficial wound infection is suspected, then a topical antibiotic or antimicrobial-impregnated dressing should be used after appropriate cultures and wound cleansing have been completed (when applicable). If deep infection is present, consider debridement and systemic antibiotics.

Lastly, if no infection is present, determine the moisture level of the wound, degree of exudate, and depth (Figure 131.6). If the exudate is dry and the wound is more superficial, then an example of an appropriate dressing would be a hydrocolloid dressing. If the wound is dry and deep, then a hydrogel dressing should be used. For wet, superficial wounds, a foam or alginate dressing would be an ideal choice. For wet, deeper wounds, an alginate dressing would be appropriate.[5] In addition, it is important to understand the phases of wound healing and understand that utilization of dressings will likely change during the course of wound healing as the wound evolves.

SIDE EFFECTS OF DRESSINGS

Any dressing has the theoretical potential to cause a localized reaction or underlying irritation, often seen as erythema in the shape of the overlying dressing material.

- Foam dressings, in our experience, can cause mild skin irritation and itching, especially in warmer temperatures and climates, as well as humid environments. Because they are also

absorptive, they may add to ongoing xerosis of the wound and any covered healthy skin.

- Dressings can also shift and shear if not adequately secured, which can cause friction and blistering. Often removing the dressings for short periods of time is curative. Making sure dressings are adequately secured can prevent friction and slippage.

- Excessive moisture and exudate under dressings can cause maceration in and around the wound bed. This can result from improper dressing choice causing ineffective exudate removal or too infrequent dressing changes.

- Dressing materials (nonorganic) can also become retained in the wound bed and impair healing when not completely removed.

- Adhesive dressings used in patients with skin fragility could actually exacerbate skin breakdown. Also, improper use of dressings could cause pain and further tissue damage, impeding healing.

- Allergic contact reactions to dressings are infrequent to rare but can especially in the case of repeated use of impregnated dressings such as those containing silver or iodine. The frequent use of topical antibiotics underneath dressings, such as polymyxin, neomycin, and bacitracin, can predispose patients to allergic contact dermatitis to these agents. The use of topical antibiotics in clean, noncontaminated wounds is not recommended to facilitate healing or prevent infection in cutaneous wounds, because of the potential for allergic sensitization as well as potential development of bacterial resistance.[7,8]

CONSIDERATIONS IN THE PEDIATRIC PATIENT

When selecting a particular dressing following a full wound assessment, it is imperative to remember that without patient adherence to the treatment plan, a wound will likely not heal as expected. In the pediatric age group, willingness to participate in dressing changes and pain and anxiety associated with dressing changes can be major barriers to care and success. Wound care can also be complex and may require a time commitment by the caregiver or patient including time spent in significant preparation and careful technique (eg, as to not soil clean dressings or wounds), knowledge of wound assessment, and communication with the wound care team or practitioner. Helpful guidelines for patients/families to reference regarding routine for dressing changes at home can be found in Table 131.3. Chapter 134. Pain Management offers suggestions on age-appropriate distractors and techniques for pain/anxiety that can be utilized in office and home dressing changes.

TABLE 131.3 : Helpful Tips for Caregivers/Patients Undertaking Home Wound Care

General Hygiene Practices When Undertaking Wound Care in the Home

- Hand hygiene: Wash hands with soap or other cleanser and water, always wash hands after removing gloves as well.
- Use gloves when handling dressings or dealing with wounds; ensure clean hands before donning gloves by hand washing or using an alcohol-based hand sanitizer.
- Use paper towels instead of fabric towels, to dry hands after hand washing, to prevent contamination.
- Handle soiled linens, clothing, and bandages using gloves, and place in a dedicated "dirty dressing" bag or bin.

Safe Practices for Dressing Changes and Wound Care at Home

- Avoid double dipping into jars of ointments or creams (prescriptions or OTC); instead use a clean/sterile wooden tongue depressor or a plastic spoon or knife to remove topicals from their containers.
- Avoid using fingers to remove ointments/creams/medications from tubes/containers, instead squeeze onto clean wooden tongue depressor, or plastic spoon or knife.
- If wounds are bleeding and/or draining, caregivers should cover their clothing with a smock or gown.
- Clean and disinfect surfaces used for dressing changes and preparation areas as well as any other reusable supplies, such as bandage scissors.
- Ensure you have adequate supplies for dressing changes, before attempting.

Preparation for Wound Dressing Changes

- Take all needed dressing supplies out and open those that will be used, laid out on a clean, disinfected surface.
- Prepare the dressings (contact layers) as directed by the doctor, applying ointments, creams, or medications as directed by the doctor, in a clean manner, so as to not contaminate the unused dressings or tubes/containers.
- Lay out any secondary dressings and retaining dressings, bandage scissors, and any other needed clean materials.
- Have a "dirty dressing" bin or bag ready to place soiled dressing materials into.
- Depending on how soiled dressings will be removed and wound will be cleansed, have supplies ready for wound cleaning.
- Keep soiled wound and dressing materials away from clean area and clean supplies.
- Address any anxiety or pain control needs in your child, before attempting the dressing change, as directed by your doctor.

Reprinted with permission from Ebnurse.org presented by AdaptHealth Patient Care Solutions. Wound care. http://ebnurse.org/wound-care. Accessed February 4, 2019.

Patient/Family Education

Patients and families should have a basic understanding of how a specifically prescribed wound dressing works, proper application technique, frequency of dressing changes and cleansing (when applicable), and when and where to report concerns or questions to the provider. To maintain adherence to a regimen, make sure the patient or caregiver can easily apply the dressing and afford the materials for the length of time required. Providing both written (eg, in the form of a handout) and verbal wound care instructions is key. Remember that a patient may not be adherent to a dressing regimen that is not aesthetically pleasing or obvious, especially if they have to maintain their daily routine. Insurance coverage, feasibility, and costs are among other significant considerations when recommending specific dressings. Care teams should also consider that dressings that have to be ordered in large quantities or for any length of time will need to be stored in the home with adequate space.

Choice of Wound Care Products for the Pediatric Population

With wound care advancements continually evolving and manufacturers constantly developing and improving products, the choices for wound care management are vast. No specific guidelines exist for wound care in the pediatric patient; however, special consideration should be taken when selecting wound care products. There are helpful review articles for wound care in specific disease states such as epidermolysis bullosa and hidradenitis suppurativa as well as in connective tissue disorders;

however, significant evidence for these guidelines is often lacking and based on expert consensus or limited literature review (see Table 132.2). Regardless of choice of wound care products, it is essential to be able to assess a wound, have a basic knowledge of various types of dressings available and their properties, and how these may aid in the healing process, so that patients can have improved outcomes with adequate wound resolution.

REFERENCES

1. Shah JB. The history of wound care. *J Am Col Certif Wound Spec.* 2011;3(3):65–66.
2. Bolton LL, Johnson CL, Van Rijswijk L. Occlusive dressings: therapeutic agents and effects on drug delivery. *Clin Dermatol.* 1991;9(4):573–583.
3. Broussard KC, Powers JG. Wound dressings: selecting the most appropriate type. *Am J Clin Dermatol.* 2013;14(6):449–459.
4. Feng QL, Wu J, Chen GQ, Cui FZ, Kim TN, Kim JO. A mechanistic study of the antibacterial effect of silver ions on Escherichia coli and Staphylococcus aureus. *J Biomed Mater Res.* 2000;52(4):662–668.
5. Jull AB, Walker N, Deshpande S. Honey as a topical treatment for wounds. *Cochrane Database Syst Rev.* 2013;(2):CD005083.
6. Schneider LA, Korber A, Grabbe S, Dissemond J. Influence of pH on wound-healing: a new perspective for wound-therapy? *Arch Dermatol Res.* 2007;298(9):413–420.
7. Rosengren H, Dixon A. Antibacterial prophylaxis in dermatologic surgery: an evidence-based review. *Am J Clin Dermatol.* 2010;11(1):35–44.
8. Elston DM. Topical antibiotics in dermatology: emerging patterns of resistance. *Dermatol Clin.* 2009;27(1):25–31.

CHAPTER 132

Wound Care and Optimizing Healing

Harper N. Price and Kellie Badger

WOUNDS ENCOUNTERED IN THE PEDIATRIC PATIENT

Pediatric dermatologists encounter various wounds in the clinic and hospital setting (Figure 132.1). Wounds can be acute or chronic in nature, and surgical or traumatic/iatrogenic. In pediatric patients, chronic wounds tend to result from congenital conditions or genetic connective tissue disorders (such as epidermolysis bullosa [EB]), other acquired or iatrogenic conditions such as pressure injuries (eg, sacral wounds in hospitalized patients), or, rarely, as a result of an underlying comorbid medical condition such as cerebral palsy and neuropathic ulcers. This is in contrast to acute wounds that can be related to an acute illness or injury. Examples of this include cutaneous drug reactions such as Stevens-Johnson syndrome/toxic epidermal necrosis (SJS/TEN), and injuries such as thermal burns and surgical wounds. Surgical wounds are often a result of excisional surgery to remove cutaneous lesions such as nevi, pyogenic granulomas, cysts, or as a result of treatment with lasers, especially resurfacing lasers such as the carbon dioxide laser. Wounds can also occur from surgical site infections, poor wound care hygiene, and dehiscence and suture reactions, among other factors. Traumatic wounds are a direct result of an accidental or intentional injury to the skin and can be seen in factitial disorders, burns, and in cases of child abuse, for example.

A common scenario when caring for pediatric patients is the development of an ulcer in a proliferating infantile hemangioma (Figure 132.1A). Ulcerated hemangiomas occur most often during the rapid growth period, which is generally during the first 1 to 6 months of life. An impending ulceration in a hemangioma will often have a grayish or bluish hue on the superficial component. The ulceration can be superficial or can extend to deeper tissues, and can have exudate and crust/eschar. Regardless of the size and depth, these ulcerations can be painful for the infant when manipulated or open to air. Ulcerated hemangiomas can have a significant amount of exudate and oftentimes are not treated appropriately until an infection or pain is noted. Thus, choosing the ideal dressing along with topical or oral antibiotics (when infected) becomes imperative to hasten healing and improve pain along with appropriate medical therapy when indicated. Exudative wounds in patients with hemangioma can be managed with foam dressings, which also add padding against friction and pressure. Hydrocolloid dressings can also be used for minimally exudative wounds, which require gentle debridement of superficial eschar/crust, in the absence of infection.

Adult and pediatric dermatologists perform cutaneous surgical excisions and punch and shave biopsies, as well as various laser procedures. Surgical wounds are many times a result of excessive bacterial colonization on the skin, and/or poor wound care compliance on the part of the patient or family. Rarely, underlying medical conditions can impede wound healing and require more diligent wound care or specialized bandages, such as in the case of skin fragility disorders. Dehiscence of surgical excision wounds and biopsies can also occur and may result from improper surgical technique and suturing (eg, a wound is under too much tension) or excessive or improper postoperative activity by the patient (Figure 132.1B). It is a rare occurrence in our experience, however, for a dermatologic surgical wound to result in infection and subsequently become a larger complicated wound in the pediatric patient.

Hereditary skin conditions with associated wounds, such as EB, account for a large portion of wounds managed by pediatric dermatologists. EB is a rare, genetic connective tissue disease that results in skin fragility and blistering with minor injury or friction. There are several subtypes of EB and varying severities and phenotypes. More severe types of EB can result in chronic nonhealing wounds and subsequent development of skin cancer (Figure 132.1C). These patients often require time-intensive and diligent daily wound care as part of their treatment plan. As the amount and type of options available for dressings constantly advances, knowing what types of dressings to use for these patients is a difficult task and often overwhelming for patients/families and practitioners alike. Patients with EB generally require a three-step process for dressing wounds. The contact layer (the layer placed directly on the skin) with a dressing that will maintain a moist environment is necessary, along with a secondary dressing, such a rolled gauze, to hold the contact layer in place, and, finally, a retention dressing to hold the contact and secondary dressings in place. Any adhesive or tape and friction should be avoided on the skin itself in patients with EB or other forms of skin fragility.

Ehlers-Danlos (ED) syndrome is another hereditary connective tissue disease resulting in skin fragility and abnormal and often delayed wound healing. Typical findings in patients with several types of ED are hyperextensibility, fragile skin with easy bruising, and poor wound healing (Figure 132.1D). There are several subtypes of ED, inherited in both dominant and recessive patterns, resulting in a defective collagen meshwork. Wounds in these patients are likely to occur on the shins, elbows, knees, and forehead and will tend to have a "fish-mouth" or gaping appearance. Wound healing often results in atrophic and abnormal scars and dehiscence is common after wound repairs. Thus, suturing after an injury must be done by a practitioner aware and proficient in multilayer closure of wounds with sutures, and wounds must be followed up closely.

Atopic dermatitis (AD) or eczema is a very common childhood condition that varies in severity, affecting 10% to 13% of children in the United States[1,2]; prevalence in other countries is variable and depends on the region. It is most often treated with topical corticosteroids and/or topical calcineurin inhibitors along with diligent use of mild skin care products and emollients. When eczema is recalcitrant to these topical medications, systemic medications such as methotrexate or cyclosporine may be utilized. Patients suffer with significant pruritus when the disease is not well controlled, with the potential to cause excoriations and open wounds, potentially leading to skin infections. Wound care can be challenging in this population because of the need to use full-body emollients, many in the

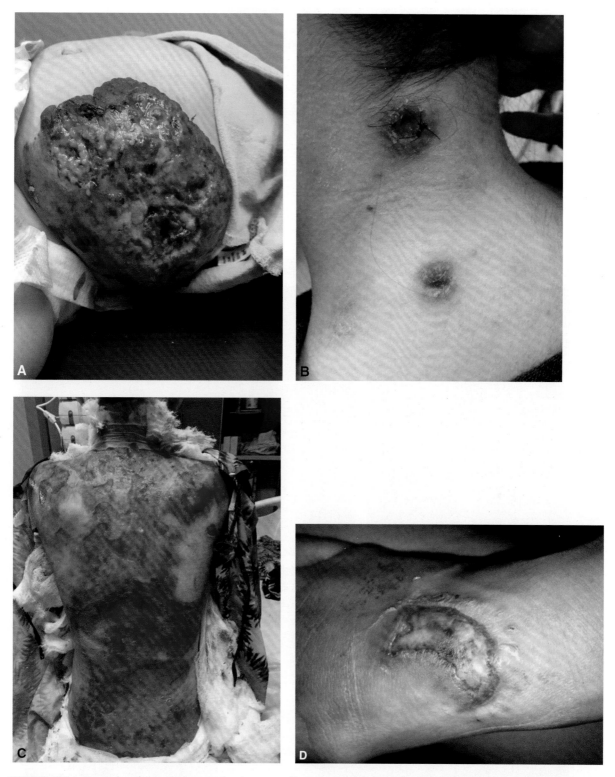

FIGURE 132.1. Examples of wounds that may be encountered in pediatric patients in the dermatology clinic. A, Development of an ulcer in a proliferating infantile hemangioma. B, Dehiscence and superficial infection of punch biopsy sites after inadequate home wound care, necessitating wound care and topical antibiotics. C, Chronic back wounds on a patient with recessive dystrophic epidermolysis bullosa. Over the mid-back is a large skin graft scar from a previous squamous cell carcinoma excision. D, Traumatic wound after a crush injury on the dorsal foot of a teenager with Ehlers-Danlos syndrome.

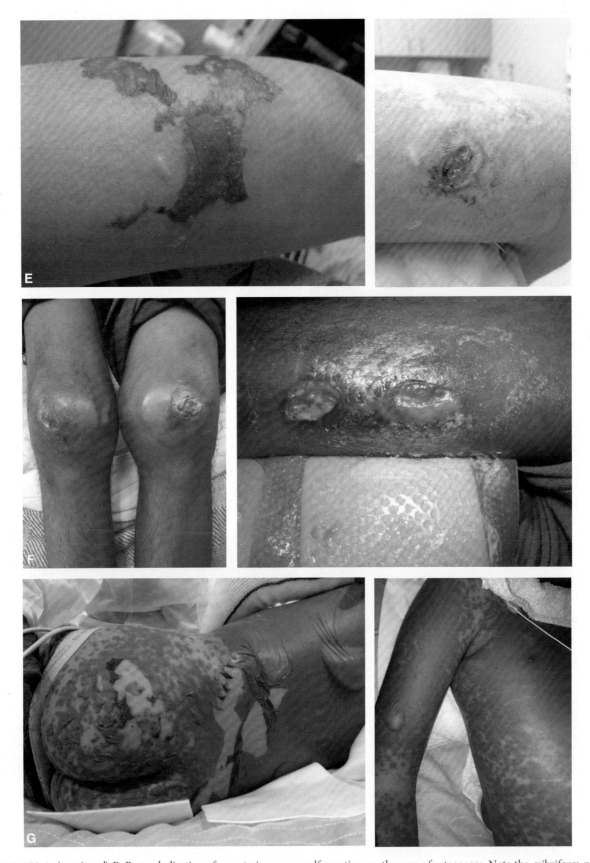

FIGURE 132.1. (*continued*) E, Postembolization of an arteriovenous malformation on the arm of a teenager. Note the cribriform necrotic plaques, the center of which resulted in an ulcer. F, Chronic nonhealing wound on the leg of a child with multiple comorbidities and undiagnosed genetic condition (left). Child with systemic scleroderma and calcinosis with numerous areas of calcinosis cutis, which extrudes from the skin and results in chronic open wounds (right). G, A child with toxic epidermal necrosis (TEN) and large areas of bullae and necrosis/epidermal sloughing on the back and buttocks (left). Dusky plaques with evolving bullae on the arms and trunk. The patient was transferred to a burn center because of the large body surface area involvement (right).

form of ointments, limiting the use of adhesive dressings; also, the potential for allergy to topical antibiotics and substances impregnated into specific bandages, as well as intolerance or irritation to adhesive materials, must be especially considered in this patient population.

Several other cutaneous conditions managed by dermatologists may involve the development and management of wounds. Vascular malformations (such as lymphatic malformations) and vascular tumors are often diagnosed and managed by dermatologists or a multidisciplinary team. Patients with certain types of vascular anomalies and associated syndromes can develop skin breakdown and ulcerations requiring wound care (primary or treatment related), especially those with arteriovenous (AV) and lymphatic malformations (Figure 132.1E). Patients with connective tissue disorders such as scleroderma and dermatomyositis may develop wounds from associated calcinosis cutis, and digital ulcerations can be seen in lupus and scleroderma as well (Figure 132.1F). Chronic forms of graft versus host disease can also result in skin ulcerations. Acute skin injuries due to medication reactions or infections, such as in the case of SJS/TEN or mycoplasma-induced mucositis and rash (MIMR) can require wound assessment, dressings, and management. Patients with SJS/TEN can develop moderate to severe skin manifestations with life-threatening full-body skin necrosis, blistering, and sloughing (Figure 132.1G). Although mortality rates are generally less than are those seen in adults, when moderate to severe reactions occur pediatric patients are often better managed in a burn unit with skilled nurses and medical staff.[3] If the reaction is mild to moderate, supportive care can be provided by a team of dermatologists, nurses, and/or wound care team, while the patient is hospitalized. Any skin blistering or skin sloughing is best managed with moist nonadhesive bandages with multiple layers to optimize fluid retention, help maintain body temperature and electrolyte abnormalities, and promote wound healing. Secondary skin infections are a common cause of morbidity in these patients and thus close monitoring with serial skin examinations is imperative. Adolescent and young adult patients with hidradenitis suppurativa (HS) may also require wound care. More advanced and chronic disease may result in draining fistulas, ulcers, and abscesses in the axilla, groin, buttocks, and inframammary areas. If these lesions have a high amount of exudate, they are best managed with absorptive dressings that are nontraumatic to the skin when removed. Lastly, arterial, venous, and diabetic wounds, seen in adult patients, are uncommon in pediatric patients and will not specifically be discussed here.

STAGES OF WOUND HEALING

The aim of wound repair is to reestablish an intact skin barrier and homeostasis as rapidly as possible. There are multiple stages involved in the wound healing process and all wounds go through the same stages to complete wound closure. There are three main phases commonly described in wound healing: inflammatory, proliferative, and remodeling phases.[4] Multiple factors (including cell and signal transduction pathways influenced by growth factors, intrinsic extracellular matrix [ECM] proteins and extrinsic mechanical forces, and biophysical forces such as electrical fields and mechanotransduction) play a role in determining the length of time a wound remains in the various stages. The process is dynamic and complex, from the inflammatory to regeneration or remodeling phases. Figure 132.2 shows the stages, key events, and typical time frames for wound healing.

The inflammatory phase begins almost immediately following the injury and can last up to 3 to 5 days. A fibrin clot is formed, which provides an initial ECM. Growth factors are released from platelets that attract inflammatory cells, including fibroblasts, macrophages, and neutrophils. Neutrophils clear the bacterial load and macrophages debride the wound and stimulate granulation tissue.[4,5] A careful balance of pro- and anti-inflammatory cytokines is needed for successful wound healing and progression into the next phase.

The proliferative phase generally begins within 24 hours of wound injury. During this phase, collagen (type III) is produced by fibroblasts and a vascular network is laid down. Remodeling ensues with the replacement of type III collagen by type I collagen in a definitive ECM in the maturation phase with regression of the vascular network and normalized cellular activity. Wound contraction often begins by day 5. The remodeling phase begins nearly 2 weeks after injury and can last weeks to years in duration.[5]

WOUND ASSESSMENT

Adequate wound healing depends on many contributing factors including the wound size and depth, location, infection/exudate, age of the patient, and other underlying medical conditions, such as poor nutrition, diabetes, anemia, hereditary skin fragility conditions, and blood supply to the wound. When assessing a wound, careful consideration and management of the abovementioned conditions will allow for optimal healing and the best patient outcomes. Several factors that should be assessed during the initial patient interview and examination are outlined in Figure 132.3.

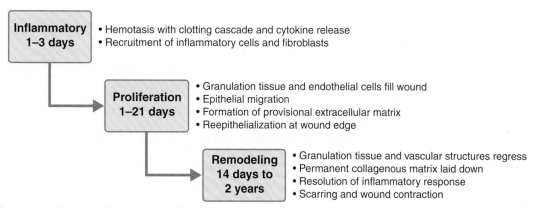

FIGURE 132.2. Illustration of the stages, key events, and typical time frames of wound healing.

Patient Interview:
1) Timing: Chronic versus acute wound: **How long has the wound been present?**
2) **What symptoms and signs noted by patient/family?**
   • Pain/tenderness/itching?
   • Increased drainage?
   • Non-healing areas?
   • Malodor?
   • Fever or other systemic signs of illness?
3) Underlying cause: Intentional versus accidental. **What events led to the wound?**
4) Comorbidities:
   • **What are the patient's underlying medical conditions, medications, etc.?**
   • **Has patient had a recent laboratory workup?**

Physical Examination:

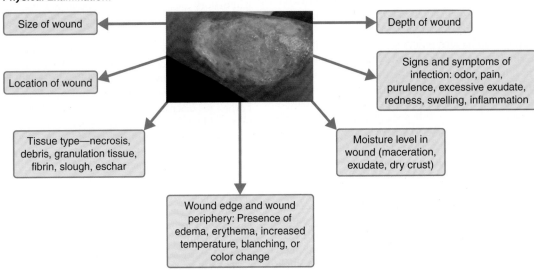

Size of wound

Location of wound

Depth of wound

Signs and symptoms of infection: odor, pain, purulence, excessive exudate, redness, swelling, inflammation

Tissue type—necrosis, debris, granulation tissue, fibrin, slough, eschar

Moisture level in wound (maceration, exudate, dry crust)

Wound edge and wound periphery: Presence of edema, erythema, increased temperature, blanching, or color change

FIGURE 132.3. Approach to the wound assessment in the pediatric patient.

Chronic Versus Acute

First, determine the nature of the wound as chronic or acute, as well as the underlying cause, including the patient's diagnosis and comorbidities, because these may affect choice of therapies. Acute wounds tend to progress through the phases of wound healing in a timely and expected manner. Chronic wounds do not progress through the stages of wound healing in an orderly or timely manner, and function and cutaneous anatomy remain distorted.[5] The length of time the wound has been present is also important to note because wounds in different anatomic locations may heal at different rates. More distal wounds may require longer wound healing times because of differences in vascularity and activity level of limbs. For example, when a wound is over a joint surface, wound healing time will likely be extended because of constant movement and tension.

Depth/Size of the Wound

The depth of the wound should be noted in wound evaluation. Erosions are superficial injuries limited to the epidermis and will not result in a scar, whereas ulcers involve a loss of the epidermis and dermis, resulting in scar formation. A "partial-thickness" wound involves loss of the epidermis and a portion of the dermis, sparing the adnexal structures and leaving the wound edges and adnexa for reepithelialization; "full-thickness" wounds extend to the subcutis and include loss of the adnexal structures, which will affect scar formation and cause wound contraction (Figure 132.4). It is also imperative to determine the size of the wound at the time

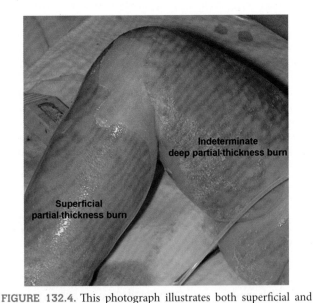

Indeterminate deep partial-thickness burn

Superficial partial-thickness burn

FIGURE 132.4. This photograph illustrates both superficial and deep partial-thickness burns. Note the white, dry, patchy appearance on the deep partial-thickness burn compared to the consistent, moist pink appearance on the superficial partial-thickness burn. Reprinted with permission from Mulholland MW, Lillemoe KD, Maier RV, et al. *Greenfield's Surgery: Scientific Principles and Practice.* 4th ed. Philadelphia, PA: Lippincott Williams & Wilkins; 2006. Figure 30.6.

TABLE 132.1 : Typical Features of Wound Infection

- Delayed healing
- Increased exudate (drainage)
- Increased redness
- Increased pain
- Increased swelling
- Increased warmth of skin compared with surrounding area
- Malodorous (unpleasant odor)
- Easy bleeding (friable

Adapted with permission from Ebnurse.org presented by AdaptHealth Patient Care Solutions. Wound care. http://ebnurse.org/wound-care.

of the initial injury, so that healing times and progress can be measured. This will help determine how often the patient should be seen for evaluation. Capturing photos for the medical record is a very useful tool when assessing wounds, and many simple and affordable options now exist for use with electronic health records.

Necrosis and Signs of Infection

Key clinical factors to note on wound evaluation include the presence of *necrosis, signs of infection, and presence and amount of exudate and moisture level* in the wound bed and periphery.

Assessment of wound periphery and rim should include presence of edema, erythema, increased temperature, and blanching/color change. Certain types of cutaneous injury and medical conditions (eg, pressure ulcers) may predispose tissues to hypoxia and toxins, causing tissue necrosis. This in turn will affect healing by impeding the granulation process and increasing the risk of microorganism colonization and potential infection. Erythema and exudate around the wound can be a sign of inflammation or infection. Inflammation is normal after any kind of wound. With adequate wound care, inflammation will often resolve within a few days to weeks. Erythema (inflammation) with pain, odor, and exudate is likely an infection and should be addressed appropriately. The presence of an infection and development of a biofilm can stall healing and result in a persistent inflammatory state. The presence of increased exudate in the wound can be a sign of infection or increased inflammation and could result in maceration of the surrounding tissues. Typical signs of infection are listed in Table 132.1. Importantly, wound infection must be differentiated from contamination (no bacterial proliferation) and colonization (proliferation of bacteria but not causing harm). Helpful acronyms have been developed to describe observed findings in assessing infection, namely, *NERDS* and *STONES*.[6] The *NERDS* acronym is applicable for assessment of superficial infection:

> *N*onhealing wound
> *E*xudative wound
> *R*ed and bleeding wound
> *D*ebris in the wound
> *S*mell from the wound

STONES is used to assess for potential deeper infection: *S*ize is bigger; *T*emperature increased; *O*s/probes to or exposed bone; *N*ew area of breakdown; *E*xudates, erythema, edema; and *S*mell.

Maintaining Moisture

Maintaining an adequate moisture level in the wound bed is critical. Contrary to common thought, studies have shown that moist wounds have quicker healing times when compared to dry or crusted wounds.[7-10] Moisture in wounds prevents desiccation, crust, and eschar formation and allows for epithelial cell migration into the wound. In addition, moisture provides an adequate environment for maintenance of important growth factors and proteins, allowing for the wound to proceed adequately through the stages of wound healing.[10] Simple and helpful acronyms have been suggested for assessment of wound characteristics,[11] such as the following:

> TIME
> *Tissue type:* granulation, necrotic, etc.
> *Infection:* heat, erythema, pain, edema, odor, increased drainage
> *Moisture*
> *Edges:* rolled, thickened, undermined, calloused

OPTIMIZING WOUND HEALING 🔘
Use of Wound Dressings and Preparation for Dressings

To maintain healing, retain a moist environment in the wound bed. This is done by utilizing wound dressings. When changing dressings from day to day or during the different stages of healing, consider choosing a dressing that will prevent maceration or trauma to the wound bed and surrounding tissues. Infection prevention in a wound is also critical. This can be accomplished in part by debriding necrotic tissue, absorbing exudate appropriately, and minimizing any external contamination.[4] There are also dressings with antimicrobial properties that can be helpful for colonized or infected wounds. See Table 131.1 for further reference on dressing products.

Wounds should be cleansed before dressing application, when appropriate. Choice of cleanser depends on the patient tolerance, the type of wound, and mobility of the patient, and, sometimes, on practitioner preference. Postsurgical wounds in dermatology are often washed gently with soap and water, avoiding disruption of superficial sutures or further tension on the wound (eg, avoid scrubbing the area). For patients who cannot shower or use soap and water, irrigation (or lavage) with sterile saline, tap water or distilled water can help remove biofilm and debris from the wound before dressing application. Warming these fluids can help decrease associated pain with lavage. Those patients with bullous skin diseases such as EB have significant pain reported when just using water. The addition of pool salt tablets to tap water can decrease pain or stinging. Care must be taken not to aggressively lavage an open wound and disrupt healthy tissue. In wounds at high risk for infection, mainly those that are not sutured and are chronic and open with critical colonization, cleansing or soaks with antiseptics/antimicrobial agents may be recommended. Antiseptics have broad antimicrobial activity but can be toxic to normal tissue. Examples include iodine-containing preparations, chlorhexidine, silver-donating products, and hydrogen peroxide. Care must be taken to limit use of these products to not compromise healthy tissues occurring in chronic wounds. The authors prefer the use of dilute sodium hypochlorite soaks, commercially available sodium hypochlorite gel cleansers, or white vinegar soaks as alternative options in patients with chronic or stalled wounds with critical bacterial colonization and as infection prophylaxis in open wounds at high risk for infection (see Chapter 138. Bleach Baths).

Wound dressing choice depends on the type of lesion, site, wound bed assessment, and any other underlying medical conditions (eg, patients with EB should not use dressings with adhesive), as well as availability and cost of dressings. See Chapter 131. Wound Dressings for an in-depth discussion on dressing choices. When selecting the appropriate dressings, it is critical to remember the importance of off-loading of the wound bed and surrounding tissue as well as limiting friction. An example where these concepts become important is the consult for a neonate with a pressure ulcer.

As with other wound care, multiple dressings and products are available, but careful consideration is recommended, especially in the neonatal population. To prevent friction on a wound, foam dressings tend to be used because they afford little to no damage to underlying skin and offer protection and padding. Clean ulcers can be covered with a hydrocolloid dressing to help off-load the wound or prevent further friction as long as significant exudate is not present.[12] In addition, layering dressings in a manner consistent with a contact layer/absorbent layer, secondary rolled gauze, and retention dressing will not only offload pressure from the wound but also help prevent friction. Constant pressure on wounds in bed-bound patients and those patients with wounds on pressure areas of the extremities and trunk may benefit from off-loading. Specialized mattresses can be utilized in the hospital setting and are sometimes needed in the home setting once the patient is discharged. Frequent turning of the patient by nursing staff or caregivers can also help limit the risk of new pressure wound development and off-load existing wounds. For wounds on the feet, use of crutches, special footwear, or other assistance devices, can alleviate pressure and allow for healing. The use of compression for extremity wounds can facilitate healing by preventing dependent edema in the tissue. This can be accomplished using an elastic wrap (such as an ACE wrap) or other compression garments. Care should be taken not to compromise circulation when using compression devices.

TREATMENT OF WOUND COMPLICATIONS
Wound Infection
The presence of bacteria on a wound can impede healing. Once the bacterial load hits a critical capacity, signs and symptoms of infection occur. These can include increased exudate, stalled healing, increased inflammation, pain, warmth, malodor and purulence, and pustule or abscess formation. On wound inspection and assessment, if infection is suspected, a swab for aerobic and anaerobic bacteria should be performed. In uncommon cases where fungal or atypical organisms are suspected, the wound should be sampled accordingly. It is ideal to gently rinse the wound with sterile water or saline first when possible, before swabbing the area. If suspicion for a localized infection is high in the absence of systemic signs/symptoms, empiric treatment with a topical antibiotic to cover the organism/s of concern (based on type of wound and location, often *Staphylococcus aureus*) could be initiated. For concern of a more moderate and/or widespread infection, empiric treatment with an oral antibiotic should be initiated until preliminary culture and sensitivities have resulted, at which time antibiotic choice could be adjusted appropriately if needed. If signs/symptoms of a more severe or life-threatening infection are present, urgent medical evaluation should be sought for intravenous antibiotics. Knowledge of local resistance patterns and common pathogenic organisms based on anatomic site and patient's medical comorbidities is often helpful. Dressings for infected wounds should be changed daily

or more often if there is a large amount of exudate. More absorptive dressings may be needed for heavily exudative wounds. Antimicrobial dressings can also be chosen for infected wounds but should not be the sole means of treatment.

A proactive approach to prevent critical bacterial colonization and subsequent infection is often pursued for more chronic wounds and acute wounds at high risk for infection, such as those in intertriginous areas and lower extremities. The use of dilute sodium hypochlorite bathes or gel cleansers (see Chapter 138. Bleach Baths) has been deemed helpful in skin conditions such as AD and EB, although significant supportive evidence is overall lacking and most evidence is based on expert consensus and opinion. However, there is little to no toxicity or side effects when these measures are performed regularly and correctly. Use of mild antiseptics, available over the counter, such as chlorhexidine gluconate can be used, with care to avoid mucosal surfaces. All of these antimicrobial agents can be used to cleanse infected wounds as well.

Necrosis
Necrotic tissue should ideally be debrided, whether surgically, mechanically, or chemically, as part of the wound care plan. Debridement is the process of removal of nonviable tissue. Autolytic debridement (process by which local factors in the wound itself are used to resolve necrotic debris) can be induced by moist, occlusive dressings, such as hydrocolloids, over a period of time. This is best for minimally necrotic wounds, tends to be painless, and is contraindicated in infected wounds. Mechanical debridement includes the use of "wet-to-dry" dressings (ie, application of a saline moistened gauze into the wound, which is allowed to dry and then removed), and surgical debridement, via resecting or scraping off necrotic tissues with a scalpel, curette, or scissors. Wet-to-dry debridement tends to be painful and does not differentiate between debridement of viable and nonviable tissues in the wound; it is often used for wounds with a large amount of necrotic tissue and is a rapid and easy technique to perform. Sharp surgical debridement is often utilized for larger and/or deeper wounds, and care should be taken to minimize injury to healthy tissue, monitor for bleeding, and address pain control. Surgical debridement for young children and those with special needs may need to occur in the operating room setting with sedation or general anesthesia because of the pain and nature of the ensuing procedure. Pediatric or Plastic Surgery will often be consulted to debride significant necrotic and large wounds. Older children and adolescents needing minor debridement and for those wounds that are analgesic, debridement may occur in the office. Clean, nonsterile techniques should be utilized to maintain optimal wound healing. For these patients, however, debridement in a clinic setting can still be quite traumatic. Distraction techniques as well as the use of child-life specialists are useful if available. Nonsurgical, chemical, or enzymatic debridement using topical proteolytic enzyme preparations (such as those containing papain-urea or collagenase) can also be tried. Topical enzyme ointments take longer to debride tissues but are less painful, incur less bleeding, and do not harm viable tissues. Familiarity with the various products available, their proper use, and side effects, is necessary before use.

Hypergranulation Tissue
Hypergranulation tissue in wounds, or those with excessive granulation tissue, will delay healing. The tissue extends above the surrounding skin surface and is often red, shiny, soft, and friable (Figure 132.5). The wound will be unable to heal because epithelial

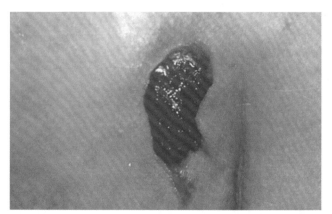

FIGURE 132.5. Hypergranulation tissue—chronic proliferative phase. Reprinted with permission from Sussman C, Bates-Jensen BM. *Wound Care.* 4th ed. Philadelphia, PA: Wolters Kluwer Health/ Lippincott Williams & Wilkins; 2011. © B.M. Bates-Jensen.

cells will not be able to migrate across the wound and contraction at the wound edge will not occur. This may occur in wounds that are excessively moist, prone to friction or irritation, highly inflamed, and those with low oxygen or high bioburden or infection. Excess granulation tissue may require treatment with topical corticosteroid preparations or silver nitrate (see Chapter 15. Injectable Corticosteroids [Intralesional Kenalog, Intramuscular]). However, caution should be taken with more potent topical corticosteroids under occlusion on wounds and prolonged use, because increased side effects such as systemic absorption and local atrophy can occur. Nonocclusive dressings can also aid in the slow removal of unwanted granulation tissue. Silver-impregnated dressings such as Mepilex Ag® (2019 Mölnlycke Health Care AB) can be used in short durations, such as 2 to 4 weeks, with daily dressing changes to aid in decrease of excess granulation tissue. These types of dressings are also known to have broad-spectrum action on bacteria, yeast, and fungi, which may also decrease excess granulation tissue that is impeding wound healing. Lastly, surgical (sharp) debridement and use of medical lasers can aid in correction of excessive abnormal granulation tissue.

Chronic Wounds: Stalled or Delayed Wound Healing

Several factors contribute to poor wound healing and the influence of the local wound environment and systemic factors should be considered (Figure 132.6). In the wound bed, poor oxygenation, chronic inflammation, bacterial colonization or infection, biofilms, poor cellular response (fibroblast senescence or impaired function), and lower levels or impairment of important growth factors and cytokines needed for wound closure can all contribute to poor wound healing. Addressing local factors affecting wound closure by methods described in this chapter can hasten wound healing. Larger and deeper wounds may also take longer periods of time to closure. Patient (systemic) factors such as lack of adequate nutrition, immune dysfunction or suppression, chronic anemia, uncontrolled diabetes, chronic steroid use, and conditions resulting in increased systemic inflammation can all contribute to abnormal and delayed wound healing. As discussed in the introduction, several congenital and genetic conditions seen in the pediatric age group can predispose patients to chronic, nonhealing wounds, such as EB. These systemic factors are often harder to control and treat in the context of chronic wounds, and adequate treatment of contributing conditions, when possible, is critical. Thankfully, chronic wounds in the pediatric population are not prolific, as compared to that in the adult population. However, experience with wound assessment and dressings and treatment of wound complications is necessary for those practitioners caring for children and adolescence. Helpful wound care reference materials for readers can be found in Table 132.2. The management of chronic wounds presents a large social, economic, and physical burden on the patient and family as well as on the health care system.

ACKNOWLEDGMENTS

Special thanks is given to Danielle Malchano, RN, of the EB Advocate Team, for her guidance and education in wound care and dressings for our patients and her amazing advocacy for and dedication to patients with EB and the EB community.

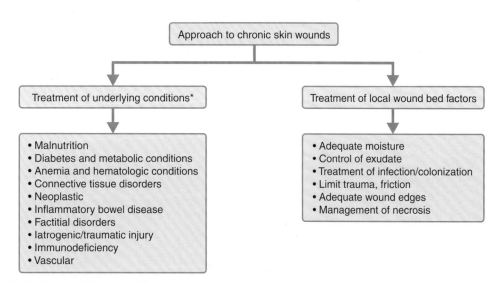

*Underlying conditions may differ by age group; those listed are those that may be seen in pediatric patients.

FIGURE 132.6. Factors contributing to poor wound healing.

TABLE 132.2 ⋮ Useful Wound Care References and Disease-Specific Guidelines

Epidermolysis Bullosa
- El Hachem M, Zambruno G, Bourdon-Lanoy E, et al. Multicentre consensus recommendations for skin care in inherited epidermolysis bullosa. *Orphanet J Rare Dis*. 2014;9:76.
- Denyer JE. Wound management for children with epidermolysis bullosa. Dermatol Clin. 2010;28(2):257–264. http://ebnurse.org.
- Denyer J, Pillay E, Clapham J. Best practice guidelines for skin and wound care in epidermolysis bullosa. An International Consensus. Wounds International, 2017. http://www.debra-international.org/clinical-guidelines/complete-eb-guidelines/wound-care.html.

Hidradenitis Suppurativa
- Antia C, Alavi A, Alikhan A. Topical management and wound care approaches for hidradenitis suppurativa. *Semin Cutan Med Surg*. 2017;36(2):58–61.
- Dini V, Oranges T, Rotella L, Romanelli M. Hidradenitis suppurativa and wound management. *Int J Low Extrem Wounds*. 2015;14(3):236–244.

General Wound Care References
- https://wwww.uptodate.com/contents/basic-principles-of-wound-management.
- Powers JG, Higham C, Broussard K, Phillips TJ. Wound healing and treating wounds: chronic wound care and management. *J Am Acad Dermatol*. 2016;74(4):607–625.
- King A, Stellar JJ, Blevins A, Shah KN. Dressings and products in pediatric wound care. *Adv Wound Care*. 2014;3(4):324–334.

REFERENCES

1. Ong PY, Leung DY. Immune dysregulation in atopic dermatitis. *Curr Allergy Asthma Rep*. 2006;6(5):384–389.
2. Williams H, Stewart A, von Mutius E, Cookson W, Anderson HR. Is eczema really on the increase worldwide? *J Allergy Clin Immunol*. 2008;121(4):947–954.
3. Waldman R, Whitaker-Worth D, Grant-Kels JM. Cutaneous adverse drug reactions: kids are not just little people. *Clin Dermatol*. 2017;35(6):566–582.
4. Broussard KC, Powers JG. Wound dressings: selecting the most appropriate type. *Am J Clin Dermatol*. 2013;14(6):449–459.
5. Morton LM, Phillips TJ. Wound and healing and treating wounds. Differential diagnosis and evaluation of chronic wounds. *J Am Acad Dermatol*. 2016;74:589–605.
6. Sibbald RG, Woo K, Ayello EA. Increased bacterial burden and infection: the Story of NERDS and STONES. *Adv Skin Wound Care*. 2006;19(8):447–461
7. Del Rosso JQ. Wound care in the dermatology office: where are we in 2011? *J Am Acad Dermatol*. 2011;64(3 suppl):S1–S7.
8. Hinman CD, Maibach H. Effect of air exposure and occlusion on experimental human skin wounds. *Nature*. 1963;200:377–378.
9. Field FK, Kerstein MD. Overview of wound healing in a moist environment. *Am J Surg*. 1994;167(1A):2S–6S.
10. Winter GD. Formation of the scab and the rate of epithelialization of superficial wounds in the skin of the young domestic pig. *Nature*. 1962;193:293–294.
11. Schultz G, Mozingo D, Romanelli M, Claxton K. Wound healing and TIME; new concepts and scientific applications. *Wound Repair Regen*. 2005;13(4 suppl):S1–S11.
12. Scheans P. Neonatal pressure ulcer prevention. *Neonatal Netw*. 2015;34(2):126–132.

CHAPTER 133

Postprocedure Antibiotics

George Hightower

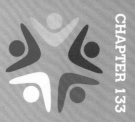

INTRODUCTION

Prospective studies of common outpatient dermatologic procedures in adults show infection rates overall are low, less than 5%.[1-3] Although few studies have specifically addressed surgical site infections (SSIs) in children following dermatologic procedures, rates are likely lower than those seen in adults, possibly explained by age-related capacity for wound healing.[4,5] Bacterial infections associated with skin flora are the most common cause of SSIs and often become clinically evident between days 5 and 10 post the procedure. The decision to initiate empiric antibiotic therapy for treatment of a suspected SSI remains a clinical decision; however, the threat of antibiotic resistance necessitates that clinicians use an evidence-based approach to ensure good antibiotic stewardship.[6]

ASSESSING PROCEDURE SITES FOR POSSIBLE BACTERIAL INFECTION

When concern is raised for possible bacterial infection of a surgical site, the primary challenge lies in distinguishing early signs of infection from the normal healing process. One of the most widely accepted approaches to the diagnosis of SSIs is the *Centers for Disease Control Guidelines for the Prevention of Surgical Site Infections*.[5] The Centers for Disease Control (CDC) guidelines specify that an SSI must involve the surgical site and occur within 30 days of the procedure. Infections may be limited to the skin (superficial), involve muscle and fascia (deep) or an organ space. Further, per CDC guidelines, the diagnosis of SSI requires one or more of the following: (1) purulent drainage, (2) suspected causative organisms isolated from surgical site, (3) signs or symptoms of infection (ie, pain or tenderness, swelling, redness, or heat), or (4) clinician having diagnosed an SSI.[7]

Wound classification has also been used as a tool for assessing infection risk. Infection risk is grouped by wound type: clean (1%-5%), clean-contaminated (3%-11%), contaminated (10%-17%), and dirty (>27%). One limitation of using wound class to make decisions about antibiotics is that it may overestimate infection risk.[8,9]

What constitutes reasonable concern for infection is a gestalt of subjective and objective factors. Warmth, edema, erythema, and tenderness are clinical features of both early infection and the normal healing process. Obvious signs of infection such as fluctuance, purulence, lymphatic streaking, and systemic symptoms are not necessarily present during the early stages of infection (Figures 133.1 and 133.2A,B). Ultimately, the decision to initiate empiric antibiotic therapy remains a clinical decision informed by the likelihood of infection, presence or absence of systemic symptoms, and patient-specific risk factors. We should expect bacterial culture patterns, along with the decision to initiate antibiotic therapy, to vary by surgical site, patient immune status, provider experience, and local rates of culture-confirmed SSIs. Although beyond the scope of this discussion, atypical presentations of presumed bacterial SSIs should raise the possibility of noninfectious processes such as hidradenitis suppurativa, cutaneous Crohn's, pyoderma gangrenosum, and other neutrophilic dermatoses.

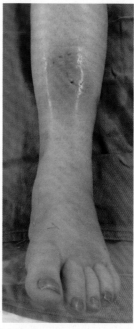

FIGURE 133.1. Clinical photograph showing the hallmark signs of infection (increasing erythema, pain, swelling, and drainage) in the lower extremity of a young woman who had a surgical procedure performed several weeks earlier; a small sinus tract has formed and can be seen at the center of the wound. Reprinted with permission from Ricci WM, Ostrrum RF. *Orthopaedic Knowledge Update: Trauma.* 5th ed. Rosemont, IL: American Academy of Orthopaedic Surgeons; 2018. Figure 13.2.

EMPIRIC TREATMENT OF SUSPECTED BACTERIAL INFECTION

Optimizing empiric therapy relies on utilizing knowledge of likely pathogenic organisms and local antimicrobial susceptibility patterns. The most common pathogens responsible for outpatient incisional SSIs are *Staphylococcus pyogene* and *Streptococcus pyogene*. For anatomic sites, such as oral/nasal mucosa, ear, axilla, groin, and perineum, difference in infection patterns is sufficient to warrant empiric coverage for organisms other than *Staphylococcus* and *Streptococcus*. *Pseudomonas aeruginosa* causes otitis externa and should be considered when selecting empiric treatment for SSIs involving the ear. *Streptococcus viridans* and anaerobes, such as Peptostreptococcus, represent important sources of infection at the oral/nasal mucosa. For infections involving the groin/inguinal folds and perineum, both *Escherichia coli* and Enterococcus should be considered.

A first-generation cephalosporin or anti-staphylococcal penicillin is first-line therapy for empiric treatment of infection in which there is high suspicion for *Staphylococcus* and *Streptococcus* species (Figure 133.3). Other considerations for empiric treatment include (1) cephalosporin in combination with metronidazole for coverage of gram-negative bacteria and anaerobes for suspected infections that involve the axilla, groin/

443

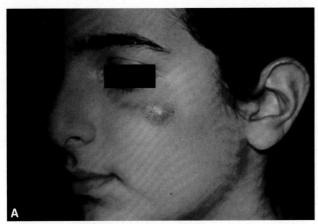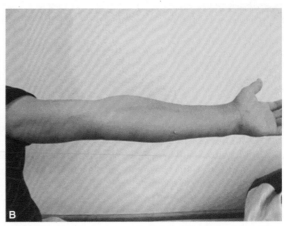

FIGURE 133.2. Lymphatic streaking (lymphangitis). A, 10-year-old female with swelling and pain on the left cheek following an insect bite a day earlier. Note the lymphatic streak, extending proximally. B, Lymphangitis presenting as a linear red streak proximal to a skin infection. A: Reprinted with permission from Salimpour RR, Salimpour P. *Photographic Atlas of Pediatric Disorders and Diagnosis*. Philadelphia, PA: Wolters Kluwer Health/Lippincott Williams & Wilkins; 2013. Chapter C UNFig 4. B: Reprinted with permission from Chung EK, Atkinson-McEvoy LR, Boom JA, et al. *Visual Diagnosis and Treatment in Pediatrics*. 3rd ed. Philadelphia, PA: Wolters Kluwer Health/Lippincott Williams & Wilkins; 2014. Figure 65.5.

inguinal folds, and the perineum, (2) clindamycin or amoxicillin-clavulanic acid for infections involving the nasal and oral mucosa, and (3) oral ciprofloxacin for infections involving the ear.[10,11] Ciprofloxacin and other fluoroquinolones have historically been avoided in children because of concern for cartilage toxicity; however, the American Academy of Pediatrics (AAP) now recommends that oral fluoroquinolones be used if no other safe and effective oral therapy exists, even if effective alternative intravenous therapy is available.[12]

As a general rule, oral, not topical, antibiotics should be used to treat SSIs. What role, if any, topical antibiotics have in preventing SSIs remains controversial. For clean and clean-contaminated wounds, the CDC recommends against the application of any topical antimicrobial agent once the surgical incision wound is closed.[13]. In settings in which there is a low baseline rate of infection,[14-16] the use of topical antibiotics does not appear to significantly reduce SSIs. The perceived benefit of using topical antibiotics should be viewed with skepticism given the infection rates observed in these studies would be considered unacceptable for outpatient dermatologic procedures.[17]

Although still uncommon, nontuberculous mycobacteria are increasingly recognized as important pathogens associated with cosmetic procedures and surgical sites and cosmetic procedures[18] (Figure 133.4A and B). A high index of suspicion is needed for diagnosis and to prevent treatment delay because of their specific nutritional requirements for culture growth and relatively slow growth. Antibiotic treatment for these organisms should be directed by susceptibility testing; however, in

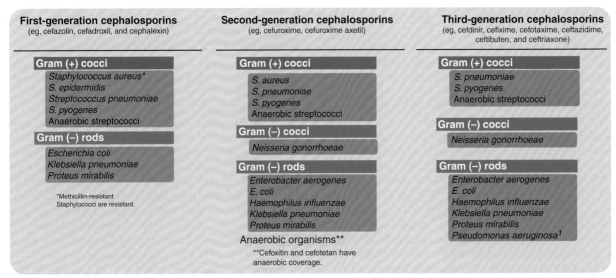

FIGURE 133.3. Summary of therapeutic applications of cephalosporins. (Note: Not shown is cefepime [a fourth-generation cephalosporin] and ceftobiprole [a fifth-generation cephalosporin], which offer potential advantages over third-generation agents, particularly against organisms with inducible, chromosomal resistance. *Pseudomonas aeruginosa* is not susceptible to ceftriaxone.) Reprinted with permission from Harvey RA, Cornelissen CN. *Lippincott's Illustrated Reviews: Microbiology*. 3rd ed. Philadelphia, PA: Wolters Kluwer Health/Lippincott Williams & Wilkins; 2012. Figure 5-12.

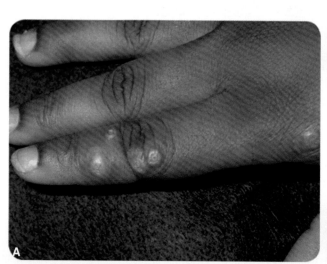

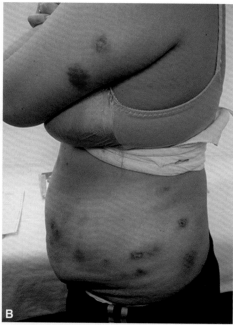

FIGURE 133.4. A, *Mycobacterium marinum* infection as firm nodules with a central crust; note the characteristic "sporotrichoid" distribution. B, Multiple draining abscesses due to *Mycobacterium chelonae*, after mesotherapy. A: Reprinted with permission from Lugo-Somolinos A, McKinley-Grant L, Goldsmith L, et al. *Visual Dx: Essential Dermatology in Pigmented Skin*. Philadelphia, PA: Wolters Kluwer Health/Lippincott Williams & Wilkins; 2012. Figure 4-571. B: Reprinted with permission from Hall JC, Hall BJ. *Sauer's Manual of Skin Diseases*. 11th ed. Philadelphia, PA: Wolters Kluwer; 2017. Figure 50.8.

vitro resistance may not predict clinical response. For otherwise healthy individuals and where feasible, complete surgical excision can provide effective treatment.[19,20] Treatment with azithromycin or clarithromycin should also be strongly considered as monotherapy or in combination with another antibiotic such as rifampin.[21,22] Antibiotic treatment may require more than 3 months and the potential for adverse effects must be taken into consideration when selecting an appropriate treatment plan.

TREATING METHICILLIN-RESISTANT *STAPHYLOCOCCUS AUREUS*

The prevalence of community-acquired methicillin-resistant *Staphylococcus aureus* (CA-MRSA) infections have significantly increased over the past decade and are expected to continue to rise.[23] The challenge in treating CA-MRSA results from resistance to β-lactam antibiotics (ie, penicillin derivatives and cephalosporins) and the relative ease with which these same organisms acquire genes that confer resistance to clindamycin, macrolides, and other antibiotics (Figure 133.5). CA-MRSA clindamycin resistance may be as high as 30% in some geographic areas. No clinical features reliably distinguish infections caused by MRSA from methicillin-susceptible *Staphylococcus aureus* (MSSA).[24] Culture and reflexive antibiotic susceptibility should be performed before starting empiric antibiotic for any suspected infection. For children and adolescents, in regions where community resistance of MRSA to clindamycin remains fairly low, oral clindamycin should be considered both for empiric and definitive treatment of superficial skin infections caused by CA-MRSA.[11,23] In adults, use of doxycycline and minocycline to treat CA-MRSA is common but not appropriate for children younger than 8 years of age because of dose-related

effects on linear bone growth, dental staining, and defects in enamel. Bactrim and linezolid also provide adequate coverage of CA-MRSA. Their usage must be weighed against the possibility of adverse complications, specifically serious drugs associated with sulfonamide/trimethoprim and hematologic toxicity for linezolid. For children, in contrast to adults, clindamycin associated *Clostridium difficile* colitis is uncommon.[11]

Adverse Reactions

There is no reliable way of predicting who will have a serious adverse reaction to a given antibiotic. Anaphylaxis associated with penicillin treatment is rare, although minor adverse reactions, such as rash, are commonly reported. Reviewing and accurately documenting patients' reported adverse events is important for preventing both unnecessary avoidance of penicillin antibiotics and preventing serious adverse reactions. For patients with a history of penicillin allergy, the risk of a serious cephalosporin allergic reaction is estimated to be less than 1%. More generally, cross-reactions between penicillin and β-lactam antibiotics are less than 5% to 20%.[25] The most common serious adverse reaction to sulfonamides is a hypersensitivity rash. Steven-Johnson syndrome, a life-threatening rash that presents as sloughing of the skin and mucosal surface, occurs in approximately 3 of 100 000 people exposed to sulfonamide/trimethoprim (Figure 133.6). Use of tetracyclines in children younger than 8 years causes dose-related dental staining and defects in enamel, as well as depression of linear bone growth (Figure 133.7). Tetracyclines should be limited to the treatment of rickettsial infections and other potentially life-threatening conditions. Fluoroquinolones generally should be avoided in children if there is a safe and effective alternative, given the potential risk of cartilage toxicity.

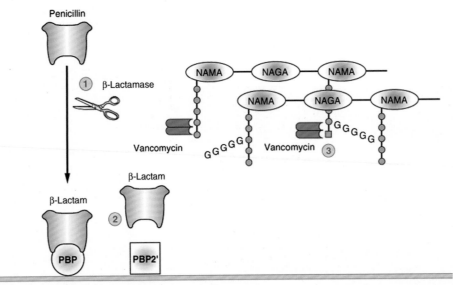

FIGURE 133.5. Mechanisms by which *Staphylococcus aureus* resists the action of antibiotics. (1) Although penicillin was initially effective against this bacterium, most strains now produce β-lactamases that cleave penicillin. For this reason, anti-staphylococcal penicillins that are resistant to cleavage by staphylococcal β-lactamases were developed. (2) Methicillin-resistant *Staphylococcus aureus* (MRSA) strains, however, produce an altered penicillin-binding protein (PBP) (referred to as PBP2′) that is not recognized by these compounds or other β-lactam agents. Vancomycin, a glycopeptide, overcomes this difficulty by binding to the terminal alanine–alanine group of the peptide side chain of peptidoglycan and thus inhibits peptidoglycan cross-linking without binding to PBPs. (3) Vancomycin-resistant strains of *S. aureus* have now been identified. Some of these strains have become resistant to vancomycin by altering the structure of the peptide side chain of newly formed peptidoglycan subunits, so that they are not recognized by vancomycin. Reprinted with permission from Hauser AR. *Antibiotic Basics for Clinicians.* 2nd ed. Philadelphia, PA: Wolters Kluwer Health/Lippincott Williams & Wilkins; 2012. Figure 10.2.

A significant, but often overlooked, component of antibiotic use is patient education. Discussions of antibiotics in the popular media are often focused on multidrug-resistant bacterial organisms and overuse. Although these discussions are important, they certainly do not provide patients and their families with adequate information to make treatment decisions. Efforts to ensure that we accurately inform our patients and provide care that we see as appropriate may necessitate an approach that incorporates emerging information from issues seemingly as disparate as an individual's gut microbiome to local *S. aureus* susceptibility patterns.

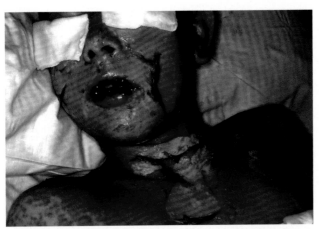

FIGURE 133.6. Typical inflammatory hemorrhagic bullae of the oral mucosa noted in Stevens-Johnson syndrome. Photo courtesy of Anne W. Lucky, MD. Reprinted with permission from Marino BS, Fine KS. *Blueprints Pediatrics.* 7th ed. Philadelphia, PA: Wolters Kluwer; 2019. Figure 3.7.

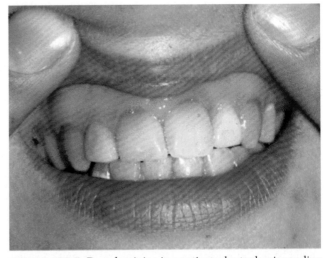

FIGURE 133.7. Dental staining in a patient who took minocycline for a prolonged period around age 5. Multiple teeth are affected bilaterally, showing characteristic discoloration. Reprinted with permission from DeLong L, Burkhart NW. *General and Oral Pathology for the Dental Hygienist.* 3rd ed. Philadelphia, PA: Wolters Kluwer; 2018. Figure 20.38.

REFERENCES

1. Cook, J. Prospective study of wound infections in dermatologic surgery in the absence of prophylactic antibiotics. *Dermatol Surg.* 2007;2007:399–400.

2. Dixon AJ, Dixon MP, Askew DA, Wilkinson D. Prospective study of wound infections in dermatologic surgery in the absence of prophylactic antibiotics. *Dermatol Surg.* 2006;32:819–826; discussion 826–827.

3. Rogers HD, Desciak EB, Marcus RP, Wang S, MacKay-Wiggan J, Eliezri YD. Prospective study of wound infections in Mohs micrographic surgery using clean surgical technique in the absence of prophylactic antibiotics. *J Am Acad Dermatol.* 2010;63:842–851.

4. Pajulo OT, Pulkki KJ, Alanen MS, et al. Duration of surgery and patient age affect wound healing in children. *Wound Repair Regen.* 2000;8:174–178.

5. Rogers SO. Surgical perspective: Centers for Disease Control and Prevention Guideline for the prevention of surgical site infection 2017. *Surg Infect.* 2017;18:383–384.

6. Moorhead C, Torres A. I PREVENT bacterial resistance. An update on the use of antibiotics in dermatologic surgery. *Dermatol Surg.* 2009;35:1532–1538.

7. Berríos-Torres SI. Evidence-based update to the U.S. Centers for Disease Control and Prevention and Healthcare Infection Control Practices Advisory Committee Guideline for the prevention of surgical site infection: developmental process. *Surg Infect.* 2016;17(2):256–261.

8. Messingham MJ, Arpey CJ. Update on the use of antibiotics in cutaneous surgery. *Dermatol Surg.* 2005;31:1068–1078.

9. Ortega G, Rhee DS, Papandria DJ, et al. An evaluation of surgical site infections by wound classification system using the ACS-NSQIP. *J Surg Res.* 2012;174:33–38.

10. Stevens DL, Bisno AL, Chambers HF, et al. Practice guidelines for the diagnosis and management of skin and soft tissue infections: 2014 update by the Infectious Diseases Society of America. *Clin Infect Dis.* 2014;59:e10–e52.

11. Bradley JS, Nelson JD, Barnett ED. *2018 Nelson's Pediatric Antimicrobial Therapy.* Itasca, IL: American Academy of Pediatrics; 2018.

12. Jackson MA, Schutze GE. The use of systemic and topical fluoroquinolones. *Pediatrics.* 2016;138(5):e20162706.

13. Berríos-Torres SI, Umscheid CA, Bratzler DW, et al. Centers for Disease Control and Prevention Guideline for the prevention of surgical site infection. *JAMA Surg.* 2017;152:784–791.

14. Dixon AJ, Dixon MP, Askew DA, Wilkinson D. Prospective study of wound infections in dermatologic surgery in the absence of prophylactic antibiotics. *Dermatol Surg.* 2006;32(6):819–826.

15. Khalighi K, Aung TT, Elmi F. The role of prophylaxis topical antibiotics in cardiac device implantation. *Pacing Clin Electrophysiol.* 2013;37(3):304–311.

16. Smack DP. Infection and allergy incidence in ambulatory surgery patients using white petrolatum vs bacitracin ointment. *JAMA.* 1996;276:972–977.

17. Heal CF, Banks JL, Lepper PD, Kontopantelis E, Driel MLV. Topical antibiotics for preventing surgical site infection in wounds healing by primary intention. *Cochrane Database Syst Rev.* 2016;(11):CD011426.

18. Wentworth AB, Drage LA, Wengenack NL, Wilson JW, Lohse CM. Increased incidence of cutaneous nontuberculous mycobacterial infection, 1980 to 2009: a population-based study. *Mayo Clin Proc.* 2013;88(1):38–45.

19. Tebruegge M, Pantazidou A, Macgregor D, et al. Nontuberculous mycobacterial disease in children—epidemiology, diagnosis & management at a tertiary center. *PLoS One.* 2016;11(1):e0147513.

20. Gonzalez-Santiago TM, Drage LA. Nontuberculous mycobacteria: skin and soft tissue infections. *Dermatol Clin.* 2015;33(3):563–577. doi:10.1016/j.det.2015.03.017.

21. Dodiuk-Gad R, Dyachenko P, Ziv M, et al. Nontuberculous mycobacterial infections of the skin: a retrospective study of 25 cases. *J Am Acad Dermatol.* 2007;57(3):413–420.

22. Kimberlin DW, Brady MT, Jackson MA, Long SS. *Red Book: 2015 Report of the Committee on Infectious Diseases.* Elk Grove Village, IL: American Academy of Pediatrics; 2015.

23. Liu C, Bayer A, Cosgrove SE, et al. Clinical practice guidelines by the Infectious Diseases Society of America for the treatment of methicillin-resistant *Staphylococcus aureus* infections in adults and children: executive summary. *Clin Infect Dis.* 2011;52(3):285–292.

24. Miller LG, Remington FP, Bayer AS, et al. Clinical and epidemiologic characteristics cannot distinguish community-associated methicillin-resistant *Staphylococcus aureus* infection from methicillin-susceptible *S. aureus* infection: a prospective investigation. *Clin Infect Dis.* 2007;44(4):471–482.

25. Shenoy ES, Macy E, Rowe T, Blumenthal KG. Evaluation and management of penicillin allergy. *JAMA.* 2019;321(2):188.

CHAPTER 134

Pain Management

Harper N. Price and Mark Popenhagen

INTRODUCTION

Inadequate pain control during and after dermatologic procedures has significant negative implications for pediatric patients, including long-term consequences of poor reactions to future painful events and acceptance of subsequent health care interventions.[1] Therefore, a pain management approach focusing on appropriate assessment and safe management in the pediatric dermatology population is a vital and essential component of perioperative care and in-office procedures.

Children and adolescents having to undergo dermatologic procedures often experience fear and anxiety related to anticipating a procedure and not knowing or understanding what the procedure will entail. This is in addition to the acute physical pain caused by the procedures performed, such as the injection of local anesthetic before a skin biopsy or cryotherapy treatment. This chapter focuses not only on assessment and management of pain during and after dermatologic procedures in the pediatric age group but also on how to manage and alleviate anxiety and fear related to in-office and operative room setting procedures.

PAIN DEFINITION AND ASSESSMENT

Pain as defined by the International Association for the Study of Pain (IASP) is "an unpleasant sensory and emotional experience arising from actual or potential tissue damage; sensation of discomfort, distress, or agony unique for that individual who is the real authority on their pain."[2] When considering the definition of pain, one of the most important and challenging factors for the practitioner is that it is unique to the individual suffering from it, thereby making it impossible to have an *exact* understanding of what, why, and how much pain the sufferer feels at any given time. Table 134.1 defines the difference between acute versus chronic pain and Table 134.2 lists the most common types of pain that present to dermatologists including specific characteristics and patient descriptors.

Because an accurate pain assessment is an important component of pain management and the subjective nature of pain

TABLE 134.1 : Definition of Acute Versus Chronic Pain and Examples

	DURATION	EXAMPLES
Acute Pain	<3 mo	Bruise, laceration, fracture
Chronic Pain	>3 mo	Complex regional pain syndrome, fibromyalgia, phantom pain
	Alternating intervals of painful and pain-free episodes	Sickle cell disease, rheumatoid arthritis, lupus

mo, months.

can make assessment in the pediatric population challenging, a multitude of assessment measures have been developed. Although it was once widely believed that neonates and infants could not feel pain because of the lack of a fully developed nervous system and that children could not accurately assess their pain because of immature cognitive development, research has repeatedly invalidated these assumptions. To the contrary, neonates and infants may feel pain more acutely; and once children are able to communicate verbally or through sign, they are able to report location, intensity, frequency, and duration in their own words with remarkable accuracy. As such, the current "gold standard" of pain assessment is the child's self-report, with the aid of parent's own assessment of their child's discomfort. It is common for patients to report a score greater than 10 (eg, "15/10") when offered a typical "0-10" option. Although this can become very frustrating for the practitioner, it should simply be taken as a statement of severe pain and the practitioner should move on.

Because self-report measures cannot be utilized with infants, preverbal young children, and those who have cognitive and/or physical impairments, observational assessment measures can be

TABLE 134.2 : Types of Pain, Potential Causes, and Descriptors

ARISES FROM	RELATED TO	DESCRIPTORS AND CHARACTERISTICS	USE	EXAMPLES
Nociceptive Pain				
Skin, bones, joints, muscles, connective tissues	Tissue injury, illness, treatment side effects	• Well-localized • Hurting, sore, aching, or throbbing • Resolves with healing	Protects from further tissue damage	Laceration, fracture, blister, abrasion
Neuropathic Pain				
Nerve damage or inflammation	Nerve disruption or injury, neuropathy, disease	Burning, stinging, pins and needles, electrical or shocking, shooting, piercing • Does not resolve with healing • Follows dermatome	None Nonprotective	Phantom pain, medication- or radiation-induced neuropathy, herpes zoster (shingles)

| 0 = no pain | 2 | 4 | 6 | 8 | 10 = much pain |

FIGURE 134.1. Faces Pain Scale—Revised, ©2001, International Association for the Study of Pain (www.iasp-pain.org/FPSR). From Hicks CL, von Baeyer CL, Spafford P, et al. Faces pain scale-revised: toward a common metric in pediatric pain measurement. *Pain.* 2001; 93(2):173-183. This Faces Pain Scale-Revised (www.iasp-pain.org/fpsr) has been reproduced with permission of the International Association for the Study of Pain® (IASP). The figure may NOT be reproduced for any other purpose without permission.

equally important and useful. Scales such as the COMFORT-B, CRIES, FLACC, Pain Assessment Tool (PAT), Premature Infant Pain Profile (PIPP), and Scale for Use in Newborns (SUN) have been widely adopted for use with these populations and are easily learned and applied in a clinical setting by physicians and support staff.[3-6] The parents' assessment of their own child's pain is an important adjunct to any pain score obtained via behavioral report because health care providers overwhelmingly tend to underestimate the patients' pain.[7]

For children who are both verbal and cognitively typical, the most commonly used pain rating scales are those that use a series of faces ranging from no pain to severe pain and the numeric pain rating scale. Children aged 3 to 16 years can use standardized visual (pictorial) scales such as the Faces Pain Scale-Revised 2001 (Figure 134.1), OUCHER, and Wong-Baker-FACES that have been endorsed and widely utilized by accreditation organizations and large health care institutions.[8-12] Children 8 years and older can be taught to use a 0 to 10 numeric scale, graded pain thermometer, or a visual analog scale (VAS)[13] (Figure 134.2). In addition, some children may prefer other methods of reporting their pain such as drawings, poker chips, or colors. It is important to explain to the child and the parents the detailed aspects of the scales before using them. Children do not always understand the words "pain" or "discomfort" but

may instead respond better to a variety of other words such as "owie," "ouchy," "boo-boo," or "hurt."[14]

Regardless of which assessment scale is chosen, it is important for the medical staff to understand that (a) to achieve the greatest clinical usefulness, the same scale should be used on an institution-wide basis and (b) pain scores obtained via any assessment measure may be arbitrary, may not necessarily be on a linear interval or ratio scale (eg, a pain score of "10" may not be twice as bad as a score "5"), and may be extremely variable depending on individual patient experience. Similarly, pain scores should not be considered to be experienced in the same way for every patient or across different measurement scales. Therefore, the practitioner may be better served by using pain scales as relative measures (eg, pre- and post the procedure) and instead focusing on the patient's ability to function in his or her own unique environment.

Once a pain assessment has been properly performed and correctly interpreted, every effort should be made to relieve identified pain as quickly as possible; this helps prevent prolonged suffering and may aid in avoiding long-term consequences of hypersensitive reactions to future painful stimuli. This includes the aggressive management of postoperative pain. Fortunately, there are many different modalities to treat pediatric pain, and it is crucial to evaluate the relative risks and benefits of each available option.

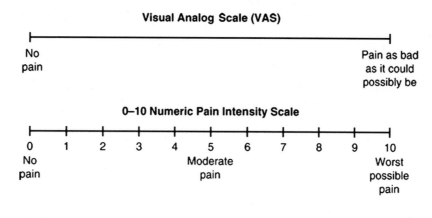

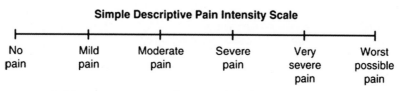

FIGURE 134.2. Pain assessment tools. Many pain intensity scales are available for ranking the pain of children and adults alike. Such scales as the visual analog, numeric pain intensity, and simple descriptive pain intensity rank pain from *no pain* to *worst pain possible.* Reprinted with permission from Aschenbrenner DS, Venable SJ. *Drug Therapy in Nursing.* 4th ed. Philadelphia, PA: Wolters Kluwer Health/Lippincott Williams & Wilkins; 2011. Figure 23.3A.

PAIN AND ANXIETY MANAGEMENT

A key to managing pain and associated anxiety with procedures is anticipation. The approach to pain and anxiety varies and is dependent on the anticipated intensity, expected duration, and type of pain. In addition, the context and meaning of pain as seen by the child and family, the coping style and temperament of the patient, the type of procedure, the child's cognitive and emotional developmental levels, the patient's history of pain, and the family support system should all be taken into consideration before proceeding with any procedure.

Preprocedure Planning for Reducing Anxiety and Pain

Procedures performed in the office setting to address common dermatologic complaints (eg, warts and molluscum) are often requested by parents and patients, may be medically indicated, and oftentimes cannot be avoided (Table 134.3). The key to the success of these procedures is the reduction of pain and anxiety, which sets the stage for an optimal outcome. Adequate pain control leads to improved patient and caregiver satisfaction as well as a more cooperative and less anxious patient during the procedure.[15]

Procedure Room Environment

Whether in the setting of a children's hospital inpatient unit or an outpatient dermatology clinic, when choosing to perform dermatologic procedures on children, the provider must begin by ensuring that the office or surrounding environment and staff are all committed to delivering a safe and comfortable experience for the pediatric patient. Even simple procedures in children often take longer and may require more staff, a thoughtful setup, and more resources for preparation, education, and pain/anxiety relief than would be utilized in an adult clinic (see Chapter 5. Surgical Procedure Room Setup). However, when done successfully, the reward is a more positive experience for everyone involved. Decreasing anxiety about potential painful procedures can begin as soon as the patient and family enter the office setting by providing a fun, upbeat, and engaging, child-friendly environment wherever possible (eg, cheerful artwork, colorful walls, toys, video games).

Once in the examination room, keep objects that may instill fear and anxiety, such as instruments, metal trays, and syringes, out of sight. Taking a few moments to establish rapport can be extremely helpful. It is important to know ahead of time whether the patient prefers to know, in detail, everything that the practitioner is doing, or that the practitioner remains silent so that they may instead focus on a video game or other active coping strategy (eg, deep breathing, imagery, self-hypnosis), or something in between.

Preparation of Parents and Patient

It is ideal to discuss procedures prior with pediatric patients, when age appropriate, in words they can understand and only if they are interested. Assessing what type and how much information a patient wants to know ahead of time can save the provider needless challenges as the procedure moves forward. Avoid using words like "cut" and "needle" or "shot" because these words can be very emotionally laden in younger children. The provider should never lie to a child about what they will experience, because doing so will destroy all trust in that provider and likely other providers as well. Instead, the patient and caregivers should be given a reasonable expectation of what the patient will feel before, during, and after the procedure. For example, saying, "This is going to be a little painful and some of my patients have told me that it feels like getting pinched by their little brother or sister; but they also say that it was really helpful to blow on this pinwheel while we do what we need to do to keep your body healthy" is much better than saying, "Hold still! This won't hurt a bit." Most children are fully aware that there will be some pain associated with almost every procedure, so getting their hopes up with a promise of "no pain" only to break that promise will only serve to damage or destroy trust moving forward.

Positive Reinforcement and Distractors

Positive reinforcement and introduction of distractors at this time while preparing for the procedure are extremely helpful and necessary. When a child is old enough, he or she should be offered age-appropriate distractors to choose from in preparation for the procedure (Tables 134.3 and 134.4). Having the parent/caregiver present during this time and engaged in the process of the procedure to follow is ideal. Often the parent and an additional staff member will be the primary designees to engage in the distractor with the child, whether this is holding a tablet, reading a book, singing a song, or playing a game (Figure 134.3).

Safe, comfortable and age-appropriate positioning should be discussed and initiated at this time as well. The age of the child, level of anxiety and coping strategies, and other medical diagnoses such as developmental delay and autism should be taken into account when considering the best approach. When a caregiver is not available, a child life specialist or trained medical support staff may be utilized instead for positioning and distraction.

TABLE 134.3 : Office Versus Operating Room Procedures and Examples[a]

IN-OFFICE, BRIEF PROCEDURES[a]	IN-OFFICE, LONGER PROCEDURES[a]	OPERATING ROOM, UNDER GENERAL ANESTHESIA[a]
• Cryotherapy • Skin biopsies • Intralesional injections (Kenalog, Candida antigen) • Wound cultures (viral/bacterial/fungal) • Curettage of molluscum • Cantharidin application	• Nonablative lasers • Small excisions • Incision and drainage • Nail procedures (nail avulsion, matrix biopsy) • Botulinum toxin for hyperhidrosis	• Excisions • Ablative lasers • Nonablative lasers • Nail procedures • Cryotherapy, skin biopsies, intralesional injections, curettage[a]

[a]The age that these procedures can be tolerated and carried out safely in the operating room and office must be determined before undertaking. Owing to developmental/intellectual delay, severe anxiety, autism, and other conditions, certain patients may require procedures in the operating room under general anesthesia or sedation.

TABLE 134.4 ⦂ Nonpharmacologic Techniques to Relieve Anticipated Pain/Anxiety for Children by Age Group[a]

NEONATES AND INFANTS	TODDLERS AND YOUNGER SCHOOL-AGE CHILDREN[a]	OLDER SCHOOL-AGE CHILDREN[a]
• Swaddling • Breastfeeding • Nonnutritive sucking • Kangaroo care (skin to skin) • Rocking/holding • Oral sucrose	• Blowing bubbles • Counting • Listening to children's books • Children's TV programs/movies on phone or tablet device • Books • Music • Toys	• Toys • Books • Music (self-selection) • Video games on phone or tablet device • Movies/videos on phone or tablet device

[a]Interventions vary with age and level of cognition.

Parents and families can also play a large role in how a child responds to painful stimuli and experiences pain. Children are astute observers of their parents and will often respond to painful stimuli similarly. Children of parents who are anxious, fearful, or overly concerned experience have poorer outcomes than do children whose parents are supportive and encourage the child to use adaptive coping strategies such as relaxation, distraction, and/or hypnosis exercises.[16-19]

Pharmacologic Interventions

Pharmacologic preprocedural interventions can be employed for those patients with significant fear and anxiety. The most common anxiolytic agent used in this manner is midazolam. This is a short-acting benzodiazepine that can be given 30 to 60 minutes before the procedure. Midazolam (anxiolytic dosing) can be especially useful in significantly anxious children and those undergoing repeated procedures such as laser treatments. This can be given before a procedure under general anesthesia or in the office setting. However, side effects of drowsiness and potential respiratory depression require familiarity for specific monitoring when administered in the outpatient realm. The presence of a parent during the induction process in children undergoing general anesthesia in the operating room for repeated procedures such as laser treatment can be helpful in reassuring the child, but only in cases where the parent remains relaxed and helps with and/or encourages the use of effective coping strategies.

Topical anesthetic creams can be applied before an anticipated painful procedure such as curettage of molluscum or intralesional injections (see Chapter 105. Molluscum Contagiosum). Refer to Chapter 14. Injectables for proper usage, application, and dosage, especially when used on very young children. In neonates and young infants younger than 1 year of age, oral sucrose solution (Sweet-Ease, Philips, Amsterdam, the Netherlands) can be used for reducing pain of a short procedure at the bedside or in clinic. However, the effect of sucrose diminishes as the child ages and overuse can lead to similar diminished effect prematurely without any prior warning.

When there is not adequate time for use of topical anesthetics or these are contraindicated, other alternatives should be considered including ice or cold devices (eg, instant ice

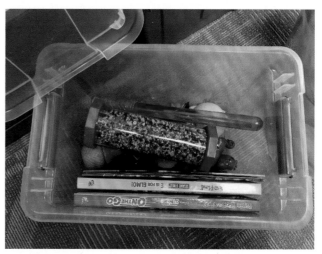

FIGURE 134.3. Age-appropriate distractors should be offered to the child to choose in preparation for the procedure. A toolbox of distractor items for various age groups can be helpful in clinic. Often a parent/caregiver or other staff member is designated to assist the child in these activities.

packs, gel ice packs, or water frozen in gloves), used for 1 to 5 minutes; these may also be combined with pressure, or vapocoolant sprays. Vapocoolant sprays such as ethyl chloride cause temporary analgesia but do involve understanding the appropriate technique and a prior explanation of what will happen to the patient. These sprays should not be used near the eyes or in the area where a specimen may be taken for histopathologic evaluation because of potential freeze artifact. Also, these sprays are flammable and must be stored accordingly in the office or hospital setting. Vibratory stimulation devices applied to or near injection sites before and during injection can decrease pain or augment pain relief (Figure 134.4). These devices can be particularly helpful for patients undergoing botulinum injections into palms and soles for hyperhidrosis, along with pressure and icing. For procedures where injectable local anesthetics are

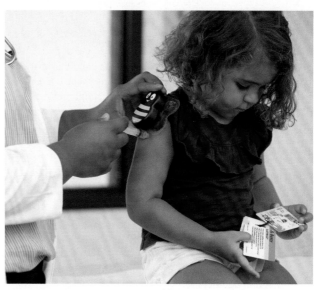

FIGURE 134.4. Buzzy Mini Healthcare Unit. Copyright © 2019 Buzzy. MMJ labs.

used, such as for biopsies and excisions, using buffered, warmed lidocaine with epinephrine can significantly help improve pain outcomes in minimally invasive procedures.[20] Using smaller needle sizes for injections (30 gauge, ½ in needle) and infiltrating local anesthetic more slowly and deeper can all contribute to a less painful experience. On the basis of the author's experience (HP), for intradermal/intralesional injections, nearby tapping/lightly scratching or pinching of the skin can also help minimize pain associated with the injection.

PROCEDURAL AND POSTPROCEDURAL SETTING

Nonpharmacologic Strategies for Pain/Anxiety

There are several adjuvant tools to aid in minimizing procedural-related pain and anxiety for children in the office and hospital setting, including nonpharmacologic approaches such as psychological strategies, physical and/or occupational therapy, proper positioning, education, and parental support. Simple distraction techniques that divert attention away from painful stimuli are often useful for short in-office procedures Figure 134.5 and Table 134.4). Additional pain and anxiety management techniques such as relaxation, hypnosis, mindfulness, and the use of more technology-driven techniques such as biofeedback and virtual reality can be extremely useful (Box 134.1). Whenever possible, these techniques should be taught before the time or date of the procedure to allow for sufficient training, practice, and mastery.

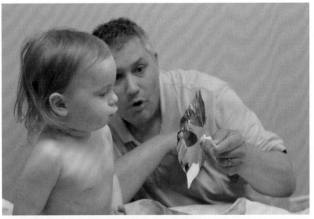

FIGURE 134.5. A toddler with epidermolysis bullosa is instructed on how to blow on a pin wheel during dressing changes to aid with pain and anxiety associated with these daily painful routines.

BOX 134.1   STRATEGIES TO MINIMIZE PROCEDURAL-RELATED PAIN/ANXIETY

- Use of topical anesthetics such as EMLA™ (AB Astra Pharmaceuticals, L.P.) or topical lidocaine
- Use of ice packs/cold packs
- Use of vapocoolant spray
- Use of vibratory stimulation devices
- Parent/caregiver at bedside when possible
- Use of age-appropriate distractors (see list earlier) such as iPad, games, books, and engaging and interactive toys
- Safe and age-appropriate, comfort positioning
- Deep breathing exercises

Postprocedure praising of the child's efforts, no matter how poorly the procedure went, and positive incentive techniques that provide a small reward (eg, stickers or small gifts) for attempts at mastery of their responses, can be effective for children undergoing procedures in the office, especially if there is a chance that they may have to undergo future procedures. For those children having repeated painful/anxiety-producing procedures, the addition of cognitive-behavioral therapy (CBT) with a licensed mental health provider can help significantly decrease anxiety, distress, and pain.

Other nonpharmacologic techniques that can help limit or alleviate postoperative pain from more invasive procedures such as excision and lasers include icing, strict limitations on activity, elevation of the affected site when a surgical excision/procedure is on an extremity, and appropriate wound care and dressings. Nonpharmacologic pain/anxiety relief strategies described earlier can also be used at home by parents and in the office for postoperative wound assessments, suture removal, and dressing changes.

Pharmacologic Pain Management and Nonopioid Analgesics

The majority of minimally or noninvasive dermatologic procedures in children do not require post procedure opioid analgesics. Nonopioid analgesics such as acetaminophen and nonsteroidal anti-inflammatory drugs (NSAIDs) should be considered first line for treating postoperative pain in children. Nonopioid analgesics are effective, have fewer side effects, and exert an opioid-sparing action through diminishing the inflammatory mediators generated at the site of injury. Potential side effects of NSAIDs include gastrointestinal upset, gastrointestinal bleeding, renal dysfunction, and hypersensitivity reactions. Patients and families should be counseled to administer NSAIDs with food and to avoid administration in those patients with dehydration and a history of hypersensitivity reactions. Patients with liver dysfunction, renal dysfunction, coagulopathies, thrombocytopenia, and active bleeding should use NSAIDs with caution.[21] Excessive doses of acetaminophen can cause hepatic failure that can lead to death. Children with diabetes, concomitant viral infections, a family history of hepatotoxic reactions, obesity, and chronic malnourishment may be at more risk for developing acetaminophen toxicity.[22]

ACETAMINOPHEN TOXICITY

Patients and families should be counseled to administer NSAIDs with food and to avoid administration in those patients with dehydration and a history of hypersensitivity reactions. Patients with liver dysfunction, renal dysfunction, coagulopathies, thrombocytopenia, and active bleeding should use NSAIDs with caution.[21] Excessive doses of acetaminophen can cause hepatic failure that can lead to death. Children with diabetes, concomitant viral infections, family history of hepatotoxic reactions, obesity, and chronic malnourishment may be at more risk for developing acetaminophen toxicity.[22]

Nonopioid analgesics are generally indicated for treatment of mild to moderate pain in children or adjuncts when opioid analgesics are prescribed for moderate to severe pain. Scheduled administration of nonopioid analgesics in the postoperative

TABLE 134.5 ⋮ Commonly Used Nonopioid Analgesics and Their Dosages[26]

DRUG	AGE	DOSING[a]	FREQUENCY	MAXIMUM DAILY DOSE
Acetaminophen	Term neonate <10 d	10-15 mg/kg/dose	Every 6 h	60 mg/kg/d
	Term neonate >10 d	10-15 mg/kg/dose	Every 4-6 h	≤75 mg/kg/d; do not exceed five doses in 24 h
	Infants, children, and adolescents	10-15 mg/kg/dose	Every 4-6 h	≤75 mg/kg/d; do not exceed five doses in 24 h; do not exceed 4000 mg/d
Ibuprofen	Infants and children 6 mo to 12 y[b]	4-10 mg/kg/dose	Every 6-8 h	40 mg/kg/d Maximum single dose: 400 mg
	Children and adolescents ≥12 y	200 mg/dose, may increase to 400 mg/dose if no response	Every 4-6 h	1200 mg/d
Naproxen	Children >2 y	5-7 mg/kg/dose	Every 12 h	
	Children >12 y	200 mg/dose	Every 8-12 h	600 mg/d

[a]Further dose adjustments must be made for patients with renal and hepatic impairment.
[b]Limited data available in infants younger than 6 months of age.

period may help further limit the need for narcotic administration.[23] Combined use of acetaminophen and NSAIDs has shown further benefits (lower pain scores, fewer side effects, and improved patient satisfaction) in the treatment of postoperative surgical pain in adults and children after tonsillectomy.[24,25] We commonly recommend combination therapy with both acetaminophen and ibuprofen in the postoperative period when anticipating moderate postoperative pain.

Acetaminophen is commonly used as a nonopioid analgesic for pediatric patients. It is available over the counter as an oral suspension and chewable tablets for children who cannot swallow tablets or capsules. See Table 134.5 for commonly available formulations and dosing instructions.[26] Maximum daily dose varies depending on age and weight, and because of the narrow therapeutic index of acetaminophen, overdose can easily occur, leading to acute liver failure or even death. Dosage should be based on ideal body weight in obese and overweight children. Ibuprofen is supplied as concentrated drops, chewable tablets, oral suspension, tablets, and caplets (Table 134.6). *Weight-based dosing is always preferred for both acetaminophen and NSAIDs.* We recommend providing caretakers with the appropriate dose as well as frequency, duration of therapy, and specific strength and formulation of over-the-counter nonopioid analgesics to ensure safe administration during the postoperative period.

Pharmacologic Pain Management and Opioid Analgesics

Pediatric patients seldom require oral opioid analgesics for postoperative pain following dermatologic procedures and these should be reserved for moderate to severe pain in the postsurgical period. Examples where this may be considered include patients undergoing nail procedures or excisions requiring extensive undermining or tissue rearrangement. Consider short-term usage of opioid analgesics in combination with nonopioid analgesics or as needed for breakthrough pain

TABLE 134.6 ⋮ Common Formulations of Acetaminophen and NSAIDs Available Over the Counter[26]

MEDICATION	FORMULATION	CONCENTRATION
Acetaminophen	Liquid	160 mg/5 mL 500 mg/5 mL 500 mg/15 mL 80/0.8 mL [drops]
	Chewable tablet ODT	80 mg 80 mg, 160 mg
	Caplet/tablet/capsule	325 mg, 500 mg
Ibuprofen	Concentrated oral drops for infants and children	50 mg/1.25 mL
	Liquid	100 mg/5 mL 40 mg/mL 50 mg/1.25 mL
	Chewable tablets	50 mg, 100 mg
	(Junior strength) Caplet and tablet	100 mg
	Capsule/tablet	200 mg
Naproxen	Liquid	125 mg/5 mL
	Capsule	220 mg
	Tablet	220 mg, 250 mg, 375 mg, 500 mg, 550 mg

NSAIDs, nonsteroidal anti-inflammatory drugs; ODT, orally disintegrating tablet.

in these circumstances; although, in our experience, these are rarely needed. When opioid analgesics are used for pain relief, their efficacy, safety, side effects, cost, and the course of recovery should be thoroughly assessed and discussed with the family before prescribing. Table 134.7 reviews opioid pain medications used in the postoperative period in the pediatric population.[26] Overall, prescribers should be familiar with important drug–drug interactions and differences in metabolism of these drugs in the pediatric population and counsel patients and families appropriately when prescribed. In 2013, the U.S. Food and Drug Administration (FDA) issued a black box warning for codeine use following outpatient tonsillectomy and adenoidectomy following several deaths in this population.[27] This has led to the removal of the drug from formularies of multiple children's hospitals. Variability in rates of metabolism of codeine could result in little to no analgesic effect as well as significant risk of severe respiratory depression. For nonmetabolizers, no analgesic effect will occur. With ultrarapid metabolizers, however, codeine is rapidly converted to morphine, leading to high drug levels that could ultimately result in respiratory depression and death. Given this information, prescribing codeine and/or hydrocodone (also a prodrug that uses CYP2D6 enzyme to produce its active form) should be done with extreme caution.

TABLE 134.7 : Oral Dosing of Opioid Analgesics in Infants Older Than 6 Months, Children, and Adolescents[26]

DRUG	DOSE	FREQUENCY
Hydrocodone[a]	<50 kg: 0.1-0.2 mg/kg/dose ≥50 kg: 5-10 mg/dose	Every 4-6 h
Hydromorphone[b] (Immediate release)	Infants >10 kg (>6 mo of age): 0.03 mg/kg/dose, range 0.03-0.06 mg/kg/dose	Every 3-4 h
	Children and adolescents <50 kg: 0.03-0.08 mg/kg/dose	Every 3-4 h
	Children and adolescents ≥50 kg: 1-2 mg/dose	Every 3-4 h
Oxycodone[c] (Immediate release)	Infants >6 mo, children and adolescents <50 kg: 0.1-0.2 mg/kg/dose	Every 4-6 h
	Children and adolescents >50 kg: 5-10 mg/dose	Every 4-6 h

All dosing should be titrated to lowest possible dose to provide appropriate analgesic effects. Dosing should be adjusted for patients with hepatic and renal impairment.
[a]Limited data available in infants and children younger than 2 years.
[b]Limited data available in children.
[c]Available as individual drugs and in combination with acetaminophen. When combined with acetaminophen, refer to Table 134.5 for maximum daily dosing of acetaminophen.

Oxycodone is an active drug without the requirement of biotransformation to take effect; however, slow metabolizers can experience increased side effects. The use of oxycodone with certain other drugs (specifically macrolide antibiotics, antifungal agents, and antiviral agents) has also led the FDA to issue a black box warning because of the risk of enhanced opioid side effects when coadministered.[28]

Clinical Caution: Opioid Analgesic Use in Children

Before prescribing opioid analgesic use in children, efficacy, safety, side effects, cost, and the course of recovery should be thoroughly assessed and discussed with the family. Prescribers should be familiar with important drug–drug interactions and differences in metabolism of these drugs in the pediatric population and counsel patients and families appropriately. Prescribing codeine and/or hydrocodone should be done with extreme caution. The use of oxycodone with certain other drugs (specifically macrolide antibiotics, antifungal agents, and antiviral agents) has also led the FDA to issue a black box warning due to risk of enhanced opioid side effects when coadministered.

Lastly, caution should be taken when prescribing codeine and oxycodone products available in combination with acetaminophen to limit risk of potential acetaminophen overdose as a side effect of therapeutic opioid dosing. Opioid analgesics' side effects include nausea, vomiting, constipation, sedation, respiratory depression, urinary retention, and pruritus. It is important to discuss these before prescribing to minimize distress and unwanted or dangerous complications.

REFERENCES

1. Taddio A, Katz J, Ilersich AL, Koren G. Effect of neonatal circumcision on pain response during subsequent routine vaccination. *Lancet*. 1997;349:599–603.
2. Merskey H, Bugduk N. *Classification of Chronic Pain. Descriptions of Chronic Pain Syndromes and Definitions of Pain Terms.* 2nd ed. Seattle, WA: IASP Press; 1994.
3. Van Dijk M, Peters WB, van Deventer P, Tibboel D. The COMFORT Behavioral scale. *Am J Nurs*. 2005;105:33–36.
4. Krechel SW, Bildner J. CRIES: a new neonatal postoperative pain measurement score. Initial testing of validity and reliability. *Paediatr Anaesth*. 1995;5:53–61.
5. Merkel SI, Voepel-Lewis T, Shayevitz JR, Malviya S. The FLACC: a behavioral scale for scoring postoperative pain in young children. *Pediatr Nurs*. 1997;23:293–297.
6. Mathew PJ, Mathew JL. Assessment and management of pain in infants. *Postgrad Med J*. 2003;79:438–443.
7. Prkachin KM, Solomon PE, Ross J. Underestimation of pain by health-care providers: towards a model of the process of inferring pain in others. *Can J Nurs Res*. 2007;39:88–106.
8. Hicks CL, von Baeyer CL, Spafford P, van Korlaar I, Goodenough B. The Faces Pain Scale—revised: toward a common metric in pediatric pain measurement. *Pain*. 2001;93:173–183.
9. Beyer JE, Villarruel AM, Denyes MJ (2009, September). The Oucher: user's manual and technical report. http://www.oucher.org/downloads/2009_Users_Manual.pdf. Accessed November 11, 2018.
10. Wong DL. Chapter 26: The child who is hospitalized. In: Whaley L, Wong D, eds. *Whaley and Wong's Nursing Care of Infants and Children*. 5th ed. St. Louis, MO: Mosby; 1995.
11. Baker CM, Wong DL. Q.U.E.S.T.: a process of pain assessment in children. *Orthop Nurs*. 1987;6:11–21.

12. Wong-Baker FACES Foundation. Resources: qualities of the Wong-Baker FACES® Pain Rating Scale. www.wongbakerfaces.org. Accessed January 5, 2015.

13. Kraemer FW, Rose JB. Pharmacologic management of acute pediatric pain. *Anesthesiol Clin.* 2009;27:241–268.

14. Gehdoor RP. Postoperative pain management in pediatric patients. *Indian J Anaesth.* 2004;48:406–414.

15. Zempsky WT, Schechter NL. Office-based pain management. The 15-minute consultation. *Pediatr Clin North Am.* 2000;47(3):601–615.

16. Calipel S, Lucas-Polomeni MM, Wodey E, Ecoffey C. Premedication in children: hypnosis versus midazolam. *Paediatr Anaesth.* 2005;15:275–281.

17. Chundamala J, Wright JG, Kemp SM. An evidence-based review of parental presence during anesthesia induction and parent/child anxiety. *Can J Anesth.* 2009;56:57–70.

18. Hoetzenecker W, Guenova E, Krug M, et al. Parental anxiety and concern for children undergoing dermatological surgery. *J Dermatol Treat.* 2014;25:367–370.

19. Yates B, Whalen J, Makkar H. An age-based approach to dermatologic surgery: kids are not just little people. *Clin Dermatol.* 2017;35:512–516.

20. Strazar AR, Leynes PG, Lalonde DH. Minimizing the pain of local anesthesia injection. *Plast Reconstr Surg.* 2013;132(3):675–684.

21. Kokki H. Nonsteroidal anti-inflammatory drugs for postoperative pain: a focus on children. *Paediatr Drugs.* 2003;5(2):103–123.

22. Dlugosz CK, Chater RW, Engle JP. Appropriate use of nonprescription analgesics in pediatric patients. *J Pediatr Health Care.* 2006;20(5):316–325.

23. Wong T, Stang AS, Ganshorn H, et al. Combined and alternating paracetamol and ibuprofen therapy for febrile children. *Cochrane Database Syst Rev.* 2013;10:CD009572. doi:10.1002/14651858. CD009572.pub2.

24. Merry AF, Edwards KE, Ahmad Z, Barber C, Mahadevan M, Frampton C. Randomized comparison between the combination of acetaminophen and ibuprofen and each constituent alone for analgesia following tonsillectomy in children. *Can J Anaesth.* 2013;60(12):1180–1189.

25. Ong CK, Seymour RA, Lirk P, Merry AF. Combining paracetamol (acetaminophen) with nonsteroidal anti-inflammatory drugs: a qualitative systematic review of analgesic efficacy for acute postoperative pain. *Anesth Analg.* 2010;110(4):1170–1179.

26. Lexicomp Online®, UpToDate®, Hudson, OH: Lexi-Comp, Inc.; June 5, 2015.

27. FDA. Safety review update of codeine use in children; new boxed warning and contraindication on use after tonsillectomy and/or adenoidectomy. https://www.fda.gov/media/85072/download. Accessed May 24, 2015.

28. O'Donnell FT, Rosen KR. Pediatric pain management: a review. *Mo Med.* 2014;111(3):231–237.

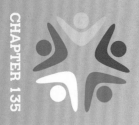

CHAPTER 135

Photoprotection

Venkata Anisha Guda and John C. Browning

Skin damage from ultraviolet (UV) rays occurs early in children because their skin is biologically different from that of adults. Infants and young toddlers have less melanin in their skin and the stratum corneum of their epidermis is thinner. In addition, children have genetic alterations in nevi. They can develop increased numbers of pigmented nevi that vary significantly from congenital nevi. Owing to these increased risk factors, it is important to provide children with sun protection early on to prevent detrimental health outcomes. Even though the American Academy of Pediatrics and the American Academy of Dermatology have promoted sun protection in the community, parents have failed to implement these practices for their children. Approximately 29% to 83% of children develop sunburn every summer. As a result, heightened efforts must be focused on enhancing parents' and children's awareness regarding sun protection.[1] The purpose of this chapter is to detail the various methods that people should use to protect themselves from the sun and the specific procedures they should follow. In addition, we present information regarding new technologies and educational programs for children in the United States and in other countries that promote sun protection. This information can help providers educate their patients in sun-protective practices that are critical to clinical outcomes many times both preprocedurally and postprocedurally and also promotes skin cancer prevention in the community.

SUNSCREEN

Sunscreen is one of the major strategies to prevent exposure to the sun's harmful UV rays and protect from skin cancer. Approximately one in five Americans will develop skin cancer in their lifetime. Sunlight consists of two types of rays, UVA and UVB. Overexposure to either can cause skin cancer. UVA rays can cause the skin to age early, resulting in wrinkles and age spots. UVB rays are the principal cause of sunburn.

The most effective sunscreens are "broad spectrum," combining agents capable of reflecting and filtering both UVA and UVB radiation. The U.S. Food and Drug Administration (FDA)'s current labeling guidelines, adopted in 2010, indicate that broad-spectrum sunscreen products with a sun protection factor (SPF) ≥15 may state, "If used as directed with other sun-protection measures, [this product] decreases the risk of skin cancer and early skin aging caused by the sun." The same labeling guidelines do not permit manufacturers to claim that products are "waterproof" or "sweatproof;" sunscreens may be labeled "water resistant" (up to either 40 or 80 minutes).[2]

Titanium dioxide and zinc dioxide are nanoparticles that are considered to be two of the most protective ingredients in sunscreens. Because of their small size, the protective capacity of these particles is enhanced. Moreover, these particles are better able to cover the skin because they have a higher level of homogeneity. They are also large enough to absorb, scatter, and reflect short-wavelength UV radiation. Other common ingredients include retinyl palmitate, which is the form of vitamin A stored by the skin, and oxybenzone, which is a synthetic estrogen and chemical filter.[3]

Important Tips Regarding Sunscreen and How/When to Apply

- Sunscreen with an SPF of 30 or higher that is water resistant and provides broad-spectrum coverage (protects from UVA and UVB rays) should be used. Sunscreen with an SPF of at least 30 will block 97% of the sun's UV rays.
- Sunscreen should be applied even on cloudy days or in the winter.
- "Water resistant" means that the sunscreen will perform well despite the presence of water or sweat and generally lasts 40 to 80 minutes. The FDA bans "waterproof" or "sweatproof" product labels because no sunscreen can protect indefinitely while swimming or sweating.[3] Sunscreen needs to be reapplied after using a towel—even if a water-resistant sunscreen is used—because the sunscreen can be removed mechanically.
- Sunscreen should be applied by hand at least 30 minutes before going outside. Generally, adults need about 1 ounce of sunscreen (a large handful), which is enough to completely cover the body (Figure 135.1).[4] The sunscreen should be

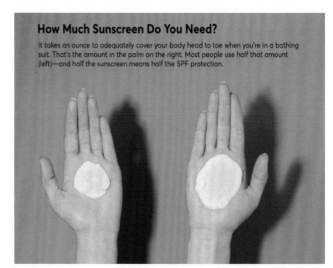

How Much Sunscreen Do You Need?

It takes an ounce to adequately cover your body head to toe when you're in a bathing suit. That's the amount in the palm on the right. Most people use half that amount (left)—and half the sunscreen means half the SPF protection.

FIGURE 135.1. How much sunscreen is enough? Reprinted with permission from Consumer Reports. The Right Way to Wear Sunscreen. May 11, 2019. Copyright © 2017 Consumer Reports, Inc. https://www.consumerreports.org/sunscreens/right-way-to-wear-sunscreen.

- *For beach/pool activities or when full body exposure:* Use a full ounce of sunscreen (blob about the size of a golf ball) per application to body and face, every 2 hours or immediately after swimming. At least 2 ounces per person required for 4 hours at pool/beach.
- *For outdoor activities when only face and arms are exposed:* 3 teaspoons needed, 1 teaspoon for the face, neck, and ears, and 2 more teaspoons for each arm.
- *When estimating how much sunscreen for vacation/trips:* If going to the pool/beach every day, estimate 8-ounce bottle to last 4 days for each person. A family of four will need four 8-ounce bottles of sunscreen for a 4-day vacation at the beach or pool activities.

rubbed into the skin and applied over all exposed skin including the neck, face, ears, and the legs and feet. Help should be asked for to apply sunscreen to the back.

- People with thinning hair should apply sunscreen to their scalp or wear a wide-brimmed hat.
- To protect the lips from the sun, lip balm with an SPF of at least 15 should be used. To continue to be protected while outdoors, sunscreen should be reapplied every 2 hours or right after swimming or sweating.
- Sunscreen should start being used in infants and toddlers after 6 months of age. Be careful when applying sunscreen on the infant's face because they can rub harmful chemicals into their eyes. In general, the teaspoon rule should be followed with children, where half a teaspoon of sunscreen is applied to each arm, a full teaspoon for each leg, a full teaspoon for their chest, abdomen, and back, and half a teaspoon for their face, head, and neck. Alternatively, a palmful (the child's palm) of sunscreen can be used to cover the child's body.
- For older teens and adults, 5 to 6 teaspoons of sunscreen should be used each application to cover the entire body.

CDC RECOMMENDATIONS FOR SUNSCREEN USE

- Before going outside, apply broad-spectrum sunscreen (SPF ≥15) to protect skin from both UVA and UVB, even on cloudy or cool days. Some professional organizations, such as the American Academy of Dermatology, recommend using sunscreens with an SPF ≥30. Apply sunscreen liberally to create a thin film on all exposed body surface areas, obtaining assistance to apply to difficult-to-reach areas.
- Reapply every 2 to 3 hours and promptly after sweating or being in the water, because sunscreens are neither waterproof nor sweatproof. U.S. Food and Drug Administration current labeling guidelines (2010) do not permit manufacturers to claim that products are "waterproof" or "sweatproof," only labeled "water resistant" (up to either 40 or 80 minutes).
- Make sure that the sunscreen is not past its expiration date.
- When also using insect repellent, apply sunscreen first, let it dry, and then apply repellent. Very limited data suggest that N,N-Diethyl-meta-toluamide (DEET) containing insect repellents can attenuate the UVB protection provided by sunscreen by as much as one-third of the reported SPF. Sunscreens may increase the absorption of DEET through the skin.
- Avoid products that contain both sunscreen and insect repellent.

From Lionetti N, Rigano L. The new sunscreens among formulation strategy, stability issues, changing norms, safety and efficacy evaluations. *Cosmetics*. 2017:4(2):15.

ORAL SUPPLEMENTATION

Oral supplementations are becoming popular in reducing risk after sun exposure. Nicotinamide is a vitamin B nutrient that has been shown to reduce the risk of skin cancer when taken as an oral supplement. In a recent study, 386 people with a history of at least two non–melanoma skin cancers received either nicotinamide twice daily or a placebo for 12 months. After 12 months, the rate of non–melanoma skin cancer was reduced by 23% in the supplemented group compared to the placebo. Nicotinamide plays a prominent role in producing adenosine triphosphate (ATP), which facilitates DNA repair in skin cells damaged by UV rays. Red orange extract is a powder derived from *Citrus sinensis*. It is rich in anthocyanins, flavanones, and hydroxycinnamic acids, which enhances the body's ability to protect against UV radiation and oxidative stress. *Polypodium leucotomos* comes from a tropical fern and is rich in polyphenols that have similar health benefits as red orange extract. The combination of these three natural ingredients can yield an oral sun-protection formula that can help protect against sun damage in children.[2]

SUN-PROTECTIVE CLOTHING AND HATS

Protective clothing and hats are another important way to shield children from the sun. The use of textiles as a form of protective clothing has not been promoted to the same extent as sunscreen (Figure 135.2). Suitable clothing can protect against skin cancer, photosensitive disorders, and premature aging. There are various factors that must be taken into account when choosing proper clothing for the sun. Textile parameters can influence the UV protection factor of clothing. The fabric type, color, weight, and thickness can impact the protection factor. Stretch, wetness, and laundering can also impact the textile. UV blocking clothes can effectively protect against the sunlight. Increased efforts need to be aimed at enhancing people's knowledge about sun-protective clothing.

UV radiation can pass through school windows, resulting in the accumulation of sun exposure and the development of skin cancer. Consequently, UV films for classroom windows are on the rise. This revolution began with automobiles in the 1990s. Researchers discovered that UV rays streamed through driver side windows causing them to develop solar damage. With the advent of UV filters, 100% of UVB and UVA rays have been screened out without reducing visibility. UVA protective films are now becoming a part of classroom windows and are able to block out up to 99.9% of UV rays. This prevents sunburn and daily UV exposure that can increase the risk of skin cancer. Moreover, UV filters are especially beneficial for children with photosensitivity conditions including xeroderma pigmentosum and lupus.[3]

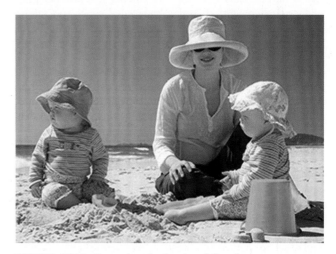

FIGURE 135.2. Protecting the head and face from sun exposure with hats and clothing is extremely important in addition to the use of sunscreen, especially for toddlers and children. NolanWynne/istockphoto.com.

ENVIRONMENTAL AWARENESS

Although children are encouraged to go outside and play to prevent childhood obesity, playgrounds can be a potentially dangerous source of sun exposure during the summer months. Triple-digit air temperatures can result in temperatures of 40° to 80° higher on equipment and surfaces. New surfaces such as rubber and green materials are not usable because of the excess heat. Many children end up in the emergency room because of playground burns. To address this problem, shade structures over playground equipment are becoming the norm. Although the shade structures keep the playground cool for children, they also help prevent long-term sun exposure. According to the Skin Cancer Foundation, one severe sunburn during childhood doubles the risk of developing melanoma. As a result, the American Academy of Dermatology created a *Shade Structure Grant program* that provides funding to schools to purchase shade structures. This has greatly helped schools create safe playgrounds for the community.[5]

Ultraviolet Indicator Wristbands

UV indicator wristbands are a type of device that is also gaining in popularity. They change color depending on whether it is safe to stay in the sun, reapply sunscreen, or avoid the sun for the rest of the day. The wristband measures the amount of UVA and UVB radiation you are exposed to during the day and will turn from yellow to beige (in certain cases) when it is time to put on sun protection. If the UV radiation is very high, the wristband will turn pink, indicating that you should go inside. This can be very helpful for children to know when it is not safe to stay outside.

In a nongovernmental school in Australia, a similar approach is taken with wristbands. Students are provided with an adhesive, disposable wristband, which is ticked every time they apply sunscreen. Students are not allowed to participate in a given event if they have not applied sunscreen hourly. This helps protect children from the sun and promotes healthy long-term behaviors.[3]

SUN-SAFE EDUCATION IN SCHOOLS AND COMMUNITIES

Education programs at a variety of schools have also been introduced to enhance children's knowledge about sun safety. The Environmental Protection Agency created the *Sun Wise School Program* to help teach sun-safe behaviors in classrooms.[6] Through the usage of school-based, classroom-based, and community-based components, the program is able to help children develop sustained sun-safe behaviors. By educating children about using sunscreen and protective clothing while also avoiding tanning booths and sunlamps, the program does an effective job at meeting its goal.

However, studies show that many schools in the United States still have not implemented sun-protection policies. Many children and staff are not protected from the sun when going outside. School principals may not be aware that skin cancer is a major health problem or what their school can do to address this problem. Enhanced public awareness regarding the dangers of sun exposure combined with increased educational awareness of school staff could potentially motivate schools to create sun-protection policies. Schools should ask parents to routinely apply sunscreen to their children before school and to have them wear protective clothing.

STRATEGIES/POLICIES TO REDUCE CHILDREN'S SUN EXPOSURE

Although there have been many campaigns to raise awareness about sun exposure in the United States, other countries are far ahead in terms of protecting their children from the sun. In many other parts of the world, sun protection is viewed as a responsibility and there are stronger initiatives to promote the sun protection strategies, most notably in Australia (particularly in Queensland), which has the highest incidence of skin cancer globally with the following campaigns/policies that have greatly helped reduce the damaging effects of children's exposure to the sun:

- Australia's Slip, Slop, Slap campaign motivates children and adults to "slip on a long sleeve shirt," "slop on some SPF 15+ sunscreen," and "slap on a broad-brimmed hat." Regular warnings promote the avoidance of the sun and the beach between 10 AM and 2 PM. Clothing is graded depending on its ability to limit sun exposure.[7,8]
- Following the success of the Slip, Slop, Slap Program, in 1988 the Cancer Council in Australia implemented the Sun-Smart program, which encourages children to wear a T-shirt, sun-suit, or swim-shirt when participating in swimming activities to provide extra protection in the water.[9]
- Australian schools have a *no-hat, no-play policy* that prevents children who are not wearing a hat from playing outdoors.[9]
- Sunscreen is offered at public swimming pools and various towns have placed shade cloths over play structures and pools in parks and community centers, resulting in 60% reduction in sun exposure.
- The Australian government has also removed taxation on sunscreens.

Compared to Australia, the United States is behind in sun-protection policies. In a study, only 36% of child care centers that were surveyed had shade in more than half of the play areas and only 56% had sufficient sun-protection policies.[10] There are very few programs in the United States compared to other countries that are geared toward spreading awareness about sun protection. The lack of well-coordinated programs in the United States is of concern because skin cancer is preventable but the incidence of melanoma is on the rise. It is essential for an implementation strategy to be arranged at the national level to protect children from the sun.

The U.S. National Weather Service and the U.S. Environmental Protection Agency have publicized about the UV index in television and weather reports across the 50 states. The index provides information regarding sun protection according to the intensity of UV light picked up that day. About 40% of Americans reported that their family had changed their sun-protection practices on the basis of the UV index. This demonstrates how important and effective it can be to spread awareness about sun protection.[11,12]

Continued efforts should be targeted toward children in summer camps, schools, outdoor pools, and health care settings. States and local governments should consider the role that they can play in implementing change by requiring daycare centers and summer camps to have sun-protection policies. Campaigns should be organized to educate the community about the detrimental effects of sun exposure and what can be done for prevention.

REFERENCES

1. Paller AS, Hawk JL, Honig P, et al. New insights about infant and toddler skin: implications for sun protection. *Pediatrics.* 2011;128(1):30–40.

2. Lionetti N, Rigano L. The new sunscreens among formulation strategy, stability issues, changing norms, safety and efficacy evaluations. *Cosmetics.* 2017:4(2):15.

3. Wanat KA, Norton SA. Sun exposure. Centers for Disease Control and Prevention. https://wwwnc.cdc.gov/travel/yellowbook/2020/noninfectious-health-risks/sun-exposure. Accessed June 2019.

4. Wadyka S. Get the facts straight about shielding your skin from damaging UV rays. Consumer Reports. 2017. https://www.consumerreports.org/sunscreens/right-way-to-wear-sunscreen/

5. Atwood E. Playground shade structures protect kids from sun. Athletic Business. 2012. https://www.athleticbusiness.com/playground-shade-structures-protect-kids-from-sun.html

6. The SunWise School Program Guide A School Program That Radiates Good Ideas Sunwise. Office of Air and Radiation 6205J EPA 430-K-03-002. May 2003. https://www.epa.gov/sites/production/files/documents/guide.pdf; www.epa.gov/sunwise

7. Turner D, Harrison SL, Bates N. Sun-protective behaviors of student spectators at inter-school swimming carnivals in a tropical region experiencing high ambient solar ultraviolet radiation. *Front Public Health.* 2016;4(168):1–11.

8. Emmons KM, Colditz GA. Preventing excess sun exposure: it is time for a national policy. *J Natl Cancer Inst.* 1999;91(15):1269–1270.

9. Sun Protection. Cancer Council Queensland. https://cancerqld.org.au/cancer-prevention/understanding-risk/sun-protection/

10. Crane L, Marcus AC, Pike DK. Skin cancer prevention in preschools and daycare centers. *J Sch Health.* 1993;63:232–234.

11. Long CS, Miller AJ, Lee HT, Wild JD, Przywarty RC, Hufford D. Ultraviolet index forecasts issued by the National Weather Service. *Bull Am Meteorol Soc.* 1996;77:729–748.

12. Geller AC, Hufford D, Miller DR, et al. Evaluation of the Ultraviolet Index: media reactions and public response. *J Am Acad Dermatol.* 1997;37:935–941.

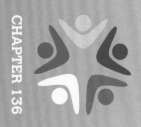

CHAPTER 136

Surgical Complications

Megan E. Shelton and Lucía Z. Díaz

INTRODUCTION

Pediatric dermatologic procedures are used to treat a wide variety of benign and, rarely, malignant conditions. Pediatric patients present unique challenges when considering surgical procedures and necessitate an individualized treatment approach. Before any procedure, the dermatologist should obtain a detailed past medical history, family history, list of current medications and supplements, medication allergies, and history of prior surgical complications. Although surgical complications occur relatively infrequently, the dermatologic surgeon should be aware of potential complications, incorporate precautions, and know how to effectively manage complications when they occur to optimize surgical outcomes.

ANESTHESIA

Topical anesthetic agents are often utilized in pediatric office procedures to minimize anxiety and pain associated with injection of local anesthesia. Topical anesthetics are effective and safe for routine use in pediatric patients, although the surgeon should be aware of potential complications. The absorption of topical anesthetic is dependent on several factors, including the anatomic location, surface area, and duration of application. In general, the risk of toxicity is increased in children because of differences in body surface area (BSA) relative to weight, as well as a nonlinear relationship between BSA and drug response.[1]

Eutectic mixture of local anesthetics (EMLA™ [AB Astra Pharmaceuticals, L.P.]) is a popular topical anesthetic, composed of the amide anesthetics lidocaine and prilocaine. Topical formulations containing prilocaine may induce methemoglobin because of iron oxidation of heme within red blood cells, thus impeding hemoglobin-mediated oxygen transport.[2] Owing to this risk, EMLA should be used cautiously in premature neonates less than 37 weeks' gestation, glucose-6-phosphate dehydrogenase deficiency, congenital or idiopathic methemoglobinemia, and in cases where other methemoglobin-inducing medications are used, including acetaminophen, sulfonamides, dapsone, and phenobarbital.[2,3] Use of EMLA on inflamed skin may enhance absorption, resulting in higher plasma levels and systemic symptoms.[2] Finally, EMLA is also known to produce purpura and petechiae in both pediatric and adult patients.[4]

Local anesthetics produce central nervous system toxicity in a dose-dependent manner. Initial symptoms of toxicity may be difficult for children to identify and vocalize; therefore, high suspicion for toxicity must be maintained when using anesthetics in pediatric patients. Such early symptoms include tinnitus, lightheadedness, circumoral numbness, metallic taste in the mouth, and diplopia. At higher levels of serum lidocaine levels, signs of lidocaine toxicity include nystagmus, slurred speech, fine tremors, seizures, and respiratory depression leading to coma and death.[2] After recognition of anesthetic toxicity, any topically applied anesthetic should be removed and further injection of anesthetics discontinued. Vitals should be closely monitored, and at higher levels of toxicity, airway and ventilation support may be required. Seizures can be controlled with benzodiazepines and intravenous infusion of lipid emulsions

may reverse the cardiac and neurologic effects of local anesthetic toxicity.[5]

True allergy or type I hypersensitivity to local anesthetics is rare, encompassing less than 1% of adverse reactions.[6] For patients with a history of true local anesthetic allergy, amide and ester anesthetics typically do not exhibit cross-reactivity, and most reported cases of cross-reactivity are secondary to paraben allergy in preservatives containing amide preparations or cosensitization.[6] In patients with a history of true anesthetic allergy, minor surgical procedures such as shave or punch biopsies can be performed with intradermal injection of 0.9% normal saline or an antihistamine such as diphenhydramine.[7] Regardless of the etiology, anaphylaxis is the most extreme presentation of type I hypersensitivity and may be fatal if not treated correctly. Prodromal signs include urticaria, diffuse swelling, and erythema, with subsequent inspiratory stridor, laryngoedema, bronchospasm, hypotension, or cardiac arrhythmias. Along with notification of emergency medical services, treatment is centered on administration of intramuscular epinephrine and supportive care with administration of oxygen, maintenance of patent airway, and initiation of cardiopulmonary resuscitation if needed.

Finally, patients may misattribute a prior episode of vasovagal syncope to a local anesthetic allergic reaction, which has been previously termed "pseudoallergy."[7] Vasovagal syncope is not an uncommon occurrence in dermatologic surgery and is usually easily recognized by the treating physician. Patients generally experience a prodromal symptoms including anxiety, diaphoresis, nausea, tachycardia, or tachypnea in response to emotional stress, pain, fear, sight of blood, or injections. Momentary clonic movements can simulate seizure activity. Transient vagally mediated bradycardia and hypotension can be corrected by repositioning the patient into a recumbent or Trendelenburg position, and applying a cool ice pack or towel to the forehead and providing reassurance can also be helpful during recovery.

INTRAPROCEDURE AND POSTPROCEDURE BLEEDING

Preoperative evaluation of every patient is critical, and past medical history, family history, review of systems, and list of current medications and over-the-counter supplements should be obtained before surgery. However, in some children, a dermatologic procedure may be the first time that difficult-to-manage bleeding is encountered. Medications, inherited syndromes, and acquired conditions may be implicated in dysfunctional hemostasis, resulting in intraoperative and postoperative bleeding. Mechanisms of such bleeding include impaired platelet adhesion and aggregation, decreased vasoconstriction, decreased coagulation, and increased fibrinolysis.[8]

Genetic and Other Disorders

Multiple inherited disorders predispose patients to experiencing intra- and postoperative bleeding. The most common inherited bleeding disorder, von Willebrand disease (VWD), manifests with easy bruising, epistaxis, gingival bleeding, menorrhagia, and prolonged surgical bleeding.[9] Although VWD affects 1 in 1000 people, bleeding is only clinically significant in a minority of patients.[10] Von Willebrand factor is a large plasma glycoprotein that is essential to both primary and secondary hemostasis because of its actions to facilitate platelet–subendothelium and platelet–platelet adhesion, aggregate platelets, and fibrinogen to form a stable plug, and protect factor VIII from proteolytic degradation.[10] Congenital coagulation disorders, the most common of which include factor VIII (hemophilia A) and factor IX (hemophilia B) deficiencies, manifest with bleeding due to decreased thrombin formation and prolonged time to clotting.[8] In cases of known inherited bleeding disorders, preoperative consultation with hematology is essential so that appropriate therapy can be instituted before surgery to minimize risk of bleeding and subsequent complications.[8]

Although often overlooked, bleeding complications may also be higher in patients with osteogenesis imperfecta, Marfan syndrome, and Down syndrome because of disordered platelet adhesion and aggregation. Finally, both Ehlers-Danlos syndrome and Osler-Weber-Rendu syndrome are associated with decreased vasoconstriction leading to difficulty in achieving hemostasis.[8]

Medications and Vitamin Supplements

Multiple medications and supplements are also associated with increased bleeding risk, although such situations are not frequently encountered in the pediatric population. Aspirin impacts primary hemostasis by irreversibly inhibiting platelet function, which only recovers following synthesis of new platelets.[11] Nonsteroidal anti-inflammatory drugs (NSAIDs) similarly affect platelet function, but effects are reversible if the drug is discontinued. In contrast, warfarin interferes with secondary hemostasis and the formation of fibrin clots as a result of vitamin K–dependent coagulation factor synthesis inhibition. Because warfarin does not impact primary hemostasis, the intra- and immediate postoperative bleeding risk is minimal; however, its effects on fibrin plug and stable clot formation may result in delayed bleeding 72 to 96 hours following surgery.[11] Finally, supplements and herbs, such as Ginkgo biloba, garlic, ginseng, ginger, feverfew, and vitamin E, have been implicated in surgical bleeding because of their antiplatelet effects.[12] Currently, it is the practice of most surgeons to continue anticoagulant therapy before, during, and after surgery. Multiple studies have found the risk of surgical bleeding from anticoagulation to be insignificant when compared to the potentially catastrophic risks of discontinuation of anticoagulant therapy.[11,13]

Strategies to Control Bleeding
Visualization of the Surgical Field

During surgery, visualization of the surgical field is critical to obtaining hemostasis. Suction, circumferential pressure (application of firm pressure on the surrounding tissue), skin hooks, cotton-tipped applicators, or sponge sticks (gauze on the end of a ring forceps) can be employed to more clearly examine the surgical wound.[11,14] When extensive bleeding is encountered intraoperatively, the surgeon should first evaluate whether the bleeding is attributable to local factors. Brisk bleeding at a local surgical site is typically due to insufficient identification and control of locally damaged blood vessels. Conversely, hemostatic defects due to previously aforementioned disorders often produce gradual oozing from the operative and injection sites.[8]

Other Approaches to Control Bleeding

Multiple approaches can be utilized to control of bleeding including electrosurgery (electrodessication and electrocoagulation—see Chapter 17. Electrosurgery/Hyfrecation) or heat cautery, although minimizing damage to normal tissue is important. If identified, bleeding from larger vessels can be stopped with application of a hemostat, allowing subsequent ligation of the vessel with absorbable suture in a figure-of-eight stitch. Although rarely required, a Penrose drain can be placed within the surgical wound to prevent hematoma formation if oozing cannot be satisfactorily managed with the aforementioned techniques (Figure 136.1). The drain is typically removed within 24 hours of placement to decrease risk of infection.[11] Finally, after hemostasis is achieved, the surgeon should utilize sutures to close any dead space within the wound, so as to decrease risk of hematoma development.

For smaller biopsy sites or wounds that will be allowed to granulate, application of topical hemostatic products can prevent or stop bleeding by creating a framework for coagulation and platelet activation to occur.[11] Such agents include absorbable gelatin foams (eg, Gelfoam®, Pfizer, US), oxidized cellulose (eg, Surgicel®, Ethicon US, LLC), and microfibrillar collagen (eg, Instat®, Ethicon US, LLC).

Following surgery, a pressure dressing should be applied to the surgical site (Figure 136.2) and the patient should be instructed to avoid extensive or strenuous physical activity. Although not necessary from a medical standpoint, we often apply large, bulky dressings following surgical procedures in our pediatric clinic (Figure 136.3A-C). Such dressings function as a visual reminder of the surgical procedure for the child and encourage the patient to minimize activity in the immediate postoperative period. It is also important to discuss the possibility of ecchymosis following surgery, especially following facial procedures, and provide reassurance that the resultant ecchymosis will improve without long-term consequence.

Bleeding in the postoperative period is anxiety provoking for the patient and family, and the risk of hemorrhagic

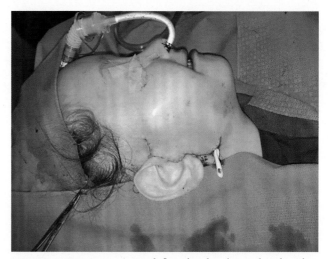

FIGURE 136.1. Large surgical flap that has been closed with a Penrose drain in the correct position to drain the area and help prevent hematoma formation. Reprinted with permission from Chung KC, Gosain AK. *Operative Techniques in Pediatric Plastic and Reconstructive Surgery*. Philadelphia, PA: Wolters Kluwer; 2020. Tech Figure 52.6C.

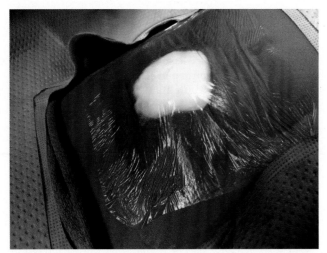

FIGURE 136.2. Large occlusive pressure dressing with sponge pad over site of repair. Reprinted with permission from Scott-Conner CE, Dawson DL. *Essential Operative Techniques and Anatomy*. 4th ed. Philadelphia, PA: Wolters Kluwer Health/Lippincott Williams & Wilkins; 2013. Figure 48.8.

complications is greatest within the first 48 hours of surgery.[11,15] In most cases, postoperative bleeding or oozing can be stopped with application of firm, continuous pressure to the surgical site for at least 15 minutes, and this process may need to be repeated to fully stop the bleeding. However, cases of uncontrolled postoperative bleeding can lead to hematoma formation, which may be further complicated by wound infection, dehiscence, and tissue necrosis. Thus, if bleeding in the postoperative period has not improved with application of direct pressure by the patient, the physician should promptly evaluate the patient for active bleeding or hematoma formation.

Strategies for Hematoma

A hematoma arises when bleeding into the subcutaneous tissue forms a localized collection of blood. Stages of evolution include early formation (stage I), gelatinous (stage II), organized (stage III), and liquefaction (stage IV).[11] A hematoma initially forms when actively bleeding vessels fill dead space within the surgical wound. Patients typically report an enlarging, warm, and painful mass in such cases. If left untreated, the mass effect exerted on normal tissue may compromise blood supply leading to tissue necrosis and wound dehiscence, and may even promote infection (Figure 136.4). Periorbital and cervical hematomas should be treated as surgical emergencies because of potential compression and subsequent damage to surrounding vital anatomic structures.

Patients with an actively expanding hematoma should be assessed by the surgeon promptly, because evacuation of the hematoma and achievement of hemostasis are essential (Figure 136.5).

Such situations require injection of local anesthesia, followed by either partial or complete opening of the surgical wound. After evacuation of coagulated blood and identification of the source of bleeding, hemostasis can be obtained with the techniques described previously. The wound should be irrigated well with saline to remove all coagulated blood and to fully inspect the surgical wound. If there is concern for more bleeding or increased risk of infection, the wound may be left open to heal by secondary intention. Otherwise, the wound can be reclosed with a layered repair. In either case, most surgeons start antibiotics to prevent surgical site infection (SSI).[11] In contrast, once fibrinolysis begins and liquefaction of the hematoma occurs, needle aspiration can be used to evacuate the hematoma contents. Smaller, uncomplicated hematomas can be allowed to resorb on their own.

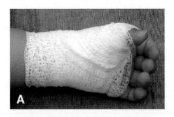

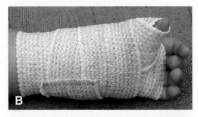

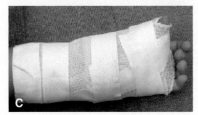

FIGURE 136.3. A-C, Postoperative pressure dressing for a dermatologic procedure involving a child's hand. Loosely wrapped gauze (A) is covered by a loosely wrapped elastic bandage (B) and a doubled-back stockinette (C) with ample tape. The multiple layers prevent premature removal by the patient. Great care must be taken to keep the dressing loose to prevent excessive swelling or even ischemia distally.

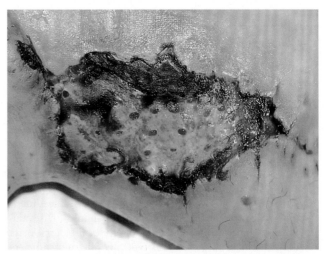

FIGURE 136.4. Partial necrosis of skin graft caused by hematoma underneath. Reprinted with permission from Chung KC, Lee GK. *Operative Techniques in Lower Limb Reconstruction and Amputation*. Philadelphia, PA: Wolters Kluwer; 2019. Figure 450.7B.

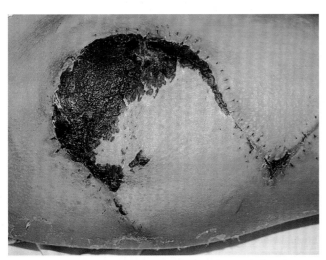

FIGURE 136.5. The distal part of an expanded flap became necrotic. Reprinted with permission from Chung KC, Lee GK. *Operative Techniques in Lower Limb Reconstruction and Amputation.* Philadelphia, PA: Wolters Kluwer; 2019. Figure 450.7C.

Dog-Ear or Standing Cone Deformity

A *dog-ear* or standing cone deformity is an excess of tissue or bunching of skin typically encountered when closing a circular wound. Prevention of a dog-ear formation can be accomplished with careful preoperative design of a fusiform or rhombic excision, with a 1:3 to 1:4 width–length ratio.[16] In addition, maintaining a 90° scalpel angle at the wound apices allows for complete removal of subcutaneous and dermal tissue, which if left behind can contribute to dog-ear formation that is less likely to regress. Sufficient undermining of the wound edges and apices before wound closure will also reduce dog-ear development.[17]

Several intraoperative surgical techniques can be utilized to correct or minimize a standing cone deformity (Figure 136.6A and B). One such approach incorporates excision of redundant tissue at the end of the wound, thereby increasing the length of the wound. In surgical wounds with unequal side lengths, the dog-ear develops on the longer side of the wound. Occasionally,

the dog-ear can be corrected by suturing through the redundancy, with wound closure accomplished with the "rule of halves." This allows the excess tissue to be dispersed evenly along the entire length of the wound without further removal of tissue. In cases where excision of the excess tissue is desired, triangular or V-shaped darts, also known as the Burrow's triangle, can be excised from the longer side of the wound.[17]

Interestingly, multiple studies have examined the likelihood of dog-ear regression without intervention. Lee et al demonstrated that standing cones were statistically more likely to regress in younger and/or female patients, and in cases where the standing cone was less than 8 mm in height. The median time to dog-ear regression in this study was 132 days.[18] Greater standing cone regression in younger patients may be due to inherently higher skin tension, whereby constant tension on the surgical incision results in widening of the scar and resolution of the standing cone.[18] A follow-up study reported that standing cones on the hands and those less than 4 mm on the trunk resolved at 6 months without intervention.[19] Given evidence of dog-ear resolution without surgical correction is frequent in pediatric patients; watchful waiting for improvement following surgery may obviate unnecessary surgical procedures.

INFECTION

The surgical wound classification system, created by the Centers for Disease Control and Prevention (CDC), categorizes surgical wounds as clean (class I), clean/contaminated (class II), contaminated (class III), and dirty-infected (class IV), with each category exhibiting varying rates of postoperative SSI.[20] Dermatologic surgery typically encompasses class I surgical wounds, given procedures are performed with aseptic surgical technique involving clean, noncontaminated skin.[21] Procedures that involve oral or nasal mucosa, however, are graded as class II surgical wounds.[21]

Per 1992 CDC definitions of nosocomial infections, superficial SSI can be diagnosed if the infection appears within 30 days of the procedure, encompasses skin or subcutaneous tissue surrounding the incision, and at least one of the following is also present:

1. Purulent discharge from the surgical site
2. An aseptically collected wound culture isolates infectious organisms

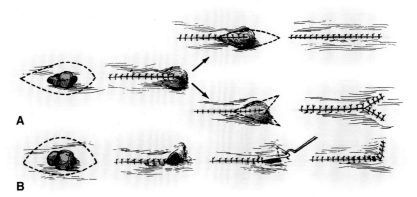

FIGURE 136.6. Repair of the "dog-ear" caused by making the elliptical excision too short. A, Dog-ear excised, making the incision longer, or converted to a "Y." B, One method of removing a dog-ear caused by designing an elliptical excision with one side longer than the other. Conversion to an "L" effectively lengthens the shorter side. Adapted with permission from Thorne CH, Guntner GC, Chung KC, et al. *Grabb and Smith's Plastic Surgery.* 7th ed. Philadelphia, PA: Wolters Kluwer Health/Lippincott Williams & Wilkins; 2013. Figure 1.4.

3. One or more of the following signs or symptoms of infection: pain, localized edema, erythema, and warmth, *and* the incision is intentionally opened by surgeon (unless wound culture finding is negative)
4. Superficial incisional SSI diagnosed by the physician[22]

Most cases of SSIs are attributed to contamination from endogenous cutaneous or mucosal microbial flora.[23] The most commonly isolated organism is *Staphylococcus aureus*, although other frequently identified bacteria include coagulase negative *Staphylococcus*, *Enterococci*, *Escherichia coli*, and *Pseudomonas aeruginosa*.[24,25]

Multiple prospective trials have reported the rate of SSI after dermatologic surgery, including Mohs micrographic surgery to be 0.7% to 1.9%.[23,26,27] A retrospective review of 872 excisions in pediatric patients identified an SSI rate of 0.3%.[28] In addition, this study reported no difference in the rate of SSI between procedures performed in the clinic and those in the operating room, after controlling for differences in preoperative antibiotic usage, surgeon, lesion type and size, and patient age. Although data are limited in pediatric patients, factors associated with increased risk of postoperative infection in adults include procedures involving the lips, ears, perineum, inguinal area, and lower extremities below the knee.[23] It is thought that the larger microbiologic burden in these areas contributes to the increased risk of infection.[21]

According to the 2008 Advisory Statement on antibiotic prophylaxis in dermatologic surgery, antibiotic prophylaxis should be administered to patients at high risk for infective endocarditis with any procedure that breaches the oral mucosa or involves infected skin.[29] Other than patients with prosthetic cardiac valves or history of previous infective endocarditis, high-risk patients include those with a history of congenital heart disease (CHD), specifically:

- Unrepaired CHD, as well as palliative shunts and conduits
- CHD repaired with prosthetic material or device within the first 6 months of the procedure
- Repaired CHD with remaining defects despite a prosthetic patch or device[29]

Regarding prevention of hematogenous prosthetic total joint infection, prophylactic antibiotics are currently indicated in patients with a history of total joint replacement in the preceding 2 years, prior prosthetic joint infection, immunosuppression, and those undergoing procedures on high-risk sites including breaches of the oral mucosa and below the knee.[29] This clinical situation is not likely to be encountered often in the pediatric population, and prophylactic antibiotics are not indicated in patients with orthopedic pins, plates, or screws. When indicated, the prophylactic antibiotic most often used is a first-generation cephalosporin, such as cephalexin, given its broad activity against gram-positive and common gram-negative organisms. Ideally, the antibiotic should be administered 60 minutes before incision, although the specific clinical scenario should dictate antibiotic selection.[29]

Ultimately, given the overall low risk of SSIs and current recommendations, preoperative prophylactic oral antibiotics are rarely indicated, and overuse may contribute to antibiotic resistance.[29,30] Additional studies have also investigated the role of topical antibiotic formulations in the prevention of SSI. A randomized control trial comparing postoperative treatment of 1249 dermatologic surgery wounds with either bacitracin ointment or white petrolatum failed to demonstrate a significant difference in infection rates (4 [0.9%] vs. 9 [2.0%], respectively).[31]

Thus, the use of white petrolatum is favored over topical antibiotics such as bacitracin in the routine care of clean surgical incisions. Finally, the role of prophylactic postoperative oral antibiotics in dermatologic surgery is also unclear. Current data have failed to demonstrate benefit of postoperative antibiotics for prevention of postoperative infection, and randomized controlled trials are lacking.[32]

When a patient presents with a concern for postoperative infection, the clinician must differentiate between normal wound healing and an SSI. Mild erythema, surgical site edema and tenderness, and serosanguinous discharge are signs of normal wound healing in the postoperative period, especially during the first 3 days following surgery. Reviewing the normal wound healing process with the patient and family before discharge from the office is important, because many patients confuse normal wound healing with infection. This may also minimize unnecessary application of topical antibiotics or other home remedies. However, when increasing pain, redness, and edema occur, especially in conjunction with a purulent discharge from the wound, an infection should be considered. Evaluation for systemic symptoms, such as fever, chills, lethargy, and decreased oral intake, is also important because patients may rarely develop bacteremia, increasing risk of infective endocarditis or hematogenous total joint infection. The signs and symptoms of infection typically appear 4 to 7 days after the procedure.[33] If possible, bacterial culture of any purulent drainage from the surgical site should be performed to confirm infection and tailor antibiotic therapy depending on sensitivities. It is important to note that wound cultures should not be used to diagnose infection and empiric treatment is warranted when SSI is suspected.

Treatment for SSI should include prompt administration of oral antibiotics to cover probable pathogens, primarily *S. aureus*. Empiric treatment with a first-generation cephalosporin, such as cephalexin, or a penicillinase-resistant penicillin, such as dicloxacillin is often selected. The recommended dose of oral cephalexin is 40 mg/kg/d, divided into doses administered three to four times daily. Azithromycin or clindamycin can be used in penicillin allergic patients. For patients presenting with an abscess or history of methicillin-resistant *Staphylococcus aureus* (MRSA) infection, antibiotic selection should include MRSA coverage, such as trimethoprim-sulfamethoxazole, clindamycin, or doxycycline. Local resistance patterns as detailed in antibiograms can direct antibiotic selection and adjustments can be rendered depending on culture results.

ALLERGIC CONTACT DERMATITIS

Allergic contact dermatitis (ACD) may present in the postoperative period, and is occasionally confused with SSI. ACD is a type IV delayed hypersensitivity reaction, with clinical presentations ranging from erythematous patches to vesicular, bullous, or indurated plaques. Reactions typically appear 48 to 96 hours after exposure to the allergen, and tend to be extremely pruritic, a key differentiating factor from SSI, which is painful. When mistaken for cellulitis, misdiagnosis of ACD results in exposure to antibiotics unnecessarily. Furthermore, exuberant inflammatory responses associated with ACD may impede wound healing and potentiate wound dehiscence.[34]

Exposure to potential allergens may occur in the preoperative, intraoperative, and postoperative settings. Although rare, there are reports of ACD occurring secondary to antiseptics in children, including chlorhexidine gluconate and benzalkonium chloride.[35] In addition, local anesthetics, whether applied topically or injected intradermally, are also known to cause ACD.[36,37] Ester anesthetics have increased allergenicity because of the metabolite para-aminobenzoic acid, with benzocaine being the most frequent anesthetic to cause ACD.[36,38] More commonly utilized as a topical anesthetic in the pediatric population, benzocaine is a component of the compounded topical anesthetic BLT® Topical Numbing Cream (Sambia Pharmaceuticals, Atlanta, GA) and the probable etiology of ACD observed with this formulation.[36] Finally, lidocaine, an amide anesthetic with comparatively reduced allergenic potential, is also associated with delayed-type hypersensitivity reactions, likely driven by widely available topical anesthetics containing lidocaine.[36]

ACD has also been associated with the use of the tissue adhesive 2-octylcyanoacrylate (Dermabond™ Topical Skin Adhesive [Ethicon US, LLC]).[37] Owing to the popularity and availability of this product and similar over-the-counter products, incidence of ACD to tissue adhesives may be increasing. In addition to cyanoacrylate adhesives, other potential sensitizers in tissue adhesives include dyes, plasticizers, polymerization inhibitors, and formaldehyde.[34]

Studies of contact dermatitis in the pediatric population indicate that neomycin sulfate, an aminoglycoside antibiotic found in over-the-counter products, is often implicated in contact dermatitis.[39] Allergy to neomycin has been documented in patients younger than 3 years old.[40] Similarly, coreactivity with bacitracin, an antipeptidoglycan cell wall antibiotic, may occur because it is present in combination with neomycin in many formulations. In contrast, mupirocin is thought to have reduced allergenic potential, and is recommended in situations where risk of infection is increased.[36]

Irritant contact dermatitis in the postoperative period may also be mistaken for SSI. Although ACD may rarely occur with antiseptics containing povidone-iodine, patients are more likely to develop irritant contact dermatitis following exposure to povidone-iodine antiseptics, especially if accidental pooling occurs under surgical drapes[37,41,42] (Figure 136.7A and B). Owing to its high irritant potential, use of povidone-iodine antiseptics should be avoided in patients with atopic dermatitis.[41] In addition, most skin reactions to wound dressings are thought to be irritant in nature. A study examining the true incidence of ACD in patients with a reported "allergy" to medical adhesive bandages found none of the subjects to have positive patch test reactions to the over-the-counter tapes and bandages. Most patients, however, exhibited an irritant reaction to at least one over-the-counter tape or bandage when left in place for 1 week.[43] Nevertheless, adhesive allergens associated with ACD include colophony, rubber accelerators, and acrylates.[44]

When ACD is suspected, at the first post-operative visit, the surgeon should throughly wash the affected area, taking care to remove any residual allergen (or irritant). The physician should obtain a detailed history of exposures, including preoperative cleansing agents, bandages, and any at-home medicaments used. A history of atopic dermatitis also increases risk of contact sensitization.[45] Diagnosis of allergic contact dermatitis can be confirmed with patch testing, with several patch test series available (see Chapter 33. Patch Testing for Allergic Contact Dermatitis). ⬅ The first of which is the Thin-layer Rapid-Use Epicutaneous (T.R.U.E. test® [Allerderm, Phoenix, AZ]) which contains 35 allergens, and is U.S. Federal Drug Administration (FDA) approved in children 6 years and older. Unfortunately, the T.R.U.E. test allergen series is not amenable to adjustments based on exposure history given its premade construction. Furthermore, the T.R.U.E. test fails to identify a significant number of relevant reactions because of the limited panel of allergens included. Previous studies indicate 25% to 33% of relevant positive reactions were missed when compared to the North American Contact Dermatitis Group (NACDG) series, and many of the allergens pertinent to surgical encounters are not included in the T.R.U.E. test.[46] The NACDG allergen series includes 70 allergens, many of which are encountered in the surgical setting. It is important to recognize

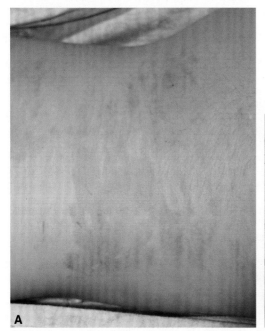
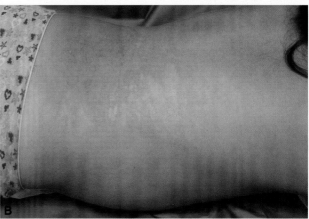

FIGURE 136.7. A, This young child developed an irritant contact dermatitis reaction from povidone-iodine used as a surgical cleanser during an extensive orthopedics surgery. B, The inflammation eventually calmed with topical steroids; however, the resultant postinflammatory dyspigmentation persisted for more than 9 months. Photos courtesy of Andrew C. Krakowski, MD.

potential limitations of the NACDG allergen series in children, specifically the smaller surface area available to apply large numbers of patches in children. Patches are typically applied to the back, but the stomach, arms, and thighs can be utilized if necessary. More recently, the Pediatric Contact Dermatitis Workgroup proposed an expert consensus–derived baseline series of 38 allergens, the Pediatric Baseline Patch Test Series.[47]

Regardless of allergen series utilized, patches are removed 48 hours after placement, followed by patch test readings 48 to 96 hours later. Of note, delayed readings beyond 7 days after patch placement may be necessary to identify reactions to specific preservatives and neomycin.[48] Any positive reaction should be evaluated for significance within the context of the patient and their exposures. Probable triggers should be strictly avoided, with subsequent assessment for improvement. Other than avoiding future exposure to the allergen, treatment of ACD is primarily accomplished with medium to high potency topical steroids, although in severe cases, an oral steroid taper over 2 to 3 weeks may be required. Scheduled antihistamines may also be of some utility in the management of pruritus associated with ACD.

HYPERTROPHIC AND KELOIDAL SCARRING

Surgical scars may significantly impact patients' physical, psychological, and social well-being. Postsurgical scar stretching, hypertrophic scars, and keloids are commonly encountered in pediatric patients, and it is important to openly discuss potential outcomes preoperatively, especially for elective procedures. In addition, patients with a personal or family history of hypertrophic or keloidal scarring may want to proceed cautiously with surgical intervention, especially if the procedure involves cosmetically sensitive locations or areas at an increased risk of abnormal scarring.

Intraoperative techniques that may optimize surgical scars include augmenting the number of dermal sutures and utilization of running subcuticular sutures with absorbable sutures such as poliglecaprone-25 (Monocryl® [Ethicon US, LLC]), especially adjacent to joints or areas subject to increased tension.[49] Excess tension on the suture line may increase the final scar width.[5] Following surgery, limiting activity and resultant mechanical stress to the surgical site is an essential aspect of postoperative wound healing. We often apply large, bulky dressings following surgical procedures in our pediatric clinic. These dressings provide a visual reminder of the surgical procedure for the child and encourage the patient to minimize activity in the postoperative period. Minimizing the risk of postoperative bleeding and infection, which may threaten wound healing, is critical, and ensuring a moist environment with white petrolatum or occlusive dressings optimizes wound healing by encouraging cell migration and shortening time to reepithelialization.[50]

Hypertrophic scars and keloids are formed from excess collagen deposition. Hypertrophic scars are raised, firm scars that remain within the border of the original wound and tend to improve with time, whereas keloids characteristically expand beyond the inciting wound and are persistent. Patients commonly experience associated pruritus, dysesthesia, and pain, and may rarely develop functional impairment. Several anatomic sites that exhibit high tension and movement, including the shoulder and anterior chest, are predisposed to abnormal scarring. In patients with a known history of abnormal scarring, topical silicone gel sheets may decrease development of hypertrophic

and keloidal scarring.[51] It is unclear whether the same benefits are observed in patients not predisposed to abnormal scarring. In addition, there is insufficient evidence to recommend topical application of vitamin E, onion extract (*Allium cepa*), or retinoids to improve appearance of surgical scars.[52]

Many approaches are utilized in the treatment of hypertrophic and keloidal scarring, and often a combination of therapies is required. The most common treatment of hypertrophic scars and keloids is intralesional corticosteroid injection. Serial injections every 2 to 6 weeks are typically required to achieve maximal results, and improvement is likely due to suppression of inflammation and collagen production, degradation of collagen, and restriction of wound oxygenation and nutrition.[53] Although several studies have demonstrated efficacy in pediatric patients, the main limitation in children is pain and anxiety associated with injection.[54,55] Localized atrophy, telangiectasia, and hypopigmentation are the most common side effects of intralesional corticosteroids.[56]

Laser therapy may also improve appearance of hypertrophic scars and keloids, and pulsed-dye laser and nonablative and ablative laser resurfacing have been utilized.[57] Finally, surgical revision may also be required in cases where adjunctive therapies have been unsuccessful.

REFERENCES

1. Cella M, Knibbe C, Danhof M, Della Pasqua O. What is the right dose for children? *Br J Clin Pharmacol.* 2010;70(4):597–603.
2. Sobanko JF, Miller CJ, Alster TS. Topical anesthetics for dermatologic procedures: a review. *Dermatol Surg.* 2012;38(5):709–721.
3. Lillieborg S, Otterbom I, Ahlen K. Topical anaesthesia in neonates, infants and children. *Br J Anaesth.* 2004;92(3):450; author reply 450–451.
4. Chen BK, Eichenfield LF. Pediatric anesthesia in dermatologic surgery: when hand-holding is not enough. *Dermatol Surg.* 2001;27(12):1010–1018.
5. Crisan D, Scharffetter-Kochanek K, Kastler S, et al. Dermatologic surgery in children: an update on indication, anesthesia, analgesia and potential perioperative complications. *J Dtsch Dermatol Ges.* 2018;16(3):268–276.
6. Bhole MV, Manson AL, Seneviratne SL, Misbah SA. IgE-mediated allergy to local anaesthetics: separating fact from perception: a UK perspective. *Br J Anaesth.* 2012;108(6):903–911.
7. Fader DJ, Johnson TM. Medical issues and emergencies in the dermatology office. *J Am Acad Dermatol.* 1997;36(1):1–16; quiz 16–18.
8. Peterson SR, Joseph AK. Inherited bleeding disorders in dermatologic surgery. *Dermatol Surg.* 2001;27(10):885–889.
9. Sharma R, Flood VH. Advances in the diagnosis and treatment of Von Willebrand disease. *Blood.* 2017;130(22):2386–2391.
10. Castaman G, Linari S. Diagnosis and treatment of von Willebrand disease and rare bleeding disorders. *J Clin Med.* 2017;6(4):45.
11. Bunick CG, Aasi SZ. Hemorrhagic complications in dermatologic surgery. *Dermatol Ther.* 2011;24(6):537–550.
12. Chang LK, Whitaker DC. The impact of herbal medicines on dermatologic surgery. *Dermatol Surg.* 2001;27(8):759–763.
13. Palamaras I, Semkova K. Perioperative management of and recommendations for antithrombotic medications in dermatological surgery. *Br J Dermatol.* 2015;172(3):597–605.
14. Bellet JS, Wagner AM. Difficult-to-control bleeding. *Pediatr Dermatol.* 2009;26(5):559–562.
15. Hurst EA, Yu SS, Grekin RC, Neuhaus IM. Bleeding complications in dermatologic surgery. *Semin Cutan Med Surg.* 2007;26(4):189–195.
16. Goldberg LH, Alam M. Elliptical excisions: variations and the eccentric parallelogram. *Arch Dermatol.* 2004;140(2):176–180.
17. Weisberg NK, Nehal KS, Zide BM. Dog-ears: a review. *Dermatol Surg.* 2000;26(4):363–370.

18. Lee KS, Kim NG, Jang PY, et al. Statistical analysis of surgical dog-ear regression. *Dermatol Surg.* 2008;34(8):1070–1076.

19. Jennings TA, Keane JC, Varma R, Walsh SB, Huang CC. Observation of dog-ear regression by anatomical location. *Dermatol Surg.* 2017;43(11):1367–1370.

20. Horan TC, Gaynes RP, Martone WJ, Jarvis WR, Emori TG. CDC definitions of nosocomial surgical site infections, 1992: a modification of CDC definitions of surgical wound infections. *Infect Control Hosp Epidemiol.* 1992;13(10):606–608.

21. Saleh K, Schmidtchen A. Surgical site infections in dermatologic surgery: etiology, pathogenesis, and current preventative measures. *Dermatol Surg.* 2015;41(5):537–549.

22. Horan TC, Gaynes RP, Martone WJ, Jarvis WR, Emori TG. CDC definitions of nosocomial surgical site infections, 1992: a modification of CDC definitions of surgical wound infections. *Am J Infect Control.* 1992;20(5):271–274.

23. Dixon AJ, Dixon MP, Askew DA, Wilkinson D. Prospective study of wound infections in dermatologic surgery in the absence of prophylactic antibiotics. *Dermatol Surg.* 2006;32(6):819–826; discussion 826–817.

24. Miner AL, Sands KE, Yokoe DS, et al. Enhanced identification of postoperative infections among outpatients. *Emerg Infect Dis.* 2004;10(11):1931–1937.

25. Rosengren H, Dixon A. Antibacterial prophylaxis in dermatologic surgery: an evidence-based review. *Am J Clin Dermatol.* 2010;11(1):35–44.

26. Maragh SL, Brown MD. Prospective evaluation of surgical site infection rate among patients with Mohs micrographic surgery without the use of prophylactic antibiotics. *J Am Acad Dermatol.* 2008;59(2):275–278.

27. Rogues AM, Lasheras A, Amici JM, et al. Infection control practices and infectious complications in dermatological surgery. *J Hosp Infect.* 2007;65(3):258–263.

28. Nuzzi LC, Greene AK, Meara JG, Taghinia A, Labow BI. Surgical site infection after skin excisions in children: is field sterility sufficient? *Pediatr Dermatol.* 2016;33(2):136–141.

29. Wright TI, Baddour LM, Berbari EF, et al. Antibiotic prophylaxis in dermatologic surgery: advisory statement 2008. *J Am Acad Dermatol.* 2008;59(3):464–473.

30. Del Rosso JQ. Wound care in the dermatology office: where are we in 2011? *J Am Acad Dermatol.* 2011;64(3 suppl):S1–S7.

31. Smack DP, Harrington AC, Dunn C, et al. Infection and allergy incidence in ambulatory surgery patients using white petrolatum vs bacitracin ointment. A randomized controlled trial. *JAMA.* 1996;276(12):972–977.

32. Levin EC, Chow C, Makhzoumi Z, Jin C, Shiboski SC, Arron ST. Association of postoperative antibiotics with surgical site infection in mohs micrographic surgery. *Dermatol Surg.* 2019;45:52–57.

33. Hurst EA, Grekin RC, Yu SS, Neuhaus IM. Infectious complications and antibiotic use in dermatologic surgery. *Semin Cutan Med Surg.* 2007;26(1):47–53.

34. Bowen C, Bidinger J, Hivnor C, Hoover A, Henning JS. Allergic contact dermatitis to 2-octyl cyanoacrylate. *Cutis.* 2014;94(4):183–186.

35. Darrigade AS, Léauté-Labrèze C, Boralevi F, Taïeb A, Milpied B. Allergic contact reaction to antiseptics in very young children. *J Eur Acad Dermatol Venereol.* 2018;32:2284–2287.

36. Butler L, Mowad C. Allergic contact dermatitis in dermatologic surgery: review of common allergens. *Dermatitis.* 2013;24(5):215–221.

37. Cook KA, Kelso JM. Surgery-related contact dermatitis: a review of potential irritants and allergens. *J Allergy Clin Immunol Pract.* 2017;5(5):1234–1240.

38. Fransway AF, Zug KA, Belsito DV, et al. North American Contact Dermatitis Group patch test results for 2007-2008. *Dermatitis.* 2013;24(1):10–21.

39. Goldenberg A, Mousdicas N, Silverberg N, et al. Pediatric Contact Dermatitis Registry Inaugural Case Data. *Dermatitis.* 2016;27(5):293–302.

40. Belloni Fortina A, Romano I, Peserico A, Eichenfield LF. Contact sensitization in very young children. *J Am Acad Dermatol.* 2011;65(4):772–779.

41. Lachapelle JM. A comparison of the irritant and allergenic properties of antiseptics. *Eur J Dermatol.* 2014;24(1):3–9.

42. Corazza M, Bulciolu G, Spisani L, Virgili A. Chemical burns following irritant contact with povidone-iodine. *Contact Dermatitis.* 1997;36(2):115–116.

43. Widman TJ, Oostman H, Storrs FJ. Allergic contact dermatitis from medical adhesive bandages in patients who report having a reaction to medical bandages. *Dermatitis.* 2008;19(1):32–37.

44. Jacob SE, Amado A, Cohen DE. Dermatologic surgical implications of allergic contact dermatitis. *Dermatol Surg.* 2005;31(9, pt 1):1116–1123.

45. Jacob SE, McGowan M, Silverberg NB, et al. Pediatric Contact Dermatitis Registry Data on contact allergy in children with atopic dermatitis. *JAMA Dermatol.* 2017;153(8):765–770.

46. Warshaw EM, Maibach HI, Taylor JS, et al. North American contact dermatitis group patch test results: 2011-2012. *Dermatitis.* 2015;26(1):49–59.

47. Yu J, Atwater AR, Brod B, et al. Pediatric baseline patch test series: Pediatric Contact Dermatitis Workgroup. *Dermatitis.* 2018;29(4):206–212.

48. Davis MD, Bhate K, Rohlinger AL, Farmer SA, Richardson DM, Weaver AL. Delayed patch test reading after 5 days: the Mayo Clinic experience. *J Am Acad Dermatol.* 2008;59(2):225–233.

49. Metz BJ. Procedural pediatric dermatology. *Dermatol Clin.* 2013;31(2):337–346.

50. Kannon GA, Garrett AB. Moist wound healing with occlusive dressings. A clinical review. *Dermatol Surg.* 1995;21(7):583–590.

51. Gold MH, Foster TD, Adair MA, Burlison K, Lewis T. Prevention of hypertrophic scars and keloids by the prophylactic use of topical silicone gel sheets following a surgical procedure in an office setting. *Dermatol Surg.* 2001;27(7):641–644.

52. Liu A, Moy RL, Ozog DM. Current methods employed in the prevention and minimization of surgical scars. *Dermatol Surg.* 2011;37(12):1740–1746.

53. Krusche T, Worret WI. Mechanical properties of keloids in vivo during treatment with intralesional triamcinolone acetonide. *Arch Dermatol Res.* 1995;287(3–4):289–293.

54. Acosta S, Ureta E, Yañez R, Oliva N, Searle S, Guerra C. Effectiveness of intralesional triamcinolone in the treatment of keloids in children. *Pediatr Dermatol.* 2016;33(1):75–79.

55. Hamrick M, Boswell W, Carney D. Successful treatment of earlobe keloids in the pediatric population. *J Pediatr Surg.* 2009;44(1):286–288.

56. Krakowski AC, Totri CR, Donelan MB, Shumaker PR. Scar management in the pediatric and adolescent populations. *Pediatrics.* 2016;137(2):e20142065.

57. Mobley SR, Sjogren PP. Soft tissue trauma and scar revision. *Facial Plast Surg Clin North Am.* 2014;22(4):639–651.

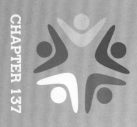

CHAPTER 137

Wet Wrap Therapy

Samantha Casselman, Judith O'Haver, and Harper N. Price

DEFINITION AND EFFECTIVENESS

Wet wrap therapy (WWT) is a therapeutic intervention that involves layering dampened gauze wrap, cotton clothing, or equivalent bandages over emollients with or without topical corticosteroids (TCSs) and a top layer of dry bandages or clothing. Typically, the moistened layer of bandages is left on overnight or for several hours throughout the day and allowed to dry before removing.

WWT has not been a widely studied treatment with defined parameters for topical medications, dressings, or timing of use; however, the clinical improvement seen with WWT has helped establish this technique as a relatively safe, clinically effective, and useful treatment for atopic dermatitis (AD) and other related inflammatory skin conditions.

UTILIZATION OF WET WRAP THERAPY

The concept of wet bandages to improve barrier dysfunction and promote wound healing was first published in 1987.[1] The act of occluding emollients and topical medications with a wet and dry layer improves penetration of topical agents and aids in passive debridement of excess scaling. WWT is also theorized to diminish transepidermal water loss and barrier dysfunction, thereby decreasing risk for opportunistic viruses, bacterial infections, and exogenous antigen exposure, lending to allergy priming.[1] Today, WWT is utilized when the skin barrier is compromised.

The utilization of TCS preparations under occlusive wet wraps improves inflammation and pruritus and aids in repair of the skin barrier. AD is the most commonly treated condition with WWT. There are small case studies highlighting the benefit of medication and emollient penetration for widespread viral conditions such as eczema coxsackium.[2] When endorsing WWT for viral conditions, you should consider the ability of the family to safely perform WWT, timing for follow-up to monitor for side effects, and socioeconomic considerations given the acute nature of viral conditions versus the chronic nature of the conditions where WWTs are more commonly utilized.

EVIDENCE FOR USE OF WET WRAPS

A systematic review and meta-analysis on the efficacy and safety of WWT for patients with AD was published in 2016 evaluating six studies that were considered low quality of evidence, and it concluded that WWT is not more effective than is standard treatment with TCS.[3] Historically, there has been a high heterogeneity in results and varying study designs, lending to the inability to assess this intervention in the context of a systematic review; however, several clinical trials have reported promising results for WWT in short-term management of severe AD flares. WWT is generally accepted as a safe, effective adjunct treatment for recalcitrant AD and is recommended in the American Academy of Dermatology (AAD) guidelines for management of AD.[3] Nicol et al[3] published an observational cohort study evaluating the effectiveness of WWT as part of a multidisciplinary AD outpatient treatment program to improve moderate to severe AD.[4] The Scoring Atopic Dermatitis (SCORAD) index was the primary measure utilized to evaluate the improvement of AD. Significant clinical improvement was observed baseline versus postprogram as a result of being treated with WWT in the cohort (mean ± SB value: 46.68 ± 17.72 baseline vs. 14.83 ± 7.45 postprogram). In this study, 72 children participated in a WWT treatment program averaging 5 to 10 days of either outpatient or inpatient management for moderate to severe AD. Subjects were managed by a multidisciplinary team of providers and assisted by registered nurses to apply low- to mid-potency TCS and moisturizer/barrier application following baths two to three times per day. Triamcinolone acetonide 0.1% ointment was the most commonly utilized corticosteroid for moderate to severe AD and desonide ointment 0.05% for the face. These formulations were not compounded or diluted with emollients. WWT was applied for a minimum of 2 hours and in some cases overnight, for an average of 7.5 ± 2.6 days. Patients had significant improvement following the outpatient program; when seen at a 1-month follow-up, AD severity remained improved and similar to the patient's discharge severity measures. Gittler et al[5] reported that many studies support WWT as an efficacious treatment and Janmohamed et al[4] conveyed that dilute TCS with WWT was more efficacious and produced results more quickly than did WWT with emollients only. In clinical practice, in an outpatient setting with pediatric patients diagnosed with AD, we find WWT with TCS a rapid and efficient therapy for acute flares and more recalcitrant disease, if applied according to recommendations.

PROCEDURE FOR WET WRAP THERAPY
(Figure 137.1A-G)

Step 1: Gather all needed equipment/items before starting the procedure, if possible. Consider planning to use distraction techniques, distraction devices, or a reward system for younger children.

Step 2: Before applying the wet wrap, review with your patient what to expect when applying, to alleviate any fear.

Step 3: On clean damp skin, apply a TCS preparation as prescribed for WWT.

Step 4: Next apply a bland, thick moisturizing cream and/or petrolatum jelly on top.

Clinical Tip

TCSs in ointment form are often utilized for infants and younger children because these may be better tolerated and cause less discomfort when applied on denuded or excoriated skin. For older children and adolescents, offering a choice of topical emollient, ointment, or a cream-based formulation is ideal for aiding in patient adherence and tolerance of wet wraps.

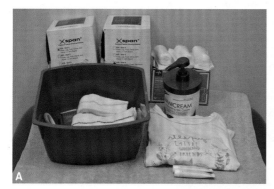
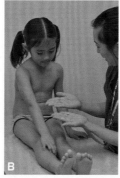
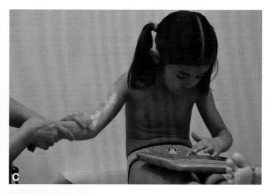

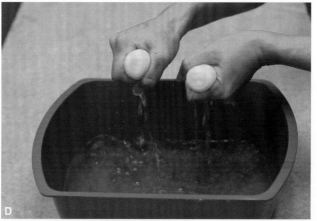

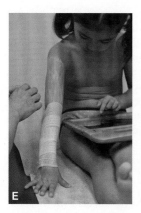
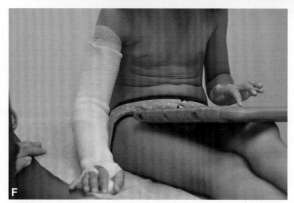
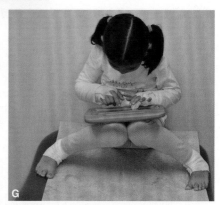

FIGURE 137.1. A, Gather your supplies to perform wet wraps to include a contact layer, dry layer, basin for warm water, medication, emollient and scissors. B, Step 1: Before applying the wet wrap, review what your patient should expect when applying the WWT to alleviate any fear. On clean, dry or damp skin apply topical medications first. C, Step 2: Next, place a thick layer of bland, thick moisturizing cream and/or petrolatum jelly. Consider using distraction techniques for children such as tablets or games. D, Step 3: Moisten your contact layer with warm water. Ring out the gauze or fabric leaving the material dampened rather than completely saturated with water. E, Step 4: Start applying the contact/wet layer directly to the affected site. Apply the contact layer adequately around the site, ensuring circulation is not compromised but that the layer remains snug. F, Step 5: Once the contact/wet layer is fully applied, apply the dry layer of gauze, stockinet or clothing on top of the damp layer. G, You can consider using pajamas or gentle fitting clothing as a final layer to help keep the dressings in place if gauze or stockinet is not available.

Step 5: Soak your chosen wrapping item in warm water and wring out until damp. If using clothing, you can consider placing in dryer for a short time before applying, to keep the moist garments warm but damp.

Step 6: Apply the wet layer of gauze or clothing around the affected site. Apply this layer snugly, while ensuring circulation is not compromised and the patient is comfortable.

Step 7: Once the contact/wet layer is fully applied, apply the dry layer of gauze or clothing on top of the damp layer. It may be helpful to have the patient wear gently fitting clothing on top to help the bandages stay in place.

Step 8: Allow the bottom layer to dry overnight or over several hours (usually 4-6 hours) and then remove.

PROCEDURE FOR PERFORMING WET WRAP THERAPY AT HOME

WWT is a reasonable and cost-effective treatment for many patients and families. Items commonly utilized for WWT are listed in Figure 137.2. Modifications should be made on the basis of the age of the child, time commitment available, and resources available for supplies. The procedure can be done quickly following a bath or shower, which is more efficacious

Wet layer options:

- Cotton socks for hands and feet, tight fitting cotton pants, tight fitting long-sleeved cotton shirts, strips of breathable cotton sheets
- Tightly woven gauze rolls
- Bland, thick emollient such as white petrolatum jelly (unscented), CeraVe™ moisturizing cream, Eucerin™ cream, or Vanicream™
- Topical steroid ointments as prescribed, appropriate for severity and location

Dry layer options:

- Cotton socks, pants, loose fitting long-sleeved shirts, loose fitting onesies for infants, toddlers and young children
- Tightly woven gauze rolls
- Specialized garments: Dermasilk™, Tubifast™, and ADRescueWear™

FIGURE 137.2. Items for wet wrap therapy.

Wet wrap instructions:

1. Apply topical medications as outlined below.
2. Apply thick layer of moisturizing cream and plain Vaseline™ (Conopco, Inc., US) jelly all over the face, neck, and body.
3. Heavily saturate a 4 inch rolled gauze in warm water (ring out excess) and wrap the wet layer tightly to arms, neck, torso, legs, and ankles while ensuring adequate circulation.
4. Wrap a dry layer of 4 inch rolled gauze over the wet layer.
5. Patient can wear their own PJs or hospital gown on top.

FIGURE 137.4. Computer-based inpatient protocol to standardize wet wrap therapy.

because the skin is dampened and clean before application. It is important to consider the risk of poor adherence if the patient does not comply with sleeping in WWT when used overnight. Alternatively, counsel patients and families that WWT can be performed when they are at home after work/school or planning to stay indoors for a few hours.

INPATIENT CONSIDERATIONS FOR WET WRAP THERAPY

In the inpatient setting, higher potency topical steroids may be utilized given the capability for medical supervision as well as accountability of accurate topical medication and emollient application by medical staff. Specialized garments (Figure 137.3) are more readily available and specifically manufactured for WWT. The inpatient setting also offers the ability for laboratory

evaluation should the patient require bacterial or viral culture, intravenous antibiotic therapy for severe skin infections, and/or serum laboratory monitoring. Appropriate bathing and/or use of dilute sodium hypochlorite baths or Dakin's solution can be facilitated in the inpatient setting (see Chapter 138. Bleach Baths). When available, creating an inpatient order set outlining instruction, typical topical medications/emollients, and nursing instruction for daily dressing changes may be valuable in standardizing care and creating a step-by-step process that is consistently utilized (Figure 137.4).

RECOMMENDED FREQUENCY OF WET WRAP THERAPY

A unified recommendation for frequency of WWT has not been established. Nicol et al[1] recommended WWT for 1 to 2 weeks under medical supervision, whereas Gonzalez-Lopez et al[6] utilized WWT daily for 4 continuous weeks. It is generally accepted that WWT with low- to mid-potency topical steroids can safely be used for 3 to 4 concurrent days, one to two times a month, as needed to manage acute flares. Patients requiring TCS with WWT for prolonged periods should be assessed at regular intervals during treatment to direct appropriate management and determine when WWT can be discontinued in favor of resuming standard care. When treating severely dry skin, WWT without TCS may be utilized as frequently as desired unless adverse events such as folliculitis or maceration occur, although the potential for adverse effects with this type of practice has not been studied thoroughly to date.

USE OF TOPICAL CORTICOSTEROIDS AND WET WRAP THERAPY

A proper understanding of the strength of TCS is essential when recommending WWT for patients. Patients should be counseled regarding risks of occluding TCS and understand the potential complications that may develop with overuse, including skin thinning, acne, pustular folliculitis, hypertrichosis, striae, telangiectasia, and abnormalities of the hypothalamic-pituitary-adrenal (HPA) axis.[3,6] For thicker, more severe areas of AD on areas of the body amendable to WWT, a mid-strength TCS such as triamcinolone 0.1% ointment may be utilized, and for thinner plaques or for areas on the body where skin thinning is at higher risk (eg, popliteal fossae or antecubital fossae), a low-potency TCS such as hydrocortisone 2.5% ointment could be utilized.

POTENTIAL COMPLICATIONS OF WET WRAP THERAPY

In addition to the TCS side effects listed earlier, WWT could cause the patient discomfort and adversely cause secondary

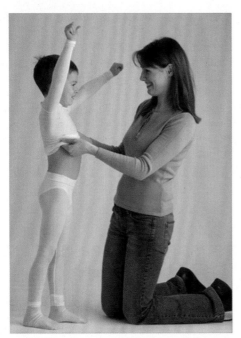

FIGURE 137.3. Specialty garments can be ordered for patients to use as dry layer options.

bacterial and viral infections, folliculitis, prickly heat, maceration, and ischemia because of diminished circulation due to tightly fitting bandages.[3] WWT with corticosteroids poses a risk of developing systemic bioactivity of corticosteroids causing HPA-axis suppression. A literature review of this potential complication by Anderson et al[7] outlined the few studies where the bioactivity of corticosteroids was measured. These studies demonstrated varying results including low serum cortisol levels immediately after treatment with a return to normalization within 2 weeks, prolonged pituitary axis suppression in long-term treated patients, as well as a single case report of prolonged HPA-axis suppression in a patient concurrently treated with inhaled corticosteroids during WWT.[7] Owing to the wide range of potential adverse effects and customized needs of each patient and clinical situation, it is the medical professional's responsibility to determine an appropriate follow-up plan to assess for these complications and determine a time to discontinuation of WWT.

From a tolerance standpoint, WWT may be uncomfortable for younger patients and, subsequently they may be defiant, fight, cry, and refuse to stay still or a combination of these obstacles. Offer suggestions to parents to utilize distraction techniques when applying WWT or a reward system for willingly participating. Although WWT is commonly applied overnight, if the patient does not tolerate this well and it is preventing restful sleep, then counsel the patient and family to perform WWT during the day for a period that allows the bandages to dry and treatment to remain effective. Warming dampened cotton pajamas in the dryer has been recommended in the literature, which may also improve compliance and comfort.[8]

Parent/caregiver adherence to WWT may also prove challenging because of the time and cost requirement of applying WWT daily. These obstacles should be addressed early on in partnership with families to anticipate appropriate patient education support such as utilizing one-on-one teaching sessions and written or video instructions. It is important to consider the socioeconomic dynamic of the patient and families to anticipate challenges in purchasing WWT items, and these patients/families should be guided to utilize items potentially already in the home, such as white tube socks and cotton pajamas and directed to purchase affordable alternatives for moisturizers and/or petrolatum jelly when needed.

TREATMENT ENDPOINTS FOR WET WRAP THERAPY

WWT should be discontinued once the prearranged time frame has lapsed; this usually corresponds to an overall decrease or significant improvement in flare of AD, improved pruritus,

sleep, and comfort level of the child or adolescent. Should complications arise, WWT should be discontinued immediately and proper treatment for adverse effects implemented on an individual basis, as guided by the health care provider. In some cases, the indication for using WWT may resolve before the prearranged time frame has lapsed and the patient/caregiver should be counseled to discontinue treatment once the predetermined endpoint has been achieved.

WET WRAP THERAPY WEB RESOURCES

Many eczema centers for children and adults have developed useful videos and handouts demonstrating application of wet wraps. In addition, patient advocacy groups such as the National Eczema Association (Nationaleczema.org) provide patient education resources and support the use of this therapy.

REFERENCES

1. Nicol NH, Boguniewicz M, Strand M, Klinnert MD. Wet wrap therapy in children with moderate to severe atopic dermatitis in a multidisciplinary treatment program. *J Allergy Clin Immunol Pract.* 2014;4:400–406.
2. Johnson VK, Hayman JL, McCarthy CA, Cardona ID. Successful treatment of eczema coxsackium with wet wrap therapy and low-dose topical corticosteroid. *J Allergy Clin Immunol Pract.* 2014;6:803–804.
3. Eichenfield LF, Tom WL, Berber TG, et al. Guidelines of care for the management of atopic dermatitis: section 2. Management and treatment of atopic dermatitis with topical therapies. *J Am Acad Dermatol.* 2014;71:116–132.
4. Janmohamed SR, Oranje AP, Devillers AC, et al. The proactive wet-wrap method with diluted corticosteroids versus emollients in children with atopic dermatitis: a prospective, randomized, double-blind, placebo controlled trial. *J Am Acad Dermatol.* 2014;6:1076–1082.
5. Gittler JK, Wang JF, Orlow SJ. Bathing and associated treatments in atopic dermatitis. *Am J Clin Dermatol.* 2017;18:45–57.
6. Gonzalez-Lopez G, Ceballos-Rodriguez RM, Gonzalez-Lopez JJ, Feito Rodríguez M, Herranz-Pinto P. Efficacy and safety of wet wrap therapy for patients with atopic dermatitis: a systematic review and meta-analysis. *Br J Dermatol.* 2017;177:688–695.
7. Anderson RM, Thyssen JP, Maibach HI. The role of wet wrap therapy in skin disorders—a literature review. *Acta Derm Venereol.* 2015;95:933–939.
8. Cooper C, DeKlotz C. Warming up to the idea of wet wraps. *Pediatr Dermatol.* 2017;34:737–738.

CHAPTER 138

Bleach Baths

Judith O'Haver, Samantha Casselman, and Harper N. Price

INTRODUCTION

Human skin has a unique microbiome that begins with the delivery of the newborn. Oh and colleagues[1] have suggested that microbial communities are not only specific to the individual but also to the sites on the body that they inhabit. A disruption of the normal host cutaneous microbiome, whether due to a skin barrier defect as seen in atopic dermatitis (AD) or ichthyosis or from a surgical wound, may result in opportunistic, nonresident organisms colonizing the skin surface and potential skin and soft-tissue infection. One potential option to address this colonization has been dilute sodium hypochlorite baths, also known hereafter as "bleach baths." Bleach baths have been in used in dermatology to manage cutaneous infections with *Staphylococcus aureus* and methicillin-resistant *S. aureus* (MRSA) infections in children with various skin conditions. Although evidence for bleach baths as an efficacious tool for treating cutaneous infections is limited, clinical experience suggests that this well-tolerated and readily available treatment may be helpful in reducing methicillin-susceptible *S. aureus* (MSSA) and MRSA infections and should be considered to augment therapy in children with AD or wound infections.

ROLE OF SODIUM HYPOCHLORITE AS A CUTANEOUS DISINFECTANT

The use of sodium hypochlorite (liquid bleach or household bleach) as a skin disinfectant began in the early 1900s. Dakin's solution was formulated by chemist Henry Drysdale Dakin and was sold as a 0.5% solution to be used after surgery for wound irrigation to prevent infection and promote healing. Dakin's solution remains commercially available today in four concentrations for the use of exudative and contaminated wounds (0.5%, 0.25%, 0.125%, and 0.0125%). There is concern regarding its use in treating open wounds, however, given the potential adverse effects on healthy tissue when other less toxic therapies are available.[2] A recent Cochrane review[3] on the use of antibiotics and antiseptics for surgical wound healing by secondary intention found limited evidence to support the effectiveness of any antiseptic, antibiotic, or antibacterial preparation. Sodium hypochlorite has received mixed reviews in the care of the pediatric patient seen in dermatology clinics. Eichenfield and colleagues[4] reviewed the available evidence in their guidelines for AD. The consensus opinion was based mostly on personal experience given the lack of objective evidence. This group suggested that bleach baths may be helpful in moderate to severe AD, particularly if the patient has a history of bacterial infections. Chopra and colleagues[5] reported that although AD severity decreased with the use of bleach baths (0.005%) or bleach-containing skin cleansers, the results were not significantly different from that of water soaks alone. The consensus of this group was that bleach baths may be helpful in moderate to severe AD, particularly if the patient has a history of bacterial infections.

In general, clinical experience with the use of dilute bleach baths for eczematous skin with suspected bacterial colonization has demonstrated similar findings in our pediatric setting, with some reported increase in overall dryness and occasional stinging; however, this is generally well tolerated and appears to be a reasonable adjunct in the therapeutic treatment plan. Families with access to chlorinated swimming pools have substituted this for bleach baths and reported this is an effective and well-tolerated substitution with an occasional report of an increase in xerosis, which responded to topical emollients. Clinic protocol includes bleach baths for suspected colonization for patients with moderate to severe AD or history of frequent skin infections (including patients with bacterial folliculitis, furunculous, epidermolysis bullosa [see Chapter 79. Epidermolysis Bullosa], and ichthyosis, among others).

PROCEDURE FOR DILUTE BLEACH BATHS

Bleach baths may be accomplished in standard household adult bathtubs (holding 80 gallons of water) using household bleach available at supermarkets (sodium hypochlorite at a concentration of around 5.25%). Adjustments should be made depending on the size of the tub and the amount of water used for bathing. The concentration of bleach may vary according to brand. The label should be checked because the desired concentration for a bleach bath is a 1:10 dilution (0.5%, 5000 ppm) (Box 138.1).[6] Bleach substitutes or alternatives such as splash-free bleach or bleach-containing detergents should not be used. It is recommended that patients soak for about 10 minutes, two to three times per week, from the neck down and then rinse with clean water before drying off, followed by an application of a bland emollient to diminish potential drying effects (Box 138.2).[7] For children too small for a standard-sized tub, the recommended dilution is 1 teaspoon per gallon of household bleach to fresh water. There is limited evidence on the use of applying diluted bleach concentrations locally (eg, such as in a compress form), and given the concern for the colonization of *S. aureus*, logic suggests that local application may not be adequate to achieve the desired purpose.

Bleach is an irritating chemical compound and both the fumes and liquids may cause damage to the skin and mucosal surfaces. Bleach should not be mixed with other chemicals, especially ammonia. Accidental exposures of any chemical substance

---

BOX 138.1. DILUTION FOR BLEACH

- Generally, 1:10 dilution is recommended for disinfection of skin and excreta (5000 ppm).
- Note: concentration of household bleach is dependent on manufacturer and can vary from 5.25% for regular bleach to 8.25% for concentrated bleach.

US Army Public Health Command. Preparing and measuring high chlorine concentration solutions for disinfection 2014. https://phc.amedd.army.mil/PHC%20Resource%20Library/TIP_No_13-034-1114_Prepare_Measure_High_Chlorine_Solutions.pdf#search=chlorine%20solutions.pdf. Accessed December 3, 2018.

to the eye requires removal of any contact lenses and the eye should be flushed with clean water either in the shower or by running tepid water over the site for 15 to 20 minutes followed by evaluation by an ophthalmologist.[8] Bleach may remove color from clothing but does not change the color of the skin or hair.

ALTERNATIVES TO BLEACH BATHS

There has been some suggestion that chlorinated pools may be an adequate substitution for dilute bleach baths, but there have been no reports to date on MRSA or MSSA bacterial counts on skin pre- and postexposure to swimming pool immersion. In a single report published by Gregg and LaCroix,[9] 25 samples of MRSA were introduced into chlorinated, saltwater, and biguanide nonchlorinated samples of pool water. Results from this study suggested that bacterial colony count was eradicated in saltwater and biguanide-treated water at 30 minutes and was eradicated or significantly diminished in the chlorine sample in 1 hour of exposure. This finding suggests that swimming in treated pool water may be effective in eradicating MRSA, but further study is indicated.

For patients who would benefit from antimicrobial therapy for eradication of *S. aureus* and prefer to shower and not immerse themselves in a pool or tub, a sodium hypochlorite gel cleanser has been developed for use in AD (sodium hypochlorite body wash 0.0061%) and other skin conditions. In the initial feasibility reports, this cleanser demonstrated a significantly reduced investigator global assessment score at all measured time points over the 12-week study period and a significant reduction in body surface area affected in the same time frame for the 18 patients with AD studied (mean reduction of 1, $P = 0.001$). During the study, no patients developed a secondary infection requiring systemic medications. Parents of the affected children reported improvement in their children's skin and felt the product was easy to use. Reported side effects included stinging and burning ($n = 2$), which improved with rinsing the product off. This study suggested that dilute sodium hypochlorite in a gel cleaner formulation was an adequate substitution for bleach baths for children who prefer showers instead of tub soaks.[10] Appropriate use of these sodium hypochlorite cleansers is important to discuss with patients and families because it differs from typical bleach baths (Box 138.3). Also, practitioners must keep in mind that these products contain surfactants and preservatives, unlike bleach baths, that may contribute to further dryness, irritation, and potential allergic contact dermatitis in susceptible patients. Use of these bleach gel cleansers has been expanded commercially for use in acne, seborrhea, folliculitis, and fungal infections, and various vehicles also exist including use as a shampoo and facial cleanser. We often recommend dilute bleach body wash formulations for older children and teens because this tends to increase compliance with therapy and be a more acceptable and time-saving option for infection prophylaxis in this population.

TOLERABILITY

The use of bleach baths appears to be well tolerated in most patients with few side effects. Wong and colleagues[11] reported findings from a randomized control trial on 36 patients with moderate to severe AD aged 2 to 30 years over a period of 2 months using 10-minute soaking baths of sodium hypochlorite 0.005% versus distilled water followed by a tap water rinse. In this study, there was no statistical difference in reported side effects between the two groups, with dry skin and mild burning and stinging reported. Both groups reported an improvement in pruritus and overall improvement of their skin and reduction in density of *S. aureus*. However, the overall Eczema Area and Severity Index (EASI score) was significantly improved in the treatment group. Similarly, Shi and colleagues[12] reported on 10 adult patients with AD, using 0.005% sodium hypochlorite on one volar forearm for 10 minutes versus tap water. Although all patients showed an increase in hydration, transepidermal water loss and pH immediately post immersion, values quickly normalized to baseline within 15 minutes with no reported irritation. This suggests that bleach baths are well tolerated on inflamed skin with minor irritation.

STABILITY OF SOLUTION

Sodium hypochlorite is not stable over time and its rate of decomposition is affected by concentration of solution, storage temperature, and whether the storage container is sealed. Although test strips are available to check to confirm the concentration of the solution, the potential for instability has led to the recommendation that preparation of the bleach solution is mixed daily to ensure desired concentration.[6]

RESOURCES

Multiple free resources are available for patients and families for education and instruction on bleach baths (see Box 138.4).

REFERENCES

1. Oh J, Byrd AL, Deming C, et. al. Biogeography and individuality shape function in the human skin metagenome. *Nature.* 2014;514:59–64.
2. Levine JM. Dakin's solution: past, present and future. *Adv Skin Wound Care.* 2013;26:410–414.
3. Dumville NG, Mohapatra DP, Owens GL, Crosbie EJ. Antibiotics and antiseptics for surgical wounds healing by secondary intention [Review]. *Cochrane Database Syst Rev.* 2016;3:1–69.
4. Eichenfield LF, Tom WL, Berger TG, et. al. Guidelines of care for the management of atopic dermatitis. *J Am Acad Dermatol.* 2014;1:116–132.
5. Chopra R, Vakharia PP, Sacotte R, Silverberg JI. Efficacy of bleach baths in reducing severity of atopic dermatitis: a systematic review and meta-analysis. *Ann Allergy Asthma Immunol.* 2017;119:435–440.
6. US Army Public Health Command. Preparing and measuring high chlorine concentration solutions for disinfection 2014. https://phc.amedd.army.mil/PHC%20Resource%20Library/TIP_No_13-034-1114_Prepare_Measure_High_Chlorine_Solutions.pdf#search=chlorine%20solutions. Accessed December 3, 2018.
7. National Eczema Association. Bleach bath recipe card. 2017. https://nationaleczema.org/wp-content/uploads/2017/06/FactSheet_BleachBath_FINAL.pdf?x59892. Accessed December 3, 2018.
8. Mayo Clinic. Chemical splash in the eye. https://www.mayoclinic.org/first-aid/first-aid-eye-emergency/basics/art-20056647. Accessed December 3, 2018.
9. Gregg M, LaCroix RL. Survival of community-associated methicillin-resistant *Staphylococcus aureus* in 3 different swimming pool environments (chlorinated, saltwater, and biguanide non-chlorinated). *Clin Pediatr (Phila).* 2010;49:635–637.
10. Ryan C, Shaw RE, Cockerell CJ, Hand S, Ghali FE. Novel sodium hypochlorite cleanser shows clinical response and excellent acceptability in the treatment of atopic dermatitis. *Pediatr Dermatol.* 2013;30:308–315.
11. Wong S, Guan T, Baba R. Efficacy and safety of sodium hypochlorite (bleach) baths in patients with moderate to severe atopic dermatitis in Malaysia. *J Dermatol.* 2013;40:874–880.
12. Shi VY, Foolad N, Ornelas JN, et al. Comparing the effect of bleach and water baths on skin barrier function in atopic dermatitis: a split-body randomized controlled trial. *Br J Dermatol.* 2016;175:212–214.

CHAPTER 139

Patient and Family Resources

Colleen H. Cotton

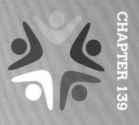

There are dozens of patient advocacy and support groups for many dermatologic conditions. Most groups have a mix of supporting patients and their families, connecting patients to registries and research opportunities, and lobbying for legislation and policies important to patients with that condition. Some groups may have a special focus. We have selected those that we feel are most applicable to the skin conditions frequently encountered in procedural pediatric dermatology. This list is by no means exhaustive, and we encourage patients and providers to explore the Internet or ask your dermatologist for the most up-to-date and relevant information. This list is updated as of April 22, 2020.

GENERAL PATIENT RESOURCES

The Alliance of Genetics Support Groups
4301 Connecticut Ave., NW, Suite 404
Washington, DC 20008-2369
Phone: 202-966-5557
Email: info@geneticalliance.orgwww.geneticalliance.org
Facebook, Twitter, Instagram

Camp Discovery
American Academy of Dermatology
Free camp for children with chronic skin conditions in
   five locations
Phone: (847) 240-1737
Email: jmueller@aad.org
www.aad.org/public/kids/camp-discovery

Canadian Skin Patient Alliance
Unit 111
223 Colonnade Rd S., Ottawa, Ontario, K2E 7K3
Phone: 613-224-4266
Email: info@canadianskin.ca
www.canadianskin.ca
Facebook, Twitter, Instagram

Genetic and Rare Diseases Information Center, National
   Institutes of Health
6100 Executive Boulevard
P.O. Box 8126
Gaithersburg, MD 20898-8126
Phone: 301-251-4925
Email: ord@od.nih.gov
www.rarediseases.info.nih.gov
Facebook, Twitter

National Organization for Rare Disorders
55 Kenosia Avenue
Danbury, CT 06810
Phone: 1-800-999-6673
   203-744-1000
Email: orphan@rarediseases.org
www.rarediseases.org
Facebook, Twitter, Instagram

Society for Pediatric Dermatology
8365 Keystone Crossing, Suite 107
Indianapolis, IN 46240
Phone: 317-202-0224
Email: info@pedsderm.net
www.pedsderm.net
Facebook, Twitter, Instagram

CONDITION-SPECIFIC RESOURCES
Albinism

National Organization for Albinism and Hypopigmentation
PO Box 959
East Hampstead, NH 03826-0959
Phone: 1-800-473-2310
603-887-2310
Email: info@albinism.org
www.albinism.org
Facebook, Twitter, Instagram

Alopecia Areata

National Alopecia Areata Foundation
65 Mitchell Boulevard, Suite 200-B
San Rafael, CA 94903
Phone: 415-472-3780
Email: info@naaf.org
www.naaf.org
Facebook, Twitter

Atopic Dermatitis/Eczema

Eczema Society of Canada
411 The Queensway South
P.O. Box 25009, Keswick, Ontario
L4P 2C7, Canada
Phone: 1-855-329-3621
Email: info@eczemahelp.ca
www.eczemahelp.ca
Facebook, Twitter

National Eczema Association
505 San Marin Drive, #B300
Novato, CA 94945
Phone: 1-800-818-7546
   415-499-3474
Email: info@nationaleczema.org
www.nationaleczema.org
Facebook, Twitter, Instagram

Basal Cell Carcinoma Nevus Syndrome

Gorlin Syndrome Alliance (formerly Basal Cell Carcinoma
   Nevus Syndrome Life Support Network/Alliance)
Phone: 267-689-6443
Email: info@gorlinsyndrome.org
www.bccns.org
www.gorlinsyndrome.org
Facebook, Twitter

Congenital Nevi (see Melanocytic Nevi)

Cutaneous T-Cell Lymphoma

Cutaneous Lymphoma Foundation
PO Box 374
Birmingham, MI 48012-0374
Phone: 248-644-9014
Email: info@clfoundation.org
www.clfoundation.org
Facebook

Ectodermal Dysplasia

National Foundation for Ectodermal Dysplasias
6 Executive Drive, Ste. 2
Fairview Heights, IL 62208-1360
Phone: 618-566-2020
Email: info@nfed.org
www.nfed.org
Facebook, Twitter

Ehlers–Danlos Syndrome

The Ehlers-Danlos Society (formerly Ehlers Danlos
   National Foundation)
P.O. Box 87463
Montgomery Village, MD 20886
Phone: 410-670-7577
www.ehlers-danlos.com
Facebook, Twitter

Epidermolysis Bullosa

**Dystrophic Epidermolysis Bullosa Research Association
   of America**
(Debra of America)
75 Broad Street, Suite 300
New York, NY 10004
Phone: 1-855-CURE-4-EB
   212-868-1573
Email: staff@debra.org
www.debra.org
Facebook, Twitter

Epidermolysis Bullosa Research Partnership
132 East 43rd St, Suite 432
New York, NY 10017
Phone: 646-844-0902
Email: info@ebresearch.org
www.ebresearch.org
Facebook, Twitter, Instagram

Epidermolysis Bullosa Medical Research Foundation
2757 Anchor Ave
Los Angeles, CA 90064
Phone: 310-205-5119
www.ebmrf.org
Instagram

Hemangiomas (see Vascular Anomalies)

Ichthyosis

Foundation for Ichthyosis and Related Skin Types
2616 N. Broad Street
Colmar, PA 18915
Phone: 215-997-9400
Email: info@firstskinfoundation.org
www.firstskinfoundation.org
Facebook, Twitter, Instagram

Mastocytosis

Mastocytosis Society
P.O. Box 416
Sterling, MA 01564
Email: info@tmsforacure.org
www.tmsforacure.org
Facebook, Twitter

Mastokids
P.O. Box 2706
Bluffton, SC 29910
www.mastokids.org
Facebook

Melanocytic Nevi

Nevus Network
Congenital Nevus Support Group
PO Box 305
West Salem, OH 44287
Phone: 419-853-4525
Email: info@nevusnetwork.org
www.nevusnetwork.org

Nevus Outreach
600 SE Delaware Ave., Suite 200
Bartlesville, OK 74003
Phone: 918-331-0595
www.nevus.org
Facebook

Melanoma (see Skin Cancers)

Morphea (see Scleroderma)

Neurofibromatosis

Children's Tumor Foundation
120 Wall Street, 16th Floor
New York, NY 10005-3904
Phone: 1-800-323-7938
   212-344-6633
Email: info@ctf.org
www.ctf.org
Facebook, Twitter, Instagram

Neurofibromatosis Network
213 S. Wheaton Ave
Wheaton, IL 60187
Phone: 1-800-942-6825
   630-510-1115
Email: admin@nfnetwork.org
www.nfnetwork.org
Facebook, Twitter

Pachyonychia Congenita

Pachyonychia Congenita Project
P.O. Box 17850
Holladay, UT 84117
Phone: 801-987-8758
Email: info@pachyonychia.org
www.pachyonychia.org
Facebook, Twitter, Instagram

Pemphigus

International Pemphigus and Pemphigoid Foundation
1331 Garden Highway, Suite 100
Sacramento, CA 95833
Phone: 855-473-6744
　　916-922-1298
Email: info@pemphigus.org
www.pemphigus.org
Facebook, Twitter, Instagram

Port Wine Birthmark (see Vascular Anomalies)

Pseudoxanthoma Elasticum

PXE International
4301 Connecticut Avenue NW
Washington, DC 20008-2369
Phone: 202-362-9599
Email: info@pxe.org
www.pxe.org
Facebook, Twitter

Psoriasis

National Psoriasis Foundation
6600 SW 92nd Avenue, Suite 300
Portland, OR 97223-7195
1800 Diagonal Road #360
Alexandria, VA 22314
Phone: 1-800-723-9166
　　503-244-7404
www.psoriasis.org
Facebook, Twitter, Instagram

Rosacea

National Rosacea Society
196 James Street
Barrington, IL 60010
Phone: 1-888-662-5874
Email: rosaceas@aol.com
www.rosacea.org
Facebook, Twitter

Scleroderma

Scleroderma Foundation
300 Rosewood Drive, Suite 105
Danvers, MA 01923
Phone: 978-463-5843
Email: sfinfo@scleroderma.org
www.scleroderma.org
Facebook, Twitter

Scleroderma Research Foundation
220 Montgomery Street, Suite 484
San Francisco, CA 94104
Phone: 415-834-9444
Email: info@srfcure.org
www.srfcure.org
Facebook, Twitter, Instagram

Skin Cancers

American Cancer Society
250 Williams Street NW
Atlanta, GA 30303
Phone: 1-800-227-2345
www.cancer.org
Facebook, Twitter, Instagram

American Melanoma Foundation
Phone: 858-412-3271
www.myamf.org
Facebook

National Cancer Institute
9609 Medical Center Drive
Bethesda, MD 20892-9760
Phone: 1-800-422-6237
www.cancer.gov
Facebook, Twitter, Instagram

Skin Cancer Foundation
205 Lexington Avenue, 11th Floor
New York, NY 10016
Phone: 212-725-5176
www.skincancer.org
Facebook, Twitter, Instagram

Tuberous Sclerosis

Tuberous Sclerosis Alliance
801 Roeder Road, Suite 750
Silver Spring, MD 20910-4487
Phone: 1-800-225-6872
　　301-562-9890
Email: info@tsalliance.org
www.tsalliance.org
Facebook, Twitter, Instagram

Vascular Anomalies

CLOVES Syndrome Community
P.O. Box 406
West Kennebunk, ME 04094
Phone: 1-833-425-6837
Email: clovessyndrome@gmail.com
www.clovessyndrome.org
Facebook, Twitter, Instagram

CLOVES Syndrome Foundation
P.O. Box 2571
Forest, VA 24551
Email: CLOVESfoundation@gmail.com
www.clovesfoundation.com
Facebook

CMTC Alliance (formerly CMTC-OVM US)
Ohio, USA
Email: president@cmtcalliance.org
www.cmtcalliance.org
Facebook, Twitter, Instagram

Hemangioma Education, From the Hemangioma Investigator Group
www.hemangiomaeducation.org

K-T Support Group (Klippel-Trenaunay syndrome and related conditions)
1471 Greystone Lane
Milford, OH 45150
Phone: 513-722-7724
Email: support@k-t.org
www.k-t.org
Facebook, Twitter, Instagram

Lymphangiomatosis and Gorham's Disease Alliance
19919 Villa Lante Place
Boca Raton, FL 33434

Phone: 561-441-9766
Email: support@igdalliance.org
www.lgdalliance.org
Facebook, Twitter, Instagram

National Lymphedema Network
411 Lafayette Street, 6th Floor
New York, NY 10003
Phone: 1-800-541-3259
Email: nln@lymphnet.org
www.lymphnet.org
Facebook, Twitter, Instagram

National Organization of Vascular Anomalies
P.O Box 38216
Greensboro, NC 27438-8216
Email: khall@novanews.orgwww.novanews.org
Facebook, Twitter

PHACES Foundation of Canada
Email: admin@phacesfoundation.com
www.phacesfoundation.ca
Facebook

PHACE Syndrome Community
3213 West Main Street #179
Rapid City, SD 57702
Phone: 678-744-3971
Email: info@phacesyndromecommunity.org
www.phacesyndromecommunity.org
Facebook, Twitter, Instagram

Proteus Syndrome Foundation
www.proteus-syndrome.org
Facebook

Sturge-Weber Foundation
P.O. Box 418
Mt. Freedom, NJ 07970
Phone: 973-895-4445
Email: swf@sturge-weber.org
www.sturge-weber.org
Facebook, Twitter, Instagram

Vascular Birthmarks Foundation
P.O. Box 106

Latham, NY 12110
Phone: 1-877-823-4646
Email: info@birthmark.org
www.birthmark.org
Facebook, Twitter, Instagram

Vitiligo

American Vitiligo Research Foundation
P.O. Box 7540
Clearwater, FL 33758
Email: vitiligo@avrf.org
www.avrf.org
Facebook

National Organization for Albinism and Hypopigmentation
PO Box 959
East Hampstead, NH 03826-0959
Phone: 1-800-473-2310
603-887-2310
Email: info@albinism.orgwww.albinism.org
Facebook, Twitter, Instagram

Vitiligo Support International
P.O. Box 3565
Lynchburg, VA 24503
Phone: 434-326-5380
www.vitiligosupport.org
Facebook

Xeroderma Pigmentosum

Xeroderma Pigmentosum Society
437 Snydertown Road
Craryville, NY 12521
Phone: 518-929-2174
Email: xps@xps.org
www.xps.org
Facebook, Twitter, Instagram

XP Family Support Group
10259 Atlantis Drive
Elk Grove, CA 95624
Phone: 916-628-3814
Email: contact@xpfamilysupport.org
www.xpfamilysupport.org
Facebook, Twitter, Instagram

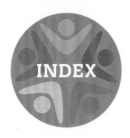

INDEX

Note: Page numbers followed by "*f*" indicate figure, and "*t*" indicate table.

A

AAD. *See* American Academy of
Dermatology (AAD)
AAP. *See* American Academy of Pediatrics
(AAP)
ABCDE detection criteria, for melanoma,
338
Ablative fractional CO_2 laser, 194
Ablative fractional laser (AFL), 101–102
for burns, 230
hypertrophic scars
postprocedural approach, 310
selecting parameters for, 308
Ablative laser skin resurfacing (ALSR),
205, 206
Ablative lasers, 99–101
Abscess, 178–180, 178–180*f*
Absorbable sutures, 55, 59
Absorbable versus nonabsorbable sutures,
34
Absorptive dressings, 425
Acanthosis nigricans (AN), 181–183, 181*f*
Accessory digits. *See* Supernumerary digits
Accessory nipple, 183–185, 184–185*f*
Accessory tragus, 186–187, 186–187*f*
ACD. *See* Allergic contact dermatitis
(ACD)
Acetaminophen toxicity, 452
Acetone-soaked gauze, 121, 122
Acetylcholine, 78
ACLS. *See* Advanced cardiac life support
(ACLS)
Acne comedones, 188–189, 189*f*
Acne cyst, 190–191, 190–191*f*
Acne inversa. *See* Hidradenitis suppurativa
(HS)
Acne scarring, 191–195, 192*f*, 193*t*, 194*f*
chemical peels, 194–195
injectables, 195
laser and energy devices
ablative fractional CO_2 laser, 194
PDL, 193–194
microneedling, 195
Acquired immunodeficiency virus (AIDS),
213
Acquired keratoderma (AK), 132, 132*f*
Acquired/functional IPPP, 385
Acral fibrokeratomas, 276
Acrochordons, 89, 196–197, 196–197*f*
ACTDs. *See* Autoimmune connective
tissue diseases (ACTDs)

Actinic keratosis (AK), 89, 198–200*f*
cryotherapy, 199–200
PDT, 200–201
special populations and
sun protection
albinism, 198
immunosuppression, 198–199
voriconazole, 199
XP, 198
topical therapy, 199
Active ingredient powder (ALA), 201
Acute versus chronic pain, 448, 448*t*
Acute wounds, 438
AD. *See* Atopic dermatitis (AD)
Adalimumab, 79
Adenoma sebaceum, 89
Adolescent, 74
Adson brown forceps, 28, 29*f*
Adson forceps, 28, 29*f*
Advanced cardiac life support (ACLS), 52
Advanced trauma life support (ATLS), 52
AFL. *See* Ablative fractional laser (AFL)
Aging, development and, 11–12, 11*f*
AIDS. *See* Acquired immunodeficiency
virus (AIDS)
Airway, 52
AK. *See* Acquired keratoderma (AK)
AK. *See* Actinic keratosis (AK)
ALA. *See* Active ingredient powder (ALA)
Albendazole, for cutaneous larva migrans,
250
Albinism, 198
patient and family resources, 475
Alcohol-based cleansers, 22, 23*f*
Aldara, 199
Alexandrite laser
for port-wine birthmarks, 377
for venous malformations, 407
Alginate dressings, 425, 427, 427*f*
Allergic contact dermatitis (ACD), 464–
466, 465*f*
patch test reactions, grading of, 152–
153, 152*f*, 153*t*
patch testing, 150
pediatric patch testing protocol, 151–
152, 152*f*
procedural Approach, 150, 151–152*f*
treatment of positive reactions, 153
T.R.U.E. test* versus comprehensive
patch testing, 150, 151*f*
Allis clamp, 31, 31*f*

Allogeneic hematopoietic stem cell
transplant (Allo-HCT), 335
Alopecia areata, 85, 142, 202–205,
203–204*f*
patient and family resources, 475
α-hydroxy acids (AHA), 120, 121
ALSR. *See* Ablative laser skin resurfacing
(ALSR)
American Academy of Dermatology
(AAD), 379, 382, 456, 468
American Academy of Pediatrics (AAP),
444, 456
American Acne and Rosacea Society, 387
American Burn Association, 231
AN. *See* Acanthosis nigricans (AN)
Anal sphincter, 75
Anesthesia, 66, 69, 70, 120, 122, 125, 157–
158, 191, 232–233, 304–305, 460
Angiofibromas, 111–112, 205–207,
205–206*f*
Angiokeratoma, 90, 207–209, 208*f*
Angioma, spider, 90, 139, 209–210,
209–210*f*
Anogenital warts. *See* Condyloma
acuminatum
Anterolateral thigh injection, 83
Anthralin, 203
Antibiotics, 79, 443–446
bacterial infection
possible, assessing procedure sites
for, 443, 443–444*f*
suspected, empiric treatment of,
443–445, 444–445*f*
methicillin-resistant *Staphylococcus
aureus* (MRSA), treatment for,
445, 446*f*
adverse reactions, 445–446, 446*f*
Antiseptic(s)
infection, guidelines to prevent and
control, 22
disinfection and sterilization, 23–
26, 24–26*t*, 24*f*
environmental infection control,
22–23, 23*f*
hand hygiene, 22, 23*f*
surgical wound classification, 22, 22*t*
Anxiety management. *See* Pain
management
Anxiolytic medication, 52
Aplasia cutis congenita, 211–213,
211–212*f*

Aquagenic wrinkling, 133–134, 133*f*
Army-Navy retractor, 31, 31*f*
Arthropod bites and stings, 213–215
    stinger removal, 215
    tick removal, 214–215
    use of epinephrine, 214
Ataxia-telangiectasia, 400
ATLS. *See* Advanced trauma life support
    (ATLS)
Atopic dermatitis (AD), 434, 437
    bleach baths for, 472–474
    patient and family resources, 475
    WWT for, 468
Atrix shave biopsy, 146–148, 147–148*f*
Atrophic disorders, 78
Atrophic scars, treatment of, 17
Atrophy, 309
Australia's Slip, Slop, Slap campaign, 458
Autoimmune bullous diseases, 223
Autoimmune connective tissue diseases
    (ACTDs), 236
Autoimmune disease, 202
Autologous fat transfer
    cautions, 127
    contraindications, 127
    postprocedural approach, 130
    preprocedural approach, 128, 128*f*
    procedural approach, 128–129,
      129–130*f*
    risks, 127
Autologous skin grafting, for large burn
    injuries, 312

B

Bacterial culture, 135–136, 135–136*f*
"BAND-AID sign", 383, 383*f*
BAND-AID™, 59, 217
Basal cell carcinoma (BCC), 91, 216–217,
    216*f*
Basal cell nevus syndrome, 218–221,
    218–219*f*
    patient and family resources, 475
Basic life support (BLS), 52
BCC. *See* Basal cell carcinoma (BCC)
Becker's nevus, 98, 221–222, 221*f*, 357*t*
Benign melanocytic nevi, 357*t*
β-hydroxy acids (BHA), 120
Billing and coding, 14
    coding evaluation/management and
      procedures when, 15
    coding procedures at different
      anatomic site, 16
    correct coding and getting paid, 14–15
    current procedural terminology (CPT)
      codes, 14
    excision of soft tissue tumors, 16–17
    laser treatment of vascular proliferative
      lesions, 17
    multimodal procedural treatment of
      warts and molluscum, 17
    "new" visits to same practice, 15

procedural coding. *See* Procedural
    coding
    treatment of atrophic scars,
      hypertrophic scars, and keloids,
      17
    use of "17999" code, 17
Bilobed flap, 66–68, 67*f*
Biopsy procedural techniques, 158–160
Biopsy site, 156–157
Biopsy technique, choice of, 156–157
Biopsy versus removal/excision, 15
Birthmarks, 12
Bleach baths, 472–474
    alternatives to, 473, 473*b*
    dilute, procedure for, 472–473, 472*b*,
      473*b*
    directions, 473*b*
    for epidermolysis bullosa, 274
    resources for, 474, 474*b*
    sodium hypochlorite as cutaneous
      disinfectant, 472
    stability of solution, 473
    tolerability, 473
Bleeding
    control strategies
      approaches to, 461–462, 461–462*f*
      surgical field, visualization of, 461
    intraprocedure and postprocedure, 460
      genetic disorders, 460–461
      hematoma, strategies for, 462–463,
        462–463*f*
      medications and vitamin
        supplements, 461
Blister
    acquired autoimmune bullous
      dermatoses, 225
    bacterial infection, 224–225
    congenital bullous dermatoses, 225
    contraindications/cautions/risks, 223,
      223*f*
    fungal infection, 225
    newborn, transient bullous disorders
      in, 225
    postprocedural approach, 225–226
    preprocedural approach, 223–224, 224*f*
    viral infection, 224
BLS. *See* Basic life support (BLS)
Blue nevus, 358*t*
Blue rubber bleb nevus syndrome
    (BRBNS), 226–228, 226*f*, 408
Blunt tenotomy, 64*f*
Body surface area (BSA), 182, 227
Bohn's nodules, 275
"BOTE" ("beginning of the end") sign, 344
BP. *See* Bullous pemphigoid (BP)
BRBNS. *See* Blue rubber bleb nevus
    syndrome (BRBNS)
Breast tissue, 183
Breathing, 52
Broad spectrum, 92, 456
BSA. *See* Body surface area (BSA)

Bullous pemphigoid (BP), 169, 225
Buried dermal suture placement, 65*f*
Burn wound care, 229–230*t*
Burns
    intralesional corticosteroids, 231
    intralesional triamcinolone acetonide,
      231
    laser therapy, 231, 232–233
    post-burn hypertrophic scar, 230*f*
    postoperative approach, 233
    scar type, treatment recommendations,
      232
    silicone-based therapy, 231
    silicone gel sheet, 230*f*
    surgery, 233
    wound care, 229–230*t*
    Z-plasty, 233
"Butterfly nevus", 368
"Buttonhole sign", 354

C

Café au lait macules (CALMs), 98–99,
    234–235, 234*f*, 372
Calcinosis cutis, 236–237
Callus, 238–239
CALMs. *See* Café au lait macules
    (CALMs)
Candida antigen immunotherapy, 79
Candidal skin infections, 225
Cantharidin application, for molluscum
    contagiosum, 346–347
Cantharidin, for verruca, 409
Carbon dioxide (CO_2) laser, 206, 221, 222,
    230, 236
    ablation, 269–271, 270*f*
    for residual anetoderma, 319–320
CCPs. *See* Code change proposals (CCPs)
CDC. *See* Centers for Disease Control
    (CDC)
CDC recommendations, for sunscreen
    use, 457
Cellulitis, 224
CelluTome device, 374
Centers for Disease Control (CDC), 2, 19,
    22, 214
Central nervous system (CNS), 175
Cephalosporins, therapeutic applications
    of, 443–444, 444*f*
Chalazion, 239–243, 240–243*f*
Chemical peels
    complications, 123, 123*f*
    deep chemical peel, 122–123
    medium-depth chemical peels, 121–122,
      121–122*f*
    postprocedure care, 123
    preprocedure preparation
      immediate patient preparation and
        anesthesia, 120
      patient assessment, 120
      priming, 120
    superficial chemical peels, 120–121

Chemovesicants-topical immunotherapy, for pediatric condyloma, 246–247
  age-specific considerations, 246
  contraindications/cautions/risks, 247
  equipment needed, 247
  postprocedural approach, 247
  preprocedural approach, 247
  procedural approach, 247
  skin color consideration, 246
  technique tips, 246
  treatment guidelines, 246
Children with mast cell disease, irritants for, 336*t*
ChloraPrep™, 217
Chlorhexidine, 23*f*
Chromophore, 107–108
Chronic wounds, 438
  stalled/delayed healing, 441, 441*f*
Circulation, 52
Circumcision adhesions, 243–245, 244*f*
  gentle traction
    age-specific considerations, 244
    contraindications/cautions/risks, 244
    equipment needed, 244
    postprocedural approach, 244–245
    procedural approach, 244
    skin color considerations, 244
    technique tips, 244
    treatment guidelines, 244
  lysis
    age-specific considerations, 245
    contraindications/cautions/risks, 245
    equipment needed, 245
    postprocedural approach, 245
    preprocedural approach, 245
    procedural approach, 245
    skin color considerations, 245
    technique tips, 245
    treatment guidelines, 245
Cladribine
  for mastocytosis, 335
Clamps, 31–32*f*
  Allis, 31, 31*f*
  Kelley, 31, 32*f*
  Kocher, 31, 32*f*
  Mosquito, 32, 32*f*
  Tonsil, 31, 31*f*
Clark's rule, 53
Clean-contaminated procedures, 22
Clean procedures, 22
Clindamycin, for miliaria pustulosa, 343
CM. *See* Cutaneous mastocytosis (CM)
CNS. *See* Central nervous system (CNS)
Code change proposals (CCPs), 14
Coding issues, 14
  coding evaluation/management and procedures when, 15

coding procedures at different anatomic site, 16
  correct coding and getting paid, 14–15
  current procedural terminology (CPT) codes, 14
  excision of soft tissue tumors, 16–17
  laser treatment of vascular proliferative lesions, 17
  multimodal procedural treatment of warts and molluscum, 17
  "new" visits to same practice, 15
  procedural. *See* Procedural coding
  treatment of atrophic scars, hypertrophic scars, and keloids, 17
  use of "17999" code, 17
Collagen dressings, 428*f*, 429–430
Common warts, 90–91
Community-acquired methicillin-resistant *Staphylococcus aureus* (CA-MRSA), 445
Complex wound repair
  bilobed flap, 66–68, 67*f*
  elliptical closure, 65, 66*f*
  general considerations, 63
  general surgical technique, 63–64
  layered closure, 64–65
  postoperative considerations, 68
  rhomboid flap, 65–66, 67*f*
  wide undermining, 64
Computed tomography (CT), 212
Condyloma acuminatum, 90, 246–249, 246*f*
  chemovesicants-topical immunotherapy, 246–247
  cryotherapy, 247
  laser treatments, 248
  surgical removal, 248–249
  tangential scissor/shave excision, 248–249
Congenital melanocytic nevus, 358*t*
Congenital nevi, patient and family resources, 476
Congenital/constitutional IPPP, 385–386
Contaminated wounds, 22
Continuous/running sutures, 56, 57*f*
Contractures, 309, 309*f*
Conventional surgery, for cSCC, 395
Cordylobia anthropophaga, 351
Corticosteroid, 202
Cotton-tipped applicator method, 141, 141*f*
CPT. *See* Current Procedural Terminology (CPT) codes
Craniofacial differences, 3
Creeping eruption. *See* Cutaneous larva migrans
CROSS technique/Dot peeling, 122, 122*f*
Croton oil, 122
Cryogen, 86
Cryosurgery, 85–87, 87*t*, 200*f*

with liquid nitrogen, for umbilical granuloma, 403
Cryotherapy, 188, 197, 199–200
  for cutaneous larva migrans, 250
  for genital warts
    age-specific considerations, 247
    contraindications/cautions/risks, 247
    equipment needed, 247
    postprocedural approach, 247
    preprocedural approach, 247
    procedural approach, 247
    skin color consideration, 247
    technique tips, 247
    treatment guidelines, 247
  for granuloma annulare, 282, 282*f*
  for molluscum contagiosum, 345, 346*f*
  for verruca, 410, 410*f*
  for xeroderma pigmentosum
    age-specific considerations, 421
    contraindications/cautions/risks, 421
    equipment needed, 422
    postprocedural approach, 422
    preprocedural approach, 422
    procedural approach, 422
    skin color considerations, 421
    technique tips, 421
    treatment guidelines, 421
cSCC. *See* Cutaneous squamous cell carcinoma (cSCC)
CT. *See* Computed tomography (CT)
CTCL. *See* Cutaneous T-cell lymphoma (CTCL)
Curettage
  for molluscum contagiosum, 346
  for xeroderma pigmentosum
    age-specific considerations, 421
    contraindications/cautions/risks, 421
    equipment needed, 422
    postprocedural approach, 422–423
    preprocedural approach, 422
    procedural approach, 422
    skin color considerations, 421
    technique tips, 421
    treatment guidelines, 421
Curettes, 32, 33*f*
  biopsy, 156, 156*f*, 158
Current Procedural Terminology (CPT) codes, 14
Cutaneous larva migrans, 249–251, 250*f*
  contraindications/cautions/risks, 250
  equipment needed, 250
  postprocedural approach, 251
  preprocedural approach, 250
  procedural approach, 251
  technique tips, 250
Cutaneous malignant melanomas, 338
Cutaneous mastocytosis (CM), 334
  types of, 334

Cutaneous squamous cell carcinoma
  (cSCC), 393–395, 394*t*
  age-specific considerations, 393
  contraindications/cautions/risks, 394
  equipment needed, 394
  postprocedural approach, 395
  preprocedural approach, 394–395
  procedural approach
    conventional surgery, 395
    Mohs micrographic surgery, 395
  skin color considerations, 393
  technique tips, 393
  treatment guidelines, 393
Cutaneous T-cell lymphoma
  patient and family resources, 476
Cutaneous T-cell lymphoma (CTCL), 115,
  116
Cysts. *See specific cysts*

D

Dakin's solution, 472
DCM. *See* Diffuse cutaneous mastocytosis
  (DCM)
DCs. *See* Dermoid cysts (DCs)
DEB. *See* Dystrophic epidermolysis
  bullosa (DEB)
Debakey forceps, 28, 29*f*
Deep chemical peel, 122–123
Deep fungal infection, 278–280, 278*f*
  age-specific considerations, 278
  contraindications/cautions/risks, 279
  equipment needed, 280
  postprocedural approach, 280
  preprocedural approach, 280
  procedural approach, 280
  skin color consideration, 278
  technique tips, 278, 279*f*
  treatment guidelines, 278
Deep-superficial-superficial-deep, 65
Deltoid injection, 83
Demerol, 120
Demodex examination, 165–166, 165–
  166*f*, 167–168, 167–168*f*
Dental lamina cysts, 275
Depigmentation, 251–256
  age-specific considerations, 251
  considerations for extent of vitiligo
    spread, 251
  contraindications/cautions/risks, 253
  equipment needed, 253
  location-specific considerations, 251
  postprocedural approach, 254
  preprocedural approach, 253
  procedural approach
    excimer laser (308-nm XeCl laser),
      253–254
    melanocyte transfer procedures. *See*
      Melanocyte transfer procedures
    narrow-band ultraviolet B, 253,
      254*t*
    phototherapy, 253

  skin color consideration, 251
  stability-based considerations, 251
  subtype-specific considerations, 251
  treatment guidelines, 251, 252*t*
Depth-enhancing agents, 121
DERMABOND Prineo™ Skin Closure
  System, 427*f*
DERMABOND™ Topical Skin Adhesive,
  397
Dermabrasion
  cautions, 124
  contraindications, 124
  postprocedural approach, 125
  preprocedural approach, 125
  procedural approach, 125, 125*f*
risks, 124
Dermal melanocytosis, 257–259, 257–258*f*
  age-specific considerations, 257
  contraindications/cautions/risks, 257
  equipment needed, 257
  postprocedural approach, 259
  preprocedural approach, 258
  procedural approach, 258–259
  skin color consideration, 257
  treatment guidelines, 257
Dermatitis herpetiformis, 169
Dermatobia hominis, 351, 351*f*
Dermatofibrosarcoma protuberans
  (DFSP), 259–261, 260*f*
  age-specific considerations, 259
  contraindications/cautions/risks, 260
  equipment needed, 260
  postprocedural approach, 261
  preprocedural approach, 260
  procedural approach, 260–261
  skin color consideration, 259
  technique tips, 259
  treatment guidelines, 259
Dermatographism, 137, 137*f*
Dermatology carrier advisory committee
  (DermCAC), 15
Dermatology, lasers, 107
DermCAC. *See* Dermatology carrier
  advisory committee
  (DermCAC)
Dermis, 11, 12
Dermoid cysts (DCs), 261–263, 261*f*
  age-specific considerations, 262
  contraindications/cautions/risks, 262
  equipment needed, 262
  postprocedural approach, 263
  preprocedural approach, 262
  procedural approach, 262–263, 263*f*
  skin color consideration, 262
  technique tips, 262
  treatment guidelines, 262
Dermoscopy, 138–139, 138–139*f*
Destructive methods, for verruca
  cryotherapy, 410, 410*f*
  laser, 411–412, 411*t*
  paring, 410–411

Development and aging, 11–12, 11*f*
DFSP. *See* Dermatofibrosarcoma
  protuberans (DFSP)
Diabetes mellitus, 63
Diclofenac sodium, 199
DIF. *See* Direct immunofluorescence (DIF)
Diffuse cutaneous mastocytosis (DCM), 334
Digital neurovascular bundle, 73
Dilute bleach baths, procedure for,
  472–473
Dimethyl sulfoxide (DMSO), 171
Diphencyclopropenone, for wart, 413–414
Direct immunofluorescence (DIF), 156,
  157, 169
Dirty wounds, 22
Disinfection, 23–26, 24–26*t*, 24*f*
DMSO. *See* Dimethyl sulfoxide (DMSO)
Dog-ears, 64, 65, 66*f*, 70, 463, 463*f*
Dorsogluteal injection, 83
Down syndrome, 461
Doxycycline, 215
Dyschromia, 309–310
Dyspigmentation, 120
Dysplastic nevus, 358*t*
Dystrophic epidermolysis bullosa (DEB),
  271–274, 272*f*

E

Ear, 71–72, 71*f*
  superficial anatomy of, 38, 38*f*
EB. *See* Epidermolysis bullosa (EB)
EBRT. *See* External beam radiation
  therapy (EBRT)
EBS. *See* Epidermolysis bullosa simplex
  (EBS)
Ectodermal dysplasia, patient and family
  resources, 476
Eczema. *See* Atopic dermatitis (AD)
  patient and family resources, 475
ED. *See* Ehlers–Danlos (ED) syndrome
Efudex, 199
Ehlers–Danlos (ED) syndrome, 434, 435*f*,
  461
  patient and family resources, 476
8-MOP, 116, 117
Either acyclovir, 120
Electrocautery, 148, 207, 209
  instruments and supplies, 29, 29*f*
  probe instrument, 28, 29*f*
Electrocoagulation, 89, 89*f*
  for xeroderma pigmentosum
    age-specific considerations, 421
    contraindications/cautions/risks,
      421
    equipment needed, 422
    postprocedural approach, 422–423
    preprocedural approach, 422
    procedural approach, 422
    skin color considerations, 421
    technique tips, 421
    treatment guidelines, 421

Electrode tip, 88
Electrodesiccation, 88
    and curettage, for epidermal nevi, 268
    for Epstein's pearls, 276
    for molluscum contagiosum, 346
Electron microscopy (EM), 223, 224
Electrosection, 89, 89*f*
Electrosurgery, 52, 88–91
    for genital warts
        age-specific considerations, 248
        contraindications/cautions/risks,
            249
        equipment needed, 249
        postprocedural approach, 249
        procedural approach, 249
        technique tips, 248
        treatment guidelines, 248
Elliptical closure, 65, 66*f*
Elliptical "football"-shaped wound, 65
EM. *See* Electron microscopy (EM)
Emancipated minors, 7
EMLA™, 53–54
Empiric antibiotic therapy, 178
Energy-based devices, for pigmentary
        mosaicism, 372–373
    pigment-specific, 373
English anvil action nail splitter, 314*f*
ENs. *See* Epidermal nevi (ENs)
Enterobius vermicularis, 154
Enucleation, for lipomas, 331
Environmental infection control, 22–23,
    23*f*
Epidermal cooling, 94–95, 94–95*f*, 108
Epidermal grafting
    for hypopigmented lesions, 373–374
    by suction blister, for depigmentation,
        254–255
Epidermal inclusion cysts
    intralesional corticosteroid
        age-specific considerations, 264
        contraindications/cautions/risks,
            264
        equipment needed, 264
        postprocedural approach, 264
        preprocedural approach, 264
        procedural approach, 264
        skin color consideration, 264
        technique tips, 264
        treatment guidelines, 264
    minimal incision technique, 266, 266*f*
    surgical excision
        age-specific considerations, 264
        contraindications/cautions/risks,
            265
        equipment needed, 265
        postprocedural approach, 266
        preprocedural approach, 265
        procedural approach, 265, 265–266*f*
        skin color consideration, 265
        technique tips, 264–265
        treatment guidelines, 264

Epidermal nevi (ENs), 267–271, 268*f*,
    358*t*, 372
    CO_2 laser ablation
        age-specific considerations, 269
        contraindications/cautions/risks,
            270
        equipment needed, 270
        postprocedural approach, 271
        preprocedural approach, 270, 270*f*
        procedural approach, 270–271, 270*f*
        skin color consideration, 270
        technique tips, 269–270
    electrodesiccation and curettage
        age-specific considerations, 268
        contraindications/cautions/risks,
            268
        equipment needed, 268
        postprocedural approach, 268
        preprocedural approach, 268
        procedural approach, 268
        skin color consideration, 268
        technique tips, 268
        treatment guidelines, 268
    surgical excision
        age-specific considerations, 269
        contraindications/cautions/risks,
            269
        equipment needed, 269
        postprocedural approach, 269
        preprocedural approach, 269
        procedural approach, 269
        skin color consideration, 269
        technique tips, 269
        treatment guidelines, 269
Epidermis, 11, 12, 64
Epidermolysis bullosa (EB), 223, 224, 225,
    271–274, 434, 435*f*
    age-specific considerations, 272
    anatomic-specific considerations, 272
    contraindications/cautions/risks, 272
    equipment needed, 272–273
    patient and family resources, 476
    postprocedural approach, 274
    preprocedural approach, 273
    procedural approach, 273–274,
        273–274*f*
    skin color consideration, 272
    subtype considerations, 272
    treatment guidelines, 272
Epidermolysis bullosa acquisita, 169
Epidermolysis bullosa simplex (EBS),
    271–274
Epstein's pearls, 275–276, 275*f*
    age-specific considerations, 275
    contraindications/cautions/risks, 276
    equipment needed, 276
    postprocedural approach, 276
    preprocedural approach, 276
    procedural approach
        electrodesiccation, 276
        incision and drainage, 276

skin color consideration, 275
technique tips, 275
treatment guidelines, 275
Erbium–yttrium argon garnet (Er:YAG)
    laser, 99, 100, 101, 102, 221, 222
Erbium–yttrium scandium gallium garnet
    (Er:YSGG), 101, 102
Erythema, 115, 116–117
Erythema toxicum neonatorum (ETN), 225
Erythrasma, 163
Erythromycin solution, for miliaria
    pustulosa, 343
Ethical dilemmas, 8–10
Etiology, 198
ETN. *See* Erythema toxicum neonatorum
    (ETN)
Eutectic mixture of local anesthetics
    (EMLA™), 356, 460
Excimer laser therapy
    for depigmentation, 253–254
    for vitiligo, 414–417
        age-specific considerations, 415
        contraindications/cautions/risks,
            415–416
        equipment needed, 416
        postprocedural approach, 417
        preprocedural approach, 416
        procedural approach, 416–417, 417*t*
        skin color considerations, 415
        technique tips, 415
        treatment guidelines, 415
Excisional biopsy, 156, 157*f*, 158, 159
External beam radiation therapy (EBRT),
    201
External genitalia, 74–75
Eye protection, 102

F
Fabry disease, 207
Face and neck, 71
Faces Pain Scale, 449, 449*f*
Facial aesthetic subunits, 40*f*
Facial expression, muscles of, 40, 41*t*
    eye, 40–41, 41*f*
    forehead and scalp, 40, 41*f*
    mouth and chin, 41, 41*f*
Fat grafting, 127, 128*f*
FDA. *See* Food and Drug Administration
    (FDA)
FDA. *See* U.S. Food and Drug
    Administration (FDA)
Fibroma, 90, 276–278, 277*f*
    age-specific considerations, 277
    contraindications/cautions/risks, 277
    equipment needed, 277
    postprocedural approach, 278
    preprocedural approach, 277
    procedural approach, 277–278
    skin color consideration, 277
    technique tips, 277
    treatment guidelines, 277

Filiform warts, 91
Fillers, 10, 78
Film dressings, 425, 427f, 429f, 431
Fitzpatrick phototype, 97, 115t
5-fluorouracil (5-FU), 199, 199f
   for verruca, 409
585-nm PDL laser
   for granuloma annulare, 282
Flap marking, 66
Flat warts, 91
Foam dressings, 425, 427f, 428f, 430
Fontanelle, 70
Food and Drug Administration (FDA), 78,
   103, 116, 118
Foot, 75–76
Forceps, 28, 29f
   Adson, 28, 29f
   Adson Brown, 28, 29f
   Debakey, 28, 29f
Fractional ablative laser resurfacing, for
   pigmented lesions, 370t, 373
Fractional carbon dioxide laser, for
   fibrofatty residua, 285
Fractionated lasers, 101
Frazier suction tip, 32, 32f
Freer nail elevator, 314f
Fulguration, 88
Fungal culture, 140–141, 140–141f
Fungal examination, 171, 171f
Fungal infections, 163
Furuncle, 178
Furuncular myiasis, 351, 351f

G

GA. *See* General anesthesia (GA)
GA. *See* Granuloma annulare (GA)
Gauze/impregnated gauze dressing, 425,
   429f, 430–431
General anesthesia (GA), 53
Genetic disorders, 460–461
Genital warts. *See* Condyloma
   acuminatum
Gentle traction, for circumcision
   adhesions, 244–245
Global Rosacea Consensus Panel, 387
Gluteal region, 45–46
Glycolic acid peels, 121
Glycolide/lactide copolymer (Vicryl), 35
GNAQ. *See* Guanine nucleotide-binding
   protein G(q) subunit alpha
   (GNAQ)
Goldenhar syndrome, 186
Gordon-Baker phenol peel, 122
Grafting, for childhood vitiligo, 415
Gram-positive bacteria, 123
Granuloma annulare (GA), 281–282, 281f
   age-specific considerations, 281
   contraindications/cautions/risks, 281
   equipment needed, 281–282
   postprocedural approach, 282
   preprocedural approach, 282

procedural approach, 282, 282f
   skin color consideration, 281
   technique tips, 281
   treatment guidelines, 281
Guanine nucleotide-binding protein G(q)
   subunit alpha (GNAQ), 109
Gut sutures, 35

H

Hair biopsy, 142
Hair, demodex examination
   diseases leading to banding of
      kwashiorkor, 167
      pili annulati, 167
      trichothiodystrophy, 167
   diseases
      loose anagen syndrome, 167
      telogen effluvium, 167, 167f
   infectious diseases
      pediculosis capitis, 167
      piedra, 167
      tinea capitis, 167
      trichomycosis axillaris, 167
   structural defects
      bubble hair, 167
      hair casts, 167
      monilothrix, 167
      pohl-pinkus constrictions, 167
      spun glass hair, 167
      trichorrhexis invaginata, 167
      trichostasis spinulosa, 167
   types of fracture
      trichoclasis, 167
      trichoptilosis, 167
      trichorrhexis nodosa, 167
      trichoschisis, 167
Hair follicle nevus, 359t
Hair pull test, 143, 143f
Hair Research Society, 142
Hairbrush method, 141
Hand hygiene, 22, 23f
Hand, upper extremity/nail bed, 72–74, 73–74f
Hats, for sun exposure, 457, 457f
Head and neck
   cosmetic subunits and free margins,
      39–40, 39t, 40f
   gluteal region, 45–46
   lymphatic drainage, 45
   median raphe, 46
   motor innervation, 41–44, 43–44f
   muscles of facial expression, 40, 41t
      eye, 40–41, 41f
      forehead and scalp, 40, 41f
      mouth and chin, 41, 41f
   nipples, 46, 46f
   sensory innervation, 44–45, 45t
   superficial musculoaponeurotic
      system, 40
   topography of, 38–39, 38–39f
   umbilicus, 46
   vasculature, 41, 42f, 43f

Healing, wound, 12
Health, definition of, 2
Heat rash. *See* Miliaria
Hemangioma, ulcerated, 434, 435f
Hemangiomas, patient and family
   resources, 476
Hematoma, 286–289, 287f
   age-specific considerations, 287
   contraindications/cautions/risks,
      287–288
   equipment needed, 288
   postprocedural approach, 288–289
   preprocedural approach, 288
   procedural approach, 287f, 288
   skin color consideration, 287
   strategies for, 462–463, 462–463f
      dog-ear or standing cone deformity,
         463, 463f
   technique tips, 287
   treatment guidelines, 287
Hematoxylin and eosin (H&E), 156
Hemifacial syndrome, 186
Hemoglobin absorption spectrum, 107f
Hemostasis
   electrosurgery, 52
   general principles, 48, 49f
   suture techniques, 52, 52f
   topical hemostatic agents, 48–52,
      50–51t, 50f
Henloch–Schönlein purpura, 169
Hereditary hemorrhagic telangiectasia
   (HHT), 400
Herpes simplex virus (HSV), 103, 125,
   175, 224
HHT. *See* Hereditary hemorrhagic
   telangiectasia (HHT)
Hidradenitis suppurativa (HS), 289–292
   age-specific considerations, 289
   contraindications/cautions/risks, 289
   equipment needed, 290
   postprocedural approach
      for all procedures, 291
      excision, 292
      incision and drainage, 291
      laser, 292
      unroofing and marsupialization,
         291
   preprocedural approach, 290, 290f
   procedural approach
      excision, 291, 292f
      incision and drainage, 290–291
      intralesional triamcinolone, 290
      laser, 291
      unroofing and marsupialization,
         290, 291f
   technique tips, 289
   treatment guidelines, 289
HIV. *See* Human immunodeficiency virus
   (HIV)
Hooks, 30–31, 30–31f
   Joseph skin, 30, 30f

Horizontal mattress suture, 58, 58f
Horizontal sectioning, 142
Hovert/Tyler techniques, 142
HPV. *See* Human papillomavirus (HPV) wart
HS. *See* Hidradenitis suppurativa (HS)
HSV. *See* Herpes simplex virus (HSV)
HTSs. *See* Hypertrophic scars (HTSs)
Human botfly. *See Dermatobia hominis*
Human immunodeficiency virus (HIV), 78, 213
Human papillomavirus (HPV) wart, 79, 408–414
   destructive methods
      cryotherapy, 410, 410f
      laser, 411–412, 411t
      paring, 410–411
   immunotherapy
      diphencyclopropenone, 413–414
      intralesional, 412–413, 412f
      squaric acid dibutylester, 413
   topical approaches
      5-fluorouracil, 409
      cantharidin, 409
      imiquimod, 409–410
      salicylic acid, 408
Human skin, embryonic development of, 11, 11f
Hydrocolloid dressings, 428f, 430
Hydrocortisone, for miliaria rubra, 343
Hydrofiber dressings, 430
Hydrogel dressings, 425, 427f, 428f, 430
Hyfrecator, 89
Hyperemia, 123f
Hypergranulation tissue, in wounds, 440–441, 441f
Hyperhidrosis, 292–294
   age-specific considerations, 293
   contraindications/cautions/risks, 293
   equipment needed, 293
   postprocedural approach, 294
   preprocedural approach, 293
   procedural approach, 293–294, 294f
   technique tips, 293
   treatment guidelines, 293
Hyperpigmentation, 294–298, 295f
   contraindications/cautions/risks, 295
   equipment needed, 295
   laser selection and parameters, 296–297t
   postprocedural approach, 298
   preprocedural approach, 295
   procedural approach, 295, 298
   skin color consideration, 295
   technique tips, 295
Hyperpigmented scars, 192
Hypertrichosis, 298–305
   age-specific considerations, 302
   contraindications/cautions/risks, 304
   equipment needed, 304
   generalized, 300–301t

localized/circumscribed, 299–300t
   postprocedural approach, 305
   preprocedural approach, 304
   procedural approach, 304–305, 304f
   skin color consideration, 302
   technique tips, 302
   treatment guidelines, 302–303t
Hypertrophic scars (HTSs), 77–78f, 306–311
   anatomic-specific considerations, 306
   case example, 310, 311f
   contraindications/cautions/risks, 306–307
   equipment needed, 307
   postprocedural approach, 310
      after AFL, 310
      after PDL, NAFLS, and 1064-nm laser treatments, 310
      between treatments, 310
   preprocedural approach, 307–308
   procedural approach, 308–310
      atrophy, 309
      changes in texture/elevation of, 308
      contractures, 309, 309f
      dyschromia, 309–310
      hypertrophy, 308–309
      red portions of, 308
      selecting ablative fractional laser parameters, 308
      textural abnormalities, 309–310
   skin color consideration, 306
   technique tips, 306, 307f
   treatment guidelines, 306
Hypertrophic scars, 466
   treatment of, 17
Hypertrophy, 308–309
Hypopigmentation, 312–313
   age-specific considerations, 312
   contraindications/cautions/risks, 312
   equipment needed, 312
   postprocedural approach, 313
   preprocedural approach, 312, 313f
   procedural approach, 312–313, 313f
   skin color consideration, 312
   technique tips, 312
   treatment guidelines, 312
Hypopigmented mycosis fungoides, 347, 347f

I

IASP. *See* International Association for the Study of Pain (IASP)
Iatrogenic injury, 69
Ichthyosis
   bleach baths for, 472
   patient and family resources, 476
IF. *See* Immunofluorescence (IF)
IFM. *See* Immunofluorescence mapping (IFM)
IG. *See* Immunoglobulin (IG)
IgA. *See* Immunoglobulin A (IgA)

IHs. *See* Infantile hemangiomas (IHs)
IIF. *See* Indirect immunofluorescence (IIF)
IL. *See* Intralesional (IL)
IM. *See* Intramuscular (IM)
Imatinib, for mastocytosis, 335
Imiquimod, 199
   for pyogenic granuloma, 384
   for verruca, 409–410
Imiquimod secrete interferon alpha (IFN-α), 199
Immediate patient preparation, 120
Immunity, 178
Immunofluorescence (IF), 169–170
Immunofluorescence mapping (IFM), 223
Immunoglobulin (IG), 169, 213
Immunoglobulin A (IgA), 156
Immunosuppression, 198–199
Immunotherapy, for wart
   diphencyclopropenone, 413–414
   intralesional, 412–413, 412f
   squaric acid dibutylester, 413
Impetigo, 224
Incision and drainage (I&D), 178
   for Epstein's pearls, 276
Incisional biopsy, 156, 157f, 158, 159
Incontinentia pigmenti (IP), 225
Indirect immunofluorescence (IIF), 169
Infancy, solitary fibrous hamartoma, 392–393, 392f
Infantile hemangiomas (IHs), 110–111, 283–286
   age-specific considerations, 283
   contraindications/cautions/risks, 283–284
   equipment needed, 284
   postprocedural approach, 285–286
   preprocedural approach, 284
   procedural approach
      fractional carbon dioxide laser, 285
      pulsed-dye laser, 284, 284f
      surgical excision, 285, 286f
   skin color consideration, 283
   technique tips, 283
   treatment guidelines, 283
Infantile perianal pyramidal protrusions (IPPPs), 385–386, 385f
   age-specific considerations, 386
   contraindications/cautions/risks, 386
   equipment needed, 386
   intraoperative technique, 386
   postoperative approach, 386
   preoperative approach, 386
   skin color considerations, 386
   technique tips, 386
   treatment guidelines, 386
   types of, 385–386
Infants, circumcision adhesions, 243–245, 244f
Infection
   surgical wound, 463–464
   wound, 440
      signs of, 439, 439t

Inflammatory linear verrucous epidermal nevus, 359*t*
Infliximab, 79
Ingenol mebutate, 199
Ingrown nail. *See* Onychocryptosis
Injectables
   antibiotics, 79
   corticosteroids
      intralesional injections, 82–83, 83*f*
      intramuscular injection, 83, 84*f*
   fillers, 78
   interferon-γ therapy/5-fluorouracil therapy, 79–80
   neuromodulators, 78
   psoriasis, 79
   use of, 77
   warts, 79
Inpatient considerations, for WWT, 470, 470*f*
Intense pulsed light (IPL) therapy, 209
   for pigmented lesions, 370*t*, 373
   for rosacea, 387
Interferon-γ therapy/5-fluorouracil therapy, 79–80, 81*f*
Interleukin 6 (IL6), 199
Intermediate versus complex repairs, 15–16
International Association for the Study of Pain (IASP), 448
The International Society for the Study of Vascular Anomalies (ISSVA), 108, 108*t*
Intralesional (IL), 77, 82, 230
Intralesional corticosteroid, 78, 231
   for epidermal inclusion cysts, 264
   for nail psoriasis
      age-specific considerations, 382
      contraindications/cautions/risks, 382
      equipment needed, 382
      postprocedural approach, 382
      preprocedural approach, 382
      procedural approach, 382, 383*f*
      technique tips, 382
      treatment guidelines, 382
   for primary JXG lesions, 318–319
Intralesional immunotherapy, for wart, 412–413, 412*f*
Intralesional injection, 82–83, 83*f*
   for mastocytoma, 336
Intralesional steroid injection, 203
   for granuloma annulare, 282
Intralesional triamcinolone acetonide, 231
   for solitary mastocytomas, 335
Intralesional triamcinolone, for hidradenitis suppurativa, 290
Intramuscular (IM), 77, 82
Intramuscular injection, 83, 84*f*
Intravenous (IV) sedation, 122
IP. *See* Incontinentia pigmenti (IP)
IPL. *See* Intense pulsed light (IPL) therapy

IPPPs. *See* Infantile perianal pyramidal protrusions (IPPPs)
Iris scissors, 29, 30*f*
Ischemia, 64, 145
Isotretinoin, for miliaria profunda, 343
ISSVA. *See* The International Society for the Study of Vascular Anomalies (ISSVA)
IV. *See* Intravenous (IV) sedation
Ivermectin
   for cutaneous larva migrans, 250
   for myiasis, 353
   for scabies, 391

J
JEB. *See* Junctional epidermolysis bullosa (JEB)
Jessner's solution, 120, 121
Joseph skin hook, 30, 30*f*
Junctional epidermolysis bullosa (JEB), 271–274, 271*f*
Juvenile xanthogranuloma (JXG), 318–320, 318*f*
   age-specific considerations, 318
   contraindications/cautions/risks, 318
   general guidelines, 318
   primary lesion, intralesional corticosteroid for, 318–319
      age-specific considerations, 319
      contraindications/cautions/risks, 319
      equipment needed, 319
      postprocedural approach, 319
      preprocedural approach, 319
      procedural approach, 319
      skin color consideration, 319
      technique tips, 319
      treatment guidelines, 318
   residual anetoderma, carbon dioxide laser for, 319–320
      age-specific considerations, 319
      contraindications/cautions/risks, 319
      equipment needed, 320
      postprocedural approach, 320
      preprocedural approach, 320
      procedural approach, 320
      skin color consideration, 319
      technique tips, 319
      treatment guidelines, 319
JXG. *See* Juvenile xanthogranuloma (JXG)

K
Kelley clamp, 31, 32*f*
Keloids, 466
   treatment of, 17
Kenalog, 77, 78, 203
Keratin proteins, 11
Keratinocytic nevus, 359*t*
Keratoacanthoma, 90
Keratosis pilaris (KP), 320–323, 321*f*

age-specific considerations, 321
   contraindications/cautions/risks, 321
   equipment needed, 321
   laser therapy and supporting case studies for, 322*t*
   postprocedural approach, 323
   preprocedural approach, 321, 323
   procedural approach, 323
   skin color consideration, 321
   technique tips, 321
   treatment guidelines, 321
Kerlix™, 201
Kindler's syndrome, 271–274
Klippel–Trenaunay syndrome (KTS), 109
Kocher clamp, 31, 32*f*
Koenen's tumor, 276
KOH. *See* Potassium hydroxide (KOH)
KP. *See* Keratosis pilaris (KP)
KTP. *See* Potassium titanyl phosphate (KTP)
KTS. *See* Klippel–Trenaunay syndrome (KTS)

L
Labial adhesion, 323–325, 324*f*
   age-specific considerations, 324
   contraindications/cautions/risks, 324
   equipment needed, 324
   postprocedural approach, 325
   preprocedural approach, 324–325
   procedural approach, 325
   skin color consideration, 324
   technique tips, 324
   treatment guidelines, 324
Laceration repair, 325–327
   contraindications/cautions/risks, 326
   equipment needed, 326
   postprocedural approach, 327
   preprocedural approach, 326
   procedural approach, 326–327, 326–327*f*
   technique tips, 325–326
   treatment guidelines, 325
Lacerations, 63
Large congenital melanocytic nevi (LCMN), 361
   serial excisions, 361
   skin grafting, 361
   tissue expansion, 361
Larvicides, for myiasis, 353
Laser
   for hair removal, 303*t*
   for hidradenitis suppurativa, 291
   selection and parameters, for hyperpigmentation, 296–297*t*
   treatments of genital warts
      age-specific considerations, 248
      contraindications/cautions/risks, 248
      equipment needed, 248
      postprocedural approach, 248

procedural approach, 248
   technique tips, 248
   treatment guidelines, 248
  for wart treatment, 411–412, 411*t*
LASER. *See* Light amplification by the
   stimulated emission of radiation
   (LASER)
Laser ablation, 99
Laser hair removal, 221
Laser surgery
  ablative and non-ablative laser
    treatments, 99–102, 100*f*
  anesthesia considerations, 103
  cooling, 94–95
  infection and prophylaxis, risk of, 103
  monitoring tissue response/clinical
    endpoints, 103
  safety, 102–103
  selective photothermolysis, 92–94,
    93–94*f*
  types
    millisecond lasers, 95–98
    QS lasers, 98–99
Laser therapy, 231, 232–233
  for keratosis pilaris, 322*t*
  for nevus, 361
Layered closure, 64–65
LCMN. *See* Large congenital melanocytic
   nevi (LCMN)
Legal definitions, 7
LET gel, 53–54
Leukemia, 213
Lichen planus (LP), 327–330, 328*f*
  age-specific considerations, 328
  contraindications/cautions/risks, 329
  equipment needed, 329
  postprocedural approach, 329–330
  preprocedural approach, 329
  procedural approach, 329
  skin color consideration, 329
  technique tips, 328–329
  treatment guidelines, 328
Lichen sclerosus et atrophicus (LSA), 385
  IPPP associated with, 385, 386
Lidocaine, 157
Light amplification by the stimulated
   emission of radiation (LASER),
   92
Light microscopy, 167
Lindane, for scabies, 391
Linear immunoglobulin A (IgA) bullous
   dermatosis, 169, 225
Linear morphea, 78*f*
Lipoma, 330–332
  age-specific considerations, 330
  contraindications/cautions/risks,
    330–331
  equipment needed, 331
  postprocedural approach, 332
  preprocedural approach, 331
  procedural approach, 331

closure, 331*f*, 332
  elliptical excision, 331–332, 331*f*
  enucleation, 331
  skin color consideration, 330
  technique tips, 330
  treatment guidelines, 330
Liposuction, for lipomas, 330
LMs. *See* Lymphatic malformations (LMs)
LMX.4™, 53, 197
LMX.5™, 208, 210
Lobular capillary hemangioma. *See*
   Pyogenic granuloma (PG)
Long-pulsed alexandrite laser, 97, 182
Long-pulsed diode laser, 98
Long-pulsed frequency-doubled Nd:YAG
   laser, 92, 97
Long-pulsed lasers, for pigmented lesions,
   370*t*, 373
Long-Pulsed Nd:YAG Laser, 98, 227, 405
Long uncut suture thread, 56
Loop technique, 178
LP. *See* Lichen planus (LP)
LSA. *See* Lichen sclerosus et atrophicus
   (LSA)
Lxodes scapularis, 215f
Lyme disease, 215
Lymphangioma, 90
Lymphatic drainage, 45
Lymphatic malformations (LMs), 332–334
  age-specific considerations, 332
  contraindications/cautions/risks,
    332–333
  equipment needed, 333
  postprocedural approach, 334
  preprocedural approach, 333
  procedural approach, 333–334, 333*f*
  skin color consideration, 332
  technique tips, 332
  treatment guidelines, 332
Lysis, for circumcision adhesions, 245

M

Macro- and microfractionated carbon
   dioxide laser, 182–183
Maculopapular cutaneous mastocytosis
   (MPCM), 334
Magnetic resonance angiogram (MRA),
   212
Magnetic resonance imaging (MRI), 212
MAL. *See* Methyl ester cream (MAL)
Mammalian target of rapamycin (mTOR)
   inhibitors, 227, 332
Mammillaria. *See* Miliaria profunda
Manual extraction
  of milium, 341–342, 341–342*f*
  for myiasis, 353
Manual extrusion method, for molluscum
   contagiosum, 345, 345*f*
Marfan syndrome, 461
Mast cell disease, children with, irritants
   for, 336*t*

Mastisol, 147, 148
Mastocytoma, 334–336
  age-specific considerations, 335
  intralesional injection, 336
  skin color consideration, 335
  surgical excision, 336
  technique tips, 335
  treatment guidelines, 335
Mastocytosis. *See also specific mastocytosis*
  patient and family resources, 476
Matrix metalloproteinases (MMPs), 12
Mature minor, 7
Mayo Clinic, 236
Mayo scissors, 29, 30*f*
McCune-Albright syndrome, 234
Measles, mumps, and rubella (MMR)
   vaccine, 79
MED. *See* Minimal erythema dose
   (MED)
Median raphe cysts, 46, 337–338, 337*f*
  age-specific considerations, 337
  contraindications/cautions/risks, 337
  equipment needed, 337
  postprocedural approach, 338
  preprocedural approach, 337
  procedural approach, 338
  skin color consideration, 337
  technique tips, 337
  treatment guidelines, 337
Median telangiectatic nevus, 368
Medium-depth chemical peels, 121–122,
   121–122*f*
Meibomian cysts, 239
Melanin, 295
Melanocyte keratinocyte transplantation
   procedure (MKTP)
  for depigmentation, 255–256
  for vitiligo, 415, 417–420, 417*f*
Melanocyte transfer procedures, for
   depigmentation
  epidermal grafting by suction blister,
    254–255
  melanocyte keratinocyte transfer
    procedures, 255–256
  punch grafts, 256
  split-thickness skin grafts, 256
Melanocytic nevi, 139
  patient and family resources, 476
Melanoma, 139, 338–340
  age-specific considerations, 338–339
  contraindications/cautions/risks, 339
  equipment needed, 339
  patient and family resources, 476
  postprocedural approach, 340
  preprocedural approach, 339
  procedural approach, 339, 340*f*
  skin color consideration, 339
  technique tips, 339
  treatment guidelines, 338
Methanol, 175
Methemoglobinemia, 157

Methicillin-resistant *Staphylococcus aureus* (MRSA), treatment for, 445, 446*f*
   adverse reactions, 445–446, 446*f*
Methicillin-susceptible *Staphylococcus aureus* (MSSA), 445
Methyl ester cream (MAL), 201
Meticulous technique, 64–65
Metzenbaum scissor, 30, 30*f*
Meyerson phenomenon, 108
MF. *See* Mycosis fungoides (MF)
Microscopic treatment zones (MTZs), 221
Microsomia syndrome, 186
Microsporum canis, 163
Microtia syndrome, 186
Migratory myiasis, 351
Mild scars, 120
Miliaria, 225, 342–343. *See also specific types*
   age-specific considerations, 343
   contraindications/cautions/risks, 343
   crystallina, 342, 342*f*
      equipment needed, 343
      postprocedural approach, 343
      preprocedural approach, 343
      procedural approach, 343
   profunda, 342
   pustulosa, 343
   rubra, 342
      skin color consideration, 343
      technique tips, 343
      treatment guidelines, 343
Milium, manual extraction of, 340–342
   age-specific considerations, 341
   contraindications/cautions/risks, 341
   equipment needed, 341
   guidelines, 341
   postprocedural approach, 342
   preprocedural approach, 341
   procedural approach, 341–342, 341–342*f*
   skin color consideration, 341
   technique tips, 341
Minimal erythema dose (MED), 115, 312–313
Minimal incision technique, for epidermal inclusion cysts, 266, 266*f*
Minoxidil, 203
MKTP. *See* Melanocyte keratinocyte transplantation procedure (MKTP)
MMPs. *See* Matrix metalloproteinases (MMPs)
MMR. *See* Measles, mumps, and rubella (MMR) vaccine
MMS. *See* Mohs micrographic surgery (MMS)
Mohs micrographic surgery (MMS), 216, 217, 218
   for cutaneous squamous cell carcinoma, 395
   for DFSP, 259–261

Moisture-retentive dressings, 425
Molluscipoxvirus, 344
Molluscum contagiosum, 90, 344–347, 344*f*
   cantharidin application, 346–347
   cryotherapy, 345, 346*f*
   curettage, 346
   electrodessication, 346
   manual extrusion, 345, 345*f*
   multimodal procedural treatment of, 17
Mongolian spot. *See* Dermal melanocytosis
Monocryl (poliglecaprone 25), 35
Morphea, patient and family resources, 476
Morphine, 120
Mosquito clamp, 32, 32*f*
Motor innervation, 41–44, 43–44*f*
Motor nerves, 39*t*
MPCM. *See* Maculopapular cutaneous mastocytosis (MPCM)
MRA. *See* Magnetic resonance angiogram (MRA)
MRI. *See* Magnetic resonance imaging (MRI)
MRSA. *See* Methicillin-resistant Staphylococcus aureus (MRSA), treatment for
MSSA. *See* Methicillin-susceptible Staphylococcus aureus (MSSA)
mTOR. *See* Mammalian target of rapamycin (mTOR) inhibitors
MTZs. *See* Microscopic treatment zones (MTZs)
Mycosis fungoides (MF), 347–351
   age-specific considerations, 348
   contraindications/cautions/risks, 348
   equipment needed, 348
   postprocedural approach, 351
   preprocedural approach, 348–349
   procedural approach, 349–350, 350*t*
   skin color consideration, 348
   technique tips, 348
   treatment guidelines, 348
Myiasis, 351–353
   age-specific considerations, 352
   clinical tips, 352
   contraindications/cautions/risks, 352
   diagnosis, 351
   equipment needed, 352
   larvicides, 353
   manual extraction, 353
   occlusion technique, 353
   postprocedural approach, 353
   preprocedural approach, 352
   procedural approach, 352
   skin color consideration, 352
   treatment guidelines, 352
   types of, 351

N
N-*2*-octylcyanoacrylate, 60
N-buty-2-cyanoacrylate, 60
NACDG. *See* North American Contact Dermatitis Group (NACDG)
NAFL. *See* Non-ablative fractional lasers (NAFL)
Nail matrix biopsy
   atrix shave biopsy, 146–148, 147–148*f*
   cautions, 144
   postprocedural approach, 149
   preprocedural approach, 144
   procedural approach, 144–146, 145*f*
   punch biopsy, 146, 146*f*
   risks, 144
Nail psoriasis, intralesional corticosteroid injections
   age-specific considerations, 382
   contraindications/cautions/risks, 382
   equipment needed, 382
   postprocedural approach, 382
   preprocedural approach, 382
   procedural approach, 382, 383*f*
   technique tips, 382
   treatment guidelines, 382
Narrow-band ultraviolet B (NB-UVB), 327
   for depigmentation, 253
   for psoriasis, 379
      age-specific considerations, 379
      contraindications/cautions/risks, 379
      equipment needed, 380
      postprocedural approach, 382
      preprocedural approach, 380
      procedural approach, 380–381
      skin color considerations, 379
      technique tips, 379
      treatment guidelines, 379
Nasal aesthetic subunits, 39, 39*f*
National Comprehensive Cancer Network, 348
National Psoriasis Foundation, 379, 382
Neck, posterior triangle of, 39, 39*f*
Necrosis, 439, 440
Needle(s)
   cutting, 36, 36*f*
   dimensions, 36, 36*f*
   holders, 31*f*, 32, 32*f*
   tapered, 36–37
Neodymium–yttrium aluminum garnet (Nd:YAG) laser, 108, 109, 110, 111, 227, 228
   for port-wine birthmarks, 377
   for telangiectasia, 401–402
   for venous malformations, 407
   for wart treatment, 411–412, 411*t*
Neonatal acne, 225
Neonatal HSV, 224
NERDS acronym, 439
Neurofibromas, 354–355, 354*f*

anatomic-specific considerations, 354
contraindications/cautions/risks, 354–355
equipment needed, 355
postprocedural approach, 355
preprocedural approach, 355
procedural approach, 355
referrals, 354
skin color considerations, 354
technique tips, 354
treatment guidelines, 354
Neurofibromatosis, patient and family
        resources, 476
Neuromodulators, 78
Nevi, 356–361
    age-specific considerations, 356
    contraindications/cautions/risks, 356
    equipment needed, 356, 360
    postprocedural approach, 361
    preprocedural approach, 360
    presentations and treatment, 357–359t
    procedural approach
        laser therapy, 361
        surgical excision, 360–361
    skin color considerations, 356
    technique tips, 356
    treatment guidelines, 356
Nevus comedonicus, 359t
Nevus flammeus. *See* Port wine birthmark
        (PWB)
Nevus of Ito, 362–364
    age-specific considerations, 363
    contraindications/cautions/risks, 363
    equipment needed, 363
    guidelines, 362
    postprocedural approach, 363–364,
        364f
    preprocedural approach, 363
    procedural approach, 363, 364f
    skin color considerations, 363
    technique tips, 362
    treatment, 362
Nevus of Ota, 357t, 362–364, 362f
    age-specific considerations, 363
    contraindications/cautions/risks, 363
    equipment needed, 363
    guidelines, 362
    postprocedural approach, 363–364, 364f
    preprocedural approach, 363
    procedural approach, 363, 364f
    skin color considerations, 363
    technique tips, 362
    treatment, 362
    types of, 362
Nevus of spilus, 357t
Nevus sebaceous, 359t, 365–367
    age-specific considerations, 365
    contraindications/cautions/risks, 365
    equipment needed, 365
    postprocedural approach, 367
    preprocedural approach, 365–366

procedural approach
    face, 367
    scalp, 366, 366–367f
    trunk and extremities, 367
    technique tips, 365
    treatment guidelines, 365
Nevus simplex, 368, 368f
Nicotine, 63
Nipples, 46, 46f
NNH. *See* The number needed to harm
        (NNH)
Nodular mastocytosis, 334
Non-ablative fractional lasers (NAFL),
        101, 230
Nonabsorbable sutures, 59
Nonadherent dressings, 425
Nonexcisional treatment, of lipomas, 330
Nononcologic applications, 119, 119f
Nonopioid analgesics, for pain
        management, 452–453, 453t
Nonsteroidal anti-inflammatory drugs
        (NSAIDs), 452–453
Normothermia, 18
North American Contact Dermatitis
        Group (NACDG), 465–466
NSAIDs. *See* Nonsteroidal anti-
        inflammatory drugs (NSAIDs)
The number needed to harm (NNH), 61
Nylon (Ethilon, Nurolon, Surgilon), 35

O

Occlusion technique, for myiasis, 353
Occlusive dressings, 425, 427f
Office versus operating room procedures,
        pain management, 450t
Omalizumab, for mastocytosis, 335
Oncologic applications, 118–119
1440-nm Nd:YAG laser
    for granuloma annulare, 282
Onychocryptosis, 313–317, 314f
    age-specific considerations, 314
    contraindications/cautions/risks, 314
    equipment needed, 314–315, 314f
    postprocedural approach, 317
    preprocedural approach, 315
    procedural approach, 315–317,
        315–317f
    technique tips, 314
    treatment guidelines, 314
Open dressings, 425
Operative markings, 64f
Opioid analgesics
    for pain management, 453–454, 454t
    use in children, 454
Oral supplementations, for sun exposure,
        457
Osler-Weber-Rendu syndrome, 461.
        See Hereditary hemorrhagic
        telangiectasia (HHT)
Otoscope, for lesions, 374–375, 375f

P

Pachyonychia congenital, patient and
        family resources, 476
Pain
    defined, 448
    types of, 448, 448t
Pain management, 448–454
    assessment, 448–449, 449f
    pharmacologic interventions, 451–452, 451f
    preprocedure planning, 450–451
        nonpharmacologic techniques, 451t
        office versus operating room
            procedures, 450t
        parents and patient, preparation
            of, 450
        positive reinforcement, and
            distractors, 450–451, 451f
        procedure room environment, 450
    procedural and postprocedural setting
        nonopioid analgesics, 452–453, 453t
        nonpharmacologic strategies, 452,
            452b, 452f
        opioid analgesics, 453–454, 454t
Parent-child relationship, 3
Paring, for verruca, 410–411
Paring/scalpel debridement, 238
PASI. *See* Psoriasis Area and Severity
        Index (PASI)
Patient and family resources, 475–478
    condition-specific, 475–478
        albinism, 475
        alopecia areata, 475
        atopic dermatitis/eczema, 475
        basal cell carcinoma nevus
            syndrome, 475
        congenital nevi, 476
        cutaneous T-cell lymphoma, 476
        ectodermal dysplasia, 476
        Ehlers–Danlos syndrome, 476
        epidermolysis bullosa, 476
        hemangiomas, 476
        ichthyosis, 476
        mastocytosis, 476
        melanocytic nevi, 476
        melanoma, 476
        morphea, 476
        neurofibromatosis, 476
        pachyonychia congenital, 476
        pemphigus, 477
        port wine birthmark, 477
        pseudoxanthoma elasticum, 477
        psoriasis, 477
        rosacea, 477
        scleroderma, 477
        skin cancers, 477
        tuberous sclerosis, 477
        vascular anomalies, 477–478
        vitiligo, 478
        xeroderma pigmentosum, 478
    general, 475

Patient assessment, 120
Patient evaluation, 52
Patient preparation/protection, 52–54,
    102–103
Patient-reported outcome (PRO)
    assessments, 4
PCR. *See* Polymerase chain reaction
    (PCR)
PDL. *See* Pulsed-dye laser (PDL)
PDS II. *See* Polydioxanone (PDS II)
PDT. *See* Photodynamic therapy (PDT)
Pediatric dermatology, procedures in, 3, 7
Pediatric patient
    wound assessment, 437–439, 438*f*
    wound dressing, considerations in, 432,
        433*t*
        patient/family education, 433
        product choice for, 433
    wounds encountered in, 434–437,
        435–436*f*
Pediatric population, 157
Pediatric provider, 69
Pediatrics, 69–70
Peel-to-skin contact, 120
PELVIS (perineal hemangioma, external
        genitalia malformations,
        lipomyelomeningocele,
        vesicorenal abnormalities,
        imperforate anus, and skin tag)
        syndrome, 386
Pemphigus
    patient and family resources, 477
Pemphigus vulgaris (PV), 169, 225
Penicillin allergy, 445
Penis, median raphe cysts, 337–338, 337*f*
Perianal region, 75
Perinatal transmission, 79
Periosteal elevator, 32, 32*f*
Peripheral vascular disease, 63
Periungual fibromas. *See* Fibroma
Permethrin, for scabies, 391
Petrolatum, 23*f*
PG. *See* Pyogenic granuloma (PG)
Phakomatosis pigmentovascularis, 257
Phenol, 122
Phenol ablation (chemical matricectomy),
    316–317, 316*f*
Photobleaching, 117, 118
Photodynamic therapy (PDT), 200–201,
    202*f*
    for lichen planus, 328
Photoprotection, 456–458
    environmental awareness, 458
    hats, 457, 457*f*
    oral supplementations, 457
    strategies/policies to reduce children's
        sun exposure, 458
    sun-protective clothing, 457, 457*f*
    sun-safe education in schools and
        communities, 458
    sunscreen, 456–457

apply tips, 456–457, 456*f*
    CDC recommendations, 457
Photosensitizer, 118
Phototherapy/photodynamic therapy,
    117*f*, 118*b*
    adverse effects of, 117–118
    for granuloma annulare, 282
    for mycosis fungoides, 349
    pediatric applications of, 118–119
    protocol considerations for
        depigmentation, 254*t*
    PUVA, 116–117
    UVA1, 115–116
    UVB, 115–116
    for vitiligo, 414–417
        age-specific considerations, 415
        contraindications/cautions/risks,
            415–416
        equipment needed, 416
        postprocedural approach, 417
        preprocedural approach, 416
        procedural approach, 416–417, 417*t*
        skin color considerations, 415
        technique tips, 415
        treatment guidelines, 415
Picato, 199
Piebaldism, 251
Pigment-specific energy-based devices, for
        pigmented lesions, 373
Pigmentary mosaicism, 369–374
    age-specific considerations, 371
    contraindications/cautions/risks, 371
    to different laser modalities,
        responsiveness of various, 370*t*
    energy-based devices, 372–373
        general considerations for, 372
        postprocedural approach, 373
        preprocedural approach, 372, 372*f*
        procedural approach, 373
    epidermal grafting, 373–374
        postprocedural approach, 374
        preprocedural approach, 374
        procedural approach, 374
    equipment needed, 371
    general preprocedural approach,
        371–372
    patterns of, 369*f*
        conditions following, examples of,
            370*t*
    skin color considerations, 371
    surgical interventions, 374
    technique tips, 371
    treatment guidelines, 371
Pigmented spindle-cell nevus, 357*t*
PIH. *See* Postinflammatory
        hyperpigmentation (PIH)
Pilar cysts, 267
    age-specific considerations, 267
    contraindications/cautions/risks, 267
    equipment needed, 267
    postprocedural approach, 267

preprocedural approach, 267
    procedural approach, 267
    skin color consideration, 267
    technique tips, 267
    treatment guidelines, 267
Pilomatricoma, 374–376, 375*f*
    age-specific considerations, 375
    anatomic-specific considerations, 375
    contraindications/cautions/risks, 375
    equipment needed, 375
    postprocedural approach, 376
    preprocedural approach, 375–376
    procedural approach, 376, 376*f*
    skin color considerations, 375
    technique tips, 375
    treatment guidelines, 375
Pilomatrixoma. *See* Pilomatricoma
Pinworm examination, 154
Platelet-rich plasma (PRP), 192, 195
Poliglecaprone 25 (Monocryl), 35
Polydioxanone (PDS II), 35
Polyester (Mersilene, Ethibond), 35
Polymerase chain reaction (PCR), 155,
    161, 246
Polypropylene (Prolene or Surgipro), 35
Porphyria cutanea tarda, 169
Port wine birthmark (PWB), 92, 95–97,
    98, 101, 108–110, 111,
    377–378
    age-specific considerations, 377
    contraindications/cautions/risks, 377
    equipment needed, 377
    patient and family resources, 477
    postprocedural approach, 378, 378*f*
    preprocedural approach, 377, 378*f*
    procedural approach, 377–378, 378*f*
    skin color considerations, 377
    technique tips, 377
    treatment guidelines, 377
Port wine stains. *See* Port wine birthmark
        (PWB)
Post-burn hypertrophic scar, 230*f*
Postaxial (ulnar) polydactyly, 396
Postinflammatory hyperpigmentation
        (PIH), 120
Postoperative approach, 233
Postoperative considerations, 68
Postoperative edema, 76
Postprocedural erythema, 122
Potassium hydroxide (KOH), 168, 171,
    171*f*, 173, 174
Potassium titanyl phosphate (KTP), 108,
    110, 111, 192
    for telangiectasia, 401
Potential complications, of WWT,
    470–471
Potential eye injuries, 102
Power settings, 90*t*
Preaxial (radial) polydactyly, 396
Prickly heat. *See* Miliaria
Primary dressing, 425

Primary JXG lesions, intralesional corticosteroid for, 318–319
  age-specific considerations, 319
  contraindications/cautions/risks, 319
  equipment needed, 319
  postprocedural approach, 319
  preprocedural approach, 319
  procedural approach, 319
  skin color consideration, 319
  technique tips, 319
  treatment guidelines, 318
Primary wound closure, 55–61
Priming, 120
Private insurers, 14
PRO. *See* Patient-reported outcome (PRO) assessments
PRO TIP, 159
Procedural coding
  biopsy versus removal/excision, 15
  intermediate versus complex repairs, 15–16
  site-specific biopsy coding, 15
  skin biopsy coding, 15
Procedural sedation, 52
Propionibacterium acnes, 119
Propranolol, 110, 111
PRP. *See* Platelet-rich plasma (PRP)
Pseudoallergy, 460
Pseudoxanthoma elasticum, patient and family resources, 477
Psoralen ultraviolet A (PUVA), 116–117, 116*b*, 327
Psoriasis, 79, 379–383
  intralesional corticosteroid injections, 382
    age-specific considerations, 382
    contraindications/cautions/risks, 382
    equipment needed, 382
    postprocedural approach, 382
    preprocedural approach, 382
    procedural approach, 382, 383*f*
    technique tips, 382
    treatment guidelines, 382
  narrow-band ultraviolet B therapy, 379
    age-specific considerations, 379
    contraindications/cautions/risks, 379
    equipment needed, 380
    postprocedural approach, 382
    preprocedural approach, 380
    procedural approach, 380–381
    skin color considerations, 379
    technique tips, 379
    treatment guidelines, 379
  patient and family resources, 477
  targeted excimer laser (308 nm) phototherapy, 379
    age-specific considerations, 379
    contraindications/cautions/risks, 379
    equipment needed, 380
    postprocedural approach, 382

    preprocedural approach, 380
    procedural approach, 381
    skin color considerations, 379
    technique tips, 379
    treatment guidelines, 379
Psoriasis Area and Severity Index (PASI), 379
Pulsed-dye laser (PDL), 95–97, 96*t*, 98, 102, 107–111, 192–194, 205–207, 209, 210, 230, 236
  for infantile hemangioma or associated telangiectasia, 284, 284*f*
  for keratosis pilaris, 321
  for port-wine birthmarks, 377
  for pyogenic granuloma, 384
  for rosacea, 387
  for telangiectasia, 401–402
  for ulcerated infantile hemangioma, 284
  for venous malformations, 407
  for wart treatment, 411*t*, 412
Punch biopsy, 146, 146*f*, 156, 158, 160*f*
Punch grafts, for depigmentation, 256
PureGraft system, 129
PUVA. *See* Psoralen ultraviolet A (PUVA)
PV. *See* Pemphigus vulgaris (PV)
PWB. *See* Port wine birthmark (PWB)
Pyogenic granuloma (PG), 383–385, 383*f*
  contraindications/cautions/risks, 384
  equipment needed, 384
  postprocedural approach, 385
  preprocedural approach, 384
  procedural approach, 384–385, 385*f*
  treatment recommendations, 383–384
Pyogenic granuloma, 90

Q

Q-switched alexandrite lasers, 370*t*, 373
Q-switched laser, 231
Q-switched Nd:YAG laser
  for pigmented lesions, 370*t*, 373
  for tattoo removal, 398, 398*f*
Q-switched ruby laser, 221
QoL. *See* Quality of life (QoL)
QS. *See* Quality-switched (QS) lasers
Quality of life (QoL), 2–5, 5*t*, 78, 79
Quality-switched (QS) lasers, 98–99
Quality-switched 1064 nm Nd:YAG, 99
Quality-switched 532 nm KTP, 98–99, 99*f*
Quality-switched 694 nm ruby, 99
Quality-switched 755 nm alexandrite lasers, 99

R

Ragnell retractor, 30, 31*f*
Rapamycin, for lymphatic malformations, 332
Reactive oxygen species (ROS), 201
Redarkening, 109
Reed nevus. *See* Pigmented spindle-cell nevus

Relative Value Scale Update Committee (RUC), 14
Residual anetoderma, carbon dioxide laser for, 319–320
  age-specific considerations, 319
  contraindications/cautions/risks, 319
  equipment needed, 320
  postprocedural approach, 320
  preprocedural approach, 320
  procedural approach, 320
  skin color consideration, 319
  technique tips, 319
  treatment guidelines, 319
Retention dressings, 425
Retractor
  Army-Navy, 31, 31*f*
  Weitlaner, 31, 31*f*
Rhomboid flap, 65–66, 67*f*, 68
Richardson retractor, 31, 31*f*
Ringer's, 129
Rongeur, 32, 33*f*
ROS. *See* Reactive oxygen species (ROS)
Rosacea, 387–389
  age-specific considerations, 387
  contraindications/cautions/risks, 388
  equipment needed, 388
  patient and family resources, 477
  postprocedural approach, 389
  preprocedural approach, 388, 388*f*
  procedural approach, 388–389, 389*f*
  skin color considerations, 388
  technique tips, 387–388
  treatment guidelines, 387
RUC. *See* Relative Value Scale Update Committee (RUC)
Rule of 25, 53
Running subcuticular, 59, 59*f*

S

SA. *See* Spider angiomas (SA)
Salicylic acid (SA) peel, 120, 121
  for verruca, 408
Salmon patch. *See* Nevus simplex
Salt bath, for epidermolysis bullosa, 274
Salt-split skin technique, 169
Sarcoptes scabiei var. hominis, 173
Saucerization biopsy, 156, 158, 159*f*
sBCC. *See* Superficial basal cell carcinomas (sBCC)
Scabies, 139, 173–174, 173–174*f*, 389–391, 390*f*
  contraindications/cautions/risks, 390
  equipment needed, 390
  postprocedure environmental management, 391
  procedural approach
    dermoscopy, 391
    microscopic examination, 390–391, 391*f*
    proper treatment, 391
  treatment guidelines, 390

Scalp, 70
Scalpels, 28, 28f
Scar. See also specific scars
    changes in texture/elevation of, 308
    red portions of, 308
Scar alopecia, 70
Scissor biopsy, 156
Scissors, 29–30, 30f
    Iris, 29, 30f
    Mayo, 29, 30f
    Metzenbaum, 30, 30f
    tenotomy, 29, 30f
Scleroderma, patient and family resources,
    477
Sclerotherapy, 227
SCORAD. See Scoring Atopic Dermatitis
    (SCORAD) index
Scoring Atopic Dermatitis (SCORAD)
    index, 468
Sebaceous papules, 90
Seborrheic keratoses, 90
Secondary dressings, 425
Selective photothermolysis, 107
Semiquantitative method, 135
Senn-Miller retractor, 30, 31f
Sensory innervation, 44–45, 45t
Sensory nerves, 39t
    of cervical plexus, 39, 39f
Septisol oil, 122
Serial excisions, for LCMN, 361
Sexual contact, 79
Shade Structure Grant program, 458
Shave biopsy, 156, 158, 159f
Shave removal followed by
        electrodessication, for pyogenic
        granuloma, 383
Silicone-based therapy, 231
Silicone gel sheet, 230f
Silver nitrate, for umbilical granuloma,
    403, 404, 404f
Simple interrupted sutures, 56, 56f
Simple wound repair, 52–61
    patient evaluation, 52
        ABC assessment, 52
        patient history, 52
        wound evaluation, 52
    patient preparation, 52–54
        anesthesia, 53–54, 54–55f
        antimicrobial treatment, 52–53, 53t
    primary wound closure, 55–61
        follow-up, 61
        layered repair, 55
        simple continuous or running
            suture, 56
        simple continuous or running
            suture technique, 56–58
        simple interrupted sutures
            technique for, 56, 56–57f
        staple technique, 60
        staples, 60, 60f

steri-strip application technique, 60
steri-strips, 59–60, 59f
suturing techniques, 55–56
technique for horizontal mattress
    sutures, 58–59
technique for running subcuticular
    sutures, 59
tissue adhesives, 60–61
vertical mattress suture technique,
    58
wound preparation, 54–55
    debridement, 54–55
    irrigation, 55
    wound trimming, 55
Situ, squamous cell carcinoma in, 91
Skin
    psoriasis. See Psoriasis
    psychological effects of, 3
    reapproximation of, 55
    and "track marks," 55
    type assessment by color and burn/tan
        characteristics, 349, 350t
Skin biopsy
    aftercare and instructions, 160
    anesthesia, 157–158
    coding, 15
    patient preparation, 157, 158f
    preprocedure strategies, 157, 158f
    procedural techniques, 158–160
    site, 156–157
    technique, choice of, 156–157
Skin cancers, patient and family resources,
    477
Skin grafting, for LCMN, 361
SM. See Systemic mastocytosis (SM)
Small congenital nevi, 372
Snip excision biopsy, 156, 158, 158f
Sodium hypochlorite
    body washes/gels, application of, 473b
    as cutaneous disinfectant, 472
    stability of solution, 473
Soft-tissue defect, 66
Soft tissue tumors, excision of, 16–17
Solaraze, 199
Solitary cutaneous mastocytoma, 334
Solitary fibrous hamartoma, of infancy,
    392–393, 392f
    age-specific considerations, 392
    contraindications/cautions/risks, 392
    equipment needed, 392
    postprocedural approach, 393
    preprocedural approach, 393
    procedural approach, 393
    skin color considerations, 392
    technique tips, 392
    treatment guidelines, 392
Solitary mastocytoma, 335f
    symptoms for, 335
    treatment of, 335
Special site surgery, 69–76

ear, 71–72, 71f
external genitalia, 74–75
face and neck, 71
foot, 75–76
hand, upper extremity/nail bed, 72–74,
    73–74f
pediatrics, 69–70
perianal region, 75
scalp, 70
Specimen, 146, 147
Speckled lentiginous nevus. See Nevus of
    spilus
Spider angiomas (SA), 110
Spindle and epithelioid cell nevus, 357t
Spitz nevus, 139. See Spindle and
    epithelioid cell nevus
Split-thickness skin grafts, for
    depigmentation, 256
Squamous cell carcinomas (SCCs),
    198, 199. See also Cutaneous
    squamous cell carcinoma
    (cSCC)
Squaric acid dibutylester, for wart, 413
SSI. See Surgical site infection (SSI)
SSSS. See Staphylococcal scalded skin
    syndrome (SSSS)
Standard surgical excisions, for nevus, 360,
    360f
Standing cone deformity, 463, 463f
Staphylococcal scalded skin syndrome
    (SSSS), 225
Staphylococcus aureus, 52, 178
Steel, 35
Steri-Strips, 68, 147, 185
Sterile water, 206
Sterilization, 23–26, 24–26t, 24f
Steven-Johnson syndrome, 445, 446f
STONES acronym, 439
Strangulation, 57
Streptococcus infections, 225
Streptococcus pyogenes, 178
Streptomyces verticillus, 79
Sturge–Weber syndrome (SWS), 108–109
Subungual fibromas. See Fibroma
Sudamina. See Miliaria crystallina
Sulfonamides, adverse reaction, 445
Sun protection, 210, 227
Sun-protective clothing, 457, 457f
Sun Wise School Program, 458
Sunlight, 456
Sunscreen, 456–457
    apply tips, 456–457, 456f
    CDC recommendations, 457
Superficial basal cell carcinomas (sBCC),
    199
Superficial chemical peels, 120–121
Superficial musculoaponeurotic system, 40
Superficial subcutaneous plane, 64
Supernumerary digits, 396–397, 396f
    age-specific considerations, 396

contraindications/cautions/risks, 396
equipment needed, 396
postprocedural approach, 397, 397f
preprocedural approach, 397
procedural approach, 397, 397f
technique tips, 396
treatment guidelines, 396
Surgery, for xeroderma pigmentosum
age-specific considerations, 421
contraindications/cautions/risks, 421
equipment needed, 422
postprocedural approach, 423
preprocedural approach, 422
procedural approach, 422
skin color considerations, 421
technique tips, 421
treatment guidelines, 421
Surgical (procedure) room set-up, 18–21, 18f, 19f, 20f
Surgical complications, 460–466
allergic contact dermatitis (ACD), 464–466, 465f
anesthesia, 460
bleeding, intraprocedure and postprocedure. See Bleeding
hypertrophic scars, 466
infection, 463–464
keloids, 466
Surgical excision
for epidermal inclusion cysts, 264–266, 265–266f
for epidermal nevi, 269
for infantile hemangioma or fibrofatty residua, 285, 286f
for lipomas, 330
for mastocytoma, 336
for median raphe cysts, 337
for melanoma, 338
for solitary fibrous hamartoma, 392
Surgical instruments, 28, 28t
categories of, 28, 28t
clamps, 31–32f
electrocautery instruments and supplies, 29, 29f
forceps, 28, 29f
hooks, 30–31, 30–31f
miscellaneous, 32–33, 32–33f
scalpels, 28, 28f
scissors, 29–30, 30f
Surgical removal
for genital warts
age-specific considerations, 248
contraindications/cautions/risks, 249
equipment needed, 249
postprocedural approach, 249
procedural approach, 249
technique tips, 248
treatment guidelines, 248
Surgical site infection (SSI), 18, 443

Surgical staples, 37
Surgical wound classification, 22, 22t
Suture techniques, 52, 52f
Sutures
absorbable versus nonabsorbable, 34
choice of needle, 35–36
cyanoacrylate glue with mesh, 37, 37f
memory, 34–35
monofilament versus multifilament/barbed/unbarbed, 34
noninvasive skin closure devices, 37, 37f
silk, 35
Suturing techniques. See also individual techniques
Sweat rash. See Miliaria
SWS. See Sturge–Weber syndrome (SWS)
Syringomas, 90
Systemic lupus erythematous, 169
Systemic mastocytosis (SM), 334
diagnostic Criteria for, 334t

T

T-cell function, 198
T-ring, 145
Tangential rhomboid, 65
Tangential scissor/shave excision, for genital warts
age-specific considerations, 248
contraindications/cautions/risks, 249
equipment needed, 249
postprocedural approach, 249
procedural approach, 249
technique tips, 248
treatment guidelines, 248
Taphylococcus aureus, 178
Targeted excimer laser (308 nm) phototherapy, for psoriasis, 379
age-specific considerations, 379
contraindications/cautions/risks, 379
equipment needed, 380
postprocedural approach, 382
preprocedural approach, 380
procedural approach, 381
skin color considerations, 379
technique tips, 379
treatment guidelines, 379
Tattoo removal, 398–400, 398f
age-specific considerations, 398
contraindications/cautions/risks, 398–399
equipment needed, 399
laser wavelengths and pulse durations for, 399t
postprocedural approach, 399–400, 400f
preprocedural approach, 399
procedural approach, 399
skin color considerations, 398
technique tips, 398
treatment guidelines, 398

TCA. See Trichloroacetic acid (TCA) peels
TCSs. See Topical corticosteroids (TCSs)
Tegaderm®, 374
Telangiectasia, 90, 400–402
age-specific considerations, 401
contraindications/cautions/risks, 401
equipment needed, 401
postprocedural approach, 402
preprocedural approach, 401
procedural approach, 401–402, 402f
skin color considerations, 401
technique tips, 401
treatment guidelines, 401
Telangiectasia macularis eruptive perstans (TMEP), 334
Telangiectasia/local hypertrichosis, 77f
Tenotomy scissors, 29, 30f
"Tent" sign, 374
Tetracyclines, adverse reactions, 445, 446f
Therapeutic method, 78
Thermal relaxation time (TRT), 92
Thin-layer Rapid-Use Epicutaneous (T.R.U.E. test®), 465
308-nm Excimer laser
for granuloma annulare, 282Tie2 gene, 227
TIME acronym, 439
Tinea versicolor, 163
Tissue expansion, for LCMN, 361
TMEP. See Telangiectasia macularis eruptive perstans (TMEP)
TNF. See Tumor necrosis factor (TNF)
Tobacco smoking, 63
Toll-like receptor 7 (TLR-7), 199
Tonsil clamp, 31, 31f
Toothbrush method, 141
Topical anhydrous lanolin, for miliaria profunda, 343
Topical approaches, for verruca
5-fluorouracil, 409
cantharidin, 409
imiquimod, 409–410
salicylic acid, 408
Topical corticosteroids (TCSs), 468
for cutaneous larva migrans, 250
for labial adhesion, 325
in ointment form, 468
and wet wrap therapy, 470
Topical estrogen, for labial adhesion, 324–325
Topical hemostatic agents, 48–52, 50–51t, 50f
Topical therapy, 199
Transposition flap, 66
Treacher Collins syndrome, 186
Treatment endpoints, for WWT, 471
Tretinoin cream, 121
Triamcinolone cream, for miliaria rubra, 343
Trichilemmal cysts. See Pilar cysts
Trichloroacetic acid (TCA) peels, 121, 122, 195

Trichophyton tonsurans, 163
Tropical anhidrosis. *See* Miliaria profunda
TRT. *See* Thermal relaxation time (TRT)
TSC. *See* Tuberous sclerosis complex (TSC)
TSC1/TSC2 genes, 111
Tuberous sclerosis complex (TSC), 111
  patient and family resources, 477
Tumbu fly. *See Cordylobia anthropophaga*
Tumescent cannula, 128f
Tumor necrosis factor (TNF), 79, 199
Type I postaxial (ulnar) polydactyly. *See* Supernumerary digits
Tzanck smear, 175, 175f

U

Ulcerated hemangioma, 434, 435f
Ultrasound-guided needle aspiration, 178
Ultraviolet (UV) rays, 198, 201, 456
  indicator wristbands, 458
  types, 456
Ultraviolet A1 (UVA1), 115–116
Ultraviolet B (UVB), 115–116
Umbilical granuloma, 403–405, 403f
  contraindications/cautions/risks, 404, 404f
  equipment needed, 404
  postprocedural approach, 405
  preprocedural approach, 404
  procedural approach, 404–405, 404f
  technique tips, 403
Umbilicus, 46
Uncooperative child, 8
Urticarial pigmentosa (UP). *See* Maculopapular cutaneous mastocytosis (MPCM)
U.S. Food and Drug Administration (FDA), 150, 157, 192, 199
Ustekinumab, 79
UV. *See* Ultraviolet (UV) rays
UVB. *See* Ultraviolet B (UVB)

V

Valacyclovir, 120
Varicella zoster virus (VZV), 175, 224
Vascular anomalies
  patient and family resources, 477–478
Vascular lesions, laser treatment of
  angiofibromas, 111–112
  IH, 110–111
  PWB, 108–110
  SA, 110
Vasculature, 41, 42f, 43f
Vasovagal syncope, 460
Venous malformations (VMs), 226, 227, 228, 405–408, 406f
  age-specific considerations, 406
  contraindications/cautions/risks, 406

equipment needed, 406
postprocedural approach, 407–408
  other associated complex disorders, 408
preprocedural approach, 406
procedural approach, 407
skin color considerations, 406
technique tips, 406
treatment guidelines, 406
Ventrogluteal injection, 83
Verruca, 139. *See* Human papillomavirus (HPV) wart
Vertical mattress suture, 58, 58f
Vertical sectioning, 142
Vicryl. *See* Glycolide/lactide copolymer (Vicryl)
Vinegar bath, for epidermolysis bullosa, 274
Viral culture, 161–162
Viral transport medium, 161f
Vitamin D, 198
Vitamin supplements, 461
Vitiligo, 78, 163, 251, 414–420
  grafting, 415
  melanocyte keratinocyte transplantation procedure, 415, 417–420, 417f
    age-specific considerations, 418
    contraindications/cautions/risks, 418
    equipment needed, 418
    postprocedural approach, 420
    preprocedural approach, 418
    procedural approach, 418–419, 419–420f
    skin color considerations, 418
    technique tips, 418
    treatment guidelines, 418
  patient and family resources, 478
  phototherapy/excimer laser procedures, 414–417
    age-specific considerations, 415
    contraindications/cautions/risks, 415–416
    equipment needed, 416
    postprocedural approach, 417
    preprocedural approach, 416
    procedural approach, 416–417, 417t
    skin color considerations, 415
    technique tips, 415
    treatment guidelines, 415
  treatment options for, 252t
VMs. *See* Venous malformations (VMs)
von Willebrand disease (VWD), 460–461
Voriconazole, 199
Vulnerable population, 7
VWD. *See* von Willebrand disease (VWD)
VZV. *See* Varicella zoster virus (VZV)

W

Warts, 79
  multimodal procedural treatment of, 17
"Water bumps", 344
Web resources, for WWT, 471
Weitlaner retractor, 31, 31f
Wet wrap therapy (WWT), 468–471
  definition, 468
  effectiveness, 468
  evidence for use of, 468
  inpatient considerations for, 470, 470f
  potential complications of, 470–471
  procedure for, 468–469, 469f
    at home, 469–470, 470f
  recommended frequency of, 470
  treatment endpoints for, 471
  use of topical corticosteroids, 470
  utilization of, 468
  web resources, 471
WHO. *See* World Health Organization (WHO)
Wide undermining, 64
Wood's lamp skin examination, 163–164, 163f
World Health Organization (WHO), 2
Wound(s)
  assessment, 437–439, 438f
    chronic versus acute, 438
    depth/size, 438–439
    infection, signs of, 439, 439t
    maintaining moisture, 439
    necrosis, 439
  complications, treatment of, 440–441
    hypergranulation tissue, 440–441, 441f
    infection, 440
    necrosis, 440
    references and disease-specific guidelines, 442t
    stalled/delayed healing, 441, 441f
  healing stages, 437, 437f
  optimizing healing, 439–440
  pediatric patient, encountered in, 434–437, 435–436f
Wound care, 213
Wound dressings, 428–433
  bandaging recommendations, 431, 431f
  history of, 425
  pediatric patient, considerations in, 432, 433t
    patient/family education, 433
    product choice for, 433
  primary characteristics and examples, 426t
  properties, 425, 427–431, 427t
    alginate, 427, 428f
    antimicrobial, 428f, 429

collagen, 428*f*, 429–430
film, 429*f*, 431
foam, 428*f*, 430
gauze/impregnated gauze, 429*f*,
    430–431
hydrocolloid, 428*f*, 430
hydrofiber, 430
hydrogel, 428*f*, 430
retention, 429*f*, 431
selection of, 431–432, 431–432*f*
side effects, 432
Wound healing, 12

Wound myiasis, 351
Wound preparation, 54–55
WWT. *See* Wet wrap therapy (WWT)

X
Xeroderma pigmentosum (XP), 198,
    420–423, 421*f*
age-specific considerations, 421
contraindications/cautions/risks, 421
equipment needed, 422
patient and family resources, 478
postprocedural approach, 422–423

preprocedural approach, 422
procedural approach, 422
skin color considerations, 421
technique tips, 421
treatment guidelines, 421
XP. *See* Xeroderma pigmentosum (XP)

Y
Yankauer suction tip, 32, 32*f*

Z
Zygomatic arch, 38